MW00715097

THE DISPENSATORY

OF THE

UNITED STATES OF AMERICA.

BY

DR. GEO. B. WOOD AND DR. FRANKLIN BACHE.

SIXTEENTH EDITION.

Rearranged, thoroughly revised, and largely rewritten.

WITH ILLUSTRATIONS.

BY

H. C. WOOD, M.D., LL.D.,

MEMBER OF THE NATIONAL ACADEMY OF SCIENCE; PROFESSOR OF MATERIA MEDICA AND THERAPEUTICS AND OF DISEASES OF THE NERVOUS SYSTEM IN THE UNIVERSITY OF PENNSYLVANIA.

JOSEPH P. REMINGTON, Ph.M., F.C.S.,

PROFESSOR OF THEORY AND PRACTICE OF PHARMACY IN THE PHILADELPHIA COLLEGE OF PHARMACY; FIRST VICE-CHAIRMAN OF THE COMMITTEE OF REVISION AND PUBLICATION OF THE PHARMACOPŒIA OF THE UNITED STATES OF AMERICA.

AND

SAMUEL P. SADTLER, Ph.D., F.C.S.,

PROFESSOR OF CHEMISTRY IN THE PHILADELPHIA COLLEGE OF PHARMACY AND OF GENERAL AND ORGANIC CHEMISTRY IN THE UNIVERSITY OF PENNSYLVANIA.

PHILADELPHIA:

J. B. LIPPINCOTT COMPANY.

1892.

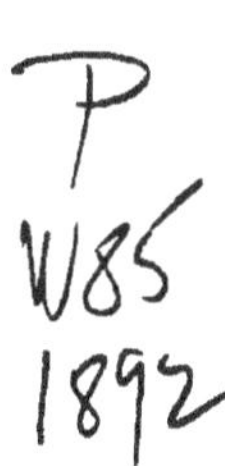

Authority to use for comment the Pharmacopœia of the United States of America, Sixth Decennial Revision, has been extended by the Committee of Revision and Publication.

PREFACE TO THE SIXTEENTH EDITION.

It was with much solicitude that the editors of the *fifteenth* edition of the United States Dispensatory offered their work as an aid and guide to their colaborers in medicine and pharmacy. The unexpectedly gratifying reception of it, and the fact that the publishers were compelled to issue more than double the number of copies required for previous editions, were convincing proofs that the work had lost nothing of its former prestige, but that substantial additions to its clientèle had been gained. These facts have acted as a powerful stimulus to the editors, who have again earnestly striven to deserve the continued favor of the two professions, by making this, the *sixteenth* revision, as thorough as possible.

The extraordinary activity in practical and theoretic research in the sciences which bear upon the Dispensatory subjects has produced so much fruit since the last revision that over six hundred pages of new matter have been incorporated in this edition; but by a very thorough elision of that which was effete, the editors have been able to restrain the net increase in the number of pages to one hundred and sixty-seven.

The serious danger of rendering the book unwieldy in size for the needs of the practical worker, has acted as an ever-present check to the natural temptation to undue expansion, and has compelled the editors to use their best judgment to avoid prolixity while yet furnishing useful detail; whilst to enhance still further the value of the information, full and accessible references, with dates, are appended whenever possible, to aid in the search for fuller knowledge. The large use now made of certain pharmaceutical preparations which have not yet secured official recognition, and the desire to aid in the organized effort now being made to furnish uniform and authoritative formulas for such, have led the editors to incorporate the National Formulary in Part II. in its entirety. The convenience of having these formulas bound in the same volume with the commentary, to facilitate easy reference, will doubtless be appreciated.

In conclusion, the editors desire to state that the labor has been partitioned among them as in the previous edition, except that the index has been prepared by Mr. A. B. Taylor, and heartily to thank their friends for the many evidences of their kind indulgence.

Philadelphia, August, 1888.

PREFACE TO THE FIFTEENTH EDITION.

JUST fifty years have gone by since Dr. Geo. B. Wood penned the preface to the first edition of the United States Dispensatory. Written from a sense of duty, and in the earnest belief that to obtain the acceptance of the newly born United States Pharmacopœia by the American professions of Medicine and Pharmacy a standard commentary was necessary, the book achieved a success which, to its authors, was as unexpected as it was gratifying. During the half-century that has elapsed, the work has passed through fourteen editions; revolutions have swept over science, the fate that awaits all men has come to the authors; and yet, with a steadiness that is unrivalled in medical literature, the United States Dispensatory has maintained its supremacy, until the copies of it which have been sold are to be numbered by the hundreds of thousands, and wherever the English language leads, it follows. Even in the last years, when it was sorely in need of revision, the demand for it has not perceptibly diminished. Such success as this must depend upon extraordinary qualities in the book. Thoroughness, accuracy, and completeness undoubtedly have had much to do with the result, but we conceive that the pre-eminent usefulness of the Dispensatory has rested largely upon the peculiar ability of its authors to perceive what facts are useful and essential to a subject, and upon their judgment and skill in utilizing and setting forth these facts.

In attempting the revision of a book which has become so necessary to the American professions, the editors have fully comprehended the difficulties and the importance of their task. They all have had the experience and the peculiar growth in the power of appreciating the proportionate fitness and importance of facts, which come with successive years of active life as a teacher. One of them has had the good fortune to have worked through the revisions of three editions under the rigid discipline of Dr. Geo. B. Wood, and to have become thoroughly familiar with his methods, not only of work, but also of thought, and with the principles which in his mind were essential to the building up of the Dispensatory. The editors come, therefore, to the work not without some especial preparation. Moreover, for the first time in the history of the volume, the original plan of Dr. Geo. B. Wood of having three editors, one for each branch of the subject-matter, has been realized.

It is evident that in the revision of a book with a history like that of the present the changes should be as few as possible. The editors have constantly borne this principle in mind, but circumstances have forced them, whilst strenuously endeavoring to retain the characteristics and essential features of the work, in great part to remodel it. The alteration in the plan of the Pharmacopœia has necessitated a parallel change in the Dispensatory. The first and second parts have therefore been alphabetically collated and formed into Part I. of the present edition. Part III. of former editions has been kept isolated as Part II.; because were it not for the great gain of space achieved by the use of the small type, two volumes would be required to contain the material now compressed between a single pair of covers. The amount of new matter added at this revision may be judged of from the fact that whilst in the index of the fourteenth edition there were about eleven thousand references, in the present index there are more than sixteen thousand titles, including in these, however, German and French synonymes, never before indexed. Part III. of the present volume contains a revision of the Appendix of former editions, with various miscellaneous new matter.

When the fourteenth edition of the Dispensatory was published, Dr. Geo. B. Wood was nearly eighty years of age, and, although he sympathized with the movement which has resulted in putting therapeutics upon the firm foundation of physiological rationalism, he could not fully apprehend the changes which had occurred in therapeutical methods during the previous decade. Consequently, in most of the more important articles the sections treating of Medical Properties and Uses have had to be rewritten. The revision of these sections, as well as of the Botany and Vegetable Materia Medica, has fallen to the senior editor, Prof. H. C. Wood.

The progress of the last decade has necessitated important changes in those sections of the Dispensatory which treat of Pharmaceutical Chemistry, whilst the Pharmacy of the present edition is almost entirely new. This part of the revision has been performed by Prof. Jos. P. Remington, by whose calculations the officinal formulæ have been adapted to the use of those pharmacists who prefer the system of measuring liquids. The alternative formulas *have been carefully tested in practice*, and we believe that they will serve a useful purpose, during the transition stage, caused by the adoption of the principle of *parts by weight.*

Dr. Franklin Bache died in 1864, at the time when the agitation was commencing in chemical science which has ended in the received nomenclature and theory. Since the death of its chemical author the portions of the Dispensatory especially within his province have had no proper revision and adaptation to the needs of the day. All of the Theoretical Chemistry of the volume has, therefore, had to be reproduced. This part of the work, with the Toxicology, has been allotted to Prof. S. P. Sadtler; and we believe that in all points the Dispensatory now represents the latest solid achievements of chemical science.

It seems proper to call attention, as novel features of the fifteenth edition, to the indication of the pronunciation of the officinal titles by diacritical marks; to the complete list of analyses of American Mineral Springs, as far as they have been published, with a number of analyses of European Springs of note; and to the illustrations. The drug illustrations are, with three minor exceptions, original; and the very accurate representations of microscopical sections will, we believe, be of service to students of structural characteristics.

In conclusion, it seems but right to state that the revision has been performed slowly and with great care, occupying most of the spare moments of the editors during the last three years. The present volume may very justly be looked upon as a new book, founded upon the old United States Dispensatory. The editors have no overweening sense of their ability: they recognise profoundly the immense responsibility that has been laid upon them; but they ask a favorable consideration for their work, because with all patience and toil, and with the love of their labor, they have honestly striven, so far as in them lay, to make the new United States Dispensatory worthy of the time when it was universally recognised as the supreme treasure-house of pharmacological lore.

PHILADELPHIA, January, 1883.

PREFACE TO THE FIRST EDITION.

THE objects of a Dispensatory are to present an account of medicinal substances in the state in which they are brought into the shops, and to teach the modes in which they are prepared for use. The importance of these objects, and the general value and even necessity of a work of this nature, will not be disputed. It may, however, be a question, how far the wants of the medical and pharmaceutical community in this country are supplied by the Dispensatories already in circulation; and whether such a deficiency exists as to justify the offer of a new one to the public attention. The great merits of the works severally entitled "The Edinburgh New Dispensatory" and "The London Dispensatory," the former edited by the late Andrew Duncan, M.D., the latter by Anthony Todd Thomson, M.D., are well known wherever the English language is spoken. Founded, as they both are, upon the excellent basis laid by Lewis, they are nevertheless entitled, from the great addition of valuable materials, and the distinctive character exhibited in the arrangement of these materials, to be considered as original works; while the style in which they have been executed speaks strongly in favor of the skill and industry of their authors. But they were calculated especially for the sphere of Great Britain, and are too deficient in all that relates exclusively to this country, to admit of being received as standards here. In the history of our commerce in drugs, and of the nature, growth, and collection of our indigenous medical plants; in the chemical operations of our extensive laboratories; and in the modes of preparing, dispensing, and applying medicines, which have gradually grown into use among us; there is much that is peculiar, a knowledge of which is not to be gained from foreign books, and is yet necessary to the character of an accomplished American pharmaceutist. We have, moreover, a National Pharmacopœia, which requires an explanatory commentary, in order that its precepts may be fully appreciated, and advantageously put into practice. On these accounts, it is desirable that there should be a Dispensatory of the United States, which, while it embraces whatever is useful in European pharmacy, may accurately represent the art as it exists in this country, and give instruction adapted to our peculiar wants. It appears due to our national character that such a work should be in good faith an American work, newly prepared in all its parts, and not a mere edition of one of the European Dispensatories, with here and there additions and alterations, which, though they may be useful in themselves, cannot be made to harmonize with the other materials so as to give to the whole an appearance of unity, and certainly would not justify the assumption of a new national title for the book. Whether, in the Dispensatories which have been published in the United States, these requisites have been satisfactorily fulfilled, it rests with the public to determine. That valuable treatises on Materia Medica and Pharmacy have been issued in this country, no candid person, acquainted with our medical literature, will be disposed to deny. In offering a new work to the medical and pharmaceutical professions, the authors do not wish to be considered as undervaluing the labors of their predecessors. They simply conceive that the field has not been so fully occupied as to exclude all competition. The pharmacy of continental Europe is ground which has been almost untouched; and much information in relation to the natural history, commerce, and management of our own drugs, has lain ungathered in the possession of individuals, or scattered in separate treatises and periodicals not generally known and read. Since the publication of the last edition of our National Pharmacopœia, no general explanation of its processes has appeared, though required in justice both to that work and to the public. The hope of being able to supply these deficiencies may, perhaps, be considered a sufficient justification for the present undertaking.

The Pharmacopœia of the United States has been adopted as the basis of this Dispensatory. It is followed both in its general division of medicines, and in its alphabetical arrangement of them under each division. Precedence is, in every instance, given to the names which it recognizes, while the explanations by which it fixes the significance of these names are inserted in immediate connection with the titles to which they severally belong. Every article which it designates is more or less fully described; and all its processes, after being literally copied, are commented on and explained wherever comment and explanation appeared necessary. Nothing, in fine, has been omitted, which, in the estimation of the authors, could serve to illustrate its meaning, or promote the ends which it was intended to subserve. This course of proceeding appeared to be due to the national character of the Pharmacopœia, and to the important object of establishing, as far as possible, throughout the United States, uniformity, both in the nomenclature and preparation of medicines. In one particular, convenience required that the plan of the Pharmacopœia should be departed from. The medicines belonging to the department of MATERIA MEDICA, instead of being arranged in two divisions corresponding with the *Primary* and *Secondary Catalogues* of that work, have been treated of indiscriminately in alphabetical succession; and the place which they respectively hold in the Pharmacopœia is indicated by the employment of the term *Secondary*, in connection with the name of each of the medicines included in the latter catalogue.

But, though precedence has thus been given to the Pharmacopœia of the United States, those of Great Britain have not been neglected. The nomenclature adopted by the different British Colleges, and their formulas for the preparation of medicines, have been so extensively followed throughout the United States, that a work intended to represent the present state of pharmacy in this country would be imperfect without them; and the fact that the writings of British physicians and surgeons, in which their own officinal terms and preparations are exclusively employed and referred to, have an extensive circulation among us, renders some commentary necessary in order to prevent serious mistakes. The Pharmacopœias of London, Edinburgh, and Dublin have, therefore, been incorporated, in all their essential parts, into the present work. Their officinal titles are uniformly given, always in subordination to those of the United States Pharmacopœia, when they express the same object; but in chief, when, as often happens, no corresponding medicine or preparation is recognized by our national standard. In the latter case, if different names are applied by different British Colleges to the same object, that one is generally preferred which is most in accordance with our own system of nomenclature, and the others are given as synonymes. The medicines directed by the British Colleges are all described, and their processes either copied at length, or so far explained as to be intelligible in all essential particulars.

Besides the medicinal substances recognized as officinal by the Pharmacopœias alluded to, some others have been described, which, either from the lingering remains of former reputation, from recent reports in their favor, or from their important relation to medicines in general use, appear to have claims upon the attention of the physician and apothecary. Opportunity has, moreover, been taken to introduce incidentally brief accounts of substances used in other countries or in former times, and occasionally noticed in medical books; and, that the reader may be able to refer to them when desirous of information, their names have been placed with those of the standard remedies in the Index.

In the description of each medicine, if derived immediately from the animal, vegetable, or mineral kingdom, the attention of the authors has been directed to its natural history, the place of its growth or production, the method of collecting and preparing it for market, its commercial history, the state in which it reaches us, its sensible properties, its chemical composition and relations, the changes which it undergoes by time and exposure, its accidental or fraudulent adulterations, its medical properties and application, its economical uses, and the pharmaceutical treatment to which it is subjected. If a chemical preparation, the mode and principles of its manufacture are indicated in addition to the other particulars. If a poison, and likely to be accidentally taken, or purposely employed as such, its peculiar toxicological effects, together with the mode of counteracting them, are indicated; and the best means of detecting its presence by reagents are explained.

The authors have followed the example of Dr. A. T. Thomson, in giving botanical descriptions of the plants from which the medicines treated of are derived. In relation to all indigenous medicinal plants, and those naturalized or cultivated in this country, the advantages of such descriptions are obvious. The physician may often be placed in situations, in which it may be highly important that he should be able to recognize the vegetable which yields a particular medicine; and the apothecary is constantly liable to imposition from the collectors of herbs, unless possessed of the means of distinguishing, by infallible marks, the various products presented to him. A knowledge of foreign medicinal plants, though of less importance, will be found useful in various ways, independently of the gratification afforded by the indulgence of a liberal curiosity in relation to objects so closely connected with our daily pursuits. The introduction of these botanical notices into a Dispensatory appears to be peculiarly appropriate; as they are to be considered rather as objects for occasional reference than for regular study or continuous perusal, and therefore coincide with the general design of the work, which is to collect into a convenient form for consultation all that is practically important in relation to medicines. The authors have endeavored to preserve a due proportion between the minuteness of the descriptions, and their value as means of information to the student; and, in pursuance of this plan, have generally dwelt more at length upon our native plants than upon those of foreign growth; but, in all instances in which they have deemed a botanical description necessary, they have taken care to include in it the essential scientific character of the genus and species, with a reference to the position of the plant in the artificial and natural systems of classification; so that a person acquainted with the elements of botany may be able to recognize it when it comes under his observation.

In preparing the Dispensatory, the authors have consulted, in addition to many of the older works of authority, the greater number of the treatises and dissertations which have recently appeared upon the various subjects connected with Pharmacy, and especially those of the French writers, who stand at present at the head of this department of medical science. They have also endeavored to collect such detached facts, scattered through the various scientific, medical, and pharmaceutical journals, as they conceive to be important in themselves, and applicable to the subjects under consideration; and have had frequent recourse to the reports of travellers in relation to the natural and commercial history of foreign drugs. The occasional references in the body of the work will indicate the sources from which they have most largely drawn, and the authorities upon which they have most relied. In relation to our own commerce in drugs, and to the operations of our chemical laboratories, they are indebted for information chiefly to the kindness of gentlemen engaged in these branches of business, who have always evinced, in answering their numerous inquiries, a promptitude and politeness which merit their warm thanks, and which they are pleased to have this opportunity of acknowledging.*

It has not been deemed necessary to follow the example of the British Dispensatories, by inserting into the work a treatise upon chemistry, under the name of Elements of Pharmacy. Such a treatise must necessarily be very meagre and imperfect; and, as systems of chemistry are in the hands of every physician and apothecary, would uselessly occupy the place of valuable matter of less easy access.

The authors may, perhaps, be permitted to observe, in relation to themselves, that they have expended much time and labor in the preparation of the work; have sought diligently for facts from every readily accessible source; have endeavored, by a comparison of authorities, and a close scrutiny of evidence, to ascertain the truth whenever practicable; and have exerted themselves to the extent of their abilities to render the Dispensatory worthy of public approbation, both for the quality and quantity of its contents, and the general accuracy of its statements. They are conscious, nevertheless, that, in so great a multiplicity of details, numerous errors and deficiencies may exist, and that the faults of undue brevity in some cases, and prolixity in others, may not have been entirely avoided; but they venture to hope that a candid public will make all due allowances; and they take the liberty to invite, from all those who may feel interested in the diffusion of sound pharmaceutical knowledge, the communication of friendly suggestions or criticisms in relation to the objects and execution of the work.

PHILADELPHIA, *January*, 1833.

* The authors deem it proper to state that they are peculiarly indebted for assistance to Mr. Daniel B. Smith, president of the Philadelphia College of Pharmacy, to whom, besides much important information in relation to the various branches of the apothecary's business, they owe the prefatory remarks on Pharmacy which are placed at the commencement of the second part of the work, and the several articles, in the Materia Medica, upon *Leeches*, *Carbonate of Magnesia*, and *Sulphate of Magnesia*.

ABBREVIATIONS.

At. Wt.—Atomic Weight.
Arab.—Arabic.
B.—Baumé's Hydrometer.
Br.—The British Pharmacopœia, 1867, and Supplement.
B. & T.—Bentley & Trimen's Medicinal Plants.
C.c.—Cubic centimetre.
Codex.—The French Pharmacopœia.
De Cand.—De Candolle.
Fr.—French.
G.—German.
Gen. Ch.—Generic Character.
Gm.—Gramme.
It.—Italian.
Juss.—Jussieu.
Linn.—Linnæus.
m.m.—Millimetre.
Mol.—Molecule.
Mol. Wt.—Molecular Weight.
Nat. Ord.—Natural Order.
Off. Prep.—Officinal Preparations.
Off. Syn.—Official Synonymes.
P. G.—The German Pharmacopœia.
Pharm. Uses.—Pharmaceutical Uses.
Sp. Gr.—Specific Gravity.
Sp.—Spanish.
U. S.—The Pharmacopœia of the United States, 1880.
Willd. Sp. Plant.—Willdenow's edition of the Species Plantarum of Linnæus.
Woodv. Med. Bot.—Woodville's Medical Botany, 2d edition.

JOURNALS FREQUENTLY REFERRED TO IN THE WORK.

A. J. P.—American Journal of Pharmacy.
Am. Journ. Med. Sci.—American Journal of the Medical Sciences.
Amer. Drug.—American Druggist.
Amer. Pract.—American Practitioner.
Ann. Ch. Phys.—Annales de Chimie et de Physique.
Ann. d. Chem.—Liebig's Annalen der Chemie.
Ann. de Thérap.—Annuaire de Thérapeutique.
Archiv d. Pharm.—Archiv der Pharmacie.
Archiv für Exp. Path. und Therap.—Archiv für Experimentalische Pathologie und Therapie.
Arch. Gén.—Archives Générales.
Ber. d. Chem. Ges.—Berichte der Deutschen Chemischen Gesellschaft.
Ber. Klin. Woch.—Berliner Klinische Wochenschrift.
Bost. Med. and Surg. Journ.—Boston Medical and Surgical Journal.
Buch. Neu. Rep.—Buchner's Neues Repertorium.
Can. Pharm. Journ.—Canadian Pharmaceutical Journal.
Chem. and Drug.—Chemist and Druggist (London).
Chem. News.—Chemical News (London).
Compt.-Rend.—Comptes-Rendus hebdomadaires des Séances.
Drug. Bull.—Druggist's Bulletin.
Drug. Circ.—Druggist's Circular.
Jahresb.—Jahresberichte (Dragendorff's).
Journ. App. Chem.—Journal of Applied Chemistry.
Journ. Chem. Soc.—Journal of Chemical Society (London).
Journ. de Pharm. d'Anvers.—Journal de Pharmacie (Antwerp).
Journ. de Pharm. et de Chim.—Journal de Pharmacie et de Chimie.
Journ. für Prakt. Chem.—Journal für Praktische Chemie.
Med. T. and G.—Medical Times and Gazette.
Nat. Drug.—National Druggist.
N. R.—New Remedies.
Pharm. Cent.—Pharmaceutische Centralhalle.
Pharm. Era.—Pharmaceutical Era.
Pharm. Rec.—Pharmaceutical Record.
Pharm. Rund.—Pharmaceutische Rundschau.
Pharm. Zeit.—Pharmaceutische Zeitung.
P. J. Tr.—Pharmaceutical Journal and Transactions (London).
Pogg. Ann.—Poggendorf's Annalen.
Proc. A. P. A.—Proceedings American Pharmaceutical Association.
Prog. Méd.—Progrès Médicale.
Répert. de Pharm.—Répertoire de Pharmacie.
T. G.—Therapeutic Gazette.
West. Drug.—Western Druggist.
Zeits. für Analyt. Chem.—Zeitschrift für Analytische Chemie.
Zeits. Oest. Apoth. Ver.—Zeitschrift des Oesterreichische Apotheker Verein.

EXPLANATORY KEY TO THE PRONUNCIATION.

The introduction of diacritical marks to indicate the pronunciation of the officinal titles in this work requires the insertion of a key to make them intelligible. The system in use in Worcester's Dictionary has been adopted.

Ā long, as in fāte.
Ă short, as in făt.
Ạ obscure, as in ạbide.
Â long before *r*, as in fâre.
Ä Italian or grave, as in fär.
Ȧ intermediate, as in fȧst.
A̤ broad, as in fa̤ll.

Ī long, as in pīne.
Ĭ short, as in pĭn.
Ị obscure, as in perịl.
Ï like long ē, as in mïen.
Ĩ obtuse, as in sĩr.

Ū long, as in tūbe.
Ŭ short, as in bŭt.
Ụ obscure, as in sụppose.
Ü as in annüal.
Û obtuse, as in bûll.
Ũ short and obtuse, as in bũr.
Ṻ long and close, as in rṻle.

Ē long, as in mēte.
Ĕ short, as in mĕt.
Ẹ obscure, as in othẹr.
Ê like â, as in hêir.
Ẽ obtuse, as in hẽr.

Ō long, as in hōpe.
Ŏ short, as in nŏt.
Ọ obscure, as in arbọr.
Ö long and close, as in möve.
Ô broad, as in nôr.
Ȯ like short ŭ, as in sȯn.

Ç soft, like s.
C̶ hard, like k.
Ģ like j.
G̶ hard, as in give.
Ş like z.
X̣ like l.

GLOSSARY.

In the following Glossary will be found short definitions of many of the terms employed in the Dispensatory to designate the medical properties of the remedies: most of the words are commonly employed as nouns and sometimes as adjectives.

ABSORBENTS.—Drugs used to produce absorption of exudates or diseased tissues.

ABSTERGENTS.—Detergents.

ALTERATIVES.—Medicines used to so modify nutrition as to overcome morbid processes.

ANÆSTHETICS.—Medicines used to produce anæsthesia or unconsciousness.

ANALEPTICS.—Restorative medicines, or food.

ANALGESICS.—Medicines used to allay pain.

ANAPHRODISIACS.—Medicines used to allay sexual feeling.

ANODYNES.—Medicines used to allay pain.

ANTACIDS.—Medicines used to neutralize acid in the stomach and intestines.

ANTHELMINTICS.—Medicines used to destroy intestinal worms.

ANTIARTHRITICS.—Medicines used for the relief of gout.

ANTIHYDROPICS.—Medicines used for the relief of dropsy.

ANTILITHICS.—Medicines used for the relief of calculous affections.

ANTIPERIODICS.—Medicines used for the relief of malarial fevers.

ANTIPYRETICS.—Medicines used for the reduction of bodily temperature in fevers.

ANTISEPTICS.—Substances which have the power of preventing putrefaction.

ANTISPASMODICS.—Medicines used for the relief of nervous irritability and minor spasms.

ANTISYPHILITICS.—Medicines used for the relief of syphilis.

ANTIZYMOTICS.—Substances which have the power of killing disease-germs.

APERIENTS.—Mild purgatives.

APHRODISIACS.—Substances used to increase sexual power or excitement.

AROMATICS.—Medicines characterised by a fragrant or spicy taste and odor, and stimulant to the gastro-intestinal mucous membrane.

AROMATIC BITTERS.—Medicines which unite the properties of the aromatics and the simple bitters.

ASTRINGENTS.—Medicines which have the power of influencing vital contractility and thereby condensing tissues.

BITTERS—SIMPLE.—Medicines which have a bitter taste and have the power of stimulating the gastro-intestinal mucous membrane, without affecting the general system.

BLISTERS.—Medicines which when locally applied cause inflammatory exudation of serum from the skin and are used as revulsants.

CALEFACIENTS.—Medicines used externally to cause a sense of warmth.

CARDIAC DEPRESSANTS.—Medicines used to lower the heart's action.

CARDIAC STIMULANTS.—Medicines used to increase the heart's action.

CARMINATIVES.—Medicines containing a volatile oil used to excite intestinal peristalsis and provoke an expulsion of flatus.

CATHARTICS.—Purgatives.

CAUSTICS.—Medicines used to destroy living tissues.

CHOLAGOGUES.—Medicines which provoke a flow of bile.

CONSTRINGENTS.—Astringents.

CONVULSANTS.—Medicines which cause convulsions.

CORRECTIVES.—Medicines used to correct or render more pleasant the action of other remedies, especially purgatives.

CORRIGENTS.—Correctives.

DEMULCENTS.—Mucilaginous principles which are used in solution to soothe and protect irritated mucous membranes or other tissues.

DEOBSTRUENTS.—(Term obsolete and not very definite.) Medicines which overcome obstruction; aperients.

DEODORANTS.—Substances which destroy or hide foul odors.

DEPILATORIES.—Substances used to remove hair.

DEPRESSANTS.—Sedatives.

DEPRESSO-MOTORS.—Medicines which lessen motor activity.

DEPURANTS.—Medicines which act upon the emunctories so as to cause excretion and thereby purify the system.

Detergents.—Medicines which cleanse wounds, ulcers, etc.
Diaphoretics.—Medicines which produce sweating.
Digestants.—Ferments and acids which have the power of aiding in the solution of food.
Diluents.—Medicines which dilute secretions and excretions.
Disinfectants.—Substances which have the power of destroying disease-germs or the noxious properties of decaying organic matter.
Diuretics.—Medicines which increase the secretion of urine.
Drastics.—Purgatives which cause much irritation.
Ecbolics.—Medicines which produce abortion.
Eccoprotics, or **Ectoprotics.**—Laxatives.
Emetics.—Medicines which cause vomiting.
Emmenagogues.—Medicines which stimulate menstruation.
Emollients.—Substances used to mechanically soften and protect tissues.
Epispastics.—Blisters.
Errhines.—Medicines which increase the nasal secretions.
Escharotics.—Caustics.
Evacuants.—Medicines which evacuate; chiefly applied to purgatives.
Excitants.—Stimulants.
Excito-Motors.—Medicines which increase motor activity.
Expectorants.—Medicines which act upon the pulmonic mucous membrane and increase or alter its secretions.
Febrifuges.—Medicines which dissipate fever.
Galactagogues.—Medicines which increase the secretion of milk.
Hæmostatics.—Medicines which arrest hemorrhages.
Hydragogues.—Purgatives which cause large watery discharges.
Hypnotics.—Medicines which cause sleep.
Laxatives.—Mild purgatives.
Local Anæsthetics.—Medicines which when applied locally destroy sensation.
Mydriatics.—Medicines which cause *mydriasis*, or dilatation of the pupil.
Myotics.—Medicines which cause *myosis*, or contraction of the pupil.
Narcotics.—Powerful anodyne hypnotics.
Neurotics.—Medicines which act upon the nervous system.
Nutriants.—Medicines which modify the nutritive processes.
Nutrients.—Substances which nourish.
Oxytocics.—Medicines which stimulate uterine contractions.
Peristaltics.—Medicines which increase peristalsis.
Prophylactics.—Medicines which prevent the taking or development of disease.
Protectives.—Medicines which protect a part when applied to it.
Ptyalagogues.—Sialagogues.
Purgatives.—Medicines which produce watery discharges from the bowels.
Refrigerants.—Medicines which lessen the bodily temperature.
Revulsants.—Medicines which by causing irritation draw nervous force and blood from a distant diseased part.
Rubefacients.—Medicines which cause irritation and redness, and are used as revulsants.
Sedatives.—Medicines which lower functional activity.
Sialagogues.—Medicines which excite the salivary glands to secretion.
Somnifacients.—Soporifics.
Soporifics.—Medicines which cause sleep.
Sorbefacients.—Medicines which cause absorption.
Specifics.—Medicines which have a direct curative influence on certain individual diseases.
Stimulants.—Medicines which increase functional activity.
Stomachics.—Stimulants to the stomach.
Styptics.—Hæmostatics.
Sudorifics.—Medicines which produce sweating.
Tænicides.—Medicines which kill the tape-worm.
Tonics.—Medicines which permanently increase the systemic tone by stimulating nutrition.
Vermicides.—Medicines which kill intestinal worms.
Vermifuges.—Medicines which cause the expulsion of intestinal worms.
Vesicatories.—Blisters.

THE

DISPENSATORY

OF

THE UNITED STATES.

PART I.

The United States Dispensatory may very properly be considered as a commentary upon the United States and British Pharmacopœias, whilst such preparations of the German Pharmacopœia and French Codex as are used generally in the United States are also commented upon. As was explained in the fifteenth edition, the changes in the arrangement of the 1880 edition of the United States Pharmacopœia necessitated corresponding alterations in the United States Dispensatory. Part I. of the present volume contains the discussion of all the remedies recognised by either of the two Pharmacopœias used by English-speaking people. In Part II. the National Formulary is introduced, to which are attached references to the pages in the other parts of the work which would prove useful to the operator whilst using the formulas; this is designated as Section I., whilst non-officinal drugs and preparations are treated, as heretofore, by themselves; they are classed now in Section II., and are printed in smaller type than that used for officinal substances, it being deemed judicious to adhere to a plan which has given so much satisfaction in the previous editions. In Part III. are considered the Tests and Test-Solutions of the two Pharmacopœias, Weights and Measures, the Art of Prescribing Medicines, and other cognate miscellaneous matters.

There can be no question as to the superiority of the alphabetical arrangement of drugs in a book of reference such as the present. Their scientific classification belongs to works which treat of them rather in their relations than their essential properties; and different systems have been adopted, according to the set of relations towards which the mind of the author has been especially directed. Thus, the naturalist classifies them according to the affinities of the several objects in nature from which they are derived; the chemist, according to their composition; the practitioner of medicine, according to their effects upon the system in a state of health and disease.

The definitions of the terms used to describe the action of remedies, which for many years occupied a place in this part of the work, are in the sixteenth edition replaced by a short glossary, which contains succinct definitions, arranged so that they may be quickly and conveniently referred to. (See the preceding pages.)

ABSINTHIUM. *U. S.* *Absinthium.*

(AB-SĬN'THI-ŬM.)

The leaves and tops of Artemisia Absinthium. Linné. (*Nat. Ord.* Compositæ.) *U. S.*

Wormwood; Absinthe commune, Grande Absinthe, Armoise amère, *Fr.;* Gemeiner Wermuth, *G.;* Assenzio, *It.;* Artemisio Axenjo, *Sp.*

Gen. Ch. *Receptacle* sub-villous, or nearly naked. *Seed-down* none. *Calyx* imbricate, with roundish converging scales. *Corollas of the ray* none. *Willd.*

Several species of Artemisia have enjoyed some reputation as medicines. The leaves of *A. Abrotanum*, or *southernwood*, are reported by Craveri to contain a crystallizable alkaloid, *abrotine;* they have a fragrant odor, and a warm, bitter, nauseous taste, and were formerly employed as a tonic, deobstruent, and anthelmintic. Similar virtues have been ascribed to *A. Santonica*. *A. pontica* has been occasionally substituted for common wormwood, but is weaker. *A. vulgaris*, or *mugwort*, formerly enjoyed considerable reputation as an emmenagoguo, and has been used in Germany in epilepsy. Along with asafetida it is also sometimes given in chorea and in amenorrhœa. *A. Ludoviciana*, a native of the southwestern regions of the U. States, is thought, when applied to the head in the state of infusion, to favor the growth of the hair. (Maisch, *A. J. P.*, 1872, p. 106.) In China, *moxa* is said to be prepared from the leaves of *A. Chinensis* and *A. Indica*. The medicine known in Europe by the name of wormseed is the product of different species.

Artemisia Absinthium. Willd. *Sp. Plant.* iii. 1844; Woodv. *Med. Bot.* p. 54, t. 22. Wormwood is a perennial plant, with branching, round, and striated or furrowed stems, which rise two or three feet in height, and are panicled at their summit. The lower portion of the stem lives several years, and annually sends up herbaceous shoots, which perish in the winter. The radical leaves are triply pinnatifid, with lanceolate, obtuse, dentate divisions; those of the stem, doubly or simply pinnatifid, with lanceolate, somewhat acute divisions; the floral leaves are lanceolate; all are hoary. The flowers are of a brownish-yellow color, hemispherical, pedicelled, nodding, and in erect racemes. The florets of the disk are numerous, those of the ray few. The plant is a native of Europe, where it is also cultivated. It is among our garden herbs, and has been naturalized in the mountainous districts of New England. The leaves and flowering summits are employed; the larger parts of the stalk being rejected. They should be gathered in July or August, when the plant is in flower. They preserve their peculiar sensible properties long when dried.

"Leaves about two inches (5 cm.) long, hoary, silky, pubescent, petiolate, roundish, triangular in outline, pinnately two- or three-cleft, with the segments lanceolate, the terminal one spatulate, bracts three-cleft or entire; heads numerous, subglobose, with numerous small, pale-yellow florets, all tubular and without pappus; odor aromatic; taste persistently bitter." *U. S.* Wormwood yields by distillation a volatile oil (*oleum absinthii*), usually dark green, sometimes yellow or brownish, having a strong odor of the plant, an acrid peculiar taste, and the sp. gr. 0·972. It is sometimes adulterated with alcohol, oil of turpentine, etc., which lessen its specific gravity. According to C. R. A. Wright, the oil is composed of a terpene boiling at 150° C., and *absinthol*, which has a specific gravity 0·926, composition $C_{10}H_{16}O$, boiling point of 200° C. (392° F.) to 205° C., and when heated with phosphorus pentasulphide or zinc chloride is split into *cymene* ($C_{10}H_{14}$) and a resinous substance. The portion of absinthol which does not distil over at about 200° C. consists chiefly of the coloring principles *azulene* of Piesse and *cœrulëin* of Gladstone (*Journ. Chem. Soc.*, Jan. 1874). The dried herb yields much more oil than the fresh. The other constituents, according to Braconnot, are a very bitter and an almost insipid azotized matter, an excessively bitter resinous substance, chlorophyll, albumen, starch, saline matters, and lignin; malic and acetic acids are also said to be present. The cold infusion becomes olive-green and turbid on the addition of ferric chloride, indicating the probable existence of a little tannic acid. (*Pereira.*) The *absinthic acid* found by Braconnot is said to be succinic acid. Caventou obtained the bitter principle *absinthin* in an impure condition. (See *U. S. D.*, 14th ed., p. 5.) Dr.

E. Luck prepared pure absinthin in 1851. (*A. J. P.*, xxiii. 358.) A. Kromayer (*Arch. Pharm.* (2), cviii. 129) considers absinthin an aldehyd, and assigns to it the formula $C_{40}H_{56}O_8 + H_2O$. He prepared it by exhausting the dry herb with hot water, evaporating the decoction, absorbing the bitter principle with animal charcoal, extracting with alcohol, partially purifying with lead acetate, precipitating with tannin, dissolving the precipitate in alcohol, mixing with lead oxide, treating the dry residue with alcohol, filtering, and evaporating to dryness. Duquesnel obtained absinthin in prismatic, odorless crystals of an intensely bitter taste. The old *salt of wormwood* (*sal absinthii*) was impure carbonate of potassium, made from the ashes of the plant.

Medical Properties and Uses. Wormwood was known to the ancients. It is highly tonic, and formerly enjoyed great reputation in debility of the digestive organs, and of the system generally. Before the introduction of Peruvian bark, it was much used in the treatment of intermittents. It has also been supposed to possess anthelmintic virtues. At present, however, it is little used in regular practice on this side of the Atlantic. It is undoubtedly capable of causing headache and other nervous disorders. The volatile oil in sufficient dose is a violent narcotic poison. In dogs and rabbits from thirty to fifty drops (1·5–3·2 C.c.) of it cause trembling, stupor, hebetude, and it may be insensibility; one to two drachms (3·75–7·5 C.c.) of it, violent epileptiform convulsions, with involuntary evacuations, unconsciousness and stertorous breathing, which may or may not end in death. (Marcé, *Bull. Thérap.*, Mai, 1864; Magnan, *L'Union Méd.*, Août, 1864; Amory, *Bost. Med. and Surg. Journ.*, March, 1868, p. 83.) In man the oil acts similarly; a half-ounce (C.c. 15) of it caused, in a male adult, insensibility, convulsions, foaming at the mouth, and a tendency to vomit; though the patient recovered under the use of emetics, with stimulants and demulcents. (*Lancet*, Dec. 6, 1862.) In large doses, wormwood irritates the stomach, and excites the circulation. The herb is sometimes applied externally, by way of fomentation, as an antiseptic and discutient. The dose in substance is from one to two scruples (1·3–2·6 Gm.); of the infusion, made by macerating an ounce in a pint of boiling water, from one to two fluidounces (30–60 C.c.).*

Off. Prep. Vinum Aromaticum.

ABSTRACTA. *Abstracts.*

(AB-STRĂC'TA.)

This new class of preparations is introduced for the first time into the Pharmacopœia. Their introduction grows out of the necessity for convenient and reliable solid preparations which bear a *definite relation to the drug*. Powdered extracts have been found in commerce for many years, but, as usually furnished, are objectionable preparations, owing to the injurious loss of strength resulting from the heating during desiccation, and to their proneness to absorb moisture and become subsequently a hard, solidified mass in the dispensing bottle. Among the advantages possessed by abstracts is that their strength bears a uniform relation with the drug, the fluid

* *Absinthe.* Under this name, a *liqueur* is much used in France, consisting essentially of an alcoholic solution of oil of wormwood containing some alcoholic extract of angelica, anise, and marjoram. According to Baudrimont (Chevallier, *Dictionnaire des Falsifications*, 6me éd.) the *absinthe ordinaire* contains 47·66 per cent. of alcohol, the *demi-fine* 50 per cent., the *fine* 68 per cent., and the *absinthe suisse* 86·66 per cent. The preparation, if manipulated properly, possesses naturally a bright-green color, brought to an olive-green by slight addition of caramel-coloring, but artificial coloring is often resorted to, and indigo, turmeric, cupric acetate, and aniline green have been used to produce the proper shade. According to the French law of 1872, the oil and other concentrated preparations of absinthe can be sold only by pharmacists, and by them only on prescription. It has for some time been noticed that the effects of this liqueur differ essentially from those of pure alcoholic drinks, constituting a series of symptoms which has been designated as *absinthism*. From a case recorded by M. Magnan, in which the patient, having habituated himself to the use of brandy, and afterwards substituted *absinthe*, gave an opportunity of comparing the effects of the two kinds of drink, it appears that the characteristic symptoms of the latter, taken in excess, are restlessness at night, with disturbing dreams, nausea and vomiting in the morning, with great trembling of the hands and tongue, vertigo, and a tendency to epileptiform convulsions, in which the patient loses consciousness, falls, bites his tongue, foams at the mouth, makes facial grimaces, throws about his limbs, etc., but from which he usually recovers.

extract, and frequently with the tincture. They are in every case twice as strong as the drug or fluid extract, and about ten times the strength of the tincture; the heat employed in evaporating does not exceed 50° C. (122° F.), and the caramel-like odor, produced by excessive heat, is absent in the finished abstract: being in the form of a dry powder, abstracts are conveniently dispensed, and the process for their preparation is simple, requiring no apparatus which is not at the command of every pharmacist. In many cases where the Fluid Extract is alcoholic and free from glycerin, the abstract may be easily made by adding about one-fourth its weight of powdered sugar of milk, drying at a low temperature, as proposed, and making up the quantity to half the weight of the Fluid Extract with more sugar of milk. As the strength of abstracts is uniform, and differs from that of extracts, it was deemed advisable to give them a new title, so that confusion should be avoided Abstracts were prepared in 1877 by Prof. Jos. P. Remington, and the process offered to the committee of the Philadelphia College of Pharmacy on the revision of the U. S. Pharmacopœia (see *Extracta*). The term "Abstractum" was proposed by Mr. A. B. Taylor as accurately defining the class, and not likely to be mistaken through abbreviation. A valuable paper on "Powdered Extracts," by C. S. Hallberg, may be found in *Proc. Am. Pharm. Assoc.*, 1879–1881. They should be kept in well-stoppered bottles in a cool and dry place.

ABSTRACTUM ACONITI. *U.S. Abstract of Aconite.*

(ĄB-STRĂC'TŲM ĂC-Ǫ-NĪ'TĪ.)

"Aconite, in No. 60 powder, *two hundred parts* [or four ounces av.]; Tartaric Acid, *two parts* [or eighteen grains]; Sugar of Milk, recently dried and in fine powder, Alcohol, each, *a sufficient quantity*, To make *one hundred parts* [or two ounces av.]. Moisten the Aconite with *eighty parts* [or one and three-quarter fluidounces] of Alcohol, in which the Tartaric Acid has previously been dissolved, and pack firmly in a cylindrical glass percolator; then add enough alcohol to saturate the powder and leave a stratum above it. When the liquid begins to drop from the percolator, close the lower orifice, and, having closely covered the percolator, macerate for forty-eight hours. Then allow the percolation to proceed, gradually adding Alcohol, until the Aconite is exhausted. Reserve the first *one hundred and seventy parts* [or three and one-half fluidounces] of the percolate, evaporate the remainder to *thirty parts* [or half a fluidounce] at a temperature not exceeding 50° C. (122° F.) and mix with the reserved portion. Place the mixture in an evaporating dish, and, having added *fifty parts* [or one ounce av.] of Sugar of Milk, cover it with a piece of thin muslin gauze, and set aside in a warm place, where the temperature will not rise above 50° C. (122° F.), until the mixture is dry. Lastly, having added enough Sugar of Milk to make the mixture weigh *one hundred parts* [or two ounces av.], reduce it to a fine, uniform powder. Preserve the powder in a well-stopped bottle." *U. S.*

Duquesnel recommended tartaric acid in alcoholic solution as the best menstruum for aconite root, and his views were confirmed by C. R. Alder Wright (*P. J. T.*, ix., 1878, p. 152) on the ground that alcohol acidulated with tartaric acid extracts a larger percentage of crystallizable aconitine than alcohol containing diluted mineral acid. Whilst the addition of a small quantity of tartaric acid to the menstruum can do no harm, there is still no difficulty in thoroughly exhausting aconite root of its virtues with alcohol alone, and a better abstract can be made without the addition of any acid. The root is preferable to the leaves on account of its greater uniformity in quality and its not containing so much soluble inert matter. The dose of the abstract is from one-half to one grain (0·03 to 0·06 Gm.).

ABSTRACTUM BELLADONNÆ. *U.S. Abstract of Belladonna.*

(ĄB-STRĂC'TŲM BĔL-LĄ-DŎN'NÆ.)

"Belladonna Root, in No. 60 powder, *two hundred parts* [or four ounces av.]; Sugar of Milk, recently dried and in fine powder, Alcohol, each, *a sufficient quantity*, To make *one hundred parts* [or two ounces av.]. Moisten the Belladonna Root with *eighty parts* [or one and three-quarters fluidounces] of Alcohol and pack firmly in a cylindrical percolator; then add enough Alcohol to saturate the powder and leave a stratum above it. When the liquid begins to drop from the percolator, close the lower orifice, and, having closely covered the percolator, macerate for forty-eight hours. Then allow the percolation to proceed, gradually adding Alcohol, until the Belladonna Root is exhausted. Reserve the first *one hundred and seventy parts* [or three and one-half fluidounces] of the percolate, evaporate the remainder to *thirty parts* [or half a fluidounce], at a temperature not exceeding 50° C. (122° F.), and mix with the reserved portion. Place the mixture in an evaporating dish, and having added *fifty parts* [or one ounce av.] of Sugar of Milk, cover it with a piece of thin muslin gauze, and set aside in a warm place, where the temperature will not rise above 50° C. (122° F.), until the mixture is dry. Lastly, having added enough Sugar of Milk to make the mixture weigh *one hundred parts* [or two ounces av.], reduce it to a fine, uniform powder. Preserve the powder in a well-stopped bottle." *U. S.*

This preparation is of a very light brownish-red color, and may be given in the dose of one-half to one grain (0·03 to 0·06 Gm.).

ABSTRACTUM CONII. *U. S.* *Abstract of Conium.*

(ĄB-STRĂC'TŲM CQ-NĪ'Ī.)

"Conium, in No. 40 powder, *two hundred parts* [or four ounces av.]; Diluted Hydrochloric Acid, *six parts* [or fifty minims]; Sugar of Milk, recently dried and in fine powder, Alcohol, each, *a sufficient quantity*, To make *one hundred parts* [or two ounces av.]. Mix the Hydrochloric Acid with *eighty parts* [or one and three-quarter fluidounces] of Alcohol, and, having moistened the Conium with the mixture, pack firmly in a cylindrical glass percolator; then add enough Alcohol to saturate the powder and leave a stratum above it. When the liquid begins to drop from the percolator, close the lower orifice, and, having closely covered the percolator, macerate for forty-eight hours. Then allow the percolation to proceed, gradually adding Alcohol, until the Conium is exhausted. Reserve the first *one hundred and seventy parts* [or three and one-half fluidounces] of the percolate, evaporate the remainder to *thirty parts* [or half a fluidounce], at a temperature not exceeding 50° C. (122° F.), and mix with the reserved portion. Place the mixture in an evaporating dish, and, having added *fifty parts* [or one ounce av.] of Sugar of Milk, cover it with a piece of thin muslin gauze, and set it aside in a warm place, where the temperature will not rise above 50° C. (122° F.), until the mixture is dry. Lastly, having added enough Sugar of Milk to make the mixture weigh *one hundred parts* [or two ounces av.], reduce it to a fine, uniform powder. Preserve the powder in a well-stopped bottle." *U. S.*

This is the best solid preparation of conium, being superior to the extract on account of the dissipation of the volatile alkaloid during the evaporation of the extract, which to a great extent is avoided in the process for the abstract. The conium seed is preferred to the leaves as more reliable; the hydrochloric acid is used to fix the alkaloid. The commencing dose is from one to two grains (0·06 to 0·12 Gm.).

ABSTRACTUM DIGITALIS. *U. S.* *Abstract of Digitalis.*

(ĄB-STRĂC'TŲM DĬG-Į-TĀ'LĬS.)

"Digitalis, recently dried and in No. 60 powder, *two hundred parts* [or four ounces av.]; Sugar of Milk, recently dried and in fine powder, Alcohol, each, *a sufficient quantity*, To make *one hundred parts* [or two ounces av.]. Moisten the Digitalis with *eighty parts* [or one and three-quarter fluidounces] of Alcohol, and pack firmly in a cylindrical percolator; then add enough Alcohol to saturate the powder and leave a stratum above it. When the liquid begins to drop from the percolator, close the lower orifice, and, having closely covered the percolator, macerate for forty-eight hours. Then allow the percolation to proceed, gradually adding Alcohol, until the Digitalis is exhausted. Reserve the first *one hundred and seventy parts* [or three and one-half fluidounces] of the percolate, evaporate the remainder to *thirty parts* [or half a fluidounce], at a temperature not exceeding 50° C. (122° F.), and mix with the reserved portion. Place the mixture in an evaporating dish, and, having added *fifty parts* [or one ounce av.] of Sugar of Milk, cover it with a piece of thin muslin gauze, and set aside in a warm place, where the temperature will not rise above 50° C. (122° F.), until the mixture is dry. Lastly, having added enough Sugar of Milk to make the mixture weigh *one hundred parts* [or two ounces av.], reduce it to a fine, uniform powder. Preserve the powder in a well-stopped bottle." *U. S.*

Abstract of Digitalis would well replace the extract, which is very variable in quality and consistence as usually dispensed. Its color is a decided, rather bright green, and it is well adapted for administration either *per se* or in pilular form. The dose is from one-half to one grain (0·03 to 0·06 Gm.), repeated with caution.

ABSTRACTUM HYOSCYAMI. *U.S. Abstract of Hyoscyamus.*

(AB-STRĂC'TUM HŸ-QS-CŸ'A-MĪ.)

"Hyoscyamus, recently dried and in No. 60 powder, *two hundred parts* [or four ounces av.]; Sugar of Milk, recently dried and in fine powder, Alcohol, each, *a sufficient quantity*, To make *one hundred parts* [or two ounces av.]. Moisten the Hyoscyamus with *eighty parts* [or one and three-quarter fluidounces] of Alcohol, and pack firmly in a cylindrical percolator; then add enough Alcohol to saturate the powder and leave a stratum above it. When the liquid begins to drop from the percolator, close the lower orifice, and, having closely covered the percolator, macerate for forty-eight hours. Then allow the percolation to proceed, gradually adding Alcohol, until the Hyoscyamus is exhausted. Reserve the first *one hundred and seventy parts* [three and one-half fluidounces] of the percolate, evaporate the remainder to *thirty parts* [or half a fluidounce], at a temperature not exceeding 50° C. (122° F.), and mix with the reserved portion. Place the mixture in an evaporating dish, and, having added *fifty parts* [or one ounce av.] of Sugar of Milk, cover it with a piece of thin muslin gauze, and set aside in a warm place, where the temperature will not rise above 50° C. (122° F.), until the mixture is dry. Lastly, having added enough Sugar of Milk to make the mixture weigh *one hundred parts* [or two ounces av.], reduce it to a fine, uniform powder. Preserve the powder in a well-stopped bottle." *U. S.*

This abstract is probably more hygroscopic and shows more evidences of coalescing than any of the others, but if it be kept in a cool and dry place and well stoppered, there will be no difficulty; it is of a green color, and when properly made, thoroughly reliable. The dose is from two to three grains (0·12 to 0·18 Gm.).

ABSTRACTUM IGNATIÆ. *U.S. Abstract of Ignatia.*

(AB-STRĂC'TUM ĬG-NĀ'TI-Æ (ĭg-nā'she-ē).)

"Ignatia, in No. 60 powder, *two hundred parts* [or four ounces av.]; Sugar of Milk, recently dried and in fine powder, Alcohol, Water, each, *a sufficient quantity*, To make *one hundred parts* [or two ounces av.]. Mix Alcohol and Water in the proportion of *eight parts* [or six fluidounces] of Alcohol to *one part* [or five fluidrachms] of Water, and, having moistened the Ignatia with *one hundred parts* [or two fluidounces] of the menstruum, pack firmly in a cylindrical percolator; then add enough of the menstruum to saturate the powder and leave a stratum above it. When the liquid begins to drop from the percolator, close the lower orifice, and, having closely covered the percolator, macerate for forty-eight hours. Then allow the percolation to proceed, gradually adding menstruum, until the Ignatia is exhausted. Reserve the first *one hundred and seventy parts* [three and one-half fluidounces] of the percolate, distil off the alcohol from the remainder, and mix the residue with the reserved portion. Place the mixture in an evaporating dish, and, having added *fifty parts* [or one ounce av.] of Sugar of Milk, cover it with a piece of thin muslin gauze, and set aside in a warm place, where the temperature will not rise above 50° C. (122° F.), until the mixture is dry. Lastly, having added enough Sugar of Milk to make the mixture weigh *one hundred parts* [two ounces av.], reduce it to a fine, uniform powder. Preserve the powder in a well-stopped bottle." *U. S.*

Abstract of Ignatia is intended to replace the extract, which is no longer officinal. Some difficulty is experienced in reducing Ignatia beans to powder, as they consist largely of an exceedingly tough, horny albumen. If they are, however, coarsely ground, and half their weight of water added, and heat applied until they have swollen, they may then be beaten into a paste, and subsequently dried and powdered without much trouble. On account of the fixed oil present in Ignatia, a slight change in the manipulation of this abstract might be advisable: the fluid extract should be evaporated to a soft extract, and allowed to stand a short time, when the fixed oil could be separated by absorbing it from the surface, or, if in sufficient quantity, poured off, and washed with diluted alcohol to separate any alkaloids which might be dissolved in the oil. This alcoholic solution should be mixed with the extract, evaporated, the sugar of milk added, and the preparation finished by the regular process given above. The yield of extract is usually about 10 per cent. The dose of abstract is from one-half to one and a half grains (0·03 to 0·10 Gm.).

ABSTRACTUM JALAPÆ. *U.S. Abstract of Jalap.*

(ĄB-STRĂC'TŲM JĄ-LĂ'PÆ.)

"Jalap, in No. 40 powder, *two hundred parts* [or four ounces av.]; Sugar of Milk, recently dried and in fine powder, Alcohol, each, *a sufficient quantity*, To make *one hundred parts* [or two ounces av.]. Moisten the Jalap with *one hundred parts* [or two fluidounces] of Alcohol, and pack firmly in a cylindrical percolator; then add enough Alcohol to saturate the powder and leave a stratum above it. When the liquid begins to drop from the percolator, close the lower orifice, and, having closely covered the percolator, macerate for forty-eight hours. Then allow the percolation to proceed, gradually adding Alcohol, until the Jalap is exhausted. Reserve the first *one hundred and seventy parts* [three and one-half fluidounces] of the percolate, distil off the alcohol from the remainder, and mix the residue with the reserved portion. Place the mixture in an evaporating dish, and, having added *fifty parts* [or one ounce av.] of Sugar of Milk, cover it with a piece of thin muslin gauze, and set aside in a warm place, where the temperature will not rise above 50° C. (122° F.), until the mixture is dry. Lastly, having added enough Sugar of Milk to make the mixture weigh *one hundred parts* [two ounces av.], reduce it to a fine, uniform powder. Preserve the powder in a well-stopped bottle." *U. S.*

This is the most useful of the abstracts, and is greatly to be preferred to the old extract of jalap, which had the fault of absorbing moisture and then drying to a hard mass in the bottle in which it was kept. It is a uniform powder, which, unlike a mixture of dry powdered alcoholic extract and powdered sugar of milk, has no tendency to form strata of varying degrees of strength in the dispensing bottle. The dose is from ten to fifteen grains (0·66 to 1 Gm.).

Off. Prep. Pilulæ Catharticæ Compositæ.

ABSTRACTUM NUCIS VOMICÆ. *U.S. Abstract of Nux Vomica.*

(ĄB-STRĂC'TŲM NŪ'CĬS VŎM'Į-ÇÆ.)

"Nux Vomica, in No. 60 powder, *two hundred parts* [or four ounces av.]; Sugar of Milk, recently dried and in fine powder, Alcohol, Water, each, *a sufficient quantity*, To make *one hundred parts* [or two ounces av.]. Mix Alcohol and Water in the proportion of *eight parts* [or six fluidounces] of Alcohol to *one part* [or five fluidrachms] of Water, and, having moistened the Nux Vomica with *one hundred parts* [or two fluidounces] of the menstruum, pack firmly in a cylindrical percolator; then add enough of the menstruum to saturate the powder and leave a stratum above it. When the liquid begins to drop from the percolator, close the lower orifice, and, having closely covered the percolator, macerate for forty-eight hours. Then allow the percolation to proceed, gradually adding menstruum, until the Nux Vomica is exhausted. Reserve the first *one hundred and seventy parts* [three and one-half fluidounces] of the percolate, distil off the alcohol from the remainder, and mix the residue with the reserved portion. Place the mixture in an evaporating dish, and, having added *fifty parts* [or one ounce av.] of Sugar of Milk, cover it with a piece of thin muslin gauze, and set aside in a warm place, where the temperature will not rise above 50° C. (122° F.), until the mixture is dry. Lastly, having added enough Sugar of Milk to make the mixture weigh *one hundred parts* [or two ounces av.], reduce it to a fine, uniform powder. Preserve the powder in a well-stopped bottle." *U. S.*

Abstract of Nux Vomica is well adapted to replace the extract, it having been the custom of late years to use the powdered extract largely in preference to the soft extract. If the fixed oil be not removed by the method noticed under Abstract of Ignatia, the abstract will be in the form of a greasy powder, which is not as sightly as the dry sabulous powder resulting when the fixed oil is removed (see *Extractum Nucis Vomicæ*). The dose is from one to two grains (0·06 to 0·12 Gm.).

ABSTRACTUM PODOPHYLLI. *U.S. Abstract of Podophyllum.*

(ĄB-STRĂC'TŲM PŎD-Q-PHȲL'LĪ.)

"Podophyllum, in No. 60 powder, *two hundred parts* [or four ounces av.]; Sugar of Milk, recently dried and in fine powder, Alcohol, each, *a sufficient quantity*, To make *one hundred parts* [or two ounces av.]. Moisten the Podophyllum with *eighty parts* [or one and three-quarter fluidounces] of Alcohol, and pack firmly in a cylindrical percolator; then add enough Alcohol to saturate the powder and leave a stratum above it. When the liquid begins to drop from the percolator, close the lower orifice, and, having closely covered the percolator, macerate for forty-eight hours. Then allow the percolation to proceed, gradually adding Alcohol, until the Podophyllum is exhausted. Reserve the first *one hundred and seventy parts* [or three and one-half fluidounces] of the percolate, distil off the alcohol from the remainder, and mix the residue with the reserved portion. Place the mixture in an evaporating dish, and, having added *fifty parts* [or one ounce av.] of Sugar of Milk, cover it with a piece of thin muslin gauze, and set aside in a warm place, where the temperature will not rise above 50° C. (122° F.), until the mixture is dry. Lastly, having added enough Sugar of Milk to make the mixture weigh *one hundred parts* [or two ounces av.], reduce it to a fine, uniform powder. Preserve the powder in a well-stopped bottle." *U. S.*

This preparation has probably no advantages over the resin of podophyllum. The yield of extract to alcohol is about 10 per cent. The dose of the abstract is from five to ten grains (0·33 to 0·67 Gm.).

ABSTRACTUM SENEGÆ. *U.S. Abstract of Senega.*

(ĄB-STRĂC'TŲM SĔN'Ę-QÆ.)

"Senega, in No. 60 powder, *two hundred parts* [or four ounces av.]; Sugar of Milk, recently dried and in fine powder, Alcohol, each, *a sufficient quantity*, To make *one hundred parts* [or two ounces av.]. Moisten the Senega with *eighty parts* [or one and three-quarter fluidounces] of Alcohol, and pack firmly in a cylindrical percolator; then add enough Alcohol to saturate the powder and leave a stratum above it. When the liquid begins to drop from the percolator, close the lower orifice, and, having closely covered the percolator, macerate for forty-eight hours. Then allow the percolation to proceed, gradually adding Alcohol, until the Senega is exhausted. Reserve the first *one hundred and seventy parts* [or three and one-half fluidounces] of the percolate, evaporate the remainder to *thirty parts* [or half a fluidounce], at a temperature not exceeding 50° C. (122° F.), and mix with the reserved portion. Place the mixture in an evaporating dish, and, having added *fifty parts* [or one ounce av.] of Sugar of Milk, cover it with a piece of thin muslin gauze, and set aside in a warm place, where the temperature will not rise above 50° C. (122° F.), until the mixture is dry. Lastly, having added enough Sugar of Milk to make the mixture weigh *one hundred parts* [or two ounces av.], reduce it to a fine, uniform powder. Preserve the powder in a well-stopped bottle." *U. S.*

This preparation is intended to take the place of the extract formerly officinal. It affords a convenient way of giving senega when a solid preparation is desired. The dose is from one to three grains (0·06 to 0·20 Gm.).

ABSTRACTUM VALERIANÆ. *U.S. Abstract of Valerian.*

(ĄB-STRĂC'TŲM VĄ-LĒ-RĮ-ĀN'Æ.)

"Valerian, in No. 60 powder, *two hundred parts* [or four ounces av.]; Sugar of Milk, recently dried and in fine powder, Alcohol, each, *a sufficient quantity*, To make *one hundred parts* [or two ounces av.]. Moisten the Valerian with *eighty parts* [or one and three-quarter fluidounces] of Alcohol and pack firmly in a cylindrical percolator; then add enough Alcohol to saturate the powder and leave a stratum above it. When the liquid begins to drop from the percolator, close the lower orifice, and, having closely covered the percolator, macerate for forty-eight hours. Then allow the percolation to proceed, gradually adding Alcohol, until the Valerian is exhausted. Reserve the first *one hundred and seventy parts* [or three and one-half fluidounces] of the percolate, evaporate the remainder to *thirty parts* [or half a fluidounce], at a temperature not exceeding 50° C. (122° F.), and mix with the reserved portion. Place the mixture in an evaporating dish, and, having added *fifty parts* [or one ounce av.] of Sugar of Milk, cover it with a piece of thin muslin gauze, and set aside in a warm place, where the temperature will not rise above 50° C. (122° F.), until the mixture is dry. Lastly, having added enough Sugar of Milk to make the mixture weigh *one hundred parts* [or two ounces av.], reduce it to a fine, uniform powder. Preserve the powder in a well-stopped bottle." *U.S.*

Abstract of Valerian is a great improvement over the former officinal extract, which was frequently found almost devoid of activity from the evaporation of the active volatile principles. An objection to it, is the large dose necessary, but it may be given enclosed in capsules. The dose is ten to twenty grains (0·67 to 1·34 Gm.).

ACACIA. *U.S. Acacia.* [*Gum Arabic.*]

(Ą-CĀ'CĮ-Ą.)

"A gummy exudation from Acacia verek, Guillemin et Perottet, and from other species of Acacia. (*Nat. Ord.* Leguminosæ, Mimoseæ.)" *U.S.*

Off. Syn. ACACIÆ GUMMI. *Gum Acacia.* "A gummy exudation from the stem and branches of Acacia Senegal, *Willd.* (A. verek, *Guill. et Per.*), and from other species of Acacia." *Br.*

Gummi Arabicum, Gummi Mimosæ; Gomme Arabique, *Fr.;* Arabisches Gummi, *G.;* Gomma Arabica, *It.;* Goma Arabiga, *Sp.;* Samagh Arabee, *Arab.*

This genus is one of those into which the old genus Mimosa of Linnæus was divided by Willdenow. The name *Acacia* was employed by the ancient Greeks to designate the gum-tree of Egypt, and has been appropriately applied to the new genus in which that plant is included.

Gen. Ch. HERMAPHRODITE. *Calyx* five-toothed. *Corolla* five-cleft, or formed of five petals. *Stamens* 4–100. *Pistil* one. *Legume* bivalve. MALE. *Calyx* five-toothed. *Corolla* five-cleft, or formed of five petals. *Stamens* 4–100. *Willd.*

The most important of the gum yielding Acacias are *A. vera* and the officinal *A. verek. A. vera* and *A. Arabica* were considered by Willdenow to be distinct species, but are now esteemed as one.

Acacia vera. Willd. *Sp. Plant.* iv. 1805; Hayne, *Darstel. und Beschreib.* x. 34. Syn. *A. Arabica.* Willd. *Sp. Plant.* iv. 1805; Hayne, *Darstel. und Beschreib.* x. 32; Carson, *Illust. of Med. Bot.* i. 31.—*Acacia Nilotica*, Delille, *Illust. Flor. de l'Égypte*, p. 79. This is a tree of middling size, with numerous scattered branches, of which the younger are much bent, and covered with a reddish-brown bark. The leaves are alternate and bipinnate, with two pairs of pinnæ, of which the lower are usually furnished with ten pairs of leaflets, the upper with eight. The leaflets are very small, oblong-linear, smooth, and supported upon very short footstalks. On the common petiole is a gland between each pair of pinnæ. Both the common and partial petiole are smooth in typical specimens of *A. vera*, but downy in the variety *A. Arabica.* Two sharp spines, from a quarter to half an inch long, of the color of the smaller branches, and joined together at their base, are found at the insertion of each leaf. The flowers are yellow, inodorous, small, and collected in globular heads, supported upon slender peduncles which rise from the axils of the leaves, in number from two to five together. The fruit is a smooth, flat, two-valved legume, divided, by contractions occurring at regular intervals, into several roundish portions, each containing one seed. This species flourishes in Southern Nubia, Egypt, and Senegal, and is probably scattered over the whole intervening portions of Africa; it is also abundant in Hindostan.

A. verek, Guillemin and Perottet, *Flore de Sénégambie*, 1830, 246, B. & T., 1877. *A. Senegal*, Willdenow, *Mimosa Senegal*, L.* This is a small tree with a grayish bark, the inner layers of which are strongly fibrous, bipinnate leaves, dense spikes of small yellow flowers longer than the leaves, and broad pods 3 to 4 inches long, containing 5 or 6 seeds. It rarely exceeds 20 feet in height, forms large forests in Western Africa, north of the river Senegal, and is abundant in Eastern Africa, Kordofan, and Southern Nubia. It is known by the natives as *Verek* or *Hashab*.

Besides the species above described, the following afford considerable quantities of gum†:—*A. Karroo* of the Cape of Good Hope, formerly considered by some as identical with *A. vera*; *A. gummifera*, seen by Broussonet in Morocco near Mogador; *A. Ehrenbergiana*, a shrub six or eight feet high, named in honor of the German traveller Ehrenberg, who observed it in the deserts of Libya, Nubia, and Dongola; *A. Seyal*, growing in the same region, and also in Upper Egypt and Senegambia; *A. Adansonii*, of the *Flore de Sénégambie*, said to contribute a portion of the Senegal gum; and *A. tortilis*, which sometimes attains the height of sixty feet, and inhabits Arabia Felix, Nubia, Dongola, and the Libyan desert. Brownish or reddish gums are also yielded by *A. stenocarpa*, *A. fistula*, and *A. Nilotica*, and probably by various undescribed species.‡ *A. decurrens* and *A. floribunda* yield gum in New Holland. Trees, moreover, not belonging to the genus, afford a similar product, especially *Feronia elephantum* of Hindostan, the gum of which, according to Ainslie, is used for medical purposes in Lower India, and *Algarobia glandulosa* of New Mexico, the source of the *mezquite gum*.§

The gum-bearing Acacias are all thorny or prickly trees or shrubs, calculated by nature for a dry and sandy soil, and flourishing in deserts where few other trees will grow. We are told that camels, attached to the caravans, derive from them their chief sustenance in many parts of those desolate regions in which Africa abounds. In these situations, they have a stunted growth, and present a bare, withered, and uninviting aspect; but in favorable situations, as on the banks of rivers, they are often luxuriant and beautiful.

Their bark and unripe fruit contain tannic and gallic acids, and are sometimes used in tanning. An extract was formerly obtained from the immature pods of *A. Arabica* and *A. vera*, by expression and inspissation. It was known to the ancients by the name of *acaciæ veræ succus*, and was highly praised by some of the Greek medical writers, but is at present little used. It is a solid, heavy, shining, reddish-brown substance, of a sweetish, acidulous, styptic taste, and soluble in water. Its

* Why the revisers of the Pharmacopœia selected the name of *A. Verek* for this plant is not clear: according to the received principles of scientific nomenclature it should be known as *A. Senegal*.

† *Constitution of Gum.* Much confusion has existed in the use of the word *gum*, which has been employed to express various concrete vegetable juices, and, at the same time, a peculiar proximate principle of plants. It is now proposed to restrict the term to the former of these applications, and to designate the principle alluded to by the name of arabin. Chemically, M. Guérin considers as characteristic of gums the property of affording mucic acid when acted on by nitric acid. He recognises in the different gums three distinct proximate principles; namely: 1, *arabin*, or the pure gum of chemical writers, which is the essential constituent of gum arabic; 2, *bassorin*, which enters largely into the composition of Bassora gum and tragacanth; and 3, *cerasin* (metarabic acid), which constitutes the portion of cherry gum insoluble in cold water. Of arabin sufficient is said in the text. Bassorin will be treated of under the head of Bassora gum. (See *Part Second.*) The gums which exude from the cherry, apricot, peach, and plum trees, and which the French call *gomme du pays*, appear to be identical in composition, consisting of a portion soluble in cold water, which is arabin, and a portion insoluble, appropriately denominated *cerasin*, and now known to be produced from the arabin by alteration.

‡ For further information in regard to gum-bearing trees of Northern Africa, see *P. J. Tr.*, Aug. 1873; *Compt.-Rendus*, t. lxxix. p. 1175.

§ *Mezquite gum* occurs in light amber-colored tears, and is soluble in three parts of water, making a slightly acid mucilage which does not precipitate with the subacetate of lead. Although the tree is very abundant in Texas and Mexico, the yield of gum is so small, not exceeding a third of a pound a season for the largest trees, that it can never be an article of commercial importance.

virtues are probably those of a mild astringent. On the continent of Europe, a preparation is said to be substituted for it called *acacia nostras*, obtained by expression and inspissation from the unripe fruit of *Prunus spinosa*, or the wild plum-tree.

The gum of the Acacias exudes spontaneously from the bark, and hardens on exposure; but incisions are sometimes made in order to facilitate the exudation. The gum is said also to be found immediately under the bark, where it is sometimes collected in regular cavities. (*Journ. de Pharm.*, t. xxiv. p. 321.) It is probably produced by a process of degeneration from the cellulose, and is incapable of serving further in plant-growth.* It is stated by Jackson that, in Morocco, the greatest product is obtained in the driest and hottest weather, and from the most sickly trees. An elevated temperature appears to be essential; for in cooler climates, though the tree may flourish, it yields no gum. According to Ehrenberg, the varieties in the characters of the gum do not depend upon difference in the species of the plant. Thus, from the same tree, it will exude frothy or thick, and clear or dark-colored, and will assume, upon hardening, different shapes and sizes; so that the pieces, when collected, require to be assorted before being delivered into commerce. Schweinfurth and other observers state, however, that the finest gum is obtained only from the *A. vera*, and perhaps one or two other species.

Commercial History and Varieties. The most common varieties of this drug are the *Turkey*, the *Barbary*, the *Senegal*, and the *India gum;* to which may be added the *Cape* and the *Australian gum.*

1. TURKEY GUM. Gum arabic was formerly procured chiefly, if not exclusively, from Egypt and the neighboring countries; and much is still obtained from the same sources. It is collected in Upper Egypt, Nubia, Kordofan, and Darfur, whence it is taken down the Nile to Alexandria. We obtain it in this country through Smyrna, Trieste, Marseilles, or some other entrepôt of the Mediterranean commerce. Two varieties have long been noticed, one more or less colored, the other white, which were formerly distinguished by the titles of *gum gedda* and *gum turic*, derived from the ports of the Red Sea, Jidda and Tor, from which the varieties were erroneously supposed to be respectively exported. The gum from Egypt is commonly called *Turkey gum*, and is the kind with which apothecaries are usually supplied. Though interspersed with roundish pieces of various sizes, it consists chiefly of small, irregular fragments, commonly whitish, or slightly tinged with yellow or reddish yellow. It is, on the whole, lighter colored, more brittle, more readily soluble, and freer from impurities than the other commercial varieties, and contains much of that form of gum arabic which is characterized by innumerable minute fissures pervading its substance, and impairing its transparency.

2. BARBARY GUM. (*Mogador Gum, Morocco Gum.*) Mogador, a port of Morocco, is the chief entrepôt of the trade. The gum is probably derived, in part at least, from *A. Nilotica.* According to Jackson, the natives call the tree which affords it *attaleh.* They gather it in July and August, when the weather is hot and very dry. Two kinds are brought to Mogador, one from the neighboring provinces, the other by caravans from Timbuctoo. This may account for the fact that Barbary gum in part resembles the Turkey, in part the Senegal. When first deposited in the warehouses, it has a faint smell, and makes a crackling noise, occasioned by the rupture of the small masses as they become more dry. Barbary gum is usually in tears, somewhat brownish, roundish or vermiform, wholly soluble in water. It reaches the United States in casks through English commerce.

* In the lower orders of life the inner cell contents or protoplasm is often set free by the rapid conversion of the cellulose wall into a substance soluble in water, and it is asserted that very frequently in the higher plants cells can be seen with one-half of their walls still cellulose, the other gum. According to Wigand, arabin is a result of a further change in bassorin. According to the independent researches of Dr. Beijerinck and of Dr. Wiesner (*P. J. Tr.*, xvi. p. 284), the change of the cell-wall is provoked by a peculiar ferment. Kraus found that the formation of gum in *Acacia Melanoxylon* takes place only in the bark and not in the wood, that it flows from the sieve-tubes and the cells of the soft bast, and he asserts that it is not a product of the degeneration of the cellulose, but a true cell-content passing out through unchanged cell-walls. (*P. J. Tr.*, 1886, p. 840.) For further information see Hofmeister, *Handbuch der physiolog. Botanik*, Bd. iv. p. 368, 1865; also Müller, *Sitzb. Akad. Wiss., Wien*, ii., Juni, 1875; Mercadante, *Gaz. Chim.; Ber. Chem. Gesell.*, 1876, p. 581; Giraud, *A. J. P.*, 1878, p. 127; also, denying explanation, Prillieux, *Compt.-Rend.*, t. lxxviii. p. 135.

3. Senegal Gum. This variety was introduced into Europe by the Dutch. The French afterwards planted a colony on the western coast of Africa, and took possession of the trade. St. Louis, at the mouth of the Senegal, and Portendic, considerably farther north, are the ports in which the commerce in gum chiefly centres. Immense forests exist in the interior, containing many species of the genus Acacia, all of which are said to yield gum; as is affirmed do also various trees belonging to other genera. (*Journ. de Pharm.*, xxiv. 318.) The juice begins to exude in November. The dry winds, which prevail after the rainy season, cause the bark to crack; the juice flows out and hardens in masses, which are often as large as a pigeon's egg, and sometimes as that of an ostrich. At this period, the Moors and negroes proceed to the forests in caravans, collect the gum in leather sacks, and convey it to the coasts, or frequently it is purchased by barter from the natives. Senegal gum is imported into the United States chiefly from Bordeaux, where it is sorted into twelve or fifteen different grades. (*P. J. Tr.*, ix. 43.) It is usually in roundish or oval unbroken pieces, of various sizes, in the finest grades whitish or colorless, but generally yellowish, reddish, or brownish red. The pieces are larger than those of Turkey gum, less brittle and pulverizable, and breaking with a more conchoidal fracture.*

4. India Gum. Most of this gum is taken to Bombay in Arab vessels from Cape Gardafui and Berbera on the northeastern coast of Africa, where it is collected, or from the ports of the Red Sea. It is in pieces of various size, color, and quality, some resembling the broken fragments of Turkey gum, though much less chinky; others large, roundish, and tenacious, like the Senegal. It is often contaminated, containing, besides genuine gum arabic, portions of a different product, having the characteristic properties of Bassora gum. This is distinguished by its insolubility in water, with which, however, it unites, swelling up, and forming a soft viscid mass. It owes its properties to the presence of *bassorin*. Besides this impurity in the India gum, there are often others more readily detected. Among these, we have observed a yellowish-white resinous substance, which has the sensible properties of the turpentines. If care be used in assorting this commercial variety, it may be employed for all the purposes of good gum arabic. India gum is brought to this country partly from Calcutta or Bombay, and partly by way of England. It usually comes in large cases. We have seen a parcel said to have come directly from the Red Sea, enclosed in large sacks made of a kind of matting, and bearing a close resemblance to the gum from Calcutta, except that it was more impure, and contained numerous large, irregular, very brittle masses, not much less than the fist in size.†

* Dr. A. Corre divides the gum Senegal into the hard gums, which are of firm consistence, with a large, clear, shining fracture, and the soft or friable gums. For an account of the grades and varieties of these the reader is referred to the *Journ. de Pharm.*, xxiv. 318. *Galam* gum (*Gommes haut-du-fleuve*) is that coming from Galam, Podor, Bakel, and Medina; it is sometimes hard, sometimes soft. For an abstract of Soubeiran's paper on Galam gums, which is scarcely applicable to the present time, see 14th ed. U. S. D. *Gommes bas-du-fleuve* are from the deserts of Bounou and the country of the Braknas.

Brittle gum, *Salabreda*, or *Sadra-beida*, is supposed to be obtained from *A. albida* of the Flora of Senegambia, which is much smaller than *A. verek*, and characterised by its white bark. The gum is usually in small, irregular pieces, like coarse salt, probably the fragments of larger lumps, but sometimes in vermicular pieces about as thick as a goose-quill, and of variable length. It is dull and often wrinkled externally, of a vitreous fracture, and of different tints of color, white, green, yellow, or orange. It is always somewhat bitter. Very easily soluble in its weight of water, it affords a mucilage of little consistence, which has but a slight effect on the tincture of litmus. When the solution is evaporated to the consistence of a paste, it absorbs moisture so as to become viscid; this property detracts much from its value. It is much less esteemed than the Galam gum.

† In the *Journ. de Pharm. et de Chim.* (Oct. 1867, p. 270), a variety of India gum, imported into France by way of London, in boxes containing about 400 pounds, is described as follows. It is a mixture of tears of various tints with impurities. In assorting it for use, the lightest-colored tears are selected. These are less perfectly transparent than gum arabic, less fissured on the surface, which is brilliant and often mammillated, and are also much less friable. But the most important distinctive character of this gum consists in its relations to water. If agitated with twice or thrice its weight of cold water, instead of forming, like ordinary gum arabic, a homogeneous, slightly mucilaginous solution, it forms a thick, transparent, very tenacious magma, which cannot be diluted with a larger quantity of water, but may, after a long time, be coarsely divided, still, however, retaining its viscid, ropy aspect, which never entirely disappears, whatever may be the quantity of water added. It imparts to syrup a very thick and very viscid consistence. It is important that the apothecary should be able to distinguish it, as it is unfit for ordinary pharmaceutic use, being employed exclusively by manufacturers in the preparation of cloths. All that is necessary is to add a few pieces to twice their weight of cold water, and allow the mixture to stand. After some hours, the peculiar, viscid mucilage above described betrays the character of the gum.

5. Cape Gum. During 1872, 101,241 pounds of this gum were imported into Great Britain from the Cape of Good Hope, where it is collected from the *Acacia horrida* of Willdenow. (*Flor. Capens.* 8.) It is of a pale yellow or amber-brown color, in tears or fragments, and is considered an inferior variety. (*A. J. P.*, xxix. 75.)

6. Australian Gum is the product of *A. pycnantha*, Benth.; *A. decurrens*, Willd.; *A. homalophylla* (A. Cunn). It occurs in hard pieces, elongated or globular; rough, varying in color from dark amber to pale yellow; entirely soluble in water, and yielding a very adhesive mucilage, which, when dry, is said not to crack. It sometimes contains tannin. The wood of *A. homalophylla* is known in commerce as *violet wood* on account of its pleasant odor. (*Amer. Drug.*, 1884, p. 204.)

7. Suakin Gum. *Talca* or *Talha Gum*, from *A. stenocarpa* and *A. Seyal*, is exceedingly brittle, and usually semipulverulent. It is a mixture of nearly colorless and brownish gum, is exported at Alexandria, and is sometimes termed *gum savakin*.

General Properties. Gum arabic is in roundish or amorphous pieces, or irregular fragments, of various size, more or less transparent, hard, brittle, pulverizable, and breaking with a shining fracture. It is usually white, or yellowish white, but frequently presents different shades of red, and is sometimes of a deep-orange or brownish color. It is bleached by exposure to the sun. In powder it is always white. It is inodorous, has a feeble, slightly sweetish taste, and when pure dissolves wholly in the mouth. The sp. gr. varies from 1·31 to 1·48 or 1·525 for the dried gum. "The aqueous solution shows an acid reaction with test paper, yields gelatinous precipitates with solution of subacetate of lead, solution of ferric chloride, or concentrated solution of borate of sodium, and is not colored blue by test solution of iodine." *U. S.* Gum arabic is a varying mixture of at least two gums, one lævo-rotatory and the other dextro-rotatory, the latter predominating. The first constituent treated with dilute sulphuric acid yields crystallized *arabinose;* the second constituent under similar conditions yields a syrupy variety of sugar. (Scheibler.) The commercial gum arabic contains 17 per cent. of water and 3 per cent. of ash, consisting almost entirely of the carbonates of calcium, potassium, and magnesium.

The gum dissolves at ordinary temperatures slowly, in an equal weight of water, forming a thick glutinous liquid of distinctly acid reaction. It is insoluble in alcohol, ether, and the oils. 100 parts of diluted alcohol containing 22 per cent. of alcohol by volume, dissolve 57 parts of gum, diluted alcohol containing 40 per cent. alcohol takes up 10 parts, and 50 per cent. alcohol only 4 parts (Flückiger). If the gum be dissolved in cold water, and the solution be slightly acidulated with hydrochloric acid, alcohol produces in it a precipitate of the *arabin* (*arabic acid*), which may also be prepared by placing a solution of gum, acidulated with hydrochloric acid, on a dialyser, when calcium chloride will diffuse out, leaving behind solution of arabin.

Arabic acid dried at 100° C. (212° F.) has the composition $C_{12}H_{22}O_{11}$, and gives up H_2O when it unites with bases. It has a decided tendency to form acid salts. Concentrated nitric acid forms with it nitro-compounds, such as $C_{12}H_{18}(NO_2)_2O_{10}$ and $C_{12}H_{16}(NO_2)_4O_{10}$; dilute nitric acid, on the other hand, gives rise to mucic and saccharic acids, together with oxalic and a little tartaric acid. Dilute sulphuric acid on prolonged boiling gives rise, according to Scheibler, to *arabinose*, or *arabin sugar* (*pectinose*, or *pectin sugar*), $C_6H_{12}O_6$, which reduces alkaline copper solution and turns the plane of polarization 121° to the right. Kiliani has, however, recently (*Ber. der Chem. Ges.*, 1887, p. 339) announced that his researches point to the formula $C_5H_{10}O_5$ for arabinose, and he considers that it is the missing pentatomic alcohol which comes in between erythrite and dextrose.

Neutral acetate of lead does not precipitate its aqueous solution, but the basic acetate forms even in a very dilute solution a precipitate.

Prolonged heating of the dry gum causes it to change readily into *metarabic* (*metagummic*) acid, which is identical with the *cerasin* found in the beet and in cherry-gum. Sulphuric acid will also change arabic into metarabic acid. 25 Gm. pure gum arabic are covered with 50 C.c. strong alcohol, 10 C.c. water, and 5 C.c. sulphuric acid, and allowed to stand 24 hours. On pouring off the fluid, and washing the residue with alcohol and with water, metarabic acid remains behind as a voluminous mass, which dries to a white, tasteless, and odorless powder of acid reaction. (*Graeger, Jahresbericht der Chem.*, 1872, p. 781.) The *metapectic* acid prepared by Scheibler from the sugar beet is identical with this.

The principle separated by cold water from the soluble arabin proves to be the same as the metarabic (metagummic) acid prepared direct from the pure gum arabic by heating, or by the action of sulphuric acid. It is also identical with gum extracted from the sugar beet by Scheibler. In the normal and sound beet this gum is insoluble in water, and merely swells up like the metarabic acid, while in altered beets there is found a portion (arabin) soluble in water. (Scheibler, *Ber. Chem. Ges.*, 1873, p. 612.)

The similarity of the reactions and composition of *arabinose* and *galactose* (from sugar of milk by inversion) led Kiliani to assert the identity of these two varieties of sugar, but later studies by himself, Claesson, and Scheibler have shown that they are distinct. Thus, galactose is fermentable, while arabinose is not; galactose yields mucic acid when oxidized with nitric acid, and dulcite when reduced with sodium amalgam, while arabinose does not yield either; the fusing-point of the crystallized galactose is given at 142–144° C., while that of arabinose is 160° C.; galactose yields with phenyl hydrazin a light-yellow compound, fusing at 170–171° C., while arabinose forms a brownish-yellow compound, fusing at 157–158° C. (Scheibler, *Ber. d. Chem. Ges.*, 17, p. 1731.) Arabinose is said to be obtainable only from those varieties of gum arabic that yield no mucic acid when treated with nitric acid. (Claesson, *Ber. d. Chem. Ges.*, 14, p. 1271.)

Gum arabic undergoes no change by age, when kept in a dry place. Its concentrated aqueous solution remains for a considerable time unaltered, but ultimately becomes sour, from the production of acetic acid. The disposition to sour is increased by employing hot water in making the solution. The tendency of a weak solution to become mouldy is said to be obviated by adding a few drops of sulphuric acid, and decanting from the sulphate of calcium deposited. (*A. J. P.*, 1872, p. 353.) Solution of gum arabic does not ferment upon the addition of yeast, saliva, or gastric juice; the addition of chalk and cheese, however, starts a fermentation which gives rise to lactic acid and alcohol, but not to mannite or glycerin. The addition of a solution of gum to an acidified albumen solution causes a precipitate, which disappears on further addition of gum, but the solution will then curdle and become flocculent on application of heat. Gum may be distinguished from dextrin by the following tests: 1. Gum contains no dextro-glucose, which, however, is present in dextrin, and may be recognized by the copper test.* 2. Gum contains a lime compound; hence its solution is rendered milky by oxalic acid, while a solution of dextrin remains almost clear. 3. Gum gives a shiny, yellow deposit when its solution is mixed with a neutral ferric salt. (Hager, *Chem. Central.*, 1873, pp. 408 and 584.)

The properties above enumerated belong to gum arabic generally. There are, however, pharmaceutic varieties with differences which deserve notice. 1. *Gum that is transparent and readily soluble.* This constitutes by far the greater portion of the commercial varieties distinguished by the names of Turkey and Senegal gum. It is characterized by its transparency, ready solubility, and the comparatively slight degree of thickness and viscidity of its solution. Under this head may be included the *gomme blanche fendillée* of Guibourt. It is distinguished by the whiteness and deficient transparency of the pieces, attributable to the minute cracks or fissures with which they abound, and which render them very brittle and easily pulverizable. This peculiar structure is generally ascribed to the influence of solar heat and light; but is conjectured by Hayne to arise from the exudation of the juice in the frothy state noticed by Ehrenberg. Though the unbroken pieces are somewhat opaque, each minute fragment is perfectly transparent and homogeneous. This variety, in consequence of its prompt and entire solubility, is usually preferred for medical use,

* *Fehling's Solution.* 40 Gm. of crystallized cupric sulphate dissolved in 200 C.c. of water; 160 Gm. of neutral potassium tartrate and 130 Gm. of fused sodium hydrate dissolved in 600 C.c. of water; mix the two solutions, dilute to 1 litre, and boil for some minutes. See also Test-Solution of Potassio-Cupric Tartrate (Part III.).

and for most purposes in pharmacy. 2. *Gum less transparent and less soluble.* Guibourt has proposed for portions of this gum the name of *gomme pelliculée*, from the circumstance that the masses are always apparently covered, on some part of their surface, by a yellowish opaque pellicle. Other portions of it have a mammillary appearance on the surface. It is less transparent than the former variety, is less freely and completely dissolved by water, and forms a more viscid solution. It melts with difficulty in the mouth, and adheres tenaciously to the teeth. It is found in all the commercial varieties of gum, but least in that from Egypt. Its peculiarities have been ascribed to variable proportions of *bassorin* or *cerasin* associated with the soluble *arabin*. Between these two varieties of gum there are insensible gradations, so that it is not always easy to classify specimens.*

Impurities and Adulterations. In parcels of gum arabic there are sometimes pieces of a dark color, opaque, and incorporated with ligneous, earthy, or other impurities. The inferior are often mixed with, or substituted for, the better kinds, especially in powder; and portions of insoluble gum, bdellium, and other concrete juices of unknown origin, are found among the genuine. Flour or starch is sometimes fraudulently added to the powder, but is easily detected by the blue color which it produces with tincture of iodine. In consequence of the impurities and difference in quality, gum arabic should generally be assorted for pharmaceutic use. A foreign substance sometimes adheres to its surface, giving it a bitter taste, from which it may be freed by washing in water.† *Dextrin*, broken into small fragments, has been mingled with parcels of gum, and may be recognized by tests already given. In Germany has been sold a gum arabic which contained yellowish and reddish pieces, some of them weighing over an ounce, mixed with pieces of tragacanth of the nodular Syrian sort, and also of opaque flakes and of the vermiform Morea variety. A substitute for acacia, made from mucilage of flaxseed, has been used satisfactorily by Trojanowsky. Another, which has recently been patented in Germany by Schumann, is prepared by the action of diluted sulphuric or nitric acid upon starch, under strong pressure. It is a colorless, transparent, gum-like substance, and is said to have the same useful properties as gum arabic. (*Pharm. Era*, 1888, p. 135.) A substitute has also been made from Irish moss. (See *Chondrus.*)

Medical Properties and Uses. This gum is used in medicine chiefly as a demulcent. By the viscidity of its solution, it serves to cover and sheathe inflamed surfaces; and, by blending with and diluting irritating matters, blunts their acrimony. Hence, it is advantageously employed in catarrhal affections and irritation of the fauces, by being held in the mouth and allowed slowly to dissolve. Internally administered, it has been found useful in inflammations of the gastric and intestinal mucous membrane; and its employment has even been extended to similar affections of the lungs and urinary organs. Whether it is beneficial, in the latter cases, in any other manner than by the dilution resulting from its watery vehicle, is doubtful. It has been used as a food, but has very little if any nutritive value. In pharmacy, gum arabic is extensively used for the suspension of insoluble substances in water, and for the formation of pills and troches. Two kinds of powdered gum arabic are used, one a coarse powder called *granulated*, the other *finely dusted*. The granulated dissolves more readily in water, according to Hager, because it has lost during desiccation only two per cent. of moisture, whilst in preparing the "finely dusted" powder the high heat necessarily used to thoroughly dry it, drives off ten per cent. of water. Its easy solubility and absence of tendency to form "lumps" cause the coarse powder to be preferred for solutions, emulsions, etc.

* A very handsome white gum was noticed in the market during 1876, which had the property of making a glairy solution with water. On allowing the mixture to stand for some days at a temperature of 95° C. (203° F.) it resumed its ordinary condition.

† M. Picciotto has proposed a method of purifying colored gum by dissolving the gum in 6 to 18 parts of water, passing the solution through linen, and then mixing it with gelatinous alumina freshly precipitated. A pap-like substance is formed; and the coloring matter is so fixed by the alumina, that, when the mixture is placed on a linen strainer, the mucilage escapes colorless; or, if not entirely so at first, becomes so on a repetition of the process. The alumina may be used a second time. To recover the alumina, it may be washed with hot water to separate the remaining gum, then treated with chlorine water, or hypochlorite of calcium, and finally washed with boiling water. (*Jour. de Pharm. et de Chim.*, Juillet, 1867, p. 55.)

Off. Prep. Mistura Amygdalæ; Mistura Glycyrrhizæ Composita; Mucilago Acaciæ; Pilulæ; Pulvis Cretæ Comp.; Trochisci.

Off. Prep. Br. Mistura Cretæ; Mistura Guaiaci; Mucilago Acaciæ; Pulvis Amygdalæ Compositus; Pulvis Tragacanthæ Compositus; Trochisci.

ACETA. *Vinegars.*

(A-CĒ'TA.)

Medicated Vinegars are solutions of medicinal substances in vinegar or acetic acid. The advantage of vinegar as a menstruum is that, in consequence of the acetic acid which it contains, it will dissolve substances not readily soluble, or altogether insoluble, in water alone. It is an excellent solvent of the alkaloids, which it converts into acetates, thereby modifying in some measure, though not injuriously, the action of the medicines of which they are ingredients. As ordinary vinegar contains principles which promote its decomposition, the Pharmacopœias now direct the substitution for it of diluted acetic acid. Even such preparations are apt to spoil in time; and a portion of alcohol is sometimes added to contribute to their preservation. A small quantity of acetic ether results from this addition; the use of alcohol is unnecessary, and in some cases injurious, as it is liable to induce precipitation. It is better to prepare the vinegars in small quantities and keep them only a short time. The vinegars now are all made of uniform strength to represent 10 per cent. of the crude drug. This change made by the Committee of Revision of Pharm., 1880, was of doubtful utility in our opinion.

ACETUM. *Br. Vinegar.*

(A-CĒ'TŬM.)

"An acid liquid, prepared from a mixture of malt and unmalted grain by the acetous fermentation." *Br.*

Acetum Crudum, Acetum Vini; Vinaigre, *Fr.;* Essig, *G.;* Aceto, *It.;* Vinagre, *Sp.*

Vinegar is a sour liquid, the product of the acetous fermentation. Viewed chemically, it is a very dilute solution of acetic acid containing certain foreign matters.

The *acetous fermentation* may be induced in all liquors which have undergone or are susceptible of the vinous fermentation. Thus sugar and water, saccharine vegetable juices, infusion of malt, cider, and wine, may be converted into vinegar, if subjected to the action of a ferment, and exposed, with access of air, to a temperature between 24° C. (75° F.) and 32° C. (90° F.). During the acetous fermentation, a microscopic vegetable, *Mycoderma* (*M. Aceti*), develops.* By the presence and influence of this plant, the germs of which exist in the atmosphere, alcohol sufficiently diluted with water is converted into acetic acid, as sugar in solution is, through the agency of an analogous growth, converted into alcohol.

Vinegar is frequently made by the *German process*, by which the time consumed in its formation is greatly abridged. A mixture is prepared of one part of alcohol of 80 per cent., four or six parts of water, and one-thousandth of honey or extract of malt, to act as a ferment. This mixture is allowed to trickle through a mass of beech shavings, previously steeped in vinegar, and contained in a deep oaken tub, called a *vinegar generator*. The tub is furnished near the top with a wooden diaphragm perforated with numerous small holes, which are loosely filled with packthread about six inches long, prevented from slipping through by a knot at one end. The alcoholic mixture, heated to between 24° C. (75° F.) and 28° C. (83° F.), is placed on the diaphragm, and slowly percolates the beech shavings, whereby it becomes minutely divided. It is essential to the success of the process that a current

* The mycoderm exists in two forms, which may be different plants or different forms of one plant, but all have the power of acetification. In one case the pellicle consists of extremely small globules (micrococci) in contiguous rows, or finally enveloped in a glue-like mass. In other instances rod-like forms (bacilli) make up the mycoderm; these vary much in size. The relations of these organisms to other plants are uncertain. Pasteur considers that they are distinct organisms, but Turpin, Berkeley, and other observers believe that they consist of the mycelium of *Penicillium glaucum*, vegetating actively and increasing also by crops of conidia or gemmæ. The action of the mycoderm seems to be an oxidizing one, so that when the supply of alcohol fails the plant probably grows at the expense of the acetic acid, converting it into carbonic acid and water.

of air should pass through the tub. In order to establish this current, eight equidistant holes are pierced near the bottom of the tub, forming a horizontal row, and four glass tubes are inserted vertically in the diaphragm, of sufficient length to project above and below it. The air enters by the holes below, and passes out by the tubes. The contact of the air with the minutely divided liquid rapidly promotes the acetification, which consists essentially in the oxidation of the alcohol. During the process the temperature rises to 37° C. (100° F.) or 40° C. (104° F.), and remains nearly stationary while the process is going on favorably. The liquid is drawn off by a discharge pipe near the bottom, and must be passed three or four times through the tub, before the acetification is completed, which generally occupies from twenty-four to thirty-six hours. According to Wimmer, pieces of charcoal, about the size of a walnut, may be substituted for the beech shavings in the process, with the effect of expediting the acetification. The charcoal must be deprived of saline matter by diluted hydrochloric acid, and afterwards washed with water. M. Pasteur denies that the more rapid acetification produced by enlarging the surface of contact with the atmosphere by means of packthread, beech shavings, etc., is owing to the direct influence of the air, and ascribes it to the presence of mycoderms upon the surface of these substances.

In his *Etudes sur la Vinaigre*, published in 1862, Pasteur proposed to substitute for the German process the sowing of the mycoderm upon the surface of a mixture of wine and vinegar, or of water, alcohol (2 per cent.) and acetic acid (1 per cent.), adding alcohol daily in small quantities after about half that contained in the original liquid had been converted into acetic acid, until a vinegar of sufficient strength was produced. In 1869, Beton-Laugier announced that he had succeeded in carrying out this method, and in 1870 he received a prize from the Société d'Encouragement de l'Industrie National. Subsequently Mr. Emanuel Wurm further elaborated this *French process* with asserted great success (for details, see *P. J. Tr.*, xi. 133).

In England, vinegar is made from the infusion of malt by the German process, which is said to have originated with Mr. Ham, of Bristol, England, as early as 1822. The fermented wort is made to fall in a shower upon a mass of fagots of birch twigs, occupying the upper part of a large vat, and, after trickling down to the bottom, is pumped up repeatedly to the top, to be again allowed to fall, until the acetification is completed. This mode of oxidizing the alcohol in the fermented wort has the advantage of rendering insoluble certain glutinous and albuminous principles, which, if not removed, would cause a muddiness in the vinegar, and make it liable to spoil.

In the United States, vinegar is often prepared from cider. When it is made on a large scale, the cider is placed in barrels with their bung-holes open, which are exposed during the summer to the heat of the sun. The acetification is completed in the course of about two years. The progress of the fermentation, however, must be watched; and, as soon as perfect vinegar is formed, it should be racked off into clean barrels. Without this precaution, the acetous fermentation would run into the putrefactive, and the vinegar be spoiled. Cider vinegar contains no aldehyd. It contains malic acid, and therefore yields a precipitate with acetate of lead. The want of such a precipitate indicates that the supposed cider vinegar is a manufactured substitute, although a fictitious article might yield a similar precipitate.

Vinegar may be clarified, without impairing its aroma, by throwing about a tumblerful of boiling milk into from fifty to sixty gallons of the liquid, and stirring the mixture. This operation has the effect at the same time of rendering red vinegar pale.

The series of changes which occur during the *acetous fermentation* is called *acetification.* During its progress, there is a disengagement of heat; the liquor absorbs oxygen and becomes turbid; and filaments form, which are observed to move in various directions, until, finally, upon the completion of the fermentation they are deposited in a mass of a pultaceous consistence. The liquor now becomes transparent, its alcohol has disappeared, and acetic acid has been formed in its place. How is this change of alcohol into acetic acid effected? Liebig supposes that it takes place in consequence of the formation of aldehyd, into which the alcohol is changed by the loss of a part of its hydrogen. The alcohol, consisting of two atoms of carbon, six of hydrogen, and one of oxygen, loses two atoms of hydrogen as the first effect

2

of oxidation, and becomes aldehyd, composed of two atoms of carbon, four of hydrogen, and one of oxygen. This, by the absorption of one atom of oxygen, becomes two atoms of carbon, four of hydrogen, and two of oxygen; that is, acetic acid (C_2H_3O,OH). Thus the conversion of alcohol into acetic acid consists in, first, the removal of two atoms of hydrogen, and afterwards the addition of one atom of oxygen. The following equation represents this change:

$$C_2H_6O + O = C_2H_4O + H_2O$$
$$C_2H_4O + O = C_2H_4O_2.$$

Aldehyd is a colorless, inflammable, ethereal liquid, having a pungent taste and smell. Its density is 0·79. It absorbs oxygen gradually, and is thus converted into acetic acid, as just stated. Its property of absorbing oxygen gives it a reducing power like that possessed by glucose. Hence, it responds to Fehling's test for that substance (page 14). It is characterized by its forming a crystalline compound with ammonia, and also with alkaline bisulphites; it is polymerised by the action of acids and some other reagents and yields *Paraldehyd* $(C_2H_4O)_n$, a liquid boiling at 124° C. The name aldehyd alludes to its relation to alcohol, *al*cohol *dehyd*rogenated. Its aqueous solution is decomposed by caustic potassa, with formation of *aldehyd resin*. This is a soft, light-brown mass, which, heated to 100° C. (212° F.), gives off a nauseous soapy smell.

Properties. Vinegar, when good, is of an agreeable penetrating odor, and pleasant acid taste. According to Magnes Lahens, wine vinegar always contains a little aldehyd. The better sorts of vinegar have a grateful aroma, probably due to the presence of an ethereal substance, perhaps acetic ether. The color of vinegar varies from pale yellow to deep red. When long kept, especially if exposed to the air, it becomes ropy, acquires an unpleasant smell, putrefies, and loses its acidity.*

The essential ingredients of vinegar are acetic acid and water; but, besides these, it contains various other substances, derived from the particular vinous liquor from which it may have been prepared. Among these may be mentioned, coloring matter, gum, starch, gluten, sugar, a little alcohol, and frequently malic and tartaric acids, with a minute proportion of alkaline and earthy salts. Vinegar should be devoid of lead and copper and of free sulphuric acid, as shown by its not being discolored by sulphuretted hydrogen, and yielding no precipitate, when boiled with a solution of chloride of calcium; and of such a strength that a fluidounce would require, for saturation, not less than thirty-five grains of bicarbonate of potassium. After saturation it should be free from acrid taste, indicating the absence of acrid substances, the taste of which may have been concealed by that of the acetic acid.

MALT VINEGAR (*Acetum Britannicum*) has a brown color, and a sp. gr. from 1·006 to 1·019. The strongest kind, called *proof vinegar*, contains from 4·6 to 5 per cent. of acetic acid. That of British manufacture usually contains sulphuric acid, which the manufacturer is allowed by law to add in a proportion not exceeding one part in a thousand. This addition was at one time thought necessary to preserve the vinegar; but it is now admitted that, if the vinegar be properly made, it does not require to be thus protected.

As ordered by the British Pharmacopœia, it is "a liquid of a brown color and peculiar odor. Specific gravity 1·017 to 1·019. 445·4 grains by weight (1 fluidounce) of it require about 402 grain-measures of the volumetric solution of soda for their neutralization, corresponding to 5·41 per cent. of real acetic acid, $HC_2H_3O_2$.†

* It is well known that, in certain kinds of vinegar, little eel-like animals, *Anguillula Aceti*, may be seen in great numbers. Their origin was unknown, until they were shown by M. Davaine to be developed in most fruits, as the apple, plum, peach, cherry, etc., in great numbers, and thus their presence in cider vinegar can easily be explained. These little animals need air for their support; and a curious contest may sometimes be noticed between them and the mycoderma upon the surface, which, as they tend to consume all the oxygen absorbed, the little eels combine their efforts to submerge, so as to expose the liquid freely to the air. They often in the French process interfere with the development of the vinegar, but are readily killed by exposing the liquid to a temperature of 60° C. (128° F.); or sometimes boracic acid is added.

† Dr. Carl Jehn published in *Archiv der Pharmacie*, May, 1877 (*N. R.*, August, 1877), a simple method of determining the percentage of acetic acid in vinegar. A quantity of sodium or potassium bicarbonate is placed in a glass jar, provided with a tightly fitting rubber stopper, carrying a glass tube for conducting off the gas. An open vial containing 10 C.c. of the vinegar to be assayed is placed inside the jar upon the sodium bicarbonate, the stopper is inserted, and by inclining the

If ten minims of solution of chloride of barium be added to a fluidounce of the vinegar, and the precipitate, if any, be separated by filtration, a further addition of the test should give no precipitate. Sulphuretted hydrogen causes no change of color." *Br.*

WINE VINEGAR (*Acetum Gallicum*) is nearly one-sixth stronger than pure malt vinegar. It is of two sorts, the white and the red, according as it is prepared from white or red wine. *White wine vinegar* is usually preferred, and that made at Orleans is the best. *Red wine vinegar* may be deprived of its color, and rendered limpid, by being passed through animal charcoal.

DISTILLED VINEGAR (*Acetum Destillatum; Vinaigre distillé, Oxéolat simple*, Fr.; *Destillirter Essig*, G.) was officinal in the U. S. Pharmacopœia, 1870, and was prepared by obtaining seven pints of distillate from eight pints of vinegar placed in a glass retort, one pint left in the retort retaining the fixed impurities, salts, etc. One hundred grains should saturate not less than seven and six-tenths grains of potassium bicarbonate. It should be wholly volatilizable by heat, yield no precipitate with acetate of lead or nitrate of silver, nor change color upon the addition of sulphuretted hydrogen or ammonia. If silver be digested with it and hydrochloric acid afterwards added, no precipitate is produced. Although preferred by some pharmacists in making medicated vinegars, it is now usually replaced by diluted acetic acid.

Adulterations. The principal foreign substances which vinegar is liable to contain, are sulphuric and sulphurous acids, certain acrid substances, and copper and lead, derived from improper vessels used in its manufacture. Tin has been found in it after standing a short time in tin vessels. Hydrochloric and nitric acids are but rarely present. A test said to have been discovered by Chevallier (*A. J. P.*, April, 1872) is as follows. Put an ounce of the suspected vinegar into a small porcelain capsule, over a water-bath, and evaporate to about half a drachm, or to the consistence of a thin extract. When cool, add half a fluidounce of stronger alcohol, and thoroughly triturate. The free sulphuric acid, if present, will be taken up by the alcohol to the exclusion of any sulphate. Filter the alcoholic solution, add one fluidounce of distilled water, evaporate off the alcohol, and filter. Acidulate the filtrate with hydrochloric acid, add a few drops of a solution of chloride of barium, and a white precipitate of sulphate of barium will result if the sample of vinegar has been adulterated with sulphuric acid. Other methods are described by O. Hehner (*Arch. der Pharmacie*, May, 1877), see *A. J. P.*, May, 1877, Nessler (*Pharm. Cent. Halle*, No. 40, 1877), *Chem. and Drug.*, April 14, 1877, *The Analyst*, 1877, p. 163, *N. R.*, Feb. 1878, F. Masset (*Jour. de Pharm. d'Anvers*, 1879, p. 88), *A. J. P.*, Feb. 1880, *Drug. Circ.*, 1882, p. 100, *Amer. Drug.*, 1885, p. 147, *Archiv d. Pharm.*, 1886, p. 597.

Chloride of barium is not a suitable test for the presence of free sulphuric acid; as it will cause a precipitate with sulphates, which are often found in vinegar when no free sulphuric acid is present. The evaporation of a sample of vinegar in contact with a piece of white sugar or on white paper will often show the presence of free sulphuric acid by the charring which ensues. A very simple method, discovered by A. Ashby, of detecting free mineral acids in vinegar is mentioned by Allen (*Com. Org. Analysis*, 2d ed., i. p. 392). A solution of logwood is prepared from boiling water and fresh logwood chips. Separate drops of this solution are spotted on the surface of a flat porcelain dish and evaporated to dryness over a water-bath. To each spot a drop of the suspected sample (concentrated first if desirable) is added, and the heating continued until it has evaporated. If the vinegar be pure the residue will be found to have a bright yellow color, but in the presence of a very small proportion of mineral acid the residue assumes a red color. The acrid substances usually introduced into vinegar are red pepper, long pepper, pellitory, grains of paradise, and mustard seed. These may be detected by evaporating the vinegar to an extract, which will have an acrid, biting taste, if any one of these substances be present. By far the most dangerous impurities in vinegar are copper and

jar the vinegar flows out, decomposing the bicarbonate. The resulting gas passes through the glass tube into a vessel of water, and by the pressure which the gas exerts upon the surface of the water it displaces a portion of the latter, which flows through an outlet into a graduated cylinder. The divisions of the latter are so arranged as to indicate at once the percentage of anhydrous acetic acid.

lead. The former may be detected by a brownish precipitate on the addition of ferrocyanide of potassium to the concentrated vinegar; the latter, by a blackish precipitate with sulphuretted hydrogen, and a yellow one with iodide of potassium. Pure vinegar is not discolored by sulphuretted hydrogen. According to Chevallier, wine vinegar, which has been strengthened with acetic acid from wood, sometimes contains a minute proportion of arsenic, which is probably derived from arseniferous sulphuric acid, employed in preparing the acetic acid.

Medical Properties. Vinegar acts as a refrigerant and diuretic. With this view it is added to diluent drinks in inflammatory fevers. It is sometimes used against seat-worms, and for other purposes, as a clyster, diluted with twice or thrice its bulk of water. Externally it is employed as a fomentation in bruises and sprains; it is a very valuable remedy in dermatitis from exposure to the sun. Diluted with water, it forms the best means of clearing the eye from small particles of lime. Its vapor is inhaled in certain states of sore throat, and it is diffused through sick-rooms under the impression that it destroys unwholesome effluvia, though, in fact, it has little other effect than to cover unpleasant smells. The dose is from one to four fluidrachms (3·75–15 C.c.); as a clyster, the quantity used is one or two fluidounces (30–60 C.c.).

Off. Prep. Emplastrum Saponis Fuscum, *Br.*

ACETUM CANTHARIDIS. *Br. Vinegar of Cantharides.*

(Ą-CĒ'TŬM CĄN-THĂR'Į-DĬS.)

Vinaigre cantharidé, *Fr.;* Canthariden-Essig, *G.*

"Cantharides, in powder, *two ounces* [Avoirdupois]; Glacial Acetic Acid *two fluidounces* [Imperial measure]; Acetic Acid sufficient for *twenty fluidounces* [Imp. meas.]. Mix thirteen fluidounces of the Acetic Acid with the Glacial Acetic Acid, and digest the Cantharides in this mixture for two hours at a temperature of 200°; then transfer the ingredients, after they have cooled, to a percolator, and, when the liquid ceases to pass, pour five fluidounces of Acetic Acid over the residuum in the apparatus. As soon as the percolation is complete, subject the contents of the percolator to pressure, filter the product, mix the liquids, and add sufficient acid to make one pint [Imp. meas.]. Specific gravity about 1·060." *Br.*

This preparation was formerly officinal in all the Pharmacopœias of the British Islands; but it was omitted in the first British Pharmacopœia, to be resumed in the present. The mode of preparation differs mainly in the partial substitution of percolation for maceration and expression. The addition of the glacial to the officinal acetic acid is simply to increase the strength of the latter.

This preparation is intended exclusively for external use, as a speedy epispastic. It is said, when lightly applied by a brush, to act as a rubefacient; and, when rubbed freely upon the skin for three minutes, to be followed, in two or three hours, by full vesication. The pain produced by the application, though more severe, is also more transient than that occasioned by the blistering cerate. From experiments made by Mr. Redwood, it may be inferred that the old Acetum Cantharidis of the London Pharmacopœia, which was prepared by maceration without heat, proved epispastic chiefly if not exclusively in consequence of its acetic acid, and that it contained little of the active principle of the flies. (*P. J. Tr.*, Oct. 1841.) Prof. Procter found that, by digestion at a temperature of 100° C. (212° F.), the active principle of the flies is readily taken up by officinal acetic acid, though a portion of the cantharidin is deposited upon cooling. (*A. J. P.*, xxiv. 299.) It would seem, therefore, that the vinegar of Spanish flies would be best prepared with the aid of heat; and, to a certain extent, this advantage is enjoyed in the present process.*

* The *vinegar of colchicum* (*acetum colchici*) was omitted in the U. S. Pharmacopœia, 1870, although a very active preparation. The following is the article on it in the 14th edition of the U. S. Dispensatory. "Take of Colchicum Root, in fine powder, *two troyounces;* Diluted Acetic Acid *a sufficient quantity.* Moisten the powder with a fluidounce of Diluted Acetic Acid, allow it to stand for half an hour, pack it firmly in a conical glass percolator, and gradually pour upon it Diluted Acetic Acid until the filtered liquid measures two pints. Vinegar of Colchicum may also be prepared by macerating the Colchicum Root, in moderately fine powder, with two pints of Diluted

ACETUM LOBELIÆ. *U. S.* *Vinegar of Lobelia.*

(A-CĒ'TŬM LO-BĒ'LI-Æ.)

Vinaigre de Lobélie enflée, *Fr.;* Lobelien-Essig, *G.*

"Lobelia, in No. 30 powder, *ten parts* [or one and three-fourths ounces av.]; Diluted Acetic Acid, *a sufficient quantity,* To make *one hundred parts* [or one pint]. Moisten the powder with *five parts* [or one fluidounce] of Diluted Acetic Acid, pack it firmly in a conical glass percolator, and gradually pour Diluted Acetic Acid upon it until *one hundred parts* [or one pint] of filtered liquid are obtained." *U. S.*

Vinegar of Lobelia may also be prepared by macerating the powder in one pint of Diluted Acetic Acid for seven days, expressing the liquid, and filtering through paper.

Vinegar of Lobelia has been reduced about 20 per cent. in strength by the above process in order to make the vinegars conform to the 10 per cent. rule adopted by the Committee of Revision of the last Pharmacopœia.

This is a good preparation of lobelia, and might well be formed into a syrup by the addition of sugar, as in the syrup of squill. It has the advantage that acetic acid gives stability to the alkaloid, which is very liable to decomposition, especially under the influence of heat. It may be used for all the purposes for which lobelia is given, either in substance or tincture, as in asthma, spasmodic catarrh, and catarrhal croup, in which it may often be advantageously conjoined with the syrups of seneka and squill. For these purposes the dose for an adult is from thirty minims to a fluidrachm (2–3·75 C.c.), repeated three or four times a day, or more frequently if required. In the paroxysm of spasmodic asthma one or two fluidrachms (3·75–7·50 C.c.) may be given every two or three hours till relief is obtained. The emetic dose would be half a fluidounce (15 C.c.).

ACETUM OPII. *U.S.* *Vinegar of Opium.*

(A-CĒ'TŬM O'PĬ-Ī.)

Black Drop; Vinaigre d'Opium, *Fr.;* Opium-Essig, *G.*

"Powdered Opium, *ten parts* [or two ounces av.]; Nutmeg, in No. 30 powder, *three parts* [or two hundred and sixty grains]; Sugar, *twenty parts* [or four ounces av.]; Diluted Acetic Acid, *a sufficient quantity,* To make *one hundred parts* [or eighteen fluidounces.] Macerate the Opium and Nutmeg in *fifty parts* [or in nine fluidounces] of Diluted Acetic Acid for twenty-four hours. Put the mixture into a conical glass percolator, and return the percolate until it passes clear. Then gradually pour on Diluted Acetic Acid until *eighty parts* [or fifteen fluidounces] of liquid are obtained. In this dissolve the Sugar by agitation without heat and strain." *U. S.*

Many will doubtless prefer to make this preparation entirely by maceration. This may be done by placing the powder in a suitable bottle and pouring on the diluted acetic acid, agitating frequently, after allowing the maceration to proceed seven days, expressing and filtering. The vinegar of opium was introduced into the Pharmacopœias as an imitation of or substitute for a preparation which has been long in use under the name of *Lancaster* or *Quaker black drop,* or simply *black drop.* The formula of the first edition of the U.S. Pharmacopœia was so deficient in precision, and so uncertain in its results, that it was abandoned in the second edition; but, as these objections were obviated in a process by Mr. Charles Ellis (*A. J. P.,* vol. ii. p. 202), it was deemed proper to restore it to its officinal rank at the subsequent

Acetic Acid, in a close glass vessel, for seven days; then expressing the liquid, and filtering through paper."

Vinegar is an excellent solvent of the active principle of colchicum; and the alkaloid of the latter loses none of its efficacy by combination with the acetic acid of the former. Of the two formulas above given, the first, directing percolation, is much preferable to the second, permitting maceration, if performed by competent hands; and the same remark will apply to all the medicated vinegars in which an alternative formula is given.

Medical Uses. This preparation has been extolled as a diuretic in dropsy, and may be given in gout, rheumatism, and neuralgia; but the wines of colchicum are usually preferred. It is recommended by Scudamore to be given in connection with magnesia, so as to neutralize the acetic acid of the menstruum. The dose is from thirty drops to two fluidrachms (1·9–7·5 C.c.).

revision of the Pharmacopœia. The preparation has, we think unfortunately, been omitted in the British Pharmacopœia with most of the other vinegars. The advantages of the black drop over laudanum are, probably, that disturbing principles contained in opium and soluble in alcohol are left behind by the aqueous menstruum employed; while the meconate of morphia is converted by the acetic acid into the acetate. In the original process, published by Dr. Armstrong, who found it among the papers of a relative of the proprietor in England, *verjuice*, or the juice of the wild crab, was employed instead of vinegar. Other vegetable acids also favorably modify the narcotic operation of opium; and lemon-juice has been employed in a similar manner with vinegar or verjuice, and perhaps not less advantageously. For the process officinal in first edition U. S. Pharm., see 14th edition U. S. Dispensatory.

The vinegar of opium may sometimes be advantageously used when opium itself, or the tincture, occasions headache, nausea, or nervous disorder. It exhibits all the anodyne and soporific properties of the narcotic, with less tendency to produce these disagreeable effects. The strength of this preparation has been more *seriously altered* than that of any other of the vinegars; it is now, in opium strength, *one-third weaker* than the black drop formerly officinal. One grain of opium was contained in 6·4 minims or 6·65 grains of the former black drop, whilst now one grain is contained in 9·6 minims or 10 grains of the present preparation. Formerly black drop was double the strength of laudanum; it has now the same strength. This alteration is in our opinion absolutely unjustifiable, and, if the preparation were more frequently used, would very probably lead to loss of life. It would be well for the present to note upon prescriptions after Acetum Opii, [*U. S. P.*, 1880,] as a safeguard, and to revise the dose accordingly. The dose may be stated at from ten to fifteen drops or minims (0·60 to 1 C.c.) of the vinegar of opium (*Pharm.*, 1880).

ACETUM SANGUINARIÆ. *U.S.* *Vinegar of Sanguinaria.*

(A-CĒ'TŬM SĂN-GUI-NĀ'RI-Æ.)

Vinaigre de Sanguinaire, *Fr.*; Blutwurzel-Essig, *G.*

"Sanguinaria, in No. 30 powder, *ten parts* [or one and three-fourths ounces av.]; Diluted Acetic Acid, *a sufficient quantity*, to make *one hundred parts* [or one pint]. Moisten the powder with *five parts* [or one fluidounce] of Diluted Acetic Acid, pack it firmly in a conical glass percolator, and gradually pour Diluted Acetic Acid upon it until *one hundred parts* [or one pint] of filtered liquid are obtained." *U. S.*

Vinegar of Sanguinaria may also be prepared by macerating the powder in one pint of Diluted Acetic Acid for seven days, expressing the liquid, and filtering through paper.

This preparation is now 20 per cent. weaker than the vinegar of bloodroot of the Pharmacopœia of 1870. It is efficient, and of a deep-red color. On standing, a deposit is always noticed upon the sides of the vessel containing it, and the color pales; the cause of this is unknown, as, according to the late Prof. Procter, the change is independent of the acetate of sanguinarina, which is formed in the process. (*A. J. P.*, May, 1864, p. 210.) A syrup may be formed from this vinegar by the addition of sugar, as in the syrup of squill. The dose of the vinegar of bloodroot as an emetic is three or four fluidrachms (11·25–15 C.c.); as an alterative and expectorant, from fifteen to thirty drops or minims (0·9–1·9 C.c.). It has been used as a local remedy in ringworm and other cutaneous diseases, and has been found by Dr. R. G. Jennings efficient as a gargle in the sore throat of scarlet fever.

ACETUM SCILLÆ. *U.S., Br.* *Vinegar of Squill.*

(A-CĒ'TŬM SCĬL'LÆ.)

Vinaigre scillitique, *Fr.*; Meerzwiebel-Essig, *G.*

"Squill, in No. 30 powder, *ten parts* [or one and three-fourths ounces av.]; Diluted Acetic Acid, *a sufficient quantity*, To make *one hundred parts* [or one pint]. Moisten the powder with *thirty parts* [or five fluidounces] of Diluted Acetic Acid, and, after the mixture has ceased to swell, transfer it to a conical glass percolator, pack it carefully, and gradually pour Diluted Acetic Acid upon it until *one hundred parts* [or one pint] of filtered liquid are obtained." *U. S.*

"Take of Squill, bruised, *two ounces and a half* [avoirdupois]; Diluted Acetic Acid, *one pint* [Imperial measure]. Macerate the Squill in the Acetic Acid for seven days, then strain with expression, and filter. Specific gravity about 1·038." *Br.*

Vinegar of Squill may also be prepared by macerating the Squill with the Diluted Acetic Acid for seven days, expressing the liquid, and filtering it through paper.

The process now officinal differs from that of the Pharmacopœia of 1860 in allowing the mixture to swell before being transferred. As pointed out by Prof. Procter (*A. J. P.*, 1864, p. 298), the old process was rendered nugatory by the tendency of the squill to swell into an adhesive mass in the percolator.

This was formerly an officinal of the Lond., Ed., and Dub. Colleges, but was omitted as a distinct preparation in the first British Pharmacopœia, being retained simply as the first step in the preparation of the syrup; but it has been introduced into the present edition. As vinegar of squill is apt to be injured by keeping, it should be prepared frequently, and in small quantities, as wanted for use. The British preparation is a trifle stronger than that of the U. S. P. 1880. As was shown by Mr. E. Gregory (*Canad. Pharm. Journ.*, Oct. 1875), the spirit added to it in the former British formula was of no use as a preservative. In the German Pharmacopœia one part of squill is macerated in a mixture of nine parts of pure vinegar and one part of alcohol for three days, with frequent shakings, expressed, and filtered. In the Codex twelve parts of white vinegar are used to macerate one part of squill for eight days. Vinegar of squill is employed chiefly in preparing the syrup. Upon standing, it deposits a precipitate, consisting, according to Vogel, of citrate of calcium and tannic acid.

Medical Uses. This preparation has all the properties of the squill in substance, and is occasionally prescribed, but the syrup is usually and very properly preferred. The dose is from fifteen minims to a fluidrachm (1–3·75 C.c.); but the latter quantity would be apt to nauseate. It should be given in cinnamon-water, mint-water, or other aromatic liquid calculated to conceal its taste and obviate nausea.

Off. Prep. Syrupus Scillæ.

Off. Prep. Br. Syrupus Scillæ; Oxymel Scillæ.

ACIDUM ACETICUM. *U.S., Br.* *Acetic Acid.*

(ĂÇ'Ĭ-DŬM Ą-CĒT'Ĭ-CŬM.)

Acidum Aceticum Dilutum, *P.G.;* Acetum Concentratum; Acide acétique, *Fr.;* Verdünnte Essigsäure, *G.*

"A liquid, composed of 36 per cent. of absolute acetic acid ($HC_2H_3O_2$; 60—HO, $C_4H_3O_3$; 60), and 64 per cent. of water." *U. S.* "An acid liquid obtained from wood by destructive distillation and subsequently purified. 100 parts by weight contain 33 parts of real acetic acid, $HC_2H_3O_2$." *Br.*

ACIDUM ACETICUM DILUTUM. *U.S., Br.* *Diluted Acetic Acid.*

(ĂÇ'Ĭ-DŬM Ą-CĒT'Ĭ-CŬM DĮ-LŪ'TŬM.)

Acetum parum, Acetum destillatum, *P.G.;* Acide acétique dilué, *Fr.;* Reiner Essig., *G.*

Contains 6 per cent. of absolute acetic acid, $HC_2H_3O_2$, sp. gr. 1·0083. *U. S.*

ACIDUM ACETICUM GLACIALE. *U.S., Br.* *Glacial Acetic Acid.*

$HC_2H_3O_2$; 60. (ĂÇ'Ĭ-DŬM Ą-CĒT'Ĭ-CŬM GLĂ-CĬ-Ā'LĒ.) $HOC_4H_3O_3$; 60.

Acidum Aceticum, *P.G.;* Acidum Aceticum Concentratum; Acetum glacialé, Acide acétique concentré, Vinaigre glacial, *Fr.;* Essigsäure, Eisessig, *G.*

"Nearly or quite absolute acetic acid," *U. S.;* "concentrated acetic acid, containing nearly 99 per cent. of real Acid, $HC_2H_3O_2$." *Br.*

Three strengths of acetic acid are now officinal in the U. S. and British Pharmacopœias. These are *Acidum Aceticum Glaciale*, of sp. gr. 1·056 to 1·058, *U. S.*, and 1·058, *Br.*, *Acidum Aceticum*, of sp. gr. 1·048, *U. S.*, and 1·044, *Br.*, and *Acidum Aceticum Dilutum*, sp. gr. 1·0083, *U. S.*, and 1·006, *Br.*

We shall consider these grades separately, in the order of their strength.

ACIDUM ACETICUM GLACIALE. A process for this preparation was given in the British Pharmacopœia of 1864, which consisted in first heating acetate of sodium so as to drive off all its water of crystallization, then, after cooling, distilling it with concentrated sulphuric acid, and, finally, if the resulting acetic acid, upon being tested with a mixture of solution of iodate of potassium and a little mucilage of starch, was found to contain sulphurous acid, agitating the distilled acid with perfectly dry black oxide of manganese, and again distilling. The object of the process was to furnish an acid of the maximum strength. But, on trial, it was not found to be satisfactory, as the resulting acid was not truly glacial, and always contained sulphurous acid. (C. H. Wood, *P. J. Tr.*, July, 1867, p. 17.) The following modification of the process does, however, yield a pure product. After the crystallized salt has been fused in an iron dish in its own water of crystallization, and has dried out, by increased heat it is again brought to fusion, whereby, if the heat applied be not too strong, no acid is decomposed or vaporized. The anhydrous salt is then treated with half a molecule of sulphuric acid (for 82 parts anhydrous acetate 49 parts of strongest sulphuric acid), which according to Mohr, *N. Rep. Phar.*, 22, p. 28 (1873), and Buchner, *N. Rep. Phar.*, 22, p. 32 (1873), suffices, instead of twice the amount, usually employed. No sulphurous acid is liberated in this case. A process to be followed on a large scale, practically the counterpart of this, is given in a foot-note, page 18, 14th ed. U. S. Dispensatory.

Acetic acid of maximum strength may also be obtained by distilling acid potassium acetate at a heat between 199° C. (390° F.) and 299° C. (570° F.). One molecule of monohydrated acetic acid distils over, and neutral acetate of potassium is left. The acid acetate may be formed by evaporating a mixture of the neutral acetate with an excess of watery acetic acid. In this process, the same acetate of potassium serves repeatedly for conversion into acid acetate, and subsequent decomposition. This process is said to be employed by manufacturers on a large scale in some parts of the continent of Europe. It originated with M. Melsens.

ACIDUM ACETICUM, *U. S.*, *Br.* (Sp. gr. 1·048, *U. S.*, 1·044, *Br.*) *Acetic Acid.* This is the acid resulting from the purification of the crude acetic acid obtained by the destructive distillation of wood. It is the acid most useful to the apothecary. As this grade of acid has its source in the impure acetic acid, obtained by the destructive distillation of wood, it will be proper to premise some account of the crude acid, called *crude pyroligneous acid.*

Wood, when charred, yields many volatile products, among which are an acid liquor, an empyreumatic oil, and tar containing creasote and some other proximate principles. When the carbonization is performed in close vessels, these products, which are lost in the ordinary process of charring, may be collected, and, at the same time, a large amount of charcoal be obtained.

Senff has furnished some comparative results in respect to the dry distillation of wood. The points worked out are a comparison of the products of distillation under similar conditions yielded by wood from various parts of the same trees, and from the same wood in a healthy and in an unsound state; also a comparison of the products from one and the same wood distilled slowly and distilled rapidly. It has been found that when similarly distilled the yield by weight of crude acid, tar, charcoal, and gas from the most diverse species of wood does not essentially differ, but that the percentage of real acid in the crude acid obtained varies considerably, and in this respect the wood from ordinary foliage trees compares favorably with that from needle-leaved trees; also that stem-wood yields more acid than branch-wood, that wood yields more acid than bark, and that sound wood yields more acid than unsound wood. In the comparison of slow with rapid carbonization, it was found that when the operation is conducted rapidly more uncondensed gas is produced, at the cost of both the total distillate and of the charcoal; that the distillate is considerably weaker in acid, and that the charcoal is much more hygroscopic than when the distillation takes place slowly. (*Ber. d. Deutsch. Chem. Ges.*, xviii. p. 60; *P. J. Tr.*, 1885, p. 696.) For older processes for making acetic acid, see 15th ed. U. S. D. Eight hundred pounds of wood afford, on an average, thirty-five gallons of acid liquor, weighing about three hundred pounds.

This is the crude pyroligneous acid, sometimes called *pyroligneous vinegar.* It is a dark-brown liquid, having a strong smoky smell, and consists of acetic acid, diluted with more or less water, and holding in solution some creasote and empyreumatic oil, with pyroxylic spirit. It is from this crude acid that the U. S. and British acetic acid, corresponding to the acetic acid of commerce, is obtained. The purification is effected as follows. The acid is saturated with milk of lime, whereby acetate of calcium is formed in solution, and thus most of the tarry matter is precipitated. The solution of acetate of calcium is then mixed with a concentrated solution of sulphate of sodium, and, by double decomposition, acetate of sodium is formed in solution, and sulphate of calcium precipitated. The solution of acetate of sodium is next subjected to evaporation, during which further impurities that separate on the surface are skimmed off. The solution, being duly concentrated, is set aside to crystallize; and the impure salt thus obtained, after having been partially purified by solution and recrystallization, is fused in an iron vessel, stirred until it dries, and, the heat being carefully raised, subjected to incipient carbonization, whereby remaining empyreumatic matters are carbonized, with little damage to the salt. The mass is then dissolved in water, and the solution, being strained and recrystallized, furnishes pure acetate of sodium. (See *Sodii Acetas.*) Finally, this salt, distilled with from 34 to 35 per cent. of its weight of sulphuric acid, yields the acetic acid of commerce, the residue being sulphate of sodium, which is reserved for decomposing fresh portions of acetate of calcium. The acid has still an empyreumatic flavor, which is removed by filtering it through animal charcoal or rectifying with potassium bichromate. The odor is due to *Furfurol*, $C_5H_4O_2$, which, as Victor Meyer has shown, can be detected even in glacial acetic acid by the red coloration it gives with aniline. It may be removed from pyroligneous acid by agitating the liquid with 2 or 3 per cent. of benzene. The aqueous layer, after separation from the benzene, is stated to give by a single distillation a very palatable table vinegar.

Acetic acid, according to Dr. Squibb, improves very much by age, and a sample examined for odor when freshly distilled would not be recognized as the same three months afterward.

An excellent quality of acetic acid is made by Dr. E. R. Squibb by an improvement on the process of Schwartz, the principal feature being the careful regulation of the heat, whereby the excessive charring of the wood is prevented and the formation of the tarry substances so reduced as to leave the acetic acid almost entirely free from empyreuma. The retorts, which are rectangular in shape, are supported by wheels secured to shafts, rotating in bearings connected with the sides, and are run upon car tracks into the ovens, after they have been loaded with small billets of oak wood from the transfer car, in an ingenious and simple manner. In the construction of the ovens, care is taken to economize the fuel and to secure control of the temperature by the use of corrugated bottoms to the retorts and dampers in the flues; when necessary the vapors are condensed in earthenware air condensers. Experience has shown that the production and liberation of acetic acid take place at a considerably lower temperature than that sufficient to convert the wood into charcoal, and, indeed, the wood which is removed from the retorts after the operation is over is sold as kindling wood, and has the color of black walnut. The crude acetic acid does not require the tedious method of purification usually employed, but is treated with soda ash, forming acetate of sodium, which is decomposed by sulphuric acid, and the acetic acid recovered in a purified condition by distillation.

The sp. gr. of the different acetic acids increases with their strength up to the density of 1·0748 (maximum), after which it decreases until it reaches 1·0553, the density of the strongest acid (*glacial acid*).

But it will be noticed by an examination of the following table of Oudemans* that the specific gravity of the glacial (100 per cent.) and the 43 per cent. acid is practically the same, and the 80, 79, 78, 77 per cent. acids have exactly the same density, the variations between 67 and 89 per cent. being very slight. It will thus

* Oudemans' more recent researches upon the specific gravities of acetic acid of varying strength are given in preference to Mohr's tables, used in previous editions of the U. S. Dispensatory, as it is believed that Mohr's experiments were conducted with an acid containing 5 per cent. of water. (Hoffmann, *Sammlung aller wichtigen Tabellen, Zahlen und Formeln*, p. 114.)

be seen that specific gravity cannot be relied upon as a criterion for strength. The glacial acid may, however, be distinguished from the 43 per cent. acid by adding 10 per cent. of water, when, if the density increases, the specimen is the stronger acid.

Percentage of Absolute Acetic Acid in Acetic Acid of Different Densities.

Per Ct.	Sp. Gr.	Per Ct.	Sp. Gr.	Per Ct.	Sp. Gr.	Per Ct.	Sp. Gr.	Per Ct.	Sp. Gr.
100	1·0553	80	1·0748	60	1·0685	40	1·0523	20	1·0284
99	1·0580	79	1·0748	59	1·0679	39	1·0513	19	1·0270
98	1·0604	78	1·0748	58	1·0673	38	1·0502	18	1·0256
97	1·0625	77	1·0748	57	1·0666	37	1·0492	17	1·0242
96	1·0644	76	1·0747	56	1·0660	36	1·0481	16	1·0228
95	1·0660	75	1·0746	55	1·0653	35	1·0470	15	1·0214
94	1·0674	74	1·0744	54	1·0646	34	1·0459	14	1·0201
93	1·0686	73	1·0742	53	1·0638	33	1·0447	13	1·0185
92	1·0696	72	1·0740	52	1·0631	32	1·0436	12	1·0171
91	1·0705	71	1·0737	51	1·0623	31	1·0424	11	1·0157
90	1·0713	70	1·0733	50	1·0615	30	1·0412	10	1·0142
89	1·0720	69	1·0729	49	1·0607	29	1·0400	9	1·0127
88	1·0726	68	1·0725	48	1·0598	28	1·0388	8	1·0113
87	1·0731	67	1·0721	47	1·0589	27	1·0375	7	1·0098
86	1·0736	66	1·0717	46	1·0580	26	1·0363	6	1·0083
85	1·0739	65	1·0712	45	1·0571	25	1·0350	5	1·0067
84	1·0742	64	1·0707	44	1·0562	24	1·0337	4	1·0052
83	1·0744	63	1·0702	43	1·0552	23	1·0324	3	1·0037
82	1·0746	62	1·0697	42	1·0543	22	1·0311	2	1·0022
81	1·0747	61	1·0691	41	1·0533	21	1·0298	1	1·0007

Temperature 15° C. (59° F.).

ACIDUM ACETICUM GLACIALE. *Br.* *Glacial Acetic Acid.* This acid, sometimes called *radical vinegar*, is a colorless, volatile, inflammable liquid, possessing a corrosive taste, and an acetous, pungent, and refreshing smell. It boils at 118.6° C. (245·5° F.). It crystallizes when cooled to 15·5° C. (60° F.), and remains crystalline until heated above 48° C. (*Br.*). Its sp. gr. is 1·056 to 1·058 at 15° C. (59° F.) *U. S.* (1·058, *Br.*). It possesses the property of dissolving a number of substances, such as volatile and fixed oils (*P. J. Tr.*, Sept. 11, 1875), camphor, resins and gum resins, fibrin, albumen, etc. As it attracts humidity from the atmosphere, it should be preserved in well-stoppered bottles. Its combinations with salifiable bases are called acetates. To neutralize 3 Gm. should require not less than 49.5 C.c. of the volumetric solution of soda, corresponding to at least 99 per cent. of absolute acetic acid. (*U. S.*) Sixty grains of it, "mixed with a fluidounce of distilled water, require for neutralization at least 990 grain-measures of the *volumetric solution of soda*. If a fluidrachm of it, mixed with half a [fluid]ounce of distilled water and half a drachm of pure hydrochloric acid, be put into a small flask with a few pieces of granulated zinc, and, while the effervescence continues, a slip of bibulous paper wetted with solution of subacetate of lead be suspended in the upper part of the flask above the liquid for about five minutes, the paper will not become discolored" (*Br.*); showing the absence of sulphurous acid. (See *Liquor Sodæ.*) One part of a decinormal solution of potassium permanganate in sixteen parts of acid gives a red color, which does not become fully brown in less than two hours (*Squibb*). The anhydride has been isolated by C. Gerhardt, who finds it to be a limpid liquid, heavier than water, and having the constant boiling point of 138° C. (279° F.) *

* *Acidum Chloraceticum*, Chloracetic Acid. Three forms of this acid are known, mono-, di-, and tri-chloracetic acids, having the following formulas respectively, $C_2H_3ClO_2$, $C_2H_2Cl_2O_2$, and $C_2HCl_3O_2$. *Monochloracetic Acid* may be prepared by acting upon glacial acetic acid containing 10 per cent. of iodine with dry chlorine, reserving the portion distilling over between 180° C. and 188° C. *Dichloracetic Acid* distils over between 189° C. and 191° C. *Trichloracetic Acid*, discovered by Dumas in 1838, may be most conveniently prepared by treating chloral hydrate with three times its volume of fuming nitric acid, and placing the whole mixture in the sunlight until the red fumes have disappeared; the liquid is then distilled, and the portion coming over at 195° C. is pure trichloracetic acid. All the chloracetic acids are powerful caustics, destroying the epidermis. They form various salts, most of which are easily soluble in water. The mono- and tri- acids are solid, crystalline, deliquescent bodies; dichloracetic acid is a colorless liquid having a suffocating odor, and crystallizing at 0° C.

Properties of the Acid of Commerce (*Acidum Aceticum*, U.S., Br.). "A clear, colorless liquid, of a distinctly vinegar-like odor, a purely acid taste, and a strongly acid reaction. It has the specific gravity 1·048 at 15° C. (59° F.). It is miscible in all proportions with water and alcohol, and is wholly volatilized by heat. Acetic acid neutralized with water of ammonia is colored deep red by ferric chloride, and decolorized again by strongly acidulating with sulphuric acid." *U. S.*

Of the British acid (sp. gr. 1·044) the strength in acetic anhydride acid is 28 per cent.; in the pure acid, according to the table, it is 33 per cent. "By weight 182 grains require for neutralization 1000 grain-measures of the *volumetric solution of soda.*" Br. "Acetic acid should not yield a precipitate with hydrosulphuric acid (lead, copper, or tin), or when supersaturated with water of ammonia (iron), or with test solution of oxalate of ammonia (calcium). When slightly supersaturated with water of ammonia, the liquid should not exhibit a blue tint (copper), nor should any residue be left on evaporating this alkaline liquid on the water-bath (other acids and fixed impurities). When supersaturated with solution of potassa, it should not have a smoky odor or taste, and when diluted with 5 volumes of distilled water, the color caused by the addition of a few drops of test solution of permanganate of potassium should not be sensibly changed by standing five minutes at the ordinary temperature (empyreumatic substances). Boiled with an equal volume of sulphuric acid, the liquid should not be darkened (organic impurities). On adding a crystal of ferrous sulphate to a cooled mixture of equal volumes of acetic and sulphuric acids, no brown or reddish-brown zone should make its appearance around the crystal (nitric acid). No precipitate should be formed on the addition of a few drops of test solution of chloride of barium (sulphuric acid), nor by adding to another portion some test solution of nitrate of silver (hydrochloric acid), nor, after the last-named addition, should the mixture turn dark on warming (sulphurous acid). 6·0 Gm. of acetic acid should require for complete neutralization 36 C.c. of the volumetric solution of soda." *U. S.* The U. S. officinal acid is somewhat stronger than the British. Phosphate of calcium has been largely detected in acetic acid sold as pure, and was copiously precipitated by ammonia added in excess. (Bruckner, *A. J. P.*, Sept. 1870, p. 389.) Victor Meyer has met with glacial acetic acid contaminated with 0·108 Gm. furfurol in a litre. (*Ber. Chem. Ges.*, 1878, p. 1870.)

It is difficult to ascertain the strength of acetic acid by saturating it with the carbonated alkalies, when the operator depends upon test-paper for ascertaining the point of neutralization. The difficulty is caused by the fact that the acetates of potassium and sodium, though neutral in composition, are alkaline to test-paper. Hence the liquid begins to be alkaline to test-paper, while some free acid yet remains, but insufficient to overcome the alkaline reaction of the salt formed. It follows, therefore, that by the use of test-paper the strength of the acetic acid will be underrated. The degree of inaccuracy, where test-paper is used, is much diminished by saturating the acid with a solution of saccharate of calcium, of a known strength, as proposed by Mr. C. G. Williams. (*P. J. Tr.*, May, 1854, p. 594.) A still better way is to add to the acid a weighed excess of carbonate of barium, and to calculate its strength by the amount of the carbonate decomposed, ascertained by deducting the undissolved from the total used. (*Redwood.*) Equally accurate results may be obtained by the use of carbonate of calcium in a similar manner. (E. C. Nicholson and D. S. Price, *Chem. Gaz.*, Jan. 15, 1856.)

Uses of Crude Pyroligneous Acid. This acid having been incidentally described as the source of the acetic acid of commerce, it may be proper in this place to notice its uses. It has been employed as an application to gangrene and ill-conditioned ulcers. It acts on the principle of an antiseptic and stimulant; the former property being in part due to the presence of creasote. Several cases in which it was successfully employed are reported in a paper by Dr. T. Y. Simons, of Charleston, S. C. (*Am. Journ. of Med. Sci.*, O. S., v. 310.)

The crude acid is advantageously applied to the preservation of animal food. Mr. William Ramsey made some interesting experiments with it for that purpose. Herrings and other fish, simply dipped in the acid and afterwards dried in the shade, were effectually preserved, and when eaten were found very agreeable to the taste. Herrings, slightly cured with salt by being sprinkled with it for six hours, then drained, next immersed in pyroligneous acid for a few seconds, and afterwards dried in the shade for two months, were found by Mr. Ramsey to be of fine quality and flavor. Fresh beef, dipped in the acid in summer for the space of a minute, was perfectly sweet in the following spring. Professor Silliman states that one quart of the acid, added to the common pickle for a barrel of hams, at the time they are laid down, will impart to them the smoked flavor as perfectly as if they had undergone the ordinary process of smoking.

ACIDUM ACETICUM DILUTUM. *U. S., Br. Diluted Acetic Acid.* "Acetic Acid *seventeen parts* [or one pint]; Distilled Water *eighty-three parts* [or five and one-eighth pints], To make *one hundred parts.* Mix them. Diluted acetic acid contains 6 per cent. of absolute acetic acid, and has the specific gravity 1·0083. It corresponds in properties to acetic acid, and should respond to the same tests of purity." *U. S.*

"To neutralize 24 Gm. of diluted acetic acid should require 24 C.c. of the volumetric solution of soda." *U. S.*

"Take of Acetic Acid *one pint* [Imperial measure]; Distilled Water *seven pints* [Imp. meas.]. Mix" *Br.* The sp. gr. of this acid is 1·006. "440 grains by weight or one fluidounce [Imp.] requires for neutralization 313 grain-measures of the *volumetric solution of soda*, corresponding to 3.63 per cent. of anhydrous acetic acid. One fluidounce [Imp.], therefore, corresponds to 16 grains of anhydrous acid." *Br.*

The object of having this preparation is to possess a weak solution of *pure* acetic acid, which may be substituted for distilled vinegar in all formulas in which nicety is required. For a long period diluted acetic acid has been made by mixing one part of acetic acid with seven of water by measure. The officinal diluted acid is now considerably stronger, as will be seen by consulting the alternative formula. This change is of doubtful utility; in our opinion it would have been better to have made the diluted acid to contain 5 per cent. of absolute acid. This would not have materially altered the strength or specific gravity, would have corresponded with the British Pharm., and would not have done violence to a very well established custom. No advantage is apparent, in the addition of one per cent. of absolute acid. Distilled vinegar contains a little organic matter, which is always darkened or precipitated when its acid is saturated with an alkali, an occurrence which does not take place when the diluted acetic acid is employed.

Medical Properties of Acetic Acid of Commerce (*Acidum Aceticum*, U. S., Br.). Acetic acid is very rarely used internally, but is refrigerant and astringent when sufficiently diluted. Owing to its volatility and pungency, its vapor is frequently applied to the nostrils as an excitant in syncope, asphyxia, and headache. When employed in this manner, it is generally added to a small portion of sulphate of potassium, so as to moisten the salt, and the mixture is put into small glass bottles with ground stoppers.*

It is a mild caustic, and has especially been used in cancer, being injected by means of a syringe into the diseased tissue, but the general result has not been favorable, and the remedy will probably be abandoned ere long. Two or three ounces of it taken internally undiluted very nearly caused death in an adult. (*Lan-*

* *Acidum Aceticum Camphoratum* (*Ed., Dub.*). *Camphorated Acetic Acid.* This is an old officinal remedy. It was prepared as follows. "Take of Camphor *one ounce* [av.]; Rectified Spirit *one fluidrachm;* Strong Acetic Acid *ten fluidounces.* Reduce the camphor to powder by means of the Spirit; then add the Acid, and dissolve." *Dub. Pharm.*

The use of the alcohol is simply to facilitate the pulverization of the camphor, and a few drops are sufficient. Acetic acid in its concentrated state readily dissolves camphor. In this preparation, the whole of the camphor is taken up by the acid. In consequence of the powerful chemical agency of the solution, and its extreme volatility, it should be kept in glass bottles accurately fitted with ground stoppers. Camphorated acetic acid is an exceedingly pungent perfume, which, when snuffed up the nostrils, produces a strongly excitant impression, and may be resorted to in fainting or nervous debility. It was an officinal substitute for Henry's *aromatic spirit of vinegar.*

A better *aromatic vinegar* is prepared by adding one and a half fluidrachms of best oil of rose geranium, and fifteen minims of oil of cloves, to four fluidounces of glacial acetic acid.

cet, July, 1867.) The prominent symptoms were at first, slight collapse, and asphyxia from closure of the glottis. Recovery was secured by tracheotomy; after the reaction, great thirst, salivation, pain in the fauces, and inability to swallow, but without any evidence of serious gastric, pulmonary, or cardiac disturbance, were present.

Medical Properties of the Glacial Acid. This acid is used only externally, and acts as a rubefacient, vesicant, or caustic, according to the length of time it is applied. Its application requires caution. It is sometimes employed as a substitute for cantharides, when a speedy blister is desired; as, for example, in croup, sore throat, and other cases of internal inflammation. It may be applied by means of blotting-paper or cambric moistened with the acid. It is a good corrosive for destroying warts and corns, and is also a valuable remedy in scaldhead.

Off. Prep. Br. Acetum Cantharidis; Acidum Aceticum Dilutum; Extractum Colchici Aceticum; Oxymel; Tinctura Ferri Acetatis.

Off. Prep. (Glacial Acetic Acid). Liquor Ferri Acetatis.

Off. Prep. Br. Acetum Cantharidis; Liquor Ferri Acetatis Fortior; Linimentum Terebinthinæ Aceticum; Mistura Creasoti.

Off. Prep. (Diluted Acetic Acid). Aceta; Emplastrum Ammoniaci; Emplastrum Ammoniaci cum Hydrargyro; Liquor Ammonii Acetatis; Mistura Ferri et Ammonii Acetatis; Syrupus Allii.

Off. Prep. Br. Acetum Scillæ; Liquor Morphinæ Acetatis.

ACIDUM ARSENIOSUM. *U.S., Br. Arsenious Acid.*

As_2O_3; 197·8. (ĂÇ'Ĭ-DŬM ÄR-SĒ-NĬ-Ō'SŬM.) AsO_3; 98·9.

[Arsenious Oxide; White Arsenic.]

"An anhydride (not a true acid), obtained by roasting arsenical ores, and purified by sublimation." *Br.*

Arsenicum Album, *Ed.;* Acidum Arsenicosum (*P. G.*)*;* Arsenious Oxide, Arsenic, Arsenious Anhydrid, White Arsenic; Acide arsénieux, Arsenic blanc, Fleurs d'Arsenic, *Fr.;* Arsenige Säure, Arsenichte Säure, Weisser Arsenik, *G.;* Arsenik, *Dan., Swed., Pol.;* Acido arsenioso, Arsenico, *It.;* Arsenico blanco, *Sp.*

Arsenious acid is prepared in Bohemia and Saxony, where it is procured on a large scale, as a collateral product, during the smelting of cobalt ores, which are almost invariably accompanied by arsenic, and in England from the mineral *arsenopyrite*, also called *mispickel* or *arsenical iron*, which is associated with the ores of tin and copper. The German process is that usually quoted as the older and better known. According to this, the ores are roasted in reverberatory furnaces with long horizontal flues. The arsenic is converted by combustion into arsenious acid, which rises in vapor, and condenses on the sides of the flues. In this state it is impure, and requires a second sublimation, which is performed in cast-iron vessels, fitted with conical heads of the same material, having an opening at the summit. The vessels are placed over a furnace, and brought to a red heat, when a portion of the impure arsenious acid is thrown in through the opening, which is immediately stopped. This portion being sublimed, a second portion is introduced in a similar manner. Finally, the vessels are allowed to cool; and, upon removing the heads, the purified acid is found attached to them in vitreous layers, at first as transparent as glass, but gradually becoming, by contact with the air, opaque at their surface. These are broken into fragments of a convenient size, and thrown into commerce. The arsenious acid so obtained is generally packed in casks, containing from two to five hundred pounds, and is shipped principally from the ports of Hamburg and Bremen. The English process differs somewhat in its details, and essentially in its final product, which is fine and crystalline rather than amorphous. In this process, the crude arsenic of the first sublimation is refined by introducing it into another furnace or series of furnaces, where it is again volatilized by the heat. When it condenses in the long series of chambers through which the vapors are carried, it is, if the process be fully successful, in the form of a perfectly white crystalline solid, which needs only to be ground and packed into kegs to be made ready for the market. The unground arsenic is, as stated, all in the *crystalline* condition, the temperature of the chambers being too low to allow of the formation of the glassy variety.

Properties. Arsenious acid is entirely volatilized by heat. As the German make of arsenic occurs in commerce, it is in masses, with a vitreous fracture, and of a milk-white color externally, but, internally, often perfectly transparent. As first sublimed, the whole mass is transparent; but it gradually becomes white and opaque, the change proceeding progressively from the surface inwards. This change has not been well explained, but probably depends upon the absorption of moisture, causing a gradual passage of the acid from the amorphous to the crystalline state. (*Pereira.*) Hence the masses "usually present a stratified appearance, caused by the existence of layers differing in degrees of opacity." *Br.* According to Guibourt, the sp. gr. of the transparent variety is 3·73, of the opaque 3·69. The experiments, however, of Dr. J. K. Mitchell and Mr. Durand make the density of the former variety from 3·208 to 3·333. The English make of arsenic is always powdered, and, under a lens, is seen to consist of small crystals perfect in form, or of small fragments of larger crystals. In a recent poisoning case (State of Conn. *vs.* Hayden) much was made to hinge upon the differences observed between this crystalline English arsenic and the commoner amorphous or German arsenic. (*Microscop. Exam. of Samples of Commercial Arsenic*, E. S. Dana. F. D. Linn & Co., Publishers, Jersey City, 1880.) As it occurs in the shops for medical use, it is often in the form of a white powder, almost as fine as flour. In this state it is sometimes adulterated with powdered lime or chalk, or sulphate or arsenite of calcium, a fraud which is easily detected by exposing the powder to a heat sufficient to evaporate the arsenious acid, when these impurities will be left behind. In consequence of the liability of the acid to contain impurities when in powder, it was directed in the U. S. Pharmacopœia of 1870 to be kept in masses; so that the apothecary may powder it for himself as it is wanted. It has been erroneously stated to have an acrid taste. Dr. Christison asserts that it possesses hardly any taste; inasmuch as it produces merely a faint sweetish impression on the palate. In strong, hot solution, it has an austere taste, most nearly resembling that of sulphate of zinc. (*Mitchell* and *Durand.*) It has no smell, even in vapor; but, when thrown on ignited charcoal, it emits a garlicky odor, in consequence of its deoxidation, and the volatilization of the reduced metal. Its point of sublimation, according to Berzelius, is at an incipient red heat; but, according to Mitchell and Durand, it is lower than that of metallic arsenic, being only 218° C. (425° F.). In the British Pharmacopœia it is said to be entirely volatilized at a temperature not exceeding 204° C. (400° F.). Dr. Taylor, in his work on Medical Jurisprudence, gives the subliming point at 188° C. (370° F.); and Mr. Wm. A. Guy, who has made careful experiments on the volatility of various substances, states that arsenious acid rises in vapor at about 138° C. (280° F.). (*P. J. Tr.*, Feb. 1868, p. 373.) "On being heated to about 218° C. (424·4° F.) it is completely volatilized, without melting (absence of non-volatile substances), and when thrown on ignited charcoal emits an alliaceous odor." *U. S.* When slowly sublimed, it condenses in regular octohedral crystals of a sparkling lustre. It may also be obtained crystallized in fine octohedrals by the slow cooling of a solution of the acid in boiling diluted hydrochloric acid. (*Journ. de Pharm.*, 1873, p. 246.) "If 0·247 Gm. of Arsenious Acid be dissolved with 2 Gm. of bicarbonate of sodium in boiling water, the solution should decolorize not less than 48·5 C.c. of the volumetric solution of iodine (corresponding to at least 97 per cent. of pure Arsenious Acid)." *U. S.* "Four grains dissolved in boiling water with eight grains of bicarbonate of soda, discharge the color of 808 grain-measures of the *volumetric solution of iodine.*" *Br.*

"Arsenious acid is soluble in 30 to 80 parts of water at 15° C. (59° F.), the solubility varying with its physical condition. It is slowly but completely soluble in 15 parts of boiling water. In alcohol it is but sparingly soluble. It is freely dissolved by hydrochloric acid, the alkalies and their carbonates, and is moderately soluble in glycerin." *U. S.* The following is given on the authority of

Bussy. The transparent acid dissolves much more rapidly than the opaque. By prolonged ebullition with water, the opaque variety attains the same solubility as the transparent, and may be supposed to be converted into the latter. Thus, at the boiling temperature, a pint of water dissolves 807 grains of either variety. The transparent variety, in cold saturated solution, gradually lessens in solubility, until it reaches the solubility of the opaque, no doubt in consequence of being changed into the latter. Pulverization lessens the solubility of the transparent variety, without affecting that of the opaque. The mixture of the two varieties of the acid in the same solution serves to explain the anomalies heretofore observed in its solubility. (*Journ. de Pharm.*, Nov. 1847.)* "An aqueous solution of arsenious acid affords a lemon-yellow precipitate with test solution of ammonio-nitrate of silver, and a grass-green one with test solution of ammonio-sulphate of copper; and if the solution is acidulated with hydrochloric acid, a bright-yellow one with hydrosulphuric acid. This latter precipitate is soluble in test solution of carbonate of ammonium and insoluble in diluted hydrochloric acid (distinction from sulphides of antimony and tin)." *U. S.*

Medical Properties. The officinal preparations of arsenic are all of them, when in sufficient concentration, violent irritants, or escharotics.† Taken internally in sufficient dose they are exceedingly poisonous to both man and the lower animals. When properly administered they are alteratives, affecting in some unknown way the nutrition, especially of the nervous system. They are often of service in simple nervous debility, but are especially useful in chorea and in chronic malaria. When given for their tonic effect only, they should be used in such small doses as not to cause any general symptoms; but when a specific action, as in chorea, is desired, it is proper to begin with small doses and rapidly increase them until the limit of tolerance is reached. Not rarely, such doses produce gastro-intestinal irritation, especially pain and diarrhœa. To avoid this as much as possible, the remedy should be given after meals. When either gastro-intestinal irritation or the more peculiar effects of arsenic are caused, the dose should at once be lessened. The specific symptoms of *arsenicalism* are a general disposition to œdema, especially of the face and eyelids, a feeling of stiffness in these parts, itching of the skin, tenderness of the mouth, loss of appetite, and uneasiness and sickness of the stomach. The peculiar swelling produced is called *œdema arsenicalis.* In some instances the internal use of arsenic causes a rash not unlike that of measles, and, as in that affection, attended with catarrhal symptoms. (Tilbury Fox, *Med. T. and Gaz.*, March, 1868.) Sometimes salivation is produced, and occasionally the hair and nails fall off. It is stated by M. Charcot that he has seen, in two cases, decided anaphrodisiac effects from the prolonged use of arsenic, which disappeared several months after its discontinuance, and in one instance returned upon its resumption. (*Ann. de Thérap.*, 1865, p. 267.)

Arsenious acid has been exhibited in a great variety of diseases, the principal of which are scirrhus and cancer, especially cancer of the lip; anomalous ulcers; various cutaneous diseases; intermittent fever; chorea; chronic rheumatism, particularly those forms of it attended with pains in the bones; rheumatic gout; diseases

* Experiments of M. L. A. Buchner on the solubility of arsenious acid in its various forms gave the following results. A litre of water saturated at 15° C. with crystallized arsenious acid contains gr. 2·821; with the amorphous and vitreous acid, gr. 9·306; while the same solutions, made by boiling and then allowed to cool for 24 hours, down to 15° C., contain of the crystallized acid gr. 27·639 per litre, and of the amorphous and vitreous, gr. 34·056 per litre. These results serve to confirm those of M. Bussy referred to in the text. (*Journ. de Pharm.*, 1873, p. 247.)

† *Kakodylic acid*, a compound of arsenic, having the formula $AsO(CH_3)_2OH$, containing 54·35 per cent. of the metal, equivalent to 71·4 per cent. of the arsenious oxide, has been stated by various investigators to be free from poisonous properties, whilst in the hands of others it has appeared to be an active toxic agent. A very elaborate research made by Drs. John Marshall and Howard Green (*Amer. Chem. Journ.*, May, 1886) appears to have settled the question. It was first found that kakodylic acid of American commerce produces in rabbits symptoms similar to those caused by arsenious acid, although in a very mild degree. Analysis, however, showed that this kakodylic acid contains free arsenious acid. Chemically pure kakodylic acid was then used. When introduced into the stomach in repeated doses of seven grains it caused in the lower animals vomiting and diarrhœa, profuse salivation, staggering, weakness, and death in one instance. Kakodylic acid is, therefore, capable of producing the ordinary symptoms of arsenical poisoning, but is remarkably free from activity, the toxic dose being extremely large.

of the bones, especially nodes, and firm swellings with deformity of the small joints of the hands; chronic syphilitic affections; frontal neuralgia; different painful affections of the head, known under the names of hemicrania and periodical headache; and intermittent neuralgic pains of the stomach and bowels. In intermittent fever it is inferior only to Peruvian bark and its alkaloids; and probably no remedy surpasses, or even equals it, in that most obstinate affection of the joints frequently called rheumatic gout. Mr. Henry Hunt, of Dartmouth, England, found it useful in mitigating the pain of ulcerated cancer of the uterus and in menorrhagia; also in irritable uterus, attended with pain and bearing down in the erect posture. He gave it in pill, in the dose of the twentieth of a grain three times a day. In this dose the remedy seldom produces unpleasant feelings, and may be continued for three or four months, for which period it must sometimes be employed in order to produce the desired effect on the uterus. In cutaneous affections, especially those of a scaly character, as lepra and psoriasis, it is an invaluable remedy. There would seem to be no objection against the very protracted use of this remedy in disease. Many years since, Tschudi drew attention to the so-called "*arsenic-eaters*" of Styria and the Tyrol. The habits of these people have been grossly exaggerated by some, whilst by others their existence has been denied, but the truth is that among the lower orders in the countries mentioned, there are many persons who habitually take small amounts of the poison. According to the report of a government commission, the dose of 0·62 grain is rarely exceeded. The "ratsbane eaters" are said not to suffer in their health, and to be unusually strong and vigorous people.

The external application of arsenic has been principally restricted to cancer, and anomalous and malignant ulcers, especially of the kind denominated *noli me tangere.* Dupuytren used with advantage a powder composed of one part of arsenious acid and 24 parts of calomel, as a topical application to herpes exedens, and to the foul ulcers occurring after repeated courses of mercury.

Arsenic is the chief ingredient in nearly all the empirical remedies for the cure of cancer by external application. *Plunket's caustic*, a remedy of this kind, of grea celebrity, consisted of the *Ranunculus acris* and *Ranunculus Flammula*, each an ounce, bruised and mixed with a drachm of arsenious acid, and five scruples of sulphur. The whole was beaten into a paste, formed into balls, and dried in the sun. When used, these balls were rubbed up with yolk of egg, and spread on pig's bladder. The use of the vegetable matter is to destroy the cuticle; for, unless this is done, the arsenic will not act. Mr. Samuel Cooper thinks that this caustic was never of any permanent benefit in genuine cancer, but has effected cures in some examples of lupus, and malignant ulcers of the lips and roots of the nails. In onychia maligna, Mr. Luke, of London, regarded an ointment composed of two grains of arsenious acid and an ounce of spermaceti ointment as almost a specific. (Pereira, *Mat. Med.*)

At Paris, an *arsenical paste* of the following composition has been used as an application to malignant ulcers:—Red sulphide of mercury 70 parts; dragon's blood, 22 parts; arsenious acid 8 parts. It is applied, made up into a paste with saliva. The pain produced by this composition is very severe, and its application dangerous. The *arsenical paste of Frère Côme* has been applied advantageously by M. Biett to the ulcerated surfaces in yaws. The precaution was used of not applying it, at one time, over a surface larger than that of half a dollar. This paste is made by mixing water with a powder consisting of ten grains of arsenious acid, two scruples of red sulphide of mercury, and ten grains of powdered animal charcoal. The practice of sprinkling unmixed arsenious acid on ulcers is fraught with the greatest danger. Mr. S. Cooper characterizes it as a murderous practice.

Febure's remedy for cancer consisted of ten grains of arsenious acid, dissolved in a pint of distilled water, to which were added an ounce of extract of conium, three fluidounces of solution of subacetate of lead, and a fluidrachm of tincture of opium. With this the cancer was washed every morning. Febure's formula for internal exhibition was, arsenious acid two grains, rhubarb half an ounce, syrup of chicory q. s., distilled water a pint. Of this mixture, a tablespoonful, containing about the sixteenth of a grain of the acid, was given every night and morning, with half a fluidrachm of the syrup of poppies. The dose was gradually increased to six tablespoonfuls.

The average dose of arsenious acid is the twentieth of a grain, three times a day, given in the form of pill. It is usually combined with opium, which enables the stomach to bear the medicine better. A convenient formula is to mix one grain of the acid with ten grains of sugar, and to beat the mixture thoroughly with crumb of bread, so as to form a pilular mass, to be divided into ten pills. The *Asiatic pills*, so called, consist of arsenious acid and black pepper, in the proportion of 1 part of the former to 80 of the latter. A preparation much used on the continent of Europe is *Boudin's solution*, which is simply an aqueous solution of arsenious acid with the addition of wine, and is made by boiling one gramme (15·4 grains) of the acid with one litre (2·1 pints) of distilled water till entirely dissolved, then cooling, filtering, adding enough distilled water to supply the loss, and finally mixing with one litre of white wine. Of this solution a fluidounce contains about one-quarter of a grain of arsenious acid.

Properties of Arsenious Acid as a Poison. Arsenious acid, in an overdose, whether internally or externally, acts with very great energy, and generally destroys life in a short time; but, in some rare instances, no well-marked symptoms are developed until eight or nine hours after the ingestion of the poison. Dr. Edward Hartshorne relates a case of recovery, in which at least a drachm of arsenious acid had been swallowed, and where the symptoms of poisoning were delayed for sixteen hours. (*Med. Examiner*, 1855, p. 707.) The symptoms produced by the poison are an austere taste; fetid state of the mouth; frequent ptyalism; continual hawking; constriction of the pharynx and œsophagus; the sensation of the teeth being on edge; hiccough; nausea; anxiety; frequent sinkings; burning pain at the præcordia; inflammation of the lips, tongue, palate, throat, bronchi, and œsophagus; irritable stomach, so as not to be able to support the blandest drinks; vomiting of matters, sometimes brown, at other times bloody; black, horribly fetid stools; small, frequent, concentrated, and irregular pulse, but occasionally slow and unequal; palpitations; syncope; insatiable thirst; burning heat over the whole body, or a sensation of icy coldness; difficult respiration; cold sweats; suppression of urine; scanty, red, bloody, and sometimes albuminous urine; change in the countenance; a livid circle round the eyelids; swelling and itching of the body; livid spots over the surface, and occasionally a miliary eruption; prostration of strength; loss of feeling, especially in the feet and hands; delirium; convulsions, often accompanied with insupportable priapism; falling off of the hair, detachment of the cuticle, etc. In some cases there is inflammation with burning pain in the urino-genital organs. It is very rare to observe all these symptoms in the same individual. Sometimes, indeed, they are nearly all wanting, death taking place without any pain or prominent symptom. Occasionally the symptoms have a perfect resemblance to those of Asiatic cholera, in the stage of collapse. After death, the morbid appearances are various. In some instances no vestige of lesion can be discovered. The appearances, however, in the generality of cases, are the following. The mouth, stomach, and intestines are inflamed; the stomach and duodenum exhibit spots resembling eschars, and perforations of all their coats; and the villous coat of the former is in a manner destroyed, and reduced to the consistence of a reddish-brown pulp. In cases of recovery, it has been a question how long it takes for the poison to be eliminated from the system. In an instance, reported by Dr. D. Maclagan, in which about two drachms of the poison had been swallowed, and in which magnesia was used successfully as an antidote, arsenic was detected in the urine by Marsh's test as late as the twentieth day.

A milder grade of arsenical poisoning, yet sometimes serious in its consequences, has resulted in many instances from the inhalation of the air of apartments lined with green wall-paper, which owes its color to arsenite of copper, and from which a fine poisonous dust sometimes escapes when the paper has not been well prepared. (See *Chem. News*, March 24, 1860.) The burning of green tapers is sometimes attended with an arsenical odor; and chemical examination has shown that, though in relatively rare instances, they do contain arsenious acid in quantities sufficient to prove injurious. (*Lancet*, 1873, p. 715.) Death has also resulted, in more than one instance, from working in the manufacture of green artificial leaves. (*Chem. News*, Nov. 30, 1861.) Ulceration of the anus has resulted from the habitual use of green paper, and has disappeared on the disuse of that material.

In view of the numerous accidents and crimes caused by the use of arsenious acid, its sale should be regulated by law in all the States of the Union. In 1851, an act for this purpose was passed by the British Parliament.

Dr. Christison divides the poisonous effects of arsenious acid into three orders of cases, according to the character and violence of the symptoms. In the first order, the poison produces symptoms of irritation and inflammation along the course of the alimentary canal, and commonly kills in from one to three days. In the second, the signs of inflammation are moderate, or even altogether wanting, and death occurs in five or six hours, at a period too early for inflammation to be always fully developed. In the third order of cases, two stages occur; the first stage being characterized by inflammatory symptoms, as in the first order; the second by symptoms referable to nervous irritation, such as imperfect palsy of the arms or legs, epilepsy, tetanus, hysterical affections, mania, and coma. It is a general character of this poison to induce inflammation of the stomach in almost all instances, provided death does not take place immediately, whatever be the part to which it is applied. Thus the poison, when applied to a fresh wound, will give rise to the same morbid appearances in the stomach and intestines, as when it is swallowed. In some cases, observed by Drs. Mall and Bailie, the rectum was much inflamed, while the colon and small intestines escaped.

There can be no doubt that, when applied to any ulcerated surface, arsenic may be absorbed with fatal result; and Roux has put on record the case of a young woman, whose death was caused, after agonizing sufferings, by the application of an arsenical paste to a cancerous breast. Death has occurred from the application of an arsenical paste to a soft tumor of the temple; the poisonous effects on the system at large being the cause of the fatal result. Sir Astley Cooper bears testimony to the dangerous effects of arsenic, externally applied. On the other hand, some writers assert the safety of the external application of this poison. Mr. Blackadder applied it in large quantities to sores, and never witnessed a single instance in which it acted constitutionally. The late Dr. Randolph, of this city, stated that Dr. Physick frequently and successfully employed arsenic by external application, without the injurious consequences which have been attributed to it. (*North Am. Med. and Surg. Journ.*, v. 257.) As indicated by Mr. Blackadder, absorption is less apt to follow the use of large than of small quantities; the larger amount probably killing the part to which it is applied, and thereby preventing absorption. If this dangerous caustic be used at all, it should be in accordance with these facts. Harles's observations also seem to show that when the surface is that of a chronic ulcer, either simple or malignant, absorption is less prone to occur than from a fresh wound.

Treatment of Poisoning by Arsenious Acid. Before the antidote, to be mentioned presently, can be obtained, the poison should be dislodged as far as possible by free vomiting, induced by the finger, the feather part of a quill, and the administration of an emetic of sulphate of copper or sulphate of zinc. The same object is promoted by the use of the stomach-pump. Demulcent drinks should be freely given, such as milk, white of eggs and water, or flour and water, which serve to encourage the vomiting and envelop the poison.

The antidote above referred to is *ferric hydrate*, in the *moist* or *pulpy* state. As soon as it is ready, it must be given in doses of a tablespoonful to an adult, of a dessertspoonful to a child, every five or ten minutes, until the urgent symptoms are relieved. It is calculated that the quantity taken should be at least twelve times the supposed amount of the poison swallowed; but, as the antidote is perfectly innocent, it is prudent to give it in larger quantities. According to the experiments of E. Riegel, one part of arsenious acid in solution is so fully precipitated by ten of the dry oxide, that, after its action, not a trace of the poison can be detected, even by Marsh's test. Its efficacy is of course greater, the sooner it is administered after the ingestion of the poison; but, even after delay, its use will prove advantageous.

so long as any portion of the poison still remains in the stomach. The antidote acts by producing with the poison, by a transfer of oxygen from the oxide to the acid, an insoluble, and therefore inert, ferrous arseniate $2(Fe_2(OH)_6) + As_2O_3 = Fe_3(AsO_4)_2 + 5H_2O + Fe(OH)_2$. The manner of preparing the antidote will be given elsewhere. (See *Ferri Oxidum Hydratum.*) This antidote for arsenious acid was discovered by Drs. Bunsen and Berthold, of Göttingen, in 1834; and its efficacy has been abundantly confirmed by experiments on inferior animals, and by its successful application to numerous cases of poisoning in the human subject. Various observations have been made as to the best forms of the oxide for use, but as long ago as 1842 Prof. William Procter (*A. J. P.*, xiv. 29) proved that the hydrate gradually decreases in its power of neutralizing arsenious acid, the longer it is kept; and that this decrease in power is more rapid when it is mixed with much water than when in the form of a thick magma. The cause of this diminution of neutralizing power, by being kept, is explained by the experiments of G. C. Wittstein. This chemist finds that ferric hydrate, recently precipitated, dissolves readily in acetic and other vegetable acids in the cold, but becomes nearly insoluble when kept for some time under water. It should be an invariable rule to prepare the antidote at the time it is wanted from materials always kept at hand for an emergency. A very efficient antidote may be made by precipitating the tincture of the chloride of iron with bi-carbonate of sodium.

Dialyzed iron has been frequently suggested as an antidote for arsenic (*Phila. Med. Times*, Dec. 8, 1877; *A. J. P.*, Jan. 1878), especially if its administration is followed by a dose of common salt, which precipitates the ferric hydrate in the stomach; but Edward Hirschsohn (Dorpat, Russia) cautions against the use of dialyzed iron, because his experiments show that the resulting combination parts with its arsenic in the presence of acids much more readily than does the *Antidotum Arsenici* of the Russian Pharmacopœia—made by diluting one ounce of solution of ferric sulphate (Monsel's solution) with four fluidounces of water, then adding a mixture of three drachms of calcined magnesia with four fluidounces of water. The presence of sulphate of magnesium, in addition to the ferric hydrate, is considered advantageous by acting as a purgative. (*See Ferri Oxidum Hydratum cum Magnesia.*)

The antidote having been faithfully applied, the subsequent treatment consists in the administration of mucilaginous drinks. Should the patient survive long enough for inflammatory symptoms to arise, these must be combated on general principles. Convalescence is generally long and distressing; and hence it is of the greatest importance to attend to the diet, which should consist exclusively of milk, gruel, cream, rice, and similar bland articles.

Dr. Köhler, of Halle, believes that saccharine oxide of iron in solution, is preferable to all other preparations, in poisoning by arsenious acid. This forms, like the hydrated powder, an insoluble compound with the acid. He bases his opinion upon experiments with the lower animals, and gives the details of a case in which it proved successful in the human subject, after the swallowing of more than half a drachm of the acid in powder. He gave a large teaspoonful of the saccharine oxide with a drachm of water immediately afterwards, which was repeated every 15 minutes for two hours, followed by an emetic dose of ipecacuanha, and then repeated every half-hour. The patient recovered. (*Br. and F. Med.-Chir. Rev.*, 1870, p. 538.)

Bussy has proposed light magnesia, or the kind which has not been too strongly calcined, as well as recently precipitated gelatinous magnesia, as an antidote for arsenious acid; and a case is given by him in which it appeared to prove efficacious. (*Journ. de Pharm.*, x. 81.) The dense kind has very little efficacy. Dr. Christison saw a case in which this antidote seemed very serviceable. A successful case is also reported by Cadet-de-Gassicourt (*Journ. de Pharm.*, Mars, 1848), and another by Dr. E. Bissell, of Norwalk, Conn. (*Am. Journ. of Med. Sci.*, July, 1848). For the full precipitation of arsenious acid, eighteen times its weight of anhydrous magnesia are required. (*E. Riegel.*) Like the ferric hydrate, the magnesian antidote is most conveniently kept, in a pulpy state, under water in stopped bottles. M. Schroff has made some experiments on rabbits, to determine the comparative efficacy, as antidotes, of the ferric hydrate and magnesia, and gives the preference to the latter. The hydrated magnesia is best prepared extemporaneously by quickly forming a solution of sulphate of magnesium, and precipitating by water of ammonia, which is preferable to potassa, as any portion of the latter, remaining in the preparation, might act injuriously by favoring the solubility of the arsenious acid. Notwithstanding these statements, however, it is asserted by T. & H. Smith of Edinburgh, on the basis of experiment, that magnesia is incapable of neutralizing arsenious acid, and is utterly useless as an antidote (*Pharm. Journ.*, 1865, p. 144), and it would be unwarrantable to rely on it when the ferruginous antidote is attainable. Probably the best antidote known is the combination of ferric hydrate with magnesia, now recognized by the U. S. Pharmacopœia. (See *Ferri Oxidum Hydratum cum Magnesia.*)

A mechanical method of counteracting the effects of arsenic is said to have been employed with complete success in several instances. It consists, after thoroughly washing out the stomach, in administering large quantities, a pound or more, of a mixture of chalk and castor oil, of the consistence of thick cream, which so envelops the particles of the poison adhering to the mucous membrane as to render them harmless while carried through the bowels and evacuated. (W. T. Fewtrell, *Chem. News*, 1860, p. 71.)

Reagents for detecting Arsenious Acid. As arsenic is so frequently employed for criminal purposes, it becomes important to detect its presence in medico-legal investigations. The tests for it may be divided into those which indicate indirectly its presence, and those which demonstrate its presence incontestably, by bringing it to the metallic state. The former embrace all the liquid reagents so called; the latter, the processes for metallization. It is necessary, however, to be aware of the fact, that many of the substances employed as tests for arsenic are themselves often contaminated with arsenic, and unless great care be exercised to select reagents perfectly free from this impurity, there will be danger that the results may be fallacious.

The most characteristic reagents are *sulphuretted hydrogen, ammoniacal nitrate of silver, and ammoniacal sulphate of copper.* In the opinion of Dr. Christison, the concurrent indications of these three tests are all-sufficient for detecting arsenious acid; but we think that, in questions involving life, the metallization of the poison should never be omitted.

In using sulphuretted hydrogen, the solution must be neutral or slightly acid. An excess of alkali may be neutralized with acetic acid, and an excess of nitric or sulphuric acid by potassa. A slight excess of acetic acid is not hurtful, but rather favors the subsidence of the precipitate, which is the tersulphide of arsenic, and is soluble in ammonia, ammonium carbonate, and potassium bisulphate, and gives, moreover, a metallic sublimate when heated in a tube with reducing agents, as described on the next page. According to Dr. Christison, this test is so exceedingly delicate that it detects the poison when dissolved in one hundred thousand parts of water. The color it produces is lemon- or sulphur-yellow; but the presence of vegetable or animal matter commonly gives it a whitish or brownish tint. If yellow, it might be mistaken for sulphide of tin or sulphide of cadmium, which are also yellow, but the latter is quite insoluble in ammonia, while the former gives no metallic sublimate when heated with reducing agents. If it be brownish, it may still contain arsenic, but must first be freed from organic matter.

The ammoniacal nitrate of silver gives a yellow precipitate of arsenite of silver, readily soluble to a clear solution in ammonia and in nitric and acetic acids.

The ammoniacal sulphate of copper is a test of very great delicacy. The precipitate occasioned by it is the arsenite of copper, of an apple-green or grass-green color. Its operation is prevented by hydrochloric, nitric, sulphuric, acetic, citric, and tartaric acids in excess; as also by ammonia.

Of the three tests mentioned, perhaps sulphuretted hydrogen is the most delicate; and it has the advantage of yielding a precipitate eligible for subsequent reduction. But they are all liable to the objection of being obscured in their indications, where the amount of poison is small, by the presence of organic matter; a complication constituting the most difficult problem for the medical jurist. As this case includes all others of more easy solution, we shall suppose it to occur, and shall indicate the steps to be pursued.

Having obtained general indications of the presence of arsenic, the first step will be to separate the organic matters; the second, to throw down the arsenic by means of sulphuretted hydrogen; and the third, to reduce the precipitate obtained to the metallic state. It is proper to state here that, in a communication to the Paris Academy, Dr. Blondlot, of Nancy, asserts, as the result of numerous experiments, that the smallest quantity of oily or fatty matter has the effect of diminishing, even to one-twentieth, the solubility of arsenious acid, and consequently of very much increasing the difficulty of detecting it. (See *A. J. P.*, 1860, p. 220.)

The following are the directions given by Prof. Wormley (*Micro-Chemistry of Poisons*, 2d ed., p. 299) for separating the organic principles. After the addition of water, if necessary, the mass is intimately mixed with about one-eighth of its volume of pure hydrochloric acid, and maintained at near the boiling temperature until the organic solids are entirely disintegrated. The mixture is then allowed to cool, transferred to a clean muslin strainer, and the matters retained by the strainer washed with water; the strainer with its contents may be reserved for future examination. The strained liquid is concentrated at a moderate heat if necessary, allowed to cool, and again filtered.

A given portion of the filtrate thus obtained is examined by the method of Reinsch (see page 41), successive slips of the copper being added as long as they receive a deposit. Any pieces of the metal that have thus become coated, after being thoroughly washed and dried, are heated in a suitable reduction tube, and the result examined in the usual manner. Another portion, or the whole of the remaining filtrate, may be exposed for several hours to a slow stream of sulphuretted hydrogen gas, then gently warmed, and allowed to stand until the supernatant liquid has become perfectly clear. The precipitate thus produced is collected upon a small filter, washed, and, while still moist, digested with pure water of ammonia; this liquid will readily dissolve any sulphide of arsenic present, whilst the organic matter may remain undissolved. The ammoniacal solution is filtered, and the filtrate carefully evaporated at a moderate heat to dryness. Should the residue contain organic matter and only a minute quantity of the sulphide, it may require further purification before its arsenical nature can be satisfactorily determined.

If, however, it be moderately pure sulphide of arsenic, it may be at once reduced to the metallic state, which can be accomplished by the method of Fresenius. The sulphide is mixed with carbonate of sodium and cyanide of potassium, and the mixture placed in the wide part of a tube of hard German glass drawn out at one end to capillary fineness. Carbonic anhydride properly dried is then passed through the tube, and the portion containing the mixture heated to redness; in this way the arsenical sulphide is reduced and the metal condensed in the capillary portion, where the smallest quantity can be recognized.

Dr. E. Davy, of Dublin, has recommended (*Chem. News*, vol. iii. p. 288) ferrocyanide of potassium previously dried at 100° C. (212° F.) as a substitute for the cyanide of potassium. It has the advantage over the latter that it does not readily absorb moisture from the atmosphere.

In order to facilitate the detection of arsenic in the solid tissues, as the liver, spleen, stomach, etc., it is necessary first to destroy the animal matter, and then to dissolve out the poison. Various agencies have been resorted to for this purpose, but the method of Fresenius and Babo is generally accepted as the best. According to this, the finely divided fragments of solid matter are heated with pure hydrochloric acid, and chlorate of potassium is added from time to time until the mass becomes homogeneous and of a light yellow color. It is then heated until the odor of chlorine has disappeared. After filtration any arsenic present will exist in the filtrate as arsenic acid. This is reduced by sulphurous acid gas or a solution of bisulphite of sodium, so that the arsenic is brought to the condition of arsenious acid, in which condition it is more readily acted upon by sulphuretted hydrogen gas.

After thorough precipitation of the sulphide and purification of this precipitate by treatment with ammonia as already described, if the residue from the evaporation of the ammonia still contain organic matter mixed with the arsenious sulphide, it is best purified as follows. Treat the residue with a small quantity of concentrated nitric acid, and evaporate the mixture again to dryness, this operation with nitric acid being repeated if necessary until the moist residue has a yellow color. The residue is then moistened with a few drops of a concentrated solution of caustic soda, a small quantity of pure powdered carbonate of soda and nitrate of soda added, and the well-mixed mass cautiously evaporated to dryness; the heat is then very gradually increased until the mass becomes colorless, when the organic matter will be entirely destroyed. The nitric acid and the soda compounds employed should be free from chlorine, or a portion of the arsenic may be volatilized as chloride. (Wormley, *Micro-Chem. of Poisons*, 2d ed., p. 303.)

Another method of separating arsenic in solution from organic matters, now frequently employed by chemists, is by the process of dialysis, invented by Prof. Graham, of London, of which a particular account is given in Part II. (See *Dialysis*.) By means of an instrument called the dialyzer, watery solutions of saline and other crystallizable substances may be separated from those not crystallizable, such as gelatinous, albuminous, mucilaginous, and amylaceous liquids, the latter refusing to pass through a diaphragm of some porous substance, which is readily permeable by the former. Thus, a circular piece of parchment paper, folded in the form of a common filter, is placed in a vessel containing distilled water; the suspected liquid, having been heated so as to effect a more complete solution of the arsenic, is poured into the filter, and the vessel set aside for twenty-four hours. At the end of this time, the crystallizable matter, including the arsenic, will have, to a great extent, passed through into the distilled water, leaving the organic matters behind, and a solution will have been obtained in a condition fit for the application of the different tests.

The passage of the arsenic through the membrane is, however, rarely a complete one, and the test cannot allow us to dispense with more thorough methods of examination.

Following up a suggestion of Dr. Clarke, of Aberdeen, that arsenic might be separated by taking advantage of the volatility of its chloride, Dr. Andrew Fyfe, of the same place, applied the principle to the detection of the metal when mixed with organic matter. For this purpose, he heated the arsenical liquid with sulphuric acid, free from arsenious acid, in a flask to which a bent tube and cooled receiver were adapted. When the mixture was brought to the boiling point, a little dried sea-salt was added, the receiver was connected, and the distillation continued for some time. Hydrochloric acid was evolved, which, by reacting with the arsenious acid, produced terchloride of arsenic, which distilled over free from organic matter. The terchloride of arsenic was then precipitated by a stream of sulphuretted hydrogen to obtain the yellow tersulphide of arsenic, or subjected to the action of Marsh's test. (*Philos. Mag.*, 4th series, ii. 487.) The distillate of terchloride, as thus obtained, is liable to contain sulphurous acid, from the action of organic matter on the sulphuric acid, with the effect of obscuring the indications of Marsh's test when subsequently applied, by giving rise to a yellow ring instead of a black stain. To prevent the formation of sulphurous acid, L. A. Buchner recommends that the chloride of sodium should be added to the arsenical liquid before the sulphuric acid, having been previously mixed with a little chlorate of potassium, the chlorine from which has the effect of promoting the formation of the arsenical terchloride, and of rendering the decomposition of the organic matter more complete. (*P. J. Tr.*, 1855, p. 38.) Much better than this method of prevention is the plan of keeping an amount of salt present larger than can be decomposed by the sulphuric acid, when the formation of sulphurous acid is avoided, and no danger is run of converting arsenious acid into the arsenic compound, as is the case in the presence of the free chlorine. Arsenic acid is not converted into a volatile chloride, and would therefore escape detection in this process. Indeed, it is proposed to distinguish between arsenious and arsenic acids in mixtures by this reaction. After all the arsenious acid has been distilled off as arsenious chloride, the arsenic acid can be reduced by sulphurous acid and then distilled for itself. (*Handwörterbuch der Chem.*, i. 746.) The reduction of arsenic acid to arsenious acid is very conveniently effected, according to E. Fischer, by ferrous chloride used in connection with hydrochloric acid. (*Ber. der Chem. Gesellschaft*, xiii. 1778.) Dr. Penny and Mr. W. Wallace bear testimony to the value of the plan of converting the arsenic into terchloride, as a means of separating the metal from organic matter, but think it will be found in practice more convenient to produce the terchloride by the direct agency of hydrochloric acid, than by sulphuric acid and chloride of sodium, as recommended by Dr. Fyfe.

One formula for reduction, that of Fresenius, has been given. Still another method, and one in which the whole process from beginning to end may take place in a single tube, is the following. The sulphide is mixed with oxalate of sodium (a salt which contains no water of crystallization), and the dry mixture is transferred to a suitable tube sealed at one end. An arsenical mirror is readily obtained. and if the heat is continued long enough no arsenic remains behind—an excellent and easy method, in which the reducing gas is carbonic oxide, in an atmosphere of carbonic annydride. (Blyth, *Poisons, Effects and Detection*, p. 542.) If any doubt be felt as to the nature of the crust, it may be driven up and down the tube, so as to convert it into sparkling octohedral crystals of arsenious acid, the triangular facets of which may be seen with a magnifying glass. Finally, the crystals may be dissolved in a drop or two of distilled water, and the solution will react characteristically with the liquid tests.

Another method of testing for arsenic was proposed by Mr. Marsh, and is perhaps the best known of the arsenic tests. It consists in taking advantage of the power, which nascent hydrogen possesses, of decomposing the acids of arsenic, with the result of forming water and arseniuretted hydrogen, as illustrated by the subjoined reaction:

$$As_2O_3 + (H_2)_6 = (H_3As)_2 + (H_2O)_3.$$

The liquid from the stomach, or obtained from its contents by boiling water, is added to the materials for generating hydrogen (pure dilute sulphuric acid and zinc), contained in a self-regulating generator of hydrogen. Dr. Canudas y Salva prevents the possible explosion of the apparatus, resulting from the ignition of the hydrogen before all the air has been expelled, by placing in the lateral exit tube two metallic meshes, enclosing between them very loose cotton. (*N. R.*, April, 1878.) Fresenius proposed the same years ago. If the liquid from the stomach contain arsenic, the nascent hydrogen will combine with the metal, and the nature of the compound gas formed may be ascertained by burning a jet of it from a fine jet-pipe connected with the generator. The flame will have a characteristic blue color; and, by holding a porcelain plate against it, a thin film of metallic arsenic, forming a black stain, will be deposited. Liebig and Mohr bear testimony to the delicacy of this test; but, to remove every source of fallacy, it is necessary to be sure of the purity of the materials for generating the hydrogen by a preliminary trial of the gas, before the suspected liquid is added; as zinc and sulphuric acid are both liable to contain arsenic. This trial is made by holding a plate against the burning hydrogen, which, if pure, will produce no stain. The pieces of zinc employed should be changed after every experiment. Magnesium might be advantageously substituted for zinc, as it contains no arsenic, or, still better, sodium amalgam (made by adding about 5 per cent. of metallic sodium to some warmed mercury), as proposed by E. W. Davy. This can be used then in a neutral solution, the evolution of nascent hydrogen being due to the decomposition of the water by the sodium.

Still another modification is Fleitmann's test, in which the use of zinc is retained, but the development of nascent hydrogen is brought about by the addition of caustic potassa or soda. Under these circumstances arseniuretted hydrogen is produced, but antimoniuretted hydrogen cannot be formed. A modification of Marsh's apparatus, which is praised by Berzelius for the certainty and distinctness of its results, consists in having the tube which delivers the hydrogen arsenide narrowed in several places. If, then, while the gas is passing, heat be applied a little this side of the narrowed place, the compound is decomposed and a bright mirror of metallic arsenic is deposited in the contraction. As ever so small a deposit can be changed subsequently into oxide or sulphide, both of which are characteristic, this test is quite delicate.

It has been objected to Marsh's test, that antimony forms a compound with hydrogen, very similar to arseniuretted hydrogen, both in the color of its flame, and in the metallic spot which it deposits during combustion on cold surfaces. Still, the two metals may be distinguished by acting on the metallic spot with a drop or two of fuming nitric acid, with the aid of heat. Arsenic will thus be converted into soluble arsenic acid, precipitable brick-red by nitrate of silver; antimony, on the other hand, into insoluble antimonic acid. Another way of distinguishing them is to apply to the stain a solution of hypochlorite of sodium, which instantly dissolves the arsenical spot, without affecting that of antimony, or solution of protochloride of tin, which has no action on metallic arsenic, while it dissolves slowly but completely the antimony stain. (Blyth, *Poisons, Effects and Detection*, p. 526.) Nitroprusside of sodium also, while it has no effect upon arsenic spots, will dissolve those of antimony completely and easily. (*Handwörterbuch der Chem.*, i. 757.) In case the metallic mirror is obtained in the tube by Berzelius's modification of Marsh's test, a stream of hydrogen sulphide may be passed, whilst immediately behind the stain a gentle heat is applied. Arsenic is changed thereby to yellow sulphide, while antimony produces an orange or black sulphide; if dry hydrochloric acid gas is now transmitted, the arsenical sulphide is unchanged, while antimony sulphide is converted into chloride of antimony, which volatilises without the application of heat. (Blyth, *loc. cit.*) Sulphide of ammonium dissolves the arsenical spot with difficulty, leaving on evaporation a yellow stain; it readily dissolves the antimonial, and yields an orange-red spot. Marsh's test may be still further modified as proposed by Lassaigne. The current of hydrogen arsenide is conducted into solution of nitrate of silver, when it is decomposed according to the reaction:

$$AsH_3 + (AgNO_3)_6 + (H_2O)_3 = H_3AsO_3 + (HNO_3)_6 + (Ag_2)_3.$$

Here arsenious acid is formed, which goes into solution, and metallic silver separates out. Hydrogen antimonide passed into nitrate of silver solution gives a black precipitate of antimonide of silver, in which all the antimony is contained.

Professor Reinsch has proposed a method for detecting arsenic in organic liquids, which is extremely delicate, and at the same time has the merits of facility and celerity. It consists in acidulating the suspected liquid with hydrochloric acid, which converts the arsenious acid into the terchloride, and boiling in it, for ten minutes, a slip of copper foil, on which the arsenic is deposited as a white alloy of arsenic and copper; and then separating it in the state of arsenious acid, by subjecting the copper, cut into small chips, to a low-red heat in the bottom of a small glass tube. The peculiar crystalline appearance of arsenious acid, mentioned in the preceding page, is conclusive of its presence; and, besides, if collected and dissolved in water, it will answer to the ordinary tests for the poison. The form of copper, preferred by Dr. Maclagan, is that of copper wire, No. 24, made bright by being rubbed with sand-paper, and rolled into a loose spiral, about an inch long, by being twisted round a small pencil. In this form, the copper affords an extensive surface for the deposition of the arsenic. The merit of Reinsch's procedure is not so much that it gives a characteristic deposit on the copper,—for bismuth, tin, zinc, and antimony also give deposits,—as that the copper collects all the arsenic from the organic liquid, and presents it in a convenient form for applying the liquid and subliming tests. Yet the gray metallic appearance of the arsenical deposit can hardly be confounded with that of any other metal, except perhaps of antimony, which can be distinguished by the tests already mentioned. But Reinsch's method is not without its fallacies. Thus, it has been ascertained that the presence of a nitrate or chlorate in the suspected material, prevents the characteristic action of the arsenic on the copper, until the whole of these substances have been consumed by reaction with the metal. Besides, both hydrochloric acid and copper, even such as have been sold in the shops as the purest, are liable to contain arsenic, and therefore to afford fallacious results. This, however, is less true of the hydrochloric acid prepared in this country than the European, as the sulphuric acid employed in its preparation is obtained generally from native sulphur, instead of from pyrites as abroad. Nevertheless, no conclusion from Reinsch's test can be certainly relied on, unless the hydrochloric acid has been ascertained to be free from arsenic. With the copper there is less risk, as the arsenic in it can act only by solution of the copper itself, and this is known by the green color imparted to the liquid; so that, if the arsenical deposit should be produced without discoloration of the liquid, the indication of the presence of the poison may be considered as satisfactory. (*Odling* and *Taylor.*)

If the process of Reinsch is to be applied to the sulphide of arsenic, it will be necessary to bring this into the liquid form. For this purpose Prof. J. C. Draper, of New York, makes use of ammonia, which dissolves the sulphide, and is also capable of attacking copper. The substance supposed to contain the sulphide having been covered, in a suitable vessel, with water of ammonia, is set aside in a warm place, and permitted to stand for a few hours. The solution of the sulphide is then separated by filtration, strips of clean, bright copper are introduced into it, and the whole gently heated. The copper gradually becomes coated with a deposit like that which is formed in Reinsch's process. (*N. Y. Med. Journ.*, 1865, p. 13.)

A modification of the methods of Marsh and Reinsch has been proposed by Dr. Alfred S. Taylor, which he has found effectual in detecting arsenic whether in liquids or solids, and whether associated with organic or inorganic substances, for an account of which, however, we must be content, from want of space, to refer the reader to the paper of that eminent toxicologist in *P. J. Tr.* (1861, p. 411).

Still another method of detecting arsenic is the *electrolytic*, consisting in exposing the suspected liquid, in connection with diluted sulphuric acid, to a voltaic current, through the influence of which, if arsenic be present, even though associated with large quantities of organic matter, arseniuretted hydrogen (*hydrogen arsenide*) is evolved. It is, however, only the arsenious acid that will respond to this test, so that if the arsenic be present as arsenic acid it must first be reduced to the arsenious condition by some reducing agent like sulphurous oxide or hydrogen sulphide. For an account of the process, and of the method of rendering arsenic acid sensible to the test, and of counteracting the influence of antimony and mercury, see papers by Mr. C. L. Bloxam in *P. J. Tr.* (1860, p. 376, and 1861, p. 528).

It has been shown by MM. Malaguti and Sarzeau that, for the detection of minute quantities of arsenic in exhumed bodies, the best method of proceeding is to distil the viscera with aqua regia, made by mixing one part of nitric with three of hydrochloric acid. The animal matter (the liver, for example), cut into small pieces, is dried by a gentle heat, and mixed with a quantity of the aqua regia equal to the weight of the matter before it was dried. The mixture is distilled, and the arsenic, if present, comes over in the form of the volatile terchloride, which may be converted into the tersulphide in the usual manner.

Arsenic may be detected in exhumed bodies long after death. M. Blondlot found it in the brain of a body that had been buried twenty years. In this case, it was ascertained that no arsenic existed in the earth of the cemetery. (See *Brit. and For. Med.-Chir. Rev.*, 1855, p. 222.) It is necessary also to be guarded against the possible presence, about the body, of metals which may contain arsenic; as, for example, brass and copper. L. A. Buchner has found, in the intestines of persons who had been poisoned with arsenious acid, examined some months after death, the poison in the state of yellow sulphide of arsenic, into which it had been converted by the sulphuretted hydrogen developed by the putrefactive process that had taken place in the bowels, showing that even in poisonous doses arsenic has not always the property of preserving the body from corruption. (*Neues Repertorium*, xvii. 21.)

Off. Prep. Liquor Acidi Arseniosi; Liquor Potassii Arsenitis.

Off. Prep. Br. Liquor Arsenicalis; Liquor Arsenici Hydrochloricus.

Off. Arseniates. Br. Ferri Arsenias; Sodii Arsenias; Liquor Sodii Arseniatis.

ACIDUM BENZOICUM. *U.S., Br.* *Benzoic Acid.*

$HC_7H_5O_2$; 122. (ĂÇ'Ĭ-DŬM BĔN-ZŌ'Ĭ-CŬM.) HO $C_{14}H_5O_3$; 122.

Acidum Benzoicum Sublimatum, Flores Benzoes; Acide benzoïque, Fleurs de Benjoin, *Fr.;* Benzoesäure, Benzoeblumen, *G.*

Both the U. S.* and Br. Pharmacopœias have omitted processes for the prepa-

* The following is the process officinal in 1870: "Take of Benzoin, in coarse powder, *twelve troyounces.* Spread the Benzoin evenly over the bottom of an iron dish eight inches in diameter,

ration of benzoic acid: the British defines it to be an "acid obtained from benzoin, and prepared by sublimation, not chemically pure."

Formerly the benzoin before sublimation was mixed with sand; but this is now usually omitted, as not only useless, but probably injurious by favoring the production of empyreumatic substances. The acid, which exists in the benzoin combined with resin, is volatilised by the heat, and condensed in the upper part of the apparatus. Unless the temperature be very carefully regulated, a portion of the resin is decomposed, and an oily substance generated, which rises with the acid, and gives it a brown color, from which it cannot be entirely freed by bibulous paper; and this result sometimes takes place even with the greatest caution. The process for subliming benzoic acid may be conducted in a glazed earthen vessel, surmounted by a cone of paper, or by another vessel with a small opening at the top, and a band of paper pasted round the place of junction. After the heat has been applied for an hour, the process should be suspended till the condensed acid is removed from the upper vessel or paper cone, when it may be renewed, and the acid again removed, and thus alternately till colored vapors rise. Mohr, after many experiments, recommends the following plan as unobjectionable. In a round cast-iron vessel, eight or nine inches in diameter and two inches deep, a pound or less of coarsely powdered benzoin is placed, and uniformly strewed over the bottom. The top of the vessel is closed by a sheet of bibulous paper, which is secured to the sides by paste. A cylinder of thick paper in the form of a hat, just large enough to fit closely around the sides of the pot, is then placed over it, and in like manner secured by paste. A moderate heat is now applied by means of a sand-bath, and continued for three or four hours. The vapors pass through the bibulous paper, which absorbs the empyreumatic oil, and are condensed within the hat in brilliant white flowers, having an agreeable odor of benzoin. (*Annal. der Pharm.*, xxix. 178.) The process officinal in U. S. P. 1870 was based upon Mohr's, but it frequently happens that the sublimed crystals, after they have formed in the cap, and whilst the sublimation is still going on, fall upon the bibulous paper, and if this paper should happen to be heated to only 120° C. (248° F.) the crystals will melt, and soon stop up the pores of the paper. If coarse muslin be substituted for the bibulous paper, it serves the purpose of retaining any empyreumatic substances, and yet permitting the vapors to pass through without becoming glazed by a deposit of melted acid. Strips of paper passed at irregular intervals across the cap prevent the falling back of crystals. The remaining acid of the benzoin may be extracted, if deemed advisable, by treating the residue of the balsam with lime or carbonate of sodium. From the mode of preparing benzoic acid by sublimation, it was formerly called *flowers of benzoin.*

Another mode of separating the acid from benzoin is by combining it with a salifiable base, and precipitating with an acid. Such is the process of Scheele. It consists in boiling the powdered benzoin with hydrate of lime and water, filtering the solution of benzoate of calcium thus obtained, and precipitating the benzoic acid with hydrochloric acid. In order to get the benzoic acid in the form to which the eye is accustomed, it has been proposed to sublime the acid after its precipitation.

Several other modes of extracting the acid have been recommended. The following is the process of Stolze. One part of the benzoin is dissolved in three parts of alcohol, the solution filtered and introduced into a retort, and the acid saturated by carbonate of sodium dissolved in a mixture of eight parts of water and three of alcohol. The alcohol is distilled off; and the benzoate of sodium contained in the residuary liquid is decomposed by sulphuric acid, which precipitates the benzoic acid. This is purified by solution in boiling water, which lets fall the

cover the dish with a piece of filtering paper, and, by means of paste, attach it closely to the rim. Then, having prepared a conical receiver or cap of thick, well-sized paper, of rather larger diameter than the dish, invert it over the latter, so as to fit closely around the rim. Next apply heat by means of a sand-bath, or of the iron plate of a stove, until, without much empyreuma, vapors of Benzoic Acid cease to rise. Lastly, separate the receiver from time to time, and remove the Benzoic Acid from it and the paper diaphragm, as long as the Acid continues to be deposited." *U. S.* 1870.

acid when it cools. By this process Stolze obtained 18 per cent. of acid from benzoin containing 19·425 per cent. By the process of Scheele he obtained 13·5 per cent.; by the agency of carbonate of sodium, 12 per cent.; by sublimation, only 7·6 per cent. Professor Scharling has prepared benzoic acid by means of heated steam, and obtained 8 per cent. (*A. J. P.*, xxiv. 236.)

The acid is manufactured very cheaply by synthetic methods. The two most commonly employed are those which start either with *toluol*, $C_6H_5CH_3$, or *naphthalene*, $C_{10}H_8$. In the first method the toluene is changed to benzotrichloride, $C_6H_5.CCl_3$, and this heated with water to 150° C. in closed vessels generates benzoic acid. By the second method naphthalene is changed first into naphthalene tetrachloride, and this by the action of nitric acid into phthalic acid, $C_6H_4(COOH)_2$. This is converted into a phthalate of calcium and strongly heated with hydrate of lime, whereby the phthalate is converted into carbonate and benzoate of calcium; this latter salt is then treated with hydrochloric acid and the benzoic acid thus set free.

Under the name of *German benzoic acid*, there has been largely imported into the United States benzoic acid prepared from the urine of cattle and horses by boiling the hippurate of calcium with hydrochloric acid. By boiling the hippuric acid thus separated with hydrochloric acid, it is split into benzoic acid and glycocoll,* according to the reaction, $C_9H_9NO_3 + H_2O = C_2H_5NO_2 + C_7H_6O_2$. It is white, has a fine lustre, and is said to be very pure, but sometimes has a slight urinous odor indicative of its origin. (*A. J. P.*, xxvii. 23; *P. J. Tr.*, July, 1875.) Owing to the scarcity in the market of benzoin yielding paying quantities of benzoic acid, it is asserted that the English manufacturers employ certain varieties of Botany Bay gum (*Gum acroides*), and obtain a larger yield of an acid which was at one time regarded as cinnamic, but has been shown to be benzoic acid. (*N. R.*, Feb. 1879.) Benzoic acid may also be prepared profitably from *suint*, the greasy substance obtained by washing wool. (*Chemist and Druggist*, 1876, p. 358.)

Properties. Sublimed benzoic acid is in white, soft, feathery crystals, of a silky lustre, and not pulverulent. From solution the acid crystallizes in transparent prisms. When quite pure it is inodorous; but prepared by sublimation from the balsam it has a peculiar, agreeable, aromatic odor, dependent on the presence of an oil, which may be separated by dissolving the acid in alcohol and precipitating it with water. Its taste is warm, acrid, and acidulous. It is unalterable in the air, but at 121·5° C. (250° F.) melts, and at a somewhat higher temperature rises in suffocating vapors. Sp. gr. 1·29. The Br. Pharmacopœia gives as its melting point 120° C. (248° F.), and boiling point 238·9° C. (462° F.). It is inflammable, burning without residue. One hundred parts of 90 per cent. alcohol dissolve about forty parts, whilst the same quantity of pure ether will dissolve about thirty parts. (*Bourgoin.*) The addition of borax or phosphate of sodium increases its solubility. It is readily dissolved by alcohol, and by concentrated sulphuric and nitric acids, from which it is precipitated by water. "Benzoic acid is soluble in 500 parts of water and 3 parts of alcohol at 15° C. (59° F.), in 15 parts of boiling water and in 1 part of boiling alcohol; also soluble in 3 parts of ether, in 7 parts of chloroform, and readily soluble in disulphide of carbon, benzol, benzin, and oils." *U. S.* The fixed oils also dissolve it. It is entirely soluble in solutions of potassa, soda, or ammonia, from which it is precipitated by hydrochloric acid. On carefully neutralizing any of these solutions and adding solution of ferric sulphate previously diluted with water, a flesh-colored precipitate is produced. Its solution reddens litmus paper, and it forms salts with salifiable bases called benzoates. "If gradually heated in a retort with 3 parts of freshly slaked lime, benzol is evolved." *U. S.*

"The solution of benzoic acid in pure cold sulphuric acid, when gently warmed, should not turn darker than light-brownish; if now poured into water, the benzoic acid should separate as a white precipitate and the liquid should be colorless. A small quantity of the acid, when taken up by some recently ignited and moistened

* Caseneuve recommends the precipitation of the acid from urine by the use of sulphate of zinc, as hippurate of zinc, decomposing with hydrochloric acid. (*Zeitschr. Oest. Ap. Ver.*, 1879, p. 2.)

cupric oxide held in the loop of a platinum wire and introduced into a non-luminous flame, should not impart a green or bluish-green color to the flame (abs. of chlorobenzoic acid). The acid should not have an odor resembling that of bitter almonds or of stale urine. On rubbing together 1 Gm. of benzoic acid and 0·5 Gm. of permanganate of potassium in a mortar with a few drops of water, the odor of oil of bitter almonds should not be evolved (cinnamic acid)." *U. S.* Benzoic acid is a characteristic constituent of the balsams, and has been found in various other vegetable and some animal products. When heated, it should sublime without residue; but the Br. Pharmacopœia allows a slight residue for impurities.

Permanganate of potassium has been depended upon more than any other reagent to distinguish between benzoic acids as obtained from different sources. Schacht proposes the following modification of the German Pharmacopœia test: if 3 grains of benzoic acid be dissolved in 96 minims of solution of potassa, sp. gr. 1·777, diluted with 96 minims of distilled water, and 10 drops of a solution made by dissolving 1 grain of permanganate of potassium in 200 grains of water be added to it and the whole heated to boiling, dark green liquids (in which brown precipitates gradually appear) are produced if the benzoic acid be obtained from urine, from toluol, or from commercial benzoin, whilst if the benzoic acid be from Siam benzoin (sublimed or made by wet process) decoloration of the liquids and brown precipitates are produced, due to the presence of cinnamic acid. (*Pharm. Centralhalle*, 1881, 565.) The odor of bitter almonds confirms the presence of cinnamic acid.

Medical Properties and Uses. Benzoic acid is irritant to the alimentary mucous membrane, and as a stimulant expectorant is of some value in chronic bronchitis and the later stages of the acute disorder. It is, however, chiefly used in connection with genito-urinary diseases. It was proposed by Dr. Alexander Ure as a remedy for uric acid deposits in the urine, and for the chalk-like concretions, consisting of urate of sodium, in the joints of gouty individuals. He supposed it to operate by converting the uric into hippuric acid, and consequently the insoluble urates into soluble hippurates. It appears, however, that such a transformation of uric acid does not take place, but that the benzoic acid is itself converted into hippuric acid, which is always found in the urine, when the former acid is taken freely. Garrod and Kletzinsky affirm that, though the uric acid is unaffected, the urea is decidedly diminished; and Kletzinsky believes that the quantity of nitrogen contained in the urea lost is almost exactly represented by the nitrogen of the hippuric acid formed; so that the benzoic acid is probably converted into the hippuric by combination with a nitrogenous body, either derived from the urea or formed at the expense of it. (*Ann. de Thérap.*, 1860, p. 110.) On the other hand, Ure, Leroy d'Etiolles, and Debouy declare that the uric acid is greatly lessened, and Keller Meissner, and Shepard have found that the elimination of urea is not affected. In consequence of the acid state of urine produced by benzoic acid, it has been found useful in the phosphatic variety of gravel; though its beneficial influence, being purely chemical, continues only during its use. It is said to have cured nocturnal incontinence of urine. It has been very highly recommended in ammoniacal cystitis by Prof. Gosselin. (*Arch. Gén.*, Nov. 1874.) The urine is rendered neutral or acid, and great relief afforded. In calculous cases a great advantage is the prevention of the formation of the ammoniaco-magnesian phosphate. It is necessary to give very large doses. One gramme a day should be exhibited in the beginning, and increased rapidly to four grammes. Relief is never afforded before the fifth day; sometimes not until the nineteenth. Prof. Gosselin employs an emulsion of one part of benzoic acid, three parts of glycerin, and one hundred and fifty parts of mucilage. Dr. Lemaire (*Phila. Med. Times*, vol. iv. p. 638) commends most highly, in acute gonorrhœa, the use of half a drachm of tincture of cannabis Indica and fifteen grains of benzoic acid in twenty-four hours. As first pointed out by Dougall in 1872, benzoic acid is a powerful antiseptic, being probably fully as poisonous to bacteria as is salicylic or carbolic acid. Bucholtz found that 0·2 per cent. of it has a decided influence upon the development of the organisms of putrefaction; and F.

Baden Benger (*P. J. Tr.*, 1875, p. 211) states that one-fourth of a grain of it added to a fluidounce of infusion of orange, buchu, or gentian, will cause it to keep unchanged for at least one month.

Benzoic acid may be readily dissolved in water by the addition to it of four parts of phosphate of sodium, or one part and a half of biborate of sodium. The dose is from 10 to 30 grains. It may be administered in pill, using soap as an excipient. It is an ingredient in some cosmetic washes, and has been employed by way of fumigation as a remedy in affections of the skin. It has also been employed as a local hæmostatic, in connection with alum, with considerable asserted success; but there can be little doubt that alum is the more efficient ingredient.

Off. Prep. Tinctura Opii Camphorata.

Off. Prep. Br. Tinctura Camphoræ Composita; Tinctura Opii Ammoniata; Trochisci Acidi Benzoici.

Off. Benzoate. Br. Ammonii Benzoas.

ACIDUM BORICUM. *U.S.* *Boric Acid.* (*Boracic Acid.*)

H_3BO_3; 62. (ĂÇ'Ĭ-DŬM BŌ'RĬ-CŬM.) $3HOBO_3$; 62.

Acidum boracicum; Acide borique. *Fr.*; **Borsäure,** *G.*

Boric acid occurs in small amount, most probably in combination as a magnesium salt, in sea-water and in certain mineral waters, as the hot springs of Wiesbaden, Aix-la-Chapelle, and Vichy; in certain minerals, such as the *borocalcite* which occurs in considerable quantities in the nitre-beds of Peru and Chili; and in the natural borax or *tincal*, first found in the basins of dried-up lagoons in Central Asia, but now obtained in large amount from Clear Lake, California. The largest amount is extracted, under the name of *sassolin*, from the lagoons of the volcanic districts of Tuscany, and from the crater of Vulcano, one of the Lipari Islands.

Preparation. In the neighborhood of Monte Rotondo, Lago Zolforeo, Sasso, and Larderello are found numerous hillocks and fissures, the latter of which emit hot aqueous vapor containing boric acid and certain gases. Around one or several of these fissures, called *suffioni*, a circular basin of masonry is built, which is filled with water and called a lagoon. By the jets of vapor constantly breaking through it, the water becomes gradually impregnated with boric acid and heated. A series of such lagoons are made to communicate with each other on the declivity of a hill, and the lowest to discharge itself into a reservoir, where the solution is allowed to rest and deposit mechanical impurities. From this reservoir the solution is made to pass into leaden evaporating pans, heated by the natural vapor, where it receives sufficient concentration to fit it for being conducted into wooden tubs, where it is allowed to cool and crystallize. The crude acid thus obtained contains, on an average, 75 per cent. of boric acid; the impurities consisting chiefly of alum, the double sulphate of ammonium and magnesium, and sulphate of calcium. The seven works belonging to Count Larderel, which are located at Castelnuovo, produced in 1882 over 3 million kilogrammes of crude acid, and a much larger production would follow increased demand.

The native borax of California supplies, at present, the entire American demand for boric acid. The production in 1884 was 7 million pounds, and in 1885 was 8 million pounds. The free acid is obtained by decomposing the salt in aqueous solution with strong hydrochloric acid.

Properties. Boric acid forms "Transparent, colorless, six-sided plates, slightly unctuous to the touch, permanent in the air, odorless, having a cooling bitterish taste and a feebly acid reaction; in solution turning blue litmus paper red and turmeric paper brown, the tint, in the latter case, remaining unaltered in the presence of free hydrochloric acid." *U. S.* They have a sp. gr. of 1·434, dissolve in 3 parts of boiling water, in 25 parts of cold water, in 6 parts of cold alcohol and 5 of boiling, and in volatile oils, but are insoluble in ether. On evaporation of the alcoholic solution, the boric acid volatilizes even more readily than from the aqueous solution. Glycerin, when heated, dissolves a very large quantity of boric acid. (See *Boroglycerinum; Boroglyceride*, Part II.*) Its aqueous solution tastes somewhat acid, colors litmus paper a wine red, and changes turmeric paper to a brown color, analogous to that produced by alkalies, even when hydrochloric acid is present. On moistening the paper so browned and then dried with caustic alkali solution, it turns first blue and then a dirty gray color. "On ignition, Boric Acid loses 43·5 per cent. of its weight, and, on cooling, becomes transparent and brittle." *U. S.*

On heating the alcoholic solution of boric acid, some boric ether (ethyl borate) is produced; to this is ascribed the green color seen when the alcohol is thus ignited. The solution in glycerin, however, yields the same green color when heated on the loop of a platinum wire, the reaction being so delicate as to cause it to be proposed as a test for glycerin. Boric acid, when heated to 100° C. (212° F.), loses a molecule of water and changes into *metaboric* acid; by prolonged heating to 140° C. (284° F.), or in a dry current of air to 160° C. (320° F.), it loses still more water and becomes *pyroboric acid;* finally, by ignition, it swells up and loses all the combined water, leaving *boric oxide*, B_2O_3. Boric acid is a weak acid, or may even act as a base. Thus, with sulphuric and phosphoric acids it forms compounds which may be considered as salts. Its compounds with bases, when in solution, are readily decomposed by other acids, but at a red heat boric oxide will displace many of the stronger but more volatile acids. "An aqueous solution of boric acid should not be precipitated by test solutions of chloride of barium (sulphate), nitrate of silver with nitric acid (chloride), sulphide of ammonium (lead, copper, iron, etc.), or oxalate of ammonium (calcium). A fragment heated on a clean platinum wire in a non-luminous flame should not impart to the latter a persistent yellow color (sodium salt)." *U. S.*

Boric acid is to be tested especially for hydrochloric acid and for common salt. Their presence is shown by acidifying the solution with nitric acid and adding silver nitrate, when a turbidity will appear. Sulphuric acid and sodium sulphate, if present, are indicated by a test with barium chloride solution. Iron is indicated by potassium sulphocyanate, which gives a red color; lead and copper by the test with sulphuretted hydrogen gas. M. Schäuffèle, of Paris, has drawn attention to a commercial boric acid containing lead. (*N. R.*, July, 1877.)

Medical Properties and Uses. The action of boric acid upon the system is not well known, but it probably is identical in its physiological and remedial powers with borax, except that it is more powerful. It has not as yet been much used internally, but is commended by Dr. Wm. Warren Greene (*Bost. Med. and Surg. Jour.*, ciii. 197) in chronic cystitis and prostatitis, in diphtheria, in chronic dyspepsia with fetid eructations, and in septic diseases. He gives it, usually, in doses of thirty grains, in cachet, and has exhibited a drachm every four hours without producing any ill effect. Whether boric acid is a poison, and, if so, in what doses, cannot yet be considered as determined. Cyon found that three-drachm doses of it produce in dogs no pronounced effects (*St. Louis Clin. Record*, Sept. 1881). Mododewkow is stated to have had two fatal cases of poisoning, but as in one case a lumbar abscess, in the other a pleuritic cavity, was freely washed out with a five per cent. solution of the acid, it is possible that the fatal collapse may have been the result of the operation. Mr. F. A. Monckton (*Cin. Lancet*, March, 1886) asserts the value of boric acid in diabetes.

When used externally, boric acid acts as a detergent, soothing, and disinfecting substance. It is said to be almost free from irritant properties, and to afford a superior substitute to carbolic acid in antiseptic surgery. In erysipelatous inflammations, foul ulcers, and similar external disorders, the saturated aqueous solution, or an ointment of the acid, may be continuously applied. Some trouble has been

* *Antibacteride.* The Antibacteride of C. Aschmann is made by heating 338 parts of borax with 198 of glucose, and a small amount of water. When the fusion is complete, 124 parts of boric acid are added, with constant stirring, until dissolved, and the liquor is evaporated at a gentle heat until it solidifies when run on a cold plate. The resulting mass is soft and translucent, forming an antiseptic said to be suitable for the preservation of provisions. Its composition is represented by the formula $C_6H_{12}O_6Na_2B_4O_7,3H_3BO_3$. (*A. J. P.*, 1884, 597.) It is, however, not proved that the habitual use of food preserved by boric compounds is free from danger.

experienced in having this ointment made properly, owing to the tendency of the crystals of boric acid to slip from under the pestle, rendering the process of pulverization very tedious. When triturating, it is very necessary to have the acid in an impalpable powder before incorporating with the fatty body; the gradual addition of ether to the acid has been suggested as a valuable aid to trituration. Boric acid ointment (Lister's) is made from one part each of boric acid and white wax, two parts each of oil of sweet almonds, and paraffin.

Off. Prep. Br. Unguentum Acidi Borici.

ACIDUM CARBOLICUM. *U.S., Br.* *Carbolic Acid.* (*Phenol.*)

C_6H_5HO; 94. (ĂÇ'Ĭ-DŬM CĂR-BŎL'Ĭ-CŬM.) $C_{12}H_6O_2$; 94.

A product of the distillation of coal-tar between the temperatures of 180°–190° C. (356°–374° F.). *U.S.*

An acid obtained from coal-tar oil by fractional distillation and subsequent purification. *Br.*

Acidum Phenicum s. Phenylicum Crystallisatum; Phenic Acid; Phenylic Acid; Phenol; Phenylic Alcohol; Acide carbolique, Hydrate de Phényle, Acide phénique, *Fr.*; Carbolsäure, Phenylsäure, Phenylalkohol, *G.*

This important medicine is officinal in the British Pharmacopœia, and was recognized by our own in 1870. It was discovered in 1834, in the tar of coal, by Runge, who gave it the name of carbolic acid. In 1841, it was thoroughly investigated by Laurent, by whom it was considered as the hydrated oxide of a peculiar compound radical called *phenyl* (from φαινω, I show), and therefore described by the name of *hydrated oxide of phenyl.* Its acid properties, however, having been subsequently recognized, it received the name of *phenic acid;* but, out of consideration for the original discoverer, chemical writers generally adhere to the title he gave it of carbolic acid. When on the subject of its composition, we shall have occasion to show that, although more closely related chemically with the alcohols than the acids, it belongs to a peculiar class known in common as *phenols.*

Preparation. For the commercial preparation of carbolic acid that portion of the heavy oil of coal-tar is taken which distils over between 165° C. (329° F.) and 190° C. (374° F.) (*Dead oil*). One or two rectifications of this oil serve to concentrate the carbolic acid greatly. A brown oil obtained in this way is used directly as crude carbolic acid. (See *Acidum Carbolicum Crudum.*) If this be well mixed with strong soda solution, a crystalline mass of sodium phenol will separate, from which fluid hydrocarbons and other impurities can be poured off. This sodium phenol can then be heated to about 170° C. (338° F.) without decomposition, whereby many of the adhering compounds distil off or are decomposed. After this roasting, the sodium phenol is dissolved in 10 parts of water, whereby still other foreign substances are separated. An amount of hydrochloric or dilute sulphuric acid calculated from a special test with a small portion, as just sufficient, is then added in order to set the carbolic acid free. It separates as an oily layer upon the surface, and, after being washed with a saturated solution of common salt, is dried over chloride of calcium and again distilled. The product so obtained crystallizes out largely on a cooled surface, and, after removing the crystals from adhering liquid, and drying them by pressure, they are again submitted to the same process of distillation. Only by such a detailed procedure can carbolic acid be separated from its homologues, like cresol (cresylic acid), $C_6H_4(CH_3)OH$, which accompany it, smell exactly like it, and boil between 185° C. (365° F.) and 200° C. (392° F.).

For the preparation of crystallized phenol, Bickerdike (*Chem. News*, xvi. 188) recommends that 1 or 2 per cent. of anhydrous cupric sulphate be added to the commercial acid distillate; this is then distilled, when the dehydrated phenol solidifies at 16° C. (60·8° F). Prof. Church (*Chem. News*, Oct. 13, 1871) proposes to prepare *pure* carbolic acid by agitating the best commercial product with 20 parts of water, siphoning off the clear solution from the undissolved portion which retains the impurities, and adding to the solution pure common salt to saturation, when the purified acid rises to the top, and may afterwards be dehydrated by distillation with lime.

Commercial Forms. In one of his publications in reference to carbolic acid, Dr. F. Crace Calvert, to whom probably, more than any other person, is owing the introduction of this substance into use in Great Britain and the United States, informed us that the carbolic acid obtained by Laurent, melting at 34° C. (93° F.), and boiling at 186° C. (367° F.), was not quite pure. By successive steps of improvement in the process employed by the manufacturing house at Manchester with which he is connected, they had at length succeeded in preparing the pure crystallized acid, without color or sulphurous odor; but, unfortunately, this statement is not accompanied with an account of the means by which the end had been attained. As the products of this factory are those now generally used, a brief notice, derived from the same source, of the forms of the drug prepared by them, and now circulating in the market, is desirable. 1. A pure acid is prepared, crystallizing in white prismatic crystals, but, as usually sold, in a white, hard, fused mass, which differs from Laurent's in being soluble in 20 parts of water instead of 33 parts, fusible at 41° C. (106° F.) instead of 34° C. (93° F.), and boiling at 182° C. (359° F.) instead of 186° C. (367° F.). This should be preferred for internal use. 2. The second form is less pure. Like Laurent's, it is white, solid, and fusible at 34° C. (93° F.), and may be employed for external purposes, whether in medicine or surgery. 3. A third quality is known in commerce as solution No. 4, which is not crystallizable at ordinary temperatures, and contains at least 10 per cent. of water, with varying quantities of homologous acids. 4. The fourth and cheapest form is that of a nearly colorless liquid, which is a mixture of carbolic and cresylic acids. Diluted with 100 parts of water or more, it may be used for the coarser antiseptic and disinfecting purposes out of doors, as in cess-pools and sewers. Besides these forms of carbolic acid, which issue from the manufacturing establishment of the Messrs. Calvert, there are others from different sources, generally in the liquid state, which are usually of a brownish color, and consist of mixtures of carbolic acid with cresylic acid, coloring matter, etc., and of which carbolic acid often constitutes but a small proportion. These are often imported from Germany. They should not be used internally; but, for disinfectant and antiseptic purposes, they are probably equal to solutions of the pure acid, as the cresylic acid is said to be quite as powerfully disinfectant as the carbolic, if not more so.

These impure liquors are sold sometimes under the improper name of *coal-tar creasote.* They are recognized in the U. S. Pharmacopœia under the name of "Acidum Carbolicum Crudum." (See the next article.)

Properties. Carbolic acid, in its pure state, is a solid at ordinary temperatures, crystallizing in minute plates or long rhomboidal needles, white or colorless, of a peculiar odor recalling that of creasote, and an acrid burning taste. Its sp. gr. is 1·065. (*Lemaire.*) It is apt to be colored pinkish or brown, under the influence of light and air. This reddening has been ascribed to various causes, such as ammonia and ammonium nitrite in the air, rust-spots in the tinned iron vessels, or alkali in glass vessels, organic matter, etc.; it is probably due to several of these causes, one or more acting at the same time. Demant recommends the removal of the red color by adding to 89 parts of the melted acid 11 parts of alcohol, subjecting the mixture to freezing, and then draining off the portion remaining liquid. Perfectly white crystals can be thus obtained. A slight discoloration does not interfere with any of the medical uses of the acid. Carbolic acid deliquesces on exposure, and becomes liquid; and the presence of water in the smallest proportion causes it to liquefy. It is customary to add 10 per cent. of water or glycerin to carbolic acid for dispensing, as it is more convenient to use in a liquid form. (See p. 54.) "When diluted it has a sweetish taste with a slightly burning after-taste, and a neutral reaction." *U. S.* When quite pure it melts at 41° C. (106° F.), forming an oily-looking, colorless liquid, and boils at 182° C. (359° F.). (*Calvert.*) But, as often met with, its point of fusion is lower, and that of volatilization higher, than those named. "The crystals melt at 36°–42° C. (96·8°–107·6° F.), and boil at 181°–186° C. (357·8°–366·8° F.), the higher melting and lower boiling points being those of the pure and anhydrous acid. On continued heating, the acid is completely volatilized." *U. S.* The British gives its melting point at 35° C. (95° F.), and its boiling point at 188°

C. (370° F.), both Pharmacopœias, therefore, admitting considerable impurity. Carbolic acid is inflammable, burning with a reddish flame. The plane of polarisation of a ray of polarised light is not affected by it. "Carbolic acid is soluble in 20 parts of water at 15° C. (59° F.). 100 parts of the crystals are liquefied by the addition of about 5 parts of water; this liquid is rendered turbid by the further addition of water, until 2000 parts have been added, when a stable and clear solution is formed. It is very soluble in alcohol, ether, chloroform, benzol, disulphide of carbon, commercial and absolute glycerin, and fixed and volatile oils." *U. S.* Its solubility in water increases on heating the water; at 84° C. (183·2° F.), both liquids are miscible in all proportions. Its solution is, if pure, colorless, and remains so; but, if impure, is colored brownish by exposure. It is but slightly soluble in cold petroleum benzin, but dissolves largely on heating.

Though neutral to test-paper, it combines feebly with salifiable bases; its salts being decomposed by carbonic acid, and those with the alkalies having an alkaline reaction. The carbolate of potassium is said to be decomposed even by water. Nitric acid converts it into picric acid, for the manufacture of which it is largely used. It reduces many metallic salts, especially those of silver and copper, and coagulates collodion. Bromine water, added in excess to a weak solution, produces a flocculent white precipitate. This precipitate, which consists of tribromphenol, is so insoluble that it separates even in the most dilute solutions, and affords an extremely delicate test. In 24 hours a solution containing but $\frac{1}{60000}$ of phenol gives the reaction. (Allen, *Com. Org. Analysis*, 2d ed., ii. p. 540.) If an aqueous solution of phenol be gently warmed with ammonium and solution of sodium hypochlorite (avoiding excess), a deep blue color is obtained, which is lasting, but turns to red on addition of acids. Solutions containing 1 part of phenol in 5000 of water react well when 20 C.c. are employed. Much smaller quantities give the reaction after a time. (*Ibid.*, p. 539.) Ferric chloride (avoiding excess) gives a fine violet color, by which 1 part of phenol in 3000 of water can be detected. The presence even of neutral salts often interferes with this reaction.

Carbolic acid in solution coagulates albumen and collodion, arrests fermentation, instantly destroys the lower forms of vegetable and animal life, and, in very small proportion, prevents mouldiness in vegetable juices, and protects animal substances against putrefaction.

The substances with which carbolic acid is most likely to be confounded are cresylic acid and creasote, the former, like it, extracted from coal-tar, the latter from wood-tar exclusively. As cresylic acid is incapable of crystallizing at ordinary temperatures, the two cannot be confounded in the solid state, and, as before observed, its presence in the liquid state is of little consequence; as its virtues are of the same kind, and at least equal. Its boiling point, however, is considerably higher than that of carbolic acid, being about 400°; and it may, therefore, be supposed to be present in any suspected liquid which will not crystallise at any common temperature, or boil under 202° C. (395° F.) to 204° C. (400° F.). It is also distinguished by being less soluble in water, ammonia, glycerin, and solution of soda than is the case with carbolic acid, but it is more soluble in petroleum benzin. (Allen.) (*A. J. P.*, Jan. 1879.) Creasote is distinguished by its lower density, its liquid form, and higher boiling point; by its insolubility in strong ammonia, or in 6 per cent. soda solution, as well as its insolubility in pure glycerin (see *Creasotum*); by not coagulating collodion and albumen; and by the different effects on it of strong nitric acid, which with carbolic acid produces pure picric or trinitrophenic acid, and with creasote, oxalic acid, resinous matter, and but a small proportion of picric acid. (Calvert, *Lancet*, 1863, p. 523.) Carbolic acid differs also in having no effect on polarized light.

The commercial carbolic acid powders and liquids all contain not only cresylic acid, but also nearly inactive and valueless neutral tar oils, and it is important to be able to determine the percentage of the *tar acids* and that of simple *tar oils* in a commercial sample. Prof. John Muter (*A. J. P.*, Nov. 1887, p. 581) has worked out a simple method for this, based upon the following four observed facts: 1st, phenol, cresol, and their homologues are completely soluble when shaken up with a 5 per cent. solution of sodium hydrate; 2d, liquefied phenol and the corresponding cresol are insoluble in a saturated solution of sodium chloride; 3d, in the presence of a sufficient excess of alkali even a largely diluted solution may be boiled down without the slightest appreciable loss of phenol or cresol; 4th, tar oils and naphthalene are only very slightly dissolved by alkali, and may be perfectly removed from the solution by agitating it with benzol.

Prof. E. W. Davy proposes as a test for carbolic acid, sulpho-molybdic acid made by dissolving 1 part of molybdic acid in 10 or even 100 parts of pure concentrated sulphuric acid; 3 or 4 drops of this solution are added to the carbolic acid placed on white porcelain: a beautiful blue coloration will be produced upon standing, particularly if gently heated; if this reagent is applied to wood creasote in aqueous solution, a brownish-red color is produced. Carbolic acid in creasote may be detected by distilling an aqueous solution of the mixture: the first portion of the distillate will give the creasote reaction, the last portion that for carbolic acid. (*P. J. Tr.*, June 22, 1878.)

"One volume of liquefied carbolic acid containing 5 per cent. of water, forms with one volume of glycerin a clear mixture, which is not rendered turbid by the addition of 3 volumes of water (abs. of creasote and cresylic acid). The amount of water contained in a solution of carbolic acid may be determined by agitating the solution in a graduated cylinder, with an equal volume of chloroform. After standing, the upper layer consists of the water contained in the mixture." *U. S.*

Composition. The view of the composition of carbolic acid, now universally accepted, is, that it is the hydroxyl (OH) derivative of benzene, C_6H_6, and its formula would therefore be C_6H_5OH. This would ally it to the alcohols, and it may be compared in fact to what are known as *tertiary* alcohols. The *primary* alcohols, like ethyl alcohol, C_2H_5OH, yield corresponding aldehyds and acids on oxidation. The counterpart of these in the aromatic series are the aromatic alcohols, like $C_6H_5.CH_2OH$, which yields benzoic acid, C_6H_5COOH, on oxidation. The name *phenols* has therefore been given to these derivatives in which H of the benzene group is replaced by OH. It is commonly called *carbolic acid*, but its claims to be considered as an acid are very feeble; as, though it combines with salifiable bases, it is incapable of neutralizing the alkalies, does not affect the color of litmus, and may be separated from its combinations with great facility, sometimes, it is asserted, even by water. Shaken in the liquid form with one-fourth of water, and cooled to 40° F., it crystallizes in the form of a hydrate, $C_6H_5OH + H_2O$, which fuses at 17° C. (62·6° F).

Medical Properties and Uses. Carbolic acid, in the liquid form, is locally powerfully irritant and anæsthetic, and, applied undiluted to the skin, causes a sharp pain followed by numbness, and accompanied with a whiteness of the surface, due to the coagulation of albumen. In contact with mucous surfaces it acts in the same way, and if continued long enough may produce a superficial caustic effect. Taken internally in large quantities, and in a concentrated state, it operates as an irritant narcotic poison, and has in a large number of cases caused death. Even when it is applied externally its absorption may lead to a fatal result. The symptoms after the ingestion of a lethal dose are usually developed very rapidly; indeed, death has occurred in two or three minutes, the patient dying in immediate collapse. After smaller amounts the symptoms, which may be delayed for several minutes, are nausea, cold sweats, marked pallor of the skin, stupor rapidly deepening into complete insensibility, a feeble pulse, which is usually rapid, but has been in some cases much slower than normal, and great disturbance of the breathing. The respirations are usually hurried and shallow, often very irregular, sometimes paroxysmally arrested. There is usually paralysis both of sensation and motion, but in some cases violent epileptiform convulsions have occurred. An almost diagnostic symptom is a blackish coloration of the urine. In severe poisoning the latter fluid is apt to contain both albumen and tube-casts. Half an ounce of carbolic acid has caused death, and one and a half ounces have been recovered from. When carbolic acid is employed externally the dark discoloration of the urine is especially marked, and its presence should be the signal for disuse of the remedy. When in sufficient concentration, carbolic acid produces a fatal paralysis of all the higher tissues of animal life. In poisoning with it the death seems to be most generally due to paralysis of the respiratory centres;

although the heart shares in the deleterious effect of the drug, and in some cases the fatal issue appears to have been produced by syncope. The lesions found after death have been whitish or blackish corrugated spots on the gastric mucous membrane, imperfect coagulability of the blood, and in some instances fatty degeneration of the hepatic cell and of the renal epithelium.

In therapeutic doses carbolic acid has no appreciable effect upon the general system. It is certainly absorbed and probably eliminated by all the emunctories, being especially abundant in the urine, and having been found by Lemaire in the breath of animals which had been poisoned with it. As an internal medicament carbolic acid is, at present, used almost solely for its sedative influence upon the gastro-intestinal mucous membrane and its antifermentative action upon the contents of the primæ viæ. It is especially useful in vomiting or diarrhœa when dependent upon excessive irritability of the gastric or intestinal mucous membrane. In yeasty vomiting, in flatulence, in diarrhœa with offensive passages, in the fermentative diarrhœa connected with intestinal dyspepsia, it is very valuable in doses of from one to three drops, not oftener than once in two hours. Dr. Kempster speaks of it as being successfully used in the State Lunatic Asylum at Utica in sluggishness of the bowels with offensive breath; and in all instances of fetid eructation, or extremely offensive flatulent discharges per anum, it would be very apt to afford relief.

By far the most important property of carbolic acid, both as a therapeutic and sanative agent, is its destructive influence over the lower grades of organic life, whether vegetable or animal. In a solution containing only one part of the acid in 500 of water, it instantly destroys vegetable mould, both plant and spores, and operates with equal destructiveness upon minute or microscopic animalcules. Hoppe-Seyler gives, as the result of his observation, that all inferior organisms perish in a liquid containing 1 per cent. of the acid. (*Arch. Gén.*, 1873, p. 633.) Rosenbach injected dogs and rabbits with unhealthy pus with and without admixture of carbolic acid; and found that death generally followed in the former case, while with the addition of 5 per cent. of carbolic acid no permanent injury resulted. (*Med. Record*, 1873, p. 427.) Through this power, it checks the different proper fermentations, including the putrefactive, and thus acts powerfully as an antiseptic or disinfecting agent. In sufficient concentration it is undoubtedly capable of destroying germs of various diseases. Experiments have determined that, mixed with vaccine matter in the proportion of 2 per cent., it entirely destroys its efficacy; while in a much smaller proportion it has no effect. (*Arch. Gén.*, 1873, p. 632.)

But it is more as a topical than as an internal and systemic remedy that carbolic acid has been used; and its employment in this way has reference in general to its antiseptic and antizymotic property. As regards the mere correction of offensive odor, by decomposition or neutralization of the effluvia on which the odor depends, there are other medicines much more energetic than carbolic acid, as chlorine, bromine, and permanganate of potassium. Indeed, the probability is that it exercises no deodorizing influence beyond that of merely disguising the smell of the offensive exhalations by its own bad odor. Its real action is upon the cause of the exhalations. Most of these offensive odors depend upon a species of fermentation, the putrefactive for example, and carbolic acid, even in very dilute solution, is powerfully destructive of the organisms which cause fermentations, and consequently acts much more by preventing putrefactive exhalations, than by destroying them. A piece of offensive animal matter is less speedily deodorized by carbolic acid than by permanganate of potassium; but the former in a short time entirely suppresses the putrefaction, and the matter consequently ceases to smell because it ceases to putrefy; whereas under the mere chemical agent it is only by its constant presence that the odor is prevented, and the putrefaction goes on unchecked.

Through its parasiticidal influence, carbolic acid is highly useful, as a local application, in all the diseases which are connected with or dependent on the presence of microscopic plants or animals. Hence its use in scabies, in which it destroys the itch insect, in the different forms of porrigo and trichosis, in pityriasis versicolor, in the thrush of infants, and in all cases of minute vermin affecting the human body. In these cases it is applied to the parts affected in weak solution, or in the form of ointment, but care must be taken to avoid poisoning by it. Offensive diphtheritic exudations, putrid ulcers wherever they can be reached, and suppuration with a similar offensive odor, whether on the outer surface, or from the mucous passages, as of the nose, bronchial tubes, external meatus, urinary outlets, the rectum, and the vagina in females, afford similar indications for its use. Its use as a vermicide is too dangerous to be justifiable. It is a very valuable remedy in the treatment of compound fractures, and other surgical or accidental wounds. As success in the so-called *antiseptic* surgery is dependent upon close attention to numerous details, the reader is referred to works upon antiseptic surgery for further information upon the subject. It has been highly recommended as a dentifrice in carious teeth with offensive breath, and to keep the teeth and gums clean from tartar or other morbid deposit, consequent upon, or at least connected with, the presence of minute parasitic organisms in these parts. Introduced on cotton, in a concentrated liquid state, into the cavity of a carious tooth, it quickly relieves pain by its local anæsthetic action; but care must be taken to prevent it from touching the lips or the internal surface of the mouth. In cases, too, of morbidly offensive secretion in the axilla and groin, between the toes, etc., it may be used in the form of solution or ointment with hope of benefit.

Independently of its disinfectant properties, it may be employed locally, in weak solution, as a gentle irritant or alterative, or concentrated, as a mild escharotic,* in chronic indolent or flabby ulcers, or in those of a specific character, as the syphilitic, in cutaneous eruptions independent of cryptogamic cause, and in non-suppurative chronic or even acute inflammation of the mucous membranes, as in common angina. In scalds and burns it is said to have proved very useful.

The treatment of carbolic acid poisoning is very important, but hitherto has usually not been satisfactory. When circumstances favor, the stomach pump or the india-rubber tube siphon should be at once employed; the benumbing of the stomach being such that emetics usually will not act. M. Husemann states, as the result of numerous experiments, that the alkaline earths, given in solution, in great excess, are the best antidotes; and the most suitable of these is lime combined with sugar, in the form of *saccharate of lime*. This may be prepared for the purpose, by dissolving 16 parts of sugar in 40 of distilled water, adding 5 parts of caustic lime, digesting it three days with occasional agitation, then filtering and evaporating to dryness. The resulting saccharate should be given in solution. (*Journ. de Pharm.*, 1873, p. 222.) More recently, Baumann and Hueter discovered that the soluble sulphates, especially the sulphate of sodium, form with carbolic acid harmless sulpho-carbolates, and are capable of neutralizing the poison even after its absorption into the blood. Dr. David Cernea has confirmed these statements by a series of experiments made in the Pharmacological Laboratory in the University of Pennsylvania, and it would seem as though we had a very sure antidote to the poison.† There is probably a union between the two acids, resulting in the formation of an innocuous sulpho-carbolate. As the sulphates used are innocuous, they should be given both promptly and in excess.

The dose of carbolic acid is one to three grains (0·065–0·20 Gm.), or of the acid in its concentrated liquid form one to three drops (0·06–0·18 C.c.), which may be given in half a fluidounce or a fluidounce of sweetened water. An excellent menstruum is glycerin, which dissolves it in all proportions; and a preparation is at present officinal in the British Pharmacopœia, consisting of an ounce of carbolic acid dissolved in four fluidounces of glycerin, of which about four minims represent a grain of the acid. From this solution formulas may be readily prepared, either for internal or external use, by diluting it with water. An emulsion also may be made by mixing

* Dr. Robert Battey, of Rome, Ga., in the *Amer. Pract.*, Feb. 1877, suggests a combination with iodine, as a uterine escharotic and alterative, under the name of *Iodized Phenol*, prepared by "gently warming one ounce of crystallised carbolic acid with half an ounce of iodine." This may be diluted, if necessary, with an equal bulk of glycerin. Under the name of *Iodated Phenol* a weaker preparation has been used, made by dissolving 4 grains each of iodine and carbolic acid in 10 drachms of glycerin. *A. J. P.*, 1886, p. 14.

† Sanftleben strongly recommends a mixture of diluted sulphuric acid 10 Gm.; mucilage of gum arabic 200 Gm.; simple syrup 30 Gm.; in tablespoonful doses. (*Ztschr. d. Allg. Oest. Ver.*, 1880, p. 10.)

one part of the acid with eight parts of water and one or two parts of sugar. (See *Glycerinum Acidi Carbolici.*)

For external use the strength varies greatly according to the object desired. When applied with a view to its superficial escharotic action, as in gangrenous or specific ulcers, it may be used in the solid state properly comminuted, or in the strongest liquid form. In this condition it may be readily obtained by placing the bottle containing it in hot water. Bufalini recommends its combination with camphor, under the name of *Camphorated Phenol*, asserting that the camphor moderates the caustic and disorganizing character of the phenol without destroying its useful effects; he prepares it by mixing one part of carbolic acid with two parts of camphor, allowing the mixture to stand some hours, and purifying by washing with water; it is a liquid of reddish yellow color, having the smell of camphor, insoluble in water, and soluble in alcohol and ether. For the skin affections one part of the acid may be dissolved in one hundred or two hundred parts of water; or the impure liquid acid may be used, diluted in the same proportion. M. Basin uses a solution of one part in forty parts of acetic acid of 8° B., and 100 of water, in tetter and psora, and states that a single application will destroy the itch insect. A solution containing a grain to the fluidounce of water may be used for application, in the form of *spray*, to the fauces, larynx, and bronchial tubes, by means of the *atomizer;* and the strength may be increased, if thought desirable, up to four or five grains or more to the fluidounce.

Various fabrics are impregnated with carbolic acid for surgical use. Prof. *Lister's gauze* may be made by soaking a loose cotton cloth with a mixture of 5 parts resin, 7 parts paraffin, and 1 part carbolic acid. Prof. Bruns improves upon this, making a more flexible dressing by dissolving 400 grammes of powdered resin in 2 litres of alcohol, adding 40 grammes castor oil and 100 grammes carbolic acid; this will impregnate 2 pounds of the gauze, which is to be dried by spreading out in the air. (See also Lund's process, *A. J. P.*, Feb. 1874.) *Carbolized jute* may be made by Rosenwasser's process by soaking in a percolator 1 pound of jute with a solution of crystallized carbolic acid 700 grains, paraffin 700 grains, resin 2800 grains, benzin 3 pints. (*Am. Journ. Med. Sci.*, 1879, p. 458. See also *N. R.*, April, 1879, and April, 1880.) For a gargle in diphtheria, the sore throat of scarlatina, etc., 20 minims of the liquid acid may be mixed with half a drachm of acetic acid (*Br.*), 2 fluidrachms of tincture of myrrh, and 6 fluidounces of water. For burns and scalds a liniment may be made by rubbing together 1 part of carbolic acid and 6 parts of olive oil, applied on lint. For the dressing of cancerous and other foul ulcers, a cerate may be used composed of five grains of the acid rubbed with an ounce of simple cerate. There is an officinal ointment. A carbolic acid paper, used in packing fresh meats, in order to preserve them, may be prepared by melting 5 parts of stearin with a gentle heat, stirring in thoroughly 2 parts of carbolic acid, adding 5 parts of melted paraffin, stirring the mixture till it cools, and finally melting, and applying in the usual manner to the paper in quires. (*Chemist and Druggist*, Dec. 1871.)

The impure liquid acid sold in the shops usually contains from 70 to 90 per cent. of carbolic and cresylic acids jointly (*Squibb*), and, as the latter acid is quite equal to the former in disinfecting power, yields, if dissolved in water in the proportion of 1 to 80 parts, a solution equivalent on the average to that produced by dissolving 1 part of the pure acid in 100 parts of water.

Off. Prep. Unguentum Acidi Carbolici.

Off. Prep. Br. Acidum Carbolicum Liquefactum; Glycerinum Acidi Carbolici; Suppositoria Acidi Carbolici cum Sapone; Unguentum Acidi Carbolici.

ACIDUM CARBOLICUM CRUDUM. *U. S. Crude Carbolic Acid.*

(ĂÇ'Ĭ-DŬM CĂR-BŎL'Ĭ-CŬM CRŪ'DŬM.)

"A liquid obtained during the distillation of coal-tar between the temperatures of 170°–190° C. (338°–374° F.), and containing carbolic and cresylic acids in variable proportions together with other substances." *U. S.*

Acide phénique cru, *Fr.;* Rohe Carbolsäure, *G.*

With great propriety, we think, the revisers of the U. S. Pharmacopœia have given a distinct heading to this form of carbolic acid, and directed it to be used only externally; for, while its impurity, and more or less uncertain composition and strength, unfit it for internal employment, it is equally efficacious with the purer acid as a local remedy, and may be very advantageously used for disinfectant purposes. In addition to what has been said of it in the preceding article, the following description of it taken from the Pharmacopœia is all that is required on the subject:

"A nearly colorless or reddish-brown liquid of a strongly empyreumatic and disagreeable odor; having a benumbing, blanching and caustic effect on the skin or mucous membrane, and a neutral reaction. Bromine water produces in an aqueous solution of carbolic or cresylic acid a white flocculent precipitate. Crude carbolic acid should not dissolve in less than 15 parts of water at 15° C. (59° F.), nor should the solution have an alkaline reaction (abs. of alkalies). If 50 volumes of crude carbolic acid be diluted with warm water to measure 1000 volumes, the mixture well shaken, cooled, and allowed to separate, the amount of undissolved impurities should not exceed 5 volumes, or 10 per cent. by volume of the crude acid. The amount of water in a solution of crude carbolic acid may be determined by agitating the solution in a graduated cylinder with an equal volume of chloroform. After standing, the upper layer consists of the water contained in the mixture." *U. S.*

ACIDUM CARBOLICUM LIQUEFACTUM. *Br. Liquefied Carbolic Acid.*

(ĂÇ'Ĭ-DŬM CĂR-BŎL'Ĭ-CŬM LĬQ-UĘ-FĂCTŲM.)

"Carbolic acid liquefied by the addition of 10 per cent. of water." *Br.*

This is a new officinal of the British Pharmacopœia, and its introduction was doubtless due to a practical use long made of the same preparation in dispensing, so as to avoid weighing the acid.

It is described as a "colorless or very slightly reddish or brownish liquid having the taste, odor, etc., of carbolic acid. Specific gravity 1·064 to 1·067 at 60° F. (15°·5 C.). Boiling point gradually rising to a temperature not higher than 371° F. (188°·3 C.). It dissolves 18 to 26 per cent. of water at 60° F. (15°·5 C.), yielding a clear or nearly clear solution, from which any slight colored impurity contained previously in the acid separates as dark oily drops." *Br.* As one minim of this preparation is practically equivalent to one grain of the pure acid, the dose is one to three minims.

ACIDUM CHROMICUM. *U. S., Br. Chromic Acid.*

CrO_3; 100·4. (ĂÇ'Ĭ-DŬM CHRŌ'MĬ-CŬM.) CrO_3; 50·2.

Chromic acid should be preserved in glass-stoppered vials.

Chromic Anhydride, Chromium Trioxide; Acide chromique, *Fr.*; Chromsäure, *G.*

This is not a true acid, but an anhydride. It may be obtained by the process officinal in the British Pharmacopœia: "Bichromate of Potassium, 30 ounces (av.); Sulphuric Acid, 57 fluidounces (Imp. meas.); Distilled Water, a sufficiency. Dissolve the bichromate of potassium in a mixture of 50 fluidounces (Imp. meas.) of the water and 42 fluidounces (Imp. meas.) of the acid. Set aside for twelve hours, and decant the liquor from the crystals of acid sulphate of potassium that have separated. Heat the liquor to about 185° F. (85° C.), and add the remainder of the acid, and water sufficient to just redissolve any crystals of chromic acid that may have been formed. Allow to cool, collect and drain the crystals, and dry them on porous tiles at a temperature not exceeding 100° F. (37°·8 C.) in an air-bath. From the mother liquor more crystals may be obtained on evaporation." *Br.*

This process yields crystals which are more or less contaminated with sulphuric acid. Dr. Vulpius (*Archiv d. Pharm.*, 1886, p. 964) shows that commercial chromic acid sometimes contains as much as 7 per cent. of sulphuric acid, and that pure chromic acid is not scarlet in color but dark brown-red and steel glistening, and not deliquescent in ordinary air.

The best yield of pure crystals is said to be according to the method of Zettnow (*Pogg. Ann.*, cxliii. 471), in which 300 Gm. of potassium bichromate are mixed with 500 C.c. of water, and 420 C.c. of concentrated sulphuric acid added, and the mixture allowed to stand for twelve hours in order that the acid potassium sulphate may crystallize out. The mother-liquor is then heated to from 80° to 90°, and 150 C.c. of sulphuric acid added, together with enough water to dissolve the crystals of trioxide which at first separate out. After standing for twelve hours the liquid is poured off from the crystals which have separated, and a second and a third crop may be obtained by concentration. The crystals having been drained upon a porous plate and washed with pure nitric acid, 1·46 gravity, are dried in a current of warm air. For a method by M. Duviller, in which chromate of barium is treated by nitric acid, and chromic acid crystallized out of the mother-liquor, see *A. J. P.*, 1873, p. 23.

Properties. Chromic acid is in the form of anhydrous, acicular crystals, of a brilliant crimson red color and an acid metallic taste, deliquescent, and very soluble in water, forming an orange red solution. "On being heated to about 190° C. (374° F.) chromic acid melts, and at 250 C. (482° F.) it is mostly decomposed with the formation of dark green chromic oxide and the evolution of oxygen. On contact, trituration, or warming with strong alcohol, glycerin, spirit of nitrous ether, and other easily oxidizable substances, it is liable to cause sudden combustion or explosion." *U.S.*

Chromic acid is a teroxide of the metal chromium, having the formula CrO_3. At a heat above the melting point, it gives off half its oxygen, and is converted into the green sesquioxide, Cr_2O_3. It is a powerful oxidizing and bleaching material, and gives up its oxygen with great facility to organic matter. The oxidation of weaker alcohol is attended with the production of aldehyd recognized by the odor, of stronger alcohol by inflaming. "If 1 Gm. of chromic acid be dissolved in 100 C.c. of cold water and mixed with 10 C.c. of hydrochloric acid, the further addition of 1 C.c. of test solution of chloride of barium should cause not more than a white turbidity (limit of sulphuric acid)." *U.S.*

Medical Properties and Uses. As an antiseptic and disinfectant, chromic acid is asserted by Dr. John Dougal (*Lancet*, Dec. 16, 1871), who founds his conclusions on experiment, to be second to none, and in some respects to surpass even carbolic acid. A piece of fresh beef immersed in a solution of chromic acid, containing only 1 part in 2000 of water, became in two days quite black, in six as hard as wood, and at the end of three months remained perfectly free from mould or taint. It is a powerful coagulant of albumen, being, according to Dougal, 10 times stronger than carbolic acid, 15 times stronger than nitric acid, and 20 times stronger than bichloride of mercury. It is, therefore, one of the best tests of the presence of albumen in a fluid; two grains dissolved in an ounce of water readily detecting albumen in a solution containing one part of a saturated solution of beef-juice in 20 of water. Besides coagulating albuminous substances, it oxidizes decaying organic matter, combines with and neutralizes the escaping ammonia, and decomposes sulphuretted hydrogen, reducing it to water and free sulphur. It is also one of the most powerfully destructive agents to inferior organic life, greatly exceeding carbolic acid in this respect. Chromic acid has been used medically only as an escharotic, in which capacity it acts by rapidly oxidizing and thus decomposing the tissues, while by the loss of one-half its oxygen it is itself converted into the inert sesquioxide. It was first employed as a caustic by Prof. Sigmund, of Vienna, on the recommendation of Dr. Heller. Used in substance, made into a paste with water, its action is exceedingly slow and gradual, but deeply penetrating. In saturated solution its action is less penetrating and less gradual. By using a solution more or less dilute, the effect may be graduated according to the degree desired. Prof. Sigmund tried the concentrated solution, with advantage, for the destruction of condylomata, occurring in his syphilitic wards. But caution is necessary in its use; as it may give rise to a deep slough if too largely applied; and, according to M. Gubler, patients have been poisoned, through absorption, by a too extensive application of the acid to the surface. (*Ed. Med. Journ.*, Sept. 1871, p. 281.) Besides these applications, it has been recommended to destroy growths in the mouth and larynx, from its combined escharotic and disinfecting properties, in hospital gangrene, scorbutic or gangrenous ulcers of the mouth, phagedænic ulcers, bites of rabid animals, poisoned wounds, etc.; as a wash to arrest fetid discharges; as an injection in ozæna, leucorrhœa, and gonorrhœa; to prevent suppuration and putrefaction in wounds, etc.; and for the disinfection of cholera and fever stools, as well as for correcting fetid odors from all sources. Care should be taken not to prescribe it in combination with glycerin, or any substance which will cause it to rapidly part with its oxygen: a compounded prescription containing 8 grains of chromic acid and 1 drachm of glycerin exploded violently. (*Zeitschr. Oester. Apoth. Verein*, June 1, 1875.) It is best to use a simple aqueous solution. The solution, or even the pure acid, is used by gynæcologists to destroy intra-uterine growths, but great care is requisite.

Chromic acid is very rarely, if ever, used internally; if employed, the dose should not exceed one-quarter of a grain (0·016 Gm.).

Off. Prep. Br. Liquor Acidi Chromici.

ACIDUM CITRICUM. *U.S., Br.* *Citric Acid.*

$H_3C_6H_5O_7$, H_2O; 210. (ĂÇ'Ĭ-DŬM CĬT'RĬ-CŬM.) **$3HOC_{12}H_5O_{11}2HO$; 210.**

Acidum Citri, s. Limonis, s. Limonum, s. Limonorum; Acide citrique, Acide du Citron, *Fr.*; Citronensäure, Citronsäure, *G.*; Acido citrico, *It.*, *Sp.*

"An acid prepared from lemon-juice or from the juice of the fruit of Citrus Bergamia, *Risso and Poit* (Citrus Limetta, D. C.), the Lime." *Br.*

Citric acid is the peculiar acid to which limes and lemons owe their sourness. It is present also in the juice of other fruits; such as the cranberry, the red whortleberry, the berry of the bittersweet, the red gooseberry, the currant, the strawberry, the raspberry, the tamarind, and the red elderberry (fruit of *Sambucus racemosa rubra*). The latter berry contains citric acid so abundantly that it has been proposed as a source of the acid by M. Thibierge, of Versailles. It is contained also largely in the fruit of *Cyphomandra botacea*, a solanaceous plant, indigenous in Mexico, Peru, and other parts of South America, where it is called *tomato de la paz*. (*Journ. de Pharm.*, Oct. 1869, p. 305.) The commercial source of citric acid is lime, lemon, and bergamot juice; large quantities of *lime-juice* are made in Sicily, concentrated, and exported to England and the United States.*

The acid is extracted from lemon or lime juice by a very simple process, for which we are indebted to Scheele; it is one requiring some careful manipulation. The boiling juice is first completely saturated with carbonate of calcium (chalk or whiting) in fine powder, and the citrate of calcium formed is allowed to subside. This is then washed repeatedly with water, and decomposed by dilute sulphuric acid. An insoluble sulphate of calcium is precipitated, and the disengaged citric acid remains in solution. This is carefully concentrated in leaden boilers until a pellicle begins to form, when it is transferred to other vessels to cool and crystallize.

The commercial lemon-juices contain free citric acid; free acids other than citric; citrates, salts of organic acids other than citric; salts of inorganic acids; and albuminous, mucilaginous, saccharine, and other indifferent bodies. Spirit is frequently added as a preservative, and mineral acids are not uncommonly employed as adulterants. Verjuice has also been used for the purpose (Allen). See also Montserrat lime-juice, *P. J. Tr.*, 1883, p. 606, and notes on manufacture, etc., *N. R.*, 1883, p. 47. In the U. S. Pharmacopœia, very properly, no process is given for making citric

* The composition of some of these commercial lime-juices is given by Allen (*Com. Org. Analysis*, 2d ed., i. p. 459), as follows:

	Density.	Oz. Free Acid per gallon.	Oz. Combined Org. Acid per gallon.
Lime-juice.			
Raw Sicilian	....	6 to 9	0·85
Raw English	1·04 to 1·05	11 to 13	0·3
Concentrated	1·20 to 1·25	56 to 72	6 to 8
Bergamot-juice.			
Concentrated	1·22 to 1·25	47 to 55	7 to 8
Lemon-juice.			
Raw	1·035 to 1·04	10·6 to 12·5	0·4 to 0·7
Concentrated	1·28 to 1·38	82 to 112	8·6

See also paper by D. H. Hassler, *A. J. P.*, 1886, p. 14.

acid, as it is always purchased from the manufacturing chemist. The British Pharmacopœia gives the following process for preparing it:

"Take of Lemon Juice *four pints* [Imperial measure]; Prepared Chalk *four ounces and a half* [avoirdupois]; Sulphuric Acid *two fluidounces and a half;* Distilled Water *a sufficiency.* Heat the Lemon Juice to its boiling point, and add the Chalk by degrees till there is no more effervescence. Collect the deposit on a calico filter, and wash it with hot water till the filtered liquor passes from it colorless. Mix the deposit with a pint [Imp. meas.] of Distilled Water, and gradually add the Sulphuric Acid previously diluted with a pint and a half [Imp. meas.] of Distilled Water. Boil gently for half an hour, keeping the mixture constantly stirred. Separate the acid solution by filtration, wash the insoluble matter with a little Distilled Water, and add the washings to the solution. Concentrate this solution to the density of 1·21, then allow it to cool, and after twenty-four hours decant the liquor from the crystals of sulphate of calcium which have formed; further concentrate the liquor until a film forms on its surface, and set it aside to cool and crystallize. Purify the crystals if necessary by recrystallization." *Br.*

Preparation on the Large Scale. The juice is placed in a large vat, closed at top, and is saturated with whiting (carbonate of calcium). Carbonic acid gas is evolved, which passes out by an exit-pipe, and may be used in the manufacture of bicarbonate of sodium; and citrate of calcium precipitates. The supernatant liquor, containing much extractive matter, is drawn off; and the citrate of calcium is decomposed by dilute sulphuric acid, liberating the citric acid, and precipitating the lime as a sulphate. The mixture of citric acid and sulphate of calcium is run off into a wooden filter back, lined with lead, furnished with a perforated false bottom, and lined throughout with stout twilled flannel. The solution of citric acid passes off through a pipe, leading from the bottom of the back to suitable reservoirs. The sulphate is washed until it becomes tasteless, and the washings are run off into the same reservoirs. The filtered acid solution is then concentrated by evaporation in wooden vessels lined with lead, through which steam is made to pass by means of coiled lead pipes. As citric acid is liable to decomposition, if subjected to too high a temperature, the use of the vacuum pan is highly advantageous in concentrating the solution. When the liquor is sufficiently concentrated, it is transferred to cylindrical sheet-lead vessels, placed in a warm situation, to crystallize. The crystals, at first obtained, are colored. In order to purify them, they are redissolved in a small quantity of water, with the assistance of heat, and the solution is digested with purified animal charcoal, filtered, and recrystallized. The crystals, after having been washed and drained, are dried on wooden trays lined with sheet-lead, in a room heated by steam. Dr. Price, Mr. Pontifex, and J. Carter Bell have made improvements in the manufacture of citric acid: for details and suggestions, see *Chem. News*, 1866, p. 100; *P. J. Tr.* (xiii. 313, and xvi. 430); *N. R.*, 1880, p. 274; *Chem. News*, 1882.

The citrate of calcium of the above process should be decomposed without delay; for, if kept, it will undergo fermentation, with the effect of destroying the citric acid. According to Personne, the products of this fermentation are acetic and butyric acids; carbonic acid and hydrogen being evolved. It is desirable to have a slight excess of sulphuric acid, as this rather favors than otherwise the crystallization of the citric acid. It is found necessary, also, to add occasionally a small proportion of sulphuric acid to the citric acid liquor, during the progress of its concentration. According to J. Carter Bell (*N. R.*, 1880, p. 274), the concentrated juice contains from sixty-four to ninety-six ounces of citric acid to the imperial gallon. The more recent the juice the better the quality. That which is stale will sometimes be quite sour, without containing any citric acid, in consequence of having undergone the acetous fermentation.

Properties. "Colorless, right rhombic prisms, not deliquescent except in moist air, efflorescent in warm air, odorless, having an agreeable purely acid taste and an acid reaction." *U. S.* Its sp. gr. is 1·6. When heated, it dissolves in its water of crystallization, and, at a higher temperature, undergoes decomposition, becoming yellow or brown, and forming a very sour syrupy liquid, which is uncrystallizable. By destructive distillation it gives rise to water, empyreumatic oil, acetic and carbonic acids, carburetted hydrogen, and a number of pyrogenous acids, among which is *aconitic*, $C_6H_6O_6$. A voluminous coal is left, which is readily combustible.

Citric acid dissolves in three-fourths of its weight of cold, and half its weight of boiling water. It is soluble also in an equal weight of alcohol and half its weight of boiling alcohol, but is nearly insoluble in pure ether, chloroform, benzol, and benzin, requiring 48 parts for its solution in common ether. A weak solution of it has an agreeable taste, but cannot be kept, as it undergoes spontaneous decomposition. It is incompatible with alkaline solutions, whether pure or carbonated, converting them into citrates; also with the earthy and metallic carbonates, most acetates, the alkaline sulphides, and soaps. It is characterised by its taste, by the shape of its crystals, and by forming an insoluble salt with lime-water when heated, and a deliquescent one with potassa. If sulphuric acid be present the acid will be hygroscopic, and the precipitate by acetate of lead will not be entirely soluble in nitric acid; the insoluble portion being sulphate of lead. Sometimes crystals of tartaric acid are substituted for or mixed with the citric, or the two acids may be mixed in powder, a fraud which is readily detected by adding a solution of potash to that of the suspected acids, when, if tartaric acid be present, a crystalline precipitate of bitartrate of potassium (cream of tartar) will be formed: "If 1 part of the acid be dissolved in 2 parts of water and treated with a solution of 1 part of acetate of potassium in 2 parts of water, the mixture should remain clear after the addition of an equal volume of alcohol (tartaric and oxalic acids)." *U. S.* See Spiller, *Journal Chemical Society*, x. 110. A still more delicate method of detecting tartaric acid is to digest the suspected acid with ferric hydrate in a test tube, afterwards to raise the heat slowly to the boiling point, and, having allowed the excess of hydrate to subside, to decant the clear liquid, and evaporate it to a syrupy consistence. If the acid be pure, the liquid remains limpid, and of a fine red color; if contaminated with the tartaric acid, even to the extent of only one per cent., it becomes cloudy, and deposits tartrate of the sesquioxide. (*Journ. de Pharm.*, 1862, p. 169.) Another test is permanganate of potassium, of which an alkaline solution is without action on citric acid; while, under the influence of tartaric acid, the peroxide of manganese is deposited. (*Ibid.*, 1867, p. 239.) "If 1 Gm. of citric acid be dissolved, without heat, in 10 C.c. of a cold, saturated solution of bichromate of potassium, no darkening of the liquid should be observed within five minutes (abs. of 1 per cent. or more of tartaric acid)." *U. S.** "When heated to 100° C. (212° F.) the acid melts and gradually loses 8·6 per cent. of its weight. At a higher temperature it emits inflammable vapors, chars, and is finally dissipated without leaving more than 0·05 per cent. of ash. On adding an aqueous solution of the acid to an excess of lime-water, the mixture remains clear until boiled, when a white precipitate separates, which is nearly all redissolved on cooling. An aqueous solution of the acid should not be darkened nor be precipitated by hydrosulphuric acid (lead and copper). If the crystals have left, on ignition, some ash (see above), this ash should not turn blue by treatment with a few drops of water of ammonia (copper); nor should the further addition of one drop of test solution of sulphide of ammonium cause any black coloration (lead, copper, and iron). 10 C.c. of a concentrated solution should show no precipitate within five minutes after the addition of 1 C.c. of test solution of chloride of barium with excess of hydrochloric acid (sulphuric acid). To neutralize 3·5 Gm. of citric acid should require 50 C.c. of the volumetric solution of soda." *U. S.* Lead is frequently found in the metallic state in citric acid in small quantity, and this arises from small portions being rubbed off in breaking off the crystals from the crystallizing vats. The presence of lead or copper may be detected as above, or by igniting in a porcelain crucible a small quantity of the acid, dissolving the ash in a few drops of nitric acid, diluting largely, and passing sulphuretted hydrogen through it; a black precipitate indicating the impurity.

* *Pusch's Method of Determining the Presence of Tartaric Acid in Citric Acid.* 1 gramme of powdered citric acid is added to 10 grammes of strong, pure, colorless, sulphuric acid in a dry test-tube, and the tube is then immersed in boiling water for an hour. The citric acid dissolves with frothing and evolution of gas, and a lemon-colored liquid is formed, which undergoes no change within half an hour if the sample be pure; but if as much as one-half per cent. of tartaric acid be present, the color is brownish and reddish-brown an hour afterward. (*Archiv d. Pharm.*, xxii. 316.

Composition. The formula of the anhydrous acid is $C_6H_5O_7H_3$. It is a tribasic acid, and may therefore yield three classes of citrates according as one, two, or three atoms of hydrogen are replaced by metal, the first two classes being acid citrates, and the third class neutral citrates. When crystallized from its solution by cooling, it contains one molecule of water. Crystals of the formula $(C_6H_8O_7)_2 + H_2O$ have also been formed. (Flückiger, *Pharm. Chem*, 1879, p. 157.) If citric acid be heated until all of its water of crystallization is driven off, there is produced *aconitic acid* ($C_6H_3O_6H_3$), which also exists naturally in aconite, larkspur, black hellebore, equisetum, yarrow, and other plants.*

Medical Properties, etc. Citric acid acts as a poison chiefly if not solely by irritating the gastro-intestinal mucous membrane. It is, however, much less irritant than is tartaric acid, and, so far as we know, no death has been caused by it. The action of therapeutic doses upon the system is not decided. In scurvy, citric acid is probably of some value, but is very inferior to lemon-juice. It is eliminated by the kidneys, and, as first stated by Bence Jones, when given in sufficient quantities renders the urine acid. In a free state it is very rarely, if ever, used internally, except as an imperfect substitute for lemon-juice. When added in the quantity of nine drachms and a half to a pint of distilled water, it forms a solution of the average strength of lemon-juice. Of this solution, or of lemon-juice, a scruple of bicarbonate of potassium saturates three fluidrachms and a half; a scruple of carbonate of potassium, four fluidrachms; and a scruple of carbonate of ammonium, six fluidrachms. Half a fluidounce of lemon-juice, or of an equivalent solution of citric acid, when saturated, is considered a dose. An agreeable substitute for lemonade may be made by dissolving from two to four parts of the acid, mixed with sugar and a little oil of lemons, in nine hundred parts of water; or a scruple of the acid may be dissolved in a pint of water, and sweetened with sugar which has been rubbed on fresh lemon-peel. The dose of the acid may be stated at from five to thirty grains (0·33–1·95 Gm.).

Off. Prep. Bismuthi Citras; Ferri et Strychninæ Citras; Liquor Ferri Citratis; Liquor Ferri et Quininæ Citratis; Liquor Magnesii Citratis; Magnesii Citras Granulatus; Liquor Potassii Citratis; Syrupus Acidi Citrici; Syrupus Hypophosphitum.

Off. Prep. Br. Succus Limonis; Syrupus Limonis; Vinum Quininæ.

Off. Citrates. Br. Liquor Ammonii Citratis Fortior; Bismuthi Citras; Liquor Bismuthi et Ammonii Citratis; Caffeina Citras; Ferri et Ammonii Citras; Ferri et Quininæ Citras; Liquor Magnesii Citratis; Lithii Citras; Potassii Citras; Sodii Citro-tartras Effervescens.

ACIDUM GALLICUM. *U. S., Br.* *Gallic Acid.*

$HC_7H_5O_5, H_2O$; 188. (ĂÇ'Ĭ-DŬM GĂL'LĬ-CŬM.) $HO\ C_{14}H_5O_9, 2\ HO$; 188.

Acide gallique, *Fr.;* Gallussäure, *G.;* Trioxybenzoic acid, Dioxysalicylic acid.

"An acid prepared from galls." *Br.*

In the last revision of the U. S. Pharmacopœia the process for the preparation of gallic acid was omitted. The British Pharmacopœia process is as follows: "Boil one part of coarsely powdered galls with four fluid parts of diluted sulphuric acid for half an hour, then strain through calico while hot; collect the crystals that are deposited on cooling, and purify with animal charcoal and repeated crystallization." *Br.*

The process based on the influence of sulphuric acid in favoring the change of tannic into gallic acid, has the merit of requiring less time than former processes.

The U. S. 1870 process† is founded upon the fact that when galls in infusion, or in the state of moistened powder, are exposed to the air, their tannic acid is gradually converted into gallic acid. The gallic acid, being freely soluble in boiling but very sparingly in cold water, is extracted from the altered galls by decoction, and is

* According to Hentschel, aconitic acid is best obtained by boiling for six hours 100 Gm. of citric acid with 50 Gm. of water mixed with 100 Gm. of pure sulphuric acid in a flask provided with a reverse condenser. Upon cooling the contents of the flask a solid cake of aconitic acid is found, which may be purified by mixing with strong hydrochloric acid, and washing until free from sulphuric acid; colorless, shining crystals are obtained. (*Archiv d. Pharm.*, 1887, p. 357.)

† See U. S. Dispensatory, 15th edition, p. 60.

deposited as the water cools. A repetition of the solution and deposition renders the acid more pure; but it cannot be obtained wholly colorless unless by the aid of animal charcoal. There are few processes in which it is more necessary that the animal charcoal should be purified. The presence of the slightest quantity of ferric salt interferes with the bleaching of the acid; and it is even advisable to examine the filtering paper, lest it may contain sufficient of this substance to vitiate the results of the process. The first crop of crystals in the process retains a very large proportion of water; and it will be found convenient to subject them to strong expression between folds of bibulous paper.

The elder Robiquet first suggested that galls contained a principle capable of converting tannic into gallic acid, with the presence of water, and in the absence of atmospheric air. M. Laroque proved that this principle acts as a ferment, and that the change referred to is the result of a *gallic acid fermentation* in the galls. M. Edmond Robiquet showed that galls contain *pectose* and *pectase*, the former of which, according to the experiments of M. Frémy, is the principle out of which pectin is formed in plants, and the latter a peculiar ferment which effects the transformation. He believed that in galls the pectase, aided by a proper temperature and the presence of water, changed not only pectose into pectin, but also tannic into gallic acid. Strecker previously advanced the opinion that tannic acid was a combination of gallic acid and sugar, the latter of which is destroyed in the process for procuring gallic acid, which is thus simply set free from the combination. M. E. Robiquet admitted the occasional transformation of tannic acid into gallic acid and sugar, but did not believe that the sugar pre-existed as such in the tannin. (*Journ. de Pharm.*, 3e sér., xxiii. 241.) Wittstein, in endeavoring to obtain gallic acid from *Chinese galls* by forming them into a paste with water, found that but a very small proportion of the acid was generated at the end of six weeks. Thinking that this might have resulted from the want of the ferment in the Chinese galls, he added to these one-eighth of their weight of common galls, and, at the end of three weeks, obtained an amount of gallic acid nearly equal to one-half the weight of the galls employed. The same result, though more slowly, followed the addition of yeast to the Chinese galls. Wittstein obtained both carbonic acid and alcohol as products of this operation, thus favoring the views of Strecker as to the constitution of tannic acid. And the idea that tannin was a glucoside convertible through exposure of galls to the air, or more rapidly by sulphuric acid, into glucose and gallic acid, was accepted without qualification, until Schiff (*Deut. Chem. Ges. Ber.*, iv. 231, 967, and *Bull. Soc. Chem.* [2], xviii. 23) proved that although crude tannic acid contains glucose, it is possible to separate a large quantity of the glucose without destroying the tannic acid. He proposes that *pure tannic acid* be called *digallic acid*, and that the term *tannin* be applied to natural tannin, *i.e.*, the *glucoside* of digallic or pure tannic acid, for when natural tannin is boiled with dilute mineral acids, or subjected to the influence of a nitrogenous ferment, it splits into digallic acid and glucose, $C_{34}H_{28}O_{22} + 4H_2O = 4C_7H_6O_5 + C_6H_{12}O_6$. Digallic acid is the first anhydride of gallic acid—$C_{14}H_{10}O_9 + H_2O = 2C_7H_6O_5$. Gallic acid is a *phenol acid*, or combination of these two classes of organic compounds, its formula being $C_6H_2(OH)_3.COOH$. It may be termed, therefore, a *trioxybenzoic acid*. It is monobasic.

Properties. Gallic acid is in delicate, silky, acicular crystals, which, as ordinarily found in the shops, are slightly brownish, but when quite pure are colorless. It is inodorous, and of a sourish, astringent taste and an acid reaction. It is soluble, according to Braconnot, in 100 parts of cold and 3 of boiling water, in 4·5 parts of alcohol, 1 part of boiling alcohol, 3 parts of absolute alcohol, and 39 parts of absolute ether. It is even less soluble in chloroform, benzol, and benzin. Mr. Thomas Weaver, of Philadelphia, has found that it is soluble in glycerin in the proportion of 40 grains to the ounce, and that the solution may be diluted to any extent with water without affecting its transparency. (*A. J. P.*, xxix. 82.) It produces a deep bluish-black color with solutions of ferric salts, which disappears when the solution is heated; a result which Dr. Mahla has shown to depend on the conversion of the gallic into *gallhumic* or *metagallic acid*, by the loss of the constituents of carbonic acid and water. (*Am. Journ. of Sci. and Arts*, Nov. 1859.) It does not precipitate gelatin, or a solution of ferrous sulphate. "When dried at 100° C. (212° F.) the crystals lose 9·5 to 10 per cent. of combined water." *U. S.* It should leave no residue when burned, and be entirely dissipated when thrown on red-hot iron. On exposure to the air, its solution undergoes spontaneous decomposition; but it is said that by the addition of a drop of oil of cloves it may be kept for a long time without change, the absence of tannin and microscopic fungi being proved. "An aqueous solution of gallic acid should not precipitate alkaloids, gelatin, albumen, gelatinized starch, or solution of tartrate of antimony and potassium with chloride of ammonium (distinction from tannic acid)." By the action of arsenic it is converted almost entirely into tannic acid without the production of arsenious acid. (Schiff, *Chem. News*, xxix. 73.) A very delicate test for gallic acid has been proposed by Henry R. Procter (*A. J. P.*, Aug. 1874.) It consists in adding the suspected solution to a faintly alkaline solution of arseniate of sodium or potassium. If gallic acid be present, an intense green color is soon developed, appearing, if the liquid be quiet, first upon the surface. Prof. Flückiger has pointed out (*P. J. Tr.*, Aug. 1, 1874) that the arseniate plays no part in this test. The change is produced by an alkali, whether caustic or not, provided it is present in very small quantity. The reaction does not occur with gallo-tannic or pyrogallic acid. A test proposed by Flückiger consists in adding to the solution of gallic acid a dilute (1 to 100) solution of pure ferrous sulphate. To the colorless solution a little acetate of sodium is to be added, when a deep violet color will appear, due to the formation of ferrous gallate. The Pharmacopœia test is as follows. "If 5 C.c. of a cold saturated solution of gallic acid be treated in a watch glass with not more than two drops of solution of potassa, a deep green color will gradually be developed. This color is changed to purple red by acids, and is prevented by an excess of alkaline hydrate or carbonate." Heated to 216° C. (420° F.), gallic acid gives out carbonic acid, and is changed into *pyrogallic acid.* (See Part II.)

Medical Properties. Gallic acid is astringent, but less powerfully so than tannic acid. As it does not coagulate albumen, it is readily absorbed when ingested, and is rapidly eliminated by the kidneys. Its presence in the urine is under these circumstances readily demonstrated by the addition of a soluble ferric salt of iron. Owing to its being more readily transported by the blood, it is more effective than tannic acid in all cases of hemorrhage (hæmoptysis, hæmaturia, etc.), in which the bleeding vessels must be reached through the route of the circulation. But in hemorrhage from the alimentary mucous membrane, or from any other part with which tannic acid can be brought into direct contact, the latter astringent is by far the more effectual. Tannic acid is also much more efficient in anginose or other relaxations in which a decided astringent action is desired, and in which a direct application can be made. Gallic acid has been employed with advantage in pyrosis, and in the night-sweats of phthisis, or exhaustion. In albuminuria, when there is a very large amount of albumen excreted, gallic acid may be employed with service to diminish the flow, and the drug has even been used in acute Bright's disease, following scarlatina, with asserted great advantage. (*N. R.*, Oct. 1875.) It is said not to constipate the bowels. The dose is from five to fifteen grains (0·33–1·0 Gm.) three or four times a day, and may be given in the form of pill or powder.

Off. Prep. Unguentum Acidi Gallici.

Off. Prep. Br. Glycerinum Acidi Gallici.

ACIDUM HYDROBROMICUM DILUTUM. *U.S., Br.* *Diluted Hydrobromic Acid.*

(ĂÇ-Ĭ-DŬM HȲ-DRO-BRŌ-MĬ-CŬM DĬ-LŪ-TŬM.)

Acidum Bromhydricum Dilutum, Acidum Bromohydricum; Acide hydrobromique, *Fr.*; Hydrobromsäure, Bromwasserstoffsäure, *G.*

"A liquid composed of 10 per cent. of absolute Hydrobromic Acid [H Br; 80·8—H Br; 80·8] and 90 per cent. of water." *U. S.* "An aqueous solution containing 10 per cent. by weight of gaseous or real hydrobromic acid, H Br." *Br.*

The U. S. Pharmacopœia does not give a process for this acid; the British process is as follows: "Bromine, 1 fluidounce [Imp. meas.]; Distilled Water, Sulphuretted Hydrogen, of each a sufficiency. Place the bromine in a glass cylinder and pour over it 15 ounces [Imp. meas.] of the water. Pass a current of sulphuretted hydrogen gas into the bromine until the red color of the aqueous liquid has disappeared. Filter the fluid and distil the filtrate. Reject the distillate until it is free from odor of sulphuretted compounds, and then collect it until sulphuric acid begins to distil. Dilute the distilled acid with water until it has a specific gravity at 60° F. (15°·5 C.) of 1·077. Preserve in glass-stoppered bottles. From the rejected distillate more hydrobromic acid may be obtained by redistillation."*

The most convenient process is undoubtedly that of Dr. Dewitt C. Wade (*Peninsular Medical Journal,* Feb. 1875), modelled after Buchanan's method of making hydriodic acid, which directs that 120 grains of bromide of potassium be dissolved in one fluidounce of water, and 153 grains of tartaric acid be added to the solution; acid tartrate of potassium is produced, the greater part of which crystallizes out on standing 12 hours at a low temperature, and a solution of hydrobromic acid is formed, sp. gr. 1·228, containing about 80 grains real hydrobromic acid to the fluidounce, equivalent to nearly 15 per cent. Fothergill's acid, although based upon Wade's formula, is weaker, the quantity of bromide of potassium being 81¼ grains and that of tartaric acid 99 grains to the fluidounce, the manipulation being the same; each fluidounce of Fothergill's acid contains about 55 grains real hydrobromic acid, or about 10 per cent. Diluted hydrobromic acid made in this way is open to the objection of containing cream of tartar, and probably some undecomposed bromide of potassium in solution, and thus is not strictly pure. To lessen this, Charles Rice proposes the addition of a double quantity of alcohol to facilitate the precipitation, recovering the alcohol by distillation subsequently. (*N. R.*, 1877, p. 107.) Other processes have been suggested for preparing hydrobromic acid. Edward Goebel (*N. R.*, Sept. 1880) proposes a method based on Glover's process, which is to decompose 148 grains barium bromide, dissolved in half an ounce of water, with 50·6 grains sulphuric acid, diluted with two drachms of distilled water; the precipitated barium sulphate is washed with distilled water until the filtrate weighs 810 grains to make the 10 per cent. acid solution. He makes bromide of barium by triturating 100 parts pure carbonate of barium with 95 parts bromide of ammonium with a little water, so as to make a damp powder, and heating in an evaporating dish until vapors of carbonate of ammonium cease to be evolved; the residue is dissolved in distilled water, filtered, evaporated, and dried. Winckler proposes a plan for making hydriodic acid, which has been adapted by Charles Rice to making hydrobromic acid. (See *N. R.*, Jan. 1880.) Bromine is dissolved in bisulphide of carbon, and hydrogen sulphide passed through the solution. The processes of Balard, Millon, and Loewig are commented upon by John M. Maisch (*Proc. A. P. A.*, 1860), who proposes some useful modifications. Prof. Markoe (*Ibid.*, 1875, p. 686) recommends an economical process, which, however, must be followed with care, and is better adapted for making the acid on a large scale.

* The following process is based upon that of Dr. E. R. Squibb.

Take of Bromide of Potassium and Sulphuric Acid, each, one hundred and fifty parts, Distilled Water, a sufficient quantity. Add the Sulphuric Acid to twenty-five parts of Distilled Water, and cool the mixture. Then dissolve the Potassium Bromide in one hundred and fifty parts of water by the aid of heat, supplying the loss of water by evaporation during the heating. Carefully pour the diluted Sulphuric Acid into the hot solution with constant stirring, and set the mixture aside for twenty-four hours, in order that the Potassium Sulphate may crystallize. Pour off the liquid into a retort, break up the crystalline mass, transfer it to a funnel, and having drained the crystals, drop slowly upon them fifty parts of cold Distilled Water so as to wash out the acid liquid. Add this liquid to that in the retort, and distil nearly to dryness at a moderate heat. If red fumes of bromine are given off during any stage of the distillation, change the receiver as soon as such fumes cease to appear. Finally determine in the distillate the amount of actual Hydrobromic Acid (16·2 Gms. should require 20 C.c. of the volumetric solution of soda), and add to the remaining weighed distillate such an amount of cold Distilled Water as shall cause the finished acid to contain 10 per cent. of actual hydrobromic acid.

This process for making solution of hydrobromic acid does not differ essentially from that of Dr. E. R. Squibb (*A. J. P.*, 1878, p. 116), except in the improvement of the rather smaller proportion of sulphuric acid used, and in the fact of the difference in strength of the two hydrobromic acids, Dr. Squibb's being 34 per cent., the above 10 per cent. The advantages possessed by both methods over those frequently used are greater purity of product and more definite strength.

He pours a pint of water into a gallon stoneware jar, and then adds one pound or more of phosphorus, distributing it over the bottom; ice is now added until the jar is half full, a gallon glass funnel is inserted in the throat of the jar, and a funnel tube adjusted, so that the end will be a short distance above the surface of the phosphorus; the funnel is about one-third filled with broken ice, and the jar placed in a larger vessel, and broken ice packed between. Three or four pounds of bromine after being chilled are *slowly* added, in order that the fumes of hydrobromic acid and bromine that may arise will be fully condensed by the ice in the funnel, and an accumulation of bromine avoided, which might produce an explosion from too sudden reaction. The excess of phosphorus is removed after all the bromine has been added, the liquid distilled, hydrobromic acid condensed, and the strength adjusted, whilst to the residue in the retort water may be added to make diluted phosphoric acid. For other processes see Wène (*Comptes-Rend.*, 1849), Bruylants (*Journ. de Pharm. d'Anvers*, 1879, p. 343, and *A. J. P.*, Jan. 1880), Hager (*Handbuch d. Pharm. Praxis*, i. 628), Grüning (*N. R.*, 1883, p. 240), Stas (*Zeitsch. f. Anal. Chem.*, 1886, p. 213).

Properties. Diluted hydrobromic acid is a colorless, transparent liquid, entirely vaporized by heat, inodorous, strongly acid to the taste, sp. gr. 1·077* at 15° C. (59° F.), containing 10 per cent. absolute hydrobomic acid. Although of a pungent and irritating odor, and fuming when in contact with the atmosphere when concentrated, in its diluted state it is odorless. On adding chlorine or nitric acid to diluted hydrobromic acid, bromine is liberated, which is soluble in chloroform or disulphide of carbon, imparting to these liquids a yellow color.

Tests. "Test solution of nitrate of silver causes a white precipitate insoluble in nitric acid, and in water of ammonia, and sparingly soluble in stronger water of ammonia. On being kept for some time, the acid should not become colored; test solution of chloride of barium should not produce a turbidity or precipitate (sulphuric acid)." *U. S.* 20 C.c. of the volumetric solution of soda should neutralize 16·2 Gm. of the diluted acid. It should be preserved in glass-stoppered bottles.

The following table by Biel will be found useful in showing from the specific gravities of solutions the percentage of absolute hydrobromic acid.

Biel's table of Percentage and Specific Gravity of Hydrobromic Acid.

Per Ct. HBr.	Specific Gravity at 15° C. (59° F.)	Per Ct. HBr.	Specific Gravity at 15° C. (59° F.)	Per Ct. HBr.	Specific Gravity at 15° C. (59° F.)	Per Ct. HBr.	Specific Gravity at 15° C. (59° F.)
1	1·0082	14	1·110	27	1·229	40	1·375
2	1·0155	15	1·119	28	1·239	41	1·388
3	1·0230	16	1·127	29	1·249	42	1·401
4	1·0305	17	1·136	30	1·260	43	1·415
5	1·038	18	1·145	31	1·270	44	1·429
6	1·046	19	1·154	32	1·281	45	1·444
7	1·053	20	1·163	33	1·292	46	1·459
8	1·061	21	1·172	34	1·303	47	1·474
9	1·069	22	1·181	35	1·314	48	1·490
10	1·077	23	1·190	36	1·326	49	1·496
11	1·085	24	1·200	37	1·338	50	1·513
12	1·093	25	1·209	38	1·350		
13	1·102	26	1·219	39	1·362		

Medical Properties and Uses. Dilute hydrobromic acid is very nearly identical with bromide of potassium in its action, but clinical experience has not yet fully tested its use as a substitute in *epilepsy* and other serious affections. In an experimental study made by Dr. Reichert, of the University of Pennsylvania, it was found to act upon animals precisely as does the bromide, and if it should be found equally serviceable in human disease it will have the advantage of the absence of the depressing effects of the potash. It has been especially commended in tinnitus

* Dr. E. R. Squibb takes exception to the sp. gr. 1·077 given for the officinal acid, and states that Biel's table is not accurate, the proper sp. gr. for a 10 per cent. acid at 15° C. (59° F.) being 1·0698. (*Ephemeris*, vol. i. p. 366.)

aurium. Two fluidrachms contain 12 grains of bromine, equivalent in this to 18 grains of the bromide of potassium, and may be given at once well diluted with syrup.

ACIDUM HYDROCHLORICUM. *U.S., Br.* *Hydrochloric Acid.*
[*Acidum Muriaticum*, Pharm. 1870.]
(ĂÇ'Ĭ-DŬM HȲ-DRO-CHLŌ'RĬ-CŬM.)

A liquid composed of 31·9 per cent. of absolute Hydrochloric Acid [HCl; 36·4—HCl; 36·4] and 68·1 per cent. of water. *U.S.* Hydrochloric Acid gas, HCl, dissolved in water, and forming about 32 per cent. by weight of the solution. *Br.*

Acidum Hydrochloratum, s. Chlorhydricum; Spirit of Sea-Salt, Marine Acid, Muriatic Acid. Chlorhydric Acid; Acide hydrochlorique, Acide chlorhydrique, ou muriatique, *Fr.;* Salzsäure, Chlorwasserstoffsäure, *G.;* Acido muriatico, *It., Sp.*

The hydrochloric acid of pharmacy and the arts is a solution of hydrochloric acid *gas* in water. The *British* Pharmacopœia gives the following process for preparing it.

"Take of Chloride of Sodium, dried, *forty-eight ounces* [avoirdupois]; Sulphuric Acid *forty-four fluidounces;* Water *thirty-six fluidounces;* Distilled Water *fifty fluidounces.* Pour the Sulphuric Acid slowly into thirty-two [fluid]ounces of the Water, and when the mixture has cooled, add it to the Chloride of Sodium previously introduced into a flask having the capacity of at least one gallon [Imp. meas.]. Connect the flask by corks and a bent glass tube with a three-necked wash-bottle, furnished with a safety tube, and containing the remaining four [fluid]ounces of the Water; then, applying heat to the flask, conduct the disengaged gas through the wash bottle, into a second bottle containing the Distilled Water, by means of a bent tube dipping about half an inch below the surface; and let the process be continued until the product measures sixty-six [fluid]ounces, or the liquid has acquired a sp. gr. of 1·16. The bottle containing the distilled water must be kept cool during the whole operation." *Br.*

Preparation. Hydrochloric acid is obtained by the action of sulphuric acid on chloride of sodium or common salt. In England it is produced in enormous quantities during the decomposition of common salt for the purpose of making sulphate of sodium, from which soda-ash and carbonate of sodium are afterwards manufactured in immense quantities. The decomposition of the sea-salt is performed in semi-cylindrical vessels, the curved part, next the fire, being made of iron, and the upper or flat surface, of stone. The acid gas is conveyed by a pipe to a double-necked stoneware receiver, half filled with water, and connected with a row of similar receivers, likewise containing water. As carried out on a larger scale, the decomposition of the salt takes place in hemispherical iron pans, 9 feet in diameter, covered by a brick-work dome; upon the mass of salt the requisite quantity of sulphuric acid is allowed to run from a leaden cistern placed above the decomposing pan. Torrents of hydrochloric acid gas are evolved, which collect in the space between the pan and the brick-work dome, whence they pass by a brick-work or earthenware flue into upright towers or condensers. These towers are filled with bricks or coke, down which a small stream of water is allowed to trickle. The gas, passing upwards, meets the water, and is dissolved by it; and as the acid liquor approaches the bottom of the tower, it becomes more and more nearly saturated with the gas.

The present annual production of soda-salt in England is 380,000 tons, and the hydrochloric acid produced reckoned on this basis would be over 1,000,000 tons. The annual production of the world is estimated at about 1,500,000 tons.

The acid, when required to be pure, is generally prepared by saturating distilled water with the gas in a Woulfe's apparatus. A quantity of pure fused common salt is introduced into a retort or matrass, placed on a sand-bath. The vessel is then furnished with an S tube, and connected with a series of bottles, each two-thirds full of water. A quantity of sulphuric acid is then gradually added, equal in weight to the common salt employed, and diluted with one-third of its weight of water. The materials ought not to occupy more than half the body of the retort. When the extrication of the gas slackens, heat is applied, and gradually increased until the water in the bottles refuses to absorb any more, or until no more gas is found to come over. As soon as the process is completed, boiling water should be added to the contents of the retort or matrass, in order to facilitate the removal of the residue. During the progress of the saturation, the water in the several bottles increases in temperature, which lessens its power of absorption. It is, therefore, expedient, in order to obtain a strong acid, to keep the bottles cool by means of water or ice. The connecting tubes need not plunge deeply into the acid.

The process of the British Pharmacopœia is substantially the same as the one here described, with the exception of the proportion of the acid and salt employed. In the process for hydrochloric acid, theory calls for a little less than 82 parts of liquid sulphuric acid to 100 of common salt. A moderate excess of the former may be useful to insure the complete decomposition of the salt; but the quantity of acid directed in the British process is sufficient to decompose twice the quantity of common salt taken. The intention obviously is to use enough of the acid to form the acid sulphate instead of the neutral sulphate of sodium; the former being more soluble and readily removed from the retort, and the reaction requiring less heat for its completion than when one mol. of sulphuric acid is taken to two of salt. The reaction for its formation is $NaCl + H_2SO_4 = HCl + HNaSO_4$. If only half the amount of sulphuric acid be used, the reaction is $(NaCl)_2 + H_2SO_4 = (HCl)_2 + Na_2SO_4$. In the first of these reactions (that of the British Pharmacopœia process), as only one mol. of salt is taken, it is obvious that there is not enough sodium furnished to neutralize the sulphuric acid completely and make the normal sulphate Na_2SO_4, so the result is the acid sulphate (bisulphate) $HNaSO_4$. On the other hand, in the second reaction, the two mols. of salt furnish just the sodium necessary to neutralize the one molecule of sulphuric acid and make the neutral sulphate Na_2SO_4.

As hydrochloric acid, prepared in the ordinary mode, often contains arsenic, so as to obscure its indications when employed in testing for that poison, it is of interest to the practical toxicologist to know that it may be obtained free from that impurity by distilling chloride of sodium or potassium with oxalic acid in equivalent proportions.

The following method of freeing hydrochloric acid from arsenious acid is recommended by M. Engel as easy and entirely efficacious. It is founded on the fact that arsenious acid is held in solution by hypophosphorous acid. Into a litre (about 2 pints) of arsenical hydrochloric acid introduce 4 to 5 grammes (about 60 or 70 grains) of hypophosphite of potassium, dissolved in a little water. At the end of an hour or two, the liquid becomes yellow and then brown; and a precipitate soon forms, more or less copious according to the amount of impurity. After the liquid becomes clear, which usually happens in 45 minutes, decant the hydrochloric acid and distil it. The acid thus obtained is entirely free from arsenic. This process should be conducted in a place where the direct rays of the sun may fall on the vessels; or, where this is impossible, the vessels should be subjected, by means of a water-bath, from 4 to 6 hours, to a heat little short of the boiling point of the acid. (*Journ. de Pharm.*, 1873, p. 10.) Traces of arsenic may also be removed by adding solution of stannous chloride, and after the precipitate of impure arsenic has settled, the clear liquid is re-distilled. (Bettendorff, *Zeit. für Chem.* [2], 5, p. 492.)

Properties of the Pure Acid. Hydrochloric acid, when pure, is a transparent colorless liquid, of a suffocating odor and corrosive taste. Exposed to the air it emits white fumes, owing to the escape of the acid gas, and its union with the moisture of the atmosphere. When concentrated, it blackens organic substances, like sulphuric acid. Its sp. gr. varies with its strength. When as highly concentrated as possible, its density is 1·21. The *U. S. acid*, as well as that of the present *British* Pharmacopœia, has the sp. gr. 1·16. "3·64 Gm. should require for complete neutralization 31·9 C.c. of the volumetric solution of soda," *U. S.*, or "114·8 grains by weight, mixed with half a [fluid]ounce of distilled water, require for neutralization 1000 grain-measures of *the volumetric solution of soda*." *Br.* When exposed to heat, it continues to give off hydrochloric acid gas, with the appearance of ebullition, until its sp. gr. falls to 1·094, when it properly boils, and may be distilled unchanged, or entirely volatilized.

Hydrochloric acid is characterized by forming, on the addition of nitrate of silver, a white precipitate (chloride of silver), insoluble in nitric acid, but readily soluble in ammonia. It is incompatible with alkalies and most earths, with oxides and their carbonates, and with sulphide of potassium, tartrate of potassium, tartar emetic, tartrate of iron and potassium, nitrate of silver, and solution of subacetate of lead.

As it is desirable to know, on many occasions, in chemical and pharmaceutical operations, the quantity of absolute acid contained in samples of acid of different densities, we subjoin the table of Kolb.

Kolb's table of Percentage and Specific Gravity of Hydrochloric Acid.

Specific Gravity.	100 Parts contain at 15° C. (59° F.) HCl.	Specific Gravity.	100 Parts contain at 15° C. (59° F.) HCl.	Specific Gravity.	100 Parts contain at 15° C. (59° F.) HCl.
1·000	0·1	1·083	16·5	1·166	33·0
1·007	1·5	1·091	18·1	1·171	33·9
1·014	2·9	1·100	19·9	1·175	34·7
1·022	4·5	1·108	21·5	1·180	35·7
1·029	5·8	1·116	23·1	1·185	36·8
1·036	7·3	1·125	24·8	1·190	37·9
1·044	8·9	1·134	26·6	1·195	39·0
1·052	10·4	1·143	28·4	1·199	39·8
1·060	12·0	1·152	30·2	1·205	41·2
1·067	13·4	1·157	31·2	1·210	42·4
1·075	15·0	1·161	32·0	1·212	42·9

Impurities. This acid, when pure, will evaporate without residue in a platinum spoon. On heating it with black oxide of manganese an abundance of chlorine gas is given off. If sulphuric acid be present, a solution of chloride of barium will cause a precipitate of sulphate of barium in the acid, previously diluted with distilled water. Iron may be detected by saturating the diluted acid with carbonate of sodium, and then adding ferrocyanide of potassium, which will strike a blue color if that metal be present, or by the simple addition of potassium sulphocyanate, when a blood-red coloration is produced. The absence of arsenic may be inferred if it does not tarnish bright copper foil when boiled with it. "If 1 C.c. of hydrochloric acid be diluted with water to make 10 C.c. and slightly supersaturated with water of ammonia, no precipitate should be formed upon gently warming, showing absence of iron or much lead; the liquid should not have a blue tint (copper). The further addition of two drops of test-solution of sulphide of ammonium should not cause a black coloration (lead, iron); the remaining liquid should leave no fixed residue on evaporation and gentle ignition (non-volatile metals). When diluted with five volumes of water it should not liberate iodine from test-solution of iodide of potassium (absence of chlorine), nor should 10 C.c. of the diluted acid be precipitated within five minutes, after the addition of 20 drops of test-solution of chloride of barium (sulphuric acid)." *U. S.* Ammonia in excess shows the absence of iron, if it produces no precipitate.

If another portion of the diluted acid be treated with test zinc, the evolved gas should not blacken paper wet with test-solution of nitrate of silver (arsenious or sulphurous acid). Free chlorine or nitric acid may be discovered by its having the power to dissolve gold-leaf. Any minute portion of the leaf which may be dissolved is detected by adding a solution of stannous chloride, which will give rise to a purplish tint. The free chlorine is derived from the reaction of nitric or nitrous acid on a small portion of the hydrochloric acid, which is thus deprived of its hydrogen. Hence it is that, when free chlorine is present, nitrous acid or some other oxide of nitrogen is also present as an impurity. The nitric and nitrous acids are derived from nitrates in the common salt, and from nitrous acid in the commercial sulphuric acid employed in the preparation of the hydrochloric acid.

Hydrochloric Acid of Commerce. This acid has the general properties of the pure aqueous acid. It has a yellowish color, owing to the presence of sesquichloride of iron, or of a minute proportion of organic matter, such as cork, wood, etc. It usually contains sulphuric acid, and sometimes free chlorine and nitrous acid. But the most injurious impurity, to those who consume it in the arts, is sulphurous acid. T. H. Savory analysed three samples of commercial hydrochloric acid, each having a sp. gr. of between 1·16 and 1·17, and found them to contain from 7 to nearly 11 per cent. of sulphurous acid. To detect this acid, M. Girardin has proposed a very delicate test, namely, stannous chloride. The mode of using the test is to take about half an ounce of the acid to be tested, and to add to it two or three drachms of the stannous chloride. The mixture having been stirred two or three times, as much of distilled water as of the stannous salt is to be added. If sulphurous acid be present, the hydrochloric acid becomes turbid and yellow immediately upon the addition of the stannous chloride; and, upon the subsequent addition of the water, a slight evolution of sulphuretted hydrogen takes place, perceptible to the smell, and the liquid assumes a brown hue, depositing a powder of the same color. The manner in which the test acts is as follows. By a transfer of chlorine, the test is converted into stannic chloride and metallic tin, the latter of which, by reacting with the sulphurous acid, gives rise to a precipitate of stannic and stannous sulphides. In case the sulphurous acid forms but one-half of one per cent. of the commercial acid, the precipitate may not be perceptible. Under these circumstances, a solution of sulphate of copper must be added to the liquid previously warmed, when a brown precipitate of sulphide of copper will be immediately formed. (*Heintz.*) Or, if weak solution of iodine is decolorized by the hydrochloric acid, sulphurous or arsenious acid may be suspected. M. Lembert has proposed the following, which he considers as a more delicate test of sulphurous acid. Saturate the suspected hydrochloric acid with carbonate of potassium, and add successively a little weak solution of starch, one or two drops of solution of iodate of potassium, and sulphuric acid, drop by drop. Sulphurous acid, if present, will be set free with iodic acid, and these, by reacting on each other, will develop iodine, which will cause a blue color with the starch. Or the addition of pure zinc will liberate nascent hydrogen, which will cause the evolution of hydrogen sulphide gas detected with acetate of lead paper.

Another impurity occasionally present in the commercial acid, as shown by Dupasquier, is arsenic. The immediate source of this impurity is the sulphuric acid used to prepare the hydrochloric acid. The sulphuric acid derives the arsenic from the sulphur used in its manufacture, and this last from pyrites containing a little of the poisonous metal. The arsenic, when present, is in the form of a terchloride, and, from its volatility in this state of combination, is transferred to the hydrochloric acid, distilled from the commercial acid. This impurity is separated by diluting the acid with an equal volume of water, and passing through it sulphuretted hydrogen, which throws down the arsenic as a tersulphide. According to Wittstein, hydrochloric acid is freed from arsenic by mercury, according to Reinsch, by copper, and in either case it may be deprived of metallic impregnation by careful distillation. (*A. J. P.*, 1851, p. 408.) M. Auguste Houzeau asserts that to deprive commercial arseniferous hydrochloric acid of arsenic it is sufficient simply to boil it, in a flat-bottomed vessel, to two-thirds of its original volume; all the arsenic escaping in the form of the terchloride. (*Journ. de Pharm. et de Chim.*, 4e sér., i. 97.) Bettendorff separates arsenious and arsenic acids from hydrochloric acid, sufficiently concentrated, by precipitating with stannous chloride, and then distilling the acid: when it is so treated, it is perfectly free from arsenic. (*A. J. P.*, 1870, p. 219.) When leaden vessels are used in preparing hydrochloric acid, it is apt to contain chloride of lead, which falls as a white precipitate on neutralizing the acid. The nature of the precipitate is verified by dissolving it in nitric acid and adding iodide of potassium, when the yellow iodide of lead will fall. (*Hainault.*) Prof. E. Scheffer proved the presence of lead in a sample used for making solution of perchloride of iron. (*A. J. P.*, Nov. 1875.) Another instance was noted by F. Reppert. (*A. J. P.*, Dec. 1875.) This impurity, being fixed, may be separated by distilling the acid. A small proportion of thallium has been detected in commercial hydrochloric acid by Mr. Wm. Crookes, being derived from sulphuric acid, in the manufacture of which pyrites were employed. (*Chem. News*, 1863, p. 194.) Selenium has been found in French hydrochloric acid, causing it to have a characteristic bad odor.

Properties of Hydrochloric Acid Gas. Hydrochloric acid gas is a colorless elastic fluid, possessing a pungent odor, and the property of irritating the organs of respiration. It destroys life and extinguishes flame. It reddens litmus powerfully, and has the other properties of a strong acid. Its sp. gr. is 1·278 (Gay-Lussac and Biot). Subjected to a pressure of 40 atmospheres, at the temperature of 10° C. (50° F.), it is condensed into a transparent liquid, to which alone the name of *liquid hydrochloric acid* properly belongs. It is absorbed by water with the greatest avidity.

Composition. Hydrochloric acid gas consists of one atom of chlorine 35·5, and one of hydrogen 1 = 36·5; or of one volume of chlorine and one of hydrogen, united without condensation.

Medical Properties. Hydrochloric acid is tonic, refrigerant, and antiseptic. It is exhibited, largely diluted with water, in low fevers, phthisis, some forms of syphilis, and to counteract phosphatic deposits in the urine. Dr. Paris has given it with success in malignant cases of typhus and scarlatina, administered in a strong infusion of quassia. It is especially valuable in gastro-intestinal indigestion when there is no tendency to diarrhœa, and may often be added with advantage to liquid preparations of columbo, gentian, and cinchona. It is also frequently given in dyspepsia, along with pepsin, to aid its solvent powers. The dose for internal exhibition is from five to ten minims (0·3–0·6 C.c.) in a sufficient quantity of some bland fluid, as barley-water or gruel. (See *Acidum Hydrochloricum Dilutum.*) It is a decided caustic when applied in concentrated form, although less powerful than nitric acid, and is frequently used to destroy small dermal growths.

Toxicological Properties. Hydrochloric acid, when swallowed, is highly irritating and corrosive, but less so than sulphuric or nitric acid. It produces blackness of the lips, fiery redness of the tongue, hiccough, violent efforts to vomit, and agonizing pain in the stomach. There is much thirst, with great restlessness, a dry and burning skin, and a small, concentrated pulse. If the acid has been recently swallowed, white vapors of a pungent smell are emitted from the mouth. The best antidote is magnesia, but soap or sufficiently dilute alkaline solutions are almost equally efficient. In the course of the treatment, bland and mucilaginous drinks must be freely given. When inflammation supervenes, it must be treated on general principles.

Off. Prep. and Pharm. Uses. Acidum Hydrochloricum Dilutum; Acidum Hydrocyanicum Dilutum; Acidum Nitro-hydrochloricum; Acidum Nitro-hydrochloricum Dilutum; Aqua Chlori; Argenti Nitras Fusus; Carbo Animalis Purificatus; Ferri Chloridum; Liquor Acidi Arseniosi; Liquor Ferri Chloridi; Liquor Pepsini; Liquor Zinci Chloridi; Resina Podophylli; Sulphur Præcipitatum; Syrupus Calcii Lactophosphatis.

Off. Prep. Br. Acidum Hydrochloricum Dilutum; Acidum Nitro-hydrochloricum Dilutum; Liquor Antimonii Chloridi; Liquor Arsenici Hydrochloricus.

Off. Chlorides. Br. Ammonii Chloridum; Apomorphinæ Hydrochloras; Calcii Chloridum; Cocainæ Hydrochloras; Hydrargyri Perchloridum; Hydrargyri Subchloridum; Liquor Antimonii Chloridi; Liquor Arsenici Hydrochloricus; Liquor Calcii Chloridi; Liquor Ferri Perchloridi; Liquor Ferri Perchloridi Fortior; Liquor Hydrargyri Perchloridi; Liquor Zinci Chloridi; Quininæ Hydrochloras; Sodii Chloridum; Tinctura Ferri Perchloridi; Zinci Chloridum.

ACIDUM HYDROCHLORICUM DILUTUM. *U. S., Br.* *Diluted Hydrochloric Acid.*

(ĂÇĮ-DŬM HȲ-DRǪ-ÇHLŌ′RĮ-ÇŬM DĮ-LŪ′TŬM.)

Acidum Muriaticum Dilutum, *Pharm.* 1870; Diluted Muriatic Acid; Acide chlorhydrique dilué, *Fr.*; Verdünnte Salzsäure, *G.*

"Hydrochloric Acid, *six parts* [or five and one-half fluidounces]; Distilled Water, *thirteen parts* [or fourteen fluidounces]. Mix the acid with the water, and preserve the product in glass-stoppered bottles." *U. S.*

"Take of Hydrochloric Acid *eight fluidounces* [Imp. measure]; Distilled Water *a sufficiency.* Dilute the Acid with 16 fluidounces [Imp. meas.] of the water; then add more water, so that, at a temperature of 60°, it shall measure 26½ fluidounces [Imp. meas.]. Or, as follows: Take of Hydrochloric acid 3060 grains; Distilled Water *a sufficiency*. Weigh the Acid in a glass flask, the capacity of which, to a mark on the neck, is one pint [Imp. meas.]; then add Distilled Water until the mixture, at 60° F. (15°·5 C.), after it has been shaken, measures a pint [Imp. meas.]." *Br.*

The existing U.S. formula differs from that of 1870 in yielding a diluted hydrochloric acid, which contains about twelve per cent. more officinal acid than the older preparation did. The change was made in order that the diluted mineral acids might have a uniform strength (ten per cent. of absolute acid). It is important to bear this fact in mind in prescribing, although the difference is not sufficient to render the present strength dangerous. "Diluted Hydrochloric Acid contains ten per cent. of absolute hydrochloric acid. It has the sp. gr. 1·049, and should respond to the same reactions and tests as Hydrochloric Acid. To neutralize, 7·28 Gm. should require 20 C.c. of the volumetric solution of soda." *U. S.*

The British preparation has the sp. gr. 1·052. "345 grains by weight (6 fluidrachms) require for neutralization 1000 grain-measures of the *volumetric solution of soda*, corresponding to 10·58 per cent. of real acid. Six fluidrachms [Imp. meas.] contain one eq. or 36·5 grains of hydrochloric acid, HCl." *Br.* The extreme precision of the British formula, though no doubt useful when the diluted acid is used as a test, is quite unnecessary in a therapeutical point of view.

For medical properties and uses, see *Acidum Hydrochloricum*. The dose of the diluted acid is from fifteen to thirty minims (0·95–1·9 C.c.), to be taken in water or other convenient vehicle.

Off. Prep. Abstractum Conii; Extractum Conii Alcoholicum; Extractum Conii Fluidum; Extractum Ergotæ Fluidum; Tinctura Conii.

Off. Prep. Br. Liquor Morphinæ Hydrochloratis; Liquor Strychninæ Hydrochloratis; Morphinæ Hydrochloras.

ACIDUM HYDROCYANICUM DILUTUM. *U.S., Br.* *Diluted Hydrocyanic Acid. Prussic Acid. Cyanhydric Acid.*

(ĂÇ'Į-DŬM HŶ-DRǪ-CŶ-ĂN'Į-CŬM DĮ-LŪ'TŬM.)

"A liquid composed of 2 per cent. of Absolute Hydrocyanic Acid [HCN; 27—HC_2N; 27] and 98 per cent. of Alcohol and Water." *U. S.* "Hydrocyanic Acid, HCN, dissolved in water, and constituting 2 per cent. by weight of the solution." *Br.*

Acidum Hydrocyanatum s. Borussicum; Acide cyanhydrique, ou hydrocyanique, *Fr.*; Cyanwasserstoff-Säure; Blausäure, *G.*

"Ferrocyanide of Potassium, in coarse powder, *twenty parts* [or four ounces av.]; Sulphuric Acid, *fifteen parts* [or one and a half fluidounces]; Diluted Alcohol, *sixty parts* [or twelve and a half fluidounces]; Water, Distilled Water, each, a *sufficient quantity* [q. s.]. Place the Ferrocyanide of Potassium in a tubulated retort, and add to it *forty parts* [or eight fluidounces] of water. Connect the neck of the retort (which is to be directed upward), by means of a bent tube, with a well-cooled condenser, the delivery tube of which terminates in a receiver surrounded with ice-cold water, and containing *sixty parts* [or twelve and a half fluidounces] of Diluted Alcohol. All the joints of the apparatus, except the neck of the receiver, having been made air-tight, pour into the retort, through the tubulure, the Sulphuric Acid previously diluted with an equal weight [or three fluidounces] of Water. Agitate the retort gently and then heat it, in a sand-bath, until the contents are in brisk ebullition, and continue the heat regularly until there is but little liquid mixed with the saline mass remaining in the retort. Detach the receiver, and add to its contents so much distilled water as may be required to bring the product to the strength of two per cent. of absolute hydrocyanic acid if tested by the method of assay given on page 72.

"*Diluted Hydrocyanic Acid* may be prepared, extemporaneously, in the following manner: Take of Cyanide of Silver *six parts* [or fifty and a half grains]; Hydrochloric Acid *five parts* [or thirty-seven minims]; Distilled Water *fifty-five parts* [or one fluidounce]. Mix the Hydrochloric Acid with the Distilled Water, add the Cyanide of Silver, and shake the whole together in a glass-stoppered bottle. When the precipitate has subsided, pour off the clear liquid." *U. S.*

"Ferrocyanide of Potassium, 2½ ounces [av.]; Sulphuric Acid, 1 fluidounce [Imp. meas.]; Distilled Water, 30 fluidounces [Imp. meas.], or a sufficiency. Dissolve the ferrocyanide of potassium in ten [fluid]ounces of the water, then add the sulphuric acid, previously diluted with four [fluid]ounces of the water and cooled. Put the solution into a flask or other suitable apparatus of glass or earthenware, to which are attached a condenser and a receiver arranged for distillation; and having put eight [fluid]ounces of distilled water into the receiver, and provided efficient means for keeping the condenser and receiver cold, apply heat to the flask, until by slow distillation the liquid in the receiver is increased to seventeen fluidounces. Add to this three [fluid]ounces of distilled water, or as much as may be sufficient to bring the acid to the required strength, so that one hundred grains (or 110 minims) of it, precipitated with a solution of nitrate of silver, and the precipitate thoroughly washed and dried, shall yield ten grains of dry cyanide of silver.

"Diluted hydrocyanic acid should be kept in well-corked bottles, tied over with impervious tissue. The bottles should be inverted when not in use, and be kept in a dark place." *Br.*

The British preparation has the sp. gr. 0·997. If 270 grains of it be made alkaline by solution of soda, they will require 1000 grain-measures of the volumetric solution of nitrate of silver to be added before a permanent precipitate begins to form, corresponding to 2 per cent. of the real acid.

When ferrocyanide of potassium is decomposed by sulphuric acid, the residue in the retort is sulphate of potassium, mixed with an insoluble compound of cyanide of iron and cyanide of potassium (*Everitt's Salt*). The reaction is expressed by the following equation:

$$2(K_4FeC_6N_6) + 3H_2SO_4 = 3K_2SO_4 + 2(KFeC_3N_3) + 6HCN.$$

Half of the cyanogen present in the ferrocyanide of potassium goes to form the hydrocyanic acid, while the other half remains in the white residue. Everitt's salt, so named from its discoverer, is a yellowish white powder. Like ferrocyanide of potassium, it is a double cyanide of iron and potassium, but of different molecular ratio. As it appears in practice, it is apt to be greenish, owing probably to the presence of a little Prussian blue.

An excess of sulphuric acid, or the use of concentrated acid, would endanger the production of hydrocyanic acid, as this is decomposed by strong sulphuric acid, with the formation of carbon monoxide (CO) and ammonium sulphate. The proportion of the acid should not exceed three-fourths of the weight of the ferrocyanide. In relation to the most convenient method of bringing the hydrocyanic acid to the standard strength, and to some other points in its preparation by the officinal formula, see Prof. Procter's paper, *A. J. P.*, xix. 259.

In the U.S. process for obtaining hydrocyanic acid extemporaneously, the reacting materials are single molecules respectively of cyanide of silver and hydrochloric acid. These, by double decomposition, generate hydrocyanic acid, which dissolves in the water, and chloride of silver, which subsides, and from which the acid is poured off when clear. (See *Argenti Cyanidum.*) The extemporaneous process is useful to country practitioners, because the acid will not generally keep. A portion of hydrocyanic acid, if purchased by a practitioner, may spoil on his hands before he has occasion to use it; but if he supply himself with cyanide of silver, he may readily at any moment prepare a small portion of the acid, by following the directions of the formula. On the other hand, it is questionable whether all of the cyanide of silver will be decomposed, except under much more careful treatment than the process is likely to receive.

It will be observed that a change has been made in the process of the Pharmacopœia of 1880, in the substitution of diluted alcohol for the distilled water formerly used as the solvent for the hydrocyanic acid. This is in accordance with the views of Gault and others, who assert that greater stability is thus secured.

Another process for obtaining medicinal hydrocyanic acid, proposed by Dr. Clark, and adopted by Mr. Laming, is by the reaction of tartaric acid on cyanide of potassium in solution. Laming's formula has been modified as follows. Potassic cyanide, pure, 65 parts; tartaric acid, 150 parts; alcohol, 675 parts; water sufficient to make 1538 parts. Mix the potassic cyanide and tartaric acid with 500 parts of water in a well-stoppered bottle, or dissolve each separately in 250 parts of water, and mix the solutions; then add the alcohol and sufficient water to make 1538 parts. After the acid potassium tartrate has subsided as a heavy crystalline powder, the clear supernatant liquid is decanted.

The yield of officinal acid is 1350 parts, but the generated cream of tartar weighs 188 parts, thus making the 1538 parts as above directed. The solution contains mere traces of the acid tartrate. (*A. J. P.*, 1883, p. 559, from *Fownes's Chemistry.*)

Great care must be observed in using this process to procure pure cyanide of potassium, the commercial article usually being adulterated.

The processes, thus far given, are intended to furnish a *dilute* hydrocyanic acid for medicinal purposes. The methods of obtaining the *anhydrous* acid are different. Vauquelin's process for the anhydrous acid is to pass a current of hydrosulphuric acid gas over cyanide of mercury contained in a glass tube, connected with a receiver kept cold by a freezing mixture of ice and salt. The first third only of the tube is filled with cyanide; the remaining two-thirds being occupied, half with carbonate of lead, and half with chloride of calcium; the carbonate being intended to detain the hydrosulphuric acid gas, the chloride to separate water.

The process of Wöhler for the anhydrous acid is the following. The cyanide of potassium selected is a black cyanide, formed by fusing together, in a covered crucible, 8 parts of dry ferrocyanide, 3 of ignited cream of tartar, and 1 of charcoal in fine powder. The cyanide, while still warm, is exhausted by 6 parts of water; and the clear solution, placed in a retort, is decomposed by cold diluted sulphuric acid, gradually added. The hydrocyanic acid is condensed first in a U-tube, containing chloride of calcium and surrounded with ice-cold water, and afterwards in a small bottle, connected with the U-tube by a narrow tube, and immersed up to the neck in a mixture of ice and salt. After the acid has been condensed and dehydrated in the U-tube, the cold water surrounding it is withdrawn by a siphon, and replaced by water at a temperature between 29·4°–32·2° C. (85°–90° F.), whereby the anhydrous acid is made to distil over into the small bottle.

M. Berthelot has made hydrocyanic acid synthetically. He first prepares, by a direct synthesis of its elements, *acetylene* (C_2H_2). He then mixes vapors of acetylene with pure nitrogen, passes a series of electric discharges from a Ruhmkorff coil through the mixture, and, when the odor of prussic acid is perceptible, agitates with a solution of potassa to get the fixed cyanide. It has also been made by heating chloroform with ammonia and caustic potash solution. (Hofmann, *Ann.*, 144, 116.)

Properties of the Medicinal Acid. Diluted hydrocyanic acid, of the proper medicinal strength, is a transparent, colorless, volatile liquid, possessing a smell resembling that of peach kernels, and a taste at first cooling and afterwards somewhat irritating. It imparts a slight and evanescent red color to litmus. If it reddens litmus strongly and permanently, some acid impurity is present. It loses strength rapidly in open vessels. It is not reddened by the iodo-cyanide of potassium and mercury. The non-action of this test shows the absence of contaminating acids, which, if present, would decompose the test, and give rise to the red iodide of mercury. The red color produced when picrate of ammonia is added to a solution of an alkaline cyanide and heated has been proposed as a test for prussic acid. (P. Guyot, *N. R.*, May, 1877.) It is liable to undergo decomposition if exposed to the light, but is easily kept in a bottle covered with black paint or black paper. "On being heated it is completely volatilized. If to the acid, rendered alkaline by potassa, a little ferrous sulphate and ferric chloride be added, and the mixture be acidulated with hydrochloric acid, a blue precipitate will make its appearance." *U. S.* From experiments carefully conducted by MM. Bussy and Buignet, it appears that, when the alteration in the acid under the influence of light has begun, it will afterward go on very rapidly in the dark; and that, after exposure for a certain time to the light, though no alteration may be apparent, an influence has nevertheless been exerted which disposes to change, and promotes decomposition even in the absence of light. Hence the necessity of immediately enclosing the acid in bottles from which the light is excluded. (*Journ. de Pharm.*, 1863, p. 475.)* Experience has shown that it is best preserved in cork-stopped bottles of amber glass; when glass and rubber stoppers were used, decomposition frequently took place rapidly. Its most usual impurities are sulphuric and hydrochloric acids; the former of which may be detected by chloride of barium, which will produce a precipitate of sulphate of barium; and the latter by precipitating with nitrate of silver, when so much of the precipitate as may be chloride of silver will be insoluble in boiling nitric acid, while the cyanide of silver is readily soluble. The presence of these acids, in slight amount, is injurious only by rendering uncertain the strength of the medicinal acid, as ascertained by its saturating power. It is now generally acknowledged that mineral acids prevent the deterioration of the dilute prussic acid. But the presence of a mineral acid is not necessary for its preservation; for Dr. Christison has known the medicinal acid from ferrocyanide of potassium to keep perfectly well, although nitrate of barium did not produce the slightest muddiness. Nevertheless it has been recently shown that much of the acid as kept in the drug-stores is often below the officinal strength. Various remedies have been proposed. (*P. J. Tr.*, July, 1871; Feb. 1, 1874; Sept. 1874.) One of these is to reduce the strength to one-tenth per cent., this weak solution being said not to undergo change. In our experience a one per cent. acid retained its properties through very severe tests of exposure. Mr. John Williams has found in a series of experiments that the addition of 20 per cent. of glycerin has a very pronounced influence in preventing deterioration. (*P. J. Tr.*, Sept. 1874; Sept. 1875.)

Formerly the medicinal acid was of different strengths, as ordered by the different pharmaceutical authorities; but happily the U. S. and Br. Pharmacopœias conform in this important point. At one time its strength was indicated by its specific gravity, which is lower in proportion as it is stronger; but this unprecise mode of estimate is not now relied on; and, though the British Pharmacopœia gives the sp. gr. of its dilute acid at 0·997, both Pharmacopœias give quantitative tests as indices of the strength. "6·75 Gm., diluted with 30 C.c. of water, and mixed with enough of an aqueous suspension of magnesia to make the mixture quite opaque, and afterward with a few drops of solution of chromate of potassium, should require 50 C.c. of the volumetric solution of nitrate of silver, before the red color caused by the latter ceases to disappear on stirring" (corresponding to the presence of two per cent. of absolute hydrocyanic acid). *U. S.* This method of assay is based upon Pappenheim's process for the determination of hydrocyanic acid in bitter almond water, as described by Vielhaber in *Archiv d. Pharm.*, 1878, p. 408; the addition of an alkali to a solution of hydrocyanic acid, previous to titration, not only prevents the volatilization of the acid, but, as has been shown by Siebold, the double cyanides of silver

* Anhydrous hydrocyanic acid sometimes undergoes an apparently spontaneous molecular change by which it is converted into a black solid body, which was supposed to be *paracyanogen* (C_3N_3), or its compounds. This change takes place more slowly in watery solutions of the acid, which are converted into a black liquid; and it is only in a state of extreme dilution, when, for example, water contains not more than one per cent. of the acid, that it is altogether prevented. It sometimes takes place in the officinal diluted acid; and Prof. Procter exhibited a bottle, which had been most carefully closed, and kept excluded from the light, and in which, nevertheless, the acid had become as black as ink. The cause of this phenomenon remained long unknown: some years ago M. E. Millon satisfied himself, by experiment, that the real agency was the presence of ammonia, which may sometimes operate even through the air. It has also been asserted that the cause of the decomposition is the presence of a microscopic plant. (*Journ. de Pharm.*, 1862, p. 48.) The preservative influence of a little sulphuric acid in the diluted hydrocyanic acid would be thus explained; and it is not impossible that the greater resistance offered to the change by the preparation made by the officinal process, in which sulphuric acid is used, than by the others, may be owing to the influence of this acid, either passing over with its vapor, or acting on the acid vapor before it leaves the retort. An important practical inference from all this is the necessity of providing, as far as possible, that ammonia should in no manner have access to the acid, during or after its preparation. The effect of ammonia in inducing changes in dilute hydrocyanic acid is denied by Pettit (*A. J. P.*, 1873.) Mr. Rimmington asserts that hydrocyanic acid acts upon the alkali of some varieties of glass. Mr. [illegible]d, who has confirmed this, declares that the addition of hydrochloric acid is perfectly usele[illegible] as a preservative, except when the prussic acid is kept in bottles which yield the alkali. (*Pharm. Journ.*, Sept. 1874.) MM. Lescolin and Rigaut (*Comptes-Rendus*, Aug. 4, 1879) state that pure hydrocyanic acid can be preserved for a long time; that the presence of potassium cyanide brings about this decomposition even in the absence of water. The substitution of diluted alcohol for water, as directed in the officinal process (1880), obviates this decomposition.

with the alkali metals are very permanent; the use of chromate of potassium as an indicator, whereby a red color, due to a combination of the chromic acid with the silver, is produced, is highly recommended. The Br. Pharmacopœia directs that 270 grains of it, when treated with solution of soda in excess, shall require the addition of 1000 grain-measures of the volumetric solution of nitrate of silver, before a permanent precipitate begins to form. To explain this test it is necessary to notice that cyanide of silver, though itself insoluble, is rendered soluble by combining with cyanide of sodium, in the proportion of one molecule of each. When, therefore, the diluted hydrocyanic acid is converted, by the addition of soda, into cyanide of sodium, no permanent precipitate will begin to appear, upon the addition of nitrate of silver, until more than sufficient cyanide of silver is produced to form the soluble compound referred to, which happens when one-half of the cyanide of sodium has been converted into cyanide of silver. An acid of the strength indicated by either of these methods contains two per cent. of anhydrous acid. The test of entire solubility in boiling nitric acid, applied to the precipitate obtained by nitrate of silver, is intended to verify its nature; for, if the hydrocyanic acid contain hydrochloric acid, part of this precipitate would be chloride of silver, not soluble in the boiling acid. Scheele's medicinal hydrocyanic acid contains about 5 per cent. of anhydrous acid; and, therefore, two minims of it are equal to five of the U. S. acid. The use of Scheele's acid should be discouraged as unnecessary and very dangerous. In view of the deterioration of hydrocyanic acid upon keeping through loss by volatilization, the following approximate practical test is recommended by Dr. Squibb. If one drop of diluted hydrocyanic acid be added to 15 C.c. of distilled water in one vessel, and one drop of test-solution of nitrate of silver (U. S. P.) be added to 7 C.c. of distilled water in a test-tube, and the first solution be dropped into the second from a pipette, and the contents be closely observed for a few seconds between the drops, a distinct opalescence should be observed before the fourth drop is added, and the opalescence become very marked as the fourth or fifth drops are added.

MM. Fordos and Gélis have proposed, as a test of the strength of the compounds containing cyanogen, an alcoholic solution of iodine of known strength; as, for example, three grains to the fluidounce. The test-solution is added, drop by drop, to the cyanogen compound, until a permanent yellowish tinge is produced. The iodine unites with the cyanogen, and with the substance in combination with the cyanogen, in the ratio of their several equivalents; and hence the cyanogen present is easily calculated from the proportion of iodine expended in uniting with it. This test is commended for its accuracy by Mr. James Roberton, of Manchester, Eng. (See *A. J. P.*, 1853, p. 551.) A. Link and R. Moeckel (*Zeitsch. f. Analyt. Chem.*, 1878, p. 455) made a series of experiments, and showed that the most delicate test for hydrocyanic acid was that of sulphocyanate of iron. (*A. J. P.*, 1879, p. 86.)

Properties of the Anhydrous Acid. Hydrocyanic acid, perfectly free from water, is a colorless, transparent, inflammable liquid, of extreme volatility, boiling at 27° C. (80° F.), and congealing at —15° C. (5° F.). Its sp.gr. as a liquid is 0·6969, at the temperature of 18° C. (64° F.); and as a vapor 0·9423. Its taste is at first cooling, then burning, with an after-taste in the throat like that of bitter almonds; but, from its extremely poisonous nature, it must be tasted with the utmost caution. Its odor is so strong as to produce immediate headache and giddiness; and its vapor so deleterious that the smallest portion of it cannot be inhaled without the greatest danger. Both water and alcohol dissolve it readily. It is much more prone to undergo decomposition than the dilute acid. In the course of a few hours it sometimes begins to assume a reddish brown color, which becomes gradually deeper, till at length the acid is converted into a black liquid, which exhales a strong smell of ammonia. It is a very weak acid in its chemical relations, and reddens litmus but slightly. It does not form solid compounds with metallic oxides, but cyanides of metals, the elements of water being eliminated. According to Sobero, hydrocyanic acid is generated, in sensible quantities, by the action of weak nitric acid on the volatile oils and resins. Wöhler affirmed in 1828 that picric acid when treated with baryta-water yields it; and Julius Post and H. Hübner have found that nitrobenzol and dinitrobenzol do also when treated, the former with fusing potassa, the latter with boiling dilute solution of potassa. It has also been formed by the slow action of carbonate of potassium on tincture of hyoscyamus, given together as a medicine. (Dr. J. T. Plummer, of Indiana, *A. J. P.*, xxv. 513.) Though a product of art, it exists in some plants, and is generated by reaction between the constituents of many vegetable products upon contact with water. These principles are usually amygdalin and emulsin, but according to Peckholt the root of *Manihot utilissima* copiously generates hydrocyanic acid with water, although he was unable in 15 analyses to find amygdalin in it. (*A. J. P.*, Oct. 1872.) (See *Amygdala Amara.*)*

Composition. Hydrocyanic acid consists of the atomic group cyanogen 26, and one atom of hydrogen 1 = 27; or, in volumes, of one volume of cyanogen and one of hydrogen without condensation, its formula being HCN or HCy. *Cyanogen* (Cy) is a colorless gas, of a strong and penetrating smell, inflammable, and burning with a beautiful bluish purple flame. Its sp. gr. is 1·8157. It was discovered in 1815 by Gay-Lussac, who viewed it as a compound radical, which, when combined with hydrogen, becomes hydrocyanic acid. Hydrocyanic acid, in a dilute state, was discovered in 1780 by Scheele, who correctly stated its elements to be carbon, nitrogen, and hydrogen; but the peculiar way in which they are combined was first pointed out by Gay-Lussac, by whom also the anhydrous acid was first obtained.

Medical and Toxical Properties. Hydrocyanic acid is one of the most deadly poisons known, and frequently exceedingly rapid in its action. According to Dr. Christison, a grain and a half of the anhydrous acid is capable of producing death in the human subject. One or two drops of the pure acid are sufficient to kill a vigorous dog in a few seconds. Sometimes death occurs almost instantaneously. Usually, however, three stages of the poisoning are manifest: a first very brief one of difficult respiration, slow cardiac action, and disturbed nervous action; a second violent convulsive stage, with dilated pupils, vomiting, often loud cries, unconsciousness, etc.; and a third closing period of asphyxia, collapse, and paralysis, sometimes interrupted by convulsions. When smaller doses are ingested, the symptoms come on more slowly, but are similar to those just described, and when paralysis is developed it affects both motility and sensation. A peculiar bloated look of the deeply suffused face and neck, with frothing at the mouth, occurring along with the symptoms previously described, is almost pathognomonic of the poisoning. The odor of hydrocyanic acid is sometimes very strong, and should always be searched for about the mouth. It is very important as an aid in the diagnosis, but is certainly not always present. Death is usually the result of asphyxia, produced by a direct paralyzant action of the poison upon the respiratory centres. The poison appears also to have a direct paralyzing action upon the heart, and sometimes to produce fatal syncope. The post-mortem appearances are glistening and staring expression of the eyes; gorged state of the venous system with fluid, dark, or bluish-black blood, especially of the veins of the brain and spinal marrow; and sometimes redness of the internal coat of the stomach. The lungs are sometimes natural, at other times turgid with blood. When the death has been very rapid, all of the blood may be found of a bright arterial hue. After a slow death the blood is cyanotic. It is rarely true that all of the muscles are insensible to the galvanic current. If the autopsy be not too long deferred, the odor of the acid is generally perceptible when the cadaver is opened. The odor after nitrobenzol poisoning resembles very closely that of the acid, but it is affirmed that the diagnosis can be made by leaving the opened body exposed, when the smell of the acid will disappear, and that of the nitrobenzol remain. Notwithstanding the tremendous energy of this acid as a poison, it has been ventured upon in a dilute state as a sedative, anodyne, and antispasmodic. Though occasionally employed as a remedy prior to 1817, it did not attract very much attention until that year, when Magendie published his observations on its use in diseases of the chest, and recommended it to the profession.

* It has been proposed to employ solutions of these vegetable products for the extemporaneous preparation of hydrocyanic acid, and in the Swedish Pharmacopœia the *Emulsio Hydrocyanata* has replaced entirely the dilute prussic acid. An emulsion is first made of 3 parts of sweet almonds, 2 of sugar, and 24 of water. To 80 parts of this emulsion is added one part of amygdalin. In an hour the mixture is ready for use; one ounce of it contains one-third of a grain of anhydrous acid Dose, one to two teaspoonfuls. (*Nat. Med. Journ.*, July, 1871.)

When given in medicinal doses gradually increased, it produces the following symptoms in different cases: peculiar bitter taste; increased secretion of saliva; irritation of the throat; nausea; disordered respiration; pain in the head; giddiness; faintness; obscure vision; and tendency to sleep. It appears to have a special action on the larynx and trachea. (*Dr. Cogswell.*) The pulse is sometimes quickened, at other times reduced in frequency. It has been extensively used in complaints of the respiratory organs, but later experience has shown that it has but little virtue, except in the quieting of cough. Its influence upon the circulation is not sufficiently pronounced to render the drug of any value as an arterial sedative in acute pulmonary or other inflammations. In phthisis it may be resorted to with advantage as a palliative for the cough. In various other affections of the chest, attended with dyspnœa or cough, such as asthma, hooping-cough, and chronic catarrh, it has often been decidedly beneficial, by allaying irritation or relaxing spasm. In certain affections of the stomach, characterized by pain and spasm, and sometimes attended with vomiting, but unconnected with inflammation, and in similar painful affections of the bowels, it has proved beneficial in the hands of several practitioners. In these cases it probably acts locally upon the nerve-endings in the stomach and intestines. It has been used with asserted good results in the paroxysmal excitement of mania. (*Ann. de Thérap.*, 1865, p. 111.) Sometimes it is used externally, diluted with water, as a wash in cutaneous diseases. The late Dr. A. T. Thomson insisted particularly on its efficacy in allaying the itching of impetiginous affections.

The dose of the diluted hydrocyanic acid is from two to four drops (0·12–0·24 C.c.), dissolved in distilled water, or mixed with gum-water or syrup. It should be administered with the greatest caution, on account of its minute dose, and its variable strength as usually found. The proper plan, therefore, is to begin with a small dose, two drops for example, and gradually to increase the quantity until some obvious impression is produced. On account of the rapidity and fugaciousness of its action, it should be given at intervals of not more than two hours; indeed, it is very improbable that the largest therapeutic dose of the substance exerts any influence whatever upon the system one hour after its ingestion. If giddiness, weight at the top of the head, sense of tightness at the stomach, or faintness come on, its use should be discontinued. In all cases in which a fresh portion of medicine is used, the dose should be lowered to the minimum quantity, lest the new sample should prove stronger than that previously employed. When resorted to as a lotion, from thirty minims to a fluidrachm may be dissolved in a fluidounce of distilled water.

Toxicology. Hydrocyanic acid is so rapidly fatal as a poison that physicians have seldom an opportunity to treat its effects. Death, if it occur at all, usually takes place in from one to forty minutes. One case has, however, been reported in which it was delayed one hour and a quarter. When recovery is brought about, the symptoms in most cases abate very rapidly. The antidotes and remedies most to be relied on are chlorine, ammonia, cold affusion, and artificial respiration. Chlorine in the form of chlorine-water, or weak solutions of chlorinated lime or soda, may be exhibited internally, or applied externally. When chlorine is not at hand, water of ammonia, largely diluted, may be given, and the vapor arising from it cautiously inhaled. A case is related, in the *Dublin Med. Journal* for Nov. 1835, of poisoning by this acid, in which the diluted aromatic spirit of ammonia applied to the mouth, and the solid carbonate assiduously held to the nostrils, produced speedy and beneficial effects. Cold affusion was first proposed in 1828, by Herbst, of Göttingen, and its utility was subsequently confirmed by Orfila. Its efficacy is strongly supported by experiments performed in 1839 by Dr. Robinson and M. Lonyet, who quickly resuscitated rabbits, apparently dead from hydrocyanic acid, by pouring on their heads and spines a stream of water artificially refrigerated. In a case of poisoning, reported by Dr. Christison in 1850, the patient recovered under a stream of cold water poured upon the head from a moderate height. In another case, reported in the *Lancet* in 1854, in which the largest reported quantity was taken to be followed by recovery (2·4 grains of anhydrous acid), the cold water douche was the principal remedy. (See *Am. Journ. Med. Sci.*, July, 1854, p. 276.) Messrs. T. & H. Smith, of Edinburgh, have recommended especially as an antidote for the medicinal acid a mixture of the ferric salts, swallowed after a solution of carbonate of potassium. So soon as the antidote comes in contact with hydrocyanic acid, sulphate of potassium is formed, and the poison is converted into Prussian blue. It may be prepared extemporaneously, by adding ten grains of sulphate of iron, and a drachm of the tincture of chloride of iron, to a fluidounce of water contained in one vial, and twenty grains of carbonate of potassium to a fluidounce of water in another vial. The patient is made to swallow the solution of carbonate of potassium, and immediately afterwards the mixed ferruginous solution. This quantity is estimated to be sufficient to render insoluble nearly two grains of the anhydrous acid.* In one instance this antidote is said to have proved very effectual. (*P. J. Tr.*, 1865, p. 139.) Atropine has been proposed as a counter-poison, on the grounds of its physiological action, and of experiments made with it on the lower animals. (See *Am. Journ. Med. Sci.*, 1868, p. 577.) It has, however, been shown by the elaborate experiments of Keen (*Proc. Phil. Acad. Nat. Sci.*, 1869), of Reese (*Am. Journ. Med. Sci.*, Jan. 1871), and of Boehm and Knie (*Archiv für Exper. Path. und Therap.*, Bd. ii.), to be of little or no antidotal value even in the case of the lower animals. Morphine has also been supposed to be antagonistic to hydrocyanic acid.

Tests. After suspected death from poison, it is sometimes necessary to ascertain whether the event was caused by this acid. At a period long after death, it would be needless to search for so volatile a poison; but it has been recognized three weeks after death, in a case reported by M. Brame, in which about six drachms of acid, containing between 8 and 9 per cent. of anhydrous acid, had been swallowed. The best test is that proposed by Liebig in 1847, consisting in the change of the hydrocyanic acid into sulphocyanate of ammonium, which salt is then tested with a ferric salt. Two drops of the acid, so dilute as not to afford the least blue tint with the salts of iron, upon being mixed with a drop of ammonium sulphydrate (yellow from dissolved sulphur), and heated upon a watch-glass until the mixture is colorless, yield a solution of sulphocyanate of ammonium, which becomes of a deep blood-red color upon the addition of ferric sulphate, in consequence of the formation of the sulphocyanate of iron. (*Chem. Gaz.*, April 1, 1847; from Liebig's *Annalen.*) This test is praised by Mr. A. S. Taylor, who found it to act characteristically on two grains of dilute hydrocyanic acid, containing only 1-3930th of a grain of anhydrous acid. To render the test thus delicate, Mr. Taylor deems it necessary to evaporate the liquid gently to dryness, after the addition of the ammonium sulphydrate, in order to bring the sulphocyanate to the solid state before adding the iron test, a fractional part of a drop of which will commonly suffice to produce the characteristic color. The red color is instantly discharged by solution of corrosive sublimate or mercuric nitrate, and is thus distinguished from that which might possibly be produced under similar circumstances by acetic acid. Should the acid be mixed with organic matters, Mr. Taylor proposes a modification of Liebig's test as follows. Place it in a watch-glass, and invert over it another, holding in the centre a drop of ammonium sulphydrate. In from half a minute to ten minutes, without heat, the sulphydrate will be converted into the sulphocyanate of ammonium; and upon removing the upper glass, and evaporating its contents to dryness, the iron test will produce the blood-red color. MM. O. Henry and E. Humbert have proposed, as a test of hydrocyanic acid, first to convert it into cyanide of silver by distilling the suspected matters into a dilute solution of nitrate of silver, and then to decompose the cyanide by iodine, so as to form iodide of cyanogen. The

* In a subsequent communication the Messrs. Smith recommend the following proportions. Mix of solution of perchloride of iron (*Br.*) 37 minims, sulphate of iron, as pure as possible and in fine crystals, 25 grains, and about half a fluidounce of water. Dissolve 77 grains of crystallized carbonate of sodium in the same measure of water. These quantities will neutralise between 150 and 200 minims of the medicinal hydrocyanic acid. (*P. J. Tr.*, 1865, p. 147.) Still more recently the authors propose to substitute magnesia for carbonate of sodium, as better fitted to neutralise any considerable quantity of gastric acid that might be present. The following is the formula now recommended. From one to two drachms of magnesia, made into a smooth cream with water, are to be first administered, and then 16 minims of solution of perchloride of iron (*Br.*) and 12½ grains of ferrous sulphate are dissolved in water. These quantities are calculated for 100 minims of medicinal hydrocyanic acid. Should more than this be supposed to have been taken, the ferruginous ingredients must be increased in proportion, but not the magnesia. (*Ibid.*, 1865, p. 276.)

dried cyanide is added to half its estimated weight of *pure* iodine, contained in a test tube. Upon the application of a gentle heat, iodide of cyanogen is formed, and characteristic crystals of it are deposited on the cool surface of the tube. (*Journ. de Pharm.*, 1857, p. 173.) Prof. Wormley (*Micro-Chemistry of Poisons*, 2d ed., p. 186) considers the nitrate of silver test as the most delicate of all when the hydrocyanic acid vapor is distilled from a mixture and received in a drop of nitrate of silver placed in a watch-glass above it.

An extremely sensitive test of hydrocyanic acid, in the state of vapor, has been offered by Schönbein. It consists of white filtering paper imbued with the resin of guaiacum, by dipping it in a solution of 3 parts of the resin in 150 of alcohol, and then drying. At the moment of use it is to be moistened with a solution of sulphate of copper containing 1 part in 500 of water. If now brought into contact with hydrocyanic acid, whether dissolved in water or diffused in the air in the form of vapor, it instantly becomes blue. According to Schönbein, it will change color in air containing only a forty-millionth part of hydrocyanic acid. (See *A. J. P.*, 1869, p. 174.) The test cannot, however, be relied on, since a similar reaction is yielded by numerous other substances, such as nitrous, nitric, and hydrochloric acids, chlorine, bromine, iodine, ammonia, dilute sulphuric acid, chromic acid, bichromate of potassium, etc. The paper should be exposed to a current of air, drawn through the suspected liquid, and, if indications be yielded, distillation practised to get the volatile acid in a state of sufficient purity to be submitted to the sulphur-iron test. This, as performed by Almén and Strieve, consists in adding ammonium sulphide, to form the sulphocyanate; converting this into the non-volatile sulphocyanate of potassium by the addition of a few drops of liquor potassæ; then evaporating nearly or quite to dryness; adding a few drops of water, acidulated with hydrochloric acid, and finally adding a drop or two of sesquichloride of iron, when the blood red of the sulphocyanate will be developed. (*Boston Med. and Surg. Journ.*, July, 1873.) Another test, which was proposed by Schönbein, and which was found to be exceedingly delicate by M. Büchner, is dependent upon the power prussic acid has of preventing the catalytic action of the red blood corpuscles. Normally, when these are brought into contact with hydrogen peroxide, the latter is decomposed and oxygen liberated; if prussic acid be present, no oxygen is set free, but the mixture becomes of a deep brown color. In this way Büchner recognised 5 milligrammes of the anhydrous acid in 600 grammes of blood and water. This test is not applicable to old blood. (*A. J. P.*, Sept. 1869.)

A very delicate test proposed for hydrocyanic acid is as follows. About one-half centigramme ($\frac{1}{12}$ grain) of ammonio-ferrous sulphate (or other pure ferrous salt), and the same quantity of uranic nitrate are dissolved in 50 C.c. of water, and 1 C.c. of this test liquid is placed in a porcelain dish. On now adding a drop of a liquid containing the smallest quantity of prussic acid, a gray purple color or a distinct purple precipitate is produced. (M. Carey Lea, *Amer. Journ. of Sci.* [3], ix. 121–123.)

Off. Prep. Br. Vapor Acidi Hydrocyanici; Tinctura Chloroformi et Morphinæ.

ACIDUM LACTICUM. *U. S., Br.* *Lactic Acid.*

(ĂÇ'Ĭ-DŬM LĂC'TĬ-CŬM.)

Oxypropionic Acid, Ethidene-lactic Acid; Acide lactique, *Fr.*; Milchsäure, *G.*

"A liquid composed of 75 per cent. of absolute Lactic Acid [$HC_3H_5O_3$; 90—$HOC_3H_5O_2$; 90] and 25 per cent. of water. *U. S.* "Lactic acid, $HC_3H_5O_3$, with about 25 per cent. of water. Produced by the action of a peculiar ferment on solution of sugar and subsequent purification of the product." *Br.*

Lactic acid was discovered by Scheele. It exists in sour milk, and has been found in a number of the secretions, including the healthy gastric juice, in which its presence has been incontestably proved by Bernard and Barreswil. Liebig has shown that a variety of lactic (sarcolactic) acid exists in the juice of flesh. It has been detected by Prof. Wittstein in the vegetable kingdom, especially in the peduncles of *Solanum Dulcamara*, and the liquid which oozes from freshly-cut vine branches. It is a product of the viscous or lactic fermentation of rice-water, or of the juices of the beet, turnip, and carrot. Indeed, it is formed whenever sugar in solution, of whatever kind, is placed in contact with an alkaline or earthy carbonate, in presence of a special ferment, as, for example, the casein of milk, or cheese which contains it. Pasteur has demonstrated that the lactic acid fermentation, like the vinous, is accompanied with the growth of a peculiar microscopic plant or mycoderm, which he is disposed to consider as the real agent of the changes produced. This fermentation is attended with the production not only of lactic acid, but of other substances also, and among them, a peculiar *gum-like substance* in abundance, which, first noticed by Kirchof, has been isolated in a pure state by Brüning. Though similar to arabin and dextrin, with the formula $C_6H_{10}O_5$, it is not exactly identical with either. (See *Chem. Gaz.*, 1858, p. 197.) The lactic acid of fermentation is one of four isomeric acids possessing the formula $C_3H_6O_3$. The *first* of these is the official lactic acid, and is inactive optically. The *second* is identical chemically with this, but physically different, being dextro-rotatory, and is found in the juice of flesh. It is called *paralactic acid*. The *third* or *ethylene lactic acid* is found mixed with the second in the so-called "*sarcolactic*" acid extracted from meat. The *fourth* acid has only been obtained synthetically, and is known as *hydracrylic* acid.

Preparation. Lactic acid may be obtained by the following process, which was recommended by M. Louradour as the first step in preparing lactate of iron. Ferment whey by keeping it at a temperature between 21·1° C. (70° F.) and 26·6° C. (80° F.), whereby it becomes charged with a considerable quantity of lactic acid. Evaporate the liquor to one-third of its bulk, decant and filter, and then saturate with milk of lime. This converts the lactic acid into lactate of calcium, which remains in solution, and throws down a precipitate, consisting principally of phosphate of calcium. The liquor is filtered again, and precipitated by oxalic acid, which throws down the lime as oxalate of calcium, and sets free the lactic acid. By a new filtration a solution of lactic acid is obtained, containing lactose (sugar of milk) and certain salts. From these it may be purified by concentrating it to a syrupy consistence, and treating it with alcohol, which dissolves the acid, and precipitates the lactose and foreign salts. The solution is filtered, and the lactic acid is obtained pure by distilling off the alcohol. Wackenroder's method is to mix 10 parts of skimmed milk, 2·5 of milk sugar, 2 of chalk, and 20 of water, to digest at about 23·8° C. (75° F.) for a month, or till the chalk is dissolved, then to express, clarify, and evaporate so as to crystallize the lactate of calcium, and, having recrystallized this salt, to decompose it with sulphuric or oxalic acid in exact saturating proportions.

Lautemann proposes a modification of this plan, consisting in substituting oxide of zinc for chalk. The fermentation is completed in eight or ten days. After boiling, the mixture is filtered, and the liquor, having been evaporated and again filtered, is allowed to stand. Lactate of zinc now separates, from which the acid may be obtained by dissolving the salt in boiling water, throwing down the zinc by sulphuretted hydrogen, filtering, and concentrating. The solution now contains mannite and lactic acid, both the result of the fermentation. By agitating with ether the acid is dissolved, and the mannite left; and by evaporating the ethereal solution the lactic acid is obtained. (See *Philos. Mag.*, 1860, p. 385.)

Another process for making lactic acid is to evaporate the water obtained from wheat starch factories, from which starch has been deposited. The extract so obtained amounts to about 1 per cent., but is rich in lactic acid (containing 87 per cent., Thenius). (*Neueste Erfind. und Erfahr.*, 1879, p. 180.) The supply of lactic acid comes almost entirely from Germany. For a report by Chas. Rice on the quality of the commercial article see *A. J. P.*, 1873, p. 388. Kiliani (*Ber. der Chem. Ges.*, xv. 136 and 699) has quite recently found that lactic acid may be readily prepared by the action of potassium or sodium hydrate upon both grape sugar and invert sugar (or cane sugar after treatment with dilute acids). He considers invert sugar to be the best material for the preparation of the acid, as it gives a better yield than ordinary glucose, and recommends caustic soda in preference to caustic potash. His procedure is the following: 500 grammes of cane sugar are placed with 150 grammes of water and 10 C.c. of the sulphuric acid, to be used later, in a stoppered flask of 2 litres' capacity and heated for 3 hours to about 50° C. (122° F.). The solution of invert sugar so obtained is colorless, or at most faintly yellow. After cooling there is to be added to it in portions of 50 C.c. at a time 400 C.c. of a caustic soda solution made by dissolving 1 part of caustic soda in 1 part of water. The strong alkali settles at first as a slimy mass on the bottom, and a new portion is only to be added when the mixture has become perfectly homogeneous by shaking. The flask should also be cooled with water while the alkali is being added. The mixture nevertheless becomes colored and greatly heated. Finally the mixture is heated to 60° or 70° C. (140° F.–158° F.) until a test heated over a boiling water-bath does not separate cuprous oxide from Fehling's solution, but gives it only a slight greenish tinge. Into the cooled mixture the calculated amount of sulphuric acid (made by mixing 3 parts of sulphuric acid with 4 of water) is then run. As soon as the acid liquid has cooled to the temperature of the room, a crystal of Glauber's salt is dropped in and the flask dipped in cold water until a thin crystalline crust forms on the sides, which is removed by a rapid shaking of the flask. Cooling and shaking are continued until a crust no longer forms, when the mixture is allowed to stand quiet for 12 to 24 hours. At the end of this time the contents of the flask appear to consist of a crystalline cake soaked with a reddish liquid. There is then added alcohol of 93 per cent., and the whole is shaken up until on further addition no precipitate separates out. The separated Glauber's salt is freed from the alcoholic solution by a vacuum filter, and can be washed with relatively very little alcohol. The half of the alcoholic solution is neutralized over the water-bath with carbonate of zinc, filtered boiling hot and united with the other half. The crystallization begins immediately upon cooling, and is complete after standing 36 hours. The lactate of zinc so obtained can be pressed free from mother-liquor and crystallized once, when it is perfectly pure. The weight of this first crystallization amounts to from 30 to 40 per cent. of the sugar used. The concentrated mother-liquor yields yet another portion of crystals, which are nearly pure, although slightly yellowish in color. For a method of making lactic acid from corn meal, see *New Rem.*, 1882, p. 235.

Properties. Lactic acid is a limpid, syrupy liquid, nearly colorless, of a slight not unpleasant odor, and a very sour taste. Its sp. gr. is 1·212, but acid of this strength is considered as containing only 75 per cent. of absolute lactic acid, the specific gravity of which is 1·248. (Allen, *Commerc. Org. Anal.*, 2d ed., i. p. 419.) It is not solidified by evaporation, and not vaporized by a heat not exceeding 160°C. (260° F.). "At a higher temperature it emits inflammable vapors, then chars, and is finally entirely volatilized, or leaves but a trace of residue." *U. S.* It unites in all proportions with water, alcohol, and ether, but is nearly insoluble in chloroform. Exposed to a heat of 150° C. (302° F.), it is for the most part converted into a new body called concrete lactic acid or *lactide*, an anhydride of the formula $C_3H_4O_2$. It coagulates albumen, and dissolves a large quantity of freshly precipitated phosphate of calcium; a property which, doubtless, renders it important in the animal economy.

"When diluted with water, Lactic Acid should afford no precipitate with test-solutions of nitrate of silver (hydrochloric acid), chloride of barium (sulphuric acid), sulphate of copper (sarcolactic acid), nor with sulphide of ammonium after addition of excess of water of ammonia (lead, iron). It should not reduce warm test-solution of potassio-cupric tartrate (sugars). When mixed and heated with excess of hydrated zinc oxide, and extracted with absolute alcohol, the latter should not leave a sweet residue on evaporation (glycerin). Cold concentrated sulphuric acid, shaken with an equal volume of Lactic Acid, should assume at most only a pale-yellow color (organic impurities). To neutralize 4·5 Gm. of Lactic Acid should require 37·5 C.c. of the volumetric solution of soda. *U. S.* "120 grains require for neutralization 1000 grain-measures of volumetric solution of soda." *Br.*

Medical Properties and Uses. Lactic acid was proposed by Magendie, on account of its being a normal constituent of gastric juice, as well of the sweat, urine, etc., as a remedy in certain forms of dyspepsia, and for the removal of phosphatic deposits in the urine. It has subsequently been employed with good effects in dyspepsia by Dr. Handfield Jones and Dr. O'Connor, both of London. The remedy should be taken at the time of meals. It is most conveniently given in solution sweetened with sugar, prepared like lemonade. From one to three drachms (3·75–11·25 C.c.) may be taken in the course of the day. Professor Cantani, of Naples, was induced by theoretical considerations to employ lactic acid in diabetes, in connection with an exclusively meat diet, and reported very remarkable success. (*Ed. Med. Journ.*, 1871, p. 533.) Certain other practitioners have achieved similar results, but the remedy has not answered the expectations formed of it, and is at present not very frequently employed. If used, half a fluidounce in a pint of water should be administered daily. Hypnotic properties have also been ascribed to lactic acid, but the claim has not been verified. In solution the acid has been found very efficacious, locally applied, in dissolving false membrane, and it has consequently been employed, with much apparent advantage, in diphtheritic affections and croup; the solution employed containing one part of the acid to five parts of the menstruum. (*Ann. de Thérap.*, 1869, p. 220.)

Prof. Hayme finds lactic acid remarkably useful in the green diarrhœa of children, a teaspoonful of a 2 to 100 solution being given to the child a quarter of an hour after nursing. (*Bull. Gén. de Thérap.*, May 30, 1887.)

Lactic acid is a useful addition to medicinal pepsin, increasing the solvent power of that agent upon the food, when taken into the stomach. Some importance has also been attached to it from the supposition that it might be the materies morbi in rheumatism, as uric acid has been supposed to be in gout; but in either case the acid is probably rather the effect than the cause of the disease.

Off. Prep. Br. Syrupus Calcii Lactophosphatis; Acidum Lacticum Dilutum.

ACIDUM LACTICUM DILUTUM. *Br.* *Diluted Lactic Acid.*

(ĂÇ'Ĭ-DŬM LĂC'TĬ-CŬM DĪ-LŪ'TŬM.)

"Lactic Acid, 3 fluidounces [Imp. meas.]; Distilled Water, sufficient to produce 1 pint [Imp. meas.]. Mix."

This is a new officinal of the British Pharmacopœia, introduced for convenience in prescribing.

Its specific gravity is 1.040, and 800 grains by weight require for neutralization 1000 grain-measures of volumetric solution of soda. Dose, one-half to two fluidrachms.

ACIDUM MECONICUM. *Br.* *Meconic Acid.*

$H_3C_7HO_7$. (ĂÇ'Ĭ-DŬM MĒ-CŎN'Ĭ-CŬM.)

"An acid obtained from opium." *Br.*

This acid has been made officinal by the British Pharmacopœia solely for the purpose of making a popular preparation used in Great Britain,—the solution of Bimeconate of Morphine.

It occurs in "micaceous crystals, nearly colorless, sparingly soluble in water, readily soluble in alcohol. The solution in water has a strongly acid taste and reaction, and is colored red by neutral solution of perchloride of iron, the color being discharged by strong but not by diluted hydrochloric acid. The aqueous solution gives no precipitate with solution of iodine and iodide of potassium." *Br.*

Its compounds with the earths and heavy metallic oxides are generally insoluble in water. Its characteristic properties are that it produces a blood-red color with ferric salts, a green precipitate with a weak solution of ammoniated sulphate of copper, and white precipitates soluble in nitric acid, with acetate of lead, nitrate of silver, and chloride of barium. It is obtained by macerating opium in water, filtering the infusion, and adding a solution of chloride of calcium. Meconate and sulphate of calcium are precipitated. The precipitate, having been washed with hot water and with alcohol, is treated with dilute hydrochloric acid at 82·2° C. (180° F.). The meconate of calcium is taken up, and, upon the cooling of the liquid, bimeconate of calcium is deposited. This is dissolved in warm concentrated hydrochloric acid, which deposits pure meconic acid when it cools. It may be freed from coloring matter by neutralizing it with potassa, decomposing the crystallized meconate thus obtained by hydrochloric acid, and again crystallizing.

Medical Properties. Meconic acid appears to be nearly free from active physiological properties. Sertürner took 4·5 grains of meconate of sodium, and Grape and Loewer 12 grains of the pure acid, without the production of any symptoms; whilst Mulder administered to dogs nearly 20 grains of the acid with similar negative results, which have also been confirmed by the researches of Pereira, Lange, and others.

Off. Prep. Br. Liquor Morphinæ Bimeconatis.

ACIDUM NITRICUM. *U. S., Br.* *Nitric Acid.*

(ĂÇ'Ĭ-DŬM NĪ'TRĬ-CŬM.)

"A liquid composed of 69·4 per cent. of absolute Nitric Acid [HNO_3; 63—$HONO_2$; 63] and 30·6 per cent. of water." *U. S.* "An acid prepared from nitrate of potassium or nitrate of sodium by distillation with sulphuric acid and water, and containing 70 per cent. by weight of real nitric acid, HNO_3." *Br.*

Acidum Nitri s. Azoticum, Spiritus Nitri Acidus; Spirit of Nitre; Aqua Fortis; Acide nitrique, Acide azotique, *Fr.;* Salpetersäure, *G.;* Zaltpeterzuur, Sterkwater, *Dutch;* Skedwater, *Sw.;* Acido nitrico, *It., Sp.*

Nitric oxide is one of the five compounds formed by the combination of nitrogen and oxygen. These are nitrogen protoxide or hyponitrous oxide (laughing gas), N_2O; nitrogen dioxide, N_2O_2 or $(NO)_2$; nitrous oxide, N_2O_3; nitrogen tetroxide or peroxide, N_2O_4; and nitric oxide, N_2O_5. From this latter by the addition of water is formed nitric acid: $N_2O_5 + H_2O = (HNO_3)_2$.

Nitric acid is now officinal in two forms; the pure acid of the sp. gr. 1·42, and the diluted. The strong acid, of the sp. gr. 1·5, which was recognized in the former Br. Pharmacopœia, has been abandoned.

Preparation. The usual practice adopted in the laboratory for obtaining nitric acid is to add to nitrate of potassium in coarse powder, contained in a retort, an equal weight of strong sulphuric acid, poured in by means of a tube or funnel, so as not to soil the neck. The materials should not occupy more than two-thirds of the capacity of the retort. A receiver being adapted, heat is applied by means of a spirit or gas-lamp, the naked fire, or a sand-bath, moderately at first, but afterwards more strongly when the materials begin to thicken, in order to bring the whole into a state of perfect fusion. Red vapors will at first arise, and afterwards disappear in the course of the distillation. Towards its close they will be reproduced, and their reappearance will indicate that the process is completed.

The proportion of equal weights, as above given, corresponding nearly to one mol. of nitrate of potassium and one of sulphuric acid, is the best for operations on a small scale in the laboratory.

A practical disadvantage in this method of obtaining very strong nitric acid is that, owing to the high heat and the presence of the crystals, the retort is frequently fractured. Prof. Trimble recommends adding one part of commercial nitric acid to two parts of strong sulphuric acid in a retort and distilling slowly until the nitric acid is all collected.

MONOHYDRATED NITRIC ACID. *Hydrogen Nitrate.* This is the strongest liquid nitric acid that can be procured, and may be supposed to be obtained by distilling one molecule of pure and dry nitre with one molecule of monohydrated sulphuric acid. One molecule of monohydrated nitric acid distils over, and one molecule of bisulphate of potassium remains behind: $KNO_3 + H_2SO_4 = HNO_3 + HKSO_4$. Acid of this strength is very difficult to make, and requires for its preparation the most elaborate attention to separate the superabundant water. According to Mr. Arthur Smith, of London, acid dehydrated as far as possible is perfectly colorless, boils at 84° C. (184° F.), has the sp. gr. 1·517 at 15·4° C. (60° F.), and nearly approaches, in composition, to a monohydrate. Acid of this strength, even at the boiling temperature, has not the slightest action on tin or iron. (*Phil. Mag.*, Dec. 1847.) According to Kolb (*Ann. Chem. Phys.* [4], x. 140), the true HNO_3 has a sp. gr. at 15° C. (59° F.) as high as 1·530.

The acid of the former Br. Pharmacopœia, having the sp. gr. 1·5, is of a yellowish color, and strongly corrosive. Strictly speaking, it is hydrogen nitrate diluted with half a molecule of water ($HNO_3 + \frac{1}{2}H_2O$). An acid of this strength is inconveniently strong, is constantly undergoing decomposition under the influence of light, and has consequently been replaced by a pure acid of the density 1·42. This substitution was made in the U. S. Pharmacopœia of 1850, and in the British of 1867.

NITRIC ACID (sp. gr. 1·42). This is the acid now officinal in both the U. S. and Br. Pharmacopœias. Acid of the density 1·5 was not found in any of the shops, and much pains was required to get it of that strength. Besides, acid of this density was not necessary for any process of the Pharmacopœia. Considerations of this kind induced the revisers of our national standard of 1850 to lower the strength of officinal nitric acid to 1·42, its purity in other respects remaining the same. "If 1 C.c. of Nitric Acid be treated with a slight excess of water of ammonia, no precipitate should be formed (absence of iron or much lead), the liquid should not have a blue tint (copper), and the further addition of 2 drops of test-solution of sulphide of ammonium should not cause a black precipitate (lead and iron). The remaining liquid should leave no fixed residue on evaporation and gentle ignition (non-volatile metals). If one part of Nitric Acid be neutralized with solution of potassa, two parts of potassa then added, and the mixture boiled with test zinc, a gas is evolved which should not blacken paper wet with test-solution of nitrate of silver (arsenic acid). A portion diluted with five volumes of water should afford no precipitate with test-solution of chloride of barium (sulphuric acid), or with test-solution of nitrate of silver (hydrochloric acid). If 5 C.c. of Nitric Acid are diluted with an equal volume of water, no blue color should be produced by the addition of a few drops of gelatinized starch (absence of free iodine), nor should the further addition, without agitation, of a layer of solution of hydrosulphuric acid cause a blue zone at the line of contact of the two liquids (abs. of iodic acid). To neutralize 3·15 Gm. of Nitric Acid should require 34·7 C.c. of the volumetric solution of soda." *U. S.* To satisfy the tests given in the U. S. Pharmacopœia, it must be colorless, and entirely volatilizable by heat; must dissolve copper with the disengagement of red vapors, and stain woollen fabrics and animal tissues a bright yellow. Acid of the density 1·42 is the most stable of the hydrated compounds of nitric acid, and boils at 121° C. (250° F.). When either stronger or weaker than this, it distils over at a lower temperature; and, by losing more acid than water in the first case, and more water than acid in the second, constantly approaches to the sp. gr. 1·42, when its boiling point becomes stationary. These facts in relation to nitric acid of this strength were first observed by Dalton, and have since been confirmed by Mr. Arthur Smith, of London. This acid may be assumed to have the composition $HNO_3 + 1\frac{1}{2}H_2O$. "Ninety grains by weight of it, mixed with half an ounce of distilled water, require, for neutralization, 1000 grain-measures of the *volumetric solution of soda.*" *Br.*

NITRIC ACID OF THE ARTS. Two strengths of this acid occur in the arts; *double aqua fortis* (sp. gr. 1·36), which is of half the strength of concentrated nitric acid, and *single aqua fortis* (sp. gr. 1·22), which is half as strong as the double. Aqua fortis is sometimes obtained by distilling a mixture of nitre and calcined sulphate of iron. By an interchange of ingredients, sulphate of potassium and nitrate of iron are formed, the latter of which, at the distilling heat, readily abandons its nitric acid. The sulphate of potassium is washed out of the residue, and the sesquioxide of iron which is left is sold, under the name of *colcothar*, to the polishers of metals. The distillation is performed in large cast-iron retorts, lined on the inside with a thick layer of red oxide of iron, to protect them from the action of the acid. The acid is received in large glass vessels containing water. A considerable portion of the acid is decomposed by the heat into reddish vapors, which subsequently dissolve in the water, and absorb the oxygen which had been disengaged. The acid thus obtained is red and tolerably strong, but is diluted with water before being sold.

The reddish acid, called *nitrous acid*, is nitric acid containing more or less nitrogen tetroxide (N_2O_4). The same acid may be formed by impregnating, to a limited extent, nitric acid with nitrogen dioxide (N_2O_2). If the saturation be complete, every two molecules of nitric oxide become three molecules of nitrogen tetroxide by the aid of one molecule of nitrogen dioxide ($2N_2O_5 + N_2O_2 = 3N_2O_4$). The commercial nitrous acid may be converted into nitric acid by exposing it to a gentle heat. As nitrogen tetroxide (N_2O_4) forms, in contact with bases, a nitrate and nitrite, there being no hyponitrates, some chemists consider it as a compound of nitric and nitrous oxides ($2N_2O_4 = N_2O_5 + N_2O_3$).

In making nitric acid on the commercial scale, sodium nitrate is substituted for nitre, as it is much cheaper, and the salt is decomposed with sulphuric acid as before. The proportions of these two substances employed are not the same in all works. If one molecule of sulphuric acid and two of sodium nitrate be taken, the following are the reactions: $H_2SO_4 + NaNO_3 = NaHSO_4 + HNO_3$. When the heat is raised, the acid sodium sulphate acts upon a second molecule of sodium nitrate; thus: $NaHSO_4 + NaNO_3 = Na_2SO_4 + HNO_3$.

In this case, however, a part of the acid is decomposed, owing to the high temperature, and nitrogen peroxide is evolved in the form of red fumes, which dissolve in the concentrated acid, giving it the red appearance usually noted in the strong commercial product. When a large excess of sulphuric acid is employed, a certain quantity of acid sodium sulphate is formed, which lowers the melting point of the residual mass so that it can be withdrawn from the retorts in a fused state, whereas in the other case the residue can only be removed in the solid state after the cylinder has cooled.

The ordinary commercial acid has a specific gravity of from 1·30 to 1·41, and is usually prepared by means of chamber (sulphuric) acid; but if a more concentrated acid is required, a stronger sulphuric acid must be employed. The strongest nitric acid occurring in commerce has a sp. gr. of 1·43, and this is obtained by distilling well-dried Chili saltpetre with sulphuric acid having a sp. gr. of 1·85.

The retorts in which nitric acid is usually prepared in England consist of cast-iron cylinders, built in a furnace in such a way that they may be heated as uniformly as possible. Some manufacturers cover the upper half of the cylinder with fire-bricks, in order to protect the iron from the action of the nitric acid vapors. This is unnecessary, however, if the retorts are so thoroughly heated that no nitric acid condenses on the surface of the iron.

M. Mallet, of Paris, has proposed to obtain nitric acid from nitrate of sodium, by distilling it with well-dried boric acid. In this case, biborate of sodium or borax is the residue. Another method, employed by Kuhlmann, is to expose a mixture of nitrate of sodium and chloride of manganese to a heat of about 232° C. (450° F.), and to pass the mixed gases which escape through water. Hyponitric acid and oxygen are disengaged, which become nitric acid when they enter the water. (See *P. J. Tr.*, 1862, p. 155.)

General Properties of Nitric Acid. Nitric acid, so called from nitre, is an extremely sour and corrosive liquid. It was discovered by Raymond Lully, in the thirteenth century, and its constituents by Cavendish, in 1784. When perfectly pure it is colorless; but, as usually obtained, it has a straw color, owing to the presence of hyponitric acid. The concentrated acid, when exposed to the air, emits white fumes, possessing a disagreeable odor. By the action of light it undergoes a slight decomposition, and becomes yellow. It acts powerfully on animal matter, causing its decomposition. On the living fibre it operates as a strong caustic. It stains the skin and most animal substances of an indelible yellow color. On vegetable fibre it acts peculiarly, abstracting hydrogen or water, and combining with its remaining elements. When diluted, nitric acid converts most animal and vegetable substances into oxalic, malic, and carbonic acids. The general character of its action is to impart oxygen to other bodies, which it is enabled to do, as oxygen in the nascent state is liberated in its decomposition. If this liberation take place while in contact with bodies capable of oxidation, the oxygen goes to effect this oxidation. Free nitric acid, however, will evolve oxygen at a red heat, according to the following reaction:

$$4HNO_3 = (N_2O_4)_2 + O_2 + (H_2O)_2.$$

It oxidises sulphur and phosphorus, giving rise to sulphuric and phosphoric acids, and all the metals, except chromium, tungsten, columbium, cerium, titanium, osmium, rhodium, gold, platinum, and iridium. It combines with salifiable bases and forms nitrates. When mixed with hydrochloric acid, mutual decomposition takes place, according to the reaction: $HNO_3 + 3HCl = NOCl + Cl_2 + 2H_2O$, and a liquid is formed, capable of dissolving gold, called nitro-hydrochloric acid.

Great care must be used in transporting nitric acid, for if the strong acid comes in contact in quantity with vegetable substances like hay, tow, excelsior, paper, etc., fire will be apt to occur. The occurrence of such accidents was proven by the official inquiry of Prof. R. Haas. (*Ber. d. Chem. Ges.*, 1881, 597.)

A trace of nitric acid has been detected in the atmosphere. It is said to be always present in the air in summer. (*Kletzinsky.*)

Tests. Nitric acid, when uncombined, is recognised by its dissolving copper with the production of red vapors, and by its forming nitre when saturated with potassa. When in the form of a nitrate, it is known by its action on gold-leaf, after the addition of hydrochloric acid, in consequence of the evolution of chlorine, or it may be discovered, according to Dr. O'Shaughnessy, by heating the supposed nitrate in a test tube with a drop of sulphuric acid, and then adding a crystal of morphine. If nitric acid be present, it will be set free by the sulphuric acid, and reddened by the morphine. The same effect is produced by brucine, by commercial strychnine, on account of its containing brucine, and still more strongly, according to M. Braun, by sulphate of anilin, which affords an exceedingly delicate test. (*Journ. de Pharm.*, 1867, p. 157.) To prevent all ambiguity arising from the accidental presence of nitric acid in the sulphuric acid employed, the operator should satisfy himself, by a separate experiment, that the latter acid has no power to produce the characteristic color with morphine. Another test for nitric acid is to add *pure* sulphuric acid to the concentrated liquid, suspected to contain it, together with a little concentrated solution of ferrous sulphate. The smallest trace of nitric acid affords, when the mixture is warmed, a pink red color; and if it be present in considerable amount, the liquid becomes almost black.* Rosa recommends the use of ammonio-ferrous sulphate, in place of ferrous sulphate, as a test for nitric acid. It is more stable than the latter, either in crystals or in solution. Equal measures of the liquid to be tested for nitric acid and of concentrated sulphuric acid are mixed, the mixture cooled, and then a layer of solution of ammonio-ferrous sulphate poured slowly on top; if even a trace of nitric acid be present, a brown zone will form at the line of contact of the liquids. (*Am. Drug.*, 1886, p. 13.)

A method, particularly useful in the determination of the nitrates contained in drinking-water, depends upon the fact that a thin zinc plate, which has been covered with a deposit of spongy metallic copper by dipping it in a solution of copper sulphate, on being heated with water containing nitrates, reduces them to ammonia, zinc hydroxide and free hydrogen being at the same time formed (*Gladstone* and *Tribe*); thus: $KNO_3 + 4H_2 = NH_3 + KOH + 2H_2O$.

The nitric acid of commerce sometimes contains iodine, probably derived from the native nitrate of sodium, in which iodate frequently occurs. This may be reduced by passing sulphuretted hydrogen into the diluted acid, taking care not to use an excess. A few drops of chloroform or bisulphide of carbon shaken up with the liquid will then show the iodine color. Still better is the test proposed by Mr. Stein, which is to introduce a stick of tin into the suspected acid, and, after red vapors have begun to escape, to withdraw the metal, add a few drops of bisulphide of carbon, and agitate. If iodine be present, the drops of the sulphide which soon separate will be colored more or less deeply red according to the amount of impurity. These impurities, however, do not affect the medical properties of the acid.

The following table, drawn up by B. J. Kolb (*Ann. Ch. Phys.*, 4, 10, 136), is the recognized standard at present:

* *A quantitative test for nitric acid* in water, first proposed by M. Boussingault, in 1857, was simplified by M. Marx, and finally perfected by M. Fischer, who substituted indigotin for indigo, on account of its solution being permanent. His method is first to prepare a test-solution by mixing 5 cubic centimetres of solution of indigotin with 30 cubic centimetres of pure sulphuric acid, and then adding a titrated solution of nitrate of potassium (5 decigrammes to the litre) until the blue color is changed to a faint green. Then the solution of indigotin is diluted until one cubic centimetre is decolorized by 0·2525 milligrammes of nitrate of potassium. In using this test-solution the temperature should always be at least 110° C. (230° F.), and the amount of sulphuric acid should always be at least double the joint volume of the indigotin solution and the water. (*Journ. de Pharm.*, Nov. 1874.)

Table showing percentage of absolute Nitric Acid in Nitric Acid of different densities, at 0° C. (32° F.) and 15° C. (59° F.).

Per Cent. HNO_3.	Specific Gravity.		Per Cent. HNO_3.	Specific Gravity.		Per Cent. HNO_3.	Specific Gravity.		Per Cent. HNO_3.	Specific Gravity.	
	At 0° C.	At 15° C.		At 0° C.	At 15° C.		At 0° C.	At 15° C.		At 0° C.	At 15° C.
0·00	1·000	0·999	40·00	1·267	1·251	61·21	1·400	1·381	83·00	1·495	1·470
2·00	1·013	1·010	41·00	1·274	1·257	62·00	1·404	1·386	84·00	1·499	1·474
4·00	1·026	1·022	42·00	1·280	1·264	63·59	1·418	1·393	85·00	1·503	1·478
7·22	1·050	1·045	43·53	1·291	1·274	64·00	1·415	1·395	86·17	1·507	1·482
11·41	1·075	1·067	45·00	1·300	1·284	65·07	1·420	1·400	87·45	1·513	1·486
13·00	1·085	1·077	46·64	1·312	1·295	66·00	1·425	1·405	88·00	1·514	1·488
15·00	1·099	1·089	47·18	1·315	1·298	67·00	1·430	1·410	89·56	1·521	1·494
17·47	1·115	1·105	48·00	1·321	1·304	68·00	1·435	1·414	90·00	1·522	1·495
20·00	1·132	1·120	49·00	1·328	1·312	69·20	1·441	1·419	91·00	1·526	1·499
23·00	1·153	1·138	49·97	1·334	1·317	69·4	....	1·420	92·00	1·529	1·503
25·71	1·171	1·157	50·99	1·341	1·323	69·96	1·444	1·423	93·01	1·533	1·506
27·00	1·180	1·166	52·33	1·349	1·331	71·24	1·450	1·429	94·00	1·537	1·509
28·00	1·187	1·172	53·00	1·353	1·335	72·39	1·455	1·432	95·27	1·542	1·514
29·00	1·194	1·179	53·81	1·358	1·339	73·00	1·457	1·435	96·00	1·544	1·516
30·00	1·200	1·185	54·00	1·359	1·341	74·01	1·462	1·438	97·00	1·548	1·520
31·00	1·207	1·192	55·00	1·365	1·346	75·00	1·465	1·442	97·89	1·551	1·523
32·00	1·214	1·198	56·10	1·371	1·353	76·00	1·469	1·445	99·52	1·557	1·529
33·86	1·226	1·211	57·00	1·376	1·358	77·66	1·476	1·451	99·72	1·558	1·530
35·00	1·234	1·218	58·00	1·382	1·363	79·00	1·481	1·456	99·84	1·559	1·530
36·00	1·240	1·225	58·88	1·387	1·368	80·00	1·484	1·460	100·00	1·559	1·530
37·95	1·253	1·237	59·59	1·391	1·372	80·96	1·488	1·463			
39·00	1·260	1·244	60·00	1·393	1·374	82·00	1·492	1·467			

Composition. The composition of the officinal acid of the density 1·42 has already been given. It contains about 75 per cent. of nitric acid, of the sp. gr. 1·5. Nitric oxide or anhydride consists of two atoms of nitrogen 28, and five atoms of oxygen 80 = 108; or, in volumes, of two volumes of nitrogen and five volumes of oxygen, supposed to be condensed to form nitric oxide vapor, into two volumes. In 1849, the interesting discovery was made by M. Deville, of Besançon, of the means of isolating nitric oxide or anhydride. The method pursued was to pass perfectly dry chlorine over nitrate of silver. The oxide is in the form of colorless, brilliant, limpid crystals, which melt at 29·5° C. (85° F.) and boil at 45° C. (113° F.). In contact with water, they form a colorless solution with evolution of heat, without the disengagement of gas. (*Journ. de Pharm.*, 1849, p. 207.)

Medical Properties. Nitric acid is tonic, antiseptic, astringent, and appears to act upon the intestinal glands in some way so as to modify their function. It is a very useful remedy in cases of intestinal indigestion: in this it resembles hydrochloric acid; the choice between the two acids in any individual case should be guided by the existence or non-existence of diarrhœa, the nitric acid being given when there is looseness of the bowels. In syphilis, and in the chronic hepatitis of India, this acid was highly extolled by Dr. Scott, formerly of Bombay. It has occasionally excited ptyalism. It cannot be depended upon as a remedy in syphilis, but, in worn-out constitutions, is often an excellent adjuvant, either to prepare the system for the use of mercury, or to lessen the effects of that metal on the economy: in hepatic troubles it is inferior to the nitro-hydrochloric acid, unless, it may be, when there is much diarrhœa. As nitric acid dissolves both uric acid and the phosphates, it was supposed to be applicable to cases of gravel in which the uric acid and the phosphates are mixed; but experience has not confirmed the opinion. Nevertheless, when the sabulous deposit depends upon disordered digestion, this acid may prove serviceable by restoring the tone of the stomach. The dose is from five to fifteen minims (0·3–0·9 C.c.) in three fluidounces or more of water, given in divided doses three or four times a day.

Externally, nitric acid has been used with advantage as a lotion to ulcers, in the strength of about twelve minims to the pint of water. This practice originated with Sir Everard Home, and is particularly applicable to those ulcers which are superficial and not disposed to cicatrize. In sloughing phagedæna, *strong* nitric acid is one of the best remedies, applied by means of a piece of lint tied round a small stick, or by the use of a glass brush. Sometimes a piece of lint is soaked with the strong acid, and pressed into the sore, being allowed to remain for several hours. In cancrum oris, concentrated nitric acid, freely applied, is one of the best local remedies that can be employed for arresting the phagedænic ulceration and disposing the sore to heal, but great care must be exercised to protect the teeth. The *strong* acid has also been found very useful as an escharotic in venereal sores and other affections.

Nitric acid vapors were formerly used as a disinfectant. Half an ounce of powdered nitre was put into a saucer, placed in an earthen dish containing heated sand, and two drachms of sulphuric acid were then poured over it.

Properties as a Poison. The swallowing of concentrated nitric acid is at once followed by burning heat in the mouth, œsophagus, and stomach, acute pain, disengagement of gas, abundant eructations, nausea, and hiccough. These effects are soon followed by repeated and excessive vomiting of matter having a peculiar odor and taste, tumefaction of the abdomen with exquisite tenderness, a feeling of coldness on the surface, horripilation, icy coldness of the extremities, small depressed pulse, horrible anxieties, continual tossings and contortions, and extreme thirst. The breath becomes extremely fetid, and the countenance exhibits a complete picture of suffering. The cases are almost always fatal. Sometimes the collapse has been immediate and has masked all the other symptoms. The best remedies are repeated large doses of alkaline solutions, soap, magnesia, chalk, as antidotes, mucilaginous drinks in large quantities, olive or almond oil in very large doses, emollient fomentations, etc.

Pharm. Uses. In the preparation of Acidum Phosphoricum, Ferri Chloridum, Hydrargyri Subsulphas Flavus, Liquor Ferri Chloridi, Liquor Ferri Subsulphatis, Liquor Ferri Tersulphatis, Liquor Zinci Chloridi, Pyroxylinum.

Off. Prep. Acidum Nitricum Dilutum; Acidum Nitro-hydrochloricum; Acidum Nitro-hydrochloricum Dilutum; Liquor Ferri Nitratis; Liquor Hydrargyri Nitratis; Spiritus Ætheris Nitrosi; Unguentum Hydrargyri Nitratis.

Off. Prep. Br. Acidum Nitricum Dilutum; Acidum Nitro-hydrochloricum Dilutum; Liquor Ferri Pernitratis; Liquor Hydrargyri Nitratis Acidus; Unguentum Hydrargyri Nitratis.

Off. Nitrates. Br. Ammonii Nitras; Argenti Nitras; Bismuthi Subnitras; Liquor Ferri Pernitratis; Pilocarpinæ Nitras; Plumbi Nitras; Potassii Nitras; Sodii Nitras; Liquor Hydrargyri Nitratis Acidus.

ACIDUM NITRICUM DILUTUM. *U.S., Br.* *Diluted Nitric Acid.*

(ĂÇ'I-DŬM NĪ'TRI-CŬM DI-LŪ'TŬM.)

Acide azotique dilué, *Fr.;* Verdünnte Salpetersäure, *G.*

"Nitric Acid, *one part* [or one and a half fluidounces]; Distilled Water, *six parts* [or twelve and a half fluidounces]. Mix the Acid with the Water, and preserve the product in glass-stoppered bottles." *U. S.*

"Take of Nitric Acid *six fluidounces* [Imperial measure], Distilled Water *a sufficiency.* Dilute the Acid with 24 fluidounces [Imp. meas.] of the Water; then add more water, so that at a temperature of 60° it shall measure 31 fluidounces [Imp. meas.]. Or, as follows:

"Take of Nitric Acid 2400 grains, Distilled Water *a sufficiency.* Weigh the Acid in a glass flask, the capacity of which, to a mark on the neck, is one pint [Imp. meas.]; then add Distilled Water until the mixture, at 60° temperature, after it has been shaken, measures a pint." *Br.*

The U. S. acid, as now directed, varies considerably from that formerly officinal. The U. S. P. 1870 diluted acid contained 18·5 per cent. of officinal nitric acid, whilst that of the present Pharmacopœia contains but 14·3 per cent., and is therefore correspondingly weaker. "Diluted Nitric Acid contains 10 per cent. of absolute Nitric Acid. It has the sp. gr. 1·059, and should respond to the same reactions and tests as Nitric Acid. To neutralize 12·6 Gm. should require 20 C.c. of the *volumetric solution of soda.*" *U. S.*

The British diluted acid is considerably stronger than our own in the same measure. It has the sp. gr. 1·101; and "361 grains by weight (six fluidrachms) require for neutralization 1000 grain-measures of the *volumetric solution of soda*, corresponding to 14·95 per cent. of real nitric acid. Six fluidrachms [Imp. meas.], therefore, correspond to one molecular weight in grains of real nitric acid, HNO_3." *Br.*

In making the U. S. diluted acid, pharmacists should be careful to use acid of the sp. gr. 1·42; or, if the acid used be weaker than this, to add proportionally less water; otherwise the diluted acid would be weaker than it is directed to be in the Pharmacopœia.

The medicinal properties of the diluted acid are the same as those of the strong acid. (See *Acidum Nitricum.*) The dose of the U. S. diluted acid is from twenty to forty drops or minims (1·25–2·5 C.c.), that of the British, from fifteen to thirty (0·9–1·9 C.c.), three times a day, properly diluted.

ACIDUM NITRO-HYDROCHLORICUM. *U. S.* *Nitro-hydrochloric Acid.*

(ĂÇ'Ĭ-DŬM NĪ-TRO-HȲ-DRO-ÇHLŌ'RĪ-CŬM.)

Acidum Chloro-nitrosum, *G.;* Acidum Nitromuriaticum, Pharm. 1870; Nitro-muriatic Acid; Acide chloro-azotique, Eau régale, *Fr.;* Saltpeter Salzsäure, Königswasser, *G.*

"Nitric Acid, *four parts* [or three fluidounces]; Hydrochloric Acid, *fifteen parts* [or thirteen fluidounces, five fluidrachms]. Mix the Acids in a capacious open glass vessel, and, when effervescence has ceased, pour the product into glass-stoppered bottles," which should not be more than half filled, and keep them in a cool place.* *U. S.*

Nitro-hydrochloric acid is the *aqua regia* of the earlier chemists, so called from its property of dissolving gold. Nitric and hydrochloric acids, when mixed together, are mutually decomposed. According to the researches of Gay-Lussac (June, 1848), the reaction gives rise to two compounds, NO_2Cl (nitroxyl chloride) and NOCl (nitrosyl chloride), mixed with free chlorine. Later researches seem, however, to show that the latter of the two chlorides exclusively is produced, the reaction for the decomposition of aqua regia being: $HNO_3 + 3HCl = 2H_2O + NOCl + Cl_2$.

The power of nitro-hydrochloric acid to dissolve gold, and similar metals having a weak affinity for oxygen, is owing exclusively to the free chlorine present, and is in no wise dependent on the compound above referred to, which remains entirely passive during the solution of the metal. According to the reaction just given, the proportion of acids needed would be 1 part of nitric for every 3 of hydrochloric acid; and this agrees very closely with the proportions in the officinal formula. It should be borne in mind, however, that the U. S. P. 1870 formula contained a large excess of nitric acid, the proportions being 3 parts of nitric to 5 parts of hydrochloric acid; it is now 1·3 parts of nitric to 5 parts of hydrochloric acid. When nitro-hydrochloric acid is made from strong acids, there is always a loss of the nitrosyl chloride and of free chlorine by effervescence, in consequence of the acids not containing sufficient water to hold the gaseous products in solution. Hence the substitution, in the U. S. Pharmacopœia of 1850, of nitric acid of 1·42 for the acid of 1·5 was an improvement.

Properties. "A golden-yellow, fuming and very corrosive liquid, having a strong odor of chlorine and a strongly acid reaction. By heat it is wholly volatilized. It readily dissolves gold-leaf, and a drop added to test-solution of iodide of potassium liberates iodine abundantly." *U. S.* Nitro-hydrochloric acid has an orange color, soon changing to a golden yellow, and the odor of chlorine. It possesses the power of dissolving gold and platinum. It should be kept in a cool dark place, on account of its liability to lose chlorine by heat, and to have its chlorine converted into hydrochloric acid by the action of light and the decomposition of water. On account of its tendency to decomposition, it should not be made in large quantities, nor be kept very long by the apothecary; and care should be taken not to transfer it to the bottle in which it is to be dispensed, until effervescence has ceased, lest the pressure within should drive out the stopper. Nitric and hydrochloric acids, as found in commerce, are sometimes so weak that when mixed they will not readily act on gold-leaf. In this case, their solvent power may be rendered effective by the addition of a little sulphuric acid, which, by its superior affinity for water, concentrates the other acids, and causes immediate action.

* For an apparatus for making nitro-hydrochloric acid upon a large scale, see *P. J. Tr.*, xi. 422.

Medical Properties and Uses. Nitro-hydrochloric acid was brought to the notice of the profession in consequence of the favorable report of its efficacy as an external remedy in hepatitis, made by Dr. Scott, formerly of Bombay. When thus employed, it produces a tingling sensation of the skin, thirst, a peculiar taste in the mouth, and occasional soreness of the gums and plentiful ptyalism; and at the same time stimulates the liver, as is evinced by an increased flow of bile. It is used either by sponging, or in the form of a local or general bath. When applied by sponging, the acid is first diluted so as to have the sourness of strong vinegar. When used as a foot-bath, three gallons of water, contained in a deep narrow wooden tub, may be acidulated with six fluidounces of the acid. In this the feet and legs are to be immersed for twenty minutes or half an hour. The bath may be employed at first daily, and afterwards twice or thrice a week; and the sponging may be used at the same time. The bath is said to be effective in promoting the passage of biliary calculi. The solution, prepared for a bath as above mentioned, may be used for a week, adding to it daily a pint of water acidulated with two fluidrachms of the acid, to make up for the waste by evaporation. The bath should have a temperature of about 97° F., which may be attained by heating part of the acid solution and throwing it back into the remainder.

Nitro-hydrochloric acid is much used internally, and it is an excellent remedy in chronic hepatic affections, in oxaluria, and in dyspepsia with a tendency to constipation. It is sometimes given also in syphilitic diseases. The strong fresh acid is preferable to the dilute, and may be given in doses of 3 to 6 drops (0·18–0·36 C.c.), well diluted, after meals, care being exercised to prevent its injuring the teeth. It should never be prescribed in combination with strong alcoholic liquids, as gases are often generated in sufficient volume to cause explosion. (See *A. J. P.*, 1878, p. 67.)

ACIDUM NITRO-HYDROCHLORICUM DILUTUM. *U. S., Br.*

Diluted Nitro-hydrochloric Acid.

(ĂÇ'Į-DŬM NĪ-TRǪ-HȲ-DRǪ-ȻHLŌ'RĮ-CŬM DĮ-LŪ'TŬM.)

Acidum Nitromuriaticum Dilutum, Pharm. 1870; Diluted Nitromuriatic Acid; Acide chlorazotique dilué, *Fr.;* Verdünnte Salpetersalzsäure, *G.*

"Contains free chlorine, hydrochloric, nitric, and nitrous acids and other compounds, dissolved in water." *Br.*

"Nitric acid, *four parts* [or three fluidrachms]; Hydrochloric Acid, *fifteen parts* [or thirteen and a half fluidrachms]; Distilled Water, *seventy-six parts* [or ten fluidounces]. Mix the Acids in a capacious, open glass vessel, and, when effervescence has ceased, add the Distilled Water. Keep the product in glass-stoppered bottles, in a cool place." *U. S.*

"Take of Nitric Acid *three fluidounces;* Hydrochloric Acid *four fluidounces* [Imperial measure]; Distilled Water *twenty-five fluidounces* [Imp. meas.]. Add the acids to the water, and keep the mixture in a glass-stoppered bottle for fourteen days before it is used. Sp. gr. 1·07. Six fluidrachms [Imp. meas.] (352 grains by weight) require for neutralization about 883 grain-measures of the *volumetric solution of soda.*" *Br.*

"A colorless, or faintly yellow liquid, odorless or having a faint odor of chlorine, a very acid taste and reaction. By heat it is wholly volatilized. On adding a few drops to test-solution of iodide of potassium, iodine is liberated." *U. S.*

Between diluted nitric and hydrochloric acids no reaction occurs; and therefore both Pharmacopœias direct that the acids shall be mixed before dilution. But according to the researches of Mr. Tilden, confirmed by Mr. Redwood (*P. J. Tr.*, x. 508), water determines a decomposition of the products resulting from the reaction between nitric and hydrochloric acids, and the reformation of hydrochloric and nitric acids, with a little nitrous acid. It would seem, therefore, that diluted nitro-hydrochloric acid is not an eligible preparation, a conclusion confirmed by clinical experience. The dose is from ten to twenty drops or minims (0·6–1·25 C.c.), properly diluted.

ACIDUM OLEICUM. *U. S.* *Oleic Acid.*

H C_{18} H_{33} O_2; 282. (ĂÇ'Ĭ-DŬM Ọ-LĒ'Ĭ-CŬM.) HO, C_{36} H_{33} O_3; 282.

Acide oléique, *Fr.;* Oleinsäure, *G.*

"A fluid fatty acid, $HC_{18}H_{33}O_2$, obtained by the saponification of olein, or by the action of superheated steam on fats, with subsequent separation from solid fats by pressure. Usually not quite pure." *Br.*

This acid is a new officinal, and, although known for many years, was not used medicinally until 1872 (*London Lancet*, 1872, p. 709), when Prof. John Marshall introduced the oleates to the profession as substitutes for some of the older ointments, stating that they are not only cleaner and more elegant, but are also much more efficacious. (See *Oleata.*)

Preparation. The difficulty in preparing oleates of good quality arises usually from the use of the commercial oleic acid, which, being obtained as a by-product in the manufacture of glycerin and candles, has a reddish brown color and a disagreeable fatty odor. It is almost always contaminated with stearic and palmitic acids with undecomposed glycerides when obtained by the autoclave process, and hydrocarbons when obtained by the distillation of the fat acids. Various processes have been suggested for the purification of oleic acid. Charles Rice (*A. J. P.*, xlv. 2) exposes the commercial acid to a temperature of 4° C. (39° F.), and expresses the liquid portion, which is oleic acid deprived of the greater part of the contaminating substances. The odorous and coloring principles are not removed by this process. A writer in *A. J. P.* (xlv. 97) prepares *oleic acid* for making oleates by saponifying almond oil with potassa; decomposing by tartaric acid, separating the precipitated bitartrate; heating for several hours on a water-bath with half its weight of finely powdered oxide of lead; after cooling, mixing with three times its volume of ether, settling, decanting, and treating the residue with ether as before; agitating the mixed ethereal solutions with dilute hydrochloric acid; skimming off the ethereal solution of oleic acid, washing it with water, skimming again, and finally recovering the ether by distillation.

L. Wolff (*A. J. P.*, 1879, p. 8) saponifies oil of sweet almond with lead oxide, agitates the plaster or lead soap in benzin, which retains lead oleate in solution, the lead palmitate being deposited. The benzin solution of lead oleate is shaken repeatedly with diluted hydrochloric acid (1 to 7), when lead chloride separates, and a benzin solution of purified oleic acid is left; finally the benzin is driven off by evaporation. The objection to this process is the difficulty of freeing the oleic acid from traces of a disagreeable benzin odor. Ernest C. Saunders (*N. R.*, June, 1880) makes a solution of 5 pounds of white castile soap in 20 pounds of boiling water, adds 10 ounces of sulphuric acid, and boils with stirring, until two clear layers are formed. The upper layer is decanted, shaken with 5 pounds of hot water, and the oily layer again decanted; 4 ounces of lead oxide are dissolved in it with a gentle heat, and while hot 5 pounds of alcohol, previously heated to 65·5° C. (150° F.), are added. It is filtered after standing 24 hours, and 1 ounce of hydrochloric acid shaken with the filtrate; 10 pounds of water are added, the acid decanted, again washed with 10 pounds of water, and finally recovered; the yield is about 2½ pounds. See also process by Chas. T. George, 1881 (*A. J. P.*, p. 379). Low grade oleic acids, obtained by the distillation of wool-grease, etc., may contain cholesterin and other unsaponifiable materials from this source (*Allen*). For a process for making oleic acid from hemp seed oil, see *Archiv d. Pharm.*, 1886, p. 804. This form of oleic acid closely resembles linoleic acid, with which it also agrees in chemical composition, $C_{18}H_{32}O_2$.

Properties. "A yellowish, oily liquid, gradually becoming brown, rancid and acid, when exposed to the air; odorless or nearly so, tasteless, and, when pure, of a neutral reaction. Sp. gr. 0·900 to 0·910. The sp. gr. of 0·800 to 0·810 as printed in U. S. Pharm., 1880, was a misprint: the British Pharmacopœia gives the specific gravity as 0·860 to 0·890. Oleic Acid is insoluble in water, but completely soluble in alcohol, chloroform, benzol, benzin, oil of turpentine, and the fixed oils. "At 14° C. (57° F.), it becomes semi-solid, and remains so until cooled to 4° C. (39·4°

F.), at which temperature it becomes a whitish mass of crystals. At a gentle heat the acid is completely saponified by carbonate of potassium. If the resulting soap be dissolved in water and exactly neutralized with acetic acid, the liquid will form a white precipitate with test-solution of acetate of lead. This precipitate, after being twice washed with boiling water, should be almost entirely soluble in ether (abs. of more than traces of palmitic and stearic acids). Equal volumes of the Acid and of alcohol, heated to 25° C. (77° F.), should give a clear solution, without separating oily drops upon the surface (fixed oils)." *U. S.*

Chemical Constitution. Oleic acid, $C_{18}H_{34}O_2$, does not belong to the "fatty acid" series, but differs from the corresponding acid of that series, stearic acid, $C_{18}H_{36}O_2$, by having two atoms of hydrogen less. It belongs to a series derived by oxidation from alcohols, which, like allyl alcohol, C_3H_5OH, have two atoms of hydrogen less than the normal monatomic alcohols, like propyl alcohol, C_3H_7OH. The alcohol from which oleic acid is in theory derivable is not, however, known. Oleic acid is monobasic, as shown in the formula $HC_{18}H_{33}O_2$.

Medical Properties. Oleic acid is not itself used in medicine, but is officinal for the preparation of oleates, which act as corresponding ointments, but are more elegant and efficient.

Off. Prep. Oleatum Hydrargyri; Oleatum Veratrinæ.

Off. Prep. Br. Oleatum Hydrargyri; Oleatum Zinci; Unguentum Zinci Oleati.

ACIDUM OXALICUM. *Oxalic Acid.*

$H_2C_2O_4, 2H_2O$; 126. (ĂÇ'Ĭ-DŬM ŎX-ĂL'Ĭ-CŬM.) **$2HO\,C_4O_6, 4HO$; 126.**

Acide oxalique ou carboneux, *Fr.;* Oxalsäure, Kleesäure, *G.*

"In small, colorless, prismatic crystals, odorless and of a very sour taste, slightly efflorescent in dry air, fusible at 98° C. (208° F.), and entirely volatile at a red heat."*

This acid is found both in animals and vegetables. It is generated occasionally in consequence of a diseased action in the kidneys, and deposited in the bladder as oxalate of calcium, forming a peculiar concretion, called the *mulberry calculus.* In vegetables, it occurs in a free state in the bristles of the chick-pea (*Cicer arietinum*), as an acid potassium oxalate in *Rumex acetosa* or common sorrel, *Oxalis Acetosella* or wood-sorrel, *Chenopodium quinoa*, *Amarantus caudatus*, *Mesembrianthemum crystallinum*, and probably many other plants. It is said to be made in the leaves. (*Journ. Chem. Soc.*, 1886.) United with lime to form raphides, it is abundant in almost every portion of the vegetable kingdom.

Preparation. The usual process for obtaining oxalic acid consists in decomposing sugar by nitric acid. Four parts of sugar are acted upon by 24 of nitric acid of the sp. gr. 1·24, and the mixture is heated so long as any nitrogen tetroxide is disengaged. A part of the carbon of the sugar is converted into carbonic acid by oxygen derived from the nitric acid, which thereby is reduced to nitrogen tetroxide. The undecomposed nitric acid, reacting with the remaining elements of the sugar, generates oxalic and saccharic acids, the former of which crystallizes as the materials cool, while the latter remains in solution. The crystals being removed, a fresh crop may be obtained by further evaporation. The thick mother-water which now remains is a mixture of saccharic, nitric, and oxalic acids; and, by treating it with six times its weight of nitric acid, the greater part of the saccharic will be converted into oxalic acid. The new crop of crystals, however, will have a yellow color, and contain a portion of nitric acid, the greater part of which may be driven off by allowing them to effloresce in a warm place. It is probable that, in the reaction occurring between nitric acid and sugar, half the carbon of the latter is converted into carbonic acid, and the other half into oxalic acid.

Oxalic acid was formerly obtained on a large scale by heating a mixture of 112 lbs. of sugar, 560 lbs. of nitrate of potassium, and 280 lbs. of sulphuric acid. The products were 135 lbs. of oxalic acid, and 490 lbs. of acid sulphate of potassium, or *sal enixum.* This process has been replaced in practice by the "sawdust process" (see p. 91).

* See test-solution of oxalic acid at the end of the volume.

Many substances, besides sugar, yield oxalic acid by the action of nitric acid; as molasses, rice, potato starch, gum, wool, hair, silk, and many vegetable acids. In every case in which it is thus generated, the proportional excess of oxygen which it contains, compared with every other organic compound, is furnished by the nitric acid. When the acid is obtained from potato starch, this is first converted into starch sugar by the action of sulphuric acid. For details of this process, see 15th edition U. S. Dispensatory, p. 90. The yield of oxalic acid from a given quantity of material has been much understated. If properly treated with nitric acid, 100 lbs. of good sugar will yield from 125 to 130 lbs. of oxalic acid, and the same weight of molasses from 105 to 110 lbs.

Certain organic substances yield oxalic acid when heated with potassa. Wood-shavings, if mixed with a solution of caustic potassa, and exposed to a heat considerably higher than 100° C. (212° F.), will be decomposed, and partly converted into oxalic acid, which then combines with the alkali. At present most of the oxalic acid of commerce is obtained by heating saw-dust with a mixture of caustic soda and potassa. Soda alone will not generate the acid, and potassa is too costly to be used by itself for the purpose; but Mr. Dale ascertained that, by mixing the two in the proportion of two molecules of soda to one of potassa, the same or an even better result was obtained than from the latter alone. The mixture of caustic alkalies and saw-dust is made in a thick paste and then heated for several hours to a temperature of 200° C. (392° F.) to 220° C. (428° F.). The gray mass is then washed with carbonate of sodium, whereby the potash is removed as carbonate, the less soluble sodium oxalate remaining. This is converted into calcium oxalate, by milk of lime, and the calcium salt then decomposed with sulphuric acid. The impure oxalic acid is then purified by recrystallization. Bohlig has suggested an improvement by precipitating the solution of potassium oxalate with magnesium chloride or sulphate. (Bayer, *N. R.*, Aug. 1877.)

As the oxalic acid of commerce often contains more or less of foreign matter, it requires for certain purposes to be purified. It has sometimes been fraudulently mixed with 25 per cent. of Epsom salt. M. E. J. Maumené gives the following process for purification, which he says answers better than the method generally recommended. Sufficient hot water is added to the crystals to leave, on the cooling of the solution, 10 to 20 per cent. undissolved, according to the degree of impurity. The first crystals are put aside. The mother-water is then concentrated; and, if the resulting crystals be submitted to two or three successive crystallizations, the acid will be obtained finally free from alkaline oxalate. (*Journ. de Pharm.*, 1864, p. 154.) Stolba prefers the method of purification by crystallization from hydrochloric acid (boiling hot). (*Journ. App. Chem.*, Aug. 1874.) Villiers (*Journ. Chem. Soc.*, 1880, p. 544) prepares anhydrous oxalic acid by dissolving 1 part of ordinary acid in about 12 parts of warm concentrated sulphuric acid, allowing the oxalic acid to crystallize out.

Properties. Oxalic acid is a colorless crystallized solid, possessing considerable volatility, and a strong, sour taste. Its crystals have the shape of slender, flattened four- or six-sided prisms, with two-sided summits; and, when exposed to a very dry atmosphere, undergo a slight efflorescence. "Soluble in 4·5 parts of absolute alcohol, in 7 parts of alcohol, and almost insoluble in ether, chloroform, benzol, and benzin. The crystals should dissolve in not less than 8 to 10 parts of distilled water at 15° C. (59° F.) (greater solubility indicating contamination with adherent nitric acid.)" *U. S.*

It fuses in its water of hydration at 98° C. (208·4° F.), although continued exposure to a heat of 60° C. (140° F.) to 70° C. (158° F.) will render it perfectly anhydrous. Solutions of oxalic acid at 100° C. (212° F.) lose acid by sublimation, and at 157° C. (314·6° F.) it sublimes rapidly. If the heat rise to 160° C. (320° F.), much loss of acid occurs. (Allen, *Commer. Org. Anal.*, 1879, p. 233.)

It combines with salifiable bases, and forms salts called oxalates. The most interesting of these are the three *oxalates of potassium*, severally called *oxalate*, *binoxalate*, and *quadroxalate* (acid potassium oxalate plus free oxalic acid), and the *oxalate of calcium*. The binoxalate and quadroxalate, both popularly called *salt of sorrel* or *essential salt of lemons*, are employed for removing iron moulds from linen, and act by their excess of acid, which forms a soluble salt with the sesquioxide of iron constituting the stain. These oxalates are sometimes met with in the market contaminated with free sulphuric acid. Oxalic acid is used for removing ink stains and iron moulds, for cleaning the leather of boot-tops, and for discharging colors in calico-printing. Prussian blue dissolves in aqueous oxalic acid to a clear blue liquid which is often employed as a *blue ink*.

This acid has a very strong affinity for lime, and makes with it an insoluble precipitate consisting of oxalate of calcium, whenever the acid and earth are brought into contact in solution. An aqueous solution forms with solution of lime a white precipitate, insoluble in an excess of oxalic or acetic acid, but dissolved by dilute hydrochloric acid. It is even capable of decomposing fluoride of calcium, evolving hydrofluoric acid. (*J. W. Slater.*) Oxalic acid and its soluble combinations are the best tests for lime; and, conversely, a soluble salt of lime for oxalic acid. In weak solution the acid is said to absorb oxygen and to be converted into carbonic acid; but a strong solution is quite permanent. (*A. J. P.*, 1870, p. 317.) When lime is searched for, oxalate of ammonium is the most convenient test. So strong is the mutual attraction between this acid and lime, that the former takes the latter even from sulphuric acid. Hence the addition of a soluble oxalate disturbs the transparency of a solution of sulphate of calcium.

Oxalic acid is distinguished from all other acids by the form of its crystals, and by its solution yielding a precipitate with lime-water, insoluble in an excess of the acid or of acetic acid.

Composition. Anhydrous oxalic acid consists of two atoms of carbon 24, two of hydrogen 2, and four of oxygen 64 = 90. It is a bibasic acid. When crystallized, two molecules of water must be added, making the molecular weight of the crystals 126. These two molecules of water may be driven off by a regulated heat, by which the acid is made to effloresce. As oxalic acid is the final oxidation product of the diatomic alcohol *glycol*, to which the formula $\begin{array}{l}CH_2,OH\\|\\CH_2,OH\end{array}$ is given, we may conclude that its structural formula is $\begin{array}{l}CO,OH\\|\\CO,OH\end{array}$, which explains the readiness with which sulphuric acid splits it up into carbon dioxide, CO_2, and carbon monoxide, CO, by withdrawing H_2O from its formula, and with which oxidizing agents like manganese and lead dioxides change it into carbonic acid.

Medical and Toxical Properties. Oxalic acid has been employed as a substitute for citric acid, but at present is never used as a medicine. Attention was first called to it as a poison by Mr. Royston in 1814, and the certainty and rapidity of its action have caused it to be largely used for suicidal purposes. Death has been produced by it in ten minutes. (Case, *Chem. News*, April 24, 1868.) The minimum fatal dose recorded is one drachm (*Taylor*).

From the general resemblance which the crystallized oxalic acid bears to Epsom salt, many fatal mistakes have occurred in consequence of its being sold for that saline purgative. It is, however, at once distinguished by its sour taste.

Oxalic acid acts on the economy in two principal ways, according as its solution is concentrated or dilute. When concentrated it causes exquisite pain, followed by violent efforts to vomit, then sudden dulness, languor, and great debility, and finally death without a struggle. When dissolved in twenty times its weight of water, it possesses no corrosive and hardly any irritating power, but causes death by acting on the brain, spinal marrow, and heart. It should be noted, however, that the acid, in weak solution, always exercises a corroding or softening power on the animal tissues.

The morbid appearances caused by oxalic acid are various. In a dissection reported by Dr. Christison, the mucous coat of the throat and gullet had an appearance as if scalded, and that of the gullet could be easily scraped off. The inner coat of the stomach was pultaceous, in many points black, in others red, and that of the intestines, similarly but less violently affected. In another case, the whole villous coat of the stomach was either softened or removed, as well as the inner membrane of the œsophagus; so that the muscular coat was exposed, and this coat exhibited a dark, gangrenous appearance, being much thickened and highly injected. The stomach usually contains a dark fluid, resembling coffee-grounds, consisting chiefly of altered blood. The tongue and mouth are sometimes white or spotted with white. In a few cases no morbid appearances have been discovered.

In the treatment of poisoning by oxalic acid, the remedial measures must be employed with great promptitude. Vomiting may be encouraged and the stomach-pump used, but unless the antidote is at hand death will rarely be averted. The proper antidote is chalk or magnesia, mixed with water; and as soon as either can be procured, it must be administered in large and repeated doses. In many cases whitewash or some other preparation of lime can be obtained sooner than chalk, and should be at once administered. These substances act by forming with the poison an insoluble, inert oxalate of calcium or of magnesium. The soluble salts of oxalic acid, as oxalate of ammonium, and oxalate of potassium, are equally poisonous, and the antidotes for them are the same as for the acid.

The best tests for the detection of oxalic acid in the contents of the stomach, or in the vomited matter, in cases of suspected poisoning, are chloride of calcium, sulphate of copper, and nitrate of silver. The first causes a white precipitate of oxalate of calcium, known by its being soluble in nitric acid; the second, a bluish-white precipitate of oxalate of copper; and the third, a dense white precipitate of oxalate of silver, which, when dried and heated, becomes brown and detonates faintly. When the antidotes have been freely used during life, the poison will be in the state of oxalate either of calcium or magnesium. In this case, the oxalate found is to be boiled with a solution of carbonate of potassium, whereby an oxalate of potassium will be generated; and this must then be examined with the reagents above indicated.

ACIDUM PHOSPHORICUM. *U. S.* *Phosphoric Acid.*

(ĂÇ'Ĭ-DŬM PHŎS-PHŎR'Ĭ-CŬM.)

"A liquid composed of 50 per cent. of Orthophosphoric Acid [H_3PO_4; 98—3HO, PO_5; 98] and 50 per cent. of water." *U. S.*

ACIDUM PHOSPHORICUM CONCENTRATUM. *Br.* *Concentrated Phosphoric Acid.*

(ĂÇ'Ĭ-DŬM PHŎS-PHŎR'Ĭ-CŬM CŎN-CĔN-TRĀ'TŬM.)

Phosphoric acid, H_3PO_4, with 33·7 per cent. of water.

"Phosphorus, *sixteen parts;* Nitric Acid, Distilled Water, each, *a sufficient quantity,* To make *one hundred parts.* Mix *one hundred parts* of Nitric Acid with *one hundred parts* of Distilled Water, in a glass retort having the capacity of *four hundred parts.* Having placed the retort upon a sand-bath or wire-gauze support, connect it loosely with a well-cooled receiver and add to the acid in the retort the Phosphorus previously cut into fine pieces. Insert a funnel through the tubulure of the retort, and then gradually apply heat until the reaction is seen to commence. Regulate the heat carefully so as to prevent the reaction from becoming too violent, or, if necessary, check it by the addition of a little Distilled Water through the funnel. From time to time return the acid liquid, which collects in the receiver into the retort, until all the Phosphorus is dissolved. Then transfer the liquid to a weighed porcelain capsule, and continue the heat, at a temperature not exceeding 190° C. (374° F.), until the excess of Nitric Acid is driven off, and an odorless syrupy liquid remains. Cool the dish and contents, and add enough Distilled Water to make the liquid weigh *one hundred parts.* Test small portions for Nitric, Phosphorous, and Arsenic Acids by the following methods. If Nitric Acid should be present, evaporate the liquid until no reaction for Nitric Acid can be obtained. Then cool the Acid and add enough Distilled Water to make the product weigh *one hundred parts.* If Phosphorous Acid be present, add to the liquid a mixture of *six parts* of Nitric Acid and *six parts* of Distilled Water, and again evaporate until no reaction for Phosphorous or Nitric Acid can be obtained. Then, having cooled the Acid, add sufficient Distilled Water to make the product weigh *one hundred parts.* If Arsenic Acid be present, dilute the Acid with *one hundred and fifty parts* of Distilled Water, heat to about 70° C. (158° F.), and pass through the liquid a stream of Hydrosulphuric Acid Gas for half an hour, then remove the heat and continue passing the gas until the liquid is cold. Close the vessel tightly, set it aside for 24 hours, filter the liquid, heat it until all the odor of the gas has been driven off, again filter, and evaporate until the residue weighs *one hundred parts.* Preserve the product in glass-stoppered bottles." *U. S.*

"Phosphorus, 413 grains; Nitric Acid, 6 fluidounces [Imp. meas]; Distilled Water, a sufficiency. Put the nitric acid, diluted with eight [fluid]ounces [Imp. meas.] of distilled water, into a glass flask, the mouth of which may be connected with a vertical glass condenser; and having added the phosphorus and connected the condenser, boil the contents at such a rate that all condensed products shall return to the flask. Continue the action until the phosphorus has entirely disappeared. Remove the condenser and concentrate the fluid, either in the flask or in a porcelain dish of hard well-enamelled ware, until it is reduced to four fluidounces [Imperial meas.]; then, transferring it to a platinum vessel, continue the evaporation until it is reduced to about two fluidounces [Imp. meas.], and orange-colored vapors are no longer formed. Mix it now with distilled water until when cold it measures three fluidounces [Imp. meas.], and has a specific gravity of 1·5.

"Phosphoric acid may also be prepared from phosphorus by treatment of the product of atmospheric oxidation with water and a little nitric acid." *Br.*

This preparation, although in common use for the last few years, is for the first time officinal in the present Pharmacopœia. It is recommended on account of its small bulk and its great convenience to the apothecary for preparing the diluted acid. The glacial phosphoric acid is no longer officinal, it having been shown that it is practically impossible to obtain it of sufficient purity to be reliable. (See *Proc. A. P. A.*, 1875, pp. 666, 672.) The present syrupy acid is a great improvement in every way, as it can be obtained of undoubted purity and strength, and by simple dilution with water diluted phosphoric acid of any desired strength can easily be produced from it.* The process for its preparation is the old and well-known one of oxidising phosphorus by the use of nitric acid, the British method not differing materially from that of the U. S. Pharmacopœia, except in the absence of the use of the hydrosulphuric acid for precipitating arsenical compounds usually found in phosphorus, and in the greater strength of the finished British product. The British concentrated phosphoric acid contains 66·3 per cent. of orthophosphoric acid, whilst the U. S. phosphoric acid contains but 50 per cent. In both, phosphorus is oxidized at the expense of the nitric acid, any excess of nitric acid and all the lower oxides of nitrogen being driven off by heat. Strong nitric acid acts too energetically on phosphorus, producing explosion and rapid combustion; but when diluted, as in the processes above given, it parts with its oxygen slowly, and it is even desirable to aid the operation with a gentle heat. Along with the nitrous fumes, a portion of the undecomposed nitric acid also rises in vapor, which, in the British process to prevent loss, is collected by means of a distillatory apparatus, and returned to the retort. In the U. S. process of 1870, the same result was effected by placing over the liquid in the capsule a glass funnel, upon the inner surface of which the acid was condensed, and returned of itself into the capsule so as to considerably simplify the operation. This modification was originally suggested by Mr. Geo. W. Andrews, of Baltimore, who, however, inverted a dish over the materials; the suggestion of the funnel being due to Prof. Procter. The operation was continued till the whole of the phosphorus was converted into phosphoric acid and dissolved, and the liquid having been deprived of any remaining acid, and reduced to a certain weight by concentration, the process was completed by adding a certain measure of water; so that an acid of definite strength was obtained. Prof. Diehl found, in carrying this process into effect, that the glass funnel

* James T. Shinn (*A. J. P.*, Oct. 1880) proposes a formula for *Liquor Acidi Phosphorici* and *Liq. Acidi Phosph. Comp.* A similar preparation under the name of Horsford's Acid Phosphates has a large use in this country. The formula is as follows. *Liquor Acidi Phosphorici* (without Iron): Calcii Phosphat. 384 gr.; Magnesii Phosphat. 256 gr.; Potassii Phosphat. 192 gr.; Acidi Phosphorici (60 per cent.) 640 minims; Aquæ, q. s. ft. 1 pint. *Liq. Acidi Phosph. Comp.* (with Iron): Calc. Phosphat. 384 gr.; Magnes. Phosphat. 64 gr.; Potassii Phosphat. 32 gr.; Ferri Phosphat. 64 gr.; Acid Phosph. (60 per cent.) 815 minims; Aquæ q. s. ft. 1 pint.

covering the capsule almost always breaks through the violence of the reaction, thus causing loss of phosphorus, besides annoyance to the operator. He, therefore, prefers using a French tubulated glass retort, and this suggestion is adopted in the present process for Phosphoric Acid (see above). (*A. J. P.*, 1867, p. 138.) Prof. G. F. H. Markoe (*Proc. A. P. A.*, 1875, p. 677) proposed a method for making phosphoric acid which is particularly adapted for making large quantities, yet works well in a smaller way. Into a flask (or stone jar) having double the capacity of the materials used, 12 troyounces of water, 2 troyounces of phosphorus, and 10 grains of iodine are placed, then 40 grains of bromine are cautiously dropped in;* when the reaction has ceased, 12 troyounces of nitric acid are added; a glass funnel is adjusted in the neck of the flask, and a smaller inverted funnel set inside of it; the apparatus is placed in a stoneware dish, and surrounded with cold water or ice; the reaction takes place slowly and regularly. In about 24 hours, if all the phosphorus be not acted upon, heat may be applied until it disappears, and the excess of bromine, iodine, and nitric acid is driven off. The acid may then be diluted to the desired specific gravity. Prof. J. U. Lloyd (*N. R.*, July, 1880) suggests the use of pure alcohol, to unite with the nitric acid to form nitrous ether, which is more volatile and thus easier to drive off.

Prof. Markoe adds a small quantity of pure oxalic acid, and heats the mixture to 300° F.; at this temperature it is asserted that all of the oxalic acid splits into carbon monoxide and carbon dioxide.

Prof. Wenzell oxidizes phosphorus with moist air, modifying the process originating with Buchols; the phosphorus is partly covered with water, care being taken to arrange the sticks so that contact with one another is avoided as much as possible; air is admitted so that slow oxidation takes place, and phosphorus and phosphoric acid are found dissolved in the water; this mixture was formerly known as *phosphatic acid*. The phosphorus acid may be converted into phosphoric acid by exposure to air, or by treatment with nitric acid in the usual way. (*Proc. A. P. A.*, 1882; *Western Druggist*, 1886, p. 1.)

Much dissatisfaction has been caused among pharmacists by the fact that diluted phosphoric acid frequently produces a white precipitate in solutions of ferric salts. An examination proved that this occurred when the glacial acid is used, or when high heat had been employed in the concentration. Experiments conducted by Louis Dohme and Prof. Remington seemed to indicate that the precipitation resulted from the presence of pyrophosphoric acid. (*Proc. A. P. A.*, 1874, pp. 431, 511; 1875, pp. 663, 670, 677.) Considerable difficulty was experienced in driving off all the nitric acid, and in the attempt to do so, the temperature became so elevated as to reconvert some of the tribasic acid to the bibasic form. This occurred slightly at 148·8° C. (300° F.), but to a much greater extent between 176·6° C. (350° F.) and 204·4° C. (400° F.). The diluted acid, made from phosphorus, can be brought to the boiling-point of 232·2° C. (450° F.), and will then only produce a slight cloud with tincture of chloride of iron, but if diluted, when cool, with about half its bulk of cold water, which causes considerable elevation of temperature, it forms a clear solution. The same acid evaporated, heated to redness, allowed to congeal, and then dissolved in water, precipitated the iron solution. The addition of twenty per cent. of pyrophosphate of sodium to the same dilute acid made a preparation which in all respects resembled that made from the glacial acid; thus giving evidence that the presence of this contamination was the cause of the difference in the two preparations.

It has been suggested that red phosphorus might be substituted for common phosphorus, as producing the same results, with less danger of explosion; but when the officinal process is carefully followed in reference to the due dilution and to the use of a moderate heat, there is no danger to be apprehended.

The following is Schiff's table exhibiting the quantity of orthophosphoric acid and phosphoric anhydride contained in solutions of different densities at 15·5° C. (60° F.), from Bayley's *Chemist's Pocket Book.*

* Dr. W. H. Pile, of Philadelphia, met with a serious accident in preparing diluted phosphoric acid by this process, by adding the bromine too rapidly. (*A. J. P.*, 1875, p. 525.)

Specific Gravity.	Per Ct. H_3PO_4.	Per Ct. of P_2O_5.	Specific Gravity.	Per Ct. H_3PO_4.	Per Ct. of P_2O_5.	Specific Gravity.	Per Ct. H_3PO_4.	Per Ct. of P_2O_5.
1·0054	1	·726	1·1262	21	15·246	1·2731	41	29·766
1·0109	2	1·452	1·1329	22	15·972	1·2812	42	30·492
1·0164	3	2·178	1·1397	23	16·698	1·2894	43	31·218
1·0220	4	2·904	1·1465	24	17·424	1·2976	44	31·944
1·0276	5	3·630	1·1534	25	18·150	1·3059	45	32·670
1·0333	6	4·356	1·1604	26	18·876	1·3143	46	33·496
1·0390	7	5·082	1·1674	27	19·602	1·3227	47	34·222
1·0449	8	5·808	1·1745	28	20·328	1·3313	48	34·948
1·0508	9	6·534	1·1817	29	21·054	1·3399	49	35·674
1·0567	10	7·260	1·1889	30	21·780	1·3486	50	36·400
1·0627	11	7·986	1·1962	31	22·506	1·3573	51	37·126
1·0688	12	8·712	1·2036	32	23·232	1·3661	52	37·852
1·0749	13	9·438	1·2111	33	23·958	1·3750	53	38·578
1·0811	14	10·164	1·2186	34	24·684	1·3840	54	39·304
1·0874	15	10·890	1·2262	35	25·410	1·3931	55	40·030
1·0937	16	11·616	1·2338	36	26·136	1·4022	56	40·756
1·1001	17	12·342	1·2415	37	26·862	1·4144	57	41·482
1·1065	18	13·068	1·2493	38	27·588	1·4207	58	42·208
1·1130	19	13.794	1·2572	39	28·314	1·4301	59	42·934
1·1196	20	14.520	1·2651	40	29·040	1·4395	60	43·660

Properties. "A colorless liquid, without odor, of a strongly acid taste and reaction. Its specific gravity is 1·347 (1·5 *Br.*). When heated the liquid loses water, and when a temperature of about 200° C. (392° F.) has been reached, the acid is gradually converted into pyrophosphoric and metaphosphoric acids, which may be volatilized at a red heat. If the diluted acid be supersaturated with ammonia, addition of test mixture of magnesium produces a white crystalline precipitate. If this precipitate be dissolved in diluted acetic acid, the solution yields a yellow precipitate with test-solution of nitrate of silver. Phosphoric Acid, diluted with 5 volumes of water, and gently warmed, should not be blackened by test-solution of nitrate of silver, nor be turned white or whitish by test-solution of mercuric chloride (absence of phosphorous acid); when heated to about 70° C. (158° F.), thoroughly saturated during half an hour, and afterward until it is cold, with hydrosulphuric acid gas, then set aside for twenty-four hours, it should not deposit a lemon-yellow sediment (absence of arsenic acid). If a crystal of ferrous sulphate be dropped into a cooled mixture of Phosphoric and Sulphuric Acids, no brown or reddish zone should make its appearance around the crystal (absence of nitric acid). After diluting the Acid with 5 volumes of distilled water, no precipitate should be produced on the addition of small portions of test-solutions of chloride of barium (sulphuric acid), or of nitrate of silver (hydrochloric acid); nor should any precipitate be formed after several hours, by the addition of an equal volume of tincture of chloride of iron (pyrophosphoric and metaphosphoric acids).

"On pouring 5 Gm. of Phosphoric Acid upon 10 Gm. of oxide of lead free from carbonate of lead and from moisture, evaporating, and igniting, a residue will be obtained which should weigh 11·81 Gm." *U. S.*

Medical Properties. This acid is rarely used medicinally. It has the same properties and uses as the diluted Phosphoric Acid (see p. 99). The dose is 5 to 10 mimims (·3–·6 C.c.), one-fifth that of the diluted acid; of the British concentrated phosphoric acid 2 to 5 minims.

ACIDUM PHOSPHORICUM GLACIALE. (*Glacial Phosphoric Acid; Metaphosphoric Acid, Monobasic Phosphoric Acid; Monohydrated Phosphoric Acid; Acide phosphorique glacial,* Fr.; *Glasige Phosphorsäure,* G.) Formula HPO_3; mol. wt., 80. Phosphoric oxide consists of two atoms of phosphorus and five atoms of oxygen, P_2O_5, and can be obtained only by the direct union of its constituents, which takes place when phosphorus is burned in perfectly dry oxygen gas. Thus procured, it is in the form of a white amorphous powder, extremely deliquescent, volatilizable at a red heat, and assuming, when it cools after fusion, a vitreous appearance. The classic researches of Prof. Graham first established clearly the character of the several varieties of phosphoric acid, which may be considered as derived from this oxide. When amorphous phosphorus is boiled with nitric acid, or when phosphoric oxide is boiled with water, the oxide takes up three molecules of water, and yields tribasic or *ordinary phosphoric* acid, according to the reaction: $P_2O_5 + 3H_2O = H_6P_2O_8$ or $(H_3PO_4)_2$. If this acid be heated for a considerable time to 215° C. (419 F.), the two molecules lose one molecule of water and yield *pyrophosphoric* acid, a tetrabasic variety, according to the reaction: $H_6P_2O_8 - H_2O = H_4P_2O_7$. Lastly, at a red heat the ordinary phosphoric acid is converted into *metaphosphoric* acid, a monobasic variety, according to the reaction: $H_3PO_4 - H_2O = HPO_3$. This last variety may also be obtained direct from the oxide by dissolving it in cold water, when it takes up one molecule of water: $P_2O_5 + H_2O = H_2P_2O_6$ or $(HPO_3)_2$. (See *Chem. News*, Jan. 7, 1876; or *A. J. P.*, 1876, p. 109.) An aqueous solution of either of the three acids, heated so long as water escapes, yields the monobasic or metaphosphoric acid; and as, upon cooling, it becomes a transparent ice-like solid, it has received in this state the name of glacial phosphoric acid. Conversely, this monobasic acid is slowly transformed, in aqueous solution, and more rapidly if the solution is heated, into the tribasic form. Prof. Maisch has ascertained that nitric acid, added to the solution of the monobasic acid, with the aid of heat, causes the change from the monobasic to the tribasic form, viz., to the common phosphoric acid, without the intermediate production of the tetrabasic variety.

Tests. The three acids are distinguishable by peculiar reactions. Thus, the *monobasic* is characterized by coagulating albumen, and giving white gelatinous uncrystallizable precipitates with the soluble salts of baryta, lime, and silver; the *tetrabasic* does not coagulate albumen, and, though it causes a *white* precipitate with nitrate of silver, must first be neutralized; the tribasic does not coagulate albumen, and until neutralized does not precipitate nitrate of silver, but after neutralization throws down a *yellow* precipitate of phosphate of silver.

Glacial phosphoric acid is most advantageously obtained from calcined bones, by first treating them with sulphuric acid, which produces an insoluble sulphate and soluble acid phosphate of calcium; then dissolving out the latter salt, and saturating it with carbonate of ammonium, which generates phosphate of ammonium in solution; and, finally, obtaining the phosphate of ammonium by evaporation to dryness, and then igniting it in a platinum crucible. The ammonia and all the water except the one molecule needed for the formation of metaphosphoric acid are driven off, and the glacial acid remains.

Properties. Thus procured, glacial phosphoric acid is in the form of a white, uncrystallizable, fusible solid, inodorous, very sour to the taste, slowly deliquescent, slowly soluble in water, and soluble also in alcohol. Its formula is HPO_3, and it is made up of 11·2 per cent. of water in combination with 88·8 per cent. of phosphoric oxide. As already stated, it is characterized by producing white gelatinous precipitates with albumen, and with the soluble salts of lime, baryta, and silver; and the precipitate produced with the chloride of barium is readily redissolved by an excess of the acid. This is the form of the acid which results when the oxide, produced by burning phosphorus in dry oxygen gas, is introduced into cold water.

Impurities. Glacial phosphoric acid is seldom prepared in this country. That found in commerce is almost all imported, and chiefly from Germany. It is often more or less impure, containing, as shown by the experiments of Prof. Maisch, silica, and the phosphates of calcium and magnesium, which are precipitated from a neutralized solution of the acid by ammonia. In one instance 8 per cent. of these impurities was found; but in some others little or none. Prof. Maisch never found nitric or hydrochloric acid, and sulphuric acid rarely; and, though the presence of ammonia might be suspected from the source whence the acid is obtained, he did not detect it. (*A. J. P.*, 1860, p. 194.) The chief impurity, however, is soda, as has been pointed out by Brescius, Remington, Dohme, Prescott, and others (see *Proc. A. P. A.*, 1875, 666, 672); of late years the acid has been found to contain occasionally as much as 60 per cent. of sodium metaphosphate, and rarely less than 55 per cent. (*N. R.*, Feb. 1879.) In consequence of its deliquescence upon exposure to the air, a portion of the monobasic acid passes into the tribasic state. This is detected, if in considerable quantity, by its giving a yellowish color to the precipitate with nitrate of silver. The U. S. Pharm. 1870 directed that the acid, in aqueous solution, should yield no precipitate with sulphuretted hydrogen, showing the absence of metals; should cause a white precipitate with chloride of barium soluble in an excess of acid; with an excess of ammonia, should cause only a slight turbidity, proving the almost total absence of earthy salts; and should yield no ammonia when treated with potassa in excess. Should the presence of arsenic be ascertained by the tests for that metal, it may be separated by boiling with hydrochloric acid, so as to convert the arsenic into its very volatile chloride, which would escape with the vapors of the hydrochloric acid.

Glacial phosphoric acid was introduced into the Materia Medica of the Pharmacopœia of 1860 as affording a convenient method of preparing the medicinal acid, but, owing to its unreliability, was very properly dismissed from the present Pharmacopœia. Thirty-eight and a half grains, dissolved in a fluidounce of water, form a solution about equal in strength to the U. S. diluted acid of Pharm. 1860.

Off. Prep. Acidum Phosphoricum Dilutum; Syrupus Ferri, Quininæ et Strychninæ Phosphatum.

Off. Prep. Br. Acidum Phosphoricum Dilutum; Syrupus Ferri Phosphatis.

Off. Phosphates. Br. Ammonii Phosphas; Calcii Phosphas; Ferri Phosphas; Sodii Phosphas.

ACIDUM PHOSPHORICUM DILUTUM. *U. S., Br.* *Diluted Phosphoric Acid.*

(ĂÇ'Ĭ-DŬM PHŎS PHŎR'Ĭ-CŬM DĪ-LŪ'TŬM.)

Acide phosphorique médicinal, *F.;* Verdünnte Phosphorsäure, *G.*

"Phosphoric acid, H_3PO_4, in solution in water to the extent of 13·8 per cent. by weight, corresponding to 10 per cent. of phosphoric anhydride, P_2O_5." *Br.*

"Phosphoric Acid, *twenty parts* [or two and a half fluidounces]; Distilled Water, *eighty parts* [or thirteen and a half fluidounces]. To make *one hundred parts* [or one pint]. Mix the Phosphoric Acid with the Distilled Water. Diluted Phosphoric Acid has a specific gravity of 1·057, and contains 10 per cent. of orthophosphoric acid. It should respond to the tests of purity required for Phosphoric Acid. On pouring 5 Gm. of Diluted Phosphoric Acid upon 5 Gm. of oxide of lead free from carbonate and from moisture, evaporating and igniting, a residue will be obtained which should weigh 5·36 Gm." *U. S.*

"Concentrated Phosphoric Acid, 3 fluidounces [Imp. meas.]; Distilled Water, a sufficiency to form 20 fluidounces [Imp. meas.]. Mix." *Br.*

It will be observed that in both Pharmacopœias, diluted phosphoric acid is made by simple dilution of the stronger acid, and that the older method of dissolving the glacial acid has been very properly abandoned. (See *Acidum Phosphoricum Glaciale.*) The officinal diluted acid is weaker than the British, the U. S. P. acid containing 10 per cent. of orthophosphoric acid, whilst the British contains 10 per cent. of phosphoric anhydride, P_2O_5, which corresponds to about 14 per cent. of orthophosphoric acid. The specific gravity of the British acid is 1·08, and 355 grains of it (6 fluidrachms) mixed with 180 grains of oxide of lead in fine powder leave by evaporation a residue (principally phosphate of lead) which after it has been heated to dull redness weighs 215·5 grains. Six fluidrachms contain one-half of the molecular weight of phosphoric acid in grains, 49 (H_3PO_4=98); equivalent to one-fourth of the molecular weight of phosphoric anhydride in grains, 35·5 (P_2O_5=142).

Properties. Diluted phosphoric acid is a colorless, inodorous, sour liquid, acting strongly on litmus, and possessing powerful acid properties. Although evaporated so as to become dense, it is not corrosive like the other mineral acids. Dr. Neubauer found that the strong acid, when pure and warm, was capable of dissolving oxalate of calcium. The officinal acid is not precipitated by chloride of barium or nitrate of silver. If precipitates are produced, chloride of barium indicates sulphuric acid or a sulphate; nitrate of silver, hydrochloric acid or a chloride. Strips of copper or silver are not affected by the acid, showing the absence of nitric acid; it is not colored by sulphuretted hydrogen, proving the general absence of metals; and albumen produces no precipitate with it, indicating the non-existence of metaphosphoric acid. If carbonate of sodium causes a precipitate, phosphate of calcium, or some other phosphate insoluble in water, is probably held in solution. It has been supposed that one-tenth of phosphorous acid would render the diluted acid dangerous to life; but experiments go far to show that this was an erroneous opinion, as half a drachm of that acid given to a dog produced no obvious poisonous effect. (See *A. J. P.*, 1858, p. 359.) Phosphorous acid may be detected by testing the medicinal acid with a solution of corrosive sublimate, which will be converted into calomel if this impurity be present. (Pagels, *Chem. Gaz.*, Jan. 15, 1857.)

When diluted phosphoric acid is kept some time it is very apt to contain microscopic plants. The presence of traces of hydrochloric acid is said to prevent their formation, according to Rother, *Drug. Circ.*, 1886, p. 99; see, also, paper by Prof. L. E. Sayre, *Proc. A. P. A.*, 1885, and one by Samuel G. Ade, *Proc. A. P. A.*, 1884.

Medical Properties and Uses. Diluted phosphoric acid is deemed tonic and refrigerant. It is free from astringency, and is certainly a valuable remedy in many cases of dyspepsia. Various properties have been ascribed to it; such as allaying pain and spasm, strengthening the sexual organs, preventing the morbid secretion of bony matter, and correcting phosphatic deposits in the urine. The last two properties are supposed to depend upon its power of dissolving phosphate of calcium. It has been recommended in hysteria, in diabetes, and in leucorrhœa when the secreted fluid is thin and acrid; it has also been used with asserted good results in low fevers, but probably has no action upon the system other than that upon the digestive organs, although Dr. A. Judson (*Ann. de Thérap.*, 1871 and 1872, p. 152) asserts that in doses of from one to three drachms it acts as a stimulant, increasing the force and frequency of the pulse, and causing headache and cerebral confusion,—effects which may be the result of gastric irritation. The dose is from twenty drops to a teaspoonful (1·25–3·75 C.c.), largely diluted with water.

ACIDUM SALICYLICUM. *U.S., Br.* *Salicylic Acid.*

$HC_7H_5O_3$; 138. (ĂÇ'Ĭ-DŬM SĂL-Ĭ-ÇȲL'Ĭ-CŬM.) $HO, C_{14}H_5O_5$; 138.

Ortho-Oxybenzoic Acid, *E.*; Acide salicylique, *Fr.*; Salicylsäure, *G.*

"A crystalline acid obtained by the combination of the elements of carbolic acid with those of carbonic acid gas and subsequent purification, or from natural salicylates such as the oils of wintergreen (Gaultheria procumbens, *Linn.*) and sweet birch (Betula lenta, *Linn.*)." *Br.*

In 1834 salicyl aldehyd (*salicylous acid*) was discovered by Pagenstecher in the flowers of *Spiræa Ulmaria.* In 1837, Piria and Ettling found that by oxidizing agents salicyl aldehyd was converted into a new body, salicylic acid, and in 1839, Löwig and Weidmann derived the latter principle directly from the flowers of the *Spiræa Ulmaria.* Shortly afterwards Prof. Procter (*A. J. P.*, 1843; Aug. 1875) discovered that the acid could be procured from the oil of wintergreen (*Gaultheria procumbens*). Modern research has shown that many essential oils contain methyl salicylate, of which ether, oil of wintergreen contains 90 per cent. When potassa is added, a new salt is formed, from which the acid is readily obtained by means of hydrochloric acid. Notwithstanding the discovery of this fact, and also the invention of still another process of manufacture by Ettling in 1845, salicylic acid remained so expensive as to be of no value in the arts until Kolbe and Lautemann discovered that it could be prepared by uniting phenol with carbonic acid through the instrumentality of sodium. The article now began to attract some attention, but remained beyond the reach of general use until Prof. Kolbe, continuing his researches, succeeded, in 1874 (*Journ. für Prakt. Chemie*, July, 1874), in producing it at a moderate cost.

Preparation. While salicylic acid may be prepared from salicin by fusion with potassium hydrate, or from oil of wintergreen by saponification with potassium hydrate solution, practically it is now obtained, according to Kolbe's patent, by treating sodium phenol (or carbolate) with carbon dioxide gas. For this purpose, the most concentrated caustic soda solution is evaporated with the corresponding amount of phenol to a dry powder, which is then heated to 100° C. (212° F.), while a stream of dry carbon dioxide gas is passed over it. The temperature is gradually raised to 180° C. (356° F.), increased to 220° C. (428° F.) as soon as phenol distils over, and finally raised to 250° C. (482° F.), until no more phenol distils. In the retort, the half of the phenol used remains as sodium salicylate, while the other half has distilled over unchanged. The reaction is as follows: $2C_6H_5ONa + CO_2 = C_6H_5OH + C_6H_4(ONa),COO,Na$.

The sodium salt thus obtained is dissolved in water, decomposed by hydrochloric acid, the salicylic acid filtered off, washed, and crystallized out of hot water, or purified by sublimation in a current of superheated steam. An important improvement has recently been made in Kolbe's process whereby all the phenol-sodium is converted into salicylate instead of half of it only. R. Schmitt has found (*Wagner's Jahresbericht für Chem. Tech.*, 1885, p. 490) that if dry sodium phenolate and dry carbon dioxide are allowed to act on each other at ordinary temperatures, as long as absorption takes place a phenyl-sodium carbonate, $CO\left\{\begin{matrix}OC_6H_5\\ONa\end{matrix}\right.$, is formed. If this is now heated for several hours in a closed vessel to 140° C., a molecular rearrangement takes place, and simple salicylate of sodium, $C_6H_4(OH)COONa$, is formed without any separation whatever of phenol. Schmitt's process has been purchased by the owners of Kolbe's patent.* Salicylic acid has been also obtained synthetically from copper benzoate and water, which, when heated together in sealed tubes, yield cuprous oxide, free benzoic acid, and salicylic acid. (E. F. Smith, *Am. Chem. Jour.*, 2, p. 338.) Dr. A. Rautert has found that the acid volatilizes with steam of 170° C. (338° F.), and has devised a process of purification based upon this, which yields at very little cost a beautiful product. Biel (*Pharm. Zeitsch. f. Russl.*, 1876) reports that the sublimed acid is liable to decompose spontaneously. Dialyzed salicylic acid of beautiful appearance has been in the market since 1876. All traces of tarry matter can be removed by dialysis, and this acid is unexceptionable. Kolbe also obtained salicylic acid from the carbolates of barium and calcium, but the yield was less than when the sodium salt was employed. The potassium phenol yielded only a trace of the salicylic acid, but an abundance of *paraoxybenzoic* acid.

Properties. Salicylic acid, when pure, occurs as a snow-white crystalline powder, free from odor, and also from taste, but leaving a sense of astringency on the tongue and of irritation in the fauces, with an increased flow of saliva. "Fine, white, light, prismatic, needle-shaped crystals, permanent in the air, free from odor of carbolic acid, but sometimes of a slight aromatic odor, of a sweetish and slightly acrid taste and an acid reaction." *U.S.* To the mucous membrane of the nose it is irritating, and will sometimes produce sneezing. It crystallizes out of its hot watery solution on cooling in slender, often very long needles, and on the spontaneous evaporation of its alcoholic solution in large four-sided prisms. It is strongly acid, acting decisively on blue litmus, and forming salts not only with alkalies, but also with metallic oxides. Salicylic acid is "soluble in 450 parts of water and in 2·5 parts of alcohol at 15° C. (59° F.); in 14 parts of boiling water; very soluble in boiling alcohol; also soluble in 2 parts of ether, in 2 parts of absolute alcohol, in 3·5 parts of amylic alcohol, and 80 parts of chloroform. When heated to about 175° C. (347° F.) the crystals melt, and at about 200° C. (392° F.) they begin to sublime; at a higher temperature they are volatilized and decomposed, with odor

* Professor J. U. Lloyd gives the following process for preparing salicylic acid from oil of wintergreen. Pure wintergreen oil, 3 parts; white caustic potash, 3 parts; hydrochloric acid, 8 parts; water, q. s. Dissolve the caustic potassa in two parts of water in a glass or porcelain vessel, and heat to the temperature of 180° F. Stir into this gradually the oil, using a glass or porcelain spatula. Into another vessel place 64 parts of cold distilled water, and add the hydrochloric acid. Then with constant stirring add the solution of salicylate of potassium. The magma of minute crystals of salicylic acid must be separated with a thin muslin strainer (previously moistened) and pressed, then dried by exposure to a temperature of 150°. The yield of this crude acid will be slightly over two parts. Dissolve this in six parts of cold alcohol and filter through a funnel stopped with cotton. Then with constant stirring pour the filtrate into 32 parts of cold water. The magma of minute crystals must be separated with a thin muslin strainer, and dried by exposure to a heat of 150 F. The yield is a trifle less than 2 parts.

of carbolic acid. The aqueous solution is colored intensely violet-red by test-solution of ferric chloride." *U. S.* When heated rapidly it is converted into carbolic and carbonic acids. It is stated that, by careful heating, glycerin can be made to dissolve 1 part in 50, and that the solution not only remains clear on cooling, but also may be diluted with water without separating. (*A. J. P.*, 1875, p. 212.) Dr. Goldsborough affirms that a mixture of the acid with alcohol, 1 to 10, may be diluted with 150 parts of water without crystallizing. By the presence of various neutral salts, its solubility is increased without its antiseptic value being interfered with. Thus:

Mixed with	1 part	potassium nitrate,	it dissolves in	50	parts	cold water.
" "	1½ "	ammonium citrate,	"	60	"	" "
" "	2 parts	sodium sulphite,	"	50	"	" "
" "	2 "	sodium phosphate,	"	50	"	" "
" "	2½ "	sodium phosphate,	"	12½	"	" "

(Allan, *Commerc. Org. Analysis*, 1879, p. 344; see, also, paper by R. Rother, *A. J. P.*, 1886, p. 420.)

On distilling salicylic acid or one of its salts with wood-spirit and sulphuric acid, acid methyl salicylate is formed, having an agreeable aromatic odor. The reaction with ferric salts is much more delicate (1 in 100,000) than that of phenol with the same reagent (1 in 3000). Commercial salicylic acid is often very impure. Chloride of sodium, carbolic acid, cresotic acid, and oxybenzoic and para-oxybenzoic acids are the usual impurities. The first of these substances remains on igniting the acid. Carbolic acid may be detected by nearly neutralizing the sample with soda and agitating the liquid with ether. On evaporating, the ethereal liquid leaves the carbolic acid recognizable by its smell and taste. (Allen, *Commerc. Org. Anal.*, p. 347.)

The most sensitive test for it is a ferric salt, with which it develops a beautiful violet color. Goldsborough states that to insure the delicacy of this reaction it is necessary that the iron salt be perfectly neutral; also that with this precaution he has clearly detected 1 part of the acid in 400,000 parts of water. On the addition of ammonia the violet color is changed to a reddish brown, then to an orange, then to a permanent greenish yellow. Sulphuric and nitric acids change the violet to a light brown (*Goldsborough*). It must be remembered that salicylous acid reacts similarly with ferric salts. Salicylous acid, however, precipitates the potassic or ammonio-nitrate of silver white, the salicylic acid yellow. Kolbe recommends a simple test to detect impurities. A little of the acid is dissolved in 10 times its weight of strong alcohol, and the solution allowed to evaporate spontaneously from a watch crystal. If the salicylic acid which remains in the dish be perfectly colorless, the acid is strictly pure; it should not be of a brown color, although a slight yellowish color would not indicate sufficient impurity to affect its medicinal value. Hager states that pure salicylic acid equal in volume to the size of a bean will yield, after agitation with about 5 C.c. of pure sulphuric acid, a colorless solution, while others which yielded a white residue from the alcoholic solution, rendered yellowish to brown-yellow solutions. (*Pharm. Centralbl.*, 1876, No. 51; *A. J. P.*, June, 1877.)

By distilling with alcohol and strong sulphuric acid, salicylic acid forms methyl- and ethyl-salicylic acids.

Tests. "A solution of 1 part of Salicylic Acid in 10 parts of alcohol, mixed with a few drops of nitric acid, should not become turbid upon the addition of a few drops of test-solution of nitrate of silver (absence of hydrochloric acid). A saturated solution in absolute alcohol, when allowed to evaporate spontaneously in an atmosphere free from dust, should leave a perfectly white crystalline residue, without a trace of color at the points of the crystals (absence of organic impurities; also of iron). On agitating a portion of Salicylic Acid with 15 parts of concentrated sulphuric acid, no color should be imparted to the latter within 15 minutes (foreign organic matter). If 5 C.c. of a saturated aqueous solution of Salicylic Acid be poured into a test tube, into which had been introduced, shortly before, a crystal of chlorate of potassium and 2 C.c. of hydrochloric acid, and some water of ammonia be now carefully poured on top, the latter should not assume a reddish or brownish tint (absence of carbolic acid)." *U. S.*

Medical Properties and Uses. Salicylic acid was originally brought to the notice of the profession on account of its inhibitory influence on putrefaction. Kolbe found that 0·04 per cent. had great influence in preventing souring of milk. Bucholz found that 0·15 per cent. of the acid is sufficient to prevent the development of bacteria in ordinary organic mixtures, and that the influence of 0·005 per cent. is plainly visible; 0·3 to 0·4 per cent. of the acid killed bacteria in vigorous growth. (*Arch. Exper. Path. u. Pharm.*, Bd. iv.) The salicylate of sodium was about equal to the pure acid, 0·4 per cent. destroying the bacteria. In the preservation of urine, Meyer and Kolbe found that one part of salicylic acid to two thousand of urine was sufficient to prevent putrefaction. (*Journ. für Prakt. Chem.*, Bd. xii.) According to Kolbe and others, salicylic acid arrests or prevents the action of the non-organized organic ferments. Thus, it will prevent the development of the hydrocyanic acid by the action of emulsin upon amygdalin in the presence of water, and will also inhibit the formation of the volatile oil of mustard. Dr. Miller found that one per cent. of salicylic acid was sufficient to check the action of ptyaline upon starch, thus equalizing in power ten per cent. of carbolic acid. He also found that 0·2 per cent. of salicylic acid affected outside of the body the digestive action of pepsin; but it must be remembered that large doses of it taken internally have no perceptible influence on gastric digestion, although in certain diseases they do seem to control fermentation of the gastro-intestinal contents. The experience of surgeons is in accord with these facts, and there can be no doubt that salicylic acid is capable of accomplishing much in antiseptic surgery, but it does not seem to be replacing carbolic acid, as it at one time bade fair to do. Its freedom from odor and comparative freedom from poisonous and irritant properties are certainly strong recommendations; nevertheless, carbolic acid is more generally employed, and Mr. Callender, after twelve months' trial in the wards of St. Bartholomew's Hospital, has formally condemned salicylic acid as much inferior to carbolic acid. (*Trans. London Clin. Soc.*, ix.) Thiersch's *salicylic acid wadding* for hermetically sealing wounds is made by dissolving two ounces of the acid in two pints of alcohol (sp. gr. 0·83), diluting with twenty pints of water at 158° to 178° F., saturating with this six pounds and eight ounces of cotton batting deprived of oily matter, and afterwards drying. This wadding contains 3 per cent. of the acid; for some purposes a stronger batting, containing 10 per cent., is prepared. When the wound or abscess is discharging profusely, jute is substituted for the cotton batting, because it is much more permeable to pus. An efficient ointment may be prepared by dissolving one and a half parts of the acid in two parts of alcohol and adding lard, or the solubility of the drug in glycerin may be taken advantage of. The following solutions are used in St. Bartholomew's Hospital. Phosphate of sodium three parts; salicylic acid one part; water fifty parts.—Salicylic acid one part; olive oil forty-nine parts.—Salicylic acid one part; bicarbonate of sodium half part; water one hundred parts.—Salicylic acid ten parts; borax eighteen parts; water one hundred parts. A 25 per cent. solution, which will bear dilution with water or alcohol may be prepared according to the following formula. ℞ Acid. salicyl. ʒii; Sodii biborat. ʒi; Glycerini q. s. Mix the acid and borax with four fluidrachms of glycerin; heat gently until dissolved; then add enough glycerin to make one fluidounce.* Prof. Thiersch has found that the drug cannot be employed for cleaning surgical instruments, because it corrodes the steel.

When salicylic acid is given to man in doses just sufficient to manifest its presence, symptoms closely resembling those of cinchonism result. These are fulness of the head, with roaring and buzzing in the ears. After larger doses, to these symptoms are added distress in the head, or positive headache, disturbances of hearing and vision (deafness, amblyopia, partial blindness), and excessive sweating. In some cases there is a decided fall of temperature without alteration of the pulse; but probably more commonly the bodily temperature remains unaltered. The actions upon the system of the acid and of its sodium, ammonium, potassium, and methyl

* *Mixture of Salicylic Acid and Iron* is largely used in hospital practice. The following is the formula of the New York Hospital. Salicylic acid, 20 gr.; pyrophosphate of iron, 5 gr.; phosphate of sodium, 50 gr.; water, sufficient to make 1½ fluidounces. Filter. (*Pharm. Rec.*, 1886, p. 115.)

(oil of gaultheria) salts appear to be identical, and, as several cases of poisoning with one or other of these agents have occurred, we are able to trace the toxic manifestations. Along with an intensification of the symptoms already mentioned, there are ptosis, deafness, strabismus, mydriasis, disturbance of respiration, excessive restlessness passing into delirium, slow laboring pulse, olive-green urine, and involuntary evacuations. In some cases the temperature has remained about normal, but in others has approached that of collapse. The respiration seems to be characteristic, it being both quickened and deepened, often sighing. Sweating usually is very free, and the urine early becomes albuminous. Various local evidences of vaso-motor weakness may supervene, such as rapidly appearing bed-sores at points subjected to pressure, and transitory dark colored maculæ on various parts of the body. In several cases death was probably produced by the acid, although there is scarcely one instance which is beyond doubt. In certain cases the mental disturbance has been strangely prolonged, lasting for eight days. In some instances it is cheerful, in others melancholic in type. It is stated that upon drunkards the acid acts very unfavorably, violent delirium being an early symptom of its influence.

Upon the lower mammals the drug acts very much as it does upon man, but we have not sufficient knowledge to enable us to frame a complete theory of its action. It undoubtedly affects very markedly the nerve centres, and, in sufficient dose, seems to be a paralyzant to all the higher nerve tissue. The earlier cerebral symptoms and the quickening of the respiration indicate that it stimulates the centres at the base of the brain before overwhelming them. Small doses seem to have very little influence upon the arterial pressure, although Danewsky affirms that moderate doses produce vaso-motor spasm of centric origin, with consequent rise of pressure. After toxic doses the force of the circulation is decreased chiefly, according to the researches of Köhler and of Danewsky, by a direct depression of the heart itself.

Salicylic acid is undoubtedly absorbed; probably in the form of a salicylate. It is eliminated chiefly by the kidneys, appearing in the urine soon after its administration, but escaping only slowly from the system. According to Byanon, it is excreted partly as salicyluric acid, partly as a form of salicin, and he believes to some extent as oxalic acid. Urine which had been passed some hours after the ingestion of a dose polarized to the left. Dr. A. E. Stuart (*Lond. Practitioner*, vol. xviii. p. 425), after so small a dose as nine grains of the acid, saw free, distinct crystals of salicyluric acid in the urine. It is possible that such of the salicylic acid as escapes unchanged from the kidney may, as first excreted, be in the form of a salicylate, but be set free by the acid of the urine. The green coloration of the urine characteristic of poisoning by this substance is stated not to be due to the presence of a derivative of the acid, but to the excessive formation of indican or allied coloring principle.

In health therapeutic doses of salicylic acid have no constant influence upon the bodily temperature, but in febrile disorders its powers are beyond question. The first effect of a single antipyretic dose in fever is usually a profuse sweat, which may appear fifteen minutes after the ingestion of the remedy. (Ewald, *London Practitioner*, vol. xvi. p. 200.) Very shortly after this the temperature begins to fall, and, according to Justi (*Centralblatt für Chirurgie*, 1876, p. 629), the depression reaches its maximum in about six hours. The sweating is profuse and exhausting, amounting, according to Ewald, not rarely to seven hundred and fifty grammes. The perspiration can scarcely be the only factor in the reduction of temperature, as there appears to be no relation between its amount and the degree of the fall, and it usually ceases before the latter reaches its maximum. The antipyretic dose employed varies somewhat. Ewald gives as a minimum to the adult seventy-five grains, repeated in five hours if necessary; Justi, from ninety to one hundred and twenty-five grains. The question as to whether good is achieved in fevers by its administration is, of course, entirely separate from that as to its power of reducing temperature. It is certainly possible for a drug to lower the fever-heat, and yet to do far more harm than good, and the evidence at hand appears to show that in typhoid and other allied febrile affections salicylic acid is not an eligible remedy. It is, indeed, no longer used, having been replaced by antipyrin. The possession of very marked antiperiodic powers has been claimed for salicylic acid, but experience has not substantiated this claim. In rheumatism the remedy is the most valuable one known. Although some cases do not seem to yield to the drug, in the great majority of instances improvement sets in within twenty-four hours, and is rapidly followed by disappearance of the pain and fever. The dangers of cardiac and cerebral complications are certainly lessened, but not altogether done away with. In excessive *rheumatic hyperpyrexia* it cannot be depended upon to the exclusion of the cold bath. Jaccoud states (*Progrès Méd.*, 1877, pp. 528, 745) that he has found it of great service in *chronic rheumatism;* but the general testimony appears to show that it is much less certain in the chronic than in the acute disorder. In accord, however, with the French professor, we have found it efficient in chronic cases. Jaccoud also states that in acute *gout* it acts with extraordinary effect. As in cases of habitual gout the kidneys are often seriously affected, the urine should always be examined, and if it be found albuminous the remedy should be withheld. The dose of salicylic acid in acute rheumatism may be set down as a drachm in the twenty-four hours, although it is employed by some practitioners in much larger doses. It may be given in powder, but is best administered in the form of the salicylate of sodium or of ammonium (fifteen grains five times in twenty-four hours), which are equally efficacious and much less irritant to the stomach than is the acid. If ringing of the ears or other evidences of intoxication appear, the remedy should at once be partially or entirely withdrawn.

Salicylic acid has been used for the preservation of various articles of food, but the employment of it should be interdicted, a commission appointed by the French government having reported that its prolonged use even in very small amounts is dangerous, especially to aged persons.

Off. Prep. Br. Unguentum Acidi Salicylici; Sodii Salicylas.

ACIDUM SULPHURICUM. *U.S., Br.* *Sulphuric Acid.*

H_2SO_4; 98. (ĂÇ'Ĭ-DŬM SŬL-PHŪ'RĬ-CŬM.) HO,SO_3; 49.

"A liquid, composed of not less than 96 per cent. of absolute Sulphuric Acid [**H_2SO_4; 98**—HO,SO_3; 49], and not more than 4 per cent. of Water." *U.S.* "An acid produced by the combustion of sulphur and the oxidation and hydration of the resulting sulphurous acid gas by means of nitrous and aqueous vapors. It contains about 98 per cent. by weight of real sulphuric acid, H_2SO_4." *Br.*

Acidum Sulfuricum, *P.G.;* Oil of Vitriol, Vitriolic Acid; Acide sulfurique, Huile de Vitriol, *Fr.;* Vitriolöl, Schwefelsäure, *G.;* Acido solforico, *It.;* Acido sulfurico, *Sp.*

Preparation. Sulphuric acid is obtained by burning sulphur or iron pyrites, FeS_2, and allowing the product of combustion, SO_2, to mix with nitrous fumes obtained from the decomposition of nitre, which change SO_2 into SO_3, and this uniting with steam yields H_2SO_4. If the sulphur were burned by itself, the product would be sulphurous oxide, which contains only two-thirds as much oxygen as sulphuric oxide. The object of the nitre is to furnish, by its decomposition, the requisite additional quantity of oxygen. To understand the process, it is necessary to remember that several of the oxides of nitrogen have oxidizing power. Thus, the main reactions of the sulphuric acid process are universally conceded to be: $2SO_2 + N_2O_4 = 2SO_3 + N_2O_2$, $SO_3 + H_2O = H_2SO_4$, $N_2O_2 + O_2 = N_2O_4$; in which the sulphurous oxide, from the burning pyrites or sulphur, is oxidized to sulphuric oxide by the nitrogen tetroxide, which readily parts with two atoms of oxygen to such bodies as sulphurous oxide, and then takes two atoms of oxygen again from the atmosphere, regenerating the original tetroxide. The nitrogen tetroxide thus acts simply as a carrier of atmospheric oxygen, whereby the SO_2 is changed into SO_3. This latter compound then unites with steam to form H_2SO_4, the final product.

If the supply of steam be insufficient, at the same time white crystals (*lead chamber crystals*) are observed to form, which have the composition $HSO_3(NO_2)$, and whose formation is explained by the following reactions: $2SO_2 + H_2O + N_2O_3 + O_2 = 2HSO_3(NO_2)$; when steam enters in larger amount they disappear with formation of sulphuric acid, while red fumes are given off, thus: $2HSO_3(NO_2) + H_2O = 2H_2SO_4 + N_2O_3$. In this case, therefore, nitrous oxide, N_2O_3, assists in the oxidation.

Preparation on the Large Scale. The manufacture of this most important chemical has grown to enormous proportions. In England, where it is manufactured in largest amount, the present annual production is over 940,000 tons, six-sevenths of which is from Spanish pyrites and one-seventh from crude sulphur (*Lunge*). In this country Sicilian sulphur is used, thereby giving a product practically free from arsenic, which is not the case with the acid made from pyrites. As carried out in England, the process is as follows. Beginning with the pyrites-kilns, or burners, the broken mineral is placed in moderate-sized lumps on the bars of the burners, which have previously been heated to redness, and when the burning is once started, the fire is kept up by placing a new charge on the top of that nearly burned out. The ordinary charge for each burner of pyrites, containing about 48 per cent. of sulphur, is 5 to 6 cwt., which is burnt out in twenty-four hours. The hot sulphur dioxide and air are drawn from the pyrites-burners through the whole system of tubes, towers, and chambers by help of the powerful draught from a large chimney, which is placed in connection with the apparatus. These gases then pass either into a tall tower (called the Glover or denitrating tower), where they meet a descending stream of strong sulphuric acid charged with nitrous fumes, which at this moment of descent is mixed with a weaker sulphuric acid, thereby liberating the nitrous fumes, and these then mix with the sulphur dioxide and air, or they are charged with nitrous fumes direct from the nitre pots, where a mixture of Chili saltpetre and sulphuric acid liberates them. The mixed gases are then delivered at a temperature of about 75° C. (167° F.) into the first of the leaden chambers. These chambers, of which there are three, are now made of much larger size than was formerly the case, having often a capacity of 38,000 cubic feet. Here the gases meet jets of steam and deposit liquid sulphuric acid, as also in the second chamber. In the third or exhaust chamber all the sulphur dioxide should have been converted into sulphuric acid, and red nitrous fumes must always be visible. These must not be lost, but are drawn into a so-called Gay-Lussac tower filled with coke, over which a finely-divided shower of strong acid is allowed to fall. The nitrous fumes are absorbed by this, and give the so-called nitrated acid used as before mentioned in the Glover tower. The acid obtained in the leaden chamber has a sp. gr. of 1·55, or contains 64 per cent. of H_2SO_4. The acid which comes from the Glover tower (or, in case this is not used, is obtained by further concentration of chamber acid in leaden pans) has a sp. gr. of 1·71, and contains 78 per cent. H_2SO_4. The strongest acid must be procured by still further concentration in glass or platinum vessels, and will contain 98 per cent. H_2SO_4. (Roscoe and Schorlemmer, *Chem.*, vol. i. pp. 321–338.)

According to theory, 100 parts of sulphur burnt should yield 305·9 parts of pure sulphuric acid. In practice the yield is 290–294. The amount of nitrate of sodium used varies very much. Manufacturers who employ Glover and Gay-Lussac towers require from 3·5 to 6·5 parts of nitrate for every 100 of sulphur burnt, while works unprovided with these appliances may take from 12 to 13 parts. (*Roscoe and Schorlemmer*, vol. i. p. 337.)

The process for making sulphuric acid by the combustion of sulphur with nitre was first mentioned by Lemery, and afterwards put in practice by an English physician, of the name of Ward. As practised by him, the combustion was conducted in very large glass vessels. About the year 1746, the great improvement of leaden chambers was introduced by Dr. Roebuck, of Birmingham, where the first apparatus of this kind was erected. In consequence of this improvement, the acid immediately fell to one-fourth of its former price.

The only way to obtain pure sulphuric acid is by distillation. Owing to the high boiling point of this acid, the operation is rather precarious, in consequence of the danger of the fracture of the retort from the sudden concussions to which the boiling acid gives rise. Dr. Ure recommends that a retort of the capacity of from two to four quarts be used in distilling a pint of acid. This is connected, by means of a wide glass tube three or four feet long, with a receiver surrounded with cold water.

All the vessels must be perfectly clean, and no luting employed. The retort is then gradually heated by a small furnace of charcoal, or, what is better, by means of a sand-bath, the retort being buried in the sand up to the neck. It is useful to put into the retort a few sharp-pointed pieces of glass, slips of platinum foil, or clay tobacco-pipe tubes, with the view of diminishing the shocks produced by the acid vapor. The distilled product ought not to be collected until a dense grayish white vapor is generated, the appearance of which is a sign that the pure concentrated acid is coming over. If this vapor should not immediately appear, it shows that the acid subjected to distillation is not of full strength; and the distilled product, until this point is attained, will be an acid water. In the distillation of sulphuric acid, M. Lembert uses fragments of the mineral called quartzite, instead of pieces of glass or platinum foil. After a time the fragments get worn, and must be changed.

What is said above relates to the mode of preparing common sulphuric acid; but there is another kind, known on the continent of Europe by the name of the *fuming sulphuric acid of Nordhausen*, so called from its properties, and a place in Saxony where it is largely manufactured. This acid is obtained by distilling dried sulphate of iron in large stoneware retorts, heated to redness, and connected with receivers of glass or stoneware. The fuming acid distils over, and ferric oxide is left in the form of *colcothar* or *polishing rouge*, a material used for polishing metals, particularly gold and silver. The formula usually given to this product is $H_2S_2O_7$ or $H_2SO_4 + SO_3$. This would demand about 45 per cent. of sulphuric oxide or SO_3. In fact, the so-called Nordhausen acid seldom contains more than 10 per cent. of SO_3, and to obtain that demanded by the formula a re-distillation is necessary. This product is semi-solid, and is now obtainable in commerce put up in sealed glass flasks. Its sale has been largely curtailed lately owing to the introduction into commerce of the *anhydride* under the name of *Solid Sulphuric Acid.* When moisture is rigidly excluded, the acid has little action on metals, and it is put up in soldered boxes of tinned sheet-iron; it is used largely in the arts in the manufacture of artificial alizarin. *Persulphuric Oxide*, S_2O_7, may be obtained in solution by carefully mixing chlorine water with strong sulphuric acid. (*Journ. de Pharm et Chim.*, 1878, p. 168.)

Properties. Sulphuric acid (*hydrogen sulphate*), commonly called *oil of vitriol*, is a dense, colorless, inodorous liquid, of an oily appearance, and strongly corrosive. On living tissues it acts as a powerful caustic. It unites with water in all proportions, and much heat is evolved on the mixture of the two fluids. When pure, and as highly concentrated as possible, as manufactured in leaden chambers, its sp. gr. is 1·840 (1·8485, Ure), a fluidounce weighing a small fraction over 14 drachms. If its density exceed this, the presence of sulphate of lead or other impurity may be inferred. Kohlrausch (*Pogg. Ann. Ergänzungs*, Bd. viii. p. 675, Lunge) found the sp. gr. of *pure sulphuric acid, real hydrate*, to be 1·8342, and believes that a higher sp. gr. than this is due to impurities (probably lead sulphate). The commercial acid is seldom of this strength. According to Mr. Phillips, it has generally the sp. gr. 1·8433, and this is about the strength of the Br. acid, of which the sp. gr. is stated to be 1·843. The sp. gr. of the officinal acid is permitted to be 1·840. Mendelejeff, after a careful determination, found that pure mono-hydrated sulphuric acid had the specific gravity 1·8371 at 15° C. (59° F.) compared with water at its maximum density, 4° C. (*Amer. Drug.*, 1885, p. 16.) The strong acid boils at 327° C. (620° F.), and freezes at —26° C. (—15° F.). When diluted, its boiling point is lowered. When of the sp. gr. 1·78, it deposits crystals of the formula $H_2SO_4 + H_2O$ at about 0° C. (32° F.), and hence it is hazardous for manufacturers to keep an acid of that strength in glass vessels in cold weather, as they are liable to burst. With salifiable bases it forms a numerous class of salts, called sulphates. It acts powerfully on organic bodies, whether vegetable or animal, depriving them of the elements of water, developing charcoal, and turning them black. A small piece of cork or wood, dropped into the acid, will for this reason render it of a dark color. It absorbs water with avidity, and is used as a desiccating agent. It has been ascertained by Professors W. B. and R. E. Rogers to be capable of absorbing 94 per cent. of carbonic acid gas, a fact having an important bearing on analytical operations. When diluted with distilled water, it ought to remain limpid;

and, when heated sufficiently in a platinum spoon, the fixed residue should not exceed one part in 400 of the acid employed. When present in small quantity in solution, it is detected unerringly by chloride of barium, which causes a precipitate of sulphate of barium. The most usual impurities in it are arsenious acid and sulphate of lead; the former derived from the presence of arsenides in the pyrites, where that has been used in the production of the sulphurous oxide; the latter from the leaden boilers in which the acid is concentrated. Sulphate of sodium or of magnesium is said to have been added to increase its specific gravity. "When heated on platinum foil, it is vaporized without leaving a residue. If the Acid be warmed with sugar, it blackens the latter; if diluted with 5 volumes of water, the liquid yields, with test-solution of chloride of barium, a white precipitate insoluble in hydrochloric acid." *U. S.* Occasionally nitre is added to render dark samples of acid colorless. This addition gives rise to the impurity of sulphate of potassium. These impurities often amount to 3 or 4 per cent. The commercial acid cannot be expected to be absolutely pure; but, when properly manufactured, it should not contain more than one-fourth of 1 per cent. of impurity. The fixed impurities are discoverable by evaporating a portion of the acid, when they will remain. If sulphate of lead be present, the acid will become turbid on dilution with an equal bulk of water. This impurity is not detected by sulphuretted hydrogen, unless the sulphuric acid be saturated with an alkali. If only a scanty muddiness arise, the acid is of good commercial quality.

Other impurities occur in the commercial sulphuric acid. The several oxides of nitrogen are always present in greater or less amount. They may be detected by gently pouring a solution of ferrous sulphate over the commercial acid in a tube, when the solution, at the line of contact, will acquire a deep red color, due to the liberation of nitrogen tetroxide. Another method is to pass into tincture of guaiac the gases proceeding from the suspected acid heated with iron filings. If nitrogen tetroxide be present, the tincture becomes blue. The commercial acid, however, is not to be rejected unless the test shows the presence of nitrogen tetroxide in unusual quantity. Nitrogen tetroxide is an injurious impurity when the sulphuric acid is employed in the manufacture of hydrochloric acid, which is decomposed by the nitrogen tetroxide with evolution of chlorine. To remove this impurity it was recommended by Wackenroder, before distilling it, to heat the acid with a little sugar. This and the N_2O_4 mutually decompose each other, and the products are dissipated by heat. For the removal of the nitrogen acids generally, Dr. J. Löwe recommends the addition, to the heated sulphuric acid, of small portions of dry oxalic acid, so long as it exhibits a yellow tinge. The oxalic acid is decomposed into carbonic acid and oxide, the latter of which, in becoming carbonic acid, deoxidizes and destroys the nitrogen acids. A slight excess of oxalic acid produces no harm, as it is immediately decomposed. Perhaps a better method of getting rid of these acids is to distil with a little sulphate of ammonium. When sulphate of potassium is fraudulently introduced into the acid to increase its density, it may be detected by saturating the acid with ammonia, and heating to redness in a crucible; when sulphate of ammonium will be expelled, and the sulphate of potassium left.

Arsenic is sometimes present in sulphuric acid. In consequence of the high price of Sicilian sulphur, most English manufacturers have employed iron pyrites for the purpose of furnishing the necessary sulphurous acid in the manufacture of oil of vitriol. As the pyrites usually contains arsenic, it happens that the sulphurous acid fumes are accompanied by arsenious oxide, and thus the sulphuric acid becomes contaminated. From 22 to 35 grains of arsenious acid have been found in 20 fluidounces of oil of vitriol, of English manufacture, by Dr. G. O. Rees and Mr. Watson, and a still larger proportion by Mr. J. Cameron, of South Wales. To detect this impurity, the acid, previously diluted with five or six measures of distilled water, must be examined by Marsh's test. (See *Acidum Arseniosum.*) But a more easy method, said to be nearly as delicate, is that of Bettendorff. A little stannous chloride is treated, in a shallow dish, with pure hydrochloric acid (sp. gr. 1·12) until dissolved. The suspected sulphuric acid is then added, drop by drop, to the solution, the vessel being shaken on each addition. Considerable heat will be produced, and the liquid, if no arsenic be present, will remain clear; but, if the acid be in the slightest degree contaminated with the poison, first a yellow, then a brown, and finally a dark grayish brown color will appear, and the liquid become turbid. (*N. R.*, April, 1873, p. 367.) To separate the arsenious acid, Dr. J. Löwe recommends that the concentrated sulphuric acid should be gently heated in a flat dish, in a place where the fumes may be carried off, and then treated with small quantities of finely powdered chloride of sodium, constantly stirred in with a glass rod. By the reaction between the arsenious acid and disengaged hydrochloric acid, ter-chloride of arsenic is formed, which, being volatile, is separated by the heat. The heat is afterwards continued, to expel the excess of hydrochloric acid. This mode of purification introduces into the oil of vitriol a little sulphate of sodium. Buchner proposes a similar process; instead of chloride of sodium, employing hydrochloric acid, or a stream of the acid gas. This plan does not introduce sulphate of sodium into the acid; but is less convenient than that of Löwe, and, when the aqueous hydrochloric acid is used, tends to weaken the oil of vitriol by introducing water. Experience, however, has shown that neither plan can be entirely relied on. An excess of sulphuric acid is said to prevent the formation of the chloride of arsenic. (See *A. J. P.*, 1860, p. 88.) For other methods of detecting arsenic in sulphuric acid, see *N. R.*, 1876, p. 297; 1880, p. 101. Until within a few years all of the sulphuric acid produced in the United States was made from sulphur. At the present time (1888) more than twenty sulphuric acid works are using pyrites. Some of the American pyrites ore is entirely free from arsenic. Dupasquier states that tin is sometimes present in commercial sulphuric acid, derived from the solderings of the leaden chambers; but this could scarcely happen now, as care is taken to avoid soldering, and to effect the union of the metal by fusion by means of the blow-pipe. It may be discovered by sulphuretted hydrogen, which precipitates sulphide of tin, convertible by nitric acid into the white insoluble stannic oxide. Should the precipitate be the mixed sulphides of arsenic and tin, the former would be converted by nitric acid into arsenic acid, and dissolved, and the latter into insoluble stannic oxide and left. Another impurity occasionally existing in French sulphuric acid is selenium, supposed to be derived from copper pyrites sometimes substituted for sulphur in the manufacture of the acid. For the mode of detecting and separating this impurity, see the *Journal de Pharmacie* (1872, p. 42). "To neutralize 2·45 Gm. diluted with about 10 volumes of water, should require not less than 48 C.c. of the volumetric solution of soda." *U. S.* As ordered by the Br. Pharmacopœia, "50 grains by weight, mixed with distilled water, require for neutralization 1000 grain-measures of *the volumetric solution of soda.*" *Br.* For a very delicate method of detecting sulphurous acid and the oxides of nitrogen in sulphuric acid, see Mr. Robert Warrington, *Chem. News* (Feb. 14, 1868).

Tests. "On pouring the acid into 4 volumes of alcohol, no precipitate should be formed (lead). If there be carefully poured upon it, in a test tube, a layer of freshly prepared test-solution of ferrous sulphate, no brownish or reddish zone should appear at the line of contact of the two liquids (nitric acid). When diluted with 10 volumes of water, no precipitate should be formed by the addition of an aqueous solution of sulphate of silver (hydrochloric acid), nor by hydrosulphuric acid (lead, arsenic, copper), nor by excess of water of ammonia (iron); nor should this liquid, containing excess of ammonia, leave any fixed residue on evaporation and gentle ignition (non-volatile metals). When considerably diluted and treated with test zinc, it evolves a gas which should not blacken paper moistened with test-solution of nitrate of silver (arsenious or sulphurous acid). To neutralize 2·45 Gm. of Sulphuric Acid, diluted with about 10 volumes of water, should require not less than 48 C.c. of the volumetric solution of soda." *U. S.*

"Evaporated in a platinum dish, it leaves little or no residue. If a few drops be mixed with about a quarter of an ounce of a solution of stannous chloride mixed with strong hydrochloric acid, and the mixture be heated to boiling and then be allowed to cool, no darkening in color and no precipitate should be produced." *Br.*

The following table by Kolb shows how much hydrated sulphuric acid of the standard specific gravity and of oxide (SO_3) is contained in acid of any given density.

Kolb's table of Percentage and Specific Gravity of Sulphuric Acid.

Specific Gravity.	100 Parts contain at 15° C. (59° F.)		Specific Gravity.	100 Parts contain at 15° C. (59° F.)	
	H_2SO_4.	SO_3.		H_2SO_4.	SO_3.
1·000	0·9	0·7	1·308	40·2	32·8
1·007	1·9	1·5	1·320	41·6	33·9
1·014	2·8	2·3	1·332	43·0	35·1
1·022	3·8	3·1	1·345	44·4	36·2
1·029	4·8	3·9	1·357	45·5	37·2
1·037	5·8	4·7	1·370	46·9	38·3
1·045	6·8	5·6	1·383	48·3	39·5
1·052	7·8	6·4	1·397	49·8	40·7
1·060	8·8	7·2	1·410	51·2	41·8
1·067	9·8	8·0	1·424	52·6	42·9
1·075	10·8	8·8	1·438	54·0	44·1
1·083	11·9	9·7	1·453	55·4	45·2
1·091	13·0	10·6	1·468	56·9	46·4
1·100	14·1	11·5	1·483	58·3	47·6
1·108	15·2	12·4	1·498	59·6	48·7
1·116	16·2	13·2	1·514	61·0	49·8
1·125	17·3	14·1	1·530	62·5	51·0
1·134	18·5	15·1	1·540	64·0	52·2
1·142	19·6	16·0	1·563	65·5	63·5
1·152	20·8	17·0	1·580	67·0	54·9
1·162	22·2	18·0	1·597	68·6	56·0
1·171	23·3	19·0	1·615	70·0	57·1
1·180	24·5	20·0	1·634	71·6	58·4
1·190	25·8	21·1	1·652	73·2	59·7
1·200	27·1	22·1	1·671	74·7	61·0
1·210	28·4	23·2	1·691	76·4	62·4
1·220	29·6	24·2	1·711	78·1	63·8
1·231	31·0	25·3	1·732	79·9	65·2
1·241	32·2	26·3	1·753	81·7	66·7
1·252	33·4	27·3	1·774	84·1	68·7
1·263	34·7	28·3	1·796	86·5	70·6
1·274	36·0	29·4	1·819	89·7	73·2
1·285	37·4	30·5	1·842	100·0	81·6
1·297	38·8	31·7			

Composition. The normal acid of the sp. gr. 1·842 (1·8485, Ure) consists of one mol. of oxide 80, and one mol. of water 18 = 98 mol. wt. As the hydrogen acts the part of a metal in the compound, the systematic name would be hydrogen sulphate. The oxide consists of one atom of sulphur 32, and three atoms of oxygen 48 = 80. The ordinary commercial acid consists, according to Phillips, of one mol. of oxide, and one and a quarter mol. of water. The hydrated acid of Nordhausen has a density as high as 1·89 or 1·9, and consists of two mols. of oxide, and one mol. of water ($2SO_3 + H_2O$). This acid is particularly adapted to the purpose of dissolving indigo for dyeing the Saxon blue. When heated gently in a retort, connected with a dry and refrigerated receiver, sulphuric oxide or anhydride distils over, and the common monohydrated acid remains behind. In performing this operation, much difficulty from concussion is avoided, and the product of oxide increased, by introducing a coil of platinum wire into the retort. The oxide may also be obtained by the action of phosphoric oxide on concentrated sulphuric acid, according to the method of Ch. Barreswil. The mixture must be made in a refrigerated retort, and afterwards distilled by a gentle heat into a refrigerated receiver. *Sulphuric oxide* (*solid sulphuric acid*) under 18° C. (64° F.) is in small colorless crystals, resembling asbestos. It is tenacious, difficult to cut, and may be moulded in the fingers like wax, without acting on them. Exposed to the air, it emits a thick opaque vapor of an acid smell. Above 18° C. (64° F.) it is a liquid, very nearly of the density 2.

Medical Properties. For the therapeutic powers and uses of sulphuric acid, when administered internally, see *Acidum Sulphuricum Dilutum*. Externally it is sometimes employed as a caustic; but, from its liquid form, it is very inconvenient for that purpose, and should be applied with caution. A plan, however, has been proposed by Prof. Simpson by which it becomes very manageable. This consists in mixing it with dried and powdered sulphate of zinc sufficient to give it a pasty consistence. *Michel's Paste* consists of strong sulphuric acid three parts, and finely powdered asbestos one part, thoroughly rubbed together. When mixed with saffron to the consistence of a ductile paste, Velpeau found it a convenient caustic, not liable to spread or be absorbed, and producing an eschar which is promptly detached.

Toxicological Properties. The symptoms of poisoning by this acid are the following. Burning heat in the throat and stomach, extreme fetidness of the breath, nausea and excessive vomitings of black or reddish matter, excruciating pains in the bowels, difficulty of breathing, extreme anguish, a feeling of cold on the skin, great prostration, constant tossing, convulsions, and death. Sometimes there is no pain whatever in the stomach; sensibility being apparently destroyed by the violence of the caustic action. The intellectual faculties remain unimpaired. Frequently the uvula, palate, tonsils, and other parts of the fauces are covered with black or white sloughs. The treatment consists in the administration of large quantities of magnesia, or, if this be not at hand, of solution of soap. The safety of the patient depends upon the greatest promptitude in the application of the antidotes. After the poison has been neutralized, mucilaginous and other bland drinks must be taken freely.

The holes burnt in linen by sulphuric acid, so long as the texture is undisturbed, are distinguished from those produced by red-hot coals, by the paste-like characters of their edges.

Uses in the Arts. Sulphuric acid is more used in the arts than any other acid. It is employed to obtain many of the other acids; to extract soda from common salt; to make alum and sulphate of iron; to refine petroleum and paraffin; to decompose the neutral fats; to dissolve indigo; to prepare skins for tanning; to prepare phosphorus, chlorinated lime, sulphate of magnesium, etc. The arts of bleaching and dyeing cause its principal consumption.

Off. Prep. and Pharm. Uses. Acidum Sulphuricum Aromaticum; Acidum Sulphuricum Dilutum; Acidum Hydrocyanicum Dilutum; Acidum Sulphurosum; Chloroformum Purificatum; Ferri Sulphas Precipitatus; Glycyrrhizinum Ammoniatum; Hydrargyri Subsulphas Flavus; Liquor Ferri Subsulphatis; Liquor Ferri Tersulphatis; Oleum Æthereum; Pyroxylinum; Spiritus Ætheris Nitrosi.

Off. Prep. Br. Acidum Sulphuricum Aromaticum; Acidum Sulphuricum Dilutum; Infusum Rosæ Acidum.

Off. Sulphates. Br. Alumen; Alumen Exsiccatum; Atropinæ Sulphas; Beberinæ Sulphas; Calcii Sulphas; Cinchonidinæ Sulphas; Cupri Sulphas; Liquor Ferri Persulphatis; Ferri Sulphas; Ferri Sulphas Exsiccata; Ferri Sulphas Granulata; Hydrargyri Persulphas; Magnesii Sulphas; Morphinæ Sulphas; Potassii Sulphas; Quininæ Sulphas; Sodii Sulphas; Zinci Sulphas.

ACIDUM SULPHURICUM AROMATICUM. *U.S., Br.* *Aromatic Sulphuric Acid.*

(ĂÇ'Ĭ-DŬM SŬL-PHŪ'RĬ-CŬM ĂR-Ọ-MĂT'Ĭ-CŬM.)

Tinctura Aromatica Acida, *P. G.;* Elixir Vitrioli Mynsichti *G.;* Elixir of Vitriol; Elixir vitriolique, Teinture (alcoolé) aromatique sulphurique, *Fr.;* Saure Aromatische Tinctur, Mynsicht's Elixir, *G.*

"Sulphuric Acid, *two hundred parts* [or two fluidounces]; Tincture of Ginger, *forty-five parts* [or one fluidounce]; Oil of Cinnamon, *one part* [or nine minims]; Alcohol, *a sufficient quantity,* To make *one thousand parts* [or twenty fluidounces]. Add the Sulphuric Acid gradually to seven hundred (700) parts [or sixteen fluidounces] of Alcohol, and allow the mixture to cool. Then add to it the Tincture of Ginger and the Oil of Cinnamon, and afterward enough Alcohol to make the product weigh *one thousand* (1000) *parts* [or measure twenty fluidounces]." *U. S.*

"Strong Tincture of Ginger, 2 fl. ozs. [Imp. meas.] (or 1 fl. part); Spirit of Cinnamon, 2 fl. ozs. [Imp. meas.] (or 1 fl. part); Rectified Spirit, 36 fl. ozs. [Imp. meas.] (or 18 fl. parts); Sulphuric Acid, 3 fl. ozs. [Imp. meas.] or 2419 grs. (or

1¼ fl. part). Mix the sulphuric acid gradually with the spirit, and add the spirit of cinnamon and tincture of ginger." *Br.*

"It should be preserved in glass-stoppered bottles. Aromatic Sulphuric Acid has the sp. gr. 0·955, and contains about 20 per cent. of officinal Sulphuric Acid, partly in the form of Ethyl-sulphuric Acid. On diluting 9·8 Gm. of Aromatic Sulphuric Acid with 20 volumes of Water, and filtering, the filtrate (with washings) should require for complete neutralization not less than 36 C.c. of the volumetric solution of soda." *U. S.*

The specific gravity of the British preparation is 0·911, and 195 grains by weight require for neutralization 500 grain-measures of the *volumetric solution of soda*, corresponding to about 12·5 per cent. of real sulphuric acid. Six fluidrachms contain about 37·5 grains of real acid, H_2SO_4.

The formula adopted at the last revision of the U. S. Pharmacopœia was that recommended by Thomas N. Jamieson, *A. J. P.*, 1867, p. 201. The change in the appearance and properties from the preparation of the U. S. P. 1870 was so marked that the wisdom of making so radical a change was doubted. Experience has proved, however, that the new preparation has not the same tendency to precipitate, and the lightness in color has thus been offset by this more substantial advantage. The British formula has also been remodelled to accord with that of the United States.

Properties. Aromatic sulphuric acid of the older Pharmacopœias was of a deep reddish brown, but it is a straw-colored liquid when freshly prepared according to the direction of the U. S. Pharmacopœia of 1880, of a peculiar aromatic odor, and, when sufficiently diluted, of a grateful acid taste. It has been supposed by some to contain ethylic ether or sulphovinic acid, its main ingredients justifying such a suspicion; but the late Dr. Duncan, of Edinburgh, who originally held this opinion, satisfied himself that the alcohol and sulphuric acid, in the proportions here employed, do not generate a single particle of ethylic ether; and Prof. Attfield has shown that there is no ethyl-sulphuric acid in the officinal preparation. (*P. J. Tr.*, 1869, p. 471.) It cannot, however, be viewed merely as a sulphuric acid diluted with alcohol and containing the essential oils of ginger and cinnamon, for the difference in odor between fresh and old preparations is quite marked, and a peculiar and agreeable ethereal odor is developed by age. Samples of fresh aromatic sulphuric acid as well as older specimens have been assayed by E. W. Clark, and all were found to be more or less deficient in sulphuric acid; the inference is quite clear that there is some decomposition of sulphuric acid in the preparation upon keeping. (*Pharm. Era*, 1887, p. 69.)

Medical Properties and Uses. This valuable preparation, commonly called *elixir of vitriol*, is a simplification of *Mynsicht's acid elixir.* It is tonic and astringent, and affords an agreeable form of sulphuric acid for administration. It acts precisely as does the *Acidum Sulphuricum Dilutum.* The dose is from ten to thirty drops (0·6–1·9 C.c.), in a wineglassful of water, repeated two or three times a day. Care must be taken that the teeth are not injured.

Off. Prep. Infusum Cinchonæ.

Off. Prep. Br. Infusum Cinchonæ Acidum.

ACIDUM SULPHURICUM DILUTUM. *U. S., Br.* *Diluted Sulphuric Acid.*

(AÇ'I-DŬM SŬL-PHŪ'RI-CŬM DI-LŪ'TŬM.)

Acide sulphurique dilué, *Fr.;* Verdünnte Schwefelsäure, *G.*

"Sulphuric Acid, *one part* [one fluidounce]; Distilled Water, *nine parts* [sixteen and a half fluidounces]. Pour the Acid gradually, with constant stirring, into the Distilled Water, and preserve the product in glass-stoppered bottles. Diluted Sulphuric Acid contains 10 per cent. of officinal Sulphuric Acid, and has the sp. gr. 1·067 nearly. It should respond to the same reactions and tests as Sulphuric Acid. To neutralize 9·8 Gm. of diluted sulphuric acid should require 19·2 to 20 C.c. of the volumetric solution of soda." *U. S.*

"Take of Sulphuric Acid 7 *fluidounces* [Imperial measure]; Distilled Water *a sufficiency*. Dilute the acid with 77 fluidounces of the Water, and when the mixture has cooled to 60° add more Water, so that it shall measure 83½ fluidounces [Imp. meas.]. Or as follows:

"Take of Sulphuric Acid 1350 grains; Distilled Water *a sufficiency*. Weigh the Acid in a glass flask, the capacity of which, to a mark on the neck, is one pint [Imp. meas.], then gradually add Distilled Water until the mixture, after it has been shaken and cooled to 60°, measures a pint [Imp. meas.]. Sp. gr. 1·094. Six fluidrachms [Imp. meas.] or 359 grains by weight require for neutralization 1000 grain-measures of the *volumetric solution of soda*, corresponding to 13·65 per cent. of real sulphuric acid. Six fluidrachms, therefore, contain half a molecular weight in grains (49) of real sulphuric acid (H_2SO_4)." *Br.*

This preparation is sulphuric acid diluted to such an extent as to make it convenient for prescription. It is not exactly coincident in strength as directed in the two Pharmacopœias, the U. S. acid being weaker than the British, and slightly weaker than that formerly officinal; but the difference is not so great as to be of practical importance. The strong acid is added gradually to the water, to guard against the too sudden production of heat, which might cause the fracture of the vessel. During the dilution, when commercial sulphuric acid is used, the liquid becomes slightly turbid, and in the course of a few days deposits a grayish white powder, which is sulphate of lead, and from which the diluted acid should be poured off. This noxious salt is thus got rid of; but sulphate of potassium, another impurity in the strong acid, still remains. The presence of a little sulphate of potassium will do no harm; but, if it should be fraudulently introduced into the strong acid to increase its specific gravity, its amount may be ascertained by saturating the acid, after dilution, with ammonia, and expelling by a red heat the sulphate of ammonium formed. Whatever sulphate of potassium is present will remain behind. If the directions of the Pharmacopœias are strictly carried out, and the kind of sulphuric acid is used which is known in commerce as chemically pure, responding to the tests given under the head of *Acidum Sulphuricum*, the officinal manipulations will be all-sufficient.

Medical Properties and Uses. Diluted sulphuric acid is tonic, refrigerant, and astringent. It is given in typhoid fevers, and often with advantage. In the convalescence from protracted fevers it acts beneficially as a tonic, exciting the appetite and promoting digestion. As an astringent, it is employed in colliquative sweats, passive hemorrhages, and diarrhœas dependent on a relaxed state of the mucous membrane of the intestines, *i.e.*, in serous diarrhœas. In 1851, Mr. Buxton, of London, called attention to its great value in choleraic diarrhœas; his assertions have received abundant confirmation both in this country and in England. (See *Med. Times and Gaz.*, Oct. 1853; *Med. and Surg. Rep.*, ix. 199; *Phila. Med. Times*, iii. 649.) In incipient *cholera* it is an efficient remedy; diluted with water, it may be given every twenty minutes in ordinary cases, every quarter of an hour in severe cases. For bilious diarrhœa the acid is not a suitable remedy. In calculous affections attended with phosphatic sediments it is the proper remedy, being preferable to hydrochloric acid, as less apt, by continued use, to disorder the stomach. The dose is from ten to thirty drops (0·6–1·9 C.c.), three times a day, in a wineglassful of plain or sweetened water. It is added with advantage to infusions of cinchona, the organic alkalies of which it tends to hold in solution. As it is apt to injure the teeth, it is best taken by sucking it through a glass tube or quill. It is much less used in the United States than the elixir of vitriol. An elegant form of administration is the Compound Infusion of Roses, *U. S.* 1870.

Off. Prep. Antimonium Sulphuratum.

Off. Prep. Br. Infusum Rosæ Acidum.

ACIDUM SULPHUROSUM, *U. S.*, *Br.* *Sulphurous Acid.*

(ĂÇ-Ĭ-DŬM SŬL-PHŪ-RŌ-SŬM.)

Acide sulfureux, *Fr.*; Schweflige Säure, *G.*

"A liquid composed of about 3·5 per cent. of Sulphurous Acid Gas [SO_2; 64.—SO_2; 32], and about 96·5 per cent. of Water." *U. S.* "Sulphurous acid gas, or sulphurous anhydride, SO_2, dissolved in water, and constituting 5 per cent. by weight of the solution; equivalent to 6·4 per cent. of real sulphurous acid, H_2SO_3." *Br.*

"Sulphuric Acid, *fourteen parts* [or five fluidounces]; Charcoal, in coarse powder, *two parts* [or one and one-quarter ounces, av.]; Distilled Water, *one hundred parts* [or four pints]. Pour the Acid upon the Charcoal which has been previously introduced into a glass flask, and mix the two well together. By means of a glass tube and well-fitting corks, connect the flask with a wash-bottle, which is one-third filled with water, and fitted with a cork having three perforations. Into one of these perforations insert a safety tube, which should reach nearly to the bottom of the bottle; into the remaining perforation fit a glass tube, and connect it with a bottle which is about three-fourths filled by the Distilled Water. This tube should dip about an inch below the surface of the water. By means of a second tube connect this bottle with another bottle containing a dilute solution of carbonate of sodium, to absorb any gas which may not be retained by the distilled water. Having ascertained that all the connections are air-tight, apply a moderate heat to the flask until the evolution of gas has nearly ceased, and, during the passage of the gas, keep the bottle containing the Distilled Water at or below 10° C. (50° F.) by surrounding it with cold water or ice. Finally, pour the Sulphurous Acid into glass-stoppered, dark amber-colored bottles, and keep them in a cool and dark place." *U. S.*

"Take of Sulphuric Acid *four fluidounces;* Wood Charcoal, broken into small pieces, *one ounce;* Water *two fluidounces;* Distilled Water *thirty fluidounces.* Put the Charcoal and the Sulphuric Acid into a glass flask, connected by a glass tube with a wash-bottle containing the two fluidounces of Water, whence a second tube leads into an [Imperial] pint bottle containing the Distilled Water, to the bottom of which the gas-delivery tube should pass. Apply heat to the flask until gas is evolved, which is to be conducted through the Water in the wash-bottle, and then into the Distilled Water, the latter being kept cold, and the process being continued until the bubbles of gas pass through the solution undiminished in size. The product should be adjusted to the strength above mentioned (6·4 per cent. of real sulphurous acid, H_2SO_3) by the method described in the following paragraph, and be kept in a stoppered bottle in a cool place." *Br.* "64 grains by weight of it mixed with one pint [Imp. meas.] of recently boiled and cooled distilled water and a little mucilage of starch do not acquire a permanent blue color with the *volumetric solution of iodine* until 1000 grain-measures of the latter have been added." *Br.*

The processes of the two Pharmacopœias are essentially the same, and both are based upon that of Wittstein. The sp. gr. of the U. S. preparation is about 1·022, of the British, 1·025.

The rationale of the process is simple. When the sulphuric acid (H_2SO_4) and charcoal are heated together, two molecules of the former give up each an atom of oxygen to the latter, and there are thus produced sulphurous and carbonic acid gases, which, having been first passed through a wash-bottle containing a little water to absorb impurities, are received into the distilled water, where the sulphurous acid is absorbed, whilst the greater part of the carbonic acid escapes, $4H_2SO_4 + C_2 = 2CO_2 + 4H_2O + 4SO_2$. The excess of sulphurous acid gas which escapes absorption is in the U. S. process received into a solution of carbonate of sodium, and condensed. In the Br. process the point of saturation is roughly indicated by the bubbles formed by the escape of the gas from the distilled water being equal in size to those formed in the wash-bottle. If there be any difficulty in getting the solution up to the officinal strength, the proportionate amount of sulphuric acid and of charcoal should be increased, and care exercised that the gas pass through the water in an abundant stream. The direction to keep the acid in well-stoppered bottles, in a cool place, is necessary in consequence of the strong tendency of the gas to escape and to undergo oxidation. An incidental advantage of the U. S. process is the production of sulphite of sodium. Old sulphurous acid often contains sulphuric acid, which may be nearly all removed by the cautious addition of sulphite of barium and the removal by filtration of the precipitated sulphate.

According to Mr. W. L. Scott (*P. J. Tr.*, Oct. 1869, p. 217), the best results are obtained when sulphuric acid containing 75 per cent. of anhydrous acid is employed; when a too concentrated acid is used, a part of it is entirely reduced and sulphur deposited, while a too dilute acid causes the evolution of sulphuretted hydrogen. The same authority also affirms that a purer gas is obtained by placing a little sulphite of lead and a few pieces of charcoal in the wash-bottles.

Prof. F. C. Calvert gives a process for preparing this acid on a large scale, by which he avoids all the inconveniences usually attendant on its manufacture, and has prepared thousands of gallons daily of a saturated solution. It consists in burning sulphur in a small furnace, and conducting the acid gas through earthenware tubes surrounded with water so as to cool them. The gas is then made to ascend through a wooden tube 40 feet high and about 4 feet wide, sometimes called a coke scrubber, filled with pumice stone previously washed first with hydrochloric acid and then with water. A certain amount of water is introduced into the tube from above, which, in its descent, meets and dissolves the gas, and runs out saturated from the bottom of the tube into an air-tight reservoir. (*P. J. Tr.*, xvii. 512.) Where sulphurous acid is to be used as a disinfectant, bisulphide of carbon, either pure or mixed with petroleum, may be burned in the room to be disinfected. Keates (*Chem. News*, Dec. 8, 1876) suggests the use of a suitable lamp. Stevenson uses an open copper dish or porcelain capsule, and simply ignites the liquid: care should be used, however, as the bisulphide is very inflammable and volatile. A purer sulphurous acid than the officinal may be made by John Kennedy's process, that of reducing sulphuric acid with metallic copper and passing the gas through a cylinder containing lumps of moist charcoal and then through a wash-bottle. The by-product is available as sulphate of copper. (*A. J. P.*, 1886, p. 226.)

Properties. The officinal sulphurous acid is a strong solution of sulphurous oxide gas. The oxide is an irrespirable gas, of a suffocating odor familiar to every one as that of burning sulphur, which is converted into it by combustion. If inhaled in the concentrated state, it proves fatal. Cold reduces it to a colorless liquid, which boils at —10·5° C. (13·1° F.). It has the sp. gr. 2·21, liquefies at —10° C. (14° F.), has a strong acid reaction, extinguishes burning bodies, has the power of bleaching many colored substances, and has a strong affinity for oxygen, with which it combines in the presence of water, forming sulphuric acid. Water at 18° C. (65° F.) takes up about 50 volumes of gas, and the solution has the sp. gr. 1·04. (*Brande and Taylor.*) Liquefied sulphurous acid gas (oxide) is now manufactured by Pictet in Geneva, and is sent into commerce in copper cylinders. It also forms the basis of the Pictet ice-making process. The Pictet machines are constructed to use either the pure SO_2 or the "Pictet fluid," a mixture of compressed carbon dioxide and sulphur dioxide.

The following table, founded on the researches of Mr. Scott (*Pharm. Journ.*, xi. 218), gives the strength of acids of various specific gravity.

Per Cent. of SO_2.	Sp. Gr. at 60°.	Per Cent. of SO_2.	Sp. Gr. at 60°.	Per Cent. of SO_2.	Sp. Gr. at 60°.
5	1·0275	7	1·0377	9	1·0474
5·5	1·0302	7·5	1·0401	9·5	1·0497
6	1·0328	8	1·0426	10	1·0520
6·5	1·0353	8·5	1·0450		

Sulphurous acid sometimes exists as an impurity in hydrochloric, acetic, and other acids; according to P. Schweitzer, the minutest quantity may be detected by dissolving zinc in the suspected acid; when, if sulphurous acid be present, the odor of sulphuretted hydrogen will be at once perceived. (*Chem. News*, xxiii. 293.)

Officinal sulphurous acid is a colorless liquid, having the smell of burning sulphur, and a sulphurous somewhat astringent taste. When exposed to the air it slowly absorbs oxygen, with the formation of sulphuric acid, and acquires a sour taste, and the property of changing vegetable blues to red. When kept in closed vessels exposed to the sunlight, a portion of it is decomposed, sulphur being deposited and sulphuric acid formed by the union of the liberated oxygen with other portions of the acid. (*A. J. P.*, xlii. 352.) It should be entirely volatilized by heat. It decolorises iodine by producing hydriodic acid, and on this fact is based the Br. test before given. It decomposes the bone phosphate of calcium.

"A colorless liquid, of the characteristic odor of burning sulphur, a very acid, sulphurous taste, and a strongly acid reaction. Sp. gr. 1·022–1·023. By heat it is completely volatilized. Litmus paper brought in contact with the acid is at first turned red, and afterward bleached. On pouring a few drops of the acid into a test tube containing diluted hydrochloric acid and some test zinc, a gas is evolved which blackens paper wet with solution of acetate of lead. If to 10 C.c. of sulphurous acid there be added 1 C.c. of diluted hydrochloric acid, followed by 1 C.c. of test-solution of chloride of barium, not more than a very slight turbidity should be produced (limit of sulphuric acid). If 1·28 Gm. of sulphurous acid be diluted with 20 volumes of water and a little gelatinized starch be added, at least 14 C.c. of the volumetric solution of iodine should be required, before a permanent blue tint is developed." *U.S.*

Medical Properties and Uses. Sulphurous acid has been introduced into use in consequence of its fatal influence upon the lower forms of animal and vegetable life. It is supposed to be thus destructive by its anti-oxygenizing or reducing influence; suffocating organic beings by denying them the oxygen necessary to their existence; but it probably acts also by a physiological property independently of its mere chemical effect. It is perhaps by the same property that it prevents fermentation, destroying the microscopic organisms essential to that process. In reference to its parasiticide property, it was brought before the notice of the profession by Dr. Jenner of London; though to Prof. Graham, we believe, belongs the first suggestion of its applicability to such purposes. In pyrosis and in cases of sarcinæ ventriculi it may be taken internally; but one of the sulphites, as sulphite of sodium, is perhaps preferable for the purpose, as it yields the acid always by decomposition in the stomach. Dr. Robt. Bird affirms that it is a powerful antipyretic. (*Amer. Journ. Med. Sci.*, lviii. 236.) As an external application, it is used in psora, the different forms of porrigo, trichosis of the scalp, pityriasis versicolor, and the thrush of children,—all parasitic affections, either animalcular or cryptogamous, generally yielding to it, if proper care be taken, by previous removal of the scabs or scales, to bring it into contact with the morbific cause. The dose for internal use is a fluidrachm (3·75 C.c.), largely diluted with water. When locally used it should be diluted with two or three measures of water or of glycerin, and applied as a lotion, or by cloths wet with it, or in the form of cataplasm. Dr. James Dewar, of Kirkaldy, has found very great advantage from the inhalation of sulphurous acid, in the form of the fumes of burning sulphur, in typhus and typhoid fevers, scarlatina, diphtheria, catarrhal fever, hay fever, gout, and rheumatism. (*N. O. Med. and Surg. Journ.*, 1867, p. 523; from *Dub. Med. Press*, Sept. 5, 1866.) Dr. Hjatelin believes that he arrested an epidemic of smallpox by the free use of the acid as a disinfectant. (*Brit. Med. Journ.*, 1871, ii. 519.) According to Rabuteau (*Neues Repert.*, xviii. 307), in the system sulphurous acid and the sulphites are converted into sulphuric acid and sulphates.

ACIDUM TANNICUM. *U.S., Br.* *Tannic Acid.*

$C_{14}H_{10}O_9$ (chiefly); 322. (ĂÇ′Į-DŬM TĂN′NĮ-CŬM.) $C_{28}H_{10}O_{18}$; 322.

Tannin, Digallic Acid, Acidum Gallo-tannicum, Tanninum; Acide tannique, Tannin, *Fr.*; Gerbsäure, Tannin, *G.*

"An acid extracted from galls." *Br.*

"Galls in powder, Ether, of each a sufficient quantity. Expose the powdered galls to a damp atmosphere for two or three days, and afterwards add sufficient ether to form a soft paste. Let this stand in a well-closed vessel for twenty-four hours, then, having quickly enveloped it in a linen cloth, submit it to strong pressure in a suitable press, so as to separate the liquid portion. Reduce the pressed cake to powder, mix it with sufficient ether, to which one-sixteenth of its bulk of water has been added, to form again a soft paste, and press this as before. Mix the expressed liquids, and expose the mixture to spontaneous evaporation until, by the aid subsequently of a little heat, it has acquired the consistence of a soft extract;

then place it on earthen plates or dishes, and dry it in a hot-air chamber at a temperature not exceeding 212° F. (100° C.)." *Br.**

The British Pharmacopœia has adopted a process which is almost identical with that of the U. S. P. 1870, both being essentially the process of Leconnet, modified by Dominé, which has been substituted, in the existing Pharmacopœias, for that of Pelouze previously employed in both.

While the Pelouze process yields the tannic acid probably in a somewhat purer state than Leconnet's, it is less easy of performance, and much less productive; and the product of the existing formula is sufficiently pure for all practical purposes. The addition of a little alcohol, 8 per cent. for example, to the ethereal menstruum, still further increases the product, and, we are informed, is practised to a considerable extent; but we doubt the propriety of this deviation from the directions given in the process, as the resulting product may not be in all respects identical. There appear to be two coloring principles in galls, one soluble in ether and not in alcohol, the other in alcohol and not in ether. Hence, while the tannic acid, in whichever way procured, is yellowish, that obtained by ether has a greenish tint, while that obtained by the addition of alcohol is slightly brownish. In consequence of the mode in which the acid is dried, in thin layers, on tinned or glass plates, and equally exposed to heat above and below, it froths up on the escape of the ether, and concretes in a soft, cellular, friable form, which is strikingly characteristic of the preparation made in strict accordance with the formula.

From a superficial examination of this process, it might appear that the result can be nothing more than an ethereal extract; but it is necessary that the ether employed should contain water, as it is directed to be washed; and yet the quantity of water is so small that it can hardly operate by its mere solvent power. The circumstances attendant upon the process of Pelouze afford the means of a satisfactory explanation, which was first suggested by M. Beral. In this, the powdered galls are submitted to percolation by watered ether, and the liquid which passes separates into two layers, a heavier which sinks to the bottom and a lighter which floats upon the surface. It is the heavier which contains the tannic acid, and from which it is obtained by evaporation. The most probable explanation is that ether, water, and tannic acid unite to form a definite compound, in which the affinities are too feeble to resist the tendency of the ether to rise in vapor, and which is, therefore, decomposed by its evaporation. The proportion of the menstruum to the galls is very small, much smaller than would be employed to obtain an extract; and the whole or nearly the whole of both liquids is probably occupied in the formation of the definite compound referred to, thus leaving little or none to act merely as solvents. Hence the exclusion from the resulting acid, in great measure, of the other soluble constituents of the galls; and the slight amount of impurity really present in the acid is probably owing to the action of that small quantity of the menstruum not occupied in forming the liquid compound. Opinion is not altogether united in this explanation; but it is that which appears to us the best to account for the phenomena of the case. It has been stated that the tannic acid obtained by either of the officinal processes has a more or less yellowish tint. From this, according to F. Kummel, it may be freed by the percolation, through recently ignited animal charcoal, of its solution in a mixture of ether and alcohol. It has, too, a slight odor, which, according to Prof. Procter, is derived from a volatile odorous principle existing in galls, which he succeeded in separating from the acid by the action of benzol. From 30 to 35 per cent. of tannic acid is obtained from galls by Pelouze's method; while that of Leconnet is said to yield 60 per cent.

The term *tannin* is applied to a class of vegetable principles, the aqueous solutions of which give blue or green colors or precipitates with ferric salts, and precipitate solutions of gelatin and albumen. They are mainly glucosides. Chemists have

* For the preparation of tannin from Chinese galls, Oscar Rothe proposes the following as a superior process. Macerate eight parts of the powdered galls with twelve of ether and three of strong alcohol for two days, decant, renew the menstruum, and finally express. Mix the liquids, and after standing decant from the sediment, add twelve parts of water, recover the alcohol and ether by distillation, rapidly filter the aqueous solution, and quickly evaporate by means of a steam bath; dry, and pulverize the residue. (*A. J. P.*, xlii. 403.)

recognized two kinds, one existing in oak bark, galls, etc., distinguished by producing a bluish-black precipitate with ferric salts, and the other existing in Peruvian bark, catechu, etc., and characterized by producing a greenish-black or dark olive precipitate with the same salts. The former is the one which has received most attention, and from an examination of which the characters of tannin have generally been given. It is the substance described in this article. See Kramer's table giving percentages of tannin found in different drugs, *A. J. P.*, 1882, p. 388; also U. S. D., 14th ed., p. 1020; *A. J. P.*, 1869, p. 194; *P. J. Tr.*, viii. p. 548. It is called, for the sake of distinction, *gallotannic acid.* According to Pettenkofer, it is found only in perennial plants, indicating some relation to the production of woody fibre. (*Buchner's Neues Repert.*, iii. 74–76.) R. Wagner (*Bull. Soc. Chim.*, 1866, ii. 461) divides tannin into two great classes, pathological, found only in diseased vegetable tissue, as gallotannic acid, etc.; and physiological, occurring in leaves, bark, wood, etc., in a natural state, as quercitannic acid, etc.

Commercial tannin from galls is an indefinite mixture of digallic acid (see *Acidum Gallicum*) and the glucoside. That this view is correct is evident from the fact that it yields from 0 to 22 per cent. of glucose when acted upon by dilute acids. The glucoside $C_{34}H_{28}O_{22}$ would yield 23 per cent. (Allen, *Com. Org. Anal.*, 2d ed., i. 283.)

Properties. Pure tannic acid is solid, uncrystallizable,* white or slightly yellowish, inodorous,† without bitterness, very soluble in water, much less soluble in alcohol and ether, especially when anhydrous, insoluble in the fixed and volatile oils.

The Pharmacopœia thus describes Tannic Acid: "light-yellowish scales, permanent in the air, having a faint, peculiar odor, a strongly astringent taste, and an acid reaction. Soluble in 6 parts of water and 0·6 part of alcohol at 15° C. (59° F.). Very soluble in boiling water and in boiling alcohol; also soluble in 6 parts of glycerin; sparingly soluble in absolute alcohol, freely in diluted alcohol; moderately in washed ether; and almost insoluble in absolute ether, chloroform, benzol, and benzin. When heated on platinum foil, it is completely volatilized. With solution of ferric chloride, Tannic Acid forms a bluish-black ink. In aqueous solution it causes precipitates with alkaloids, gelatin, albumen, gelatinized starch, and solution of tartrate of antimony and potassium (distinction from gallic acid)." *U. S.*

Exposed to heat, tannic acid partly melts, swells up, blackens, takes fire, and burns with a brilliant flame. Thrown on red-hot iron, it is entirely dissipated. Its solution reddens litmus, and it combines with most of the salifiable bases. It forms with potassa a compound but slightly soluble, and is, therefore, precipitated by this alkali or its carbonates from a solution which is not too dilute, though a certain excess of alkali will cause the precipitate to be redissolved. Its combination with soda is much more soluble; and this alkali affords no precipitate, unless with a very concentrated solution of tannic acid. With ammonia its relations are similar to those with potassa. Lime and magnesia, added in the state of hydrates, form with it compounds of little solubility. The same is the case with most of the metallic oxides, when presented, in the state of salts, to a solution of the tannate of potassium. Tannic acid even in the uncombined state precipitates many of the metallic salts, especially those of lead, copper, silver, uranium, chromium, mercury, teroxide of antimony, and stannous oxide. With ferric salts it forms a black precipitate, which is a compound of tannic acid and the iron, and is the basis of ink. It does not disturb the solutions of the pure salts of ferrous oxide. Several of the alkaline salts precipitate it from its aqueous solution, either by the formation of

* E. Schering has put upon the market a "*crystalloid*" tannin which has a very deceptive appearance, leading a careless observer to believe that tannin is crystallizable. It is produced by dropping a small portion of a concentrated solution a distance of about 16 feet through a warmed atmosphere, upon a revolving cylinder. It is thus practically spun into threads more or less fine, which are afterwards scraped carefully off the cylinder. (*Neueste Erfind. und Erfahr.*, 1880.)

† Commercial tannic acid often has a decided odor, which Prof. Procter, after a practical investigation, believed to be owing chiefly to the presence of the odorous principle of the galls, though sometimes to matter derived from the ether with which it is prepared. (*A. J. P.*, 1865, p. 53.) According to M. Heinz, the odor is due to a greenish resinous principle, which may be separated by dissolving the acid in twice its weight of hot water, adding one-fourth part of ether, agitating slowly, allowing the coagulated coloring matter to precipitate, filtering, and evaporating. (*Journ. de Pharm.*, xv. 308.) Commercial tannic acid is often impure; in 9 samples tested by T. Maben (*P. J. Tr.*, xv. 851) the percentage of pure tannic acid varied from 54 to 86 per cent.

insoluble compounds, or by simply abstracting the solvent. Chlorate of potassium when rubbed up with it explodes with great violence, and several serious accidents have occurred during the attempt to dispense such a mixture.

Tannic acid unites with all the vegetable alkaloids, forming compounds which are for the most part of a whitish color, and but very slightly soluble in water; though they are soluble in the vegetable acids, especially acetic, and in alcohol. In this latter respect they differ from most of the compounds which tannic acid forms with other vegetable principles. On account of this property of tannic acid, it has been employed as a test of the vegetable alkaloids; and it is so delicate that it will throw down a precipitate from their solution, even when too feeble to be disturbed by ammonia.

It has an affinity for several acids, and when in solution affords precipitates with sulphuric, nitric, hydrochloric, phosphoric, and arsenic acids, but not with oxalic, tartaric, lactic, acetic, or citric. The precipitates are considered as compounds of tannic acid with the respective acids, and are soluble in pure water, but insoluble in water with an excess of acid. Hence, in order to insure precipitation, it is necessary to add the acid in excess to the solution of tannic acid. Strecker, however, denies that the precipitates are compounds of the tannin with the acid, and maintains that they are tannin imbued with free acid. (*Chem. Gaz.*, No. 287, p. 370.)

When tannic acid, iodine, and water are mixed, a reaction takes place, by which the water is decomposed; its hydrogen forming with the iodine hydriodic acid, which combines with a portion of the tannic acid and remains in solution; while the oxygen of the water combines with another portion of the tannic acid, to form a compound, which, being insoluble, is precipitated. The iodized solution thus obtained is capable of dissolving more iodine, and holding it in permanent solution, however much diluted. (Socquet and Guilliermond, *Journ. de Pharm.*, xxvi. 280.) Iodine in a liquid containing tannic acid cannot be detected by starch; but if the liquid is placed in a watch-glass, sulphate of iron added, and the glass covered with a starched paper, tannate of iron being precipitated, the blue color soon appears. (*A. J. P.*, xlvii. 398.)

Griessmayer (*Zeitschr. f. Chemie*, 1873) proposes a test for tannin and free alkalies. On mixing a drop of a solution of tannin with 1 C.c. of $\frac{1}{100}$ normal solution of iodine, the reddish color of the iodine solution instantly disappears; if one drop of solution of ammonia be now added (previously diluted with ten times its bulk of water), a brilliant red color is produced which is quite permanent.

Tannic acid precipitates solutions of starch, albumen, and gluten, and forms with gelatin an insoluble compound, which is the basis of leather.

Liebig first gave it the formula $C_{18}H_8O_{12}$. Mulder, however, considered it isomeric with gallic acid, and gave for its formula $C_{14}H_{10}O_9$; and both Julius Löwe and Hugo Schiff confirmed the correctness of this formula. (*A. J. P.*, xxv. 223; xlvii. 208.) Strecker looked upon it as a compound of gallic acid and glucose, the latter of which is destroyed in the spontaneous change that moistened galls undergo by time. (See *Acidum Gallicum.*) Hugo Schiff, however, asserts that it is not a glucoside; that glucose exists in commercial tannic acid as an impurity, and is not a necessary part of it, and that it is a "first anhydride," formed from two molecules of gallic acid by the abstraction of water, according to the reaction, $2C_7H_6O_5 - H_2O = C_{14}H_{10}O_9$, and is consequently digallic acid, and this view at this time prevails. (See *Acidum Gallicum.*) (*Chem. News*, xxix. 73; also *A. J. P.*, xlvi. 234.)*

Medical Properties and Uses. Tannic acid is the chief principle of vegetable astringents, and has an advantage over the astringent extracts in the comparative smallness of its dose, which renders it less apt to offend an irritable stomach. In most of the vegetable astringents it is associated with more or less bitter extractive,

* Various plans have been proposed of estimating the quantity of tannic acid, which is an object of importance to tanners, as enabling them to judge of the value of their tanning materials; but on this point we must content ourselves, from want of space, with referring to *A. J. P.* (1859, p. 427; 1861, p. 164; 1863, p. 519; 1864, p. 314); also a paper by Mr. John Watts in the *P. J. Tr.* (1867, p. 515); also one by H. R. Procter, in the *Chem. News* (1874, p. 51); and one by MM. A. Muntz and Ramspacher (*Journ. de Pharm.*, xx. 287): also *Journ. de Pharm.*, 1874, pp. 445–447; *A. J. P.*, March, 1874, and Aug. 1877; *N. R.*, Aug. 1878; *N. R.*, 1882, pp. 150, 185; *P. J. Tr.*, 1885, pp. 121, 850.

or other principle which modifies its operation, and renders the medicine less applicable than it otherwise would be to certain cases in which there is an indication for pure astringency without any tonic power. Such is particularly the case in the active hemorrhages; and tannic acid, in its separate state, is here preferable to the native combinations in which it ordinarily exists. In diarrhœa it is probably more beneficial than ordinary astringents, as less liable to irritate the stomach and bowels. Owing to its very powerful coagulant action upon albumen, it is, however, absorbed only after conversion into gallic acid, and consequently has been superseded by the latter agent in all cases in which it must reach the diseased surface through the blood, or in which a general astringent action is desired. Locally applied, it is much more powerful than gallic acid, and is very largely employed (see *Collodium Stypticum*), as in hemorrhages from external surfaces or from mucous membranes which can be reached from without, relaxation of the uvula, coryza, chronic inflammation of the fauces, diphtheria, toothache, aphthæ, excessive salivation, leucorrhœa, chapped nipples, gleet, gonorrhœa, flabby and phagedænic ulcers, piles, chilblains, etc. It may be applied in solution of varying concentration according to the necessities of the case. When a very powerful influence is desired, the solution in glycerin may be used, either the *glycerite of tannin*, formerly officinal, made by dissolving two troyounces of tannic acid in half a pint of glycerin with the aid of a gentle heat, or a still stronger preparation. In affections of the rectum it may be used in the form of a suppository. In diseases of the uterus it has been recommended in the form of a cylindrical pencil about an inch long and two lines thick, made with 4 parts of the acid to 1 part of tragacanth, with a little crumb of bread to give the mixture due flexibility. Dose, from three to ten grains (0·20–0·67 Gm.).

As already stated, tannic acid is probably converted into gallic acid before absorption · it is eliminated through the kidneys in the form of gallic and pyrogallic acids. (*Chem. Gaz.*, No. 136, p. 231.) In the largest amounts it is very feebly poisonous, producing only a mild gastro-intestinal irritation.

Off. Prep. Collodium Stypticum; Trochisci Acidi Tannici; Unguentum Acidi Tannici.

Off. Prep. Br. Glycerinum Acidi Tannici; Suppositoria Acidi Tannici; Suppositoria Acidi Tannici cum Sapone; Trochisci Acidi Tannici.

ACIDUM TARTARICUM. *U.S., Br.* *Tartaric Acid.*

$H_2C_4H_4O_6$; 150. (ĂÇ'ĭ-DŬM TĂR-TĂR'ĭ-CŬM.) $2HO, C_8H_4O_{10}$; 150.

"An acid prepared from the acid tartrate of potassium." *Br.*

Sal Essentiale Tartari; Acide du Tartre, Acide tartrique, *Fr.*; Weinsteinsäure, Weinsäure, *G.*; Acido tartarico, *It.*, *Sp.*

No formula for the preparation of tartaric acid is given in the U. S. Pharmacopœia. In the Br. Pharmacopœia a process is given for its preparation. It is extracted from *tartar*, a peculiar substance which concretes on the inside of wine casks, being deposited there during the fermentation of the wine. Tartar, when purified and reduced to powder, is the cream of tartar of the shops, and consists of acid potassium tartrate. (See *Potassii Bitartras.*) The following is the British process.

"Take of Acid Tartrate of Potassium *forty-five ounces* [av.]; Distilled Water, *a sufficiency*; Prepared Chalk *twelve ounces and a half* [av.]; Chloride of Calcium *thirteen ounces and a half* [av.]; Sulphuric Acid *thirteen fluidounces*. Boil the Acid Tartrate of Potassium with two gallons [Imp. measure] of the Water, and add gradually the Chalk, constantly stirring. When the effervescence has ceased, add the Chloride of Calcium dissolved in two pints [Imp. meas.] of the Water. When the tartrate of calcium has subsided, pour off the liquid, and wash the tartrate with Distilled Water until it is rendered tasteless. Pour the Sulphuric Acid, first diluted with three pints [Imp. meas.] of the Water, on the tartrate of calcium, mix thoroughly, boil for half an hour with repeated stirring, and filter through calico. Evaporate the filtrate at a low temperature until it acquires the sp. gr. of 1·21, allow it to cool, and then separate and reject the crystals of sulphate of calcium which have formed. Again evaporate the clear liquor till a film forms on its surface, and allow it to cool and crystallize. Lastly, purify the crystals by solution, filtration (if necessary), and recrystallization." *Br.*

Tartaric acid was first obtained in a separate state by Scheele in 1770. The process consists in saturating the excess of acid in bitartrate of potassium or cream of tartar with carbonate of calcium, and decomposing the resulting insoluble tartrate of calcium by sulphuric acid, which precipitates in combination with the lime, and liberates the tartaric acid. The equivalent quantities are two mols. of the acid tartrate and one of carbonate of calcium. The process, when thus conducted, furnishes the one half only of the tartaric acid. The other half may be procured, as in the British process, by decomposing the neutral tartrate of potassium, remaining in the solution after the precipitation of the tartrate of calcium, by chloride of calcium in excess. By double decomposition, chloride of potassium will be formed in solution, and a second portion of tartrate of calcium will precipitate, which may be decomposed by sulphuric acid together with the first portion. The process, when thus conducted, will, of course, furnish twice as much tartaric acid as when the acid salt only is decomposed.

The reactions are as follows: $2\ KHC_4H_4O_6 + CaCO_3 = K_2C_4H_4O_6 + CaC_4H_4O_6 + H_2O + CO_2$, then $CaC_4H_4O_6 + H_2SO_4 = CaSO_4 + H_2C_4H_4O_6$, and $K_2C_4H_4O_6 + CaCl_2 = (KCl)_2 + CaC_4H_4O_6$, then $CaC_4H_4O_6 + H_2SO_4 = CaSO_4 + H_2C_4H_4O_6$.

Formerly all of the tartaric acid used in America was imported from England and France, the amount in some years being as much as 500,000 lbs. annually. Scarcely any is imported now. In 1877 the amount was only 183 lbs. It is now made in the United States, not only of better quality, but actually cheaper than the imported acid costs in bond.

Preparation on the Large Scale. The process pursued on the large scale is different from that above given. The decompositions are effected in a wooden vessel, closed at the top, called a generator, of the capacity of about 2000 gallons, and furnished with an exit-pipe for carbonic acid, and with pipes, entering the sides of the generator, for the admission of steam and of cold water respectively. Into the generator, about one-fourth filled with water, 1500 pounds of washed chalk (carbonate of calcium) are introduced, and the whole is heated by a jet of steam, and thoroughly mixed by an agitator, until a uniform mass is obtained. About two tons of tartar are now introduced by degrees, and thoroughly mixed. The carbonate of calcium is decomposed, the carbonic acid escapes by the exit-pipe, and the lime unites with the excess of tartaric acid to form tartrate of calcium, which precipitates; while the neutral tartrate of potassium remains in solution. The next step is to decompose the tartrate of potassium, so as to convert its tartaric acid into tartrate of calcium. This is effected by the addition of sulphate of calcium in the state of paste, which, by double decomposition, forms a fresh portion of tartrate of calcium, while sulphate of potassium remains in solution. The solution of sulphate of potassium, when clear, is drawn off into suitable reservoirs, and the remaining tartrate of calcium is washed with several charges of cold water, the washings being preserved. The tartrate of calcium, mixed with sufficient water, is now decomposed by the requisite quantity of sulphuric acid, with the effect of forming sulphate of calcium, and liberating the tartaric acid, which remains in solution. The whole is now run off into a wooden back, lined with lead, furnished with a perforated false bottom, and covered throughout with stout twilled flannel. Through this the solution of tartaric acid filters, and the filtered liquor passes through a pipe, leading from the bottom of the back to suitable reservoirs. The sulphate of calcium is then washed until it is tasteless, and the whole acid liquor is evaporated, in order to crystallize. The evaporation is effected in wooden vessels, lined with lead, by means of steam circulating in coils of lead-pipe, care being taken that the heat does not exceed 93·8° C. (165° F.). The vacuum-pan is used with advantage in evaporating the acid solution; as it furnishes the means of concentration at a lower temperature. When the acid liquor has attained the sp. gr. of about 1·5, it is drawn off into sheet-lead, cylindrical crystallizing vessels, capable of holding 500 pounds of the solution. These crystallizers are placed in a warm situation, and, in the course of three or four days, a crop of crystals is produced in each, averaging 200 pounds. These crystals, being somewhat colored, are purified by redissolving them in hot water. The solution is then digested with purified animal charcoal, filtered, again concentrated, and crystallized. The crystals, having been washed and drained, are finally dried on wooden trays, lined with thin sheet-lead, placed in a room heated by steam. The mother-liquors of the first crystallization are again concentrated, and the crystals obtained, purified by animal charcoal as before. When the residuary liquors are no longer crystallizable, they are saturated with chalk, and converted into tartrate of calcium, to be added to the product of a new operation. In order to obtain fine crystals of tartaric acid, it is necessary to use a slight excess of sulphuric acid in decomposing the tartrate of calcium. The merit of this process consists in the greater economy of sulphate of calcium over chloride of calcium for decomposing the tartrate of potassium.

Dr. Price, of England, has made some improvements in the above process (for details see *P. J. Tr.*, Jan. 1854). The main point in his improvements is to convert the crude tartar into tartrate of potassium and ammonium by means of ammoniacal liquor, which gives a soluble double salt, comparatively free from organic coloring matter and other impurities, and, therefore, favorable for conversion into tartrate of calcium by the usual methods. Mr. Pontifex, of England, has obtained a patent for an improvement in manufacturing tartaric acid, which consists in evaporating in vacuo. (*Ibid.*, Feb. 1857, p. 430.)

Liebig has succeeded in preparing tartaric acid artificially by the oxidation of sugar of milk, and other substances, by nitric acid; and the resulting product has been found to be identical in all respects, even in its influence on polarized light, with the acid derived from grapes.

Oscar Ficinus, of Bensheim, proposes the following process to procure a pure tartaric acid. Saturate the crude tartar with carbonate of calcium, and decompose the resulting calcium tartrate with solution of zinc chloride, whereby calcium chloride and tartrate of zinc are produced. The latter is almost insoluble, and is completely decomposed by sulphuretted hydrogen. The residuary sulphide of zinc may again be converted by means of hydrochloric acid into chloride of zinc and sulphuretted hydrogen, so that the expense of the process is very small. The liquid filtered from the precipitated sulphide of zinc, containing tartaric and sulphydric acids in solution, is heated for some time to 60°–80° C. (140°–176° F.), in order to dissipate the latter acid, filtered from the precipitated sulphur, and concentrated to the point of crystallization. (*Arch. d. Pharm.*, April, 1879, p. 310.) It is asserted that in Hungary and Southern Italy tartaric acid of extreme purity is prepared; that occurring in flat, crystalline crusts being chemically pure, that in pointed crystals containing a little sulphuric acid.

Properties. "Nearly or entirely colorless, transparent, monoclinic prisms, permanent in the air, odorless, having a purely acid taste and an acid reaction. Soluble in 0·7 part of water and 2·5 parts of alcohol at 15° C. (59° F.); in 0·5 part of boiling water, and 0·2 part of boiling alcohol; also soluble in 36 parts of absolute alcohol, in 23 parts of ether and 250 parts of absolute ether, and nearly insoluble in chloroform, benzol, and benzin. When heated for two hours at 100° C. (212° F.), the crystals do not lose more than a trace in weight. On ignition they should not leave more than 0·05 per cent. of ash." *U. S.* The powder is generally directed to be kept in well-stoppered vials; but Prof. Otto has shown that this direction tends to spoil rather than to preserve it, by preventing the evaporation of some water of crystallization which is set free by a commencing chemical reaction. A better plan is to keep the powder in ordinary boxes. (*Proc. A. P. A.*, 1856, p. 52.)

As found in the shops, it is in the form of a fine white powder, prepared by pulverizing the crystals. A weak solution undergoes spontaneous decomposition by keeping, becoming covered with a mouldy pellicle; but, if boiled and filtered, it is said to lose this tendency. (W. H. Wood, *Chem. News*, 1871, p. 246.) It is asserted that the addition of $\frac{1}{1000}$ of salicylic acid will effectually preserve solutions of tartaric acid. In uniting with bases it has a remarkable tendency to form double salts, several of which constitute important medicines. It combines with several of the vegetable organic alkalies, so as to form salts. It is distinguished from all other acids by forming a crystalline precipitate, consisting of bitartrate of potassium, when added to a neutral salt of that alkali. When associated with an excess of boric acid, it is detected with difficulty; potassa not precipitating it, even with the addition of acetic or hydrochloric acid. Its separation, however, may be effected, according to Barfoed, by means of fluoride of potassium, which detaches the boric acid, to form the fluoborate of potassium, and renders free the tartaric acid, which then responds to the ordinary test. (*Journ. de Pharm. et de Chim.*, 4e sér., ii. 70.) Its most usual impurity is sulphuric acid, which may be detected by the solution affording with acetate of lead a precipitate only partially soluble in nitric acid. When incinerated with red oxide of mercury, it leaves no residuum, or a mere trace. The British Pharmacopœia directs that it should give no precipitate with solution of sulphate of calcium, showing the absence of racemic and oxalic acids, or with solution of oxalate of ammonium, which would detect lime, sometimes present in minute proportion. Its solution should not be affected by sulphuretted hydrogen. "An aqueous solution of 1 part of Tartaric Acid in 3 parts of cold water, when mixed with a solution of 1 part of acetate of potassium in 3 parts of cold water, followed by the addition of a volume of alcohol equal to the whole mixture, yields a white crystalline precipitate. If, after standing two hours at the ordinary temperature, the liquid is separated by filtration, and the precipitate well washed with diluted alcohol and dried at 100° C. (212° F.), in an air-bath, it should weigh between 1·25 and 1·26 parts. A concentrated aqueous solution should not be blackened, at the line of contact, by the careful addition of test-solution of hydrosulphuric acid (lead and copper). If the crystals have left, on ignition, some ash (see above), this ash should not turn blue by treatment with a few drops of water of ammonia (copper), nor should the further addition of one drop of test-solution of sulphide of ammonium cause any black coloration (lead, copper, iron). 10 C.c. of a concentrated solution should show no precipitate within 5 minutes after the addition of 1 C.c. of test-solution of chloride of barium with an excess of hydrochloric acid (sulphuric acid). To neutralize 3·75 Gms. of Tartaric Acid should require 50 C.c. of the volumetric solution of soda." *U. S.* "Twenty-five grains dissolved in water require for neutralization 330 grain-measures of *the volumetric solution of soda.*" *Br.*

Tartaric acid is incompatible with salifiable bases and their carbonates; with salts of potassa, with which it produces a crystalline precipitate of bitartrate; and with the salts of lime and lead, with which it also forms precipitates. It consists of four atoms of carbon 48, six of hydrogen 6, and six of oxygen 96 = 150. Of the six hydrogen atoms, however, only two are replaceable by metal, so that it is dibasic, and can form both acid and neutral salts with monad elements like potassium and sodium. Thus, cream of tartar is the acid potassium tartrate (bitartrate of potassium), and so-called "soluble tartar," the neutral potassium tartrate.

MODIFICATIONS OF TARTARIC ACID. Five distinct modifications of tartaric acid exist. Their chief physical and chemical differences are as follows:

a. *Dextro-tartaric* acid, or ordinary tartaric acid, forms anhydrous, hemihedral, rhombic crystals, the aqueous solution of which turns the plane of polarization of a luminous ray to the *right*. The crystals fuse at 135° C. (275° F.), have a sp. gr. of 1·74 to 1·75, and are readily soluble in absolute and in aqueous alcohol.

b. *Lævo-tartaric* acid forms anhydrous, hemihedral, rhombic crystals, the aqueous solution of which turns the plane of polarisation of a luminous ray to the *left*.

c. *Racemic* or *para-tartaric* acid forms hydrated, holohedral, triclinic crystals of $H_2C_4H_4O_6 + H_2O$, which are optically *inactive*. The crystals have a sp. gr. of 1·69, and are soluble in five parts of cold water and with difficulty in cold alcohol. The calcium racemate is less soluble in water than calcium dextro-tartrate, and is also distinguished by its insolubility in acetic acid and in chloride of ammonium solution. Racemic acid can be prepared by mixing *a* and *b* tartaric acids, and can be resolved into them by appropriate methods. Racemic acid exists naturally in small proportion in the juice of grapes growing in particular localities, and was first obtained artificially in 1853 by M. Pasteur.

d. *Inactive* or *meso-tartaric* acid, optically inactive, but not resolvable into *a* and *b* acids.

e. Meta-tartaric acid, produced by fusing the ordinary variety. It is deliquescent and uncrystallizable. Its solution and the solutions of its salts are converted by boiling into those of the ordinary modification.

Medical Properties. Tartaric acid, being cheaper than citric acid, forms, when dissolved in water and sweetened, an available substitute for lemonade. It may be improved by adding a drop of fresh volatile oil or a few drops of essence of lemon. Dried by a gentle heat, and then mixed with bicarbonate of sodium, in the proportion of thirty-five grains of the acid to forty of the bicarbonate, it forms a good effervescing powder, the dose of which is a teaspoonful (3·75 C.c.) stirred in a tumbler of water. Tartaric acid resembles citric acid in its medical properties, but is more irritant, and taken in large amount and concentrated form has caused fatal gastro-intestinal inflammation. It is chiefly used in medicine in the preparation of effervescing draughts.* Dose, five to thirty grains (0·33–1·95 Gm.).

Off. Prep. and Pharm. Uses. Abstractum Aconiti; Extractum Aconiti; Extractum Aconiti Fluidum; Ferri et Ammonii Tartras; Pulvis Effervescens Compositus; Tinctura Aconiti.

Off. Tartrates. Br. Antimonium Tartaratum; Ferrum Tartaratum; Potassii Tartras; Potassii Tartras Acida; Sodii Citro-tartras Effervescens; Soda Tartarata.

ACONITINA. *Br.* *Aconitine.*

(A-CŎN-I-TĪ'NA.)

"An alkaloid obtained from aconite root." *Br.*

Aconitia, Aconitina, Aconitinum; Aconitin, *E.*; Aconitine, *Fr.*; Aconitin, *G.*

Formerly a process for the manufacture of aconitine was given in the U. S. Pharmacopœia, but in the 1880 revision the so-called alkaloid was dropped from the officinal preparations, because the process of 1870 does not yield a definite proximate principle. The British officinal process is as follows:

"Take of Aconite Root, in coarse powder, *any convenient quantity;* Rectified Spirit, Distilled Water, Solution of Ammonia, Pure Ether, Diluted Sulphuric Acid, of each *a sufficiency.* Mix the aconite root with twice its weight of the spirit, and apply heat until ebullition commences; then cool and macerate for four days. Transfer the whole to a displacement apparatus, and percolate, adding more spirit, when requisite, until the root is exhausted. Distil off the greater part of the spirit from the tincture, and evaporate the remainder over a water-bath until the whole of the alcohol has been dissipated. Mix the residual extract thoroughly with twice its weight of boiling distilled water, and when it has cooled to the temperature of the atmosphere, filter through paper. To the filtered liquid add solution of ammonia in slight excess, and heat them gently over a water-bath. Separate the precipitate on a filter, and dry it. Reduce this to coarse powder, and macerate it

* *Solution of Tartrate of Magnesium as a Purgative.* From the relatively high price of citric acid, attempts have been made to substitute for that acid, in the solution of citrate of magnesium, a cheaper acid, which might yield with magnesia an equally acceptable solution. M. E. Leger thinks he has accomplished this object by means of tartaric acid. The ordinary tartaric acid, however, will not answer; as the solution of the magnesian tartrate made with it, though at first limpid, soon becomes turbid, and most of the salt is deposited. But by employing a metatartaric acid he prepared a solution having all the desired properties. He prepares the *metatartaric acid* in the following manner.

Heating over a gentle fire, in a porcelain or preferably silver capsule, a little tartaric acid until it melts, stirring carefully from time to time, he adds successively small portions of fresh acid, taking care not to use so much as to cause the liquid to cool and solidify, and continuing to add until the vessel is two-thirds full. The heat is maintained until the mass, at first pasty and puffed up, becomes completely liquid. When bubbles are formed on the surface, the acid assumes a slight amber hue, and the desired modification has been effected. The vessel is now removed from the fire, and the contents allowed to cool until the acid can be handled without adhering to the fingers, when it is pressed into cakes, quickly cooled, and put into stopped bottles.

In the preparation of the magnesian solution, three-fourths of the water to be used is poured, cold, on a mixture of the acid and carbonate of magnesium (two parts of the former and one of the latter); a very brisk reaction takes place, and in less than ten minutes the solution is complete. Heat must be avoided; as otherwise the acid returns to the former state, and the salt is precipitated. When the acid has been completely modified, the solution will keep unchanged for several weeks. The cathartic action of the tartrate of magnesium is, according to M. Leger, much more certain than that of the citrate, and nearly equal to that of the sulphate. The solution is without unpleasant taste. (*P. J. Tr.*, 12, 1873, p. 29; from *Répertoire de Pharm.*, Juin 25, 1873.)

in successive portions of the pure ether with frequent agitation. Decant the several products, mix, and distil off the ether until the extract is dry. Dissolve the dry extract in warm distilled water acidulated with the sulphuric acid; and, when the solution is cold, precipitate it by the cautious addition of solution of ammonia diluted with four times its bulk of distilled water. Wash the precipitate on a filter with a small quantity of cold distilled water, and dry it by slight pressure between folds of filtering paper and subsequent exposure to air." *Br.**

This process was given to the Pharmacopœia Committee of the British Council by a manufacturer who had been in the habit of preparing the alkaloid, but it does not yield a reliable, medicinally pure alkaloid. The English aconitine is frequently in great part composed of pseudo-aconitine, originally discovered by Von Schroff, of Vienna.

Pure aconitine may exist in an amorphous or in a crystalline form. The officinal product is always amorphous, but even of amorphous aconitine there are two varieties, the hydrated and the anhydrous. When, as in the officinal processes, the alkaloid is dried at ordinary temperature, it retains 20 (Hager) or 25 (Hottot) per cent. of water; but when dried at the temperature of the water-bath it is anhydrous, and is then *not* soluble in 50 parts of boiling water. (Hager, *A. J. P.*, xlvii. 210.) For Hottot's process of preparing aconitine, see 15th ed. U. S. Dispensatory, p. 123.

Aconitine as obtained by the Br. Pharmacopœia process is "A white, usually amorphous, solid; soluble in 150 parts of cold, and 50 of hot water, and much more soluble in alcohol, in ether, and in chloroform; strongly alkaline to reddened litmus, neutralizing acids, and precipitated from solutions of its salts by the caustic alkalies, but not by carbonate of ammonium or the bicarbonates of sodium or potassium. It melts when heated, and burns with a smoky flame, leaving no residue if ignited with free access of air. When rubbed on the skin it causes a tingling sensation, followed by prolonged numbness." *Br.* It restores the blue color of litmus reddened by acids, and neutralizes the acids, forming crystallizable salts. The solution of these salts produces a white precipitate with bichloride of platinum, a yellowish with terchloride of gold, and a yellowish brown with free iodine. Aconitine is precipitated from the solution by the caustic alkalies, but not by carbonate of ammonium, or the bicarbonates of potassium and sodium. A spurious substance has sometimes been sold under the same name, which is nearly or quite inert; and at best the alkaloid is apt to be of uncertain strength, as found in commerce.

Crystallized aconitine was first made known by the researches of Mr. Groves (*P. J. Tr.*, 2d ser., viii. 121), but it was elaborately studied by Duquesnel. The methods of obtaining it differ, but, according to Patrouillard (*Journ. de Pharm.*, 4e sér., xix. 151), that of Duquesnel gives much the larger yield.† It occurs in regular rhombic tables, sometimes having the angles modified so as to look like hexagons, or else in small, short, four-sided prisms; it is anhydrous, nearly insoluble in water, insoluble in glycerin, but soluble in alcohol, ether, acetic acid, and benzin, and freely so in chloroform, inodorous, of an intensely bitter taste, followed by the characteristic tingling, not volatile at 100° C. (212° F.), and forms with most acids crystallizable salts. Juergens states that aconitine is soluble in 64 parts of absolute ether, 37 parts of absolute alcohol, 2800 parts of light petroleum of 0·670 sp. gr., 5·5 parts of chloroform or benzin, and 750 parts of water. (See *Jour. Chem. Soc.*, June, 1886.)

* See U. S. Dispensatory, 15th ed., p. 122.

† The method of Duquesnel is as follows. 100 parts of the powdered roots having been mixed with one part of tartaric acid, and the whole exhausted by repeated percolation with cold alcohol, the liquid is evaporated at a low temperature on a water-bath to the consistence of a fluid extract. To this distilled water is added, and the precipitated resinous and oily matters removed by filtration. The solution of tartrate of aconitine is then precipitated with a slight excess of bicarbonate of potassium, agitated with washed ether, and the two fluids separated with the siphon. The ethereal solution is shaken four or five times with a 10 per cent. solution of hydrochloric acid, which takes up the alkaloids from the ethereal solution. The acid liquids are treated with calcium carbonate to saturation in order to prevent the prolonged and injurious action of the acid upon the crystallizable aconitine, the mixture is evaporated at a very gentle heat, filtered, and while still warm mixed with a solution of sodium nitrate (2 of salt to 3 of water) having the same temperature. The whole is allowed to cool slowly during several hours, and set away for several days' rest, when the crystals separate out as a crust on the bottom (*N. R.*, 1883, p. 265; see, also, a paper by Williams, *Year-Book of Pharmacy*, 1886, p. 428.)

For Dr. Squibb's physiological tests for aconitine and aconite preparations, see page 130. Its only peculiar color reaction is obtained with difficulty by dissolving in dilute phosphoric acid and evaporating; at a certain degree of concentration a violet coloration appears.

The most elaborate investigations upon the *Aconitum* species are those which have been made by Dr. C. R. A. Wright during the years 1876–80, with grants made by the British Pharmaceutical Conference.

In *Aconitum Napellus* he found two distinct alkaloids; *aconitine*, a crystalline base possessing the formula $C_{33}H_{43}NO_{12}$, which possesses high physiological activity. It is crystallizable, anhydrous, and melts at 185° C. (365° F.); it is readily dehydrated by heating in contact with acids (preferably tartaric), forming *apo-aconitine*, $C_{33}H_{41}NO_{11}$, which closely resembles the parent alkaloid; on saponification with alkali it splits up into benzoic acid and a new base, *aconine*, $C_{26}H_{39}NO_{11}$, according to the reaction: $C_{33}H_{43}NO_{12} + H_2O = C_7H_6O_2 + C_{26}H_{39}NO_{11}$; and *picraconitine*, $C_{31}H_{45}NO_{10}$, an uncrystallizable base, which, however, forms crystallized salts of an intensely bitter taste but comparatively inert. This base also splits up upon saponification into benzoic acid and a new base, *picraconine*, much resembling aconine: $C_{31}H_{45}NO_{10} + H_2O = C_7H_6O_2 + C_{24}H_{41}NO_9$.

Besides these well-defined alkaloids, *Aconitum Napellus* yields a considerable quantity of non-crystalline alkaloids, which contain more carbon and are of lower molecular weight than aconitine. These are very likely in great part alteration products. In *Aconitum ferox*, he found chiefly the alkaloid *pseudaconitine*, $C_{36}H_{49}NO_{12}$. It crystallizes in transparent needles and sandy crystals, but is apt to separate as a varnish if not evaporated extremely slowly. It forms crystallized salts with difficulty. It can be dehydrated, forming *apo-pseudaconitine*, $C_{36}H_{47}NO_{11}$, and when saponified yields dimethyl-protocatechuic acid instead of benzoic and a new base, *pseudaconine*: $C_{36}H_{49}NO_{12} + H_2O = C_9H_{10}O_4 + C_{27}H_{41}NO_9$. Wright considers that pseudaconitine is closely related to the opium alkaloids narceine, narcotine, and oxy-narcotine, which all give rise to derivatives of dimethyl-protocatechuic acid. Pseudaconitine crystallizes with H_2O and melts at 104°–105° C. (220° F.). In Japanese aconite roots (species not certainly known) Wright found a larger percentage of active alkaloids than in either of the other varieties. He also considers that he has obtained here a new base, *japaconitine*, $C_{66}H_{88}N_2O_{21}$. This base on saponification splits up into benzoic acid and a base, *japaconine*, $C_{26}H_{41}NO_{10}$.

Aconitine exists in the root in combination with aconitic acid. Dragendorff and Spohn (*Jour. Pharm.* (5), 10, 361–368) find in the *Aconitum Lycoctonum* two alkaloids; *lycaconitine*, $C_{27}H_{34}N_2O_6 + 2H_2O$, which is not crystalline, nor does it yield a crystalline aurochloride or platinochloride, and *myoctonine*, $C_{27}H_{30}N_2O_8 + 5H_2O$, which is amorphous. The former alkaloid, heated with water under pressure, gives rise to two acids, a volatile one and a crystalline one, *lycoctonic acid*, $C_{17}H_{18}N_2O_7$, while two alkaloids remain dissolved, one, *lycaconine*, soluble in ether, the other soluble in chloroform, and apparently Hübschmann's acolytine. (See p. 126, foot-note.)

Medical Properties and Uses. It is practically true that the various products which are sold under the name of aconitine represent the activity of aconite, but it is well known that commercial aconitine is a very improper remedy for internal use, varying immensely in its purity, its composition, and its powers.* Two and a half grains have been taken almost with impunity, and 1-50th of a grain has nearly proved fatal. M. Hottot found that 0·46 of a grain of alkaloid, prepared by his process, produced very serious symptoms, and gave the fifth of a milligramme ($\frac{1}{325}$ of a grain) as the dose. So uncertain and powerful a remedy as is commercial aconitine ought not to be used at all internally, especially as it possesses no advantages over the other preparations of aconite, which are sufficiently concentrated for all practical purposes. Even as an external remedy, as first

* Even different specimens of apparently pure crystallized aconitine made by the same chemist in the same manner vary greatly in toxic property. For an elaborate discussion of this subject the reader is referred to the following papers: K. F. Mandelin, *Archiv d. Pharm.*, 1885, xxiii.; abstracted, *P. J. Tr.*, xvi.; Bunzen and Madsen, *Trans. Internat. Congress*, Copenhagen, 1884.

recommended by Dr. Turnbull, aconitine is of very limited value. It produces in the skin a sensation of heat and prickling, followed by numbness, lasting, according to the quantity applied, from two to twelve hours or more. Applied much diluted and in minute quantity to the eye, or even to the upper eyelid, it causes contraction of the pupil, with an almost intolerable sense of heat and tingling. Dr. Turnbull employed it with benefit in neuralgia, gout, and rheumatism. If the alkaloid be pure, the ointment should not exceed the officinal strength (8 grains to the ounce), and even then must be used with great caution by friction over the part affected, to be continued till the peculiar sensation above described is produced, and to be repeated three or four times, or more frequently, during the day. No good can be expected unless the sensation alluded to be experienced in a greater or less degree. Care should be taken not to apply the medicine to an abraded surface, or to a mucous membrane, for fear of dangerous constitutional effects.

Off. Prep. Unguentum Aconitinæ, *Br.*

ACONITI FOLIA. *Br.* *Aconite Leaves.*

(ĂC-O-NĪ'TĪ FŌ'LI-Ă.)

The fresh leaves and flowering tops of Aconitum Napellus, gathered when about one-third of the flowers are expanded, from plants cultivated in Britain. *Br.*

Herba Aconiti; Feuilles d'Aconit, Coqueluchon, *Fr.;* Eisenhutblätter, Sturmhutblätter, Aconit Napel, Capuchon, Pistolet, Akonitblätter, Wolfstormhut, Mönchskappeblätter, *G.*

ACONITUM. *U.S., Br.* *Aconite.*

(ĂC-O-NĪ'TŬM.)

"The tuberous root of Aconitum Napellus, *Linné.* (*Nat. Ord.* Ranunculaceæ.)" *U. S.* "The root of Aconitum Napellus, *Linn.*, collected in winter or early spring before the leaves have appeared, from plants cultivated in Britain, and carefully dried; or imported in a dried state from Germany." *Br.*

Aconiti Radix, *Br.*, Aconite Root; Tubera Aconiti, *P. G.;* Racine d'Aconit, *Fr.;* Eisenhut, Eisenhutknollen, Mönchskappe, *G.;* Aconito Napello, *It.;* Aconito, *Sp.;* Monkshood, Wolfsbane, Aconit, Coqueluchon, Sturmhut, Akonitknollen.

As Aconite Leaves are no longer officinal in the U. S. Pharmacopœia, the former titles of "Aconiti Folia" and "Aconiti Radix" have been abandoned, and "Aconitum" substituted. The Br. Pharmacopœia has also adopted the latter term for the root.

Gen. Ch. Calyx none. *Petals* five, the highest arched. *Nectaries* two, peduncled, recurved. *Pods* three or five. *Willd.*

The plants belonging to this genus are herbaceous, with divided leaves, and violet, yellow, or white flowers, in spikes, racemes, or panicles. In the Paris Codex three species were recognized as officinal, *A. Anthora*, *A. Cammarum*, and *A. Napellus;* but the French authorities unite at present with our own and the British in acknowledging only *A. Napellus*. There has been much difference of opinion as to the plant originally employed by Störck. Formerly thought to be *A. Napellus*, it was afterwards generally believed to be *A. neomontanum* of Willdenow, and by De Candolle was determined to be a variety of his *A. paniculatum*, designated as *Störckianum*. It is probable that this species, which is not infrequent in the Alps, yields much of the aconite of commerce, as probably does also *A. lycoctonum.** But, according

* M. Hubschmann is said to have extracted two alkaloids from *A. lycoctonum;* one in the form of a white powder, insoluble in ether, but soluble in water and alcohol, which he names *acolytine;* the other crystallizable, very soluble in alcohol, and but slightly so in ether or water, and named by him *lycoctonine*. (*A. J. P.*, 1866, p. 376.) According to Prof. Flückiger, *lycoctonine* is in white acicular crystals, melting like aconitine in boiling water, though at a somewhat higher heat. On cooling it crystallizes only when moistened with water, when the amorphous mass is converted into tufted crystals. It leaves no water upon melting, and combines with none on crystallizing. It readily dissolves in chloroform, and upon evaporation is left as an amorphous varnish, which, on the addition of a little water, becomes strikingly crystalline. It is largely dissolved by sulphide of carbon, ether, alcohol, the fixed and volatile oils, amylic alcohol, and petroleum spirit; but requires 600 parts of boiling water for solution. The solution is bitter and has an alkaline reaction, and with bromine water produces fine yellow crystals; and this effect results, though the solution contain only one part of the alkaloid in 30,000. Lycoctonine is an alkaloid quite distinct from

to Geiger, *A. neomontanum* is possessed of little acrimony; and Dr. Christison states that *A. paniculatum*, raised at Edinburgh from seeds sent by De Candolle himself, was quite destitute of that property. Neither of these, therefore, could have been Störck's plant, which is represented as extraordinarily acrid. Dr. Christison found *A. Napellus*, *A. Sinense*, *A. Tauricum*, *A. uncinatum*, and *A. ferox* to have intense acrimony; and Geiger states that he has found none equal, in this respect, to *A. Napellus*. This species is said to yield aconitine most largely. (*Répert. de Pharm.*, Nov. 1859.) *A. uncinatum* and *A. reclinatum* (Gray) are our only indigenous species. Most of the others are natives of the Alpine regions of Europe and Siberia. Those used in medicine appear to be indiscriminately called by English writers *wolfsbane* or *monkshood*. Under the name of Bish or Bikli, *Nepaul aconite** is largely sold in the bazaars in India. It is probably often a mixed product of a number of indigenous species, such as *A. lucidum*, *A. Napellus*, and *A. palmatum*, but is chiefly derived from *A. ferox*, which grows in the Himalayas, attaining a height of 3 to 6 feet, and having large dull blue flowers. The tuberous roots of *A. heterophyllum* are also met with in the bazaars. This native of the Himalayas has dull yellow flowers veined with blue or purple.

Aconitum Napellus. Linn., *Flor. Suec.*, ed. 1755, p. 168.—*A. neubergense*. De Candolle, *Prodrom.* i. 62.—*A. variabile neubergense*. Hayne, *Darstel. u. Beschreib.*, etc., xii. 14. This is a perennial herbaceous plant, with a spindle-shaped, tapering root, seldom exceeding at top the thickness of the finger, three or four inches or more in length, brownish externally, whitish and fleshy within, and sending forth numerous long, thick, fleshy fibres. When the plant is in full growth, there are usually two roots joined together, of which the older is dark brown and supports the stem, while the younger is of a light yellowish brown, and is destined to furnish the stem of the following year, the old root decaying. The stem is erect, round, smooth, leafy, usually simple, and from two to six or even eight feet high. The leaves are alternate, petiolate, divided almost to the base, from two to four inches in diameter, deep green upon their upper surface, light green beneath, somewhat rigid, and more or less smooth and shining on both sides. Those on the lower part of the stem have long footstalks and five or seven divisions; the upper, short footstalks and three or five divisions. The divisions are wedge-form, with two or three lobes, which extend nearly or quite to the middle. The lobes are cleft or toothed, and the laciniæ or teeth are linear or linear-lanceolate and pointed. The flowers are of a dark violet blue color, large and beautiful, and are borne at the summit of the stem upon a thick, simple, straight, erect, spike-like raceme, beneath which, in the cultivated plant, several smaller racemes arise from the axils of the upper leaves. Though without calyx, they have two small calycinal stipules, situated on the peduncle within a few lines of the flower. The petals are five, the upper helmet-shaped and beaked, nearly hemispherical, open or closed, the two lateral roundish and internally hairy, the two lower oblong-oval. They enclose two pediceled nectaries, of which the spur is capitate, and the lip bifid and revolute. The fruit consists of three, four, or five pod-like capsules.

The plant is abundant in the mountain forests of France, Switzerland, and Germany. It is also cultivated in the gardens of Europe, and has been introduced into

aconitine and pseudaconitine; and is much less poisonous than ether. (Flückiger, *P. J. Tr.*, 1870, p. 122.) Dr. Wright and Luff concluded that lycoctonine and acolytine are identical with *aconine* and *pseudaconine*, decomposition-products respectively of aconitine and pseudaconitine, but, according to Dragendorff and Spohn, they are really decomposition-products of two previously unnoticed alkaloids of *A. Lycoctonum*, namely, *lycaconitine* and *myoctonine*. (See p. 125, also *P. J. Tr.*, viii. 169, and xv. 104.) Jacobowsky found lycaconitine to resemble curare in its physiological action, but to be of no value in practical medicine.

* Under the name of *Utees*, *Atees*, or *Atis*, the root of *Aconitum heterophyllum* is said to be largely used in India as an antiperiodic. It is stated that it is free from poisonous properties, and is given in doses of 20 grains. The plant grows in the western Himalaya, at an elevation of 8000 to 13,000 feet. The roots are ovoid, oblong, or conical, $\frac{1}{2}$ to $1\frac{1}{2}$ inches in length, $\frac{4}{10}$ to $\frac{6}{10}$ of an inch in diameter, bitter without acridity, of a light ash-color. Their transverse section shows a white, farinaceous, homogeneous tunic, traversed by 4 to 7 yellowish vascular bundles. According to Wasowicz, the root yielded $\frac{6}{100}$ of 1 per cent. of *atesine*, an amorphous, very slightly poisonous alkaloid (the same alkaloid was previously pointed out by Broughton), aconitic acid, an acid similar to tannic acid, a soft fat, cane sugar, mucilage, and pectinous substances. *Wakhma*, another Indian drug, appears to be a variety of Atis. (See *P. J. Tr.*, xvi. 86.)

this country as an ornamental flower. All parts of the plant are acrid and poisonous. The leaves and root are used. The leaves should be collected when the flowers begin to appear, or shortly before. After the fruit has formed, they are less efficacious. The root is much more active than the leaves; and an extract from the latter is said to have only one-twentieth of the strength of one made from the former. It should be gathered in autumn or winter after the leaves have fallen, and is not perfect until the second year. It has been mistakenly substituted for horseradish root, as a condiment, with fatal effect. The wild plant is said to be more active than the cultivated. (*Schroff.*) Prof. Wm. Procter found the roots of the plant cultivated in this country richer in the active alkaline principle than the imported roots; having obtained as much as 0·85 per cent. from the former. (*Proc. A. P. A.*, 1860.)

The aconite root is brought into market in packages or bales, originally, in general, either from the continent of Europe or from India. It is of variable quality; some parcels being unobjectionable, while others contain a considerable proportion of inert or defective roots. Among these roots that of *Imperatoria ostruthium* has been expressly noted. (*P. J. Tr.*, vii. 749.) The best test is the taste; and roots should be rejected which have not in a fair degree the characteristic properties in this respect described below, especially the sensation of numbness and tingling on the tongue, lips, and fauces.

Nepaul aconite is composed of elongated, conical, tuberous, or nearly cylindrical roots, 3 to 4 inches long, ½ to 1¼ inches in diameter at the base; unbranched; often abruptly broken off below; more or less flattened; shrivelled chiefly in a longitudinal direction, and sparsely marked with the scars of rootlets. *Japanese aconite* has also been largely sold in London.* It consists of plump, oblong or ovoid, dark grayish or blackish tubers, from half an inch to an inch in length, and ⅓ to ⅔ of an inch in diameter.

Properties. The *fresh leaves* have a faint narcotic odor, most sensible when they are rubbed. Their taste is at first bitterish and herbaceous, afterwards burning and acrid, with a feeling of numbness and tingling on the inside of the lips, tongue, and fauces, which is very durable, lasting sometimes many hours. When long chewed, they inflame the tongue. The *dried leaves* have a similar taste, but the acrid impression commences later. Their sensible properties and medicinal activity are impaired by long keeping. They should be of a green color, and free from mustiness. The *root* has a feeble earthy smell. Though sweetish at first, it has afterwards the same effect as the leaves upon the mouth and fauces. It shrinks much in drying, and becomes darker, but does not lose its acrimony. Those parcels, whether of leaves or roots, should always be rejected which are destitute of this property. As found in commerce, the aconite root is described as being "from a half to three-quarters of an inch (12 to 20 m.m.) thick at the crown; conically contracted below; from two to three inches (50 to 70 m.m.) long, with scars or fragments of radicles; dark brown externally; whitish internally; with a rather thick bark, enclosing a star-shaped pith about seven-rayed; without odor; taste at first sweetish, soon becoming acrid, and producing a sensation of tingling and numbness." *U. S.*† The seeds also are acrid. For an account of the chemistry of aconite, see *Aconitina*, page 123.

Medical Properties and Uses. Aconite was well known to the ancients as a

* *Japanese Aconite.*—Seven varieties of aconite tubers are said by Dr. Langaard to be found in the Japanese drug stores, usually preserved in vinegar or child's urine, or by drying. The botanical source of these aconite roots is not accurately determined, but they are probably, at least in part, yielded by *A. japonicum*, Thunb., and *A. Fischeri*, Reich., believed by many botanists to be respectively identical with *A. lycoctonum*, Linn., and *A. Chinense*, Sieb. Several alkaloids have been separated, but have not been studied at all, with the exception of *Japaconitine*, which is said to be the most poisonous of the known aconite alkaloids. (See *P. J. Tr.*, 3 ser., xi. 149, 1021.)

† Prof. Joseph Schrenk observes that the aconite root is not correctly described in our Pharmacopœia, and that the *nucleus sheath* or endodermis of the aconite root is found quite close to the surface; it is nearly circular, and consists of a single layer of tangentially elongated cells. It is the *cambium zone*, consisting of about eight rows of cells, which presents on the cross-section the appearance of an irregular star, with from five to nine rays. The cambium line encloses the entire woody portion of the fibro-vascular bundles, not the pith only, as the Pharmacopœia might lead the reader to believe by speaking of the "seven-rayed pith." (*Amer. Drug.*, April, 1887, 61.)

powerful poison, but was first employed as a medicine by Baron Störck, of Vienna, whose experiments with it were published in the year 1762. In moderate doses, it produces warmth in the stomach and sometimes nausea, general warmth of the body, numbness and tingling in the lips and fingers, muscular weakness, diminished force and frequency of the pulse, and diminished frequency of respiration. From larger doses all these effects are experienced in an increased degree. The stomach is more nauseated; the numbness and tingling extend over the body; headache, vertigo, and dimness of vision occur; the patient complains occasionally of severe neuralgic pains; the pulse, respiration, and muscular strength are greatly reduced; and a state of general prostration may be induced, from which the patient may not quite recover in less than two or three days. The effects of remedial doses begin to be felt in twenty or thirty minutes, are at their height in an hour or two, and continue with little abatement from three to five hours.

In poisonous doses, besides the characteristic tingling in the mouth and elsewhere, aconite occasions burning heat of the œsophagus and stomach, thirst, violent nausea, vomiting and purging, severe gastric and intestinal spasms, headache, dimness of vision, with contracted or expanded pupils, numbness or paralysis of the limbs, diminished sensibility in general, stiffness or spasm of the muscles, great prostration, pallid countenance, cold extremities, an extremely feeble pulse, and death in a few hours, sometimes preceded by delirium, stupor, or convulsions. All these effects are not experienced in every case; but there is no one of them which has not been recorded as having occurred in one or more instances. The proper treatment of aconite poisoning consists in the maintenance of absolute rest in a position horizontal, or with the head lower than the feet; the evacuation of the stomach by the siphon tube or stomach-pump, if free vomiting do not occur; the administration of stimulus, and the use of external heat to keep up the bodily temperature. Whisky or brandy should be given freely in a concentrated form by the mouth and rectum; when the symptoms are very urgent, it may be injected under the skin. Ammonia should be employed *pro re nata*. In severe cases the tincture of digitalis should be given hypodermically (gtt. xv to xxv); and ammonia may be injected into the veins. We have known life to be apparently saved by laudanum given in drachm doses; and there is sound reasoning as well as some clinical experience (*Boston Med. and Surg. Jour.*, Sept. 1861) in justification of the use of tincture of nux vomica in combination with that of digitalis. If the bodily temperature decreases, it should be maintained by external heat.

The symptoms produced by aconite are chiefly due to its action upon the circulation and the nervous system. It is a direct and powerful depressant of the heart, if in sufficient amount completely paralyzing the cardiac muscle. The lowering of the force of the circulation is certainly in large part due to this action; but it is probable, although not proved, that it also paralyzes the vaso-motor system. Upon the cerebrum the drug exerts very little if any direct influence. Upon the peripheral sensory nerves it acts as a powerful depressant, thereby causing the characteristic tingling and numbness of aconite poisoning. The influence upon the spinal marrow seems to be less pronounced than that upon the sensory nerves; but, if in sufficient amount, the poison depresses the motor centres of the cord. To this, and not to any effect upon the motor trunks or the muscles, is due the loss of reflex activity and of voluntary power caused by toxic doses.

As an internal remedy, aconite is very valuable in sthenic fever from any cause; when the condition is asthenic it should never be administered. It is also useful in some cases for the purpose of benumbing sensitive nerves; thus it will sometimes arrest the vomiting of pregnancy, and has often been used with excellent results in rheumatic neuralgia. To obtain such effects it must be given boldly. Applied locally to a sensitive or painful part, it is very efficient, owing to its being brought in a concentrated state into contact with the irritated nerves. It is a favorite application in neuralgias, and will probably achieve good more often than any other narcotic local remedy. Applied to the skin, aconite occasions heat and prickling or tingling, followed by numbness, and, if in contact with a wound, produces its peculiar constitutional effects. Applied to the eye, it causes decided contraction of the pupil.

It may be administered in powder, extract, or tincture.* The dose of the powdered leaves is one or two grains (0·065–0·13 Gm.), of the extract from half a grain to a grain (0·03–0·065 Gm.), of the tincture of the leaves twenty or thirty drops (1·25–1·9 C.c.), to be repeated twice or three times a day, and gradually increased till the effects of the medicine are experienced. The preparation now almost exclusively employed is the tincture of the root, *Tinctura Aconiti. U. S.* Of this, from 3 to 5 drops (0·18–0·3 C.c.) may be given every two to four hours until its effects become obvious. It is very important to distinguish between the tincture of the leaves formerly officinal and still used and the much stronger tincture of the root just referred to. Few patients will bear at first more than four minims of the latter. Very properly, we think, the tincture of the leaves was abandoned at the revision of the U. S. P. 1860. Aconite may be used externally in the form of the saturated tincture of the root, of extract mixed with lard, of a plaster or liniment, or of aconitine ointment. The tincture may be applied by means of a soft piece of sponge on the end of a stick.

Off. Prep. of the Root. Abstractum Aconiti; Extractum Aconiti; Extractum Aconiti Fluidum; Tinctura Aconiti.

Off. Prep. of the Leaves. Br. Extractum Aconiti.

Off. Prep. of the Root. Br. Aconitina; Linimentum Aconiti; Tinctura Aconiti.

ADEPS. *U. S.* *Lard.*

(Ă'DĔPS.)

"The prepared internal fat of the abdomen of Sus scrofa, Linné (Class, *Mammalia;* Ord., *Pachydermata*), purified by washing with water, melting, and straining." *U. S.*

ADEPS PRÆPARATUS. *Br.* *Prepared Lard.*

(Ă'DĔPS PRÆ-PA-RĀ'TŬS—prē-pa-rā'tŭs.)

"The purified fat of the hog, *Sus Scrofa.*" *Br.*

Adeps Præparatus, *Br.* Adeps Suillus, *P. G.;* Axungia Porci, s. Porcina, Axungia, *Lat.;* Prepared Lard, Hog's Lard, *Eng.;* Axonge, Graisse, Graisse de Porc, Saindoux, *Fr.;* Schweineschmalz, *G.;* Grasso di Porco, Lardo, *It.;* Manteca de Puerco, Lardo, *Sp.*

Preparation. Lard is the prepared fat of the hog. The Br. Pharmacopœia gives a process for its preparation; but in this country it is generally purchased by the druggists already prepared. The adipose matter of the omentum and mesentery, and that around the kidneys, are usually employed; though the subcutaneous fat is said to afford lard of a firmer consistence. In the crude state it contains membranes and vessels, and is more or less contaminated with blood, from all which it must be freed before it can be fit for use. For this purpose, the fat, having been deprived as far as possible by the hand, of membranous matter, is cut into pieces, washed with water till the liquor ceases to be colored, and then, after carefully separating the water, it is melted in a copper or iron vessel, over a slow fire.† The

* *Squibb's Test for Aconite and its Preparations.*—In the absence of any reliable chemical tests for aconitine, Dr. Squibb suggests that a fluidrachm of a solution of the various preparations be taken into the anterior part of the mouth (after the latter has been thoroughly rinsed), and held there for one minute by the watch, and then discharged. The peculiar numbing sensation should be experienced within fifteen minutes, and it should continue for fifteen or thirty minutes. Tested in this way, he found the commercial aconitines, in solution of the strength of $\frac{1}{350}$ grain in 1 fluidrachm of water, to have the following relative strengths; 1 grain good powdered aconite root is equal to 1 grain ordinary commercial aconitine, $\frac{1}{4}$ grain Merck's ordinary aconitine, $\frac{1}{13}$ grain Merck's pseudaconitine, $\frac{1}{111}$ grain Duquesnel's aconitine crystallised (really nitrate of aconitine). He also found by this approximate method that 1 grain of powdered aconite root was equivalent to 1 minim of fluid extract, $\frac{1}{4}$ grain alcoholic extract of aconite root, 2·66 minims of U. S. P. tincture of aconite root, 8·43 minims of British tincture of the root, 11·8 minims of German tincture of the root, 1·5 minims of Fleming's tincture, 9 grains of powdered aconite leaf, 1·5 grains of alcoholic extract of dried aconite leaf, 1 grain of Allen's English extract of fresh plant, and 72 minims of tincture of aconite leaf.

† Prof. Procter recommends the following method of operating. After careful removal of the membranes and adhering flesh, the crude lard is to be cut into small pieces, malaxated with successive portions of cold water until this remains clear, and then heated moderately, in a tinned vessel, until the melted fat becomes perfectly clear and anhydrous. Lastly, it is to be strained into earthen pots, being occasionally stirred as it cools; and the pots should be securely covered with waxed or varnished paper, and kept in a cool, dry cellar. (*A. J. P.*, xxxv. 114.)

heat is continued till all the moisture is evaporated, which may be known by the transparency of the melted fat, and the absence of crepitation when a small portion of it is thrown into the fire. Care should be taken that the heat be not too great; as otherwise the lard might be partially decomposed, acquire a yellow color, and become acrid. This may be guarded against by using a water-bath in melting the lard. The process is completed by straining the liquid through linen, and pouring it into suitable vessels, in which it concretes upon cooling. To render it, however, perfectly free from particles of membrane and tissue, which are often the cause of rancidity, and unfit lard for its finer and more permanent uses, Mr. Ed. Smith, of Torquay, insists on the necessity of filtering the lard through paper, after freeing it from its coarser impurities by straining through linen. By this author it is recommended that the process of purification should be completed by remelting the lard, by means of a water-bath, and then carefully filtering it through paper in a warm closet. (*P. J. Tr.*, 1869, p. 131.) Lard may be rendered quite inodorous by melting it, when fresh, by means of a salt-water bath, adding a little alum or common salt, continuing the heat till a scum rises which is to be skimmed off, and, after the lard has concreted, separating the saline matter by washing it thoroughly with water. For a particular account of the process, see *A. J. P.*, xxviii. 176.

The following is the process of the British Pharmacopœia for preparing lard. "Take of the internal fat of the abdomen of the hog, perfectly fresh, *any convenient quantity*. Remove as much of the external membranes as possible, and suspend the fat so that it shall be freely exposed to the air for some hours; then cut it into small pieces, and beat these in a stone mortar until they are thus, or by some equivalent process, reduced to a uniform mass in which the membranous vesicles are completely broken. Put the mass thus produced into a vessel surrounded by warm water, and apply a temperature not exceeding 130° F. (54·4° C.) until the fat has melted and separated from the membranous matter. Finally, strain the melted fat through flannel." *Br.*

The process of the British Pharmacopœia differs from that formerly used, and is modelled upon the suggestions of Prof. Redwood, that the use of water be especially avoided, and that the selected fat be exposed freely to air and light before rendering. (*P. J. Tr.*, 1883, p. 364; also *Ephemeris*. 1884, p. 504.)

Lard, as offered for sale, often contains common salt, which renders it unfit for pharmaceutic purposes. This may be detected, when the quantity is insufficient to be sensible to the taste, by means of nitrate of silver, which will produce a precipitate of chloride of silver with water in which the salted lard has been boiled, after cooling and filtration. To free it from this impurity, it may be melted with twice its weight of boiling water, the mixture well agitated and set aside to cool, and the fat then separated. Lard is sometimes adulterated with water, starch, and a small proportion of alum and quicklime, which render it whiter, but unfit for medical use. But by far the most common adulteration of lard at this time (1888) is through the use of cotton-seed oil. Indeed, some specimens of lard consist almost wholly of mixtures of stearin and cotton-seed oil. Lard of this kind can easily be detected by the disagreeable and characteristic odor of cotton-seed oil which is evolved when it is heated.

Properties. Lard is "a soft, white, unctuous solid, of a faint odor, free from rancidity, having a bland taste and a neutral reaction. Entirely soluble in ether, benzin, and disulphide of carbon. Sp. gr. about 0·938. It melts at or near 35° C. (95° F.) to a clear, colorless liquid, and at or below 30° C. (86° F.) it is a soft solid. Distilled water, boiled with lard, should not acquire an alkaline reaction, (abs. of alkalies), nor should another portion be colored blue by solution of iodine (abs. of starch). A portion of the water, when filtered, acidulated with nitric acid, and treated with test-solution of nitrate of silver, should not yield a white precipitate soluble in ammonia (abs. of common salt). When heated for several hours on the water-bath, under frequent stirring, lard should not diminish sensibly in weight (abs. of water)." *U. S.* When melted, it readily unites with wax and resins. Like most animal fats and oils, it consists of stearin, palmitin, and olein; its consistence, when pure, depending largely upon the relative proportions of these principles; olein, being the liquid principle, can readily be separated from the other two, by subjecting lard in cold weather to strong pressure, when the *olein* (*lard oil*) is pressed out, the solid residue (*stearin*) being used for various purposes, more particularly the manufacture of candles. Olein may also be separated by means of boiling alcohol, which, on cooling, deposits the concrete principles of the lard. It is extensively employed for burning in lamps, and other purposes in the arts. Vast quantities of it are prepared in Cincinnati, Ohio, and much is exported. In France it is said to be largely used for adulterating olive oil, and is itself now often adulterated by a heavy lubricating petroleum.

Exposed to the air, lard absorbs oxygen and becomes rancid. It should, therefore, be kept in well-closed vessels, or procured fresh when wanted for use. In the rancid state, it irritates the skin, and sometimes exercises an injurious reaction on substances mixed with it. Rancidity in lard and other fats is prevented by digesting them with benzoin or poplar buds, and rancid lard may often be greatly improved by washing it with lime-water. (See *Unguenta.*) Lard even when fresh is slightly acid, as was proved by Dieterich, *Arch. d. Pharm.*, 1887, p. 494.

Medical Properties and Uses. Lard is emollient, and is occasionally employed by itself in frictions, or in connection with poultices to preserve their soft consistence; but its chief use is in pharmacy as an ingredient of ointments and cerates. It is frequently added to laxative enemata.

Off. Prep. Adeps Benzoinatus; Ceratum; Ceratum Cantharidis; Ceratum Extracti Cantharidis; Ceratum Resinæ; Unguentum; Unguentum Hydrargyri; Unguentum Mezerei; Unguentum Simplex.

Off. Prep. Br. Adeps Benzoatus; Emplastrum Cantharidis; Unguentum Iodi; Unguentum Terebinthinæ; Unguentum Hydrargyri Nitratis.

ADEPS BENZOINATUS. *U.S.* *Benzoinated Lard.*

(Ă′DĔPS BĔN-ZŌ-Ĭ-NĀ′TŬS.)

Adeps Benzoatus, *Br.;* Benzoated Lard; Unguentum Benzoini, *U. S.* 1870; Axungia Balsamica, s. Benzoinata, s. Benzoata; Ointment of Benzoin, *E.;* Axonge (Graisse) benzoinée (balsamique), *Fr.;* Benzoinirtes Schmalz, *G.*

Preparation. "Benzoin in coarse powder *two parts* [or one hundred and forty grains]; Lard *one hundred parts* [or sixteen ounces, av.] Melt the Lard by means of a water-bath, and, having loosely tied the Benzoin in a piece of coarse muslin, suspend it in the melted Lard, and, stirring them together frequently, continue the heat for two hours, covering the vessel and not allowing the temperature to rise above 60° C. (140° F.). Lastly, having removed the Benzoin, strain the Lard and stir while cooling." *U. S.*

"Take of prepared Lard *one pound;* Benzoin reduced to coarse powder *one hundred and forty grains;* melt the lard by the heat of a water-bath, add the benzoin, and, frequently stirring them together, continue the application of heat for two hours; finally remove the residual benzoin by straining." *Br.* That the balsamic or resinous principles, in certain substances like benzoin, exercise a valuable function in preserving fats has been proved by abundant experience. It has been shown that when made, as originally suggested by Doliber and directed in the U. S. Pharmacopœia of 1870, by incorporating the tincture with lard, ointment of benzoin was irritating to the skin in certain diseases; hence the return to the old process of digesting the benzoin in lard, kept at a temperature of 60° C. (140° F.). The present U. S. formula does not differ materially from the British, except in the directions to enclose the benzoin in a muslin bag and the regulation of the temperature; the first improvement has for its object the prevention of the hard cake of benzoin, which otherwise collects at the bottom of the water-bath, and is apt to be imperfectly acted upon. A much pleasanter and more agreeable product is insured by heeding the U. S. directions as to limiting the temperature, a high heat volatilizing the odorous principles, and communicating an empyreumatic odor.

Off. Prep. Unguentum Acidi Gallici; Unguentum Acidi Tannici; Unguentum Belladonnæ; Unguentum Chrysarobini; Unguentum Gallæ; Unguentum Hydrargyri

Ammoniati; Unguentum Iodi; Unguentum Iodoformi; Unguentum Plumbi Carbonatis; Unguentum Plumbi Iodi; Unguentum Potassii Iodidi; Unguentum Stramonii; Unguentum Sulphuris; Unguentum Sulphuris Alkalinum; Unguentum Veratrinæ; Unguentum Zinci Oxidi.

Off. Prep. Br. Unguentum Aconitinæ; Unguentum Atropinæ; Unguentum Belladonnæ; Unguentum Calaminæ; Unguentum Chrysarobini; Unguentum Gallæ; Unguentum Hydrargyri Subchloridi; Unguentum Iodoformi; Unguentum Plumbi Acetatis; Unguentum Potassii Iodidi; Unguentum Sabinæ; Unguentum Simplex; Unguentum Staphisagriæ; Unguentum Sulphuris; Unguentum Zinci.

ÆTHER. *U. S., Br.* *Ether.*

(Æ′THẸR—ē′thẹr.)

Æther Sulphuricus, *Ed., Dub.;* Ether, Hydric Ether, Naphtha Vitrioli, Hydrate of Ethylen, Oxide of Ethyl; Ether hydrique, ou vinique, ou sulfurique, *Fr.;* Æther, Schwefeläther, *G.*

"A liquid composed of about 74 per cent. of Ethyl Oxide [$(C_2H_5)_2O$; 74.—C_2H_5O; 37] and about 26 per cent. of Alcohol containing a little water. Sp. gr. about 0·750 at 15° C. (59° F.)." *U. S.* "A volatile liquid prepared from Alcohol, and containing not less than 92 per cent. by volume of pure ether, $(C_2H_5)_2O$, or $C_4H_{10}O$." *Br.*

Preparation. The present U. S. Pharmacopœia has abandoned the process for preparing ether.*

"Take of Rectified Spirit *fifty fluidounces* [Imp. meas.]; Sulphuric Acid *ten fluidounces* [Imp. meas.]; Chloride of Calcium *ten ounces* [avoird.]; Slaked Lime *half an ounce* [avoird.]; Distilled Water *thirteen fluidounces* [Imp. meas.]. Mix the Sulphuric Acid with twelve fluidounces of the Spirit in a glass flask having a wide neck and capable of containing at least two pints [Imp. meas.], and not allowing the mixture to cool, connect the flask by means of a bent glass tube with a Liebig's condenser, and distil at a temperature sufficient to maintain the liquid in brisk ebullition. As soon as the ethereal fluid begins to pass over, supply fresh Spirit through a tube into the flask in a continuous stream, and in such quantity as to equal the volume of the fluid which distils over. For this purpose use a tube furnished with a stop-cock to regulate the supply, connecting one end of the tube with a vessel containing the Spirit raised above the level of the flask, and passing the other end into the acid fluid through a cork fitted into the flask. When the whole of the Spirit has been added, and forty-two fluidounces have distilled over, the process may be stopped. Dissolve the Chloride of Calcium in the Water, add the Lime, and agitate the mixture in a bottle with the impure ether. Leave the mixture at rest for ten minutes, pour off the light supernatant fluid, and distil it until a glass bead of specific gravity 0·735 placed in the receiver begins to float. The ether and spirit retained by the chloride of calcium, and by the residue of each rectification, may be recovered by distillation and used in a subsequent operation." *Br.*

The preparation of ether embraces two stages: its generation, and its subsequent rectification to remove impurities. The formulas agree in obtaining it by the action

* The following is the process of U. S. P. 1870. "Take of Stronger Alcohol *six pints;* Sulphuric Acid *thirty-six troyounces;* Potassa *three hundred and sixty grains;* Distilled Water *three fluidounces.* To two pints of the Alcohol, contained in a six-pint tubulated retort, gradually add the Acid, stirring constantly during the addition. By means of a cork fitted to the tubulure, adapt a long funnel-shaped tube, with the lower end drawn out so as to form a narrow orifice, and reaching nearly to the bottom of the retort, and also a thermometer tube, graduated from 260° F. [126·6° C.] to 300° F. [148·8° C.], with its bulb reaching to the middle of the liquid. Having placed the retort on a sand-bath, connect it with a Liebig's condenser, and this with a well-cooled receiver. Then raise the heat quickly until the liquid boils, and attains a temperature between 266° F. [130° C.] and 280° F. [137·7° C.]. By means of a flexible tube, connected with the stop-cock of an elevated vessel containing the remainder of the Alcohol, introduce that liquid into the retort, through the funnel-shaped tube, in a continuous stream; the quantity supplied being so regulated that the temperature of the boiling liquid shall continue between the degrees mentioned. After all the Alcohol has been added, proceed with the distillation until the temperature rises to 286°, when the process should be discontinued. To the distilled liquid add the Potassa, previously dissolved in the Distilled Water, and shake them occasionally together. At the end of twenty-four hours, pour off the supernatant liquid, introduce it into a retort, and, with a gentle heat, distil into a well-cooled receiver three pints, or until the liquid attains the specific gravity 0·750. Lastly, keep the Ether in a well-stopped bottle."

of sulphuric acid on alcohol. In the former United States process, which was adopted, with modifications, from the French Codex, one-third of the alcohol taken is mixed with the acid, and, while still hot from the reaction, distilled from a glass retort, by a heat quickly applied, into a refrigerated receiver. When the heat of the mixture has risen to between 130° C. (266° F.) and 137·7° C. (280° F.), the remainder of the alcohol is allowed to enter the retort in a continuous stream, the supply being so regulated that the heat shall be maintained between the degrees mentioned. By a complicated reaction which is explained on page 137, the acid converts the alcohol into ether; and, were it not that the acid becomes more and more dilute as the process proceeds, it would be able to etherize an unlimited quantity of alcohol. Although the acid, before it becomes too dilute, is capable of determining the decomposition of a certain amount of alcohol, yet it is not expedient to add this amount at once; as a considerable portion of it would distil over undecomposed with the ether. The proper way of proceeding, therefore, is that indicated in the formulas; namely, to commence the process with the use of part of the alcohol, and, when the decomposition is fully established, and a portion of ether has distilled, to add the remainder in a gradual manner, so as to replace that which, every moment of the progress of the distillation, is disappearing by its conversion into ether.

In the U. S. process of 1850, the point at which the distillation should cease was determined by the proportion of the ether distilled to that of the alcohol employed, or by the appearance in the retort of white vapors, which indicate the generation of other products besides the ether; but, in the 1870 plan, arrangements having been made by which the temperature can be determined, the degree of heat has been adopted as a better criterion; as it is only when the temperature exceeds the point of 141·1° C. (286° F.) indicated, that the production of injurious impurities is to be apprehended. The modifications of the old process were made in conformity with suggestions by Dr. Squibb, contained in a paper published in the *Proc. A. P. A.*, 1858, p. 390. The direction in the 1850 process to reserve a small portion of acid, to be added gradually with the reserved alcohol, upon the supposition that the acid in the retort might be too much weakened to perform its part duly, has been found upon trial to result in no practical advantage. As the proper proportion between the acid and alcohol is that which requires for ebullition a temperature somewhat above 130° C. (266° F.), or that at which the ether is formed, there is an obvious propriety in supplying the alcohol just so rapidly as may be sufficient to maintain this temperature in the liquid of the retort. If the alcohol be supplied so rapidly as to reduce the temperature below the point mentioned, alcohol will distil over in undue proportion; if too slowly supplied, the temperature will rise so high as to produce other reactions in the materials than that required for etherification, and various other products will result. The rising of the temperature to 141·1° C. (286° F.), after all the alcohol has been added, is, therefore, an indication that the process should be suspended. Nevertheless, the caution to check the process when white vapors appear in the retort is not amiss, as affording an additional security that it shall not be carried too far. At the temperature of 160° C. (320° F.), there would be generated sulphurous acid, heavy oil of wine, olefiant gas, and a large quantity of resino-carbonaceous matter, blackening and rendering thick the residuary liquid; all of them products arising from the decomposition of a portion of sulphuric acid, alcohol, and ether.

The *British* process is that of the Edinburgh Pharmacopœia slightly modified. The principles are the same as those of the U. S. 1870 process; but the directions about temperature are wanting; and the regulation of the supply of alcohol, and the cessation of the operation, are made to depend on the less reliable method of determining the measure of liquid, in the first place in the retort, and in the second place in the receiver; as in the U. S. process of 1850.

In both processes, whatever care may be taken in conducting them, and to stop them in due time, the ether obtained is apt to be contaminated with sulphurous acid, heavy oil of wine, alcohol, and water; and hence its purification becomes necessary. The U. S. Pharmacopœia of 1870 directed for this purpose an aqueous solution of potassa, the British a saturated solution of chloride of calcium, to which a portion of recently slaked lime has been added. In both cases, the crude ether is agitated with the purifying agent, and submitted to a new distillation at a gentle heat, called the *rectification.*

The purifying substances are potassa for sulphurous acid and water, and water for alcohol in the U. S. formula; lime for acid, and a saturated solution of chloride of calcium for alcohol and water, in the British. The British substances for purifying are stated by Dr. Christison to be convenient, and to act perfectly and promptly. The chloride of calcium solution, after having been used, yields on distillation a further portion of ether of the officinal density; and, by concentrating it, filtering while hot, and separating the crystals of sulphite of calcium which form on cooling, the chloride may be recovered for future operations.

In the apparatus employed by Dr. Squibb the ether is made in one operation; the vapors of ether and unchanged alcohol are first washed by a solution of caustic potash maintained at a temperature above the boiling point of alcohol, the latter liquid is then condensed in a worm kept at a suitable temperature and runs back into the still, while the ether vapor, retaining about 4 per cent. of alcohol, is condensed in a well-cooled arrangement. 360 lbs. of concentrated sulphuric acid are sufficient to etherify 120 barrels of clean spirit; the acid has then to be changed, chiefly because the impurities of the spirit render the mixture dark and tarry and liable to froth in the still. (*Ephemeris*, ii. p. 590.)

Properties of Officinal Ether. "The properties of Ether are given under Stronger Ether (see *Æther Fortior*). It dissolves in about five times its volume of water. Tested, as directed under Stronger Ether, the reaction should be neutral; on evaporation it should leave no fixed residue, and the last portion should have not more than a very slight foreign odor; a volume of 10 C.c., upon agitation with an equal volume of glycerin, should not be reduced to less than 7·5 C.c." *U. S.* Notwithstanding the officinal directions for purifying ether, it is not absolutely pure as obtained by either of the formulas here given. Both contain a considerable portion of alcohol, the U. S. about 26 per cent., or, according to Dr. Squibb, 25 per cent. of 88 per cent. alcohol, the British, according to the Pharmacopœia, 8 per cent. of alcohol by measure. In both, there is a little of the light oil of wine. They should, however, be free from various impurities, which are too often found in commercial ether, the result of careless operation, or the employment of imperfect processes. As the Br. Pharmacopœia gives special directions for the purification of ether, we shall postpone an account of the chemical and remedial properties of the medicine till the pure preparation is treated of. (See *Æther Fortior.*) In the mean time, it will be proper to indicate the means of determining the purity of the proper officinal ethers. Commercial ether varies in sp. gr. from 0·733 to 0·765. The impurities found in it are excess of alcohol, water, sulphurous and other acids, heavy oil of wine, and various fixed substances.

The U. S. ether should have the sp. gr. 0·750, and, if heavier than this, must contain too much alcohol or water. When shaken with an equal bulk of water it should not lose more than from one-fifth to one-fourth of its volume. The statement that water takes up only one-tenth has been shown by Dr. Squibb to be erroneous. If it take up more than one-fourth, the ether must contain an excess of alcohol or water, or of both. If the alcohol be in excess, it may be removed by agitating the liquid with twice its bulk of water, which unites with the alcohol, forming a heavier stratum, from which the ether may be poured off. The ether, however, takes up about one-tenth of water, which may be removed by agitation with freshly burned lime, and subsequent distillation. An easy method for detecting and measuring any alcohol present in ether, was given by the Edinburgh College; namely, to agitate it, in a minim measure, with half its volume of a concentrated solution of chloride of calcium. This will remove the alcohol; and the reduction of the volume of the ether, when it rises to the surface, will indicate the amount. The use of glycerin to separate the alcohol and water is for the first time officinal. Heavy oil of wine may be discovered by the ether becoming milky upon being mixed with water. If the ether is pure, it wholly evaporates in the air, leaving no solid residue. All non-volatile impurities are thus detected. It should not redden litmus, showing the absence of acids. The point of ebullition is also an indication of the strength of the ether. When evaporating from bibulous paper, it should offer only a slight degree of foreign odor, aromatic and free from pungency, and should leave the paper, when dry, nearly or quite odorless. This test proves the absence of volatile impurities, except a slight and not inadmissible proportion of light oil of wine. (*Squibb.*)

"Ether should be preserved in well-stopped bottles, or in soldered tins, in a cool place remote from lights and fire." *U. S.*

The British ether should have the sp. gr. 0·735. Fifty measures, agitated with an equal volume of water, are reduced to 45 by an absorption of 10 per cent. It boils below 105°. It is, therefore, considerably stronger than the U. S. ether. In other respects it should answer to the tests above given.

Officinal ether may answer for external application, and may even be given by the mouth, yet for purposes of inhalation it is entirely unfitted without further purification.

Pharm. Uses. In preparing Extractum Lactucarii Fluidum; Hydrargyrum cum Creta; Tinctura Opii Deodorata.

Off. Prep. Br. Æther Purus; Collodium; Collodium Flexile; Spiritus Ætheris; Spiritus Ætheris Compositus; Tinctura Chloroformi et Morphinæ.

ÆTHER ACETICUS. *U. S., Br. Acetic Ether. Acetate of Ethyl.*

$C_2H_5, C_2H_3O_2$; 88. (ÆTHER A-CĒT'I-CŬS.) $C_4H_5O, C_4H_3O_3$; 88.

Naphtha Aceti; Ethyl Acetate; Ether acétique, Naphte acétique, *Fr.*; Essigaether, Essignaphtha, *G.*

Preparation. A process for preparing this ether is for the first time given in the last British Pharmacopœia. It is a modification of the process recommended by W. I. Clark (*P. J. Tr.*, 1883, p. 777), and is as follows. "Take of Rectified Spirit, 32½ fluidounces [Imp. meas.]; Sulphuric Acid, 32½ fluidounces [Imp. meas.]; Acetate of Sodium, 40 ounces [av.]; Carbonate of Potassium, freshly dried, 6 ounces [av.]. To the spirit slowly add the acid, keeping the fluid cool, and, the product being cold, add the acetate, mixing thoroughly. Distil forty-five fluidounces [Imp. meas.]. Digest the distillate with the carbonate of potassium for three days in a stoppered bottle. Separate the ethereal fluid, and again distil until all but about four fluidounces have passed over. Preserve the resulting acetic ether in a well-closed bottle and in a cool place." *Br.* In addition to this method, acetic ether may be made by several processes, the chief of which are the following. 1. Mix 100 parts of alcohol (sp. gr. 0·83) with 63 parts of concentrated acetic acid, and 17 parts of strong sulphuric acid, and distil 125 parts into a receiver, kept cold with wet cloths. 2. Distil to dryness a mixture of three parts of acetate of sodium, three of alcohol, and two of sulphuric acid, mix the distilled product with one-fifth of sulphuric acid, and distil a second time an amount of ether equal to the alcohol employed. 3. Distil two parts of effloresced acetate of lead with one part of alcohol, and a little more than one part of sulphuric acid. In the last two processes, the acetic acid is set free by the action of the sulphuric acid on the acetate employed. J. A. Pabst has devised a process for acetic ether in imitation of that for the preparation of common ether. 50 C.c. of sulphuric acid and the same quantity of alcohol are heated together in a retort to 140° C. (284° F.), and then a mixture of one litre of 96 per cent. alcohol and one litre acetic acid (93 per cent.) is allowed to flow in slowly. At first some ethyl ether goes over, and then a liquid which contains, with considerable uniformity, 85 per cent. acetic ether. The reaction takes place between 130° C. (266° F.) and 135° C. (275° F.); at 145° C. (293° F.) some sulphurous acid is produced. The yield is about 1350 grammes, or 78 per cent., which is 90 per cent. of the theoretical amount. With reference to the solubility of acetic ether in saturated calcium chloride solution, it is to be remarked that pure acetic ether is not dissolved, although it is if mixed with 90 per cent. alcohol. One volume acetic ether, one volume alcohol, and two volumes calcium chloride solution give a homogeneous liquid. The methyl acetic ether can be prepared exactly as the ethyl compound, but in the attempt to prepare the amyl acetic ether in an analogous manner side reactions were found to interfere. In order to study the proportional power of combination possessed by the two alcohols, Mr. Pabst allowed a mixture of 100 C.c. methyl alcohol and 100 C.c. acetic acid to flow into a mixture of 50 C.c. sulphuric acid and 50 C.c. ethyl alcohol. The first distillates contained essentially methyl acetate and the latter pure ethyl acetate. In the flask were found remaining nearly equal amounts of sulphuric and ethyl sulphuric acids, and in addition alcohol, acetic acid, and some residual ethyl acetate. (*Bull. Soc. Chim.*, vol. xxxiii. pp. 350, 351; *A. J. P.*, 1880.)

"A transparent and colorless liquid, of a strong, fragrant, ethereal, and somewhat acetous odor, a refreshing taste, and neutral action. Soluble, in all proportions, in alcohol, ether, and chloroform, and in about 17 parts of water. Sp. gr. 0·889 to 0·897. It boils at about 76° C. (168·8° F.). It is inflammable, burning with a bluish-yellow flame, and acetous odor. Acetic Ether should not change the color of blue litmus paper previously moistened with water, nor leave any fixed residue upon evaporation. When 10 C.c. are agitated with an equal volume of water, in a graduated test-tube, the upper, ethereal layer, after its separation, should not measure less than 9 C.c." *U. S.* It should be kept away from lights or fire. The British Pharmacopœia gives its specific gravity at about 0·900, boiling point about 166° F. (74·4° C.). One part by weight dissolves in about 10 parts of water at 60° F. (15·5° C.).

Medical Properties and Uses. Acetic ether is occasionally used in medicine as a stimulant and antispasmodic. Its action upon the system is probably very similar to that of ether; but as it is less volatile it is less rapidly absorbed and eliminated, and consequently is much less prompt and fugacious in its influence than is ether. It is locally irritating. It has been found by Dr. H. C. Wood to be capable of being used as an anæsthetic, but to be too slow in its action for practical purposes. The dose by the mouth is from fifteen to thirty drops (0·9–1·9 C.c.), sufficiently diluted with water. It is sometimes employed externally, by friction, as a resolvent, and for rheumatic pains.

Off. Prep. Spiritus Odoratus; Tinctura Ferri Acetatis.
Off. Prep. Br. Liquor Epispasticus.

ÆTHER FORTIOR. *U. S.* *Stronger Æther.*

(ÆTHER FŎR'TI-OR.)

"A liquid composed of about 94 per cent. of Ethyl Oxide [$(C_2H_5)_2O$; 74—C_4H_5O; 37] and about 6 per cent. of Alcohol containing a little Water. Sp. gr. not higher than 0·725 at 15° C. (59° F.), or 0·716 at 25° C. (77° F.)." *U. S.**

ÆTHER PURUS. *Br.* *Pure Æther.*

(Æ'THER PŪ'RUS.)

"Ether $(C_2H_5)_2O$ free from alcohol and water." *Br.*

Ether hydrique, *Fr.*; Reiner Æther, *G.*

"Take of Ether, Distilled Water, of each, *two pints* [Imperial measure]; Lime, recently burned, *one ounce* [avoirdupois]; Chloride of Calcium, *four ounces* [av.]. Put the Ether with one pint [Imp. meas.] of the Water into a bottle, and shake them together; allow them to remain at rest for a few minutes, and, when the two liquids have separated, decant off the supernatant ether. Mix this with the remainder of the Water, and again, after separation, decant as before. Put now the washed ether, together with the Lime and Chloride of Calcium, into a retort to which a receiver is closely attached, let them stand for 24 hours, then distil with the aid of a gentle heat. Sp. gr. not exceeding 0·720." *Br.*

The formula of 1870 and the above are nearly the same; the U. S. limiting the amount distilled by the measure, the British by the sp. gr. The ether is first shaken

* "The following is the process of U. S. P. 1870. "Take of Ether, Water, each, *three pints*; Chloride of Calcium, in fine powder, Lime, in fine powder, each, *a troyounce*. Shake the Ether and the Water thoroughly together, and when the Water has subsided, separate the supernatant ether. Agitate this well with the Chloride of Calcium and the Lime in a well-stopped bottle, and allow the mixture to stand for twenty-four hours. Then decant the Ether into a retort, and, having adapted thereto a Liebig's condenser, distil a pint and a half of Stronger Ether into a receiver refrigerated with ice-cold water. Lastly, keep the liquid in a well-stopped bottle. By continuing the distillation, a portion of weaker ether may be obtained." *U. S.*

with the water, in order that the latter, by its superior affinity for alcohol, may take it from the former; and afterwards with the chloride of calcium and lime, to separate from the ether the water with which it has itself united in the first step of the process. Of course, the lime, for this purpose, must be in its freshly calcined state, so that it may have had no opportunity to absorb water from the air. The subsequent distillation is intended still further to strengthen the ether, the less volatile liquids being left in the retort. The lime answers the further purpose of neutralizing any sulphurous or other acid which the ether may have happened to contain. The weaker ether obtained at the end of the process may be kept for subsequent purification. It will be noticed that this separate process accomplishes more perfectly what is effected by the British formula for ether.

Even thus prepared, however, the ether, though sufficiently pure for all pharmaceutical or remedial purposes, is not absolutely pure, still containing a little alcohol. To meet the intentions of the U. S. process, it must have the sp. gr. 0·725 (0·720, *Br.*).

Properties. "A thin and very diffusive, clear, and colorless liquid, of a refreshing characteristic odor, a burning and sweetish taste, with a slightly bitter after-taste, and a neutral reaction. It is soluble, in all proportions, in alcohol, chloroform, benzol, benzin, fixed, and volatile oils, and dissolves in eight times its volume of water at 15° C. (59° F.). It boils at 37° C. (98·6° F.). Ether is highly inflammable, and its vapor, when mixed with air and ignited, explodes violently. If a piece of pale blue litmus paper moistened with water be immersed ten minutes in a portion of the Ether, the color should not change. On evaporating at least 50 C.c. in a glass vessel, no fixed residue should appear, and, on evaporating a portion dropped upon blotting paper no foreign odor should be developed. When 10 C.c. are agitated with an equal volume of glycerin in a graduated test-tube, the Ether layer, when fully separated, should not measure less than 8·6 C.c. It should boil actively, in a test-tube half filled with it and held a short time in the hand, on the addition of small pieces of broken glass. It should be preserved in well-stopped bottles, or in soldered tins in a cool place remote from lights or fires." *U. S.*

The requirement of the British Pharmacopœia, that "when ether is shaken with a fourth of its bulk of solution of iodide of potassium and a little starch paste no blue color is produced," has provoked some criticism, Boerrigter showing that Warden, Werner, Buchner, and others were correct in stating that pure ether would liberate iodine from iodide of potassium. This change is said to be due to hydrogen peroxide by Dunstan and Dymond (*P. J. Tr.*, 1887, p. 841), but others attribute the change to ozone or aldehyd.

Its extreme volatility causes it to evaporate speedily in the open air, with the production of considerable cold. Its inflammability is very great, and the products of its combustion are water and carbonic acid. In consequence of this property the greatest care should be used not to bring it in the vicinity of flame, as, for example, a lighted candle. One of the great advantages of using steam as the source of heat is that it obviates, in a great measure, the danger of its accidental inflammation. When too long kept it undergoes decomposition, and is converted in part into acetic acid. It dissolves iodine and bromine freely, and sulphur and phosphorus sparingly. Its power to dissolve corrosive sublimate makes it a useful agent in the manipulations for detecting that poison. It is also a solvent of volatile and fixed oils, many resins and balsams, tannic acid, caoutchouc, and most of the organic vegetable alkalies. It does not dissolve potassa and soda, in which respect it differs from alcohol. It was formerly believed that when water dissolves more than a tenth of its volume, the ether is shown to contain an undue quantity of water or alcohol, or of both; but according to Dr. Squibb this is not correct, water readily taking up one-fourth of its volume of ether. Ether unites in all proportions with alcohol. According to Prof. R. Boettger, water may be detected in ether by agitating the suspected liquid with bisulphide of carbon; if water be present the mixture becomes milky and turbid, otherwise it remains clear. Stefanelli (*Ber. d. Chem. Ges.*, 8, 439) proposes to shake ether with a small fragment of anilin-violet, which does not impart color to ether free from alcohol. One per cent. of alcohol may be thus detected.

The most delicate test for the presence of alcohol in ether is that of Lieben, founded on the formation of iodoform by alcohol but not by ether. (See p. 144.) The mere keeping of ether in presence of moisture is said to generate traces of alcohol sufficient to produce the reaction. (Allen, *Com. Org. Anal.*, 2d ed., i. p. 125.)

On filtering an ethereal liquid with free access of air, a frost-like congelation is observed on the upper part of the filter, its appearance and quantity depending upon the temperature and the hygrometric state of the atmosphere. Tauret has collected some of this *hydrate of ether*, and found that after it had been completely freed from ether by strongly blowing upon it, it had the temperature 3·5° C. (25·7° F.), and on fusion yielded 17 to 18 parts of water for 37 of ether; the formula $(C_2H_5)_2O,2H_2O$ requires 18 parts. (*A. J. P.*, 1878.)

Composition and Theory of its Production. The empirical formula of ether is $C_4H_{10}O$, and this is the result both of analysis and a determination of its vapor density, whereby the molecular weight is established. This formula, however, is better understood when we examine the conditions of its formation. Ether is then found to be the oxide of ethyl (C_2H_5). This is the group which gives character to common alcohol and all its salts, whether with organic or inorganic acids. The group C_2H_5 acts as a monad radical, and common alcohol is its hydrate, C_2H_5,OH. Its oxide then would be $(C_2H_5)_2O$, and all the reactions by which ether is produced show it to be this oxide. It is commonly formed from common alcohol (ethyl hydrate) by the action of sulphuric acid, according to the following reactions:

$$C_2H_5,OH + SO_2,OH,OH = SO_2,OH,OC_2H_5 + H_2OH;$$

that is, alcohol reacting with sulphuric acid yields ethyl-sulphuric acid (sulphovinic acid) and water. In the presence of an excess of alcohol and at the proper temperature the ethyl-sulphuric acid then reacts with another molecule of alcohol as follows:

$$C_2H_5,OH + SO_2,OH,OC_2H_5 = C_2H_5,OC_2H_5 + SO_2,OH,OH,$$

whereby ethyl oxide (ether) is formed, and sulphuric acid is regenerated. These reactions take place best at a temperature of about 140° C. (284° F.), and if the mixture in the flask is kept at this temperature a steady stream of alcohol can be converted into ether, whence the process has been called "the continuous etherification process."

Medical Properties and Uses. The chief use of ether in medicine is as an anæsthetic; although when taken into the stomach, it is absorbed and exerts its narcotic powers. Locally applied it acts at first as a stimulant and afterwards as a narcotic. If it be on an exposed surface its evaporation occurs so rapidly as to mask by refrigeration the direct action of ether. It was at one time employed for freezing parts about to be operated upon, but has been superseded by the more volatile and cheaper petroleum products. It is frequently employed in nausea dependent upon gastric depression, and also in flatulent or even biliary colic; it is sometimes effective in gastrodynia, in neuralgia of the gums, earache, etc. When applied locally its evaporation should be prevented if possible. When ether is taken into the general system it produces an increase of the force and frequency of the pulse, which appears to be due to a stimulant action both upon the heart and vaso-motor system. The augmentation of the force of the circulation is remarkably well maintained even during profound etherization, and after death from ether poisoning the heart is usually, if not always, found to be beating. When the drug causes a fatal result, it is almost always by paralyzing the centres of respiration. In sufficient amount ether acts powerfully as a narcotic, suspending consciousness and also lessening reflex activity. In some subjects there is a stage of etherization in which sensibility is destroyed, although consciousness is preserved. The influence of ether upon the nervous system is a direct one, and the usual order of the involvement of the nerve centres as shown by Flourens is: first the cerebrum, next the sensory centres of the cord, next the motor centres of the cord, next the sensory centres of the medulla, and finally the motor centres (including that of respiration) of the medulla.

For external use, the unrectified ether is sufficiently pure. The internal dose of ether is from fifty drops to a teaspoonful, to be repeated frequently when the full effect of the remedy is desired. It may be given in capsules, or simply floating upon the surface of ice-cold water or incorporated in an aqueous mixture, to be made by first rubbing it up with spermaceti, employed in the proportion of two grains for each fluidrachm of the ether.

A *syrup of ether* is directed by the French Codex. MM. J. Regnault and Adrian, after a thorough investigation of the solubility of ether in solutions of sugar, offer the following formula. Take of sugar 440 parts, distilled water 490 parts, alcohol at 90° 50 parts, pure ether 20 parts. Put into a bottle, shake, and preserve. The whole of this might be given at a dose, if the parts taken are represented by grains.

Capsules of ether, also called *pearls of ether*, are inodorous, will keep for a year at least without loss, and furnish the means of introducing ether into the stomach without irritating the mouth and throat. In a few seconds after they arrive in the stomach, they burst and diffuse their effects with singular rapidity. Analogous effects are produced when they are introduced into the rectum or vagina. Ether may be gelatinized by the process of M. Grimault. This consists in briskly shaking, in a stoppered bottle, four measures of ether, free from alcohol and acid, with one measure of white of egg. *Gelatinized ether* is an opaline trembling jelly, which may be spread with the greatest facility. It may be used as a local anæsthetic, applied to the seat of pain, spread on linen, and covered with a piece of cloth or of sheet caoutchouc. Gelatinized ether will not keep, but must be prepared at the time it is wanted.

Etherization. Ether may be exhibited by inhalation. Many years ago, its use in this way was proposed by Drs. Beddoes, Pearson, and Thornton, of England, in certain diseases of the lungs. As early as 1805, the late Dr. Warren, of Boston, employed ethereal inhalation to relieve the distress attending the last stage of pulmonary inflammation. About the year 1812, in Philadelphia, at a time when the nitrous oxide was the subject of popular lectures, the vapor of ether was frequently breathed from a bladder for experiment or diversion; and its effects in producing transient intoxication, analogous to that caused by the nitrous oxide, were observed. It was not, however, until October, 1846, that attention was particularly drawn to ethereal inhalation as a remedy for pain. In that month, Dr. Warren, of Boston, was applied to by Dr. W. T. G. Morton, dentist of that city, to ascertain by trial whether an agent which he had successfully employed to render painless the extracting of teeth would be equally successful in preventing the pain of surgical operations. This agent was the vapor of ether. Dr. Warren acceded to this request, and shortly afterwards, at the Massachusetts General Hospital, performed a severe operation, without pain to the patient, under the influence of ether, administered by Dr. Morton. A few days subsequently, Dr. C. T. Jackson, of Boston, in conversation with Dr. Warren, claimed to have first made known to Dr. Morton the use of ethereal vapor for the prevention of pain in dental operations.

From this beginning, the employment of ether by inhalation for the prevention and removal of pain has spread throughout the civilized world. The effect produced, called *etherization*, is usefully resorted to in all severe operations, not merely for the prevention of pain, but also of the shock which the system would otherwise suffer as a consequence of the pain, and also as a means of producing muscular relaxation in dislocation, strangulated hernias, etc. It has been employed for the detection of feigned diseases, by suspending the operation of the will; in neuralgia, biliary or renal colic, dysmenorrhœa, etc., as a palliative; in tetanus, and in the spasms produced by an overdose of strychnia, as an antispasmodic; and in asthma and chronic bronchitis, as an antispasmodic expectorant. In midwifery it is extensively employed; and, while it does not seem materially to interfere with the due contraction of the uterus, it promotes the relaxation and lubricating secretions of the soft parts. In vivisections, humanity calls for the use of it as an anæsthetic.

Ethereal vapor is most conveniently inhaled through a soft sponge, hollowed out on one side to receive the projection of the nose, and saturated with ether of the purest quality. The sponge, thus prepared, is applied over the nostrils, through which the inhalation should be made in preference to the mouth. When the inhalation is thus conducted through a sponge, the ethereal vapor is copiously mixed with air, and there is no fear of inducing asphyxia. At first a short cough is generally produced, but this soon disappears; and, after the lapse of from two to five minutes, and the expenditure of about two fluidounces of ether, the quantity being very variable in different cases, the patient becomes insensible, and appears as if in a deep, almost apoplectic sleep. The usual signs of the full effect of the ether are the closure of the eyelids, muscular relaxation, and inability to answer questions. During the whole process of etherization, the fingers should be kept on the pulse; and, if it become feeble, or very slow, or very rapid, the sponge should be removed until the circulation improves. At first there is redness, afterwards paleness of the face and neck, succeeded by cold perspirations. The danger in etherization is very rarely, if ever, through failure of the circulation, but by arrest of the respiration, and the state of the latter function should be closely watched; should it become very slow, or shallow, or irregular, the anæsthetic should be withdrawn, and, if necessary, appropriate measures of relief adopted. This is the mode of proceeding in surgical operations; in midwifery cases, partial etherization is often sufficient. One of the drawbacks to the use of ether is that vomiting is very apt to occur and be severe during the recovery from the narcosis. To lessen the gastric disturbance as much as possible, no food should be allowed for some hours before etherization, and a moderate dose of brandy or whisky should be administered at the beginning of the latter process. In a few instances etherization has produced alarming remote effects. Dr. F. D. Lente has reported three cases of this kind. (*New York Journ. of Med.*, Nov. 1856.) Sometimes death has ensued; but the instances are extremely rare in which a fatal result could be clearly traced to the direct influence of ether.

Pharm. Uses. Oleoresina; Opium Denarcotisatum; Pilulæ Ferri Iodidi; Pilulæ Phosphori; Pyroxylinum.

Off. Prep. Collodium; Collodium Stypticum; Oleum Æthereum; Oleum Phosphoratum; Spiritus Ætheris; Spiritus Ætheris Compositus.

ALCOHOL. *U.S.* *Alcohol.*

(ĂL′CO-HŎL.)

"A liquid, composed of 91 per cent. by weight (94 per cent. by volume) of Ethyl Alcohol [C_2H_5HO; 46 — C_4H_5O,HO; 46], and 9 per cent. by weight (6 per cent. by volume) of Water. Sp. gr. 0·820 at 15·6° C. (60° F.), and 0·812 at 25° C. (77° F.). Alcohol should be preserved in well-closed vessels, in a cool place, remote from lights or fire." *U.S.* "Alcohol, C_2H_5HO, with 16 per cent. of water obtained by the distillation of fermented saccharine fluids, of the sp. gr. 0·838." *Br.*

Spiritus Rectificatus, *Br.*, Rectified Spirit; Spiritus, *P. G.;* Spiritus Vini Rectificatissimus, Alcohol Vini; Spirit of Wine; Alcool, Esprit de Vin, *Fr.;* Rectificirter Weingeist, *G.;* Alcoole, Aquavite rettificata, *It.;* Alcohol, Espiritu rectificado de Vino, *Sp.*

ALCOHOL DILUTUM. *U.S.* *Diluted Alcohol.*

(ĂL′CO-HŎL DI-LŪ′TŬM.)

"A liquid composed of 45·5 per cent. by weight (53 per cent. by volume) of Ethyl Alcohol and 54·5 per cent. by weight (47 per cent. by volume) of Water. Sp. gr. 0·928 at 15·6° C. (60° F.) and 0·920 at 25° C. (77° F.)." *U.S.* "Made by mixing five pints of Rectified Spirit with three pints of Distilled Water. Sp. gr. 0·920." *Br.*

Spiritus Tenuior, *Br.*, Proof Spirit; Spiritus Dilutus, *P. G.;* Spiritus Vini Rectificatus; Alcool dilué, *Fr.;* Verdünnter Spiritus, *G.*

ALCOHOL ETHYLICUM. *Br.* *Ethylic Alcohol, Absolute Alcohol.*

(AL′CO-HŎL Ē-THYL′I-CŬM.)

From the titles and definitions above given, which include all the forms of alcohol recognized by the U. S. and Br. Pharmacopœias, it will be perceived that there are three officinal strengths of Alcohol, those being considered the same which approach nearly in specific gravity and are employed for similar purposes.

In the present U. S. Pharmacopœia, 1880, the title *Alcohol* now means a spirit of the sp. gr. 0·820; this replaces both the *Alcohol Fortius* (stronger alcohol, sp. gr. 0·817), and the *Alcohol* (sp. gr. 0·835) of the Pharmacopœia of 1870. This change is undoubtedly a wise one, as the use of two comparatively strong alcohols led to some confusion in practice. The consolidation, as it may be termed, makes officinal an alcohol as strong as can easily be obtained, and strong enough for all pharmaceutical purposes. Absolute alcohol is made officinal in the British Pharmacopœia as Ethylic Alcohol. (See page 145.)

Alcohol, in the chemical sense, is a peculiar liquid, generated for the most part in vegetable juices and infusions by a *fermentation*, called the *vinous* or *alcoholic*. The liquids which have undergone it are called vinous liquors, and are of various kinds. Thus, the fermented juice of the grape is called wine; of the apple, cider; and the fermented infusion of malt, beer.

With regard to the nature of the liquids susceptible of the vinous fermentation, however various they may be in other respects, one general character prevails; that, namely, of containing sugar in some form or other. It is found, further, that, after they have undergone the vinous fermentation, the sugar they contain has either wholly or in part disappeared; and it was long believed that the only new products are alcohol which remains in the liquid, and carbonic acid which escapes during the process; and that these, when taken together, are equal in weight to the sugar lost. It was hence inferred that sugar is the subject-matter of the changes that occur during the vinous fermentation, and that it is resolved into alcohol and carbonic acid. More recently, however, it has been shown by M. Pasteur that, along with alcohol and carbonic acid, glycerin and succinic acid are generated in small amount, and that the process is not so simple as at first supposed.

Sugar will not undergo the vinous fermentation by itself; but requires to be dissolved in water, subjected to the influence of a ferment, and kept at a certain temperature. Accordingly, sugar, water, the presence of a ferment, and the maintenance of an adequate temperature may be deemed the prerequisites of the vinous fermentation. The water acts by giving fluidity, and the ferment and temperature by commencing and maintaining the chemical changes. The precise manner in which the ferment operates has not been positively determined; but the fermentative change seems to be intimately connected with the multiplication of a microscopic vegetable, *torula cerevisiæ*. Pasteur has shown that the yeast plant lives and grows at the expense of the sugar, which is converted partly into the tissue of the plant, partly into alcohol and other products. The proper temperature for conducting the vinous fermentation ranges from 15·5° C. to 32·2° C. (60° to 90° F.).

Certain vegetable infusions, as those of potatoes and rice, readily undergo vinous fermentation, on account of the ease with which their starch is changed into sugar under the influence of certain ferments. Taking the formula of starch as $(C_6H_{10}O_5)_3$, as at present accepted, it is first changed under the influence of dilute acids or ferments according to the reaction,

$$(C_6H_{10}O_5)_3 + H_2O = C_{12}H_{22}O_{11} + C_6H_{10}O_5,$$

and these products are both changed under the continued action of the same agents into a *glucose* sugar, $C_6H_{12}O_6$, which is then fermentable:

$$C_{12}H_{22}O_{11} + H_2O = (C_6H_{12}O_6)_2, \text{ and}$$
$$C_6H_{10}O_5 + H_2O = C_6H_{12}O_6.$$

The intermediate product, $C_{12}H_{22}O_{11}$, known as *maltose*, is not directly fermentable. According to Berthelot, mannit, glycerin, and similar substances may be made to ferment by contact, for several weeks, with chalk and cheese at 40° C. (104° F.); and the change takes place without the production of sugar, provided chalk be present. M. Arnoult has succeeded in obtaining alcohol by fermenting sugar (glucose), formed by the action of sulphuric acid on poplar wood sawdust, which yielded from 70 to 80 per cent. of this kind of sugar.

Alcohol, being the product of the vinous fermentation, necessarily exists in all vinous liquors, and may be obtained from them by distillation. Formerly it was supposed that these liquors did not contain alcohol, but were merely capable of furnishing it, in consequence of a new arrangement of their ultimate constituents, the result of the heat applied. Brande, however, disproved this idea, by showing that alcohol may be obtained from all vinous liquors without the application of heat, and therefore must pre-exist in them. His method of separating it consists in precipitating the acid and coloring matter from each vinous liquor by subacetate of lead, and removing the water by carbonate of potassium. According to Gay-Lussac, litharge, in fine powder, is the best agent for precipitating the coloring matter.

In vinous liquors, the alcohol is largely diluted with water, and associated with coloring matter, volatile oil, extractive, ethereal substances, and various acids and salts. In purifying it, we take advantage of its volatility, which enables us to separate it by distillation, combined with some of the principles of the vinous liquor employed, and more or less water. The distilled product of vinous liquors forms the different *ardent spirits of commerce.* When obtained from wine, it is called brandy; from fermented molasses, rum; from cider, malted barley, or rye, whisky; from malted barley and rye-meal with hops, and rectified from juniper berries, Holland gin; from malted barley, rye, or potatoes, and rectified from turpentine, common gin; and from fermented rice, arrack.* These spirits are of different strengths, that is, contain different proportions of alcohol, and have various peculiarities by which they are distinguished by the taste. Their strength is accurately judged of by the specific gravity, which is always less in proportion as their concentration is greater.† When they have the sp. gr. 0·920 (0·91984, *Drinkwater*), they are designated in commerce by the term *proof spirit.* If lighter than this, they are said to be above proof; if heavier, below proof; and the percentage of water, or of spirit of 0·825, necessary to be added to any sample of spirit to bring it to the standard of proof spirit, indicates the number of degrees the given sample is above or below proof. Thus, if 100 volumes of a spirit require 10 volumes of water to reduce it to proof spirit, it is said to be "10 over proof." On the other hand, if 100 volumes of a spirit require 10 volumes of spirit of 0·825 to raise it to proof, it is said to be "10 under proof."

Proof spirit is still very far from being pure; being a dilute alcohol, containing about half its weight of water, together with a peculiar oil and other foreign matters. It may be farther purified and strengthened by redistillation, or *rectification* as it is called. Whisky is the spirit usually employed for this purpose; and from every hundred gallons, between fifty-seven and fifty-eight may be obtained, of the average strength of rectified spirit (sp. gr. 0·835), corresponding very nearly with the *Spiritus Rectificatus* of the British. When this is once more cautiously distilled, it will be further purified from water, and the sp. gr. attained will be about 0·825, which is the lightest spirit that can be obtained by ordinary distillation, and is the pure spirit of the British system of excise. It still, however, contains 11 per cent. of water. In the mean while, the spirit, by these repeated distillations, becomes more and more freed from the contaminating oil, called *grain oil* or *fusel oil.* (See *Alcohol Amylicum*, p. 150.) We shall first consider the general properties of alcohol, and afterwards the different officinal forms.

Properties. Alcohol, using this term in a generic sense, is a colorless, transparent, volatile liquid, of a penetrating, agreeable odor, and burning taste. It should be free from foreign odor, which, when present, is owing to fusel oil. When free from water, it is called *anhydrous* or *absolute alcohol.* It is inflammable, and burns without smoke or residue, forming water and carbonic acid. Its flame is bluish when strong, but yellowish when weak. It combines in all proportions with water and ether; and, when diluted with distilled water, preserves its transparency. Its density varies with the proportion of water it contains. (See table on p. 145.) Its value depends upon the quantity of absolute alcohol contained in it; and, as this is greater in proportion as the sp. gr. is less, it is found

* It is stated that in Eastern commerce, under the name of *toddy*, *arrack*, *saki*, and *tsin*, is sold a liquid which has only once been distilled; whilst *sam-shu* is a thrice-distilled rice spirit, and contains from 33 to 52 per cent. of absolute alcohol. (*Journ. Am. Chem. Soc.*, 1885.)

† H. Grouven (*Vortr. über Agriculturchemie*, i. 425; *N. R.*, May, 1879) gives the following average percentages of alcohol, as contained in the ordinary liquors:

	Vol. per cent.	Weight per cent.
Scotch Whisky	50·3	42·8
Irish "	49·9	42·3
American " (old)	60·0	52·2
English "	49·4	41·9
French Cognac (Brandy)	55·0	47·3
Rum	49·7	42·2
Gin	47·8	40·3
German "Schnapps"	45·0	37·9
Russian "Dobry Wutky"	63·0	54·2

The percentage of alcohol in American whisky is usually lower than that given above.

convenient to take the density of a sample in estimating its strength. This is done by instruments called hydrometers, which, when allowed to float in the spirit, sink deeper into it in proportion as it is lighter. Each hydrometer strength has a corresponding specific gravity; and, by referring to tables constructed for the purpose, the percentage of absolute alcohol is at once shown. Dr. W. H. Pile & Son, makers of hydrometers in Philadelphia, graduate instruments showing specific gravity and Baumé's degrees upon the same scale in parallel columns, with a thermometer taking the place of the bulb; these are exceedingly convenient.

Alcohol is capable of dissolving a great number of substances; as, for example, sulphur and phosphorus in small quantity, iodine and ammonia freely, and the hydrates of potassium, sodium, and lithium, but not the carbonates of these metals. Among organic substances, it is a solvent of the organic vegetable alkalies, urea, tannic, citric, and tartaric acids, sugar, mannite, camphor, resins, balsams, volatile oils, and soap. It dissolves the fixed oils sparingly, except castor oil, which is abundantly soluble in it. It reacts chemically with some acids, forming the ethyl ethers, but with others acts only as a solvent. All deliquescent salts are soluble in alcohol, except carbonate of potassium; while the efflorescent salts, and those either insoluble or sparingly soluble in water, are mostly insoluble in it. It dissolves ammonium chloride, and most of the chlorides readily soluble in water; also some nitrates, but none of the metallic sulphates.

A method of detecting alcohol in small proportions has been proposed by M. Carstanjin. The liquid supposed to contain it, having been mixed with platinum black in a small flask, is heated to 51·1° C. (124° F.), well shaken, and filtered. To the filtrate a few drops of solution of potassa are added, and the liquor evaporated to dryness on a water-bath. The residue is then heated with a little arsenious acid; when, if alcohol be present, a garlicky odor will be perceived, owing to the production of cacodyl. According to M. Nickles, however, propylic alcohol would produce the same result. (*A. J. P.*, 1865, p. 334.) A very delicate test for small quantities of alcohol is that of Lieben as modified by Hager. (*Zeitsch. Anal. Chem.*, ix. 492.) It depends on the fact that alcohol under the influence of iodine and an alkali yields iodoform, CHI_3, the properties of which are very characteristic. To 10 C.c. of the clear suspected liquid five or six drops of a 10 per cent. solution of caustic potash or soda are added, and the liquid is warmed to about 50° C. (122° F.). A solution of iodide of potassium fully saturated with free iodine is next added drop by drop, with agitation, until the liquid becomes permanently yellowish brown, when it is carefully decolorized by a further cautious addition of the caustic alkali solution. If alcohol be present, iodoform is gradually deposited at the bottom of the tube in yellow crystals, which, after standing, may be examined with a lens. Spirit diluted with 2000 parts of water, when treated as above and allowed to stand twelve hours, gives a distinct dust-like deposit of iodoform. Unfortunately, the above delicate reaction is not peculiar to alcohol, being produced by acetone, aldehyde, propylic and butyric alcohols, various ethers, etc. On the other hand, it is not given by pure methyl or amyl alcohol, chloroform, chloral, glycerin, or ether, nor by acetic, formic, or oxalic acid. (Allen, *Commercial Org. Anal.*, 2d ed., i. p. 59; see, also, *A. J. P.*, Feb. 1877, Feb. 1879, Nov. 1879; *N. R.*, Aug. 1876.) Prof. Barfoed, of Copenhagen, recommends for an approximate simple test, to moisten small slips of filtering paper thoroughly with the alcohol, and set fire to them. If, when the alcohol has burned out, the paper slip catches fire readily, the latter must be stronger than 80 per cent.; if the paper barely catches fire, the strength may be presumed to be between 75 to 80 per cent.; if it does not catch fire at all, the alcohol cannot be stronger than 73 to 75 per cent. (*A. J. P.*, Jan. 1875.)

The following table, compiled from that of Dr. A. B. Lyons, will be found useful, because it gives the specific gravities and proportions of *officinal* alcohol and water required to make 100 measures at the temperature of 15·5° C. (60° F.) Condensation is taken into account in these figures. Corresponding specific gravities and percentages of mixtures of *absolute* alcohol and water may be found by referring to the alcoholmetrical tables in the Appendix. For criticisms upon these tables, see *A. J. P.*, 1884, pp. 71, 251.

For 100 Measures use		Sp. Gr. of Mixture.	For 100 Measures use		Sp. Gr. of Mixture.	For 100 Measures use		Sp. Gr. of Mixture.	For 100 Measures use		Sp. Gr. of Mixture.
Alc. U.S.P. 0·820.	Water.		Alc. U. S. P. 0·820.	Water.		Alc. U. S. P. 0·820.	Water.		Alc. U. S. P. 0·820.	Water.	
1	99·04	·9986	26	75·83	·9717	51	52·02	·9387	76	26·34	·8871
2	98·08	·9972	27	74·91	·9707	52	51·02	·9369	77	25·28	·8847
3	97·12	·9958	28	73·99	·9697	53	50·02	·9351	78	24·21	·8822
4	96·17	·9945	29	73·07	·9687	54	49·02	·9333	79	23·18	·8799
5	95·23	·9933	30	72·15	·9677	55	48·02	·9315	80	22·09	·8774
6	94·28	·9920	31	71·22	·9666	56	47·01	·9296	81	21·02	·8749
7	93·34	·9908	32	70·30	·9656	57	46·00	·9277	82	19·95	·8724
8	92·41	·9897	33	69·37	·9645	58	44·99	·9258	83	18·88	·8699
9	91·46	·9884	34	68·44	·9634	59	43·97	·9239	84	17·79	·8673
10	90·54	·9874	35	67·51	·9623	60	42·95	·9219	85	16·73	·8648
11	89·61	·9863	36	66·56	·9610	61	41·93	·9199	86	15·65	·8622
12	88·67	·9852	37	65·61	·9597	62	40·91	·9179	87	14·58	·8597
13	87·75	·9842	38	64·67	·9585	63	39·88	·9158	88	13·49	·8570
14	86·82	·9832	39	63·72	·9572	64	38·86	·9138	89	12·39	·8542
15	85·90	·9821	40	62·77	·9559	65	37·83	·9117	90	11·28	·8513
16	84·98	·9811	41	61·81	·9545	66	36·79	·9095	91	10·19	·8486
17	84·05	·9802	42	60·84	·9531	67	35·75	·9073	92	9·05	·8455
18	83·16	·9793	43	59·87	·9516	68	34·72	·9052	93	7·97	·8429
19	82·25	·9784	44	58·90	·9501	69	33·68	·9030	94	6·86	·8400
20	81·34	·9775	45	57·93	·9486	70	32·65	·9009	95	5·72	·8368
21	80·43	·9766	46	56·95	·9470	71	31·60	·8986	96	4·60	·8338
22	79·51	·9756	47	55·97	·9454	72	30·55	·8963	97	3·46	·8306
23	78·59	·9746	48	54·99	·9438	73	29·51	·8941	98	2·32	·8274
24	77·67	·9736	49	54·00	·9421	74	28·46	·8818	99	1·16	·8240
25	76·74	·9726	50	53·01	·9404	75	27·40	·8895	100	0·00	·8206

1. **Absolute Alcohol.** *Anhydrous Alcohol, Ethylic Alcohol.* No process is given in the U. S. Pharmacopœia for the preparation of absolute alcohol; the following is that of the British Pharmacopœia: "Rectified Spirit, 1 pint [Imp. meas.]; Carbonate of Potassium, anhydrous, 2 ounces [av.]; Chloride of Calcium, fused, a sufficiency. Add the carbonate of potassium to the spirit in a stoppered bottle, and macerate for twenty-four hours with frequent agitation. Put the chloride of calcium into a covered crucible, and subject it to a red heat for half an hour; then pour the fused salt on to a clean stone slab, cover it quickly with an inverted porcelain dish, and when it has congealed, break it up into small fragments, and enclose in a dry stoppered bottle. Put one pound [av.] of this fused chloride of calcium into a flask, pour over it the spirit decanted from the carbonate of potassium, and, closing the mouth of the flask with a cork, shake them together and allow them to stand for twenty-four hours with repeated agitation. Then attaching a dry condenser closely connected with a receiver from which free access of air is excluded, and applying the flame of a lamp to the flask, distil about two fluidounces [Imp. meas.], which should be returned to the flask, after which the distillation is to be continued until fifteen fluidounces [Imp. meas.] have been recovered." *Br.* By the term absolute alcohol is meant pure alcohol, entirely free from water. In this state it cannot be obtained by ordinary distillation alone; the purest alcohol thus procured still containing 11 per cent. of water. To separate this it is customary to have recourse to substances having a very strong affinity for water, sufficient not only to abstract it from the alcohol, but to retain it at a temperature at which alcohol will distil over. Soubeiran recommends the following method for obtaining it, and the British process is largely based upon his plan. 1st. Rectify alcohol marking 86° of the centesimal alcoholmeter of Gay-Lussac (rectified spirit), by distilling it from carbonate of potassium. This operation raises its strength to 94° or 95°. 2d. Raise this alcohol to 97° by distilling it with fused chloride of calcium, or by digesting it with quicklime (from which it must be afterwards poured off), in the proportion of a pint of the alcohol to 1½ ounces of the chloride, or 2½ ounces of the lime. 3d. Distil the product of this operation slowly with quicklime, in the proportion of 3¾ ounces to the pint. The product will be absolute alcohol. The operation may be shortened

10

to two steps, by distilling the alcohol of 94° or 95° with an excess of quicklime (7½ ounces to the pint). In all cases, before decanting or distilling, the alcohol must be digested for two or three days with the lime, at a temperature between 95° and 100° F. Lime will not answer as a substance to be distilled from, unless it be in sufficient excess; for otherwise, towards the end of the distillation, the hydrate of lime formed will yield up its water to the alcohol, and weaken the distilled product. Prof. J. Lawrence Smith (*Amer. Chemist*, Oct. 1874) procures an alcohol of 98 to 100 per cent. by macerating 3 pints of alcohol, 94 per cent., in a four-pint bottle with about six troyounces of well-burned lime; well corked and agitated at intervals for ten days, the strengthened alcohol, at the end of this time, is drawn off by a siphon, and may be freed, if desired, of the small trace of lime by redistillation.

Properties. Absolute alcohol is a colorless, volatile liquid, of an agreeable odor and burning taste. It boils at 78·4° C. (173·1° F.), and is congealed at —130·5° C. Its sp. gr. is 0·7978 at 68°, according to Regnault; 0·79381 at 60°, according to Drinkwater; 0·797 to 0·800, by the British Pharmacopœia; while Dr. Squibb has shown that pure alcohol is obtainable of as low a density as 0·7935, and possibly lower. (*Ephemeris*, ii. p. 522.) The sp. gr. of its vapor is 1·59. The tests usually given to prove the absence of water by dropping into the absolute alcohol anhydrous baryta or anhydrous sulphate of copper are not reliable, as Dr. Squibb has demonstrated that when half of one per cent. of water was added to absolute alcohol no change in either the baryta or the anhydrous sulphate of copper took place. Görgen's test of forming a clear solution when mixed with an equal bulk of pure benzol is more delicate, but a test for determining the presence of at least one per cent. of water is badly needed. Absolute alcohol should be free from fusel oil.

Absolute alcohol burns with a pale flame without residue, the products being carbonic acid and water. Its vapor, passed through a porcelain tube filled with pumice-stone and heated to redness, yields carbon, gaseous hydrocarbons, aldehyde, naphthalen, benzen, phenol, and various other substances. (*Berthelot.*) It unites in all proportions with ether and water. Its union with water is attended by condensation and a rise of temperature. When 52·6 volumes of alcohol are mixed with 47·4 of water, corresponding with one mol. of the former to three of the latter, the decrease of volume is at the maximum, amounting to 3·4 per cent. Berthelot has announced the formation of alcohol synthetically, by the union of olefiant gas with water. In this discovery he was anticipated by the late Mr. Hennel, who published it in 1828.

Composition. Absolute alcohol consists of two atoms of carbon 24, six of hydrogen 6, and one of oxygen 16 = 46. Its empirical formula is, therefore, C_2H_6O. It is, however, recognized as the hydrate of the radical ethyl (C_2H_5), so that its rational formula would be C_2H_5OH.

During the vinous fermentation sugar disappears, and the sole products were supposed to be alcohol and carbonic acid, which, taken together, were believed to equal in weight the lost sugar. Now, the comparative composition of the substances concerned supports the opinion that these are the sole derivatives of a portion of the sugar lost. Preparatory to the fermentation, the cane sugar is changed into *grape sugar*, or into a mixture of equal molecules of *dextrose* and *levulose*, called *invert* sugar, according to the reaction given on the preceding page. These two sugars, dried at 100° C. (212° F.), consist of $C_6H_{12}O_6$. Supposing one mol. of this fermentable sugar to be the subject of the change, it will be found to have a composition which admits of its being broken up into two mols. of alcohol and two of carbonic acid; for $C_6H_{12}O_6 = 2(C_2H_6O) + 2(CO_2)$. But it does not follow that all the sugar has been converted into alcohol and carbonic acid; and Pasteur, as before stated, has shown that a portion lost has not been thus converted, but has been partly appropriated to the growth of the yeast plant of the ferment, and partly changed into glycerin and succinic acid.

2. ALCOHOL. *U. S. Alcohol*, sp. gr. 0·820. This was an officinal of the Dublin College, which gave a formula for its preparation, and stated its sp. gr. at 0·818. The Stronger Alcohol introduced into the Materia Medica of the U. S.

Pharmacopœia, at the revision of 1860, though of the sp. gr. 0·817, and therefore a little stronger than the late Dublin preparation, may for all practical purposes be considered as identical with it. To prepare it on a small scale, carbonate of potassium, previously ignited in a heated mortar, may be mixed with ordinary alcohol (sp. gr. 0·835) in a bottle, and shaken occasionally for about four hours; the mixture being, in the mean time, maintained at the temperature of about 100°. Upon resting, the liquid divides into two strata, the lower consisting of a watery solution of carbonate of potassium, the upper of the stronger alcohol, which is to be separated, and distilled so as to obtain the measure of about nine-tenths of the original alcohol employed.

It is described as "a transparent, colorless, mobile and volatile liquid, of a characteristic, pungent and agreeable odor, and a burning taste. It should not change the color of blue or red litmus paper, previously moistened with water. It boils at 78° C. (172·4° F.), and is readily inflammable, giving a blue flame without smoke.

"If a portion of at least 50 C.c. be evaporated to dryness in a glass vessel, no residue or color should appear. If mixed with its own volume of water, and one-fifth its volume of glycerin, a piece of blotting-paper, on being wet with the mixture, after the vapor of Alcohol has wholly disappeared, should give no irritating or foreign odor (fusel oil). And if a portion be evaporated to one-fifth its volume, the residue should not turn reddish upon the addition of an equal volume of sulphuric acid (amyl alcohol). When treated, in a test-tube, with an equal volume of solution of potassa, there should not be an immediate darkening of the liquid (methyl alcohol, aldehyde, and oak tannin). If a portion of about 150 C.c. be digested for an hour with 20 Gm. of carbonate of lead, and filtered, the filtrate then distilled from a water-bath, and the first 20 C.c. of the distillate treated with 1 C.c. of test-solution of permanganate of potassium, the color should not disappear within one or two minutes (abs. of methyl alcohol). If 20 C.c. are shaken in a glass-stoppered vial, previously well rinsed with the same Alcohol, with 2 C.c. of test-solution of nitrate of silver, the mixture should not be rendered more than faintly opalescent during one day's exposure to direct sunlight (abs. of more than traces of foreign organic matters, fusel oil, etc.)." *U. S.*

On a large scale, we are informed that alcohol of this strength is now prepared in the United States, very abundantly, by simple distillation by means of a modified distillatory apparatus. The modification consists in substituting for a single refrigerated receiver, a series of receivers, kept at such temperatures that, in the first of them, the watery vapor shall condense with comparatively little of the alcoholic, which, as it passes through the successive recipients, is more and more deprived of water, until, when condensed in the last, it yields a spirit at least as strong as the officinal Alcohol of the sp. gr. 0·820. At the same time that the spirit is thus strengthened, it becomes, on the same principle, more and more freed from fusel oil, until at length almost wholly deprived of it.

The British preparation contains 16, the U. S. only 9 per cent. of water. Officinal alcohol, though of standard strength, may still be impregnated with a volatile principle, called *fusel oil.* This is usually removed by digesting the alcohol with charcoal. It may also be removed, as well as other impurities, by passing the impure spirit through a filtering bed, composed of sand, wood-charcoal, boiled wheat, and broken oyster-shells, arranged in layers according to the method of Mr. W. Schaeffer. (*A. J. P.*, 1854, p. 536.) Another method, proposed by M. Breton, is to add a few drops of olive oil to the spirit in a bottle, which is then to be shaken, allowed to settle, and decanted. The olive oil dissolves and retains the fusel oil. (*Chem. Gaz.*, April 15, 1859, p. 160.) If 5 C.c. of alcohol be mixed with 6 times its volume of water and then agitated with about 20 drops of chloroform, the latter will, if separated and allowed to evaporate spontaneously, leave the fusel oil perceptible by its odor; and by treating with a little sulphuric acid and potassium acetate, its peculiar ether may be recognized by its odor. (*Ber. Chem. Ges.*, viii.; *A. J. P.*, 1875, p. 304.) If a little of the solution of nitrate of silver be added to alcohol, and the mixture exposed to a bright light, a black powder will be precipitated, if fusel oil be present. Officinal alcohol will not withstand this test; as the best contains a little of the foreign oil. According to Mr. E. N. Kent, of New York, nitrate of silver will not detect fusel oil, but affords its indications by reacting with other organic substances. For detecting fusel oil, Mr. Kent finds pure sulphuric acid the best test. To apply it he half fills a test-tube with the spirit to be tested, and then fills it up very slowly with pure concentrated sulphuric acid. If the spirit be pure, it will remain colorless, otherwise it will become colored, the tint being deeper in proportion to the amount of the impurity. (*New York Journ. of Pharm.*, Aug. 1854.) "Four fluidounces, with thirty grain-measures of *the volumetric solution of nitrate of silver*, exposed for 24 hours to bright light, and then decanted from the black powder which has formed, undergoes no further change when again exposed to light with more of the test." *Br.* This admits the presence of a small but limited proportion of fusel oil. The U. S. Pharmacopœia directs that officinal alcohol, when diluted with 20 parts of distilled water, should have little or no foreign odor; the Br. Pharmacopœia, that its odor and taste should be purely alcoholic.

The best alcohol is that manufactured under Atwood's patent process, in which manganic acid or permanganate of potassium or sodium is used to destroy the fusel oil and other foreign substances. This alcohol withstands the tests of nitrate of silver and sulphuric acid remarkably well. Pure fused sodium acetate has been proposed as a substance particularly adapted to retain fusel oil, and has been used by adding it to the alcohol to be rectified in the proportion of about 10 pounds to the barrel of forty-five gallons, and redistilling. *Perfumers' alcohol* can now be had, which is very much cleaner than *cologne spirit*, as the purest alcohol attainable was formerly called. It is termed perfumers' alcohol because it was found necessary to prepare a very high grade of alcohol for those who need a solvent for fine odors, on the score of economy and to insure greater excellence of product.

Medical Properties and Uses. Probably all the soft tissues of the body are capable of being impressed by alcohol, if it be in sufficient amount and concentration. Locally applied it is irritant even to the skin, and much more so to the more delicate organs: hence the various abdominal inflammations which are so frequent in habitual drunkards. When it is taken internally in proper quantity, it causes a feeling of exhilaration, with distinct increase in the force and frequency of the pulse. When larger amounts are ingested, the well-known phenomena of drunkenness follow. A single dose of it, if large enough, may produce death, preceded by loss of consciousness, profound muscular relaxation, and diminished respiration. The temperature of the body may be elevated slightly by small doses of the drug, the rise being due to the excitement of the circulation and not to any direct action. After toxic amounts the temperature is usually lowered, and the fall may be very marked. The action of the drug upon the bodily temperature of those who use it habitually is very slight. The nervous symptoms caused by alcohol show that it has a very powerful and direct influence upon the nerve centres. This action, at first stimulant, after large doses soon becomes depressant, many of the phenomena of intoxication being really due to a loss of control by the paralyzed will over the lower nerve centres. The order of involvement by the nerve centres is probably the same as in etherization. The arterial pressure and the pulse rate are both increased by moderate doses of alcohol; the way in which this increase is produced is not positively determined, but it is probably by a direct influence upon the heart itself. After toxic amounts the force of the circulation is greatly lessened, partly by vaso-motor paralysis and partly by a direct depression of the heart. Alcohol is undoubtedly absorbed, and is in part burnt up in the system and in part eliminated by the lungs, skin, and especially the kidneys. The organism seems to have the power of destroying only a certain amount of the drug, and consequently elimination increases disproportionately with the dose. The amount of alcohol that the system can consume varies very greatly not only with the individual, but in different bodily conditions of the same individual: in conditions of exhaustion, and especially in the "typhoid state," very much more can be appropriated than in health. There is good ground for believing that alcohol lessens the excretion of nitrogenous material from the body; it would seem most probable that this is achieved by checking tissue waste; but it may be that, as suggested by Dr. Geo. B. Wood, alcohol simply renders the digestion of the food more perfect and lessens the production of food urea.

In acute diseases associated with debility, alcohol is often an invaluable remedy. Of all medicines it is the one most frequently employed as a stimulant. Taken along with food in small quantity, it favors digestion by its local effect upon the stomach, and possibly also by stimulating the nerve and arterial centres. It does not directly elevate temperature, and hence is not contraindicated by fever; in typhoid and other low fevers it is of great value. In all conditions of depression the system tolerates much more of it than in health: hence in snake-bite, typhoid and typhus fever, diphtheria, etc., enormous quantities are often exhibited with great benefit. So long as it is not perceptible in the breath, and does not cause nervous or circulatory excitement, alcohol in these cases is probably not in excess. In chronic diseases great care is necessary in the exhibition of the remedy for fear of begetting intemperate habits. This is especially the case in neuralgia and other painful affections in which the narcotic influence of alcohol may be very soothing; under these circumstances there is a constant tendency to an increase of the frequency and size of the dose. Taken habitually in excess, alcohol produces the most deplorable results, and is a very common cause of fatal maladies. For the symptoms and treatment of chronic alcoholism, the reader is referred to H. C. Wood's Treatise on Therapeutics. In acute poisoning, the stomach should be at once emptied, the respiration be maintained by the use of atropia and other methods (see *Opium Poisons*), and the bodily heat sustained by external warmth. In some cases it may be well to employ ammonia or digitalis to act upon the nearly paralyzed heart. Locally, alcohol is sometimes used for the purpose of hardening the skin and as an antiseptic dressing for wounds, the wound being washed out with it until all bleeding has ceased, the edges then united, and the whole surrounded by an alcoholic dressing. As an internal remedy alcohol is very rarely employed in the pure state, but only in the form of spirits, wines, or fermented liquors, which are described elsewhere.

3. ALCOHOL DILUTUM. *U. S.* "A liquid composed of 45·5 per cent. by weight (53 per cent. by volume) of Ethyl Alcohol, and 54·5 per cent. by weight (47 per cent. by volume) of Water. Sp. gr. 0·928 at 15·6° C. (60° F.) and 0·920 at 25° C. (77° F.).

"Alcohol *fifty parts* [or seventeen fluidounces]; Distilled Water *fifty parts* [or fourteen fluidounces], To make *one hundred parts*. Diluted Alcohol of this strength may be prepared from Alcohol of any higher percentage by the following rule, in which all terms denote weight. Divide the alcoholic percentage of the alcohol to be diluted by 45·5, and subtract 1 from the quotient. This gives the number of parts of water to be added to *one* (1) *part* of the alcohol. Diluted Alcohol should respond to the tests of purity given under *Alcohol*." *U. S.*

Spiritus Tenuior, *Br.*, Proof Spirit.

The U. S. preparation consists of equal weights of officinal alcohol and water, and has the sp. gr. 0·9303; the British, for which a process is given, is made by mixing five pints of Rectified Spirit with three pints of Distilled Water, and has the sp. gr. 0·920. The latter is the stronger of the two, containing only 51 per cent. of water, while the U. S. preparation contains nearly 55 per cent., both by weight.

The purer forms of alcohol, whether strong or diluted, are employed almost exclusively in pharmacy; as in the preparation of medicines, such as ether, into the composition of which they enter; for the preservation of organic substances; in the extraction of the active principles of vegetables, as in the tinctures; for dissolving bodies soluble in alcohol much more readily than in water, or insoluble in the latter fluid; and for various other pharmaceutic purposes. Nélaton, however, uses rectified spirit as a local application to wounds to be healed by the first intention, washing the surface with the liquid, before bringing them together, until hemorrhage ceases. Dr. Sempleton, in the *British Medical Journal*, 1879, proposes an undiluted benzoated alcohol, made by dissolving half an ounce of benzoic acid prepared from gum benzoin in a pint of alcohol, to be used as a lotion, gargle, or in the form of spray.

Diluted alcohol is employed as an addition to some infusions and decoctions, and to some of the distilled waters and preparations of vinegar, in order to preserve them from decomposition; as a menstruum for extracting the virtues of plants, preparatory to the formation of extracts and syrups; and in preparing many of the spirits, and a few of the medicated wines. But it is in forming the tinctures that diluted alcohol is chiefly used. Some of these are made with officinal alcohol (rectified spirit), but the majority with diluted alcohol (proof spirit) as the menstruum. As the latter contains more than half its weight of water, it is well fitted for acting on organic substances, the virtues of which are partly soluble in water and partly in alcohol. The apothecary, however, should never substitute the commercial proof spirit for diluted alcohol, on account of the impurities in the former, even though it may be of the same strength; but, when it is recollected how variable the so-called proof spirits are in strength, the objection to their use in pharmacy becomes still stronger. The use of alcohol for making fluid extracts, tinctures, and other preparations is so extensive and universal that it has not been deemed necessary to specify the particular preparations into which it enters.

ALCOHOL AMYLICUM. *Br.* *Amylic Alcohol.*

$C_5H_{11}HO$; 88. (ĂL'CO-HŎL Ą-MȲL'Ĭ-CŬM.) $C_{10}H_{11}O, HO$; 88.

"Amylic alcohol, $C_5H_{11}HO$, with a small proportion of other spirituous substances. A liquid of oily consistence, contained in the crude spirit produced by the fermentation of saccharine solutions with yeast and separated in the rectification or distillation of such crude spirit. It should be redistilled, and the product passing over at 253° to 260° F. (122·8° to 126·7° C.) be alone collected for use." *Br.*

Hydrated Oxide of Amyl, Amylic Alcohol, Grain Oil, Potato Spirit Oil; Alcohol Amylique, Huile de Grain, *Fr.*; Amylalcohol, Fuselöl, *G.*; Fousel Oil; Hydrate of Amyl.

This oil is always present in the products of alcoholic fermentation. It is an ingredient in the ardent spirit obtained from various grains, but is most abundant in that procured from fermented potatoes. In grain spirit it is present in the proportion of about one part in five hundred by measure. When grain or potato whisky is distilled for the purpose of obtaining alcohol, the pure spirit will continue to come over for a certain time, after which, if the distillation be continued, a milky liquid will be obtained, which, upon standing, will be covered with a stratum of this peculiar oil. Subjected to distillation, the milky liquid will at first boil at a comparatively low temperature, and yield water and a little of the oil; but after a time the boiling point will rise to 132° C. (269° F.), when the oil will come over pure. By changing the receiver when the oil begins to distil free from water, the oil is collected separate.

Properties. Amylic alcohol is an oily, colorless liquid, of a strong, offensive odor, and acrid, burning taste. As usually prepared it has a pale yellow color. Its sp. gr. is 0·818; that of its vapor 3·15. It boils at 132° C. (269° F.), and congeals at —25° C. (—13° F.) in the form of crystalline leaves. It is very sparingly soluble in water, but unites in all proportions with alcohol, ether, and essential oils. It dissolves iodine, sulphur, and phosphorus, and is a good solvent for fats, resins, and camphor. When dropped upon paper it does not leave a permanent greasy stain. It does not take fire like alcohol by the contact of flame, but requires to be heated to a temperature of about 54·5° C. (130° F.) before it begins to burn. Pasteur first observed that the ordinary amyl alcohol of fermentation was a mixture of two distinct alcohols, one present in smaller amount optically active, lævogyrate, and the other, the main portion, optically inactive. Their boiling points are very close, but they may be separated by the difference in solubility of the barium amyl-sulphates, and yield different sets of derivatives. (*Compt.-Rend.*, 41, p. 296.) Amyl alcohol consists of five atoms of carbon 60, twelve of hydrogen 12, and one of oxygen 16 = 88. It is recognized as the hydrate of the radical amyl (C_5H_{11}), and its formula is, therefore, $C_5H_{11}.OH$. Heated with phosphoric oxide, it loses a molecule of water, and forms a hydrocarbon, C_5H_{10}, homologous with ethylen, called *amylen* or *valeren*, which has been proposed as an anæsthetic. Amyl alcohol should not affect the color of litmus paper, previously moistened with water, should leave no fixed residue upon evaporation, should require to dissolve it about 40 parts of distilled water at 15° C. (59° F.), and should become not more than slightly turbid upon mixture with benzin (absence of more than a little alcohol, or water). (See *Amylen* in Part II.) When subjected to oxidizing agents, it loses two atoms of hydrogen and gains one of oxygen, and becomes $C_5H_{10}O_2$, or *amylic acid*, which is identical with *valerianic acid*, the acid found in valerian. Hence the test given in the Br. Pharmacopœia; "exposed to the air in contact with platinum-black, it is slowly oxidized, yielding valerianic acid." *Br.* This acid bears the same relation to amylic alcohol that acetic acid does to ethylic alcohol, and formic acid to methylic alcohol. The free amyl, $(C_5H_{11})_2$, has been isolated by Dr. E. Frankland. It is a colorless pellucid liquid, of the sp. gr. 0·7704. (*Chem. Gaz.*, March 15, 1850.) Its hydride, $C_5H_{11}H$, has been discovered to be an energetic anæsthetic by Dr. Simpson, of Edinburgh.

Crude fusel oil may be obtained from the alcohol distillers. Mr. Kent, of New York, found in it, as impurities, water, alcohol, acetic and amylic acids, oxide of iron, and an amyl compound, analogous to œnanthic ether. According to Messrs. T. and H. Smith, the crude oil is a mixture of propylic, butylic, and amylic alcohols, and of other alcohols much higher in the series. Fusel oil is now used largely by the manufacturers of cinchona alkaloids as a solvent.

Fusel oil was made officinal by the Dublin College, in its Pharmacopœia of 1850, as an artificial source of valerianic acid, to be used in forming valerianate of sodium, from which, by double decomposition, three other valerianates, namely, those of iron, zinc, and quinia, were directed by the College to be prepared. It was introduced into the U. S. Pharmacopœia for a similar purpose, but at the late revision, valerianic acid was dismissed, and amylic alcohol being no longer wanted for its preparation, shared its fate.

Amylic alcohol is an active irritant poison.

Pharm. Uses. Br. In making Amyl Nitris; Sodii Valerianas.

ALLIUM. *U.S.* *Garlic.*

(ĂL'LĬ-ŬM.)

"The bulb of Allium sativum. Linné. (*Nat. Ord.* Liliaceæ.)" *U. S.*

Bulbus Allii; Ail, *Fr.;* Knoblauch, *G.;* Aglio, *It.;* Ajo, *Sp.*

Gen. Ch. Corolla six-parted, spreading. *Spathe* many-flowered. *Umbel* crowded. *Capsule* superior. *Willd.*

This is a very extensive genus, including more than sixty species, most of which are European. Of the nine or ten indigenous in this country, none are officinal. Dr. Griffith states that the bulb of *A. Canadense* has been substituted for the cultivated garlic, and found equally efficient. (*Med. Bot.*, p. 653.) Of the European species several have been used from a very early period, both as food and medicine. *A. sativum*, or garlic, is the only one now officinal; and to this we shall here confine our observation, simply stating that there are few genera of which the several species resemble one another more closely in sensible and medical properties than the present. For an account of *A. cepa*, or onion, and *A. Porrum*, or leek, see Part II.

Allium sativum. Willd. *Sp. Plant.* ii. 68; Woodv. *Med. Bot.* p. 749, t. 256. This is a perennial plant, and, like all its congeners, bulbous. The bulbs are numerous, and enclosed in a common membranous covering, from the base of which the fibres that constitute the proper root descend. The stem is simple, and rises about two feet. The leaves are long, flat, and grass-like, and sheathe the lower half of the stem. At the termination of the stem is a cluster of flowers and bulbs mingled together, and enclosed in a pointed spathe, which opens on one side and withers. The flowers are small and white, and make their appearance in July. This species of garlic grows wild in Sicily, Italy, and the south of France, and is cultivated in all civilized countries.

The part employed, as well for culinary purposes as in medicine, is the bulb, which is described in the U. S. Pharmacopœia as follows. "Bulb subglobular, compound, consisting of about eight compressed, wedge-shaped bulblets, which are arranged in a circle around the base of the stem, and covered by several dry, membranaceous scales. It has a pungent, disagreeable odor, and a warm, acrid taste. It should be preserved in a dry place, and used only in the fresh state." The bulbs are dug up with a portion of the stem attached, and, having been dried in the sun, are tied together in bunches, and thus brought to market. They are said to lose, by drying, nine parts of their weight out of fifteen, with little diminution of their sensible properties. This species of Allium is commonly called *English garlic*, to distinguish it from those which grow wild in our fields and meadows. Garlic bulbs are apt to germinate and thus to undergo serious injury. Mr. A. P. Sharp preserves them by placing them in a bottle, pouring on them a little alcohol, about two fluidounces to a quart, and securely closing the bottle by a stopper of glass or cork. All tendency to germinate is thus destroyed, and the bulbs will retain their peculiar smell and taste unchanged for years. (*Proc. A. P. A.*, 1864.)

Properties. Garlic, as found in the shops, is somewhat spherical, flattened at the bottom, and drawn towards a point at the summit, where a portion of the stem several inches in length projects. It is covered with a white, dry, membranous envelope, consisting of several delicate laminæ, within which the small bulbs are arranged around the stem, having each a distinct coat. These small bulbs, commonly called *cloves* of garlic, are usually five or six in number, of an oblong shape, somewhat curved, and in their interior are whitish, moist, and fleshy.* They have a disagreeable pungent odor, so peculiar as to have received the name of *alliaceous*. Their taste is bitter and acrid. The peculiar smell and taste, though strongest in the bulb, are found to a greater or less extent in all parts of the plant. They depend on an *essential oil*, which is very volatile, and may be obtained by distillation, passing over with the first portions of water. As first obtained, the oil is of a dark brownish yellow color, heavier than water, and decomposed at its boiling temperature. It may be purified by repeated distillation in a salt-water bath, and is then lighter than water, of a pale yellow color, and not decomposed by boiling. According to Wertheim, it consists of a peculiar organic radical, called *allyl*, (C_6H_5), combined with sulphur, and is therefore sulphide of allyl, $(C_6H_5)_2S$. From one hundred-weight of garlic Wertheim obtained from three to four ounces of the impure oil, and about two-thirds as much of the rectified. (*Chem. Gaz.*, iii. 177.) The impure oil has an exceedingly pungent odor, and strong acrid taste, and, when applied to the skin, produces much irritation, and sometimes even blisters. The pure oil combines with nitrate of silver, forming a precipitate, soluble in heated alcohol and afterwards separating in crystals. This compound consists of one eq. of the oil and two eqs. of the salt, and on the addition of ammonia gives up the oil unchanged. (*Journ. de Pharm. et de Chim.*, 4e sér., v. 237, 1867.) Besides this oil, fresh garlic, according to Cadet-Gassicourt, contains, in 1406 parts, 520 of mucilage, 37 of albumen, 48 of fibrous matter, and 801 of water. Bouillon-Lagrange mentions, among its constituents, sulphur, a saccharine matter, and a small quantity of fecula. The fresh bulbs yield upon pressure nearly a fourth part of juice, which is highly viscid, and so tenacious as to require dilution with water before it can be easily filtered. When dried, it serves as a lute for porcelain. It has the medical properties of the bulbs. Water, alcohol, and vinegar extract the virtues of garlic. Protracted boiling renders it inert.

Medical Properties and Uses. The use of garlic as a medicine and condiment ascends to the highest antiquity. When it is taken internally, and even when applied externally, the oil is absorbed, and imparts its odor to the breath, urine, and perspiration, etc. Its effects on the system are those of a general stimulant. It quickens the circulation, excites the nervous system, promotes expectoration in debility of the lungs, produces diaphoresis or diuresis according as the patient is kept warm or cool, and acts upon the stomach as a tonic and carminative. It is said also to be emmenagogue. Applied to the skin, it is irritant and rubefacient, and moreover exercises, in some degree, its peculiar influence upon the system, in consequence of absorption. Moderately employed, it is beneficial in enfeebled digestion and flat-

* A variety of garlic, sometimes seen in the market, having larger and fewer cloves or small bulbs than the officinal, has been shown by Prof. Robert P. Thomas to be the product of a hybrid, probably between *A. sativum* and *A. Porrum*. (*Proc. A. P. A.*, 1860.)

ulence; and by many it is habitually used as a condiment. It has been given with advantage in chronic catarrh, and other pectoral affections in which the symptoms of inflammation have been subdued, and a relaxed state of the vessels remains. We have used it habitually, and with great benefit, in such affections in children, as well as in the nervous and spasmodic coughs to which the very young are peculiarly liable. It is thought also to be an excellent anthelmintic, especially in cases of ascarides, in which it is given both by the mouth and the rectum. The juice is said sometimes to check nervous vomiting in the dose of a few drops. If taken too largely, or in excited states of the system, garlic is apt to occasion gastric irritation, flatulence, hemorrhoids, headache, and fever. As a medicine, it is at present more used externally than inwardly. Bruised, and applied to the feet, it acts very beneficially, as a revulsive, in disorders of the head, and is especially useful in the febrile complaints of children, by quieting restlessness and producing sleep. Its juice mixed with oil, or the garlic itself bruised and steeped in spirit, is frequently used as a liniment in infantile convulsions and other spasmodic or nervous affections in children. The same application has been made in cutaneous eruptions.

Garlic clove may be swallowed either whole, or cut into pieces of a convenient size, but the officinal syrup has replaced all other methods of administration. The dose in substance is from half a drachm to two drachms (1·95–7·8 Gm.) of the fresh bulb. That of the juice is half a fluidrachm (1·9 C.c.).

Off. Prep. Syrupus Allii, *U. S.*

ALOE. *U. S. Aloes.*

(ĂL′Q-Ē.)

"The inspissated juice of the leaves of Aloe Socotrina. Lamarck. (*Nat. Ord.* Liliaceæ.)" *U. S.*

ALOE SOCOTRINA, *Br. Socotrine Aloes.*

"The juice, when inspissated, which flows from the transversely cut bases of the leaves of Aloe Perryi, *Baker;* and probably other species. Imported principally by way of Bombay and Zanzibar, and known in commerce as Socotrine and Zanzibar Aloes." *Br.*

Aloès socotrin, ou sucotrin, *Fr.;* Socotora, oder Socotrinische Aloe, *G.;* Musebber, *Ar.*

ALOE BARBADENSIS. *Br. Barbadoes Aloes.*

(ĂL′Q-Ē BĂR-BA-DĔN′SIS.)

"The juice, when inspissated, which flows from the transversely cut bases of the leaves of the Aloe vulgaris, *Lam.* Imported from Barbadoes and the Dutch West Indian Islands, and known in commerce as Barbadoes and Curaçoa Aloes." *Br.*

Aloès hépatique des Barbades, *Fr.;* Barbadoes Aloe, *G.*

Most of the species belonging to the genus Aloe are said to yield a bitter juice, which has all the properties of the officinal aloes. It is impossible, from the various and sometimes conflicting accounts of writers, to determine exactly from which of the species the drug is in all instances actually derived. *Aloe spicata*, however, is generally acknowledged to be an abundant source of it. In Lindley's Flora Medica, *A. purpurascens*, *A. arborescens*, *A. Commelyni*, and *A. multiformis*, all natives of the Cape of Good Hope, are enumerated as yielding aloes; *A. leptocaulon* and *A. Sahnudra*, found in Madagascar (*P. J. Tr.*, July 16, 1881), and other species are, without doubt, occasionally resorted to. We shall confine ourselves to a description of the three species which probably yield most of the aloes of commerce.

Gen. Ch. Corolla erect, mouth spreading, bottom nectariferous. *Filaments* inserted into the receptacle. *Willd.*

Aloe spicata. Willd. *Sp. Plant.* ii. 185. This species of Aloe was first described by Thunberg. The stem is round, three or four feet high, about four inches in diameter, and leafy at the summit. The leaves are spreading, subverticillate, about two feet long, broad at the base, gradually narrowing to the point, channelled upon their upper surface, and with remote teeth upon their edges. The flowers are bell-shaped, and spread horizontally in very close spikes. Beneath each flower is a broad, ovate, acute bract, white, with three green streaks, and nearly as long as the corolla.

Of the six petals, the three inner are ovate, obtuse, white, with three green lines, and broader than the outer, which otherwise resemble them. The stamens are much longer than the corolla. The *spiked aloe* is a native of Southern Africa, growing near the Cape of Good Hope, and, like all the other species, preferring a sandy soil. In some districts of the colony it is found in great abundance, particularly at Zwellendam, near Mossel Bay, where it almost covers the surface of the country. Much of the Cape aloes is said to be derived from this species.

A. Socotrina. Lamarck, *Encycl.* i. 85; De Cand. *Plantes Grasses, fig.* 85; Curtis's *Bot. Mag. pl.* 472; Carson's *Illust. of Med. Bot.* ii. 48, *pl.* 92.—*A. vera.* Miller, *Dict., ed.* 8, *No.* 55. The stem of this species is erect, eighteen inches or more in height, woody, and leafless below, where it is very rough from the remains of former leaves. At top it is embraced by green, sword-shaped, ascending leaves, somewhat concave on their upper surface, convex beneath, curved inward at the point, with numerous small white serratures at their edges. The flowers, which are in a cylindrical, simple raceme, are scarlet near the base, pale in the centre, and greenish at the summit, and have unequal stamens, of which three are longer than the corolla. This plant was supposed to be a native of Socotra and the source of the Socotrine aloes, but was shown by Mr. Bolus to be indigenous to the Cape of Good Hope.

A. vulgaris. Lamarck, *Encycl.* i. 86; Carson's *Illust. of Med. Bot.* ii. 46, *pl.* 90. —*A. vera.* Linn. *A. Barbadensis.* Miller. This species has a very short woody stem, and lanceolate embracing leaves, which are first spreading, then ascending, of a glaucous green color, somewhat mottled with darker spots, flat on the upper surface, convex beneath, and armed with hard reddish spines, distant from each other, and perpendicular to the margin. The flower-stem is axillary, of a glaucous reddish color, and branched, with a cylindrical-ovate spike of yellow flowers, which are at first erect, then spreading, and finally pendulous, and do not exceed the stamens in length. *A. vulgaris* is a native of southeastern Europe, the north of Africa, and Madagascar. It is cultivated in Italy, Sicily, Malta, and especially in the West Indies, where it contributes largely to furnish the Barbadoes aloes.

A. Perryi. J. G. Baker, *Journ. Linn. Soc.*, xxviii. The true Socotrine aloes plant was first described from specimens sent to Kew Gardens by Mr. Wykeham Perry, and was subsequently found by Prof. Balfour, of Edinburgh, growing abundantly upon the island of Socotra, especially in the limestone tracts, from the sea-level to an altitude of 3000 feet; along with it, but much less abundant, was a dwarf species with spotted leaves. *A. Perryi* resembles in its general habit the Barbadoes aloe, but differs in its shorter leaves, and especially in its flowers, which are arranged in looser racemes on longer pedicels and have the tube much longer than the segments.

The proper aloetic juice was formerly thought to exist in longitudinal vessels beneath the epidermis of the leaves, and readily flows out when these are cut transversely; but, according to M. Edmond Robiquet, who has made elaborate researches in relation to this drug, these vessels are air-ducts, and the juice flows in the intercellular passages between them. The liquid obtained by expression from the parenchyma is mucilaginous, and possessed of little medicinal virtue. The quality of the drug depends much upon the mode of preparing it. The finest kind is that obtained by exudation, and subsequent inspissation in the sun. Most of the better sorts, however, are prepared by artificially heating the juice which has spontaneously exuded from the cut leaves. The chief disadvantage of this process is the conversion of a portion of the soluble active principle into an insoluble and comparatively inert substance, through the influence of an elevated temperature. The plan of bruising and expressing the leaves, and boiling down the resulting liquor, yields a much inferior product; as a large portion of it must be derived from the mucilaginous juice of the parenchyma. The worst plan of all is to boil the leaves themselves in water, and evaporate the decoction. The quality of the drug is also affected by the careless or fraudulent mixture of foreign matters with the juice, and the unskilful management of the inspissation.

Commercial History and Varieties. Three chief varieties of aloes are known in commerce; the Cape aloes, the Socotrine, and the Barbadoes, of which the first two are most used in this country.

1. Cape Aloes (*Shining Aloes*) was dropped from the U. S. Pharmacopœia at the recent revision. It is imported from the Cape of Good Hope, either directly, or through the medium of English commerce. It is collected by the Hottentots and Dutch boors indiscriminately from *A. spicata* and other species, which grow wild in great abundance. Mr. Backhouse (1838), Dr. L. Pappe, of Cape Town, and Mr. P. MacOwan (1871), all state that the best aloes is derived from *Aloe ferox* (*Lam.*), and, according to Dr. L. Pappe, a weaker product is obtained from *A. Africana* and *A. plicatilis* of Miller. (*Flor. Capens.* 28.) The process is very simple. As stated by Hallbeck, a Moravian missionary who resided at the Cape, a hole is made in the ground, in which a sheep-skin is spread with the smooth side upward. The leaves are then cut off near the stem, and arranged around the hole, so that the juice which runs out may be received into the skin. The juice flows most freely in hot weather. (*United Breth. Mission. Intelligencer, N. Y.*, vi. 436.) When a sufficient quantity of the liquor has been collected, it is inspissated in iron caldrons, and, when sufficiently concentrated, is poured into boxes or skins, where it concretes upon cooling. The finest kind is collected at the Missionary Institution at Bethelsdorp, and hence called *Bethelsdorp aloes.* Its superiority is owing exclusively to the greater care observed in its preparation.

According to the recent descriptions in *Pharmacographia*, the process just described is still followed in its essential details throughout the Cape. Cape aloes differs from Socotrine aloes especially in its brilliant conchoidal fracture and peculiar odor, which is strong, but neither nauseous nor aromatic. When freshly broken, it has a very dark olive or greenish color approaching to black, presents a smooth bright almost glassy surface, and, if held up to the light, appears translucent at its edges. The small fragments also are semi-transparent, and have a tinge of yellow or red, mixed with the deep olive of the opaque mass. The same tinge is sometimes observable in the larger pieces. The powder is of a fine greenish yellow color, and, being generally more or less sprinkled over the surface of the pieces as they are kept in the shops, gives them a somewhat yellowish appearance. Cape aloes, when quite hard, is very brittle, and readily powdered; but in very hot weather it is apt to become somewhat soft and tenacious, and the interior of the pieces is occasionally more or less so even in winter. It is usually imported in casks or boxes. Dr. Pereira says that a variety is sometimes imported into England from the Cape, of a reddish brown color like hepatic aloes. *Natal aloes* is a variety coming from Natal, on the southeast coast of Africa, which occurs in irregular pieces, with a fracture much less shining than that of Cape aloes and a totally different color, having a greenish slate hue. It is less soluble than Cape aloes, and has a peculiar composition, which will be adverted to under the chemistry of the drug.

2. Socotrine Aloes. This aloes, which has been very long known and highly esteemed under its present name, is nominally produced in the island of Socotra, which lies in the Straits of Babelmandel, about forty leagues to the east of Cape Guardafui; but we are told by Ainslie that the greater part of what is sold under that name is prepared in the kingdom of Melinda, upon the eastern coast of Africa; and Wellsted states that the aloes of the neighboring parts of Arabia is the same as that of Socotra. The commerce in this variety of aloes is carried on chiefly by the maritime Arabs, who convey it either to India, or up the Red Sea by the same channel through which it reached Europe before the discovery of the southern passage into the Indian Ocean. Mr. Vaughan states that nearly the whole product of the island is carried to Maculla, on the southern coast of Arabia, and thence transhipped to Bombay. (*P. J. Tr.*, xii. 263.) The whole produce was formerly monopolized by the Arabian Sultan of Kisseeu; but at present the business of collecting the drug is entirely free to the inhabitants. The leaves are plucked at any period of the year, and are placed in skins, into which the juice is allowed to exude. In what way the inspissation is effected we are not informed by Wellsted; but, according to Hermann, it is by exposure to the heat of the sun. The aloes is exported in skins, or in kegs or tin-lined boxes. Its quality differs much according to the care taken in its preparation.

Socotrine aloes is in pieces of a yellowish or reddish-brown color, wholly different from that of the former variety. Sometimes the color is very light, especially in the fresh and not fully hardened parcels; sometimes it is a deep brownish red like that of garnets. It is rendered much darker by exposure to the air; and the interior of the masses is consequently much lighter-colored than the exterior. Its surface is somewhat glossy, and its fracture smooth or ragged, but not conchoidal, often with sharp and semi-transparent edges, which show with transmitted light in the finest grades a ruby-red color. The color of its powder is a bright golden yellow. It has a peculiar, not unpleasant odor, and a taste which, though bitter and disagreeable, is accompanied with an aromatic flavor. Though hard and pulverulent in cold weather, it is somewhat tenacious in summer, and softens by the heat of the hand. "When moistened with rectified spirit and examined in a thin stratum under the microscope, it exhibits numerous crystals." *Br.* "It is almost entirely soluble in alcohol and in 4 times its weight of boiling water." *U. S.*

Under the name of Socotrine aloes, are occasionally to be met with in the market small parcels beautifully semi-transparent, shining, and of a yellowish, reddish, or brownish-red color. These, however, are very rare, and do not deserve to be considered as a distinct variety. They are probably portions of the juice carefully inspissated in the sun, and may accompany the packages brought from any of the commercial sources of aloes. When in mass, as imported from the East, Socotrine aloes is usually soft and plastic, and of a very light yellowish-brown color in the interior. At present it reaches the United States in casks, tubs, or boxes, and not rarely in a semi-liquid state. Very liquid specimens are sometimes of the consistence of molasses, of an orange or yellowish color, and of a strong fragrant odor. It separates, upon standing, into a transparent liquid, and an opaque, lighter-colored, granular portion which subsides. Pereira found the latter portion to consist of innumerable minute prismatic crystals, which he believed to be identical with or closely analogous to the aloin of the Messrs. Smith. When the juice is heated, the deposit dissolves, and the whole being evaporated yields a solid, transparent product, having the properties of fine Socotrine aloes. (*P. J. Tr.*, xi. 439.)

Much of the aloes sold as Socotrine consists simply of superior specimens of other varieties falsely labelled to enhance the value.

Much confusion and uncertainty have prevailed in relation to the term *Hepatic Aloes.* The name was originally applied to a product from the East Indies, of a reddish brown or liver color, and has been extended to similar aloes from the West Indies. The hepatic aloes of the present London markets is simply a dark, opaque, liver-colored Socotrine aloes.

3. Barbadoes Aloes. This is the name by which the aloes produced in the West Indies is generally designated. The aloe plants are largely cultivated in the poorer soils of Jamaica and Barbadoes, especially of the latter island. The species from which most of the drug is procured is *A. vulgaris;* but *A. Socotrina*, *A. purpurascens*, and *A. arborescens* are also said to be cultivated. The process employed appears to be somewhat different in different places, or at least as described by different authors. A fine kind was formerly prepared by the spontaneous inspissation of the juice, placed in bladders or shallow vessels, and exposed to the sun. The common Barbadoes aloes, however, is now made either by boiling the juice to a proper consistence, or by first forming a decoction of the leaves, chopped and suspended in water in nets or baskets, and then evaporating the decoction. In either case, when the liquor has attained such a consistence that it will harden on cooling, it is poured into calabashes and allow to concrete. A gentleman from Barbadoes, who had seen the aloes prepared, informed Mr. Squire that the leaves are cut transversely, and so placed that the juice flows from the incised surfaces into a trough, which inclines to the boiler. (*Med. T. and Gaz.*, Jan. 1868, p. 75.) It is imported into England in gourds weighing from 60 to 70 pounds, or even more, or sometimes in boxes. A variety known as "*Capey Barbadoes*," having a smooth glassy fracture, occurs in the London markets. In consequence of the great demand for it in veterinary practice, it commands a high price in Great Britain.

The color of Barbadoes aloes is not uniform. Sometimes it is dark brown or almost black, sometimes of a reddish brown or liver color, and again of some intermediate shade. It has usually a dull fracture, and is almost perfectly opaque, even at the edges; "in thin films translucent and of an orange-brown tint." *Br.* It is also distinguishable by its odor, which is disagreeable and even nauseous. The powder is of a dull olive-yellow. According to Mr. Giles, it yields 80 per cent. of aqueous extract, and is even more active than the Socotrine. (*P. J. Tr.*, Dec. 1860, p. 301.) "When moistened with rectified spirit and examined in a thin stratum under the microscope, it exhibits numerous crystals." *Br.* "The Curaçoa variety is commonly more glassy and translucent than the ordinary Barbadoes aloes, and has a distinctive odor." *Br.* According to M. Marais, Barbadoes aloes, from whatever part of the West Indies derived, and however differing in color, when dissolved in distilled water in the proportion of one part to 100,000 parts, has, in a high degree, the property of giving rise to a fine rose-color on the addition of chloride of gold or tincture of iodine; while all other varieties, whether African or Indian, with the exception of the hepatic, produce with these reagents either a feeble color, slow in occurring, or no change of color whatever. (*Journ. de Pharm.*, 4e sér., v. 326.)

Besides these varieties of aloes, others are mentioned by authors. A very inferior kind, supposed to consist of the dregs of the juice which furnished the better sorts, almost black, quite opaque, hard, of a rough fracture and very fetid odor, and full of various impurities, was formerly sold under the name of *fetid*, *caballine*, or *horse aloes*. It was used exclusively for horses; but, in consequence of the cheapness of better kinds, it has been banished from veterinary practice, and is not now found in the market. Aloes has been imported from Muscat, and a considerable quantity came over in a vessel sent by the Sultan to the United States. Some of a similar origin has been called *Mocha aloes* in London. *Jafferbad aloes*, supposed to be the same as *Mocha aloes* (*A. J. P.*, 1881, p. 175), has been shown to be the product of *A. Abyssinica*, and is said by Shenstone to contain β-barbaloin. (*A. J. P.*, 1883, p. 92.) *Curaçoa aloes*, resembling Barbadoes aloes but having a different odor, comes into European commerce through Holland from the Dutch West Indies.

General Properties. The odor of aloes is different in the different varieties. The taste is in all of them intensely bitter and very tenacious. The color and other sensible properties have been sufficiently described.* Several distinguished

* Hugo Borntrager claims that one part of aloes in 5000 can be detected in the following manner. A little of the suspected liquid is shaken with about twice its bulk of benzin, which is allowed to separate, decanted, and shaken with a few drops of strongest water of ammonia. On separation the ammonia will be of a clear red color. With solids a tincture should first be made. According to Mr. R. H. Groves (*P. J. Tr.*, 3d ser., xi. 1045), this test will never succeed with a less concentration than 1 part in 250, and with some aloes 1 in 100, and is due to the tannin-like substance of aloes; he also states that extreme care is necessary to have the benzin solution perfectly clear. R. A. Cripps and T. S. Dymond have given the testing of aloes a lengthy investigation, and they recommend the following method. Place 1 grain of the substance in a glass mortar standing on white paper, now add 16 drops of strong sulphuric acid and triturate until dissolved, then add 4 drops of nitric acid, sp. gr. 1·42, and then 1 ounce of distilled water. If aloes be present, a color varying from deep orange to crimson will be produced, according to the kind of aloes that has been used; the color is deepened by the addition of ammonia. The following table illustrates the application of the tests:

Variety of Aloes.	Borntrager's Test.	H_2SO_4 and vapor of HNO_3.	Cripps and Dymond's Test.	Cripps and Dymond's Test with Ammonia.
Barbadoes	Pale rose color.	Faint blue color.	Crimson.	Deep claret.
Natal	Very faint pink.	Deep blue color.	Deep crimson.	Intense brownish-red.
Curaçoa	Fine rose color.	Faint blue color.	Crimson.	Intense claret.
Hepatic	Faint color after 24 hours.	Nil.	Orange-red.	Claret.
Hepatic (Indian)	Faint color after 24 hours.	Nil.	Orange-red.	Pale claret.
Cape	Faint color after 24 hours.	Nil.	Orange-red.	Pale claret.
Socotrine (true)	Pale rose color.	Very faint blue color.	Pale crimson.	Deep claret.
Socotrine (commercial), three samples.	Pale rose color after 24 hours.	Nil.	Orange-red.	Claret.
Socotrine (Mocha or Zanzibar).	Pale rose color.	Faint blue color.	Crimson.	Deep claret.
Aloes juice (Natal)	Pale brownish-pink.		Crimson.	Intense brownish-red.

(*P. J. Tr.*, 1885, p. 653. For Hager's quantitative method for determining the percentage of aloin in aloes, see *A. J. P.*, 1885, p. 287.)

chemists have investigated the nature and composition of aloes. Braconnot found a bitter principle, which he named *resino-amer* (*resinous bitter*), and another substance in smaller proportion, which he designated by the name of *flea-colored principle*. These results were essentially confirmed by Trommsdorff, Bouillon-Lagrange, and Vogel. Berzelius considers aloes to be made up of a *bitter extractive* and products from this by the alterations in the air. Robiquet obtained a product which he called *aloëtin*. (For details, see 14th ed. U. S. D.)

ALOÏNS. The bitter substances noticed above, viz., the *resino-amer* of Braconnot, the *bitter extractive* of Berzelius and others, and the *aloetin* of Robiquet, probably contain the active principle of aloes, but combined with impurities which render it insusceptible of crystallization. It is probable that there exists not one compound, but a set of three closely related compounds, to which the general name of *aloïns* is now given. The first of these, found exclusively in Barbadoes aloes, and discovered by T. and H. Smith, is called *barbaloïn;* the second, discovered by Flückiger in Natal aloes, is called *nataloïn;* the third, found by Histed and Flückiger in Socotrine aloes, is called *socaloïn*.

Barbaloïn. This is a neutral substance crystallizing in tufts of small yellow prisms. These crystals represent hydrated aloïn, and part with one mol. of water (= 2·69 per cent.) by desiccation in vacuo, or by the prolonged heat of a water-bath. Barbaloïn, $C_{17}H_{18}O_7 + \frac{1}{2}H_2O$, dissolves sparingly in water or alcohol, but very freely if either liquid be even slightly warmed; it is insoluble in ether.

By oxidation with nitric acid, barbaloïn yields, as Tilden has shown, about one-third of its weight of *chrysammic acid*, besides aloëtic, oxalic, and picric acids. It combines easily with bromine to form yellow needles of *tribromaloïn*, $C_{17}H_{15}Br_3O_7$; *trichloraloïn*, $C_{17}H_{15}Cl_3O_7$, has also been obtained. (*Pharmacographia*, 2d ed., p. 687.) According to Tilden, from 20 to 25 per cent. of barbaloïn can be extracted from good qualities of the drug, by agitating with seven or eight parts of boiling water slightly acidulated with hydrochloric acid, allowing to stand for twenty-four hours, filtering, setting aside for a day or two, putting the resulting mass in a calico bag, and squeezing out the liquid. The barbaloïn thus obtained is purified by solution in alcohol and crystallization. (*P. J. Tr.*, ii. 845.)

Nataloïn. This exists naturally in Natal aloes, from which it can be easily prepared in the crude state if the drug be triturated with an equal weight of alcohol at a temperature not exceeding 48° C. This will dissolve the amorphous portion, from which the crystals should be separated by a filter and washed with a small quantity of cold spirit. From 16 to 25 per cent. of crude nataloïn in pale yellow crystals may be thus extracted. Its formula is $C_{25}H_{28}O_{11}$. It is scarcely more soluble in warm than in cold spirit of wine, so that to obtain crystals it is best to allow the solution to evaporate spontaneously. Water, hot or cold, dissolves it very sparingly. Nataloïn gives off no water when exposed over oil of vitriol, or to a temperature of 100° C. By the action of nitric acid it affords both oxalic and picric acids, but no chrysammic acid.

Socaloïn. In the Socotrine or Zanzibar aloes, the crystals are of comparatively large size, such as are not seen in Natal aloes. They cannot, however, be so easily separated as the nataloïn, since they are nearly as soluble as the amorphous matter surrounding them. Histed recommends treating the powdered crude drug with a little alcohol, sp. gr. 0·960, and strongly pressing the pasty mass between several thicknesses of calico; then dissolving the yellow crystalline cake in warm weak alcohol, and collecting the crystals which are formed by cooling and repose.

Socaloïn forms tufted acicular prisms, which by solution in methylic alcohol may be obtained 2 to 3 millimetres in length. It is much more soluble than nataloïn. Socaloïn is a hydrate, losing, when dried over oil of vitriol, 11 to 12 per cent. of water, but slowly regaining it if afterwards exposed to the air. Its elementary composition is $C_{34}H_{38}O_{15} + 5H_2O$.

The three aloïns, *Barbaloïn*, *Nataloïn*, and *Socaloïn*, are easily distinguished by the following beautiful reaction, first noticed by Histed. A drop of nitric acid on a porcelain slab gives, with a few particles of barbaloïn or nataloïn, a vivid crimson (rapidly fading in the case of barbaloïn, but permanent with nataloïn unless heat be applied), but produces little effect with socaloïn. To distinguish barbaloïn from nataloïn, test each by adding a minute quantity to a drop or two of oil of vitriol, then allowing the *vapor* from a rod touched with nitric acid to pass over the surface. Barbaloïn (and socaloïn) will undergo no change, but nataloïn will assume a fine blue. (*Pharmacographia*, 2d ed., p. 688.) E. von Sommaruga and Egger consider that the three aloïns form a homologous series possessing the formulas: barbaloïn, $C_{17}H_{20}O_7$; nataloïn, $C_{16}H_{18}O_7$; socaloïn, $C_{15}H_{16}O_7$, and that they are all derived from *anthracene*, $C_{14}H_{10}$. Tilden subsequently assigned a different composition to the aloïns: barbaloïn and socaloïn, each $C_{16}H_{18}O_7$; for nataloïn, the formula $C_{25}H_{28}O_{11}$. He further states that barbaloïn and socaloïn differ in physical and chemical properties on account of the variation in the molecules of water which are associated with them.

Aloes yields its active matter to cold water, and when good is almost wholly dissolved by boiling water; but the inert portion, or apothême of Berzelius, is deposited as the solution cools. It is also soluble in alcohol, rectified or diluted. Long boiling impairs its purgative properties by oxidizing the aloïn and rendering it insoluble. The alkalies, their carbonates, and soap alter in some measure its chemical nature, and render it of easier solution. It is inflammable, swelling up and decrepitating when it burns, and giving out a thick smoke which has the odor of the drug.

Those substances only are incompatible with aloes which alter or precipitate the soluble matter; as the insoluble portion is without action upon the system. Among these is the infusion of galls, which we have found, probably through its tannic acid, to afford a copious precipitate with an aqueous solution of aloes. It is said that such a solution will keep a long time, even for several months, without exhibiting mouldiness or putrescence, though it becomes ropy.

Medical Properties and Uses. Aloes was known to the ancients. It is mentioned in the works of Dioscorides and Celsus, the former of whom speaks of two kinds. The varieties are similar in their mode of action. They are all cathartic, operating very slowly but certainly, and having a peculiar affinity for the large intestine, and especially its pelvic portion. Their action, moreover, appears to be directed rather to the muscular coat than to the exhalant vessels; and the discharges which they produce are, therefore, seldom very thin or watery. In a full dose they quicken the circulation, and produce general warmth. When frequently repeated, they are apt to irritate the rectum. Aloes has a decided tendency to the uterine system. Its emmenagogue effect, which is often very considerable, is generally attributed to a sympathetic extension of irritation from the rectum to the uterus; but we can see no reason why the medicine should not act specifically upon this organ; and its influence in promoting menstruation is by no means confined to cases in which its action upon the neighboring intestine is most conspicuous. A peculiarity in the action of this cathartic is, that an increase of the quantity administered, beyond the medium dose, is not attended by a corresponding increase of effect. Its tendency to irritate the rectum may be obviated, in some measure, by combining with it soap or an alkaline carbonate; but it does not follow, as supposed by some, that this modification of its operation is the result of increased solubility; for aloes given in a liquid state produces the same effect as when taken in pill or powder, except that it acts somewhat more speedily. Besides, when externally applied to a blistered surface, it operates exactly in the same manner as when internally administered, thus proving that its peculiarities are not dependent upon the particular form in which it may be given, but on specific tendencies to particular parts. (Gerhard, *N. Am. Med. and Surg. Journ.*, x. 155.) With its other powers, aloes combines the property of slightly stimulating the stomach. It is, therefore, in minute doses, an excellent remedy in habitual costiveness attended with torpor of the digestive organs. It has been supposed to stimulate the hepatic secretion, and certainly acts sometimes very happily in jaundice, producing bilious stools even after calomel has failed. From its special direction to the rectum, it has been found peculiarly useful in the treatment of ascarides, and is useful in hemorrhoids without inflammation. In amenorrhœa it is perhaps more frequently employed than any other remedy, entering into almost all the numerous empirical preparations habitually resorted to by females in that complaint. It is much used in regular practice, and is frequently combined with more irritating cathartics, in order to regulate their liability to excessive action. In amenorrhœa it is said to be peculiarly efficacious, when given, in the form of enema, about the period when the menses should appear. Aloes is unsuitable, unless modified by combination, to the treatment of inflammatory diseases.

The medium dose is 10 grains (0·65 Gm.); but as a laxative it will often operate in the quantity of 2 or 3 grains (0·13–0·20 Gm.); and when a decided impression is required, the dose may be augmented to 20 grains (1·3 Gm.). In consequence of its excessively bitter and somewhat nauseous taste, it is most conveniently administered in pills.

Off. Prep. Aloe Purificata; Extractum Aloes Aquosum; Extractum Colocynthidis Compositum.

Off. Prep. Br. Aloin; Decoctum Aloes Compositum; Enema Aloes; Extractum Aloes Barbadensis; Extractum Aloes Socotrinæ; Extractum Colocynthidis Compositum; Pilula Aloes Barbadensis; Pilula Aloes et Asafœtidæ; Pilula Aloes et Ferri; Pilula Aloes et Myrrhæ; Pilula Aloes Socotrinæ; Pilula Cambogiæ Compositæ; Pilula Colocynthidis Compositæ; Pilula Colocynthidis et Hyoscyami; Pilula Rhei Composita; Tinctura Aloes; Tinctura Benzoini Composita; Vinum Aloes.

ALOIN. *Aloin. Br.*

$C_{16}H_{18}O_7$. (ĂL'Q-ĬN.)

"A crystalline substance extracted from aloes by solvents and purified by recrystallization. As obtained from the different varieties of aloes, the products differ slightly, but their medicinal properties are similar." *Br.*

Preparation. Aloïn may be prepared by W. A. Tilden's process, as follows. 1 part of aloes is dissolved in 10 parts of boiling water, acidulated with hydrochloric acid, and allowed to cool. The liquid is then decanted from resinous matter, evaporated to about 2 parts, and set aside two weeks for crystals to form; the liquid portion is poured off, the crystals pressed, and the adherent resinous matter separated by shaking with acetic ether, which dissolves the resin. This process answers fairly well for obtaining aloïn from Barbadoes, Curaçoa, or Bonaire aloes.

Aloïn from Socotrine aloes is best obtained by digesting the aloes in 3 parts of alcohol for 24 hours, then transferring to a water-bath, and boiling for 2 hours. After cooling, the liquid is filtered and set aside to crystallize. The crystals are washed with a little alcohol and dried. The yield is about 10 per cent. (H. C. Plenge, *A. J. P.*, 1884, p. 507.)

Aloïn is officinally described as "Usually in tufts of acicular crystals, yellow, inodorous, and having the taste of aloes. Sparingly soluble in cold water, more so in cold rectified spirit, freely soluble in the hot fluids. Insoluble in ether. Not readily altered in acidified or neutral solutions; rapidly altered in alkaline fluids."

Medical Properties and Uses. The earlier experimenters with aloïn obtained results which were strangely at variance and difficult of explanation. The numerous recent investigations of Craig, Nelson, Dobson, W. A. Tilden, etc., have shown, however, that socaloïn, barbaloïn, and nataloïn are all active purgatives in doses of 2 to 4 grains. Barbaloïn is affirmed to be the most powerful. In combination with belladonna and strychnine, aloïn is one of the most serviceable and pleasantly active laxatives that we have. The ordinary laxative dose may be set down as 1 grain; the full purgative dose, 3 grains. Fronmüller (*Lond. Med. Rec.*, 1879, p. 70) affirms that aloïn dissolved in 25 times its weight of water acts as an efficient though slow purgative, when given hypodermically, without causing any local irritation.

ALOE PURIFICATA. *U. S. Purified Aloes.*

(ĂL'Q-Ē PŪ-RĮ-FĮ-CĀ'TA.)

Aloès dépuré, *Fr.;* Gereinigte Aloe, *G.*

"Aloes, *one hundred parts* [or sixteen ounces av.]; Alcohol, *fifteen parts* [or three fluidounces]. Heat the Aloes, by means of a water-bath, until it is completely melted. Then add the Alcohol, and, having stirred the mixture thoroughly, strain it through a fine sieve, which has just been dipped into boiling water. Evaporate the strained mixture by means of a water-bath, constantly stirring, until a thread of the mass becomes brittle on cooling. Lastly, break the product, when cold, into pieces of a convenient size, and keep it in well-stopped bottles." *U. S.*

Aloes, even of good quality, is so often mixed as found in the market with various accidental impurities, such as fragments of wood, vegetable remains, pieces of leather, and earthy matter, that it has been thought advisable to have an officinal process by which it may be freed from these, should its purification be found necessary in any particular instance. The use of alcohol in the formula is simply to render the melted aloes more liquid, and thus facilitate the straining; and it is subsequently got rid of by evaporation; but care should be taken not to use too great a heat, or to continue it too long, for fear of impairing the virtues of the drug.

Thus prepared, purified aloes is in irregular, brittle pieces of a dull brown or reddish brown color, and having the peculiar aromatic odor of Socotrine aloes. It is almost entirely soluble in alcohol.

Off. Prep. Pilulæ Aloes; Pilulæ Aloes et Asafœtidæ; Pilulæ Aloes et Ferri; Pilulæ Aloes et Mastiches; Pilulæ Aloes et Myrrhæ; Tinctura Aloes; Tinctura Aloes et Myrrhæ; Vinum Aloes.

ALTHÆA. *U.S.* *Althæa. Marshmallow.*

(ĂL-THÆ'Ą.)

"The root of Althæa officinalis. Linné. (*Nat. Ord.* Malvaceæ.)" *U. S.*

Radix Althææ, *P.G.;* Racine de Guimauve, Guimauve, *Fr.;* Althäewurzel, Eibischwurzel, Eibisch, *G.;* Altea, *It.;* Altea, Malvavisco, *Sp.*

Gen. Ch. Calyx double, the exterior six or nine-cleft. *Capsules* numerous, one-seeded. *Willd.*

Althæa officinalis. Willd. *Sp. Plant.* iii. 770; Woodv. *Med. Bot.* p. 552, t. 198. Marshmallow is an herbaceous perennial, with a perpendicular branching root, and erect woolly stems, from two to four feet or more in height, branched and leafy towards the summit. The leaves are alternate, petiolate, nearly cordate on the lower part of the stem, oblong-ovate and obscurely three-lobed above, somewhat angular, irregularly serrate, pointed, and covered on both sides with a soft down. The flowers are terminal and axillary, with short peduncles, each bearing one, two, or three flowers. The corolla has five spreading, obcordate petals, of a pale purplish color. The fruit consists of numerous capsules united in a compact circular form, each containing a single seed. The plant grows throughout Europe, inhabiting salt marshes, the banks of rivers, and other moist places. It is found also in this country on the borders of salt marshes. In some parts of the continent of Europe, it is largely cultivated for medical use. The whole plant abounds in mucilage. The flowers, leaves, and root are mucilaginous, and were formerly officinal; but the last only is employed to any considerable extent in this country.

The roots should be collected in autumn from plants at least two years old. They are usually prepared for the market by removing the epidermis. The article in commerce is supplied from Europe.

Properties. Althæa occurs "in cylindrical or somewhat conical pieces, from three to six inches (7 to 15 centimetres) long, about half an inch (12 millimetres) in diameter, deeply wrinkled; deprived of the brown, corky layer and small radicles; externally white, marked with a number of circular spots, and of a somewhat hairy appearance from the loosened bast-fibres; internally whitish and fleshy. It breaks with a short, granular and mealy fracture, has a faint aromatic odor, and a sweetish mucilaginous taste." *U. S.* Sections of the root assume a bright yellow tint when an alkali is added to them. Those pieces are to be preferred which are plump and but slightly fibrous. The woody part, on examination with the microscope, is seen to consist of scalariform or pitted vessels, and a few ligneous cells embedded in a loose parenchymatous tissue. The bark is composed of numerous branched liber cells, in bundles of 3 to 30 fibres separated by parenchymatous tissue. The abundant mucilage is situated chiefly in the parenchymatous cells, and can be seen to be in layers when alcohol is added. It, with starch and saccharine matter, is taken out by boiling water. The mucilage, without the starch, is extracted by cold water, which thus becomes ropy. Marshmallow is said to become somewhat acid by decoction. Those pieces should be rejected which are woody, discolored, mouldy, of a sour or musty smell, or of a sourish taste. A principle was discovered in the root by M. Bacon, which has been ascertained to be identical with *asparagin*, $C_4H_8N_2O_3+H_2O$. MM. Boutron-Charland and Pelouze found it to belong to that class of organic principles which are convertible by strong acids, and other agencies, into ammonia and organic acids, and which are designated by the termination *amide*, being compounds of acid radicals with the group NH_2 derived from ammonia by the withdrawal of an atom of hydrogen. When such an amide is acted upon by acids, it is decomposed, the acid radical taking OH to form the free acid and the amide group taking H to form ammonia. Thus asparagin, which in this view should be called *asparamide*, is converted into ammonia and *aspartic acid*, $C_4H_7NO_4$, and one mol. of the resulting aspartate of ammonium corresponds with one mol. of asparamide and one of water. (*Journ. de Pharm.*, xix. 208.) Asparagin, being now recognized as a derivative of succinic acid, is called *amido-succinamide*, and the aspartic acid is called *amido-succinic* acid. It is found in various other plants besides the marshmallow, as in the shoots of asparagus, in vetches grown in the dark, in all the varieties of the potato, and in the roots of the comfrey and liquorice plant. According to Professor Pira, asparagin has acid properties. It has no therapeutic value.

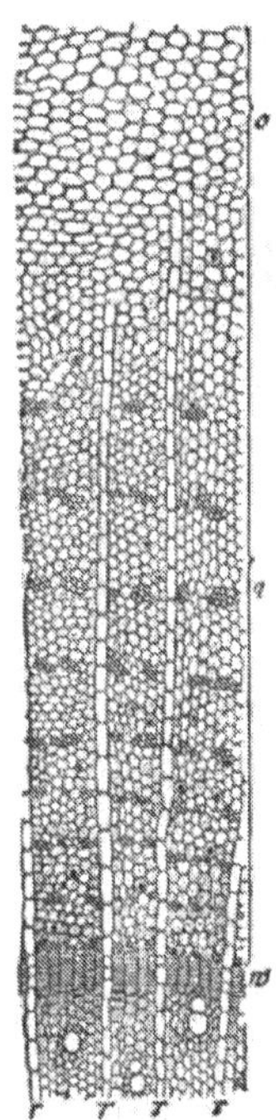

A segment of althea-root after removal of the starch (after Berg). *w*, cambium layer; *x*, wood; *r*, medullary rays; *q*, bast tissues; *o*, middle bark.

The roots of other Malvaceæ are sometimes substituted for that of marshmallow, without disadvantage, as they possess similar properties. Such are those of *Althæa rosea*, or *hollyhock*, and *Malva Alcea*. The dark purple flowers of a variety of *A. rosea* are proposed by Professor Aiken, formerly of the University of Maryland, as a test for acids and alkalies. A strong infusion of these flowers imparts to slips of white filtering paper immersed in it, a permanent purplish-blue color, which is reddened by acids, and rendered bluish green by alkalies.

Medical Properties and Uses. The virtues of marshmallow are exclusively those of a demulcent. The decoction of the root is much used in Europe in irritation and inflammation of the mucous membranes. A syrup of althæa is officinal in the German Pharmacopœia, and was introduced into the last U. S. Pharmacopœia. The roots themselves, as well as the leaves and flowers, boiled and bruised, are sometimes employed as a poultice. In France, the powdered root is much used in the preparation of pills and electuaries.

Off. Prep. Syrupus Althææ.

ALUMEN. *U.S., Br.* Alum.

$K_2Al_2(SO_4)_4, 24H_2O$; 948. (A-LŪ'MEN.) $KO, SO_3, Al_2O_3, 3SO_3, 24HO$; 474.

Sulphate of aluminium and potassium (Potassium Alum or Potash Alum), or of aluminium and ammonium (Ammonium Alum or Ammonia Alum), crystallized from solution in water. $Al_23SO_4,K_2SO_4,24H_2O$ or $Al_23SO_4,(NH_4)_2SO_4,24H_2O$. *Br.*

Aluminii et Potassii Sulphas, *U. S.* 1870, Potassa Alum; Sulphas Aluminico-potassicus; Alun, *Fr., Dan., Swed.;* Sulfate d'Alumine et Potasse, *Fr.;* Alaun, *G.;* Allume, *It.;* Allumbre, *Sp.*

Aluminii et Ammonii Sulphas, Sulphas Aluminico-Ammonicus; Alumen, *U. S.* 1870; Ammonia Alum; Alum, *U.S.* 1870; Alun ammoniacal, *Fr.;* Ammoniak Alaun, *G.*

The name alum has been applied indifferently to two salts, one consisting of tersulphate of aluminium combined with sulphate of ammonium, the other of the same salt of alumina combined with sulphate of potassium; and distinguished as *ammonia-alum* and *potassa-alum*. The former was officinal in the U. S. P. 1870, but has been replaced by *potassa-alum*. *Ammonia-alum* is still retained with potassa-alum under the title *Alumen* in the British Pharmacopœia.

ALUM (SULPHATE OF ALUMINIUM AND POTASSIUM. *U. S.* 1870). Potassa-alum is manufactured occasionally from earths which contain it ready formed, but most generally from minerals which, from the fact of their containing most or all of its constituents, are called *alum ores*. The principal alum ores are the *alum stone*, which is a native mixture of sulphate of aluminium and sulphate of potassium, found in large quantities at Tolfa and Piombino in Italy; certain natural mixtures of bisulphide of iron with alumina, silica, and bituminous matter, called *aluminous schist* or *alum-slate;* and *cryolite.* (See *Sodii Carbonas.*)

At the Solfaterra, and other places in Southern Italy, alum was formerly extracted from earths containing it ready formed. The ground being of volcanic origin, and having a temperature of about 104°, an efflorescence of pure alum formed upon its surface. This was collected and lixiviated, and the solution crystallized by slow evaporation in leaden vessels sunk in the ground.

The alum stone is manufactured into alum by calcination, and subsequent exposure to the air for three months; the mineral being frequently sprinkled with water, in order that it may be brought to the state of a soft mass. This is lixiviated, and the solution obtained crystallized by evaporation. The alum stone may be considered as consisting of alum united with a certain quantity of hydrate of alumina. The latter, by the calcination, loses its water, and becomes incapable of remaining united with the alum of the mineral, which is consequently set free. Alum of the greatest purity is obtained from this ore.

Alum-slate, when compact, is first exposed to the air for a month. It is then stratified with wood, which is set on fire. The combustion which ensues is slow and protracted. The sulphur is in part converted into sulphuric acid, which unites with the alumina; and the sulphate of aluminium thus formed generates a portion of alum with the potassa derived from the ashes of the wood. The iron, in the mean time, is almost wholly converted into sesquioxide, and thus becomes insoluble. The matter is lixiviated, and the solution crystallized into alum by evaporation. The mother-waters, containing sulphate of aluminium, are then drawn off, and made to yield a further portion of alum by the addition of sulphate of potassium or chloride of potassium; the latter being obtained from the soap-boilers, or from the native potassium chloride of the Stassfurt deposits.

When the alum-slate is easily disintegrated, it is not subjected to combustion, but merely placed in heaps, and occasionally sprinkled with water. The bisulphide of iron gradually absorbs oxygen, and passes into ferrous sulphate, which effloresces on the surface of the heap. Part of the sulphuric acid formed unites with the alumina; so that, after the chemical changes are completed, the heap contains both the sulphate of iron and the sulphate of aluminium. At the end of about a year, the matter is lixiviated, and the solution of the two sulphates produced is concentrated to the proper degree in leaden boilers. The sulphate of iron crystallizes, while the sulphate of aluminium, being a deliquescent salt, remains in the mother-waters. These are drawn off, and treated with sulphate of potassium in powder, heat being at the same time applied. The whole is then allowed to cool, that the alum may crystallize. The crystals are then separated from the solution, and purified by a second solution and crystallization. They are next treated with water, just sufficient to dissolve them at the boiling temperature; and the saturated solution is run into casks or tubs, so constructed as to be easily taken to pieces, and set up again. In the course of ten or fifteen days, the alum concretes into a crystalline mass, from which the mother-liquor is let off. The vessel is then taken to pieces, and the salt, having been broken up, is packed in barrels for sale. This process for forming the alum in large masses is called *rocking*.

Alum is now largely manufactured by the direct combination of its constituents. With this view, clays are selected as free from iron and carbonate of calcium as possible, and calcined to sesquioxidize the iron, and render them more easily pulverisable; after which they are dissolved, by the assistance of heat, in weak sulphuric acid. Advantage has been found from mixing the clay, previous to calcination, with powdered charcoal, coke, or other carbonaceous matter, in the proportion of about one to six of the clay, and then applying heat by a reverberatory furnace till all the carbon is consumed. It is asserted that the alumina is thus rendered more soluble in the acid. (*P. J. Tr.*, Dec. 1857, p. 328.) The sulphate of aluminium, thus generated, is next crystallized into alum by the addition of sulphate of potassium in the usual manner. Alum is made in this way from the ashes of the Boghead cannel-coal, which occurs near Edinburgh. These ashes, which form the residue of the combustion of the coke derived from the coal used for making gas, contain a considerable quantity of alumina in a state readily soluble in acids.

The elements *rubidium* and *cæsium* are found in lepidolite, and, as much of the alum in continental Europe is made from this mineral, Salzer found samples of commercial potash alum which contained a considerable quantity of rubidium alum; this contaminated potash alum is less soluble in water than ordinary alum. (*Archiv d. Pharm.*, 1887, p. 217.)

ALUMEN, *Br.* ALUMINII ET AMMONII SULPHAS. *Sulphate of Aluminium and Ammonium. Ammonia-alum.* Besides the potassa-alum, which is now the only U.S. officinal variety of this salt, there are several others, in which the potassa is replaced by some other base, as, for example, ammonia or soda. Of these, *ammonia-alum*, or the sulphate of aluminium and ammonium, was introduced into the U. S. Pharmacopœia at its revision in 1860; and in the Pharmacopœia of 1870, and Br. Pharmacopœia it was adopted under the name of alumen. It is made by adding sulphate of ammonium to the solution of sulphate of aluminium. This kind of alum has come into very general use, owing to the comparative cheapness of ammonia, obtained in the process for ferrocyanide of potassium, or derived from the liquor of gas-works. Ammonia-alum is extensively manufactured by Powers & Weightman of this city. *Scotch alum*, made near Paisley, generally contains both potassa and ammonia. Ammonia-alum resembles potassa-alum so exactly that it cannot be distinguished by simple inspection; and in composition it is perfectly analogous to the potassa-salt. It may, however, be distinguished by subjecting it to a strong calcining heat, after which alumina will be the sole residue; or by rubbing it with potassa or lime and a little water, when the smell of ammonia will be perceived.

Properties. Alum, as usually seen, is in "large, colorless, octahedral crystals, sometimes modified by cubes, acquiring a whitish coating on exposure to air, odorless, having a sweetish, astringent taste, and an acid reaction, soluble in 10·5 parts of water at 15° C. (59° F.) and in 0·3 part of boiling water; insoluble in alcohol. When gradually heated, the salt loses water; at 92° C. (197·6° F.) it melts, and if the heat be gradually increased to 200° C. (392° F.), it loses 45·57 per cent. of its weight (water of crystallization), leaving a bulky, white residue. The aqueous solution of the salt dissolves zinc and iron with evolution of hydrogen. Water of Ammonia produces a bulky, white precipitate, which is nearly insoluble in an excess of ammonia. With solutions of potassa or soda, Alum yields a white precipitate which is completely soluble in excess of the alkali, no odor of ammonia being evolved (difference from, and absence of ammonia-alum). The clear alkaline solution should yield no precipitate with test-solution of sulphide of ammonium (zinc or lead). A solution of 1 Gm. of Alum in 30 C.c. of water should not assume more than a bluish coloration on the addition of a drop of test-solution of ferrocyanide of potassium (limit of iron)." *U. S.* Its sp. gr. is 1·71. It reddens litmus, but changes the blue tinctures of the petals of plants to green. When heated a little above 100° C. (212° F.), it undergoes the aqueous fusion; and, if the heat be continued, it loses its water, swells up, becomes a white, opaque, porous mass, and is converted into the officinal *dried alum.* (See *Alumen Exsiccatum.*) Exposed to a red heat, it gives off oxygen, together with sulphurous and sulphuric oxides, and the residue consists of alumina and sulphate of potassium. When calcined with finely divided charcoal, it forms a spontaneously inflammable substance, called *Homberg's* *pyrophorus*, which consists of a mixture of sulphide of potassium, alumina, and charcoal.

The characters of the ammonia-alum, as stated in the British Pharmacopœia, are that its solution gives with caustic potassa or soda a white precipitate, soluble in an excess of the reagent and an immediate precipitate with chloride of barium; and does not acquire a blue color from the addition of ferrocyanide or ferricyanide of potassium, proving the absence of iron.

Several varieties of alum are known in commerce. *Roche alum*, so called from its having come originally from Rocca, in Syria, is a sort which occurs in fragments about the size of an almond, and of a pale rose color, which is given to it, according to Pereira, by bole or rose-pink. *Roman alum*, which is the purest variety found in commerce, also occurs in small fragments, covered with a reddish brown powder, resembling ochre, which is put on by the manufacturers. It has been supposed that the powder contains iron; but this is probably a mistake. Roman alum crystallizes in cubes, from the fact that the crystals are deposited from a solution always containing an excess of alumina, which decomposes any iron salt that may be present. This crystalline form of alum is, therefore, an index of its freedom from iron.

All the alums of commerce contain more or less sulphate of iron, varying from five to seven parts in the thousand. The iron is readily detected by adding to a solution of the suspected alum a few drops of the ferrocyanide of potassium, which will cause a greenish blue tint, if iron be present. It may be detected also by precipitating the alumina as a subsulphate with a solution of potassa, and afterwards adding the alkali in excess. This will redissolve the precipitate, with the exception of any iron, which will be left in the state of sesquioxide. The proportion of iron usually present, though small, is injurious when the salt is used in dyeing. It may, however, be purified, either by dissolving it in the smallest quantity of boiling water, and stirring the solution as it cools, or by repeated solutions and crystallizations.*

Incompatibles. Alum is incompatible with the alkalies and their carbonates, lime and lime-water, magnesia and its carbonate, tartrate of potassium, and acetate of lead.

Composition. Alum was regarded as a sulphate of aluminium, until it was proved by Descroizilles, Vauquelin, and Chaptal to contain also sulphate of potassium, sulphate of ammonium, or both these salts. When its second base is potassa, it consists of one mol. of aluminium sulphate 343, one of sulphate of potassium 174·2, and twenty-four of water 432 = 949·2. In the ammonia-alum, the mol. of sulphate of potassium is replaced by one of the sulphate of ammonium. *Alumina* is classed as an earth, and may be obtained by subjecting ammonia-alum to a strong calcining heat. It consists of two atoms of a metal called *aluminium* 55, and three of oxygen 48 = 103. It is, therefore, a sesquioxide. The existence of this metal was rendered probable by Sir H. Davy in 1808; but it was not fairly obtained until 1828, when Wöhler procured it in an impure state, in globules of the size of a pin's head, by the action of potassium on chloride of aluminium. In 1854, Deville succeeded in obtaining the pure metal in ingots by decomposing the same chloride with sodium. The process of Deville remained the only practical process for its manufacture until 1886, when the Messrs. Cowles, of Cleveland, Ohio, succeeded in effecting the reduction of corundum, the native oxide, by charcoal, with the aid of a powerful electric current from a Brush dynamo-electric machine, using large carbon electrodes. They now manufacture the pure aluminium and the alloys of copper known as aluminium bronzes. A German process, that of Graetzel, for electrolizing the fused chloride, is also in successful use. Aluminium is silver-white, sonorous, unalterable in the air, and lighter than glass, having the sp. gr. 2·56 only. Its fusing point is somewhat lower than that of silver. It is not

* A preparation called *chloralum*, or solution of chloride of aluminium, has been largely vaunted as an antiseptic. According to Mueller (*Berichte d. Chem. Gesellsch. zu Berlin*, 1872, p. 519), it contains 16·1 per cent. chloride of aluminium, 1·7 per cent. chloride of calcium, 0·1 per cent. sulphates of alkalies, 1·2 per cent. hydrochloric acid, 80·9 per cent. water. It is made by acting upon slightly roasted porcelain clay with crude hydrochloric acid, and is inferior to many antiseptics now in use. (See *Chloride of Aluminium*, Part II.)

attacked by sulphuric or nitric acid, nor tarnished by sulphuretted hydrogen. Its proper solvent is hydrochloric acid. After silver, gold, and platinum, it is the least alterable of the metals.

Medical Properties, etc. Alum is a powerful astringent, with very decided irritant qualities, owing to which, when taken internally in sufficient quantity, it is emetic and purgative, and may even cause fatal gastro-intestinal inflammation. It may be employed in passive relaxations of the mucous membranes or skin, hemorrhages, serous diarrhœa, colliquative sweats, etc., but is not much used internally, except in *colica pictonum.* The latter employment of it was introduced by Grashuis, a Dutch physician, in 1752, was imitated by Dr. Percival with great success, and has been revived in recent times with the happiest results. It allays nausea and vomiting, relieves flatulence, mitigates the pain, and opens the bowels with more certainty than any other medicine. Sometimes it is advantageously conjoined with opium and camphor. It is also efficacious in nervous colic. Sir James Murray found it a useful remedy in gastrorrhœa. He gave it in doses of ten or twelve grains (0·65–0·809 Gm.) three or four times a day, mixed with an equal quantity of cream of tartar to prevent constipation, and a little ginger to obviate flatulence. By Dr. C. D. Meigs alum has been strongly recommended, in doses of a teaspoonful (3·9 Gm.), in pseudo-membranous croup as a mechanical emetic, but it is not as certain or powerful as is the sulphate of zinc.

Alum is a powerful astringent when topically applied, and has been largely used as such. In various anginas it has been a favorite remedy, but on account of its destructive influence upon the teeth it should never be used in gargles, but be applied in powder or concentrated solution with the brush. Bretonneau, Vulpian, etc., strongly recommend it in pseudo-membranous angina, applied by insufflation in the case of children. When used in the latter way, a drachm of finely powdered alum may be placed in one end of a tube, and then blown by means of the breath into the throat of the child. Alum coagulates blood very rapidly and firmly, and is frequently used as a local styptic in external hemorrhages and in epistaxis and other bleedings from mucous membranes to which it can be applied directly. In hæmoptysis its saturated solution may be used by atomization. It is sometimes applied locally in the form of *cataplasm*, made by coagulating the whites of two eggs with a drachm of alum. In *colica pictonum* from 20 to 30 grains of alum in molasses (or thick syrup) may be given three or four times a day. The emetic dose is one to two teaspoonfuls, repeated, if necessary, in fifteen minutes. An elegant mode of giving alum in solution is in the form of *alum-whey*, made by boiling two drachms of alum with a pint of milk, and then straining to separate the curd. The dose is a wineglassful (60 C.c.), containing about 15 grains (1 Gm.) of alum. As a collyrium, the solution is made of various strengths; as 4, 6, or 8 grains to the fluidounce of water. A solution, containing from half an ounce to an ounce in a pint of water, and sweetened with honey, is a convenient gargle. Solutions for gleet, leucorrhœa, ulcers, etc., must vary in strength according to the state of the parts to which they are applied.*

In a case recorded by Dr. Ricquet, of Liège, death resulted from about an ounce of alum taken in solution by mistake for Epsom salts. A sensation of burning in the mouth, throat, and stomach occurred immediately upon the swallowing of the poison, followed by bloody vomiting, and death in the midst of inexpressible suffering. Upon post-mortem examination there was found a grayish yellow coating covering the mucous membrane of the mouth, pharynx, and œsophagus; the tongue and uvula were swollen; and the stomach, bowels, and kidneys were injected. (*Journ. de Pharm.*, Oct., 1873, p. 333.)

* Alum enters as an ingredient into the famous *Wickersheimer Preserving Liquid.* The formula, as purchased by the German government from the originator, is as follows. Alum 100 grammes, sodium chloride 25 grammes, potassium nitrate 12 grammes, potassium carbonate 60 grammes, arsenious acid 10 grammes; these are to be dissolved in 3000 grammes (3 litres) of boiling water, the solution allowed to cool, filtered, and to every 10 litres of the liquid 4 litres of glycerin and 1 litre of wood naphtha added. Owing to the precipitation of the alumina in this preparation, it is frequently the practice to substitute for the alum the same quantity of potassium sulphate.

Alum is sometimes used to adulterate bread, with the view to increase its whiteness, and to conceal the defects of the flour.

Off. Prep. Alumen Exsiccatum; Aluminii Hydras.

Off. Prep. Br. Glycerinum Aluminis.

ALUMEN EXSICCATUM. *U.S., Br.* *Dried Alum.*

$K_2 Al_2 (SO_4)_4$; 516. (A-LŪ'MEN EX-SIC-CĀ'TŬM.) KO, SO_3 $Al_2 O_3$ $3SO_3$; 258.

Alumen Ustum, Burnt Alum; Alun calciné, desséché, brûlé, *Fr.*; Gebrannter Alaun, *G.*

"Alum, in small pieces, *one hundred and eighty-four parts*, To make *one hundred parts*. Expose the Alum for several days to a temperature of about 80° C. (176° F.) until it has thoroughly effloresced. Then place it in a porcelain capsule, and gradually heat it to a temperature of 200° C. (392° F.), being careful not to allow the heat to rise above 205° C. (401° F.). Continue heating at the before-mentioned temperature until the mass becomes white and porous, and weighs *one hundred parts*. When cold, reduce it to a fine powder, and preserve it in well-stopped vessels." *U. S.*

"Take of Alum *four ounces*. Heat the Alum in a porcelain dish, or other suitable vessel, till it liquefies, then raise and continue the heat, not allowing it to exceed 400° F. (204·4° C.), till aqueous vapor ceases to be disengaged, and the salt has lost between 45 and 46 per cent. of its weight. Reduce the residue to powder, and preserve it in a well-stoppered bottle." *Br.*

The object of these processes is to obtain the alum free from its water of crystallization, without otherwise in the least decomposing it. For this purpose a certain degree of heat is necessary; and yet, if the heat be too great, the salt itself is decomposed, and the desired end is not attained. If the alum employed be the potassa-alum, the old indefinite directions will generally be sufficient to secure the requisite result, as this salt will resist a heat short of redness; but this is not the case with the ammonia-salt, which is officinal in the Br. P. To guard against failure from this cause, the Pharmacopœias prescribe about 205° C. (400° F.) as the highest heat to be employed, and check the operation when nearly all the water has been driven off, as indicated by the weight of the residue. Prof. John M. Maisch has satisfactorily determined by experiment that, whichever alum may be used, this temperature is quite high enough; and the direction of the Pharmacopœias, as to the weight of the residue, insures that a sufficient heat will be employed. By the officinal process there is left behind about 4 per cent. of the water of crystallization, when potassa-alum is used.

Properties. Dried alum is officinally described as "a white, granular powder, attracting moisture when exposed to the air, odorless, having a sweetish, astringent taste, very slowly but completely soluble in 20 parts of water at 15° C. (59° F.), and quickly soluble in 0·7 part of boiling water. It answers to the same reactions as Alum. (See *Alumen.*)" *U. S.* Before pulverization, it is a light, white, opaque, porous mass. During the exsiccation, alum loses from 41 to 46 per cent. of its weight in dissipated water. Dried alum resists the action of cold water for a long time, showing its altered aggregation. In composition it differs from crystallized alum merely in the absence of water.

Medical Properties and Uses. Dried alum has the same medical properties as ordinary alum, excepting that it is more powerful and irritant. It is used as a mild escharotic to destroy exuberant granulations, on which it should be freely dusted.

ALUMINII HYDRAS. *U. S.* *Hydrate of Aluminium. Hydrated Alumina.*

$Al_2 (HO)_6$; 156. (ĂL-Ū-MĬN'I-Ī HȲ'DRĂS.) $Al_2 O_3$, 3HO; 78.

Hydrate de l'Alumine, *Fr.*; Thonerdehydrat, *G.*; Argilla Pura, s. Hydrata, *P. G.*

"Alum, *eleven parts*; Carbonate of Sodium, *ten parts*; Distilled Water, *a sufficient quantity*. Dissolve each salt in *one hundred and fifty* (150) *parts* of Distilled Water, filter the solutions and heat them to boiling. Then having poured the hot solution of Carbonate of Sodium into a capacious vessel, gradually pour in the hot solution of Alum with constant stirring, and add about *one hundred* (100) *parts* of boiling Distilled Water. Let the precipitate subside, decant the clear liquid and pour upon the precipitate *two hundred* (200) *parts* of hot Distilled Water. Again decant, transfer the precipitate to a strainer, and wash it with hot Distilled Water until the washings give but a faint cloudiness with test-solution of chloride of barium. Then allow it to drain, dry it with a heat not exceeding 40° C. (104° F.), and reduce it to a uniform powder." *U. S.*

This new officinal is identical with the "Alumina Hydrata" of the German Pharmacopœia, and has been introduced probably out of respect to the large number of German practitioners in this country who may use it.

Properties. It is "a white, light, amorphous powder, permanent in dry air, odorless and tasteless, and insoluble in water or alcohol. Soluble, without residue, in hydrochloric and sulphuric acids, and also in solution of potassa or soda. When heated to redness it loses 34·6 per cent. of its weight (water of hydration)." *U. S.*

Tests. "A solution of 1 Gm. of Hydrate of Aluminium in 30 C.c. of diluted hydrochloric acid should not be colored blue by a drop of test-solution of ferrocyanide of potassium (iron), and should not give more than a faint cloudiness with test-solution of chloride of barium (limit of sulphate). When dissolved in solution of potassa or of soda, it should yield no precipitate with test-solution of sulphide of ammonium (zinc or lead). When Hydrate of Aluminium is boiled with 20 parts of water, and filtered, the filtrate should not leave more than a slight residue on evaporation (limit of salts of alkalies)." *U. S.*

Medical Properties. This is a very feebly astringent and desiccant powder, sometimes used externally as an application in inflammatory affections of the skin. So far as our experience goes, it is very rarely employed in this country.

ALUMINII SULPHAS. *U. S.* *Sulphate of Aluminium.*

$Al_2(SO_4)_3$. $18H_2O$; 666. (ĂL-Ū-MĬN'Ĭ-Ī SŬL'PHĂS.) Al_2O_3, $3SO_3$. 18HO; 333.

Sulfate d'Alumine, *Fr.*; Schwefelsaure Thonerde, *G.*

A process was given in the U. S. P. 1870 for the preparation of this salt:* the Committee of Revision, 1880, have very properly omitted the process, merely giving a description and tests for the salt. In the process of 1870, the soda of the carbonate unites with the sulphuric acid of the aluminium sulphate, with the escape of the carbonic acid, and the precipitation of the alumina in the form of a hydrate; while the undecomposed sulphate of ammonium of the alum, and the newly formed sulphate of sodium, remain in solution. The alumina is then washed in order to separate any portion of the sulphates adhering to it, the absence of which is shown by the non-action of chloride of barium on the washings. It now remains to unite the hydrate of alumina and sulphuric acid, which is effected by heating them with water; and the salt, which is formed in solution, is obtained by evaporating the solution to dryness. It may also be obtained from the solution by the addition of alcohol, which precipitates it. In the process the several substances are used in very nearly saturating proportions. See paper on Sulphate of Aluminium by Prof. J. U. Lloyd. (*N. R.*, Aug. 1879, p. 237.) Sulphate of aluminium may be prepared also by the process of MM. Huria and Brunel, which consists in exposing, in an iron cylinder, sulphate of aluminium and ammonium (ammonia-alum), first dried to separate its water of crystallization, to a cherry-red heat. Sulphate of aluminium remains in the cylinder, and the volatilized products are collected in water. The chief of these is sulphite of ammonium, which serves for the preparation of a fresh portion of alum, after having been changed into the sulphate by

* "Take of Alum, Carbonate of Sodium, each, *four troyounces*; Sulphuric Acid *a troyounce and one hundred and fifty grains*; Water *a sufficient quantity*. Dissolve the salts separately, each in six fluidounces of boiling water, and pour the solution of the Alum gradually into that of the Carbonate of Sodium; then digest with a gentle heat until the evolution of carbonic acid ceases. Collect upon a filter the precipitate formed, and wash it with water, until the washings are no longer affected by chloride of barium. Next, with the aid of heat, dissolve the precipitate in the Sulphuric Acid, previously diluted with half a pint of Water, and, having filtered the solution, evaporate it until a pellicle begins to form. Then remove it to a water-bath, and continue the evaporation, with constant stirring, until a dry salt remains. Lastly, preserve this in a well-stopped bottle." *U. S.* 1870.

oxidation in the air. (*Chem. Gaz.*, Sept. 15, 1852, p. 359.) It is now also obtained in enormous quantities, for use in the place of alum as a mordant in dyeing, as one of the by-products in the manufacture of soda from cryolite.

Sometimes free sulphuric acid exists in sulphate of aluminium. It may be recognized by the salt imparting a strongly acid reaction to alcohol, also by the fact that the dark violet color imparted to decoction of logwood by sulphate of aluminium changes to brown in the presence of free acid. (*A. J. P.*, Nov. 1873.) Prof. Wittstein treats the finely powdered salt with absolute alcohol; if the latter does not become acid, no free acid is present.

Properties. As procured by the process of 1870, sulphate of aluminium is in the form of a white powder. It may, however, be obtained in lamellar crystals. As seen in commerce, it is usually in flattened crystalline cakes, which appears as though formed by the cooling of soft masses of minute crystals. It has a sour as well as sweet and very astringent taste, is soluble in twice its weight of water, and has an acid reaction.

The salt is "soluble, without leaving more than a trifling residue, in 1·2 parts of water at 15° C. (59° F.), and very soluble in boiling water; almost insoluble in alcohol. When heated, the salt melts in its water of crystallization, and at or near 200° C. (392° F.) it loses the whole of it, amounting to 48·6 per cent. of its weight. The aqueous solution of the salt yields with water of ammonia a white, gelatinous precipitate, soluble in solution of potassa or soda, and, with test-solution of chloride of barium, a white precipitate insoluble in hydrochloric acid." *U. S.*

It is formed by the union of one mol. of alumina, which is a sesquioxide of aluminium, and three mols. of sulphuric acid, $Al_2(SO_4)_3$, and, when crystallized, contains eighteen mols. of water. The salt is, therefore, a tersulphate of aluminium. It is known to be a sulphate by giving a precipitate with chloride of barium insoluble in nitric acid, and a salt of alumina by forming octahedral crystals of alum when its solution is evaporated with sulphate of potassium or ammonium. In consequence of its strong affinity for potassa, it is coming into use in the arts as a means of separating that alkali.

Tests. "A solution of 1 Gm. of the salt in 30 C.c. of water should not give more than a faint blue coloration with a drop of test-solution of ferrocyanide of potassium (limit of iron). If 1 Gm. of the salt be dissolved in 50 C.c. of water, a slight excess of water of ammonia added, the liquid heated until all odor of ammonia has disappeared, and then filtered, the precipitate well washed with water, and the filtrate and washings evaporated to dryness and gently ignited, the residue should not weigh more than 0·05 Gm. (abs. of more than 5 per cent. of sulphates of alkalies)." *U. S.*

Medical Properties and Uses. The soluble simple salts of alumina have the property of opposing animal putrefaction, but the sulphate is probably the most powerful and certainly the most used. It is often employed in solution (ʒiiss–f℥vi up to saturation *pro re nata*) as an antiseptic, detergent application to foul ulcers, and as an injection in fetid discharges from the vagina. M. Homolle employs a saturated solution with much advantage as a mild caustic in enlarged tonsils, nasal polypi, nævi, scrofulous and cancerous ulcers, diseases of the os uteri, and various chronic enlargements. He applies it daily by means of a hair pencil. He has sometimes found the solution to answer still better by the addition of oxide of zinc. Solution of sulphate of aluminium is capable of dissolving a considerable quantity of recently precipitated gelatinous alumina. Such a solution, impregnated with benzoin, has been proposed by M. Mentel as a hæmostatic, under the name of *benzoinated solution of alumina.* It resembles the *styptic liquid* of *Pagliari.* It is prepared by saturating, with gelatinous alumina, a solution made of eight ounces of sulphate of aluminium dissolved in a pint of water. To the saturated solution six drachms of bruised amygdaloid benzoin are added, and the whole is kept at a temperature of about 150° F. for six hours, with occasional agitation; so that the liquid, after filtration, may have about the density 1·26. This liquid, put in a cool place for several days, so as to deposit some crystals of alum, forms the benzoinated solution, remarkable for its very sweet odor and astringent balsamic taste. Benzoinated solution of alumina, diluted in the proportion of from two to five fluidrachms to the pint of water, has been found useful as an injection in leucorrhœa, and in ulcerations of the neck of the uterus, accompanied by fetid discharges. (See *A. J. P.*, 1857, p. 128.)

Sulphate of alumina has been used to preserve cadavers for dissection, but is much inferior to the chloride of zinc. The solution for injection should be a pound to the quart.

AMMONIACUM. *U. S., Br.* *Ammoniac.*

(ĂM-MO̧-NĪ'Ą-CŬM.)

"The gum-resin obtained from Dorema Ammoniacum. Don. (*Nat. Ord.* Umbelliferæ Orthospermæ.)" *U. S.* "A gum-resinous exudation obtained from the stem (after being punctured by beetles) of Dorema Ammoniacum. Don." *Br.*

Gummi-resina Ammoniacum; Ammoniacum; Ammoniaque, Gomme-résine ammoniaque, Gomme ammoniaque, *Fr.;* Ammoniak, Ammoniakgummi, *G.;* Gomma ammoniaco, *It.;* Gomma amoniaco, *Sp.;* Ushek, *Ar.;* Semugh belsheren, *Pers.*

Much uncertainty long existed as to the ammoniac plant. It was generally believed to be a Ferula, till Willdenow raised, from some seeds mixed with the gum-resin found in the shops, a plant which he ascertained to be a Heracleum, and named *H. gummiferum*, under the impression that it must be the source of the medicine. On this authority the plant was adopted by the British Colleges, and recognized in former editions of our national Pharmacopœia. Willdenow expressly acknowledged that he could not procure from it any gum-resin, but ascribed the result to the influence of climate. The Heracleum, however, did not correspond exactly with the representations given of the ammoniac plant by travellers; and Sprengel ascertained that it was a native of the Pyrenees, and never produced gum. Mr. Jackson, in his account of Morocco, imperfectly described a plant of that country, supposed to be a *Ferula*, from which gum-ammoniac is procured by the natives. This plant was ascertained by Dr. Falconer to be *Ferula Tingitana* (Royle's *Mat. Med.*), and its product is thought to be the ammoniacum of the ancients, which was obtained from Africa; but this is not the drug now used under that name, which comes exclusively from Persia.* M. Fontaniér, who resided many years in Persia, saw the ammoniac plant growing in the province of Fars, and sent a drawing of it with specimens to Paris. From these it was inferred to be a species of Ferula; and Mérat and De Lens proposed for it the name, originally given to it by Lemery, of *F. ammonifera*. It was subsequently, however, ascertained, from specimens obtained in Persia by Col. Wright, and examined by Dr. David Don, that it belonged to a genus allied to Ferula, but essentially different, which was named by Dr. Don, *Dorema*. It is described in the 16th vol. of the Linn. Transactions, under the name of *Dorema Ammoniacum*. This is now acknowledged by the officinal authorities. The same plant was described and figured by Jaubert and Spach, in their "*Illustrations of Oriental Plants*" (Paris, 1842, t. 40, p. 78), by the name of *Diserneston gummiferum*, under the erroneous impression that it belonged to a previously undescribed genus.

The ammoniac plant grows spontaneously in Farsistan, Irauk, Chorassan, and other Persian provinces. Dr. Grant found it abundantly in Syghan near Bameean, on the northwest slope of the Hindoo-Koosh Mountains. It attains the height of six or seven feet, and in the spring and early part of summer abounds in a milky juice, which flows out upon the slightest puncture. From the accounts of travellers, it appears that, in the month of May, the plant is pierced in innumerable places by an insect of the beetle kind. The juice, exuding through the punctures, concretes upon the stem, and when quite dry is collected by the natives. M. Fontanier states that the juice exudes spontaneously, and that the harvest is about

* The *African Ammoniac*, which is said to have appeared in the London market only in the years 1857 and 1871, has been described by Mr. Daniel Hanbury as follows. It is "in large, compact, dark, heavy masses, formed of agglutinated tears of a gum-resin of hard, waxy consistence. The tears are opaque, white or of a pale greenish yellow, mixed with others of a blackish brown, which, with vegetable and earthy impurities, constitute a large portion of the mass." The odor of the drug is feeble, and quite different from that of the Persian gum-resin; its taste slightly acrid and very persistent. (*P. J. Tr.*, March, 1873, p. 741.) Examined by Mr. John Moss, it was found to consist of 67·76 per cent. of resin, 9·014 of gum, 4·29 of water and volatile oil, and 18·85 of bassorin and insoluble matters. (*Ibid.*, p. 742.) It is used chiefly for incense in Mohammedan countries, and sent eastward by the caravans, or in vessels from the ports of Morocco to Alexandria.

the middle of June. According to Dr. Grant, the drug is collected in Syghan, like asafetida, from the root of the plant. The gum-resin is sent to Bushire, whence it is transmitted to India, chiefly to Bombay. A small portion is said to be taken to the ports of the Levant, and thence distributed. The name of the drug is thought to have been derived from the temple of Jupiter Ammon in the Libyan desert, where the ammoniac of the ancients is said to have been collected; but Dr. Don considers it a corruption of *Armeniacum*, originating in the circumstance that the gum-resin was formerly imported into Europe through Armenia.

Properties. Ammoniac comes either in the state of tears, or in aggregate masses, and in both forms is frequently mixed with impurities. That of the tears, however, is preferable, as the purest may be conveniently picked out and kept for use. These are of an irregular shape, usually more or less globular, from two to eight lines in diameter, opaque, yellowish on the outside, whitish within, compact, homogeneous, brittle when cold, and breaking with a conchoidal, shining, waxy fracture. The masses are of a darker color and less uniform structure, appearing, when broken, as if composed of numerous white or whitish tears, embedded in a dirty-gray or brownish substance, and frequently mingled with foreign matters, such as seeds, fragments of vegetables, and sand or other earth. We have seen masses composed of agglutinated tears alone.

The smell of ammoniac is peculiar, and stronger in the mass than in the tears. The taste is slightly sweetish, bitter, and somewhat acrid. The sp. gr. is 1·207. When heated, the gum-resin softens and becomes adhesive, but does not melt. It burns with a white flame, swelling up, and emitting a smoke of a strong, resinous, slightly alliaceous odor. It is partly soluble in water, alcohol, ether, vinegar, and alkaline solutions. Triturated with water, it forms an opaque milky emulsion, which becomes clear upon standing. The alcoholic solution is transparent, but is rendered milky by the addition of water. Braconnot obtained 18·4 per cent. of gum, 70·0 of resin, 4·4 of a gluten-like substance (bassorin), and 6·0 of water, with 1·2 per cent. of loss. Martius found 0·4 per cent. of ethereal oil, Flückiger 0·33 per cent. (*Pflanzenstoffe*, 2d ed., p. 962.) Plugge's analysis gives 1·27 per cent. of volatile oil, 5·10 per cent. of water, 2 per cent. of ash, 65·53 per cent. of resin, and 26·10 per cent. of gum. Hager succeeded in procuring the volatile oil in a separate state by repeated distillation with water. It has a penetrating disagreeable odor, and a taste at first mild, but afterwards bitter and nauseous. Flückiger says that the oil contains no sulphur, and this result was confirmed by Przeciszewski, while, on the other hand, Vigier asserts that it blackens silver, and that when oxidised with nitric acid it yields sulphuric acid. The resin ammoniacum usually amounts to about 70 per cent. Unlike the gum-resin of allied plants, ammoniacum yields no umbelliferone. When melted with caustic potash it affords protocatechuic acid and resorcin. The resin of ammoniac is dissolved by alcohol, and by the fixed and volatile oils; but it is divided by ether into two resins, of which one is soluble, the other insoluble in that menstruum. P. C. Plugge states that hypobromite of sodium, made by dissolving 30 grammes of pure caustic soda in water, adding 20 grammes of bromine, cooling the mixture, and adding distilled water until the whole measures 1 litre, is a sensitive reagent for ammoniac resin. (*Archiv d. Pharm.*, 1883, p. 801.)

Medical Properties and Uses. This gum-resin is stimulant and expectorant, in large doses cathartic, and, like many other stimulants, may be so given as occasionally to prove diaphoretic, diuretic, or emmenagogue. It has been employed in medicine from the highest antiquity, being mentioned in the writings of Hippocrates, but is now seldom administered. The complaints in which it was most frequently used were chronic catarrh, asthma, and other pectoral affections attended with deficient expectoration without acute inflammation, or with a too copious secretion from the bronchial mucous membrane, dependent upon debility of the vessels. It is usually administered in combination with other expectorants, with tonics, or with emmenagogues. Externally applied, in the shape of a plaster, it is thought to be useful as a discutient or resolvent in white swellings of the joints, and other indolent tumors. (See *Emplastrum Ammoniaci.*) It is given in substance, in the shape of pill or emulsion. The latter form is preferable. (See *Mistura Ammoniaci.*) The dose is from ten to thirty grains (0·65–1·95 Gm.).

Off. Prep. Emplastrum Ammoniaci; Emplast. Ammoniaci cum Hydrargyro; Mistura Ammoniaci.

Off. Prep. Br. Emplastrum Ammoniaci cum Hydrargyro; Emplastrum Galbani; Mistura Ammoniaci; Pilula Scillæ Composita; Pilula Ipecacuanhæ cum Scilla.

AMMONII BENZOAS. *U.S., Br.* *Benzoate of Ammonium.*

$NH_4, C_7H_5O_2$; 139. (ĄM-MŌ'NĮ-Ī BĔN'ZǪ-ĂS.) **$NH_4O, C_{14}H_5O_3$; 139.**

Ammoniæ Benzoas, Ammonium Benzoicum, Benzoas Ammonicus; Benzoate d'Ammoniaque, *Fr.*; Benzöesaures Ammonium, *G.*

The process for the preparation of this salt was omitted in the last U. S. revision.* The British process is as follows. "Take of Solution of Ammonia *three fluidounces* [Imperial measure], or *a sufficiency;* Benzoic Acid *two ounces* [avoirdupois]; Distilled Water *four fluidounces.* Dissolve the Benzoic Acid in three fluidounces of Solution of Ammonia previously mixed with the Water; evaporate at a gentle heat, keeping ammonia in slight excess; and set aside that crystals may form. $NH_4C_7H_5O_2$." *Br.*

Although the amount of ammonia ordered in the formula is in excess, yet, from the feeble affinity between the constituents, and the consequent escape of ammonia during the evaporation, a portion of the acid benzoate would be formed, if it were not that a little solution of ammonia is from time to time added during or near the close of the evaporation, so as to maintain the alkali in slight excess. The crystals, for the same reason, should be dried without heat. If slightly evaporated, and then allowed to cool, the solution becomes a mass of crystals, retaining so much water as to render it necessary to dry them by bibulous paper.

Properties. "Thin, white, four-sided, laminar crystals, permanent in the air, having a slight odor of benzoic acid, a saline, bitter, afterwards slightly acrid taste and a neutral reaction. Soluble in 5 parts of water and 28 parts of alcohol at 15° C. (59° F.); in 1·2 parts of boiling water and 7·6 parts of boiling alcohol. When strongly heated, the salt melts, emits vapors having the odor of ammonia and of benzoic acid, and is finally wholly dissipated. The aqueous solution of the salt, when heated with potassa, evolves ammonia. On mixing the aqueous solution with a dilute solution of ferric sulphate, a flesh-colored precipitate is thrown down. If the benzoic acid be separated from the salt by precipitating with diluted nitric acid and thoroughly washed, it should answer to the reactions of purity mentioned under *Acidum Benzoicum.*" *U. S.* Gmelin states that, if the solution be boiled, the salt is converted into the acid benzoate, which crystallizes in feathery tufts of needles. (*Handbook*, xii. 38.) According to Lichtenstein, it deliquesces in the air. It gives a copious yellow precipitate with ferric salts; and is known to contain benzoic acid and ammonia, by depositing the former when the solution is acidulated with hydrochloric acid, and giving off the latter when it is heated with potassa. According to Mr. Squire, it is the acid salt that is commonly met with in the shops, which is less soluble than the officinal salt, requiring 60 parts of water and 12 of alcohol for solution. This is a decided objection to it.

Medical Properties and Uses. Benzoate of ammonium is a slightly stimulant diuretic, which acts chiefly through its benzoic acid; it being decomposed by the gastric acids, which combine with the ammonia, while the benzoic acid is absorbed, and passes out through the kidneys in the form of hippuric acid. (See *Benzoic Acid.*) The salt has been found useful as a diuretic in defective action of the kidneys, as an alterative to the mucous membrane of the urinary passages in chronic inflammation of that tissue, and as a solvent of the phosphatic deposits, through the hippuric acid into which it is converted. It has been employed in gouty affections with a view to the removal of the deposits of urate of sodium about the joints; but it has been shown to have no effect on the elimination of uric acid. The salt does

* "Take of Benzoic Acid *two troyounces;* Water of Ammonia *three fluidounces and a half*, or *a sufficient quantity;* Distilled Water *four fluidounces.* Dissolve the Acid in three fluidounces and a half of the Water of Ammonia, previously mixed with the Distilled Water; evaporate with a gentle heat, occasionally adding Water of Ammonia, if necessary, to maintain a slight excess of the alkali; then set aside to crystallize, and dry the crystals without heat." *U. S.* 1870.

not appear to produce any injurious effects even in considerable quantities. (Garrod, *Med. Times and Gaz.*, Feb. 1864, p. 146.) The dose is from 10 to 30 grains (0·65–1·95 Gm.), which may be taken dissolved in water.

AMMONII BROMIDUM. *U.S., Br.* *Bromide of Ammonium.*

NH_4Br; 97·8. (AM-MŌ'NI-I BRO-MĪ'DŬM.) NH_4Br; 97·8.

Ammonium Bromatum; Bromure d'Ammonium, *Fr.;* Brom-Ammonium, *G.*

The U. S. Pharmacopœia gives no directions for the preparation of this salt; the Br. Pharmacopœia neutralizes hydrobromic acid with ammonia. The salt may be made by dissolving bromine in water of ammonia; but, in accordance with the researches of Prof. Procter, the U. S. Pharmacopœia of 1870* preferred the method of first forming bromide of iron, precipitating with water of ammonia, separating by filtration the oxide of iron, and obtaining by evaporation the bromide of ammonium from the solution. This process, it will be seen, is completely parallel with that by which bromide of potassium is prepared. According to Prof. Procter, a still better method consists in adding to bromine and water sufficient solution of sulphide of ammonium to discharge the color, filtering to separate the sulphur, and then evaporating to dryness. Charles Rice (*A. J. P.*, 1873, p. 249) recommends making bromide of ammonium by double decomposition between hot solutions of bromide of potassium and sulphate of ammonium, assisting the precipitation of sulphate of potassium by alcohol. Dr. W. H. Pile (*Proc. A. P. A.*, 1874, p. 434) published a simple process for this salt. Pour the bromine (one pound) carefully into four times its weight of distilled water in a stone jar, add *very gradually* about one quart of solution of ammonia, cover the top of the jar with a glass plate when vapors arise, and when all of the ammonia has been added, and the solution is free from the smell of bromine, it is evaporated and the salt granulated; the yield is about twenty ounces.

Properties. Bromide of ammonium may be obtained in colorless crystals, but the officinal salt is a white, granular powder. Whether in crystal or powder, on exposure to the air it gradually becomes yellowish, in consequence of a partial decomposition, by which hydrobromic acid appears to be liberated, as it now changes litmus red. The salt has a saline, pungent taste. Exposed to heat, it sublimes unchanged. It is "soluble in 1·5 parts of water, and in 150 parts of alcohol at 15° C. (59° F.); in 0·7 part of boiling water and in 15 parts of boiling alcohol." *U.S.* It is sparingly soluble in ether, and is incompatible with acids, acid salts, and spirit of nitrous ether.

Tests. The Br. Pharmacopœia directs "that 5 grains dissolved in an ounce of distilled water to which 2 drops of solution of yellow chromate of potassium have been added, require not more than 514·5 and not less than 508·5 grain-measures of the *volumetric solution of nitrate of silver* to produce a permanent red precipitate."

"The aqueous solution, when heated with potassa, evolves ammonia. If disulphide of carbon be poured into the solution, then chlorine water added drop by drop, and the whole agitated, the disulphide will acquire a yellow or yellowish brown color without a violet tint. If diluted sulphuric acid be dropped on the salt, the latter should not at once assume a yellow color (bromate). If 1 Gm. of the salt be dissolved in water, some gelatinized starch added, and then a few drops of chlorine water carefully poured on top, no blue zone should make its appearance at the line of contact of the two liquids (iodide). On adding to 1 Gm. of the salt dissolved in 20 C.c. of water, 5 or 6 drops of the test-solution of chloride of barium,

* "Take of Bromine *two troyounces;* Iron, in the form of wire and cut in pieces, *a troyounce;* Water of Ammonia *four fluidounces and a half;* Distilled Water *a sufficient quantity.* Add the Iron and then the Bromine to half a pint of Distilled Water, contained in a glass flask having the capacity of two pints; loosely cork the flask, and agitate the mixture until the odor of Bromine can no longer be perceived, and the liquid assumes a greenish color. Mix the Water of Ammonia with half a pint of Distilled Water, and add it to the mixture in the flask; agitate the mixture, and heat it by means of a water-bath for half an hour; then filter, and, when the liquor ceases to pass, wash the precipitate on the filter with boiling distilled water. Evaporate the solution, in a porcelain capsule, until a pellicle begins to form, then stir it constantly with a glass rod, at a moderate heat, until it granulates." *U. S.* 1870.

no immediate cloudiness or precipitate should make its appearance (limit of sulphate). If 3 Gm. of the well-dried salt be dissolved in distilled water to 100 C.c. and 10 C.c. of this solution treated with a few drops of test-solution of bichromate of potassium, and then volumetric solution of nitrate of silver be added, not more than 31·4 C.c. of the latter should be consumed, before the red color ceases to disappear on stirring (abs. of more than 3 per cent. of chloride). 1 Gm. of the powdered and dry salt, when completely precipitated by nitrate of silver, yields, if perfectly pure, 1·917 Gm. of dry bromide of silver." *U.S.*

Medical Properties and Uses. This bromide resembles the bromide of potassium in its physiological powers, but probably has a less depressing effect upon the arterial muscular system. It has been used by various practitioners for exactly the same purposes as is the bromide of potassium. Brown-Séquard claims that it does not produce bromism; and commends very highly the combination of it with the potassium salt in epilepsy. It may be substituted for the latter in various functional disorders (see *Potassii Bromidum*), and has been specially recommended by Dr. Gibbs in the milder forms of ovaritis. (*Lancet*, Jan. 3, 1863, p. 121.) The dose is one to two drachms a day (3·9–7·8 Gm.) in dilute solution.

AMMONII CARBONAS. *U.S., Br.* *Carbonate of Ammonium.*

(ĄM-MŌ'NĮ-Ī CÄR-BŌ'NĂS.)

$NH_4HCO_3.NH_4NH_2CO_2$; 157. $NH_4O, HO, 2CO_2. 2NH_3CO_2$; 157.

"A volatile and pungent ammoniacal salt, produced by submitting a mixture of sulphate or chloride of ammonium and carbonate of calcium to sublimation and re-sublimation. It is considered to be a compound of acid carbonate of ammonium (NH_4HCO_3) with carbamate of ammonium ($NH_4NH_2CO_2$), and the compound molecule is usually regarded as containing one molecule of each of these salts." *Br.*

Ammoniæ Carbonas, *Br.*, 1867; Ammoniæ Sesquicarbonas, *Lond.*, *Dub.*; Ammonium Carbonicum, *P.G.*; Carbonas Ammonicus, Sal Volatile Siccum, Volatile Salt; Sal Volatile; Carbonate d'Ammoniaque, Alkali volatil concret, Sal volatil d'Angleterre, *Fr.*; Kohlensaures Ammonium, Flüchtiges Laugensalz, Reines Hirschhornsalz, *G.*

There have been many methods of obtaining carbonate of ammonium, in all of which the ammonia originated in organic decomposition. It was probably originally prepared from putrid urine, and it is sometimes made in Scotland now from this source. A patent was taken out in England for manufacturing it from guano, and another for making it by the direct combination of its constituents; the carbonic acid and ammoniacal gases being introduced simultaneously into leaden chambers. (*Chem. News*, Dec. 29, 1865.) But at present the salt is manufactured by subliming a mixture of either the chloride or sulphate with chalk. Chloride of ammonium and chalk (carbonate of calcium) are heated together in iron pots or retorts, and sublimed into large earthen or leaden receivers. By the reciprocal action of the salts employed, the carbonic acid of the chalk unites with the ammonia of the chloride, generating carbonate of ammonium, and the hydrochloric acid with the lime, forming water and chloride of calcium. The carbonate and water sublime together as hydrated carbonate of ammonium, and the residue is chloride of calcium. The relative quantities of chalk and chloride of ammonium, for mutual decomposition, are 50 of the former, and 53·5 of the latter, or one mol. of each. But a great excess of chalk is usually taken, in order to insure the perfect decomposition of the chloride of ammonium, any redundancy of which would sublime with the carbonate and render it impure.

Sulphate of ammonium may be substituted for the chloride with much economy, as was shown by Payen. This double decomposition between sulphate of ammonium and carbonate of calcium takes place in the dry way only, that is, by sublimation. In the wet way, the double decomposition is reversed; carbonate of ammonium and sulphate of calcium reacting so as to form sulphate of ammonium and carbonate of calcium. Large quantities of this carbonate are manufactured indirectly from *coal-gas liquor* and *bone-spirit;* the ammoniacal products in these liquors being converted successively into sulphate, chloride, and carbonate of ammonium. (See *Ammonii Chloridum.*) The salt as first obtained has a slight odor of tar, and leaves a blackish carbonaceous matter when dissolved in acids. Hence it requires to be purified, which is effected in iron pots surmounted with leaden heads. The American carbonate has almost supplanted the English article, formerly exclusively used.

Properties. Commercial carbonate of ammonium, recently prepared, is in "white, translucent masses, consisting of Bicarbonate (Acid Carbonate) and Carbamate of Ammonium, losing both ammonia and carbonic acid gas on exposure to air, becoming opaque and finally converted into friable porous lumps, or a white powder (Acid Carbonate of Ammonium). The salt has a pungent ammoniacal odor, free from empyreuma, a sharp, saline taste, and an alkaline reaction. Soluble in 4 parts of water at 15° C. (59° F.), and in 1·5 parts at 65° C. (149° F.). Alcohol dissolves the carbamate and leaves the acid carbonate of ammonium. When heated the salt is wholly dissipated, without charring. If the aqueous solution is heated to near 47° C. (116·6° F.), it begins to lose carbonic acid gas, and at 88° C. (190·4° F.) it begins to give off vapor of ammonia. Dilute acids wholly dissolve the salt with effervescence. On acidulating the aqueous solution with nitric acid, no turbidity should be produced by test-solution of chloride of barium (sulphate), or nitrate of silver (chloride), nor by hydrosulphuric acid (metals). If 1 Gm. of the salt be supersaturated with diluted sulphuric acid, then diluted to 20 C.c. with distilled water, and treated with a few drops of test-solution of permanganate of potassium, the color should not be perceptibly changed by standing for five minutes, at the ordinary temperature (abs. of empyreumatic substances). To neutralize 2·616 Gm. of Carbonate of Ammonium should require 50 C.c. of the volumetric solution of oxalic acid." *U. S.* If commercial ammonium carbonate be treated with 90 or 91 per cent. alcohol, it is decomposed into the two salts of which it is composed, ammonium carbamate going into solution while the acid ammonium carbonate remains undissolved. This latter compound also remains undissolved when the commercial carbonate is treated with an amount of water insufficient for complete solution. The result of the complete solution of the commercial salt in water is a mixture of acid and neutral carbonates, the carbamate having been decomposed according to the reaction, $(NH_4)HCO_3 + CO\begin{cases} ONH_4 \\ NH_2 \end{cases} + H_2O = (NH_4)HCO_3 + (NH_4)_2CO_3$. When long or insecurely kept, it gradually passes into the state of bicarbonate, becoming opaque and friable, and falling into powder. When heated on a piece of glass, the commercial carbonate should evaporate without residue, and, if turmeric paper held over it undergoes no change, it has passed into bicarbonate. As prepared from coal-gas liquor, it sometimes contains traces of tarry matter, which give a dark color to its solution in acids, but a refined carbonate, made by resubliming the commercial article, is now in the market, and this alone should be dispensed in preparations for internal use. When it is saturated with nitric acid, neither chloride of barium nor nitrate of silver causes a precipitate. The non-action of these tests shows the absence of sulphate and chloride of ammonium. It is decomposed by acids, the fixed alkalies and their carbonates, lime-water and magnesia, solution of chloride of calcium, alum, acid salts such as bitartrate and bisulphate of potassium, solutions of iron (except the tartrate of iron and potassium and analogous preparations), corrosive sublimate, the acetate and subacetate of lead, and the sulphates of iron and zinc. "Fifty-nine grains dissolved in one [fluid]ounce of distilled water, will be neutralized by 1000 grain-measures of *the volumetric solution of oxalic acid.* Twenty grains neutralize 23·5 grains of citric acid and 25·5 grains of tartaric acid." *Br.* Traces of chlorine have been noticed in some samples of commercial carbonate, and a sublimed salt which had been sold as carbonate, was *devoid of odor*, hard, crystalline, yet having the external appearance of carbonate, was proved by Prof. Bridges to be anhydrous bicarbonate of ammonium. (*A. J. P.*, Nov. 1874.) Although much inferior to the officinal compound, this salt is still to be found in the market. (Kraut, *Archiv d. Pharm.*, 1885, p. 21.)

Composition. This salt, which used to be considered a sesquicarbonate of ammonium of the formula $2(CO_2(NH_4)H) + CO_2(NH_4)_2 + H_2O$, is now generally recognized as a mixture of either one or two mols. of acid ammonium carbonate,

$(NH_4)HCO_3$, with one mol. of *carbamate* of ammonium, $CO\left\{\begin{matrix}ONH_4\\NH_2\end{matrix}\right.$. When the salt is dissolved in water, the reaction given above converts it into a mixture of acid and neutral carbonates, and when water of ammonia is added in sufficient amount, it converts the acid carbonate into neutral carbonate, which is used frequently as a laboratory reagent, or by passing carbonic acid gas into a solution of the commercial salt, the whole may be converted into acid carbonate or bicarbonate.

Medical Properties and Uses. Locally applied, carbonate of ammonium is an irritant, and when taken internally in sufficient amount it acts as an irritant poison. When administered in therapeutic doses it is a powerful cardiac stimulant, acting not so rapidly and fugaciously as the solutions of ammonia, but still in a very prompt and temporary manner. It is employed in low conditions of the system as a stimulant, but it should always be remembered that its influence lasts only for a short time, and that there is reason for believing that when continuously given it is apt to impair the crasis of the blood. It is probably eliminated in part by the lungs, and certainly is a stimulant to the respiratory centres. It seems also to exert some influence upon the pulmonary mucous membrane, and is largely employed in adynamic pneumonias and bronchitis, in the last stages of phthisis, etc. In some of these cases it does good by increasing muscular power and aiding in the expulsion of the sputa.

Coarsely bruised with the addition of half its bulk of strongest water of ammonia, and scented with oil of lavender, it constitutes the common smelling salts, so much used as a nasal stimulant in syncope and hysteria.* The ordinary dose is five grains (0·33 Gm.), given in mixture, and repeated at not longer intervals than two hours. It should never be given in powder or in pill, on account of its volatile nature, and its irritant action on mucous membranes.

Carbonate of ammonium is sometimes employed to make effervescing draughts, 20 grains of the salt requiring for this purpose 6 fluidrachms of lemon-juice, 24 grains of citric acid, or 25½ grains of tartaric acid.

Off. Prep. Ferri et Ammonii Tartras; Liquor Ammonii Acetatis; Spiritus Ammoniæ Aromaticus.

Off. Prep. Br. Bismuthi Carbonas; Liquor Ammonii Acetatis Fortior; Spiritus Ammoniæ Aromaticus.

AMMONII CHLORIDUM. *U. S.*, *Br.* *Chloride of Ammonium.*

NH_4Cl; 53·4. (AM-MŌ′NĬ-Ī CHLŌ′RĬ-DŬM.) NH_4Cl; 53·4.

Muriate of Ammonia, Ammonium Muriaticum s. Hydrochloratum, Chloruretum Ammonicum, Sal Ammoniacum, Ammoniæ Hydrochloras s. Murias; Sal Ammoniac, Hydrochlorate of Ammonia; Hydrochlorate d'Ammoniaque, Muriate d'Ammoniaque, Sel Ammoniac, Chlorure d'Ammonium, Clorure d'Ammonium pur; Ammonium Muriaticum Depuratum, Sal Ammoniacum Depuratum, *Fr.*; Ammonium Chloratum, *P. G.*; Salmiak Chlorammonium; Reiner (gereinigter) Salmiak, *G.*; Sale Ammoniaco, *It.*; Sal Ammoniaco, *Sp.*

In the Pharmacopœia of 1870 both the crude and the purified chloride of ammonium were officinal, under the names *Ammonii Chloridum* and *Ammonii Chloridum Purificatum.* The Pharm. 1880 recognizes but one, *Ammonii Chloridum*, but it transfers this title, which formerly was given to the crude sal ammoniac, to the purified salt without giving a process for preparing it.† It originally came from Egypt, where it was obtained by sublimation from the soot resulting from the burning of camels' dung, which is used in that country for fuel, and it is still to be

* In Mounsey's recipe for the English *Preston salts*, the essence to be added to the carbonate is made as follows. Take of oil of cloves ℥ss; oil of lavender ℥j; oil of bergamot ℥iiss; stronger water of ammonia (sp. gr. 0·880) f℥x. Mix. The bottles are to be filled with carbonate of ammonium, half with the salt coarsely bruised, and the remainder with it in fine powder; and then as much of the above essences as the salt will absorb is to be added. (*P. J. Tr.*, xiii. 628.)

† The process (Pharm. 1870) for purifying sal ammoniac is here given as found in 14th ed. U. S. D.

"Take of Chloride of Ammonium, in small pieces, *twenty troyounces*; Water of Ammonia *five fluidrachms*; Water *two pints*. Dissolve the Chloride of Ammonium in the Water, in a porcelain dish, with the aid of heat; add the Water of Ammonia, and continue the heat for a short time; filter the solution while hot, and evaporate to dryness, with constant stirring, at a moderate heat, until it granulates." *U. S.* 1870.

The object of this process is to free the drug from chloride of iron, which is a frequent impurity of the crude salt, derived from the subliming vessels.

found in the Indian bazaars in an impure state, as it has been obtained from the unburnt extremity in the interior of brick-kilns in which camels' manure is used for fuel. It has long been known in China, where it is obtained from the water of certain volcanic springs, and exists in commerce in various states of purity. It is found in the fumeroles of Vesuvius, Etna, Hecla, and other volcanoes, as well as in the cracks and fissures in recent lava streams.

Preparation. At present chloride of ammonium is derived from two principal sources, the ammoniacal liquor, called *gas liquor*, found in the condensing vessels of coal-gas works, and the brown, fetid ammoniacal liquor, known under the name of *bone-spirit*, which is a secondary product, obtained from the destructive distillation of bones, in the manufacture of bone-black. These two liquors are the chief sources of ammoniacal compounds; for they are both used to procure chloride of ammonium, and this salt is employed directly or indirectly for obtaining all the other salts of ammonia. Other sources are stale urine, coal soot, guano, peat, and bituminous schist.

Gas liquor contains carbonate, cyanide, sulphide, and sulphate of ammonium, but principally the carbonate. It is saturated with sulphuric acid, and the solution obtained, after due evaporation, furnishes brown crystals of sulphate of ammonium. These are then sublimed with chloride of sodium in iron pots, lined with clay, and furnished with a leaden dome or head. By the mutual action of the sulphate, water, and chloride, there are formed chloride of ammonium which sublimes, and sulphate of sodium which remains behind. Thus $(NH_4)_2SO_4$ and $(NaCl)_2$ become $(NH_4Cl)_2$ and Na_2SO_4. Sometimes, instead of the ammonia of the gas liquor being first converted into the sulphate, it is made at once into chloride by the addition of hydrochloric acid or chloride of calcium. When chloride of calcium is employed, the chief reaction takes place between carbonate of ammonium and the chloride, whereby chloride of ammonium is formed in solution, and carbonate of calcium precipitated. The solution is duly evaporated, whereby brown crystals of the chloride are obtained. These, after having been dried, are purified by sublimation in an iron subliming pot, coated with a composition of clay, sand, and charcoal, and covered with a dome of lead. These pots are sometimes sufficiently large to hold five hundred pounds. "A gentle fire is kept up under the subliming pot for seven or eight days, when, the dome having cooled down, and the sal ammoniac somewhat contracted, so as to loosen from the sides, the dome is thrown off from the iron pot, and about two or three hundred weight of white, semi-transparent sal ammoniac are knocked off in cakes." (Pereira, *Mat. Med.*, 3d ed., p. 446.)

In the destructive distillation of bones for making bone-black, the distilled products are the bone-spirit already mentioned, being chiefly an aqueous solution of carbonate of ammonium, and an empyreumatic oil, called *animal oil*. Chloride of ammonium may be obtained from the bone-spirit in the manner just described for procuring it from gas liquor. Sometimes, however, the sulphate of ammonium is not made by direct combination, but by digesting the bone-spirit with ground plaster of Paris. By double decomposition, sulphate of ammonium and carbonate of calcium are formed. The sulphate of ammonium is then converted into the chloride by sublimation with common salt. The chloride "may be formed by neutralising hydrochloric acid with ammonia or carbonate of ammonium, and evaporating to dryness." *Br.*

Other processes have been proposed or practised for obtaining chloride of ammonium. For an account of the manufacture of ammoniacal salts, and for a list of the patents issued in Great Britain, since 1827, for their preparation, the reader is referred to the *P. J. Tr.* (xii. 29, 63, and 113).

Commercial History. Nearly all the chloride of ammonium used in the United States is obtained from abroad. Its commercial varieties are known under the names of the *crude* and *refined*. The crude is imported from Calcutta in chests containing from 350 to 400 pounds; and is consumed almost exclusively by coppersmiths and other artisans in brass and copper, being employed for the purpose of keeping the metallic surfaces bright, preparatory to brazing. The refined comes to us exclusively from England, packed in casks containing from 5 to 10 cwt.

Properties. Commercial chloride of ammonium is a white, translucent, tough, fibrous salt, occurring in large cakes, about two inches thick, convex on one side and concave on the other, due to the shape of the dome of the subliming apparatus: the pieces frequently are tinged on the surface with iron stains, owing to the contact with the iron dome. It has a pungent, saline taste, but no smell. Its sp. gr. is 1·45. This salt is very difficult to powder in the ordinary way. Its pulverization, however, may be readily effected by making a boiling saturated solution of the salt, and stirring it as it cools. The salt is thus made to granulate, and in this state, after having been drained from the remaining solution and dried, may be easily powdered. At a red heat it sublimes without decomposition, and without residue. Exposed to a damp atmosphere it becomes slightly moist. It has the property of increasing the solubility of corrosive sublimate in water. It is decomposed by the strong mineral acids, and by the alkalies and alkaline earths; the former disengaging hydrochloric acid, the latter ammonia, both sensible to the smell. Chloride of ammonium is usually employed for obtaining gaseous ammonia, which is conveniently disengaged by lime. It is incompatible with acetate of lead and nitrate of silver, producing precipitates respectively, of the chlorides of lead and silver.

Chloride of ammonium is little subject to adulteration. If not entirely volatilized by heat and soluble in water, it contains impurity. Still, as ordinarily prepared, it contains ferrous chloride. This metal may be detected by boiling a small portion of a saturated solution of the salt with a drop or two of nitric acid, and then adding ferrocyanide of potassium, when the characteristic blue color occasioned by iron will be produced. If the salt is entirely volatilized by heat, and yet produces a precipitate with chloride of barium, the presence of sulphate of ammonium is indicated. The description and tests of the officinal purified salt are as follows.

"A snow-white crystalline powder, permanent in the air, odorless, having a cooling saline taste and a slightly acid reaction. Soluble in 3 parts of water at 15° C. (59° F.) and in 1·37 parts of boiling water; very sparingly soluble in alcohol. On ignition, the salt volatilizes, without charring, and without leaving a residue. The aqueous solution of the salt, when heated with potassa, evolves vapor of ammonia. Test-solution of nitrate of silver added to the aqueous solution previously acidulated with nitric acid, produces a white precipitate soluble in ammonia. The aqueous solution of the salt should remain unaffected by diluted sulphuric acid (abs. of barium), hydrosulphuric acid, or sulphide of ammonium (metals), and, after being acidulated with hydrochloric acid, it should not be rendered turbid by test-solution of nitrate of barium (sulphate). A one per cent. aqueous solution should not be rendered blue by test-solution of ferrocyanide of potassium (iron)." *U.S.*

Composition. Chloride of ammonium consists of one atom of chlorine and one of ammonium, $(NH_4) = NH_4Cl$. Viewed as *hydrochlorate of ammonia or muriate of ammonium*, it is composed of one mol. of hydrochloric acid 36·5, and one of ammonia 17 = 53·5.

Medical Properties. Chloride of ammonium has the stimulant properties of ammonia, and probably differs little in its physiological powers from the carbonate, but it is believed by many to be less fugacious in its action, and to be less stimulant to the circulation than is the latter salt. Clinical experience has also led to a somewhat particular use of it in diseases. It is one of the most employed of the stimulant expectorants in the advanced stages of acute bronchitis and in chronic bronchitis, also in catarrhal pneumonia. It has been very highly recommended of late years in chronic hepatic torpor and engorgement, and even in acute hepatitis, by Dr. W. Stewart, who gives 20 grains of it three times a day, and continues its use for weeks. We have seen catarrhal jaundice apparently very much benefited by it. Many years ago it was a favorite remedy as a resolvent in chronic glandular enlargements, but at present is rarely so employed. There is much testimony as to the value of chloride of ammonium in various obscure nervous affections, especially hemicrania, ovaralgia, dysmenorrhœa, sciatica, and various other neuralgic disorders. The usual expectorant dose of the chloride is 5 to 10 grains (0·33–0·65 Gm.) every two hours, administered in sweetened mucilage; but formerly in prostatic and other glandular enlargements it was recommended to increase the dose until half an ounce a day was ingested. When such amounts are given, the remedy is prone to produce disordered digestion, a miliary eruption, profuse sweats, and scorbutic symptoms.

Externally, chloride of ammonium is used in solution, as a stimulant and resolvent, in contusions, indolent tumors, etc. An ounce of the salt, dissolved in nine fluidounces of water and one of alcohol, forms a solution of convenient strength. When the solution is to be used as a wash for ulcers, or an injection in leucorrhœa, it should not contain more than from one to four drachms of the salt to a pint of water. Such a solution, with addition of wine of opium, had been advantageously employed by M. Guinau de Mussy in milky engorgement and scrofulous swellings of the breast, being applied upon cataplasms. A case of decided senile gangrene in a woman of 83 has been recorded, in which the immersion of the feet in a pediluvium consisting of half a pound of chloride of ammonium dissolved in water, afforded relief in two hours; and, being followed by fomentations with the same solution, resulted in cure. (*Annuaire de Thérap.*, 1868, p. 105.)

The vapor of chloride of ammonium has been administered by inhalation, employed several times a day, in chronic catarrh, with marked advantage, by Dr. Gieseler, of Germany. Dr. Hermann Beigel, of London, strongly recommends its inhalation in the nascent state, resulting from a mixture of the two gases composing it. Three bottles are used, one containing water of ammonia, the second an equivalent quantity of liquid hydrochloric acid, and the third half filled with water, connected with the first two by tubes, and supplied itself with a tube for inhalation. By inhalation the patient draws the two gases from their respective bottles into the third, where they combine to form the chloride of ammonium, which is freed from any excess of either gas by the water. The greater or less force of the inspiration will determine the depth to which the medicine will penetrate; and this will depend on the part of the respiratory passages specially affected. (*Lancet*, Oct. 1867, p. 512.) Another mode of inhaling chloride of ammonium is in *spray*, by means of the atomizer; from 10 to 20 grains being dissolved for the purpose in a fluidounce of water.

Off. Prep. Trochisci Ammonii Chloridi.

Pharm. Uses. Br. Liquor Ammoniæ Fortior; Liquor Hydrargyri Perchloridi.

AMMONII IODIDUM. *U.S.* *Iodide of Ammonium.*

NH_4I; 144·6. (AM-MŌ'NI-Ī Ī-ŎD'I-DŬM.) NH_4I; 144·6.

Iodure d'Ammonium, *Fr.;* Ammonium Jodatum, Ioduretum Ammonicum, Jodammonium, *G.*

No process is given in the Pharm. 1880 for this salt; that of the Pharm. 1870 will be found below.*

This salt was formerly prepared according to the method of Mr. Jno. A. Spencer, of London, the formula for which is as follows. Add to a portion of iodine, placed in a flask with a little water, a solution of ammonium sulphydrate, until the mixture loses its red color, and is turbid from the separation of sulphur only. Shake the flask, which causes the sulphur, for the most part, to agglomerate; and, having poured off the liquid, boil it until all odor of sulphuretted hydrogen and of ammonia is lost. Then filter the liquid, and, constantly stirring, evaporate it, first with a naked flame until it becomes pasty, and then in a water-bath until it forms a dry salt. In 1864 (*A. J. P.*, May, 1864), Dr. Jacobson proposed a plan in which double decomposition between the sulphate of ammonium and the iodide of potassium was brought about. Mr. James F. Babcock (*Proc. A. P. A.*, 1866) stated that on trial of the first of the above processes, and of all others in which sulphuretted hydrogen or an alkaline sulphide was employed, the resulting iodide of ammonium retained a portion of sulphur, which caused its color to change with time to yellow and ultimately to brown, and rendered it unfit for the accurate preparations required in

* "Take of Iodide of Potassium, in coarse powder, *four troyounces;* Sulphate of Ammonium, in coarse powder, a *troyounce* [this should be 867 grains]; Boiling Distilled Water *two fluidounces;* Alcohol, Water, each, a *sufficient quantity*. Mix the salts, add them to the Boiling Water, stir well, and allow the mixture to cool; then add a fluidounce of Alcohol, mix well, and reduce the temperature, by a bath of iced water, to about 40°; throw the mixture into a cool glass funnel, stopped with moistened cotton, and, when the clear solution has passed, pour upon the salt a fluidounce of a mixture containing two parts of Water and one part of Alcohol. Lastly, evaporate the solution rapidly to dryness, stirring constantly; and preserve the residue in a well-stopped bottle." *U. S.*, 1870.

photography. Having tried also other formulas, which he found objectionable on the score of time, cost, etc., he at length satisfied himself that the process of Dr. Jacobson above described was the best in use, and with slight modifications would yield an absolutely pure product.

In a former edition of the Dispensatory may be found the exact process finally adopted by Mr. Babcock. It is substantially that which was officinal in Pharm. 1870, and is in close accord with that of Dr. Jacobson. The object of the first step of the process is sufficiently evident. After the double decomposition has occurred, the alcohol is added to complete the precipitation of the sulphate of potassium; the pouring of alcohol upon the cotton filter is to remove completely from the sulphate all of the iodide. As made by this process, iodide of ammonium always contains a minute proportion of sulphate of potassium. Charles Rice (*A. J. P.*, 1873, p. 249) calls attention to the fact that the process officinal in U. S. Pharm. 1870 is deficient in the amount of sulphate of ammonium required, and therefore wasteful of the more expensive iodide; instead of one ounce of sulphate of ammonium the quantity should be 867 grains. The view taken by Mr. Rice, however, is that the reaction takes place between single molecules of the respective salts, which is no doubt correct, whereas the view of the Pharmacopœia committee was that two mols. of the iodide reacted with one of sulphate of ammonium, $2KI + (NH_4)_2SO_4 = K_2SO_4 + 2NH_4I$.

Properties. Iodide of ammonium is "a white, granular salt, or minute crystalline cubes, very deliquescent, and soon becoming yellow or yellowish brown on exposure to air; odorless when white, but emitting a slight odor of iodine when colored, having a sharp, saline taste and a neutral reaction. Soluble in 1 part of water and in 9 parts of alcohol at 15° C. (59° F.), in 0·5 part of boiling water, and in 3·7 parts of boiling alcohol. When heated on platinum foil, the salt evolves vapor of iodine and volatilizes without melting. The aqueous solution of the salt, when heated with potassa, evolves vapor of ammonia. If disulphide of carbon be poured into the solution, then chlorine water added drop by drop, and the whole agitated, the disulphide will acquire a violet color." On adding to 1 Gm. of the salt, dissolved in 20 C.c. of water (with a few drops of diluted hydrochloric acid), 5 or 6 drops of test-solution of nitrate of barium, no immediate cloudiness or precipitate should make its appearance (limit of sulphate). If 1 Gm. of the salt be dissolved in 10 Gm. of water of ammonia, then shaken with a solution of 1·3 Gm. of nitrate of silver in 20 Gm. of water, and the filtrate be supersaturated with 8 Gm. of nitric acid, no cloudiness should make its appearance within 10 minutes (abs. of more than about 0·5 per cent. of chloride and bromide)." *U. S.* Prof. Prescott states, in connection with the last test, that it is based on the careful trial tests of Biltz, who "found the time reaction to exclude more than 0·5 per cent. of bromine and chlorine," although, as the test stands, it would theoretically indicate as much as 6 per cent. (nearly) of chlorine. But the *dilution*, the *acid*, and the *short time* operate as retarding or preventive measures.

100 parts of NH_4I require of $AgNO_3$ 117·3 parts.
100 parts of $NH_4I + 1\ NH_4Cl$ require of $AgNO_3$ 119·38 parts.
94 parts of $NH_4I + 6\ NH_4Cl$ require of $AgNO_3$ 128·91 parts.

"A one per cent. aqueous solution should not be colored blue by test-solution of ferrocyanide of potassium (abs. of iron), nor, after being mixed with gelatinized starch, should it assume a deep blue color (limit of free iodine). 1 Gm. of the dried salt, when completely precipitated with nitrate of silver, yields, if perfectly pure, 1·62 Gm. of dry iodide of silver." *U. S.* The salt should be preserved in small well-stopped vials, protected from the light. "When deeply colored it should not be dispensed, but it may be deprived of all but traces of free iodine by washing with stronger ether and rapidly drying." *U. S.*

Medical Properties. Iodide of ammonium is employed, both externally and internally, as a resolvent, and resembles closely, in its action, iodine and iodide of potassium. Dr. B. W. Richardson, of London, has prescribed it, in the dose of from one to three grains, with considerable success, in secondary syphilis, chronic rheumatism, incipient phthisis, and in a variety of forms of scrofulous disorder, attended with glandular enlargements. Dr. Richardson found a liniment, made by dissolving half a drachm of the iodide in an ounce of glycerin, very efficacious in enlarged tonsils, applied every night with a large camel's-hair brush, and his practice has been followed to some extent by other members of the profession.* Externally, this salt has been used as a substitute for iodide of potassium. By Dr. Pennock it is considered as a good remedy in certain cases of lepra and psoriasis, in the form of ointment, applied by friction in the quantity of half an ounce, morning and evening. The proportions employed are from a scruple to a drachm of the salt to an ounce of lard; the weaker preparation being used when the disease is recent, the stronger when it is chronic. As the iodide is decomposed by the air, the ointment should be kept in well-stopped bottles. For internal use, the dose of iodide of ammonium is from three to five grains (0·20–0·33 Gm.).

AMMONII NITRAS. *U. S., Br.* *Nitrate of Ammonium.*

NH_4NO_3; 80. (AM-MŌ'NI-Ī NĪ'TRĂS.) NH_4O, NO_5; 80.

Ammoniæ Nitras, *Br.*, 1867; Nitrate of Ammonia; Ammonium Nitricum, Nitrum Flammans; Azotate d'Ammoniaque, Nitre inflammable, Nitre ammoniacal, Sal ammoniacal nitreux, *Fr.*; Salpetersaures Ammon, Ammonium, Ammoniak, *G.*

An extraordinary property possessed by this salt of absorbing ammoniacal gas, and giving it out again at a moderate heat unchanged, renders it capable of useful pharmaceutical application; but the chief cause of its introduction into the U. S. Pharmacopœia was its being the source whence nitrogen monoxide is produced.

Nitrate of ammonium may be prepared by treating commercial ammonium carbonate by nitric acid so long as effervescence takes place, or to saturation, filtering, and evaporating the solution. By careful evaporation and slow refrigeration, the salt may be obtained in well-defined crystals. If crystallized after rapid concentration by boiling, and sudden cooling, it forms long flexible and elastic threads. If the solution be heated till all the water is driven off and the fused mass kept at a temperature not exceeding 320° F. (160° C.), the commercial fused salt is produced. It may also be made by double decomposition between solutions of ammonium sulphate and potassium nitrate.

Properties. "Colorless crystals, generally in the form of long, thin, rhombic prisms, or in fused masses, somewhat deliquescent, odorless, having a sharp, bitter taste and a neutral reaction. Soluble in 0·5 part of water and 20 parts of alcohol at 15° C. (59° F.); very soluble in boiling water and in 3 parts of boiling alcohol. When gradually heated, the salt melts at 165° C.–166° C. (329° F.–331° F.), and at about 185° C. (365° F.) it is decomposed into nitrous oxide gas and water, leaving no residue. The aqueous solution of the salt, when heated with potassa, evolves vapor of ammonia. On heating the salt with sulphuric acid, it emits nitrous vapors." *U. S.*

At all temperatures between —15° C. (5° F.) and 25° C. (77° F.), if exposed to a current of dry ammoniacal gas, its crystals absorb the gas and melt, yielding a colorless liquid, which, if the absorption has taken place at —10° C. (14° F.), contains two mols. of the gas for each mol. of the salt, and would be represented by the formula $NH_4NO_3 + 2NH_3$. It is not frozen by a mixture of salt and snow. Its sp. gr. is 1·05. Heated moderately it boils, with loss of ammonia, and is changed into a crystalline mass, containing 21·25 parts of the gas in 100 of the salt by weight, and corresponds with the formula, $NH_4NO_3 + NH_3$, thus retaining one-half the gas absorbed. By exposure to increased heat, this loses ammonia, and at 80° C. (176° F.) has been reconverted to pure nitrate of ammonium. This preparation may be used for obtaining small quantities of pure ammonia, when wanted, by exposing it to a gentle heat in a small retort. To be fit for this purpose, it must be kept at a low temperature. (*P. J. Tr.*, June, 1872.)

* Theodore G. Davis (*A. J. P.*, 1877, p. 305) gives a formula for *Liniment of Iodide of Ammonium* which he says closely corresponds with a proprietary liniment largely sold at one time; but it cannot be regarded as correctly named, for it contains but 2 grains of iodide in a *pint* of liniment. Water of Ammonia 10 per cent. f℥ij, Soap Liniment f℥ij, Tinct. Iodine f℥viij, Alcohol f℥iv. Mix the soap liniment with the tincture of iodine, and add the alcohol and ammonia; shake, and add alcohol to make 1 pint. Let it stand two or three days before using.

Tests. "The aqueous solution, when acidulated with nitric acid, should not be rendered cloudy by test-solutions of nitrate of silver (chloride), or of nitrate of barium (sulphate)." *U. S.*

For the mode of preparing nitrogen monoxide (hyponitrous oxide) or nitrous oxide gas from nitrate of ammonium, the reader is referred to the article on Nitrogen Monoxide in Part II. of this work.

AMMONII PHOSPHAS. *U. S., Br.* *Phosphate of Ammonium.*

$(NH_4)_2HPO_4$; 132. (AM-MŌ'NI-Ī PHŎS'PHĂS.) $2NH_4O, HO, PO_5$; 132.

Phosphate of Ammonia; Ammonium Phosphoricum, *P.G.;* Phosphas Ammonicus; Phosphate d'Ammoniaque, *Fr.;* Phosphorsaures Ammoniak, *G.*

This salt was introduced into the U. S. Pharmacopœia at the late revision without a process for making it. The following is the British process. "Take of Diluted Phosphoric Acid *twenty fluidounces;* Strong Solution of Ammonia, *a sufficiency.* Add the Ammonia to the Phosphoric Acid, until the solution is slightly alkaline, then evaporate the liquid, adding more Ammonia from time to time, so as to keep it in slight excess, and when crystals are formed on the cooling of the solution, dry them quickly on filtering paper placed on a porous tile, and preserve them in a stoppered bottle. $(NH_4)_2HPO_4$." *Br.*

The variety of phosphoric acid employed in this formula is the tribasic, which forms three salts with ammonia, one containing three atoms of ammonium without basic hydrogen, which is called the neutral phosphate, the second, two mols. of ammonium and one of basic hydrogen, forming an acid phosphate, and the third, one mol. of ammonium and two of basic hydrogen, forming also an acid phosphate. The second of these is the one intended by the U. S. and British Pharmacopœias, and is represented by the formula $(NH_4)_2HPO_4$. To prepare it, a constant excess of ammonia must be maintained, and this is done by compliance with the process, if the materials are of due strength. Without such a precaution, more or less of the more acid phosphate would be generated, in consequence of the escape of the alkali.

Properties. Hydrogen di-ammonium phosphate, which is the officinal salt, occurs in "colorless, translucent, monoclinic prisms, losing ammonia on exposure to dry air, without odor, having a cooling, saline taste and a neutral or faintly alkaline reaction. Soluble in 4 parts of water at 15° C. (59° F.), in 0·5 part of boiling water, but insoluble in alcohol. When strongly heated, the salt fuses, afterward evolves ammonia, and at a bright red heat is wholly dissipated." *U. S.* The salt commonly found in commerce is either this acid phosphate, or a mixture of the two acid salts. The officinal salt may be made by saturating the excess of acid in acid phosphate of calcium by means of carbonate of ammonium. Phosphate of calcium is precipitated, and phosphate of ammonium obtained in solution, which, being duly concentrated by a gentle heat, affords the salt in crystals upon cooling. The method of obtaining the acid phosphate of calcium is given under the head of phosphate of sodium. (See *Sodii Phosphas.*) Phosphate of ammonium prepared in this way is a white salt, crystallizing in six-sided tables, derived from oblique quadrangular prisms, efflorescent, insoluble in alcohol, and soluble in 4 parts of cold water. The solution has an alkaline somewhat saline taste, and an alkaline reaction, and gives out ammonia when heated.

The other acid phosphate, $NH_4H_2PO_4$, is obtained by boiling a solution of either of the other salts so long as ammonia escapes, and then crystallizing. Its crystals are four-sided prisms, permanent in the air, of an acid taste and reaction, and soluble in 5 parts of cold water. (*Bridges.*) In a specimen of the common phosphate of ammonium of commerce which came under our notice, we recognized both the tabular crystals of the phosphate with two mols. of ammonium, having a saline slightly acrid taste, and neutral in reaction, and the prisms of the acid salt, with a sour and saline taste and decided acid reaction.

Tests. "The aqueous solution of the salt, when heated with potassa, evolves vapor of ammonia. Addition of test-solution of nitrate of silver to the aqueous solution produces a canary-yellow precipitate, soluble in nitric acid and in ammonia. The aqueous solution should remain unaffected by sulphide of ammonium, or, after being acidulated with hydrochloric acid, by hydrosulphuric acid (abs. of metals), or by test-solution of chloride of barium (sulphate). When acidulated with nitric acid, it should not be rendered turbid by test-solution of nitrate of silver (chloride). 2 Gm. of the salt dissolved in water and precipitated with test-mixture of magnesium, yields a crystalline precipitate, which, when washed with diluted water of ammonia, dried, and ignited, should weigh 1·68 Gm." *U. S.* This quantitative test is intended as a means of identifying the hydrogen di-ammonium salts. The British Pharmacopœia gives the following quantitative test. "If 20 grains be dissolved in water, and solution of ammonio-sulphate of magnesium be added, a crystalline precipitate falls, which, when well washed on a filter with solution of ammonia, diluted with an equal volume of water, dried, and heated to redness, leaves 16·08 grains." *Br.* The residue is pyrophosphate of magnesium, and its amount indicates the quantity of phosphoric acid contained in the salt.

Medical Properties and Uses. This salt was first brought to the notice of the profession, as a remedy for gout and rheumatism, by Dr. T. H. Buckler, of Baltimore, in a paper published in the *Am. Journ. of the Medical Sciences* for Jan. 1846. Since the publication of Dr. Buckler's paper, several practitioners, both in this country and in Europe, have employed the remedy with apparently useful results in chronic gout, and certain urinary diseases. The dose of the salt is from ten to forty grains (0·65–2·6 Gm.), three or four times a day, dissolved in a tablespoonful of water.

AMMONII SULPHAS. *U. S.* *Sulphate of Ammonium.*

$(NH_4)_2SO_4$; 132. (ĂM-MŌ'NĬ-Ī SŬL'PHĂS.) NH_4O, SO_3; 66.

Ammonium Sulphuricum, Sal Ammonium Secretum Glauberi; Sulfate d'Ammoniaque, Sel secret de Glauber, *Fr.;* Schwefelsaures Ammon, Ammonium, Ammoniak, *G.*

The impure salt resulting from the sublimation of gas liquor or fetid bone-spirit, saturated with sulphuric acid, is submitted repeatedly to solution and crystallisation until obtained pure, or the gas liquor is distilled with lime and the gas received in sulphuric acid, which yields a purer product. Most of the ammoniacal liquor is worked up into sulphate of ammonium at present. According to Lunge (*Coal-Tar and Ammonia*, 2d ed., 1887, p. 667), the annual production of Great Britain and Ireland is 100,000 tons; of Germany, 10,000 tons; of France, 12,500 tons; of Holland and Belgium, about 3000 tons; and of the United States, 11,000 tons. "Colorless, transparent, rhombic prisms, permanent in the air, odorless, having a sharp, saline taste and a neutral reaction. Soluble in 1·3 parts of water at 15° C. (59° F.) and in 1 part of boiling water; insoluble in absolute alcohol, but slightly soluble in alcohol of sp. gr. 0·817; when heated to about 140° C. (284° F.), the salt fuses, is gradually decomposed, and on ignition is wholly dissipated. The aqueous solution of the salt, when heated with potassa, evolves vapor of ammonia. With test-solution of chloride of barium it yields a white precipitate insoluble in hydrochloric acid. A one per cent. solution of the salt should not be blackened by test-solution of sulphide of ammonium (lead and iron), nor, when acidulated with nitric acid, should it be rendered more than opalescent by test-solution of nitrate of silver (limit of chloride)." *U. S.* It is not used as a medicine, but enters into the composition of ammonia-alum and the sulphate of iron and ammonium.

AMMONII VALERIANAS. *U. S.* *Valerianate of Ammonium.*

$NH_4C_5H_9O_2$; 119. (ĂM-MŌ'NĬ-Ī VĂ-LĒ-RĬ-Ā'NĂS.) $NH_4O, C_{10}H_9O_3$; 119.

Valérianate d'Ammoniaque, *Fr.;* Baldriansaures (Valeriansaures) Ammonium, *G.*

A process for preparing this salt is no longer officinal; that of the Pharm. 1870 is found below.*

* "Take of Valerianic Acid *four fluidounces;* Chloride of Ammonium, Lime, each, *a sufficient quantity.* From a mixture of Chloride of Ammonium, in coarse powder, and an equal weight of Lime, previously slaked and in powder, contained in a suitable vessel, obtain gaseous ammonia, and cause it to pass, first through a bottle filled with pieces of Lime, and afterward into the Valerianic Acid, in a tall, narrow, glass vessel, until the Acid is neutralized. Then discontinue the process, and set the vessel aside that the Valerianate of Ammonium may crystallise. Lastly, break the salt into pieces, drain it in a glass funnel, dry it on bibulous paper, and keep it in a well-stopped bottle." *U. S.*

Valerianate of ammonium was a new officinal of the U. S. Pharmacopœia of 1860; much difficulty was experienced by manufacturing chemists in procuring a crystallized valerianate of ammonium, until, after a series of experiments, Mr. B. J. Crew, of Philadelphia, ascertained that it was necessary to employ the *monohydrated* valerianic acid, as the ordinary acid with three mols. of water could not be successfully used for the purpose. The officinal formula is based upon that of Mr. Crew, published in the *A. J. P.* (1860, p. 109). In this formula the monohydrated valerianic acid, procured by a special process (see *Acidum Valerianicum*), is saturated with gaseous ammonia obtained in the usual manner from a mixture of chloride of ammonium and lime. The saturation is known to have been effected when litmus paper is no longer acted on. During the operation heat is developed sufficient to prevent premature crystallization, and, when the saturation is completed, nothing more is necessary than to allow the solution to cool. Crystallization soon begins, and in a few hours the contents of the vessel become a nearly solid mass of crystals; these should be thoroughly drained, and, without unnecessary exposure, at once transferred to well-stoppered bottles.

Properties. Thus prepared, valerianate of ammonium is in snow-white, pearly, four-sided, tabular crystals, perfectly dry, of an offensive odor like that of valerianic acid, and a sharp sweetish taste. Instead of liquefying whenever exposed to the air, as happened to the salt formerly procured, it undergoes this change only in a moist atmosphere, and effloresces when the air is dry. It is very soluble both in water and alcohol. Exposed to heat it is in great measure volatilized unchanged; but a small portion, by giving off a part of its ammonia, is converted into the acid valerianate. Hager (*Pharm. Centralb.*, 1879, p. 465) states that commercial valerianate of ammonium is always the acid salt, as is proved by the acid reaction and the strong rotation of the crystals, when placed upon cold water; the neutral salt is only obtained with difficulty, is in prismatic crystals, and is easily liquefied by moderate temperatures. Its formula is $NH_4C_5H_9O_2$. "The aqueous solution, if heated with potassa, evolves vapor of ammonia, and, if supersaturated with sulphuric acid, separates an oily layer of valerianic acid on the surface. If this mixture be neutralized with ammonia, the clear liquid should not be rendered deep red by test-solution of ferric chloride (abs. of acetate). The aqueous solution, when acidified by nitric acid, should not be precipitated by test-solution of nitrate of barium (sulphate), nor of nitrate of silver (chloride)." *U. S.*

Medical Properties. Valerianate of ammonium is not poisonous. Given to dogs in the dose of 150 grains, it produced no inconvenience. As a therapeutic agent it was first brought to the notice of the profession, in 1856, by M. Déclat, of Paris. The preparation which he used was a solution of valerianate of ammonium of uniform strength, made according to the recipe of M. Pierlot, an apothecary of Paris, which had been extensively given to the epileptics of the Salpêtrière and the Bicêtre. Since then it has been used in various diseases, principally of the nervous system, such as hysteria, epilepsy, chorea, neuralgia, and is certainly useful in various mild functional nervous affections, but in such grave maladies as epilepsy it is powerless. The dose of the salt is from two to eight grains (0·13–0·52 Gm.), dissolved in water. As now prepared, it may be made into pills without inconvenience; and, properly coated so as to conceal their disagreeable odor, they are probably the best form for the administration of the salt. *Pierlot's solution*, mentioned above, should be made by dissolving a drachm of valerianic acid in thirty-two drachms of distilled water, saturating the solution with carbonate of ammonium, and adding to the salt formed two scruples of the alcoholic extract of valerian. According to M. Pierlot, the latter addition is necessary in order to preserve the preparation from change; for a simple solution of the ammoniacal salt is rapidly decomposed. It will keep still better if the extract, when added to the solution, be mixed with a fluidounce of diluted alcohol, while but 24 drachms of distilled water are used, so as to preserve the measure. The solution of M. Pierlot is neutral, of a brown color, and a strong odor of valerian. It contains 1-25th of its weight of the pure salt. The dose is from six to thirty drops (0·36–1·9 C.c.), given in water or on a lump of sugar. (*Ann. de Thérap.*, 1857, p. 55.)

AMYGDALA AMARA. *U. S., Br.* *Bitter Almond.*

(A-MYG'DA-LA A-MA'RA.)

"The seed of Amygdalus communis, *var.* amara. Linné. (*Nat. Ord.* Rosaceæ, Amygdaleæ.)" *U. S.*

"The seed of the bitter almond tree, Prunus Amygdalus, Stokes, *var.* amara. Baillon (Amygdalus communis, Lin., *var.* amara. D. C.)." *Br.*

Amygdalæ Amaræ, *P. G.;* Semen Amygdali Amarum; Amande amère, *Fr.;* Bittere Mandeln, *G.;* Mandorle amare, *It.;* Almendra amarga, *Sp.*

Bitter Almonds. These are smaller than the sweet almonds, and are thus described in the U. S. Pharmacopœia. "About one inch (25 m.m.) long, oblong lanceolate, flattish, covered with a cinnamon-brown scurfy testa, marked by about sixteen lines emanating from a broad scar at the blunt end. The embryo has the shape of the seed, is white, oily, consists of two plano-convex cotyledons, and a short radicle at the pointed end, has a bitter taste, and, when triturated with water, yields a milk-white emulsion, which emits an odor of hydrocyanic acid." They have the bitter taste of the peach kernel, and, though when dry inodorous or nearly so, have, when triturated with water, the fragrance of the peach blossom. They contain the same ingredients as sweet almonds, and like them form a milky emulsion with water. It was formerly supposed that they also contained hydrocyanic acid and volatile oil, to which their peculiar taste and smell, and their peculiar operation upon the system, were ascribed. It was, however, ascertained by MM. Robiquet and Boutron that these principles do not pre-exist in the almond, but result from the reaction of water; and Wöhler and Liebig proved, what was suspected by Robiquet, that they are formed out of a peculiar substance denominated *amygdalin,* which is the characteristic constituent of bitter almonds. This substance, which was discovered by Robiquet and Boutron in 1830, is white, crystallizable, inodorous, of a sweetish bitter taste, unalterable in the air, freely soluble in water and hot alcohol, very slightly soluble in cold alcohol, and insoluble in ether. It is decomposed by the action of dilute acids or in the presence of water by the nitrogenous ferments, like emulsin, which accompany it in the bitter almond. The reaction is as follows:

$$\underset{\text{Crystallized amygdalin.}}{C_{20}H_{27}NO_{11}} + 3H_2O = 2(\underset{\text{Dextro-glucose.}}{C_6H_{12}O_6}) + \underset{\text{Hydrocyanic acid.}}{HCN} + \underset{\text{Oil of bitter almonds.}}{C_7H_6O} + H_2O.$$

It is recognized as belonging to the *glucoside* class, compounds which, when decomposed by dilute acids, alkalies, or ferments, yield glucose and some other characteristic decomposition product. They may be considered as compound ethers of glucose analogous to the compound ethers of glycerin which exist in the fats under the name of *glycerides.* Liebig and Wöhler give the following process for obtaining amygdalin, in which the object of the fermentation is to destroy the sugar with which it is associated. Bitter almonds, previously deprived of their fixed oil by pressure, are to be boiled in successive portions of alcohol till exhausted. From the liquors thus obtained all the alcohol is to be drawn off by distillation; care being taken, near the end of the process, not to expose the syrupy residue to too great a heat. This residue is then to be diluted with water, mixed with good yeast, and placed in a warm situation. After the fermentation which ensues has ceased, the liquor is to be filtered, evaporated to the consistence of syrup, and mixed with alcohol. The amygdalin is thus precipitated in connection with a portion of gum, from which it may be separated by solution in boiling alcohol, which will deposit it upon cooling. If pure, it will form a perfectly transparent solution with water. Any oil which it may contain may be separated by washing with ether. One pound of almonds yields at least 120 grains of amygdalin. (*Annal. der Pharm.,* xxii. 329.)*

Amygdalin, mixed with emulsion of *sweet* almonds, gives rise, among other products, to the volatile oil of bitter almonds and hydrocyanic acid—the emulsin of the

* Amygdalin appears to be extensively diffused in plants, having been noticed not only in the different genera of the Amygdaleæ, as *Amygdalus, Cerasus,* and *Prunus,* but also by Wicke in various Pomaceæ, as *Pyrus Malus, Sorbus Aucuparia, Sorbus hybrida, Sorbus torminalis, Amelanchier vulgaris, Cotoneaster vulgaris,* and *Cratægus Oxyacantha.* (*Ann. der Chem. und Pharm.,* lxxix. 79.) It may be advantageously procured from peach kernels, which have been found to yield 80 grains for each avoirdupois pound, or more than 1 per cent. (*A. J. P.,* xxvii. 227.)

sweet almonds acting the part of a ferment, by causing a reaction between the amygdalin and water; and the same result is obtained when pure *emulsin* is added to a solution of amygdalin. It appears then that the volatile oil and hydrocyanic acid, developed in bitter almonds when moistened, result from the mutual reaction of amygdalin, water, and emulsin. Certain substances have the effect of preventing this reaction, as, for example, alcohol and acetic acid. It is asserted that emulsin procured from other seeds, as those of the poppy, hemp, and mustard, is capable of producing the same reaction between water and amygdalin, though in a less degree. (*Annal. der Pharm.*, xxviii. 290.) Amygdalin appears not to be poisonous when taken pure into the stomach, unless there be emulsin in food in stomach.

Bitter almonds yield their fixed oil by pressure, and at the present time this oil is an article of commerce, and is frequently sold as oil of sweet almonds, being produced in England from North African bitter almonds; the volatile oil, impregnated with hydrocyanic acid, may be obtained from the residue by distillation with water. (See *Oleum Amygdalæ Amaræ.*)

Confectioners employ bitter almonds for communicating flavor to the syrup of orgeat. (See *Syrupus Amygdalæ.*) The kernel of the peach possesses similar properties, and is frequently used as a substitute. It has been ascertained that bitter almond paste, and other substances which yield the same volatile oil, such as bruised cherry-laurel leaves, peach leaves, etc., have the property of destroying the odor of musk, camphor, most of the volatile oils, creasote, cod-liver oil, the balsams, etc.; and M. Mahier, a French pharmacist, has employed them successfully to free mortars and bottles from the odor of asafetida, and other substances of disagreeable smell. All that is necessary is first to remove any oily substance by means of an alkali, and then to apply the paste or bruised leaves.

Medical Properties and Uses. (See *Amygdala Dulcis.*)

Off. Prep. Syrupus Amygdalæ.

Off. Prep. Br. Oleum Amygdalæ.

AMYGDALA DULCIS. *U.S., Br.* *Sweet Almond.*

(Ą-MY̆G'DĄ-LĄ DŬL'CĮS.)

"The seed of Amygdalus communis, *var.* dulcis. Linné. (*Nat. Ord.* Rosaceæ, Amygdaleæ.)" *U.S.* "The ripe seed of the sweet almond tree, Prunus Amygdalus, Stokes, *var.* dulcis. Imported from Malaga and known as the Jordan Almond." *Br.*

Amygdalæ Dulces, *P. G.*; Semen Amygdali Dulce; Amande douce, *Fr.*; Süsse Mandeln, *G.*; Mandorle dolci, *It.*; Almendra dulce, *Sp.*

Gen. Ch. *Calyx* five-cleft, inferior. *Petals* five. *Drupe* with a nut perforated with pores. *Willd.*

Amygdalus communis. Willd. *Sp. Plant.* ii. 982; Woodv. *Med. Bot.* p. 507, t. 183. The almond tree rises usually from fifteen to twenty feet in height, and divides into numerous spreading branches. The leaves stand upon short footstalks, are about three inches long and three-quarters of an inch broad, elliptical, pointed at both ends, veined, minutely serrated, with the lower serratures and petioles glandular, and are of a bright green color. The flowers are large, of a pale red color varying to white, with very short peduncles, and petals longer than the calyx, and usually stand in pairs upon the branches. The fruit is of the peach kind, with the outer covering thin, tough, dry, and marked with a longitudinal furrow, where it opens when fully ripe. Within this covering is a rough shell, containing the kernel or almond.

There are several varieties of this species of Amygdalus, differing chiefly in the size and shape of the fruit, the thickness of the shell, and the taste of the kernel. The two most important are *Amygdalus (communis) dulcis* and *Amygdalus (communis) amara*, the former bearing sweet, the latter bitter almonds. Another variety is the *fragilis* of De Candolle, which yields the *paper-shelled almonds.*

The almond-tree is a native of Persia, Syria, and Barbary, and is very extensively cultivated in various parts of the south of Europe. It has been introduced into the United States; but in the northern and middle sections the fruit does not usually come to perfection. We are supplied with sweet almonds chiefly from Spain and the south of France. They are separated into the soft-shelled and hard-shelled, the former of which come from Marseilles and Bordeaux, the latter from Malaga. From the latter port they are sometimes brought to us without the shell. In British commerce, the two chief varieties are the *Jordan* and *Valencia* almonds, the former imported from Malaga, the latter from Valencia.* The former are longer, narrower, more pointed, and more highly esteemed than the latter. The bitter almonds are obtained chiefly from Morocco, and are exported from Mogador.

Properties. The shape and appearance of almonds are too well known to require description. Each kernel consists of two white cotyledons, enclosed in a thin yellowish brown, bitter skin, which is easily separable after immersion in boiling water. Deprived of this covering, they are called *blanched almonds.* On exposure to the air, they are apt to become rancid; but, if thoroughly dried, and kept in well-closed glass vessels, they may be preserved unaltered for many years. The two varieties each require a separate notice.

Sweet almonds are without smell when blanched, and have a sweet, very pleasant taste, which has rendered them a favorite article of diet in all countries where they are readily attainable. They are, however, generally considered difficult of digestion. The Pharmacopœia thus describes them. "Closely resembling the bitter almond (see *Amygdala Amara*), but having a bland, sweetish taste. When triturated with water, it yields a milk-white emulsion, free from the odor of hydrocyanic acid." *U.S.* By the analysis of M. Boullay, it appears that they contain, in 100 parts, 5 parts of pellicle, 54 of fixed oil, 24 of albumen, 6 of uncrystallizable sugar, 3 of gum, 4 of fibrous matter, 3·5 of water, and 0·5 of acetic acid comprising loss. The albumen is somewhat peculiar, and is called *emulsin.* It may be obtained separate by treating the emulsion of almonds with ether, allowing the mixture, after frequent agitation, to stand until a clear fluid separates at the bottom of the vessel, drawing this off by a siphon, adding alcohol to it so as to precipitate the emulsin, then washing the precipitate with fresh alcohol, and drying it under the receiver of an air-pump. In this state it is a white powder, inodorous and tasteless, soluble in water, and insoluble in ether and alcohol. Its solution has an acid reaction, and, if heated to 100° C. (212° F.), becomes opaque and milky, and gradually deposits a snow-white precipitate, amounting to about 10 per cent. of the emulsin employed. (*A. J. P.*, xxi. 354.) Its distinguishing characteristic is that of producing certain changes, noticed previously, in amygdalin, which property it loses when its solution is boiled, though not by exposure in the solid state to a heat of 100° C. (212° F.). (*Ibid.*, 357.) It consists of nitrogen, carbon, hydrogen, and oxygen, with a minute proportion of sulphur, and is probably identical with the *synaptase* of Robiquet. Mr. L. Portes announced the discovery of *asparagin* in sweet almonds. (*N. R.*, January, 1877.) The fixed oil is described under the head of *Oleum Amygdalæ*, to which the reader is referred. Sweet almonds, when rubbed with water, form a milky emulsion, free from the odor of hydrocyanic acid, the insoluble matters being suspended by the agency of the albuminous, mucilaginous, and saccharine principles.

Medical Properties and Uses. *Sweet almonds* have no other influence on the system than that of a nutrient and demulcent. The emulsion formed by triturating them with water is a pleasant vehicle for the administration of other medicines, and is itself useful in catarrhal affections. From their nutritive properties, and the absence of starch in their composition, they are much used in the diet of diabetic patients, as originally recommended by Dr. Pavy. (*Guy's Hosp. Rep.*, 1862, p. 213.) *Bitter almonds* are more active, and might be employed with advantage in pectoral

* In 1861, Dr. Geo. B. Wood was informed, when at Valencia, that the thin, paper-shelled almonds were produced, not in the immediate neighborhood, but chiefly in the Balearic Islands, and the province of Alicante, whence they are sent to Valencia; and, in a journey through the interior from Valencia to Alicante, he noticed that the almond-tree was very abundant in the region back of the latter city, while there were comparatively few near the former.

and other complaints to which hydrocyanic acid is applicable. In some persons almonds produce urticaria, in the smallest quantities. Largely taken, they have sometimes proved deleterious. Landerer mentions the case of a lady, who was alarmingly affected by a bath, made from the residue of bitter almonds after expression of the fixed oil. (See *A. J. P.*, xxviii. 321.)

Wöhler and Liebig propose, as a substitute for cherry-laurel water, which owes its effects to the hydrocyanic acid it contains, but is objectionable from its unequal strength, an extemporaneous mixture, consisting of seventeen grains of amygdalin, and one fluidounce of an emulsion made with two drachms of *sweet* almonds, and a sufficient quantity of water. This mixture contains, according to the above named chemists, one grain of anhydrous hydrocyanic acid, and is equivalent to two fluidounces of fresh cherry-laurel water. If found to answer in practice, it will have the advantage of certainty in relation to the dose; as amygdalin may be kept any length of time unaltered. If the calculation of Wöhler and Liebig is correct as to the quantity of acid it contains, not more than a fluidrachm (3·75 C.c.) should be given as a commencing dose.

Off. Prep. Mistura Amygdalæ; Syrupus Amygdalæ.

Off. Prep. Br. Oleum Amygdalæ; Pulvis Amygdalæ Compositus.

AMYL NITRIS. *U. S., Br.* *Nitrite of Amyl.*

$C_5H_{11}NO_2$; 117. (Ā'MȲL NĪ'TRĬS.) $C_{10}H_{11}O,NO_3$; 117.

"A liquid produced by the action of nitric or nitrous acid on amylic alcohol which volatilizes between 262° and 270° F. (or about 128° to 132° C.). It consists chiefly of nitrite of amyl, $C_5H_{11}NO_2$. It should be stored in hermetically-sealed vessels or in well-stoppered bottles, and in a cool dark place." *Br.*

Amylium Nitrosum, Amylæther Nitrosus; Azotite d'Amyl, *Fr.*; Amyl Nitrit, *G.*; Amylo-nitrous Ether.

This substance, which was discovered by M. Balard in 1844, should not be confounded with *nitrate of amyl*, $C_5H_{11}NO_3$, which is not used as a medicine.

Preparation. Nitrite of amyl may be prepared by passing a stream of nitrous acid (hyponitric acid) gas through purified amylic alcohol at a temperature of 132° C. (269·6° F.), or by acting upon amylic alcohol with nitric acid, as originally suggested by Balard. The alcohol should always first be purified according to the method of Hirsch (*A. J. P.*, 1862, pp. 139, 328), by agitating with an equal bulk of strong solution of common salt, then distilling in a retort with a thermometer, collecting what comes over between 125° C. (257° F.) and 140° C. (284° F.), and redistilling this until it has a boiling point near 132° C. (269·6° F.). The purified alcohol should be mixed with about an equal bulk of nitric acid in a capacious glass retort, being gradually heated until it approaches boiling, when the fire is to be removed. As soon as a thermometer inserted into the tubulures rises above 100° C. (212° F.) the receiver is changed, because both ethyl-amylic ether and nitrate of amyl at such temperatures come over freely and would contaminate the product. The distillate obtained below 100° C. (212° F.) is agitated with a solution of carbonate of potassium, and the oily liquid which separates is very slowly heated in a clean retort to 96° C. (204·8° F.), then the receiver is changed and the distillate collected as before, until the thermometer reaches 100° C. (212° F.). That which comes over between the two temperatures is pure nitrite of amyl. It is essential to this process that in every case the heating be very gradual. (*A. J. P.*, 1871, p. 148.) Allen states (*Commerc. Org. Anal.*, 2d ed., i. p. 159) that the use of nitric acid is certain to result in the formation of much valeric aldehyde and more or less amyl nitrate, and the boiling point of the former of these bodies precludes the possibility of subsequently separating it by fractioning the crude product. He therefore prefers the passing of nitrous acid gas into purified amyl alcohol. Prof. Maisch attempted to produce nitrite of amyl by Redwood's process (*A. J. P.*, 1867, p. 330) for the production of nitrous ether, substituting amylic for ethylic alcohol. He found that the reactions occurred with such excessive violence as to render the preparation of the nitrite in this way impracticable. Subsequently, however, Mr. Alfred Tanner pointed out (*P. J. Tr.*, Nov. 1871, also *A. J. P.*, 1872, p. 21) that

Prof. Maisch used a nearly anhydrous amylic alcohol, and that the reactions are equally violent with ethylic alcohol of similar strength. He finds no difficulty when the fusel oil is diluted with water, and prefers the process, especially for the production of the drug upon a small scale. Having introduced the purified amylic alcohol into a tubulated retort containing copper wire, he adds one-tenth of its bulk of strong sulphuric acid, and then the same quantity of nitric acid, previously diluted with an equal bulk of water, and heats gently to 63° C. (145·4° F.). At this temperature the reaction commences, and goes on very manageably, until a bulk about equal to double the quantity of nitric acid collects in the receiver. The chemical movement now ceases, and the temperature, which has risen to near 100° C. (212° F.), begins to fall. More dilute nitric acid is added, and the process carried out as before. These additions are repeated until the amylic alcohol is exhausted, which is known by the appearance of red fumes in the retort. The whole product is washed with caustic soda, to remove hydrocyanic and other acids, and rectified over carbonate of potassium, to get rid of moisture. The portion which distils over between 95° C. (203° F.) and 100° C. (212° F.) is medicinally pure nitrite of amyl. John Williams (*Year-Book of Pharmacy*, 1885) recommends the method of passing nitrous acid, obtained by acting upon lump arsenious acid with nitric acid, sp. gr. 1·350, into purified amylic alcohol until the latter has assumed a brownish-green color, the product is then washed and distilled fractionally; the distillate under 100° C. and 105° C. amounted to nearly 95 per cent. Mr. D. B. Dott (*P. J. Tr.*, Aug. 31, 1878) called attention to the difficulties in the way of fixing a standard boiling point for nitrite of amyl, and Dr. W. H. Greene (*A. J. P.*, 1879, p. 65) shows that nitropentane (an isomer of nitrite of amyl) is almost invariably a constituent of nitrite of amyl, and he believes that commercial nitrite of amyl is frequently put upon the market unrectified, specimens examined having boiling points varying from 70° C. (158° F.) to 180° C. (356° F.).

Properties. "A clear, pale yellowish liquid, of an ethereal, fruity odor, an aromatic taste, and a neutral or slightly acid reaction. When freely exposed to the air it decomposes, leaving a large residue of amyl alcohol. It is insoluble in water, but soluble, in all proportions, in alcohol, ether, chloroform, benzol, and benzin. Its sp. gr. is 0·872 to 0·874, and it boils at about 96° C. (205° F.), giving an orange-colored vapor. It burns with a fawn-colored flame. Warmed with excess of solution of potassa it gives the odor of amyl alcohol. If this alkaline mixture be treated with a little test-solution of iodide of potassium, and then with acetic acid to an acid reaction, there is an immediate separation of iodine, and on the addition of gelatinized starch a deep blue color appears (distinction from nitrate). It should remain transparent, or nearly so, when exposed to the temperature of melting ice (abs. of water). On shaking 10 C.c. of Nitrite of Amyl with 2 C.c. of a mixture of 1 part of water of ammonia and 9 parts of water, the liquid should not redden blue litmus paper (limit of free acid). Nitrite of Amyl should be preserved in small glass-stoppered vials, in a cool and dark place." *U. S.*

Medical Properties and Uses. Owing to its excessive volatility and the ease with which it is absorbed, nitrite of amyl acts with great quickness upon the organism. As early as 1859, Guthrie investigated, to some extent, its physiological action; but the attention of the profession was really first directed to the drug by the researches of Dr. Richardson, of London, in 1865. Since this time elaborate studies of its physiological action have been made by various investigators. Want of space forbids more than a summarizing of them in this book; for a full account the reader is referred to Dr. H. C. Wood's Treatise on Therapeutics. When inhaled in doses of from 5 to 10 drops, nitrite of amyl produces in man violent flushing of the face, accompanied with a feeling as though the head would burst, and a very excessive action of the heart. Along with these symptoms, after a larger quantity, there is a sense of suffocation, and more or less marked muscular weakness. As no case of serious poisoning from nitrite of amyl has occurred in man, for a further knowledge of its action we are dependent upon the study made on the lower animals. In dogs, rabbits, cats, etc., it induces effects similar to those occurring in man, followed, after toxic doses, by violently hurried, panting respiration, progressive loss of muscular power and of reflex activity, and finally death from failure of respiration; sensation and consciousness being preserved to the last. Although the frequency of the pulse may be increased, the force of the circulation is always diminished. This decrease of the arterial pressure is in a great measure due to a dilatation of the capillaries. The vaso-motor palsy appears to be chiefly produced by a direct action upon the coats of the capillaries, but may in part be caused by an influence exerted upon the vaso-motor centres. The cause of the acceleration of the pulse has not been made out, but there is some evidence for the belief that the rise is due to a depressing action upon the inhibitory cardiac nerves, and it is also possible that small quantities of the drug are primarily stimulant to the cardiac muscle.

The diminution of voluntary movements and of reflex action is chiefly owing to a powerful depressing influence exerted upon the spinal centres, although the drug does act to some extent upon both motor nerve and muscle, lowering their functional activity. Upon the perceptive and conscious portions of the nervous system nitrite of amyl has almost no influence, so that, as already stated, both consciousness and sensation are preserved in poisoning by it almost to the close.

After toxic doses the animal temperature falls to a most remarkable degree. Very small doses produce in man a slight (½° F.) temporary increase of the bodily heat, probably caused by the vascular dilatation. The vapors of nitrite of amyl outside of the body have a very extraordinary power of checking oxidation, and the results of numerous experiments seem to show that in the body the drug lessens very decidedly the chemical interchanges. With the exception of the decrease of temperature, the general symptoms produced by the poison do not seem to be due to this lowered oxidation, but to a direct influence exerted upon the various tissues.

Locally applied, nitrite of amyl causes a progressive loss of power in every highly organized tissue; this may end in a total cessation of function, but, even after this, recovery is possible, provided the poison be withdrawn sufficiently early.

The chief indication for the employment of nitrite of amyl is to relax spasm, either of the vaso-motor muscular fibres or of the voluntary or involuntary muscles. A disease, probably associated with vaso-motor spasm, but whose pathology is not established, in which experience has demonstrated the extreme value of nitrite of amyl, is angina pectoris. Immediate and great relief is nearly always afforded, whether the heart-pain is or is not connected with organic cardiac disease. So far as experience goes, the cautious use of the remedy is safe, even when there is severe organic cardiac disease. In these cases it should always be administered by inhalation. Experience has also justified the use of the drug in many spasmodic diseases. In asthma the relief is often immediate; in convulsions occurring after labor the nitrite affords quiet, but its employment is dangerous, on account of its tendency to produce uterine relaxation and consequent flooding. In spasmodic dysmenorrhœa good may be expected from its use; in tetanus it will frequently temporarily arrest the spasm and aid other remedies in obtaining recovery; in strychnine poisoning, in hysterical convulsions, indeed, in almost any convulsive disorder, much is to be expected from its employment. The convulsive stage of the ordinary epileptic paroxysm is so short that the nitrite is usually not available; when, however, there is a marked epileptic stasis and the patient passes from one convulsion to another, the drug may be used with benefit. In those cases in which there is an aura of sufficient length, the epileptic attacks may be arrested by the patient carrying in the pocket a tightly-corked homœopathic vial containing five or ten drops of the remedy, and, as soon as the aura commences, inhaling deeply from the opened mouth of the bottle.

Nitrite of amyl is generally administered by inhalation, usually in doses of from three to five drops, although much larger quantities have been given without bad results. The rule is to commence with three drops on a handkerchief held close to the nose, and then gradually to increase *pro re nata*. The handkerchief should always be withdrawn so soon as the face flushes or the heart begins to become excited, as the effects always increase for some time, even if no more be inhaled. The best method, however, of administering the very volatile liquid is by the use of the glass pearls,—small flask-shaped vessels containing 2, 5, or 10 minims of the nitrite;

these are crushed in a handkerchief or towel when wanted for inhalation, the very thin and friable glass causing no inconvenience. The drug may also be given by the mouth, in doses of three to five drops (0·18–0·3 C.c.) on sugar or dissolved in alcohol.

AMYLUM. *U.S., Br.* *Starch.*

(ĂM'Y̆-LŬM.)

"The fecula of the seed of Triticum vulgare. Villars. (*Nat. Ord.* Graminaceæ.)" *U.S.* "The starch procured from the grains of common wheat, Triticum sativum, *Lam.*; Triticum vulgare, *Villars*; maize, Zea mays, *Linn.*, and rice, Oryza sativa, *Linn.*" *Br.*

Amylum Tritici; Wheat Starch, *E.*; Fécule (Amidon) de Froment, de Blé, Amidon, *Fr.*; Stärkmehl, Stärke, Kraftmehl, Weizenstärke, *G.*; Amido, *It.*; Almidon, *Sp.*

Starch is a proximate vegetable principle contained in most plants, and especially abundant in the various grains, such as wheat, rye, barley, oats, rice, maize, etc.; in other seeds, as peas, beans, chestnuts, acorns, etc.; and in numerous rhizomes and tuberous roots, as those of the potato (*Solanum tuberosum*), the sweet potato (*Convolvulus Batatus*), the arrow-root, etc. The starch is always in the form of grains, which are contained within the parenchymatous cells, and is procured by reducing the substances in which it exists to a state of minute division, agitating or washing them with cold water, straining or pouring off the liquid, and allowing it to stand till the fine fecula which it holds in suspension has subsided. This, when dried, is starch, more or less pure, according to the care taken in conducting the process. The starch of commerce is procured chiefly from potatoes and the cheaper grains.

Starch is white, pulverulent, opaque, and, as found in the shops, is usually in columnar masses, and produces a peculiar sound when pressed between the fingers. Its specific gravity is 1·505 at 67° F. (*Payen.*) "Under the microscope appearing as granules, mostly very minute, more or less lenticular in form, and indistinctly, concentrically striated." *U.S.* When exposed to a moist air, it absorbs a considerable quantity of water, which may be driven off by a gentle heat. It is insoluble in alcohol, ether, and cold water; but unites with boiling water, which, on cooling, forms with it a soft semi-transparent paste, or a gelatinous opaline solution, according to the proportion of starch employed. The paste placed on folds of blotting-paper, renewed as they become wet, abandons its water, contracts, and assumes the appearance of horn. If the proportion of starch be very small, the solution, after slowly depositing a very minute quantity of insoluble matter, continues permanent, and upon being evaporated yields a semi-transparent mass, which is partially soluble in cold water. The starch has, therefore, been modified by the combined agency of water and heat; nor can it be restored to its original condition. Heating with glacial acetic acid to 100° C., or glycerin to 190° C., will also make starch soluble. "Triturated with cold water it gives neither an acid nor an alkaline reaction with test-paper. When boiled with water, it yields a white jelly having a bluish tinge, which, when cool, acquires a deep blue color on the addition of test-solution of iodine." *U.S.* At a temperature of 160° C. (320° F.) for air-dried starch, and 200° C. (392° F.) for starch previously dried at 100° C., it is changed into *dextrin* (British gum), and at 200° C. (392° F.) to 215° C. (419° F.) forms a transparent fused mass, which consists exclusively of dextrin (*Payen*); at 220° C. (428° F.) to 230° C. (446° F.) it undergoes further change and yields chiefly *pyrodextrin*, a brown, tasteless, and odorless compound, readily soluble in water, insoluble in alcohol and ether. (Gelis, *Ann. Chim. Phys.*, (3) lii. 388.)

Composition and Nature. The formula of starch is generally taken as $C_6H_{10}O_5$, or a multiple of this. Musculus, in 1861, showed that by the action of dilute acids or *diastase*, starch is resolved into *dextrin*, $C_{12}H_{20}O_{10}$, and *dextrose*, $C_6H_{12}O_6$, so that its formula is most probably $C_{18}H_{30}O_{15}$ or $(C_6H_{10}O_5)_3$, although Pfeiffer and Tollens make it $(C_6H_{10}O_5)_4$, and Brown and Heron say the molecule contains C_{72}. Iodine forms with starch, whether in its original state or in solution, a blue compound; and the tincture of iodine is the most delicate test of its presence. The color varies somewhat according to the proportions employed. When the two substances are about equal, the compound is of a beautiful indigo blue; if the iodine is in excess, it is blackish blue; if the starch, violet blue. A singular property of the iodide of starch is that its solution becomes colorless if heated to about 93·5° C. (200° F.), and afterwards recovers its blue color upon cooling. By boiling, the color is permanently lost, whilst Puchot states that certain nitrogenised organic bodies, as albumen, prevent the reaction of iodine on starch or destroy it. (*N. R.*, Nov. 1876.) Alkalies unite with starch, forming soluble compounds, which are decomposed by acids, the starch being precipitated. It is thrown down from its solution by lime-water and baryta-water, forming insoluble compounds with these earths. The solution of subacetate of lead precipitates it in combination with the oxide of the metal. Starch may be made to unite with tannin by boiling their solutions together; and a compound results, which, though retained by the water while hot, is deposited when it cools. By long boiling with diluted sulphuric, hydrochloric, or oxalic acid, it is converted into *dextrin** and glucose or grape sugar. A similar conversion into dextrin and glucose is effected by means of a principle called *diastase*, discovered by MM. Payen and Persoz in the seeds of barley, oats, and wheat, after germination. (See *Hordeum*.) Strong hydrochloric and nitric acids dissolve it; and the latter, by the aid of heat, converts it into oxalic and malic acids. By the action of strong nitric, sulphuric, or crystallizable acetic acid, used with certain precautions, the starch is rendered soluble, and may be obtained in this state by separating the acid by means of alcohol. (*Chem. Gaz.*, Dec. 1, 1854, p. 450.) By the continued action of concentrated sulphuric acid it is decomposed. When it is dissolved in strong nitric acid, and precipitated by water, a white powder is thrown down, called *xyloidin*, $C_6H_9(NO_2)O_5$ (*Braconnot*), in which one atom of the hydrogen of the starch is replaced by one group, NO_2, furnished by the nitric acid. Mixed with hot water and exposed to a temperature of 27° C. (80° F.), it undergoes chemical changes, which result in the formation of several distinct principles, among which are sugar, a gummy substance (perhaps *dextrin*), and a soluble modification of starch. With yeast, starch undergoes the vinous fermentation, being, however, first converted into sugar. Mixed with cheese and chalk it is said to yield alcohol without the previous saccharine conversion. (Berthelot, *Journ. de Pharm.*, 3e sér., xxxii. 260.) All plants which contain chlorophyll have the power of using the chemical rays of sunlight in producing from inorganic compounds and elements a substance which is organic. There is first formed in the centre of the chlorophyll granule a minute speck, which is believed to be starch; this new starch granule is incapable of solution, but by conversion into sugar or dextrin is rendered soluble, and in this form is carried in the juices of the plant. One of two destinies there awaits it. It may be converted into the permanent compound cellulose which constitutes the woody tissue, or it may be reconverted to its original form and be deposited in some part of the plant. These stores of starch are usually accumulated for future growth, and are especially seen in plants which flower in the

* *Dextrin* is a substance resembling gum in appearance and properties, but differing from it in not affording mucic acid by the action of nitric acid. It is largely dissolved by water, hot or cold, and forms a mucilaginous solution, from which it is precipitated by alcohol. Large quantities of dextrin are now made both here and abroad, and employed for various purposes in the arts, under the name of *artificial gum*. It is found in the market in the form of mucilage, in that of a white brilliant powder, and in small masses or fragments resembling natural gum. According to M. Emil Thomas, it may be distinguished from gum arabic by the taste and smell of potato oil which it always possesses. It is made by the action either of acids or of diastase on starch. For particulars as to the manufacture, the reader is referred to a paper by M. Thomas, republished in *A. J. P.* (vol. xix. p. 284). Recent researches of Nägili and Musculus seem to show that the change of starch into dextrin takes place in several phases, and they name the several products *amylodextrin, erythrodextrin, achrodextrin α and β*. For a fuller account of these products see Husemann, *Pflanzenstoffe*, 2d ed., 1882.

Dextrin, according to Payen, is converted into glucose, through the action of diastase; but the glucose impedes the action unless removed; as, however, during the alcoholic fermentation the glucose is consumed, no obstacle prevents the influence of diastase. Hence dextrin by conversion into sugar may contribute to the alcoholic product. (*Journ. de Pharm.*, 4e sér., i. 863.)

Adulteration and purification of dextrin.—Commercial dextrin is said to be occasionally very impure. Several parcels, analyzed by Dr. H. Hayes, were found to contain an average of about 45 per cent. of impurities, consisting mainly of insoluble matter with sugar and water. He recommends, as the best method of purifying it, to dissolve 10 parts of the impure dextrin, with agitation, in 18 parts of distilled water, in a cylindrical vessel; to decant the solution when it has become clear on standing, and mix it with 1·5 or 2 per cent. of alcohol of 95. The liquid is then decanted from the doughy precipitate formed, which is dissolved in a little distilled water; and the solution spread on glass or porcelain plates to dry, in a warm place. (*A. J. P.*, 1870, p. 327.)

spring before the leaves are put forth, or which reproduce the species without seeding. When the potato is planted by the farmer, the starch is converted into a soluble form, passes into the growing "eye" or bud, and, as cellulose, forms the new shoot. Different opinions have been held as to the precise structure of the starch granules. The one first adopted is that they consist of a thin exterior coating, and of an interior substance; the former wholly insoluble, the latter soluble in water. The former constitutes, according to M. Payen, only 4 or 5 thousandths of the weight of starch. In relation to the interior portion, there is not an exact coincidence of opinion. M. Guérin supposed that it consisted of two distinct substances, one soluble in cold water, the other soluble at first in boiling water, but becoming insoluble by evaporation. Thus, when one part of starch is boiled for fifteen minutes in one hundred parts of water, and the liquid is allowed to stand, a small portion, consisting of the broken teguments, is gradually deposited. If the solution be now filtered and evaporated, another portion is deposited which cannot afterwards be dissolved. When wholly deprived of this portion, and evaporated to dryness, the solution yields the part soluble in cold water. According to MM. Payen and Persoz, the interior portion of the globules consists only of a single substance, which is converted into the two just mentioned by the agency of water; and Thenard is inclined to the same opinion. An appropriate name for the interior soluble portion of starch is *amidin*, which has been adopted by some chemists. Starch, in its perfect state, is not affected by cold water, because the exterior insoluble teguments prevent the access of the liquid to the interior portion; but, when the pellicle is broken by heat, or by mechanical means, the fluid is admitted, and the starch partially dissolved.

Another view of the structure of the starch granule, founded on microscopic observation, was advanced by Schleiden. According to this observer, it consists of concentric layers, all of which have the same chemical composition; but the outer layers, having been first formed, have more cohesion than the inner, and are consequently more difficult of solubility. The rings observed upon the surface of the granules, in some varieties, are merely the edges of these layers; and the point or hylum about which the rings are concentrically placed, is a minute hole, through which probably the substance of the interior layers was introduced. (*Pharm. Centralb.*, 1844, p. 401.)

Mr. J. J. Field thinks he has demonstrated that the granule consists, as at first supposed, of an interior matter surrounded by a distinct membranous envelope. Having saturated some canna starch with glycerin, and then added a little water, an endosmose of the thinner outer liquid took place into the granules, distending them so as to rupture their investing membrane, which was distinctly visible, under the microscope, in longitudinal wrinkles. The concentric rings he thinks nothing more than folds of the membrane, produced probably by the contraction of the granules. (*P. J. Tr.*, xiv. 253.)

The tegumentary portion of starch, for which the name of *amylin* has been proposed, is, when entirely freed from the interior soluble matter, wholly insoluble in water even by prolonged boiling, insoluble in alcohol, and said to suffer no change by the action of diastase. The acids, however, act upon it as they do upon starch. It is thought to approach nearer in properties to lignin than to any other principle. Musculus (*Comptes-Rendus; Journal Franklin Institute*, June, 1879) believes that starch may exist in an amorphous and crystallizable form. In its amorphous state it is soluble in water, capable of being acted on by diastase, soluble in diluted mineral acids, but easily rendered insoluble by undergoing modifications. In its crystalline condition it can be obtained in isolated crystals, which can be readily dissolved in cold water, but when these crystals are united they become less soluble, and then it largely has the properties of the amorphous variety. Sulkowsky (*Ber. d. Chem. Ges.*, xiii. 1395) states that starch may be rendered soluble by heating with glycerin to 190° C. (374° F.), and pouring whilst hot into water, filtering, and adding alcohol to the filtrate, which causes precipitation of the soluble starch.

The view that is held in most esteem at present (1888) is that the granules of starch consist of two substances, *granulose* and *amylo-cellulose*. The latter occurs in largest proportion in the outer layers of the granule, and probably so envelops and protects the granule as to prevent the action of cold water upon it, the granulose or inner portion being slightly soluble. When the granules are ruptured by being triturated with sand, water acts upon them, and the liquid will yield a blue color with iodine. The insoluble amylo-cellulose may be obtained pure by treating starch paste with extract of malt; it gives then a brownish-yellow color (not a blue) with iodine. Granulose is acted on by ptyalin (the ferment from saliva), pepsin, organic acids, diluted hydrochloric or sulphuric acid, whilst amylo-cellulose is unaffected. The solid starch granules become blue when touched by tincture of iodine, because the liquid penetrates through the fissures of the amylo-cellulose to the granulose.

Varieties. Starch, as obtained from different substances, is somewhat different in its characters. *Wheat starch*, when examined with a microscope, is found to consist of granules varying from about $\frac{1}{1000}$ of an inch in diameter to a mere point, the smaller being spheroidal, the larger rounded and flattened, with the hylum in the centre of the flattened surface, and surrounded by concentric rings, which often extend to the edge. The granules are mixed with loose integuments, resulting from the process of grinding. This variety of starch has a certain degree of hardness and adhesiveness, owing, according to Guibourt, to the escape of a portion of the interior substance of the broken granules, which attracts some moisture from the air, and, thus becoming glutinous, acts as a bond between those which remain unbroken. Another opinion attributes this peculiar consistence to the retention of a portion of the gluten of the wheat flour, which causes the granules to cohere. Under the name of *corn starch*, a variety of fecula obtained from the meal of maize or Indian corn is much used for nutritive purposes in the United States. It is an excellent preparation. The granules of maize starch are very small, with a diameter not exceeding, according to Payen, one-sixth of that of the potato, and little more than one-half that of the wheat granules. (*Gmelin*, xv. 79.) *Potato starch* is employed in various forms, being prepared so as to imitate more costly amylaceous substances, such as arrow-root and sago. In its ordinary state, it is more pulverulent than wheat starch, has a somewhat glistening appearance, and may be distinguished, with the aid of the microscope, by the size of its granules, which are larger than those of any other known fecula, except canna or *tous les mois*.* They are exceedingly diversified in size and shape, though their regular form is thought to be ovate. The characters of other kinds of fecula will be given under the heads of the several officinal substances of which they constitute the whole or a part.

According to Chevallier, starch is sometimes adulterated with carbonate and sulphate of calcium; and the fraud is also practised of saturating it with moisture, of which it will absorb 12 per cent. without any obvious change.

* CANNA was dropped at the last U. S. revision. Although not used as much as formerly, it merits a notice. (*Amylum Cannæ; Tous les Mois, Amidon de Canne, Fécule de Tolomane*, Fr.; *Cannastärke*, G.) It is yet somewhat uncertain from what species of Canna the fecula is derived, though it is generally believed to be *C. edulis*. The tubers of *Canna Achiras* (Gillies), growing in Central and South America, are said to be used as food in Peru and Chili (Lindley, *Med. and Econom. Bot.* p. 50); and a root or rhizome, closely resembling turmeric, and used by the native Africans at Sierra Leone for dyeing yellow, was found by Dr. Wm. F. Daniell to be the product of a species of Canna, believed to be the *C. speciosa* of Roscoe. (*P. J. Tr.*, Nov. 1859, p. 258.)

Canna edulis. Lindley, *Flor. Med.* p. 569, figured in *Fl. Med. and Econ.* of the same author, p. 49, also *B. and T.* 266. This is a tuberous plant, with erect, smooth, purplish stems, from four to six feet high, and invested with sheathing leaves, which are ovate-oblong, tapering towards each end, smooth, and of a deep glaucous green, with purplish edges. The flowers are few, and in compact racemes, of a red and yellow color. The plant is a native of the West Indies, and is cultivated in the islands of St. Kitts and Trinidad, and perhaps others. The tubers are first rasped, by means of a machine, into a pulp, from which the starch is extracted in the usual manner, by washing and straining, and, after the washings have been allowed to stand, so as to deposit the fecula, decanting the clear liquid. (Pereira, *Mat. Med.*)

Properties. Canna starch is in the form of a light, beautifully white powder, of a shining appearance, very unlike the ordinary forms of fecula. Its granules are said to be larger than those of any other variety of starch in use, being from the 300th to the 200th of an inch in length. Under the microscope they appear ovate or oblong, with numerous regular unequally distant rings; and the circular hilum, which is sometimes double, is usually situated at the smaller extremity. (*Pereira.*) This fecula has the ordinary chemical properties of starch, and forms, when prepared with boiling water, a nutritious and wholesome food for infants and invalids. It may be prepared in the same manner as *arrow-root*, and is said to form even a stiffer jelly with boiling water. (See *Maranta.*)

Medical Properties, etc. Starch is nutritive and demulcent, but in its ordinary form is seldom administered internally. Powdered and dusted upon the skin, it is sometimes used to absorb irritating secretions, and prevent excoriation. Dissolved in hot water and allowed to cool, it is often employed in enemata, either as a vehicle, or as a demulcent application in irritated states of the rectum. It may be used as an antidote to iodine taken in poisonous quantities.

Off. Prep. Amylum Iodatum; Glyceritum Amyli.

Off. Prep. Br. Glycerinum Amyli; Mucilago Amyli; Pulvis Tragacanthæ Compositus; Suppositoria Acidi Tannici cum Sapone; Suppositoria Morphinæ cum Sapone.

AMYLUM IODATUM. *U.S.* *Iodized Starch.*

(ĂM'Y̆-LŬM Ī-O-DĀ'TŬM.)

Amyli Iodidum, Iodide of Starch; Iodure d'Amidon, *Fr.;* Jodstärke, *G.*

"Starch, *ninety-five parts* [or four hundred and eighteen grains]; Iodine, *five parts* [or twenty-two grains]; Distilled Water, *a sufficient quantity*, To make *one hundred parts* [or one ounce av.]. Triturate the Iodine with a little distilled water, add the starch gradually, and continue triturating until the compound assumes a uniform blue color, approaching black. Dry it at a temperature not exceeding 40° C. (104° F.), and rub it to a fine powder. Iodide of Starch should be preserved in glass-stoppered vials." *U.S.*

This is a new officinal. The view taken by our Pharmacopœia is that of Liebig and Duclaux, that iodized starch is not a definite chemical compound, hence the name *iodized.* Bondonneau, on the other hand, assigns to it the formula $(C_6H_{10}O_5)_5I$, whilst Payen and Fritzsche give it $(C_6H_{10}O_5)_{10}I$. If it is a definite compound, it is one of the most feeble known; sunlight, boiling water, alcohol, potash, and hydrosulphuric acid decomposing it easily. The officinal formula is substantially that of Dr. Andrew Buchanan, of Glasgow, who proposed iodized starch as a means of administering iodine in large doses without causing irritation of the stomach. He prepares it by triturating twenty-four grains of iodine with a little water, adding gradually an ounce of very finely powdered starch, and continuing the trituration until the compound assumes a uniform blue color. The iodide is then dried by a gentle heat, and kept in a well-stopped bottle.

M. Magnes-Lahens, of Toulouse, first employed torrefied starch, but subsequently abandoned its use, and now contents himself with making an intimate mixture of iodine and starch, slightly moistened, which he subjects to the heat of a water-bath, until it is converted into the iodide of starch, forming a solution with water of a magnificent blue color. The heat, thus regulated, disaggregates the starch, without completely transforming it into dextrin, and gives a preparation in the form of a black powder. M. Seput, of Constantinople, has also given a formula for this soluble iodide, and for a *syrup* to be made from it. (See *Journ. de Pharm.*, Mars, 1852, p. 202.) M. Soubeiran reported upon these preparations to the Paris Society of Pharmacy, and deemed them ineligible on account of their variable strength in iodine, arising from the greater or less loss of this element during the necessary exposure to heat. Nevertheless, as the syrup is called for, he recommended the following process for making it, availing himself of the observations of his predecessors, which he had occasion to cite in his report. Triturate thoroughly, in a porcelain mortar, 36 grammes of nitric starch with 4½ grammes of iodine, dissolved in three times its weight of ether, and added in successive portions, until, after the evaporation of the greater part of the ether, a blue powder remains. Introduce this into a weighed, stoppered flask, and, having added 520 grammes of water, expose the whole to the heat of a water-bath, with the stopper at first removed, in order to complete the dissipation of the ether. Afterwards the stopper is replaced, being loosely tied with a packthread, so as to permit of its being raised without being driven out; and the heat is continued for about an hour and a half, when the iodide of starch will be completely formed. The flask is then weighed, and a quantity of water added to it, equal to that lost by evaporation. Lastly, 1040 grammes of sugar are added to the liquid, and dissolved by a gentle heat. By this formula a syrup is prepared, containing a quarter of one per cent. of iodine, a small part of which is in the state of hydriodic acid. The *nitric starch* is used by M. Soubeiran, because it unites with the iodine in much less time than the ordinary starch. It is made by mixing ordinary starch, in the cold, with 150 parts of water, to which 1 part of nitric acid has been added, and allowing the whole to dry in the open air. Three grains of this syrup, diluted with a pint of water, communicate to the liquid a sensible blue tint. This test may serve to determine whether the preparation is of full strength. (*Journ. de Pharm.*, Mai, 1852, p. 329.) The dose of the syrup is from one to four tablespoonfuls a day.

M. Quesneville, for whom it is claimed that he first introduced iodide of starch into therapeutics, recommends the following method of preparing it. Take of the finest starch, unmixed with that from the potato, 1050 grammes; iodine, in very fine powder passed twice through a sieve of silk, 100 grammes. Carefully mix the powders, and, when the mixture is complete, sprinkle into it gradually, agitating constantly, a mixture of 400 grammes of water and 100 of alcohol. The powder becomes gradually more and more deeply colored, and soon of a beautiful black. It is to be allowed to stand 15 or 20 days, and is then dried, first by a current of air and then in a stove. When well dried, the powder has no smell of iodine, of which it contains exactly one-tenth of its weight. It is quite insoluble in cold water; but to render it soluble, it is sufficient to heat it in an enamelled pan over a very gentle fire with constant agitation; the heat must be removed when a pungent odor is emitted. The powder thus procured is sufficient for pharmaceutical use. If it be desired to obtain it purer and extremely soluble in cold water, and always of a fine violet-blue, it will be necessary to make with heat a concentrated solution, so as to mark 7 or 8 degrees on the areometer for saline solutions, allow it to stand and settle for several days, then decant the liquor, add a quantity of alcohol just sufficient to precipitate the iodide of starch, put the magma which forms upon a linen cloth, press it as strongly as possible, and dry it by a stove-heat upon shallow dishes. (*Journ. de Pharm.*, Juillet, 1868, p. 30.)

Medical Properties. This preparation has been highly recommended by Drs. A. Buchanan, J. C. Dalton, and others, as affording a means of introducing iodine very largely into the general system without causing local irritation. Dr. Buchanan thinks that, by means of the starch, the iodine is converted into hydriodic acid, and in this state enters the circulation. Prof. Dalton, of New York, found that nearly all the animal fluids decompose iodide of starch, and destroy its blue color. (*Am. Journ. of Med. Sci.*, April, 1856, p. 327.) This result is owing, no doubt, to the alkaline nature of most of the animal fluids, especially those of the duodenum, alkaline iodides being formed at the expense of the starch. The dose is a heaped teaspoonful, given in water-gruel, three times a day, and afterwards increased to a tablespoonful. No nicety is necessary in apportioning the dose. In some cases Dr. Buchanan has given half ounce (15·6 Gm.) doses of the iodide three times a day, immediately increased to an ounce (31·1 Gm.).

ANETHI FRUCTUS. *Br.* *Dill Fruit.*

(A-NĒ'THĪ FRŬC'TŬS.)

"The dried fruit of Peucedanum graveolens. Hiern. (Anethum graveolens. Linn.)" *Br.*

Aneth, Fenouil puant, *Fr.*; Dill, *G.*

Gen. Ch. Fruit nearly ovate, compressed, striated. *Petals* involuted, entire. *Willd.*

Anethum graveolens. Willd. *Sp. Plant.* i. 1469; Woodv. *Med. Bot.* p. 125, t. 48. Dill is an annual plant, three or four feet high, with a long spindle-shaped root; an erect, striated, jointed branching stem; and bipinnate or tripinnate, glaucous leaves, which stand on sheathing footstalks, and have linear and pointed leaflets. The flowers are yellow, and in large, flat, terminal umbels, destitute of involucre. The plant is a native of Spain, Portugal, and the south of France; and is found growing wild in various parts of Africa and Asia. It is cultivated in all the countries of Europe, and has been introduced into our gardens. The seeds, as the fruit is commonly called, are the only part used. They are usually rather more than a line in length, and less than a line in breadth, of an oval shape, thin, concave on one side, convex and striated on the other, of a brown color, and surrounded by a yellowish membranous expansion. Each mericarp has three sharply keeled dorsal ridges, besides two marginal thin membranous projections or ridges. The vittæ or oil tubes are six in number, two upon the face and one in each furrow between the ridges. The odor is strong and aromatic, but less agreeable than that of fennel seed; their taste, moderately warm and pungent. These properties depend on a volatile oil, which may be obtained separate by distillation. The bruised seeds impart their virtues to alcohol and to boiling water. The oil will be found described under the heading of *Oleum Anethi.*

Medical Properties. Dill seeds have the properties common to the aromatics, but are very seldom used in this country. They may be given in powder or infusion. The dose of the fruit is from fifteen grains to a drachm (1–3·9 Gm.), of the oil three or four drops (0·18–0·24 C.c.).

Off. Prep. Br. Aqua Anethi; Oleum Anethi.

ANISUM. *U.S.* *Anise.*

(A-NI'SŬM.)

"The fruit of Pimpinella Anisum. Linné. (*Nat. Ord.* Umbelliferæ, Orthospermæ.)" *U.S.* "The dried fruit of Pimpinella Anisum. Linn." *Br.*

Anisi Fructus, *Br.;* Fructus (Semen) Anisi, s. Anisi vulgaris; Aniseed, *E.;* Anis, Anisvert, Graines d'Anis, *Fr.;* Anissame, Anis, *G.;* Semi d'Aniso, *It.;* Simiente de Anis, *Sp.;* Anison, *Ar.*

Gen. Ch. *Fruit* ovate-oblong. *Petals* inferior. *Stigma* nearly globular. *Willd.*

Pimpinella Anisum. Willd. *Sp. Plant.* i. 1473; *B. and T.* 122. This is an annual plant, about a foot in height, with an erect, smooth, and branching stem. The leaves are petiolate, the lower roundish-cordate, lobed, incised-serrate, the middle pinnate-lobed with cuneate or lanceolate lobes, the upper trifid, undivided, linear. The flowers are white, and in terminal compound umbels, destitute of involucres.

The anise plant is a native of Egypt and the Levant, but has been introduced into the south of Europe, and is cultivated in various parts of that continent. It is also cultivated occasionally in the gardens of this country. The fruit is abundantly produced in Malta and Spain; in Romagna, in Italy, whence it is largely exported through Leghorn; and in Central and Southern Russia. The Spanish is smaller than the German or French, and is usually preferred; the Russian fruit is very short. It is said also to be extensively cultivated in India and South America, although we are not aware that the product ever comes into American commerce.

It is one of the oldest aromatics, having been spoken of by Theophrastus and cultivated in the imperial German farms of Charlemagne. In 1305, Edward I. granted a patent giving the right to levy tolls upon it at the Bridge of London for the purpose of repairing the bridge itself.

Anise seeds (botanically, fruit) are about a line in length, oval, striated, somewhat downy, attached to their footstalks, and of a light greenish brown color, with a shade of yellow. "About one-sixth of an inch (4 mm.) long, ovate, compressed at the sides, grayish, finely hairy, and consisting of two mericarps, each with a flat face, and five light brownish filiform ridges, and about fifteen thin oil tubes." *U.S.* Their odor is fragrant, and increased by friction; their taste, warm, sweet, and aromatic. These properties, which depend upon a peculiar volatile oil, are imparted sparingly to boiling water, freely to alcohol. The volatile oil exists in the envelope of the seeds, and is obtained separate by distillation. (See *Oleum Anisi.*) Their internal substance contains a bland fixed oil. By expression, a greenish oil is obtained, which is a mixture of the two. The seeds are sometimes adulterated with small fragments of argillaceous earth, which resembles them in color; and their aromatic qualities are occasionally impaired by a slight fermentation, which they are apt to undergo in the mass, when collected before maturity.

When examined by the microscope, anise is seen to contain a very great but variable number of small oil tubes, which are well represented in the accompanying figure,—from fifteen to thirty to each mericarp. The epidermis is supplied with short, simple hairs, easily detached in making a section, and not represented in the cut.

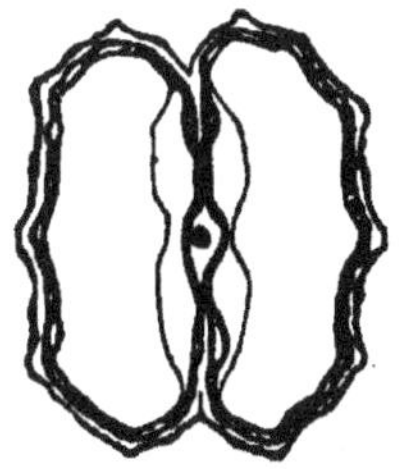

A case of poisoning is on record from the accidental admixture of the fruits of *Conium maculatum*, which bear some resemblance to those of anise, but may be distinguished by their crenate or notched ridges and the absence of oil tubes. They are, moreover, broader in proportion to their length, and are generally separated into half fruits, while those of anise are whole.

Star aniseed, the *Cardamomum Siberiense* or *Annis de Sibérie* of the seventeenth century and the *badiane* of the French writers, is the product of the *Illicium anisatum*, and is fully described under the heading of *Illicium*. They contain about 4 per cent. of a volatile oil, very closely resembling that of anise. There are no known chemical differences between these oils, although dealers distinguish them by their smell and taste.

Dr. Ruschenberger, U.S.N., has shown that oil of anise has a remarkable power of deodorizing sulphide of potassium; a drop of the oil having entirely deprived of offensive odor a drachm of lard with which five grains of the sulphide had been incorporated. (*Am. Journ. of Med. Sci.*, N. S., xlviii. 419.)

Medical Properties and Uses. Anise is a grateful aromatic carminative; and is supposed to have the property of increasing the secretion of milk. It has been in use from the earliest times. In Europe it is much employed in flatulent colic, and as a corrigent of griping or unpleasant medicines; but in this country fennel seed is preferred. Anise may be given bruised, or in powder, in the dose of twenty or thirty grains (1·3–1·95 Gm.) or more. The infusion is less efficient. The volatile oil may be substituted for the seeds in substance. Much use is made of this aromatic for imparting flavors to liquors.

Off. Prep. Syrupus Sarsaparillæ Compositus; Tinctura Rhei Dulcis.

Off. Prep. Br. Aqua Anisi; Oleum Anisi.

ANTHEMIS. *U.S., Br.* *Anthemis.*

(ĂN'THE-MĬS.)

Anthemidis Flores, *Br.;* Flores Chamomillæ Romanæ, *P. G.;* Roman or English Chamomile, *E.;* Camomille Romaine, *Fr.;* Römische Kamille, *G.;* Camomilla Romana, *It.;* Manzanilla Romana, *Sp.;* Chamomile, Chamomile Flowers.

"The flower heads of Anthemis nobilis. Linné. (*Nat. Ord.* Compositæ.) Collected from cultivated plants." *U. S.* "The dried single and double flower heads or capitula of Anthemis nobilis. Linn. From cultivated plants." *Br.*

Gen. Ch. Receptacle chaffy. *Seed-down* none or a membranaceous margin. *Calyx* hemispherical, nearly equal. *Florets of the ray* more than five. *Willd.*

Several species of Anthemis have been employed in medicine. *A. nobilis*, which is the subject of the present article, is by far the most important. *A. Cotula*, or mayweed, was formerly recognized by the U.S. Pharmacopœia. *A. Pyrethrum*, which affords the pellitory root, is among the officinal plants. (See *Pyrethrum*.) *A. arvensis*, a native of this country and of Europe, bears flowers which have an acrid bitter taste, and possess medical properties analogous though much inferior to those of common chamomile. They may be distinguished by their want of smell. *A. tinctoria* is occasionally employed as a tonic and vermifuge in Europe. *Matricaria suaveolens* is said to yield the chamomile of the Indian bazaars.

Anthemis nobilis. Willd. *Sp. Plant.* iii. 2180; *B. and T.* 154. This is an herbaceous plant with a perennial root. The stems are from six inches to a foot long, round, slender, downy, trailing, and divided into branches, which turn upwards at their extremities. The leaves are bipinnate, the leaflets small, threadlike, somewhat pubescent, acute, and generally divided into three segments. The flowers are solitary, with a yellow convex disk, and white rays. The calyx is common to all the florets, of a hemispherical form, and composed of several small imbricated hairy scales. The receptacle is convex, prominent, and furnished with rigid bristle-like paleæ. The florets of the ray are numerous, narrow, and terminated with three small teeth. The whole herb has a peculiar fragrant odor, and a bitter aromatic taste. The flowers only are officinal.

This plant is a native of Europe, and grows wild in all the temperate parts of that continent. It is also largely cultivated for medicinal purposes.* In France, Germany, and Italy, it is generally known by the name of *Roman chamomile.* By cultivation the yellow disk florets are often converted into the white ray florets. Thus altered, the flowers are said to be *double*, while those which remain unchanged are called *single;* but, as the conversion may be more or less complete, it generally happens that with each of the varieties there are intermingled some flowers of the other kind, or in different stages of the change. The double flowers are generally preferred; though, as the sensible properties are found in the greatest degree in the disk, the single are the most powerful. It is rather, however, in aromatic flavor than in bitterness that the radical florets are surpassed by those of the disk. If not well and quickly dried, the flowers lose their beautiful white color, and are less efficient. The flowers which are largest, most double, and whitest should be preferred. They are thus described officinally. "Subglobular, about three-quarters of an inch (2 c.m.) broad, consisting of an imbricated involucre, and numerous white, strap-shaped, three-toothed florets, inserted upon a chaffy, conical, solid receptacle. It has a strong, agreeable odor, and an aromatic bitter taste." *U. S.* The seeds yield by expression a fixed oil, which is said to be applied in Europe to various economical uses.

Though not a native of America, chamomile grows wild in some parts of this country, and is occasionally cultivated in our gardens for family use; the whole herb being employed. The medicine, as found in our shops, consists chiefly of the double flowers, and is imported from Germany and England. From the former country the flowers of *Matricaria Chamomilla* are also occasionally imported, under the name of chamomile. (See *Matricaria.*) In France, the flowers of two other plants are sold in the shops, indiscriminately with those of *Anthemis nobilis;* viz., those of *Pyrethrum Parthenium* (the *Chrysanthemum Parthenium* of Persoon) or *feverfew*, and those of *Anthemis parthenoides*, De Cand., or the *Matricaria parthenoides*, Desf. (*Journ. de Pharm.*, Mai, 1859, p. 347.) For the peculiar character by which these two flowers may be distinguished from the chamomile, see *Pyrethrum Parthenium* in Part II.

Properties. Chamomile flowers, as usually found in the shops, are large, almost spherical, of a dull white color, a fragrant odor, and a warmish, bitter, aromatic taste. When fresh, their smell is much stronger, and was fancied by the ancients to resemble that of the apple. Hence the name *chamæmelum* (*χαμαι*, on the ground, and *μηλόν*, an apple); and it is somewhat singular that the Spanish name *manzanilla* (a little apple) has a similar signification. The flowers impart their odor and taste to water and alcohol, the former of which, at the boiling temperature, extracts nearly one-fourth of their weight. The investigations of several chemists performed in 1878–1879, in Fittig's laboratory at Strassburg, have shown the oil of chamomile to contain the following constituents:—a fraction distilling at 147°–148° C. (296°–298° F.) consisting of *isobutylic ethers* and hydrocarbons; *angelicate of isobutyl* at 177° C. (350·5° F.); *angelicate of isoamyl* at 200°–201° C. (392°–394°

* Mr. Jacob Bell, of Mitcham, in Surrey, England, stated that the plant is usually propagated by dividing the root, though the seeds are employed when it is desired to introduce new varieties. Each root will serve as the source of thirty or forty plants. They are set in rows a yard apart, at intervals of about eighteen inches. The proper period for planting is March; and the flowers are in perfection in July, but continue to appear throughout the season. Extremely wet or extremely dry weather is injurious to the crop. It is more productive in a rather heavy loam, than either in light sandy soil, or in stiff clay. It requires little manure, but attention to weeding is necessary. Over-manuring increases the leaves at the expense of the flowers. When gathered, the flowers are dried upon canvas trays in a drying-room, artificially warmed, where they remain about a day. The crop varies from three to ten hundredweight per acre. The single flowers are more productive than the double by weight; but, as they command a less price, the value of the crop is about the same. (*P. J. T.*, x. 118.)

F.); *tiglinate of isoamyl* at 204°–205° C. (399°–401° F.) (both these compound ethers answering to the formula $C_5H_{11}, C_5H_7O_2$). In the residual portion, hexylic alcohol, $C_6H_{13}OH$, and an alcohol of the formula $C_{10}H_{18}O$ are met with, both probably occurring in the form of compound ethers. By decomposing the angelicates and the tiglinate above mentioned with potash, *angelic acid*, $C_5H_8O_2$, and *tiglinic acid* (or *methyl-crotonic*) isomeric with the former are obtained to the extent of about 30 or more per cent. of the crude oil. In the oil examined by Fittig, angelic acid prevailed; from another specimen E. Schmitt (1879) obtained but very little of it, tiglinic acid prevailing. For an examination of the oil from *Anthemis Cotula*, which closely resembles that from *A. nobilis*, see *A. J. P.*, 1885, p. 376, and *A. J. P.*, 1885, p. 381. Flückiger performed some experiments in order to isolate the *bitter principle*, but did not succeed in obtaining it in a satisfactory state of purity; it formed a brown extract, apparently a glucoside. He also confirms the statement that no alkaloid is present.

Medical Properties and Uses. Chamomile is a mild tonic, in small doses acceptable and corroborant to the stomach, in large doses capable of acting as an emetic. In cold infusion it is often advantageously used in cases of enfeebled digestion, whether occurring as an original affection, or consequent upon some acute disease. It is especially applicable to that condition of general debility, with languid appetite, which often attends convalescence from idiopathic fevers. As a febrifuge it formerly enjoyed much reputation, and was employed in intermittents and remittents; but we have remedies so much more efficient, that it is now seldom used in this capacity. The tepid infusion is very often given to promote the operation of emetics, or to assist the stomach in relieving itself when oppressed by its contents. The flowers are sometimes applied externally in the form of fomentation, in cases of irritation or inflammation of the abdominal viscera, and as a gentle incitant in flabby, ill-conditioned ulcers. The dose of the powder as a tonic is from half a drachm to a drachm (1·95–3·9 Gm.) three or four times a day, or more frequently. The infusion is usually preferred. The decoction and extract cannot exert the full influence of the medicine; as the volatile oil is driven off.

Off. Prep. Br. Extractum Anthemidis; Infusum Anthemidis; Oleum Anthemidis.

ANTIMONIUM. *Antimony.*

Sb; 120. (ĂN-TĬ-MŌ'NĬ-ŬM.) Sb; 120.

Stibium, *Lat.;* Antimoine, *Fr.;* Antimon, Spiessglanz Metall, *G.;* Antimonio, *Sp., It.*

Metallic antimony, sometimes called *regulus of antimony*, is not officinal in the British or United States Pharmacopœias; but, as it enters into the composition of a number of important pharmaceutical preparations, we have thought it proper to notice it under a distinct head.

Antimony exists in nature—1, uncombined; 2, as an oxide; 3, as antimonious sulphide (tersulphide) and 4, as an oxysulphide. It is found principally in France and Germany; but has been discovered also in the province of New Brunswick and in Ontario, Canada.

Extraction. All the antimony of commerce is extracted from the native sulphide. The ore is first separated from its gangue by fusion. It is then reduced to powder, and placed on the floor of a reverberatory furnace, where it is subjected to a gentle heat, being constantly stirred with an iron rake. This process of roasting is known to be completed, when the matter is brought to the state of a dull grayish white powder, called *antimony ash.* By this treatment the antimony is partly teroxidized, and partly converted into antimonious acid; while nearly all the sulphur is dissipated in the form of sulphurous acid gas; a portion of tersulphide, however, remains undecomposed. The matter is then mixed with charcoal impregnated with a concentrated solution of carbonate of sodium, and the mixture heated in crucibles, in a melting furnace. The charcoal reduces the teroxide of antimony, while the alkali unites with the undecomposed tersulphide, and forms melted scoriæ, which cover the reduced metal, and diminish its loss by volatilization. Antimony is more generally obtained by the reduction of the native sulphide by iron. The reduction of the antimony sulphide by iron takes place at a red heat, but as sulphide of iron needs a higher temperature for its fusion, and its specific gravity is not much less than that of the metallic antimony, the mass must be heated to a white heat to effect a perfect separation, and this occasions a loss of the antimony. In order to avoid this, sodium sulphide is added in practice, which unites with the sulphide of iron to form a more fusible and lighter slag of double sodium and iron sulphide. To 100 parts of antimony sulphide is taken 42 parts of iron, 10 parts of anhydrous sulphate of sodium, and 2½ to 3½ parts of carbon.

The purest commercial antimony is not entirely free from foreign metals, chiefly iron, lead, and arsenic. M. Lefort purifies it for the purposes of pharmacy, by gradually adding twenty-five parts of the metal, in fine powder, to fifty parts of nitric acid, by the action of which the antimony is precipitated as antimonious acid, while the foreign metals remain in solution. The precipitate is then thoroughly washed with water, containing a hundredth part of nitric acid, drained completely, mixed with three or four parts of powdered sugar, and reduced to the metallic state by being heated to redness in a Hessian crucible. (*Journ. de Pharm.*, Août, 1855, p. 93.)

Antimony is imported into the United States principally from France, packed in casks. A portion is also shipped from Trieste, from Holland, and occasionally from Cadiz. The Spanish antimony is generally in the form of pigs; the French, in circular cakes of about ten inches in diameter, flat on one side and convex on the other; the English, in cones. The French is most esteemed.

Properties, etc. The time of the discovery of antimony is not known; but Basil Valentine was the first to describe the method of obtaining it, in his work entitled *Currus Triumphalis Antimonii*, published towards the end of the fifteenth century. It is a brittle, brilliant metal, ordinarily of a lamellated texture, of a silver-white color when pure, but bluish white as it occurs in commerce. Its atomic weight is 120 (or, according to some authorities, 122), symbol Sb, sp. gr. 6·7, and fusing point 425° C. (797° F.), or about a red heat. On cooling, after fusion, antimony assumes an appearance on the surface bearing some resemblance to a fern leaf. When strongly heated, it burns with the emission of white vapors, consisting of teroxide, formerly called *argentine flowers of antimony*. A small portion, being fused, and then thrown upon a flat surface, divides into numerous globules, which burn rapidly as they move along. It forms three combinations with oxygen, *antimony trioxide* (antimonous oxide), Sb_2O_3, *antimony tetroxide*, Sb_2O_4 (by some considered to be an antimonate of the teroxide of antimony, Sb_4O_8), and *antimony pentoxide* (antimonic oxide), Sb_2O_5. The first of these unites with water to form antimonous acid, the salts of which are called *antimonites*, the third unites with water to form antimonic acid, the salts of which are called *antimonates*. The trioxide will be noticed under the head of *Antimonii Oxidum*. The tetroxide is a white powder, yellowish when hot, and difficultly soluble in acids. It forms when either of the other two oxides is strongly heated in air. *Antimony ash* described above is also an impure tetroxide. *Antimonic acid* is a lemon-colored powder, which may be prepared by oxidizing the metal by digestion in nitric acid, and then driving off the excess of the acid by a heat not exceeding 315·5° C. (600° F.). When exposed to a red heat, it parts with oxygen, and is converted into the *antimony tetroxide* just described. This, though medicinally inert, frequently forms a large proportion of the preparation called antimonial powder. (See *Pulvis Antimonialis*.)

The antimonial preparations are active in proportion to their solubility in the gastric juice. According to Mialhe, those antimonials which contain the hydrated teroxide, or are easily converted into it, are most active. Hence metallic antimony in fine powder, and tartar emetic, act with energy. The teroxide is much more active when prepared in the moist than in the dry way. According to Serullas, all the antimonial preparations, except tartar emetic and butter (or terchloride) of antimony, contain a minute proportion of arsenic. Tartar emetic is an exception, because it separates entirely, in the act of crystallizing, from any minute portion of arsenic in the materials from which it is prepared; the poisonous metal being left behind in the mother-water of the process.

ANTIMONII ET POTASSII TARTRAS. *U.S., Br.* *Tartrate of Antimony and Potassium.* [*Tartar Emetic.*]

(ĂN-TĮ-MŌ'NĮ-Ī ĔT PǪ-TĂS'SĮ-Ī TĂR'TRĂS.)

$2KSbO\ C_4H_4O_6.\ H_2O$; 664. $KO, SbO_3, C_8H_4O_{10}. HO$; 332.

"An oxytartrate of antimony and potassium." *Br.*

Antimonium Tartaratum, *Br.;* Antimonium Tartarizatum, Tartarised Antimony, Tartrated Antimony; Antimonii Potassio-Tartras, Tartarus Stibiatus, *P. G.;* Tartarus Emeticus, Stibio-Kali Tartaricum; Tartrate de Potasse et d'Antimoine, Emétique, Tartre stibié, *Fr.;* Brechweinstein, *G.*

"Take of Oxide of Antimony *five ounces* [avoirdupois]; Acid Tartrate of Potassium, in fine powder, *six ounces* [av.]; Distilled Water *two pints* [Imperial measure]. Mix the Oxide of Antimony and Acid Tartrate of Potassium with sufficient Distilled Water to form a paste, and set aside for twenty-four hours. Then add the remainder of the Water and boil for a quarter of an hour, stirring frequently. Filter, and set aside the clear filtrate to crystallize. Pour off the mother-liquor, evaporate to one-third, and set aside that more crystals may form. Dry the crystals on filtering paper at the temperature of the air." *Br.*

A process for Tartar Emetic not being given in the new U. S. Pharmacopœia, that of 1870 is inserted below.* This compound is a normal tartrate. Tartaric acid is dibasic. In acid potassium tartrate (cream of tartar) one of the two replaceable hydrogen atoms is replaced by potassium, while the other is unreplaced; in neutral potassium tartrate (soluble tartar) both are replaced by potassium; in tartar emetic, one is replaced by potassium, while the other is replaced by the group (SbO) antimonyl, which is a univalent group, exactly replacing one hydrogen atom.

In the preparation of tartar emetic several circumstances should be taken into view. The cream of tartar should not be in excess; as in that case it is apt to crystallize, upon cooling, with the tartar emetic. To avoid such a result it is better to have a slight excess of antimonial oxide. No rule is applicable to the determination of the proper proportion of water, except that it should be sufficient to dissolve the tartar emetic formed. The hot filtration, directed in the U. S. Pharmacopœia of 1870, may be conveniently performed by a jacketed funnel filled with hot water. In all cases the salt should be obtained in well-defined crystals, unmixed with those of cream of tartar, as the best index of its purity. The practice of some manufacturing chemists of boiling the filtered liquor to dryness, whereby an impure mass is obtained, consisting in part only of the antimonial salt, is very reprehensible.

It is not easy to decide as to the relative eligibility of the different forms of antimonial oxide, used for preparing tartar emetic. The preference, however, was given to the oxychloride (*powder of Algaroth*) by Berzelius; and M. Henry, an eminent pharmaceutist of Paris, after a careful comparison of the different processes, declared also in its favor.

M. Henry has given a process for preparing tartar emetic with the oxychloride on a large scale; and, as his formula may be useful to the manufacturing chemist, we subjoin it, converting French weights into the nearest *apothecaries'* weights and measures. Take of prepared sulphide of antimony, in very fine powder, three pounds four ounces; hydrochloric acid, marking 22° (sp. gr. 1·178), eighteen pounds and a half; nitric acid, two ounces and a half. Introduce the sulphide into a glass matrass, of a capacity double the volume of the mixture to be formed; and add to it from three to five pounds of the acids previously mixed; so that the sulphide may be thoroughly penetrated by them; then add the remainder of the acids. Place the matrass on a sand-bath, and heat the mixture gradually to ebullition, avoiding the vapors, which are disengaged in large quantity. Continue the heat until the vapors given off are so far deprived of sulphuretted hydrogen as not to blacken white paper moistened with solution of acetate of lead; after which allow the liquor to cool, and to remain at rest until it has become clear. Decant the clear liquor, and, in

* "Take of Oxide of Antimony, in very fine powder, *two troyounces;* Bitartrate of Potassium, in very fine powder, *two troyounces and a half;* Distilled Water *eighteen fluidounces.* To the Water, heated to the boiling point in a glass vessel, add the powders, previously mixed, and boil for an hour; then filter the liquid while hot, and set it aside that crystals may form. Lastly, dry the crystals, and keep them in a well-stopped bottle. By further evaporation the mother-water may be made to yield more crystals, which should be purified by a second crystallization." *U. S.* 1870.

order to procure the portion of liquid which may be retained by the moist residue, add to this a small portion of hydrochloric acid, and again decant. Mix the decanted liquids, which consist of a solution of terchloride of antimony, and add them to a large quantity of water, in order that the oxychloride may be precipitated; taking care, during their addition, to stir constantly in order that the precipitated powder may be more minutely divided, to facilitate its subsequent washing. To determine whether the water has been sufficient to decompose the whole of the terchloride, a part of the supernatant liquid, after the subsidence of the powder, is to be added to a fresh portion of water; and, if a precipitate take place, more water must be added to the mixture, so as to obtain the largest possible product of oxychloride. The precipitation being completely effected, wash the powder repeatedly with water, until this no longer affects litmus, and place it on linen to drain for twenty-four hours. The quantity of oxychloride thus obtained will be about three pounds and a half in the moist state, or two pounds nine ounces when dry. Assuming it to be this quantity, mix it with three pounds eleven ounces of cream of tartar in fine powder, and add the mixture to two gallons and five pints of boiling water, contained in an iron kettle. Concentrate the liquor rapidly until it marks 25° of Baumé's hydrometer for salts, and then filter. By repose the liquor furnishes a crop of very pure crystals, which require only to be dried. The mother-waters are treated in the following manner. Saturate the excess of acid with chalk, filter, and concentrate to 25°. By cooling, a second crop of crystals will be obtained; and by proceeding in a similar manner, even a third crop. But these crystals are somewhat colored, and must be purified by recrystallization.*

In relation to the above process, it may be observed that the proportion of oxychloride and cream of tartar must be adjusted according to the numbers given, on the assumption that the former is dry; but it by no means follows that the whole of the oxide should be dried. To proceed thus would be a waste of time. The mode of proceeding is to weigh the whole of the moist oxide, and afterwards to weigh a small part of it, and ascertain how much this loses in drying. Then, by a calculation, it is easy to determine how much the whole of the moist oxide would weigh if dry.

Tartar emetic is not usually prepared by the apothecary, but made on a large scale by the manufacturing chemist. Different processes are pursued in different manufactories; and it is not material what plan is adopted, provided the crystals of the antimonial salt are carefully purified. In an extensive manufactory in London, antimony ash is employed for boiling with the cream of tartar, and it is stated to form the cheapest material for making tartar emetic. (*Pereira's Mat. Med.*) Mohr prefers the use of a *moist* oxide, prepared by adding gradually an intimate mixture of one part, each, of tersulphide of antimony and nitrate of potassium, to a boiling mixture of one part of sulphuric acid and two of water. The liquid is boiled down nearly to dryness and allowed to cool. The grayish white mass, thus formed, is then washed thoroughly with water. The details of this process are given by Soubeiran, by whom it is praised, in the *Journ. de Pharm.*, 3e sér., iii. 327.

Properties, etc. It is in the form of "small, transparent crystals, of the rhombic system, becoming opaque and white on exposure to air, or a white, granular powder, having a sweet, and afterwards disagreeable metallic taste, and a feebly acid reaction. Soluble in 17 parts of water at 15° C. (59° F.) and in 3 parts of boiling water. Insoluble in alcohol, which precipitates it from its aqueous solution in the form of a crystalline powder. When heated to redness, the salt chars, emits the odor of burnt sugar, and leaves a blackened residue of an alkaline reaction. The aqueous solution of the salt yields with hydrochloric acid, a white precipitate soluble in an excess of the acid; but no precipitate occurs if tartaric acid has been previously added. In a solution of the salt acidulated with hydrochloric acid, hydrosulphuric acid causes an orange-red precipitate. A dilute solution at once becomes permanently turbid on the addition of a little carbonate of potassium." *U.S.* Tartrate of antimony and potassium was discovered in 1631 by Adrian de Mynsicht. When prepared from the oxychloride it crystallizes in tetrahedrons. As it occurs in the shops, it is often in the

* For still another method of preparing tartar emetic, which we omit from want of space, see *Journ. de Pharm.*, 4e sér., xi. 404.

form of a white powder, resulting from the pulverization of the crystals. They are insoluble in alcohol, but dissolve in proof spirit or wine.* (See *Vinum Antimonii.*) Its aqueous solution slightly reddens litmus, and undergoes decomposition by keeping. If one-fifth of its bulk of alcohol be added to the water, the decomposition is prevented. It is incompatible with acids, alkalies and their carbonates, some of the earths and metals, chloride of calcium, and acetate and subacetate of lead. It is incompatible also with astringent infusions and decoctions, as of rhubarb, cinchona, catechu, galls, etc.; but these substances, unless galls be an exception, do not render it inert, though they lessen its activity to a greater or less extent.

Characteristics and Tests of Purity. "A one per cent. aqueous solution of the salt previously acidulated with acetic acid, should not be clouded by the addition of a few drops of test-solution of chloride of barium (sulphate), or of ferrocyanide of potassium (iron and other metals), or of oxalate of ammonium (calcium), or of nitrate of silver (chloride). If 1 Gm. of the salt and some pieces of aluminium wire be added to strong solution of soda (sp. gr. about 1·260), contained in a long test-tube, a gas is given off which should not impart any color to filter paper wet with test-solution of nitrate of silver, and held over the mouth of the test-tube (abs. of more than traces of arsenic)." *U. S.* Tartar emetic, when pure, exhibits its appropriate crystalline form. A crystal or two, dropped into a solution of hydrosulphuric acid, will be covered with an orange-colored deposit of tersulphide of antimony. "Twenty-nine grains dissolve slowly but without residue in an [Imperial] fluidounce of distilled water at 60°; and the solution gives with sulphuretted hydrogen an orange precipitate, which, when washed and dried at 212°, weighs 15·1 grains." *Br.* Entire solubility in water is not a character belonging exclusively to the pure salt, for, according to the late Mr. Hennell, tartar emetic may contain 10 per cent. of uncombined cream of tartar, and yet be wholly soluble in the proper proportion of water. Hennell's method of detecting uncombined bitartrate, is to add a few drops of a solution of carbonate of sodium to a boiling solution of the antimonial salt. If the precipitate formed be not redissolved, no bitartrate is present.

The impurities found in tartar emetic are uncombined cream of tartar from faulty preparation or fraudulent admixture, tartrate of calcium, iron, sulphates, and chlorides. The mode of detecting cream of tartar has been indicated above. Tartrate of calcium is derived from the cream of tartar, which always contains this impurity. It is apt to form on the surface of the crystals of tartar emetic in crystalline tufts, which are easily brushed off. Iron is sometimes present, especially when the antimonial salt has been prepared from glass of antimony. It is detected by a blue color being *immediately* produced by ferrocyanide of potassium, added after a little acetic acid. If the blue color be *slowly* produced, it may arise from reactions on the iron of the ferrocyanide itself. If much iron be present, the solution of the tartar emetic will be yellow instead of colorless. According to Serullas, tartar emetic, except when well crystallized, and all the other antimonial preparations usually contain a minute proportion of arsenic, derived from the native tersulphide of antimony, which almost always contains this dangerous metal. Subsequently, however, Mr. Thos. Williams (*P. J. Tr.*, July, 1874, p. 63) examined a number of samples of various antimonial preparations and found them remarkably free from arsenic. Tartar emetic should always be bought by the apothecary in good crystals, in which state the salt is pure, or very nearly so, and entirely free from arsenic. Its powder is perfectly white; and, when it is yellowish white, iron is probably present. A. H. Jackson found some samples of commercial tartar emetic to contain from 40 to 70 per cent. of potassium sulphate. (*Year-Book of Pharmacy*, 1885, p. 459.)

It has been already stated, in general terms, that tartar emetic in solution is incompatible with acids and alkalies, and with some of the earths; but this salt is so important, that some details in regard to the effects of particular reagents, included under these titles, seem to be necessary. Hydrochloric and sulphuric acids, added to a

* Alcohol precipitates it from its aqueous solution, and Mr. T. S. Wiegand proposes as a method of obtaining it in fine powder, to boil an ounce in four times its weight of water, and to pour the solution into a pint and a half of 95 per cent. alcohol. (*A. J. P.*, 1858, p. 407.)

solution of the antimonial salt, not too dilute, throw down a white precipitate of terchloride or subsulphate of antimony, mixed with cream of tartar, which is redissolved by an excess of the precipitant. Nitric acid throws down a subnitrate, which is taken up by an excess of it. When caustic potassa is added to a tolerably concentrated solution, it produces at first no effect, then a precipitate of teroxide, and afterwards the solution of this precipitate, if the addition of the alkali be continued. Lime-water acts in a weaker solution, and throws down a white precipitate, consisting of the mixed tartrates of calcium and antimony. Carbonate of potassium affects still weaker solutions, throwing down a white precipitate of teroxide; but this test does not act in solutions containing less than a quarter of a grain to the fluidounce. Ammonia, both pure and carbonated, precipitates a solution of tartar emetic, throwing down the pure teroxide. To these reagents may be added infusion of galls, which, when fresh and strong, causes a dirty yellowish white precipitate of tannate of antimony.

Medical Properties and Uses. When tartar emetic is given in minute doses to the healthy man (gr. $\frac{1}{12}$), it produces only a slight lessening of the force of the pulse and a tendency to increased secretion from the skin. After somewhat larger amounts these symptoms are more pronounced and have nausea added to them. If a grain be ingested, the nausea and vomiting are usually severe and persistent, and are accompanied by marked prostration, both of the circulation and of the muscular strength. Symptoms of acute poisoning by the drug are an austere metallic taste; excessive nausea; copious vomiting; frequent hiccough; burning pain in the stomach; colic; frequent stools and tenesmus; fainting; small, contracted, and accelerated pulse; coldness of the skin, and even of the internal organs; difficult and irregular respiration; cutaneous anæsthesia; loss of sense; convulsive movements; very painful cramps in the legs; prostration, and death. Ten grains is the smallest dose reported to have proved fatal. In the lower animals antimony causes symptoms similar to those which it produces in man. It has been experimentally proven that the fall of the arterial pressure is produced, at least in part, by a direct action upon the heart. The loss of muscular power, of reflex activity and of sensibility, are believed to be due to depression of the spinal centres, and the disturbance of respiration to a direct influence upon the nerve centres which preside over that function. The purging and vomiting are connected with an effort at elimination, the poison escaping through the gastro-intestinal mucous membrane, as well as through the kidneys. After death from antimony, fatty degeneration of the liver, kidneys, and other organs has been found, indicating that the poison has a powerful influence upon nutrition.

The above summary shows that in small doses tartar emetic is powerfully depressant to the circulation and stimulant to the secretion of the skin. It has been very largely used as a sedative, antiphlogistic, diaphoretic, and expectorant. It is, however, at present much less frequently administered than formerly; in *small* doses (gr. $\frac{1}{12}$ to $\frac{1}{8}$), mostly associated with saline, alkaline, or diaphoretic remedies, and assisted by copious dilution, it is still resorted to in febrile complaints, for the purpose of producing perspiration, which is often freely induced, especially if the remedy gives rise to nausea. It also proves useful, on many occasions, in the first stages of bronchitis; and with a view to its action in this way, it is conjoined with expectorant remedies. In *full* doses it acts as an emetic, and is characterized by certainty, strength, and permanency of operation. It remains longer in the stomach than ipecacuanha, produces more frequent and longer-continued efforts to vomit, and exerts a more powerful impression on the system. The nausea and attendant prostration are often very considerable. As an emetic its use is indicated where the object is not merely to evacuate the stomach, but to agitate and compress the liver and other abdominal viscera; its employment is contraindicated by debility or gastro-intestinal irritability, and it is very badly borne by children. By the extension of its action to the duodenum, it often causes copious discharges of bile, and may thus prove useful when there is a morbid excess of that secretion.

The so called contra-stimulant use of large doses of antimony originated with Dr. Rasori, professor of clinical medicine at Milan, who published his views in 1800, but has gone entirely out of vogue. The principal diseases in which it was practised were pneumonia, pleurisy, bronchitis, and acute rheumatism. The medicine was directed in doses, varying from a grain to two grains or more, every two hours, dissolved in a small quantity of water; the patient being restricted in the use of drinks whilst under its operation. It is stated that, when the remedy is thus given in diseases of high action, it seldom produces vomiting, an effect which the author of the practice wished to avoid. The power of the system to bear large doses of tartar emetic, during the existence of acute diseases, was considered by Rasori to depend upon the coexisting morbid excitement, and the capability of bearing them was expressed by the term *tolerance*.

Externally, tartar emetic is employed as a counter-irritant, mixed with lard, or cerate, or in the form of a plaster. (See *Unguentum Antimonii* and *Emplastrum Antimonii.*) It causes, after a longer or shorter interval, a burning sensation, accompanied by a peculiar and painful pustular eruption. This mode of producing counter-irritation is serviceable when a very powerful and persistent effect is desirable. Care must be taken, when the salt is applied by means of a plaster, that the pustular inflammation does not proceed too far; as, in that event, it produces deep and very painful ulcerations, difficult to heal. According to M. Guérin, inflamed parts exhibit a condition of tolerance to the local effects of tartar emetic, evinced by the absence of pustulation.

Tartar emetic is generally given in solution, and in an amount which varies with the object in view in its administration. Its dose as an alterative is from the thirty-second to the sixteenth of a grain (0·002–0·004 Gm.); as a diaphoretic or expectorant, from the twelfth to the sixth of a grain (0·005–0·01 Gm.); and as a nauseating sudorific, from a sixth to a quarter of a grain (0·01–0·016 Gm.); repeated, according to circumstances, every hour, two, or four hours; as an emetic, half a grain (0·03–0·065 Gm.), repeated every fifteen or twenty minutes till it vomits; the operation being aided by warm water or chamomile tea.

Poisoning. The general symptoms of acute tartar emetic poisoning have been sufficiently described. In rare cases vomiting and purging do not take place; and, when they are absent, the other symptoms are aggravated. Sometimes a pustular eruption is produced, like that caused by the external application of the antimonial; as in a case reported by Dr. J. T. Gleaves, of Tennessee.

The effects of slow poisoning by tartar emetic on inferior animals have been carefully studied by Dr. B. W. Richardson, of London, and Dr. Nevins, of Liverpool. All the surfaces absorb the solution of the salt, and the metal is found in all the tissues after death, except that of the brain; but most abundantly in that of the liver. The elimination of the poison is effected by all the secreting organs, but especially by the kidneys. The tolerance of antimony is attributed by Dr. Richardson to the eliminating action of these glands. The pathological appearances are general congestion, marked fluidity of the blood, and intense vascularity of the stomach and sometimes of the rectum, but without ulceration. No other pulmonary lesion occurs but simple congestion. (*Am. Journ. of Med. Sci.*, 1857, p. 266.) The general results obtained by Dr. Richardson were confirmed by Dr. Nevins. (*P. J. Tr.*, 1857, p. 415.)

In treating a case of poisoning by tartar emetic, if it be found that the patient has not vomited, immediate recourse must be had to tickling the throat with a feather, and the use of abundance of warm water. Usually, however, the vomiting is excessive and distressing; and here it is necessary to use remedies calculated to decompose the poison, and to allay the pain and irritation. Tannic acid should be freely administered, in order to form the insoluble and inactive, if not absolutely inert, tannate of antimony. A case of poisoning with half an ounce of tartar emetic, successfully treated with copious draughts of green tea and large doses of tannin, is reported by Dr. S. A. McCreery, of the U. S. Navy. (*Am. Journ. of Med. Sci.*, 1853, p. 131.) To stop the vomiting and relieve pain, laudanum should be given, either by the mouth or by injection; and to combat consecutive inflammation, leeches to the epigastrium and other antiphlogistic measures may be resorted to.

After death from suspected poisoning by tartar emetic, it is necessary to search for the poison in the body. The contents of the stomach should be digested in water, acidulated with hydrochloric and tartaric acids. The former acid will serve to coagulate organic matter; the latter to give complete solubility to the antimony. The solution obtained, after having been filtered, should be subjected to a stream of sulphuretted hydrogen, which, if tartar emetic be present, will throw down the orange red tersulphide of antimony, distinguished from tersulphide of arsenic and all other precipitates by forming with hot hydrochloric acid a solution, from which a white curdy precipitate of oxychloride of antimony (powder of Algaroth) is thrown down upon the addition of water. Sulphuretted hydrogen is by far the most delicate test for tartar emetic.

Sometimes the antimony is not in the stomach and bowels, and yet may exist in other parts, especially in the liver and kidneys, and their secretions. The mode of extracting the antimony, recommended by Orfila, is to carbonise the dried viscera with pure concentrated nitric acid in a porcelain capsule, to boil the charred mass obtained for half an hour with hydrochloric acid, assisted with a little nitric acid, to filter the liquor, and introduce it into Marsh's apparatus. Antimoniuretted hydrogen will be formed, which, being inflamed, will deposit the antimony on a cold surface of porcelain as a black stain, distinguishable from the similar stain produced by arsenic by its slighter volatility, by its forming, with hot hydrochloric acid, a solution which affords a white precipitate of oxychloride of antimony when added to water, its insolubility in solution of bleaching powder or chlorinated soda, and its solubility in solution of stannous chloride. (See *Acidum Arseniosum*, p. 41.)

Reinsch's process is a good one for separating antimony from the tissues, and was first used for that purpose by Dr. Alfred Taylor, of London. The tissues are boiled in hydrochloric acid, and a bright slip of copper is immersed in the hot solution. The metallic film, deposited on the copper, must be proved to be antimony. This is done by Dr. Odling by first boiling the coated copper in a solution of permanganate of potassium, with a little excess of potassa, for a few minutes, whereby the antimony becomes oxidised and dissolved, and then passing sulphuretted hydrogen through the filtered and acidulated solution. The characteristic orange red precipitate of tersulphide of antimony is produced, which may be tested for antimony as above mentioned. Mr. H. H. Watson has simplified Dr. Odling's process by dispensing with the use of the permanganate of potassium. He subjects the coated copper slip, in a tube, to a boiling very dilute solution of caustic potassa, the metal being alternately drawn out of and immersed in the solution, by the aid of a copper wire, until the whole of the coating is oxidized and dissolved. The solution is then treated as directed by Dr. Odling. (*Med. Times and Gaz.*, July, 1857, p. 613.) Antimoniuretted hydrogen (evolved either by galvanic processes or from zinc and sulphuric acid), when passed over sulphur, is decomposed, slowly in diffused daylight, very rapidly in sunlight, antimonous sulphide forming, with liberation of hydrogen sulphide. The orange red sulphide can be freed from excess of sulphur by exhaustion with bisulphide of carbon. (Jones, *Journ. Chem. Soc.*, i., 1876.)

Off. Prep. Syrupus Scillæ Compositus; Vinum Antimonii.

Off. Prep. Br. Unguentum Antimonium Tartarati; Vinum Antimoniale.

ANTIMONII OXIDUM. *U. S., Br.* *Oxide of Antimony.*

Sb_2O_3; 288. (ĂN-TĮ-MŌ′NĮ-Ī ŎX′Į-DŬM.) SbO_3; 144.

Stibium Oxydatum, Oxydum Antimonicum s. Stibicum; Oxyde d'Antimoine, *Fr.;* Antimonoxyd, *G.*

A process for this salt is no longer officinal. Below is that of the Pharm. 1870.*

* "Take of Sulphuret of Antimony, in very fine powder, *four troyounces;* Muriatic Acid *eighteen troyounces;* Nitric Acid *a troyounce and one hundred and twenty grains;* Water of Ammonia *a fluidounce and a half;* Water, Distilled Water, each, *a sufficient quantity.* Introduce the Sulphuret into a flask, of the capacity of two pints, and, having added the Muriatic Acid, digest, by means of a sand-bath, until effervescence ceases. Then, having removed the flask from the sand-bath, add the Nitric Acid gradually; and, when nitrous acid vapors cease to be given off, and the liquid has grown cold, add to it half a pint of Water, and filter. Pour the filtered liquid gradually into twelve pints of Water, constantly stirring, and allow the precipitate to subside. Decant the supernatant liquid, and wash the precipitate twice by decantation, using, each time, eight pints of Water. Then transfer it to a muslin filter to drain, and, after the draining is completed, wash it with Water until the washings cease to have an acid reaction. Next introduce it into a suitable vessel, and subject it to the action of the Water of Ammonia for two hours; at the end of which time transfer it to a moistened muslin filter, and wash it with Distilled Water as long as the washings produce a precipitate with nitrate of silver. Lastly, dry the precipitate upon bibulous paper with the aid of a gentle heat." *U. S.* 1870.

"Take of Solution of Chloride of Antimony *sixteen fluidounces;* Carbonate of Sodium *six ounces* [avoird.]; Water *two gallons* [Imperial measure]; Distilled Water *a sufficiency.* Pour the Antimonial Solution into the Water, mix thoroughly, let the precipitate settle, remove the supernatant liquid by a siphon, add one gallon [Imp. meas.] of Distilled Water, agitate well, let the precipitate subside, again withdraw the fluid, and repeat the process of affusion of Distilled Water, agitation, and subsidence. Add now the Carbonate of Sodium previously dissolved in two pints [Imp. meas.] of Distilled Water, leave them in contact for half an hour, stirring frequently, collect the deposit on a calico filter, and wash with boiling distilled water until the washings cease to give a precipitate with a solution of nitrate of silver acidulated by nitric acid. Lastly, dry the product at a heat not exceeding 212° (100° C.)" *Br.*

In the U. S. 1870 formula the solution of terchloride is prepared as the first step of the proceeding; in the British it is taken already formed, as the result of a distinct process. When tersulphide of antimony is digested with hydrochloric acid, a chemical reaction takes place as follows: $Sb_2S_3 + 6HCl = (SbCl_3)_2 + (H_2S)_3$; the hydrogen of the acid uniting with the sulphur of the antimonial, and escaping as sulphuretted hydrogen, while the chlorine and antimony combine to form terchloride of antimony which is held in solution. The effect of the nitric acid is supposed to be to render the oxide whiter, by decomposing any remaining sulphuretted hydrogen, and thus preventing it from contaminating the product. Though the result thus far is an aqueous solution of the terchloride, this cannot be diluted beyond a certain degree without decomposition. Hence, if largely diluted, as when poured into an excess of water, decomposition takes place, and a white powder is precipitated,[1] formerly called *powder of Algaroth*, which is mainly an oxychloride. The composition of the powder, however, is not uniform; as it contains more teroxide, the greater the proportion of water used in the decomposition. The pure oxychloride, SbOCl, is formed when the proportion of 4 mols. of water to 1 mol. of antimony chloride exists, but with a relatively larger proportion of water the average composition of the powder is $Sb_4O_5Cl_2$, which may be considered as made up of $(SbOCl)_2 + Sb_2O_3$. The oxychloride is first washed with abundance of water to separate adhering hydrochloric acid, and then acted upon by a solution of alkali (Ammonia, *U. S.*, Carbonate of sodium, *Br.*) to decompose the oxychloride, with the effect of adding to the amount of teroxide; after which the teroxide only requires to be washed with water in order to render it pure. The last washing separates the chloride of ammonium or of sodium resulting from the decomposition of the oxychloride; and the water of this washing is tested, in both formulas, by nitrate of silver, until the presence of chlorine ceases to be indicated.

Properties. Teroxide of antimony is a heavy, grayish white powder, permanent in the air, almost insoluble in water, insoluble in alcohol and nitric acid, readily soluble in hydrochloric or tartaric acid, or in boiling solution of bitartrate of potassium. Heated in close vessels it becomes yellow, fuses at a full red heat, and finally sublimes in crystalline needles. When cooled from a state of fusion it forms a fibrous crystalline mass, of pearl color. Heated in open vessels it suddenly becomes red hot, and, by the absorption of oxygen, changes into Sb_2O_4 (antimony antimonate), which differs from the teroxide in being insoluble in hydrochloric acid, less fusible, and not volatile. This oxide is the active ingredient of all the medicinal preparations of antimony. "By dropping its solution in hydrochloric acid into water, a white precipitate is formed, which is at once changed to orange by hydrosulphuric acid. A solution of Oxide of Antimony in an excess of tartaric acid should yield no precipitate with test-solutions of nitrate of silver (chloride), chloride of barium (sulphate), or ferrocyanide of potassium (iron and other metals)." *U. S.* It is frequently impure from the presence of the before-mentioned antimonate of antimony, in which case it is not *entirely* soluble in hydrochloric acid. If it contain oxychloride, which it is apt to do from the imperfect action of the alkaline solutions employed in its purification, its solution in tartaric acid will be precipitated by nitrate of silver. When antimonate of antimony is substituted for it, the fraud may be detected by the spurious preparation being entirely insoluble in hydrochloric acid.

Medical Properties. This oxide, which must not be confounded with the powder of Algaroth, has the general therapeutic properties of the antimonials. Like antimonial powder, it is unequal in its effects, sometimes vomiting, at other times being apparently inert. The inequality of action is plausibly explained by the state of the stomach as to acidity, the presence of acids giving the medicine activity; and this explanation is confirmed by the experiments of Dr. Osburn, of Dublin, with the Dublin oxide. As to the French Codex oxide, prepared by boiling the oxychloride with a solution of bicarbonate of potassium, the inequality is attributed by M. Durand, of Caen, to the presence of more or less terchloride, which is separated with difficulty. Objecting to the Codex oxide, M. Durand proposes to prepare the teroxide by precipitating tartar emetic with ammonia in excess. Thus obtained it contains no terchloride, and does not vomit. (*Journ. de Pharm.*, 3e sér., ii. 364.) The dose of teroxide of antimony is set down as three grains (0·20 Gm.), every two or three hours, but the drug should not be employed as a medicine. It was introduced into the U. S. Pharmacopœia, to be used in the preparation of tartar emetic.

Off. Prep. Pulvis Antimonialis.

Off. Prep. Br. Antimonium Tartaratum; Pulvis Antimonialis.

ANTIMONII SULPHIDUM. *U. S.* *Sulphide of Antimony.*

Sb_2S_3; 336. (AN-TI-MŌ'NI-Ī SŬL-PHĪ'DŬM.) **Sb, S_3; 168.**

[Antimonii Sulphuretum, Pharm. 1870.]

"Native sulphide of antimony, purified by fusion and as nearly free from arsenic as possible." *U. S.* "Native sulphide of antimony, Sb_2S_3, purified from silicious matter by fusion, and afterwards reduced to fine powder." *Br.* (See page 210.)

Antimonium Nigrum, *Br.* 1864; Black Antimony. (Prepared Sulphuret of Antimony, *Br.*) Stibium Sulfuratum Crudum et Lævigatum, *P. G.;* Antimonium Crudum, Stibium Sulfuratum Nigrum, Sulfuretum Stibicum; Artificial Sulphuret of Antimony; Antimoine sulfuré, Sulfure d'Antimoine, Antimoine cru, *Fr.;* Schwefelantimon, Schwefelspiessglanz, *G.;* Solfuro d'Antimonio, *It.;* Antimonio crudo, *Sp.*

Preparation, etc. The sulphide of antimony of the Pharmacopœias is obtained from the native sulphide, called *antimony ore*, by different processes of purification; the following being an outline of that generally pursued. The ore is placed in melting-pots in a circular reverberatory furnace, and these are made to connect, by means of curved earthen tubes, with the receiving pots, situated outside the furnace. This arrangement affords facilities for removing the residue of the operation, and allows of the collection of the melted sulphide without interrupting the fire, and, consequently, without loss of time or fuel. In the U. S. Pharmacopœia it is directed to be melted in order to purify it from infusible substances; in the British, to be reduced to fine powder, to fit it for pharmaceutic use. In order to bring it to this state, it should be submitted to the process of levigation. (See *Antimonii Sulphidum Purificatum.*) Much of the "Black Antimony" of commerce has been shown by Prof. Warder to contain no antimony whatever, but to be simply powdered coal and marble, and such can be easily distinguished by a rough test, as follows. Fill a dry, tared one-ounce bottle with the powder, after shaking it down it will be found that it will hold two and a quarter ounces of powdered black antimony, but only one and a quarter ounces of powdered coal. (*Proc. A. P. A.*, 1885, p. 479; see, also, S. W. McKeown's paper, *Proc. Ohio State Pharm. Assoc.*, 1885.)

Properties. Sulphide of antimony is mostly prepared in France and Germany. It is called, in commerce, antimony, or *crude antimony*, and occurs in fused conical masses, denominated loaves. "Steel-gray masses of a metallic lustre and a striated crystalline fracture, forming a black or grayish black, lustreless powder, without odor or taste, and insoluble in water or alcohol. When heated, it fuses at a temperature below red heat. One part of the powdered sulphide, when boiled with 10 parts of hydrochloric acid, dissolves without leaving more than a slight residue, hydrosulphuric acid being evolved. The solution when added to water gives a white precipitate, which is soluble in a solution of tartaric acid. After separation of the precipitate by filtration, the filtrate gives an orange red precipitate with hydrosulphuric acid." *U. S.* The quality of the sulphide cannot well be judged of, except in mass; hence it ought never to be bought in powder. Arsenic, which is often present in considerable quantities, may be detected by the usual tests for that metal. (See *Acidum Arseniosum*, p. 41.)

Composition. The officinal sulphide of antimony is a tersulphide consisting of two atoms of antimony 240, and three of sulphur 96 = 336.

When prepared by pulverization and levigation, it is in the form of an insoluble powder, without taste or smell, usually of a dull blackish color, but reddish brown when perfectly pure. By exposure to the air, it absorbs, according to Buchner, a portion of oxygen, and becomes partially converted into teroxide.

Medical Properties and Uses. This preparation is very uncertain in its operation; being sometimes without effect, at other times, if it meet with acid in the stomach, acting with violence by vomiting and purging. The effects attributed to it are those of a diaphoretic and alterative; and the principal diseases in which it has been used are scrofula, glandular obstructions, cutaneous diseases, and chronic rheumatism. It is employed in the United States solely in veterinary practice. The dose is from ten to thirty grains (0·65–1·95 Gm.), given in powder or bolus.

Off. Prep. Antimonii Sulphidum Purificatum.

ANTIMONII SULPHIDUM PURIFICATUM. *U.S.* *Purified Sulphide of Antimony.*

Sb_2S_3; 336. (ĂN-TĮ-MŌ′NĮ-Ī SŬL-PHĪ′DŬM PŪ-RĮ-FĮ-CĀ′TŬM.) $Sb\ S_3$; 168.

"Sulphide of Antimony, *ten parts;* Water of Ammonia, *five parts.* Reduce the Sulphide of Antimony to a very fine powder. Separate the coarser particles by elutriation, and, when the finely divided sulphide has been deposited, pour off the water, add the Water of Ammonia, and macerate for five days, agitating the mixture frequently. Then let the powder settle, pour off the Water of Ammonia, and wash the residue by repeated affusion and decantation of water. Finally dry the product by the aid of heat." *U. S.*

ANTIMONIUM NIGRUM PURIFICATUM. *Br.* *Purified Black Antimony.*

(ĂN-TĮ-MŌ′NĮ-ŬM NĪ′GRŬM PŪ-RĮ-FĮ-CĀ′TŬM.)

"Native sulphide of antimony, Sb_2S_3, purified from siliceous matter by fusion, reduced to fine powder, and, if, on testing as described below, any soluble salt of arsenium is present, purified by the following process. Take of Native Sulphide of Antimony, in fine powder, 1 pound; Solution of Ammonia 8 fluidounces; Distilled Water a sufficiency. Macerate the sulphide of antimony with the solution of ammonia for five days, stirring frequently. Then allow the powder to subside, pour off the supernatant liquid, and thoroughly wash the residue with the water. Dry the powder by the aid of heat." *Br.*

The test for arsenium is as follows. "If one grain be dissolved in hydrochloric acid, and the solution, slightly diluted, be gently warmed with a piece of bright copper foil, the copper being washed, dried, and heated in a dry, narrow test-tube, no crystalline sublimate (of arsenious anhydride) should form on the upper cool part of the tube."

These are new officinal processes, which are intended to furnish a black sulphide of antimony better fitted for the manufacture of the officinal preparations of antimony and for internal administration. Copper, a common impurity in the crude sulphide, is rendered soluble by the water of ammonia, whilst the subsequent washing and decantation effectually remove all soluble impurities.

Properties. "A dark gray powder, odorless and tasteless, and insoluble in water or alcohol. It fuses at a temperature below red heat. When boiled with 10 parts of hydrochloric acid it is nearly all dissolved, hydrosulphuric acid being evolved. The solution when added to water yields a white precipitate, which is soluble in a solution of tartaric acid. After separation of the precipitate by filtration, the filtrate gives an orange red precipitate with hydrosulphuric acid." *U. S.*

Tests. "If 2 Gm. of the salt be mixed and cautiously ignited, in a porcelain crucible, with 8 Gm. of pure nitrate of sodium, and the fused mass boiled with 25 Gm. of water, there will remain a residue which should be white or nearly so, and not yellowish or brownish (abs. of other metallic sulphides). On boiling the filtrate with an excess of nitric acid, until no more nitrous vapors are evolved, then dissolving in it 0·1 Gm. of nitrate of silver, filtering again if necessary, and cautiously pouring a few drops of Water of Ammonia on top, not more than a white cloud, but no red or reddish precipitate should appear at the line of contact of the two liquids (abs. of more than traces of arsenic)." *U. S.*

Medical Properties and Uses. This preparation was introduced into the British Pharmacopœia for pharmaceutical purposes, and should not itself be used in medical practice.

Off. Prep. Antimonium Sulphuratum.

Off. Prep. Br. Antimonium Sulphuratum; Liquor Antimonii Chloridi.

ANTIMONIUM SULPHURATUM. *U. S., Br.* *Sulphurated Antimony.*

(ĂN-TI-MŌ′NI-ŬM SŬL-PHŮ-RĀ′TŬM.)

Antimonii Oxysulphuretum, *Lond.;* Antimonii Sulphuretum Aureum, *Ed.;* Precipitated Sulphide of Antimony; Stibium Sulfuratum Aurantiacum, *P. G.;* Sulphur Stibiatum Aurantiacum, Sulphur Auratum Antimonii; Golden Sulphuret of Antimony, Golden Sulphur; Soufre doré d'Antimoine, *Fr.;* Goldschwefel, *G.*

"Chiefly Antimonious Sulphide [Sb_2S_3; 336—SbS_3; 168] with a very small amount of Antimonious Oxide." *U. S.* "A mixture containing sulphide and oxide of antimony, Sb_2S_5 and Sb_2O_3." *Br.*

"Purified Sulphide of Antimony, *one part* [or four ounces av.]; Solution of Soda, *twelve parts* [or two pints and thirteen fluidounces]; Distilled Water, Diluted Sulphuric Acid, each, *a sufficient quantity.* Mix the Purified Sulphide of Antimony with the Solution of Soda and *thirty parts* [or eight pints] of Distilled Water, and boil the mixture over a gentle fire, for two hours, constantly stirring, and occasionally adding distilled water so as to preserve the same volume. Strain the liquid immediately through a double muslin strainer, and drop into it, while yet hot, Diluted Sulphuric Acid so long as it produces a precipitate. Wash the precipitate with hot Distilled Water until the washings are at most but very slightly clouded by test-solution of chloride of barium; then dry the precipitate and rub it to a fine powder." *U. S.*

"Take of Purified Black Antimony 10 ounces [av.]; Sublimed Sulphur 10 ounces [av.]; Solution of Soda 4½ pints [Imp. meas.]; Diluted Sulphuric Acid, Distilled Water, of each a sufficiency. Mix the Purified Black Antimony with the Sublimed Sulphur and the Solution of Soda, and boil for two hours with frequent stirring, adding distilled water occasionally to maintain the same volume. While still hot add nine pints [Imp. meas.] of boiling distilled water. Strain the liquor through calico, and, before it cools, add to it by degrees the Diluted Sulphuric Acid till the latter is in slight excess. Collect the precipitate on a calico filter, wash with distilled water till the washings no longer precipitate with chloride of barium, and dry at a temperature not exceeding 212° F. (100° C.)" *Br.*

There are three preparations containing antimony and sulphur, viz.: the *amorphous precipitated antimonious sulphide*, Sb_2S_3, which while orange red in color corresponds to the black native sulphide; a reddish brown mixture known as "*kermes mineral,*" which contains both antimonious sulphide and oxide, and has an average composition $(Sb_2S_3)_2 + Sb_2O_3$;* and the *golden sulphide*, which is antimonic sul-

* ANTIMONII OXYSULPHURETUM. *U. S.* 1870. *Oxysulphuret of Antimony. Kermes Mineral. Kermes mineral* was officinal in 1870. The following is the process. "Take of Sulphuret of Antimony, in very fine powder, *a troyounce;* Carbonate of Sodium *twenty-three troyounces;* Water *sixteen pints.* Dissolve the Carbonate of Sodium in the Water previously heated to the boiling point, and, having added the Sulphuret of Antimony, boil for an hour. Then filter rapidly into a warm earthen vessel, cover this closely, and allow the liquid to cool slowly. At the end of twenty-four hours, decant the supernatant liquid, drain the precipitate on a filter, wash it with boiled water previously allowed to become cold, and dry it without heat. Lastly, preserve the powder in a well-stopped bottle, protected from the light." *U. S.*

Though very long in use as a medicine, and much employed on the continent of Europe, it was only recently that this preparation was admitted into the U. S. Pharmacopœia, having been superseded by the precipitated sulphide, which was supposed to have very similar if not identical properties.

phide, Sb_2S_5, and is obtained by decomposing sulph-antimoniates like *Schlippe's salt* (SbS_4Na_3) by the addition of a strong mineral acid.

The first of these is obtained by dissolving the powdered native sulphide in caustic potash solution with the aid of heat and then adding to this solution, which contains the antimony combined as potassium antimonite and sulph-antimonite, sulphuric acid, when a reddish precipitate is formed which dries to a reddish brown powder.

The second is obtained by boiling the native sulphide or the red amorphous sulphide just described with sodium carbonate, and then allowing the compound to settle out from the hot filtered liquid as it cools.

The third is obtained by first forming a sulph-antimoniate by boiling finely powdered antimonious sulphide and caustic soda with sulphur (or carbonate of sodium and

Kermes mineral, according to Thenard, may be obtained by treating the tersulphide of antimony in three ways; 1st with a boiling solution of the carbonated alkalies, 2d with a boiling solution of the caustic alkalies, and 3d with the carbonated alkalies at a red heat. These several processes give brown powders, which vary in their shade of color, and which, though usually considered as identical, differ in composition. The kermes obtained by means of the carbonated alkalies in solution is an oxysulphide, that is, a compound of hydrated tersulphide of antimony with the teroxide; while the product, when either the caustic alkalies in solution or the carbonated alkalies at a red heat are used, is essentially a hydrated tersulphide, though containing occasionally a little oxysulphide. It is the first of these methods that was adopted in the U. S. process of 1870. It is in fact the formula of Cluzel (see U. S. D., 11th ed., p. 926), and is substantially that of the French Codex of 1837.

The rationale of the formation of kermes by this process is as follows. A portion of the carbonate of sodium is converted, by a transfer of carbonic acid, into caustic soda and sesquicarbonate. By a double decomposition taking place between a part of the tersulphide of antimony and the caustic soda, sulphide of sodium and teroxide of antimony are formed. The undecomposed portion of the tersulphide then dissolves in the solution of sulphide of sodium, and the teroxide in that of the remaining carbonate of sodium. The tersulphide and teroxide, being both more soluble in these menstrua hot than cold, precipitate together as the liquid cools, and constitute this variety of kermes. Thus obtained it is light, velvety, of a dark reddish purple color, brilliant in the sun, and of a crystalline appearance. It consists, according to M. Henry, jun., of tersulphide of antimony 62·5, teroxide 27·4, water 10, and soda a trace; proportions which correspond most nearly with two mols. of tersulphide, one of teroxide, and six of water. From the presence of so large a proportion of teroxide of antimony in this variety of kermes, it must be far more active than the other kinds, and ought, therefore, to be preferred for medical use.

Kermes, when obtained by means of the caustic alkalies, may be formed by the use of either potassa or soda. When the former alkali is selected, it may be prepared by boiling, for a quarter of an hour, two parts of the tersulphide of antimony with one part of caustic potassa dissolved in twenty-five or thirty parts of water, filtering the liquor, and allowing it to cool; whereupon the kermes precipitates. In this process one portion of the tersulphide, by reacting with a part of the potassa, gives rise to teroxide of antimony and sulphide of potassium. A second portion dissolves in the solution of sulphide of potassium formed, and a third forms an insoluble compound with a part of the teroxide. The remainder of the teroxide unites with the undecomposed potassa, forming a compound, which, being but sparingly soluble, is only in part dissolved. The hot filtered liquor, therefore, contains this compound dissolved in water, and tersulphide of antimony dissolved in the solution of sulphide of potassium. By refrigeration, the tersulphide in a hydrated state falls down, free or nearly free from teroxide, this latter being still held in solution by means of the caustic alkali.

Kermes may be obtained by the third method, that is, in the dry way, by the use of the carbonated alkalies at a red heat. If carbonate of potassium* be selected, the process is as follows. Rub together two parts of tersulphide of antimony and one of carbonate of potassium, fuse the mixture in a crucible by a red heat, reduce the fused mass to powder, boil it with water, and strain. As the strained liquor cools the kermes is deposited. The rationale of its formation is nearly the same with that of the formation of the second variety of kermes. An inferior kermes, prepared in the dry way, and intended for use in veterinary medicine, is directed in the French Codex of 1837 to be prepared by fusing together, well mixed, 500 parts of tersulphide of antimony, 1000 of carbonate of potassium, and 30 of washed sulphur, reducing the fused mass to powder, and boiling it with 10,000 parts of water. The liquor, upon cooling, lets fall the kermes, which must be washed with care and dried.

Kermes mineral is an insipid, inodorous powder, of a purplish brown color, and soft and velvety to the touch. By the action of air and light it gradually becomes lighter colored, and at last yellowish white. It is readily and wholly dissolved by hydrochloric acid, with escape of hydrosulphuric acid gas, and is partly soluble in a hot solution of potassa, leaving a residue soluble in tartaric acid. It is sometimes adulterated with ferric oxide. In Paris, in 1849, a number of the shops contained a spurious kermes of very handsome appearance, which was little else than this oxide. Kermes mineral first came into use as a remedy in France about the beginning of the last century. Its mode of preparation was possessed as a secret by a French surgeon named La Ligerie. In 1720, the recipe was purchased by the French government and made public. Its remedial properties are considered above.

---

* According to the researches of M. A. Terreil (*Journ. de Pharm.*, 4e sér., xix. 131), carbonate of potassium if absolutely pure will not yield kermes by the moist way, but by the dry way will give a larger yield than will carbonate of sodium.

chalk instead of the caustic soda), and then adding the solution of this to dilute hydrochloric or sulphuric acid, when yellow Sb_2S_5 separates according to the reaction—

$$2(SbS_4Na_3 + 9H_2O) + 3H_2SO_4 = 3Na_2SO_4 + Sb_2S_5 + 3H_2S + 18H_2O.$$

Ten parts of Schlippe's salt yield in theory 4·17 parts of pentasulphide of antimony. E. G. Eberhardt recommends the more direct preparation of sulphurated antimony by treating the native sulphide with hydrochloric acid and precipitating the solution with sulphuretted hydrogen. The objection that arsenic might be found in the product was met by an examination which showed that traces of arsenic were present, but not more than when made by the officinal process. (*A. J. P.*, 1886, p. 229.)

Properties of the Precipitated Sulphide of Antimony. (*Sulphurated Antimony, U. S., Br.*) "A reddish brown, amorphous powder, odorless and tasteless, and insoluble in water and in alcohol. When heated with 12 parts of hydrochloric acid, it is nearly all dissolved with evolution of hydrosulphuric acid. The residue, after having been washed and dried, burns, on the application of a flame, with the characteristic odor of sulphur, and should leave not more than a scanty ash. On dropping a solution of Sulphurated Antimony in hydrochloric acid into water, a white precipitate is produced, which, after washing and drying, should weigh not less than 85 per cent. of the sulphide. The liquid filtered from this precipitate yields an orange red precipitate with hydrosulphuric acid. Distilled Water boiled with Sulphurated Antimony, filtered and acidulated with hydrochloric acid, should be rendered not more than slightly opalescent by test-solution of chloride of barium (limit of sulphate)." *U. S.* Water in which this preparation has been boiled, should not yield a white precipitate with oxalate of ammonium. The non-action of this test shows the absence of lime. When pure, precipitated sulphide of antimony is completely soluble in a hot solution of potassa; but, as it is found in commerce, a white matter is usually left undissolved. When boiled with a solution of cream of tartar, about 12 per cent. of teroxide is dissolved; but, according to H. Rose, this method of determining the proportion of the teroxide cannot be relied on. Exposed to heat it takes fire, and burns with a greenish blue flame, giving off sulphurous acid; while the metal remains behind in the state of a grayish oxide.

The London precipitated sulphide of antimony, as analyzed by Mr. Phillips, consisted, in the 100 parts, of tersulphide 76·5, teroxide 12, and water 11·5; proportions corresponding nearly with five mols. of tersulphide, one of teroxide, and fifteen of water. It usually contained a portion of pentasulphide, as shown by the action of hydrochloric acid, which, when heated with this antimonial, forms the terchloride with disengagement of sulphur. (*Gmelin's Handbook*, iv. 989.) Its active ingredient is the teroxide; and, in reference to its presence, the London College called the preparation *oxysulphuret of antimony*. The Edinburgh College named it incorrectly *golden sulphuret of antimony;* this name being properly applicable to the precipitate produced by the sole action of acids, and not to that obtained by the action of acids and refrigeration conjointly.

Sulphurated Antimony, in the British Pharmacopœia, is defined to be "a mixture containing sulphide and oxide of antimony, Sb_2S_3 and Sb_2O_3," and is described as "an orange-red powder, readily dissolved by caustic soda, also by hot hydrochloric acid with the evolution of sulphuretted hydrogen and the separation of sulphur. Boiled in water with acid tartrate of potassium, the resulting solution is precipitated orange red with sulphuretted hydrogen." "Sixty grains, moistened and warmed with successive portions of nitric acid until red fumes cease to be evolved, and then dried and heated to redness, give a white residue weighing about forty grains." *Br.* Mr. John Moss asserted, before the London Pharmaceutical Society, that the British process always yields a dark reddish or reddish-brown powder; but that the kermes mineral, in English commerce, is golden yellow or yellowish red, and must be prepared by some other method. He was confirmed in both statements by Profs. Redwood and Attfield; the latter explaining that the officinal kermes contains the tersulphide, the commercial the pentasulphide of antimony.

Medical Properties. *Precipitated sulphide of antimony* (*sulphurated antimony*) is alterative, diaphoretic, and emetic. It is, however, an uncertain medicine, and is very little used. In combination with calomel and guaiac (*Plummer's pill*), it was formerly employed in secondary syphilis and cutaneous eruptions. (See *Pilulæ Antimonii Compositæ.*) During its use the patient should abstain from acidulous drinks. Its dose as an alterative is from one to two grains given twice a day, in the form of pill; as an emetic, from five grains to a scruple.

Kermes mineral, when prepared by means of the carbonated alkalies in the moist way, contains between two and three times as much teroxide as the precipitated sulphide, and is a more active preparation, to be used in a smaller dose.

Golden sulphide acts like kermes mineral, but is much weaker, and must be given in a larger dose.

Off. Prep. Pilulæ Antimonii Compositæ.

Off. Prep. Br. Pilula Hydrargyri Subchloridi Composita.

APOCYNUM. *U. S.* *Apocynum.* [*Canadian Hemp.*]

(A-PÖC'Y-NÜM.)

"The root of Apocynum cannabinum. Linné. (*Nat. Ord.* Apocynaceæ.)" *U. S.*

Chanvre du Canada, *Fr.;* Canadische Hanfwurzel, *G.*

Gen. Ch. *Calyx* five-parted, the lobes acute. *Corolla* bell-shaped, five-cleft, bearing five triangular appendages in the throat opposite the lobes. *Stamens* five, inserted on the very base of the corolla. *Filaments* flat, shorter than the arrow-shaped anthers, which converge round the ovoid, obscurely two-lobed stigma, and are slightly adherent to it by their inner face. *Style* none. *Stigma* large, ovoid, slightly two-lobed. *Fruit* of two long slender follicles. *Gray's Manual.*

There are two indigenous species of this genus, *A. cannabinum*, L., and *A. androsæmifolium*, L., of very similar general aspect. Both plants abound in a milky juice, and have a tough fibrous bark, which, by maceration, affords a substitute for hemp. From this circumstance the common name has been derived.

In the officinal species the stem and branches are upright or ascending, terminated by erect and close, many-flowered cymes, which are usually shorter than the leaves, and the corolla has nearly erect lobes, with the tube not longer than the lanceolate divisions of the calyx. In *A. androsæmifolium* the branches are divergently forked, the cymes loose and spreading, the open bell-shaped corolla with revolute lobes and a tube much longer than the ovate-pointed divisions of the calyx. The two plants grow together, although *A. cannabinum* seems to be proportionately more common in the West, and frequently they are gathered indiscriminately by the herbalists. *A. androsæmifolium* was formerly included in the U. S. secondary list, but seems to have almost disappeared from the market. According to Mr. Edward A. Manheimer, it can be distinguished from that of *A. cannabinum* on microscopic examination by the thick-walled bast-cells, which are arranged somewhat in a circle near the middle of the bark. (*A. J. P.*, Nov. 1881.)

The root of *A. cannabinum* is horizontal, five or six feet in length, about one-third of an inch thick, dividing near the end into branches which terminate abruptly, of a yellowish brown color when young, but dark chestnut when old, of a strong odor, and a nauseous, somewhat acrid, permanently bitter taste. The internal or ligneous portion is yellowish white, and less bitter than the exterior or cortical part. "Long, cylindrical, somewhat branched, one-fourth to one-third of an inch (6 to 8 m.m.) thick, pale brown, longitudinally wrinkled and transversely fissured; brittle; fracture short, white; the bark rather thick; the wood porous, spongy, with delicate, medullary rays and a thin pith; inodorous; taste bitter, disagreeable." *U. S.* The fresh root, when wounded, emits a milky juice, which concretes into a substance resembling caoutchouc. In the dried state, it is brittle and readily pulverized, affording a powder like that of ipecacuanha. Schmiedeberg and te Water (*Pflanzenstoffe*, 2d ed., p. 1332) found two principles acting like digitalin; one, an amorphous resinous substance, not a glucoside, easily soluble in alcohol and ether, almost insoluble in water, which he names *apocynin*, and the other, a glucoside, easily soluble in water, which he names *apocynein*. Neither of the principles gives any color reaction with sulphuric acid and bromine. The root yields its virtues to water and alcohol, but, according to Dr. Griscom, most readily to the former. Prof. J. U. Lloyd noticed a white, tasteless, crystalline, waxy precipitate, formed in a fluid extract of *A. cannabinum.*

Medical Properties and Uses. Apocynum (or, as it is frequently improperly called, *Indian Hemp*) is powerfully emetic and cathartic, sometimes diuretic, and, like other emetic substances, promotes diaphoresis and expectoration. It produces much nausea, diminishes the frequency of the pulse, and appears to induce drowsiness independently of the exhaustion consequent upon vomiting. The disease in which it has been found most beneficial is dropsy. From fifteen to thirty grains (1–1·95 Gm.) of the powdered root will generally produce copious vomiting and purging. The decoction is a more convenient form for administration. It may be prepared by boiling half an ounce of the dried root in a pint and a half of water to a pint, of which from one to two fluidounces (30–60 C.c.) may be given twice or thrice daily, or more frequently. The watery extract, in doses of three or four grains (0·20–0·26 Gm.), three times a day, will generally act on the bowels.

APOMORPHINÆ HYDROCHLORAS. *U. S., Br.* *Hydrochlorate of Apomorphine.*

(ĂP-Q-MŎR-PHĪ'NÆ HȲ-DRQ-ȻHLŌ'RĂS.)

$C_{17}H_{17}NO_2, HCl$; 303·4. $C_{34}H_{17}NO_4, HCl$; 303·4.

Chlorhydrate d'Apomorphine, *Fr.;* Apomorphinum Hydrochloricum, *G.*

"The hydrochlorate of an artificial alkaloid prepared from morphine. It should be kept in small well-stopped vials, in a dark place." *U. S.* "The hydrochlorate of an alkaloid, obtained by heating morphine or codeine in sealed tubes with hydrochloric acid." *Br.*

Apomorphine was discovered by Dr. Matthiessen and Mr. C. A. Wright. It is prepared by heating morphine in a closed tube with a great excess of hydrochloric acid for two or three hours to the temperature of 140° and 150° C. The contents of the tube are then dissolved in water, an excess of the bicarbonate of sodium added, and the precipitate exhausted with ether or chloroform. On the addition to the solution of a very small quantity of hydrochloric acid, crystals of the chloride of apomorphine form. The process is one of dehydration; the morphine parting with one molecule of water, the formula of apomorphine being $C_{17}H_{17}NO_2$. Apomorphine may also be made by the action of hydrochloric acid upon codeine, and it is affirmed that the best method in practice is that of E. Mayer, in which morphine is treated with a solution of chloride of zinc, at 120° C. (*Berichte Deutsch. Chem. Gesell.*, Berlin, 1871, iv. 121.) Codeine, $C_{18}H_{21}NO_3$, when treated with hydrochloric acid, yields first $C_{18}H_{20}ClNO_2$, and then splits off methyl chloride, CH_3Cl, and leaves apomorphine, $C_{17}H_{17}NO_2$.

Properties. Hydrochlorate of apomorphine is usually in "minute, colorless, or grayish white, shining crystals, turning greenish on exposure to light and air, odorless, having a bitter taste, and a neutral or faintly acid reaction. Soluble in 6·8 parts of water and in 50 parts of alcohol at 15° C. (59° F.); slowly decomposed by boiling water or boiling alcohol; almost insoluble in ether or chloroform, and should it impart color to either of these liquids, it should be rejected, or it may be purified by thoroughly agitating it with either liquid, filtering, and then rapidly drying the salt on bibulous paper, in a dark place. The aqueous solution, on gentle warming, rapidly turns green, but retains a neutral reaction. Solution of bicarbonate of sodium, added to an aqueous solution of the salt, throws down the white, amorphous alkaloid, which soon turns green on exposure to air, and forms a bluish green solution with alcohol, a purple one with ether or pure benzol, and a violet or blue one with chloroform. Addition of test-solution of nitrate of silver to an aqueous solution of the salt produces a white precipitate insoluble in nitric acid, but instantly reduced to metallic silver by water of ammonia." *U. S.* The alkaloid is colored dark red by nitric acid and rose-red by ferric chloride, changing to violet, and finally black on exposure. The aqueous and alcoholic solutions are at first colorless, but change rapidly to greenish, finally becoming deep emerald-green in color. This change in color has been attributed to oxidation, and it has been noticed that the solution on standing loses its power: for this reason it is best not to keep the solution, but to make it as wanted. Mr. C. Bernbeck has observed that the change in the solution to a green color may be prevented by the addition of a small quantity of hydrochloric acid, he having proved that the cause of the green coloration is due to ammonia, either resulting from partial decomposition of the solution or from absorption from the atmosphere. (*Pharm. Zeitung*, 1885.) According to Max Quehl and H. Koehler, apomorphine is precipitated from its solutions greenish by tannic acid, lemon-yellow by picric acid, bluish white, and turning to sap-green on boiling, by sulphate of copper, purplish by chloride of gold, white, turning to blackish violet on boiling, by ferricyanide of potassium, blood-red by iodine in solution of iodide of potassium, the precipitate disappearing on boiling, white and curdy by sulphocyanate of potassium. (*A. J. P.*, 1873, p. 166.) With bichromate of potassium and concentrated sulphuric acid it turns a dark red; with the potassium salt alone, a deep yellow-orange; with neutral chloride of iron, an amethyst color.

Medical Properties and Uses. Apomorphine was first brought forward as a prompt and safe emetic by Dr. Gee. It has the great advantages of smallness of dose and freedom from irritating properties, so that it can be used hypodermically. When from $\frac{1}{16}$ to $\frac{1}{10}$ of a grain (0·004–0·006 Gm.) of it is injected under the skin of a man, in from 5 to 20 minutes free emesis usually occurs; the dose may be repeated at intervals if necessary. The effects upon the general system are usually not marked; but in some cases very alarming syncopal symptoms have been produced, and death is said to have resulted from $\frac{1}{16}$ of a grain (0·004 Gm.) in a feeble adult, worn out with chronic bronchitis and emphysema. (*Med. Rec.*, 1877, p. 664.) According to Harnack, young children bear the remedy very badly. Apomorphine has also been used to some extent as a sedative expectorant in the earlier stages of acute bronchitis, and if given in such small doses ($\frac{1}{25}$ to $\frac{1}{35}$ of a grain) as not to cause vomiting, is said by various clinicians to act happily. As an emetic, it has been employed in narcotic poisoning, to dislodge foreign bodies from the œsophagus, in suffocative catarrh, etc. Very alarming symptoms have followed the use of a solution which has undergone change, and fresh solutions only should be administered. Under no circumstances should more than ¼ grain (0·016 Gm.) be given at a dose; indeed, except to the strongest adults and in narcotic poisoning, it is not safe to administer more than $\frac{1}{10}$ of a grain (0·006 Gm.).

Off. Prep. Br. Injectio Apomorphinæ Hypodermica.

AQUÆ. *U. S.* *Medicated Waters.*

(Ā'QUÆ—ā'kwē.)

Aquæ Destillatæ; Distilled Waters, *E.*; Eaux distillées, Hydrolats, *Fr.*; Destillirte Wässer, *G.*

Under this head are included, in the U. S. Pharmacopœia, all preparations consisting of water holding volatile or gaseous substances in solution, many of which were formerly obtained by distillation, and some of which still continue to be so. They include the preparations formerly specially designated as "Distilled Waters," having been made by distilling water from plants or parts of plants containing volatile oil.

The Distilled Waters, as thus defined, hold a much more prominent position in the pharmacy of Europe, particularly of continental Europe, than in that of the United States; and a great deal of thought and elaborate investigation has been bestowed there upon the various conditions calculated to furnish the best products in the most convenient method. It would be doing injustice to the subject not to give it a distinct consideration in a work like the present.

Many vegetables impart to water distilled from them their peculiar flavor, and more or less of their medical properties. The Distilled Waters chiefly used are those prepared from aromatic plants, the volatile oils of which rise with the aqueous vapor, and are condensed with it in the receiver. But, as water is capable of holding but a small proportion of the oil in solution, these preparations are generally feeble, and are employed chiefly as pleasant vehicles or corrigents of other medicines.

In the preparation of the Distilled Waters, dried plants are sometimes used, because the fresh are not to be had at all seasons; but the latter, at least in the instance of herbs and flowers, should be preferred if attainable. Flowers which lose their odor by desiccation may be preserved by incorporating them intimately with one-third of their weight of common salt, and in this state afford Distilled Waters of delicate flavor. Some pharmacists prefer to employ the salted flowers in certain instances, believing that the waters distilled from them keep better than when prepared from the fresh flowers. Mr. C. R. Tichborne has discovered a method of preserving flowers, which is said to answer even better than the use of salt. It consists simply in immersing the fresh flowers in glycerin, which preserves them with all their aromatic properties wholly unimpaired. The flowers, as of the elder, rose, and orange, should be gathered after full expansion, and packed firmly in wide-mouthed bottles or jars, but without crushing them. The glycerin is then to be poured on until it covers them, and the vessel closed. Mr. Tichborne has kept flowers in this way for two years, and at the end of that time procured from them distilled waters, of which the perfume has equalled that of the waters prepared from recent flowers. It is not necessary that the glycerin should be perfectly pure; but it should be without smell. (*P. J. Tr.*, 2d ser., vii. 135.)

The idea at one time prevailed, to a considerable extent, that Waters kept better distilled from dried herbs than from fresh; and the opinion was true in regard to those prepared with the defective alembics of former times, and by a naked fire; but experiment has sufficiently established the fact, that, with a suitable apparatus, and a regular heat, the fresh herbs yield products which, while they have a more agreeable odor of the plant, keep quite as well as those from dried herbs.

It is necessary to observe certain practical rules in conducting the process of distillation. When the substance employed is dry, hard, and fibrous, it should be mechanically divided, and macerated in water for a short time previous to the operation. The quantity of materials should not bear too large a proportion to the capacity of the alembic, as the water might otherwise boil over into the receiver. The water should be brought quickly to the state of ebullition, and continued in that state till the end of the process. Care should be taken to leave sufficient water undistilled to cover the whole of the vegetable matter; lest a portion of the latter, coming in contact with the sides of the vessel, might be decomposed by the heat, and yield empyreumatic products. Besides, when the operation is urged too vigorously, or carried too far, a slimy matter is apt to form, which adheres to the sides of the still above the water, and is thus exposed to igneous decomposition. To obviate these disadvantages, the heat may be applied by means of an oil-bath, regulated by a thermometer, or of a bath of solution of chloride of calcium, by which any temperature may be obtained between 100° C. (212° F.) and 132·2° C. (270° F.), according to the strength of the solution; or, when the process is conducted upon a large scale, by means of steam introduced under pressure into a space around the still. To prevent the disagreeable effects of charring, and the excessive empyreumatic odor frequently noticed in distilled waters, caused by the solid contents of the still coming into direct contact with the heated bottom, we have devised an expedient which prevents the herb from touching the bottom, and yet permits the water and steam to have free access to all parts of it. (See Pharmaceutical Still under *Extracta.*) A hemispherical No. 12 sieve of copper with a loosely-fitting lid and handle is filled with the herb and placed in the water in the still. If the bottom of the still be flat or nearly so, the rounded bottom of the cage must have a very slight point of contact, and thus charring will be prevented. A convenient mode of applying heat by steam, is by means of a coil of leaden tube placed in the bottom of the still, having one end connected with a boiler, and the other passing out beneath or at the side, and furnished with a stop-cock, by which the pressure may be increased, or the condensed water drawn off at will. If any volatile oil float upon the surface of the Distilled Water, it may be separated.*

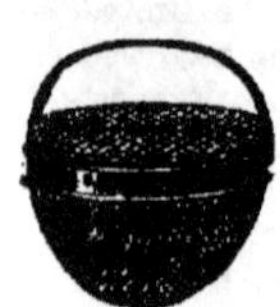

* This direction is generally given; but, in a communication to the Pharmaceutical Society of England, Mr. Haselden recommends the excess of oil to be well shaken with the water, and the whole to be transferred to the stock vessel, where it may be allowed to rest, and the oil to separate. He thinks the water keeps better when thus treated; and the full strength is always insured. The stock vessel he prefers made of stoneware, and furnished with a tap placed two inches from the bottom, whereby the water may be drawn off clear when wanted for the ordinary shop bottles; the oil rising to the top, or sinking to the bottom, according to its sp. gr. (*P. J. Tr.*, xvi. 14, 15.)

From a series of experiments made in Paris in reference to the best mode of applying heat, it was concluded that, as regards the great majority of aromatics, the direct application of steam was preferable, because the Distilled Waters prepared by means of it have a freshness of aroma that is wanting in the others, are always free from the odor of the still, are much more limpid, are less apt to deposit mucilaginous matter, and keep better; but that exceptions to the general rule are afforded by bitter almonds, cherry-laurel leaves, mustard, and horse-radish, in all of which the oil does not pre-exist in the plant, but is formed upon contact with water; by woods, barks, and roots, the tissue of which cannot be sufficiently penetrated by steam; and by roses. (*Journ. de Pharm.*, Mai, 1861, p. 364.) Later experiments have led to the conclusion that even these substances are most advantageously treated by distillation with steam; and that, in fact, there is no exception to the general rule.

But, however carefully the process may be conducted, the Distilled Waters prepared from plants always have at first an unpleasant smoky odor. They may be freed from this by exposure for a short time to the air, before being enclosed in well-stopped bottles, in which they should be preserved. When long kept, a viscid ropy matter is apt to form in them, and they become sour. This result has been ascribed to other principles, which rise with the oil in distillation, and promote its decomposition. To prevent this decomposition, rectified spirit is sometimes added to the water employed in the distillation. But this addition is inadequate, and is in fact injurious, as the alcohol by long exposure to the air undergoes the acetous fermentation. A better plan is to redistil the Waters. When thus purified, it is said that they may be kept for several years unchanged.

Robiquet considered the mucosity which forms in Distilled Waters to be the result of a vegetative process, for which the presence of air is essential. He has found that, so long as the water is covered with a layer of essential oil, it undergoes no change; but that the oil is gradually altered by exposure to the air, and, as soon as it disappears, the water begins to be decomposed. He states that camphor exercises the same preservative influence over the Distilled Waters by resisting the vegetation, and that those in which the odor of camphor is developed keep better on that account. Finally, he has observed that the more Distilled Water is charged with volatile oil, the more abundant is the mucosity when it has begun to form. Robiquet unites with Henry and Guibourt, and with Virey, in recommending that all these Waters, when intended to be kept for a considerable time, should be introduced, immediately after distillation, into bottles of a size proportionate to the probable consumption of the water when brought into use; and that the bottles should be quite filled, and then sealed or otherwise well stopped, so as entirely to exclude the air. It is best that they should be small, and be closed with well-fitting glass stoppers. Thus treated, the Waters may be preserved without change for many years. (*Journ. de Pharm.*, xxi. 402.) We have frequently noticed microscopic plants belonging to the *Confervoideæ* in the Distilled Waters contained in shop bottles standing on the shelves in the dispensing room, and if it be desired to keep Distilled Waters, the only sure way is to destroy the spores and prevent the admission of fresh ones by placing the bottles filled to the lip with the Distilled Water into a bath of boiling water, and when thoroughly heated, corking and sealing.*

Another mode of preparing the Distilled Waters is to substitute the volatile oil, previously separated from the plant, for the plant itself in the process. This mode is directed in the British Pharmacopœia, in several instances. It is said to afford a more permanent product than the preceding, but does not always preserve the flavor of the plant.

In relation to most of the aromatic waters, the U. S. Pharm. formerly directed

* It is of some importance to know the proportion which the aromatic submitted to distillation ought to bear to the amount of Distilled Water obtained. The following statement upon this point, based upon experiments, is contained in the *Journ. de Pharm.* (Mai, 1861, p. 367). Fresh aromatic plants requiring one part of the plant for one of product, wormwood, black cherry, scurvy-grass, hyssop, cherry-laurel, lavender, balm, mint, peach-leaves, roses, and sage;—fresh and dry aromatics requiring one part of the plant to two of product, bitter almonds, orange-flowers, melilot, horseradish, elder, and tansy;—dry and very aromatic plants requiring one part to four of product, angelica, green anise, juniper berries, chamomile, canella, cascarilla, fennel, sassafras, linden flowers, and valerian.

that water should be impregnated with the volatile oil by trituration with carbonate of magnesium, and subsequently filtered. This was by far the most simple and easy process. The resulting solution is nearly pure and permanent, and is perfectly transparent, the carbonate of magnesium being separated by the filtration. Carbonate of magnesium is preferable to the pure earth; as the latter sometimes gives a brownish color to the liquid, and requires to be used in larger proportion. But both these substances are dissolved in minute quantities, and are apt to occasion a slight flocculent precipitate. They may also possibly prove injurious by decomposing certain substances given in very small doses, as salts of the alkaloids, bichloride of mercury, and nitrate of silver. The object of the magnesia or its carbonate is simply to enable the oil to be brought to a state of minute division, and thus presented with a larger surface to the action of the solvent. Precipitated phosphate of calcium has been used as a substitute for carbonate of magnesium, but this has been shown to be slightly soluble in water and also objectionable. W. S. Thompson, of Washington, D.C., suggests the use of absorbent cotton as being free from all of these objections, and his views have been substantially adopted by the Committee of Revision of the present Pharmacopœia. Mr. E. V. Zoeller proposes to use a hand cotton-card to aid in pulling the filaments of cotton apart when a large quantity of medicated water is needed. (*New Rem.*, 1883, p. 56.) A very good way to make medicated waters when a volatile oil is directed, is that proposed by Percival, which is to heat the water required, pour it in a bottle and add the oil, cork tightly, shake occasionally until cool, then pour off and filter; this secures a medicated water free from foreign substances, and a saturated solution; most oils being more soluble in hot than in cold water. According to Mr. Robert Warington, this object may be better accomplished by porcelain clay, finely powdered glass, or pumice stone, which are wholly insoluble; and the London College employed finely powdered silica for the purpose. Talcum or soapstone in powder, purified by washing with diluted hydrochloric acid, has been adopted by the Committee on National Formulary (1888). (See *Talcum Purificatum*, Part II.; also paper recommending it by Prof. Curtman. *Proc. A. P. A.*, 1887.) The *Dublin College* prepared its Waters by agitating an alcoholic solution of the oil with distilled water, and filtering. They consequently contained alcohol, and were liable to the objection, already mentioned, against the medicated waters thus impregnated. They were, besides, feeble in the properties of their respective oils. In the preparation of the aromatic waters by these processes, it is very important that the water should be pure. The presence of a sulphate causes a decomposition of the oil, resulting in the production of sulphuretted hydrogen and a carbonate; and the aromatic properties are quite lost. (See *A. J. P.*, xix. 303.) Hence the propriety of the officinal direction to employ distilled water.*

The Distilled Waters are liable to contain various metallic impurities, derived from the vessels in which they are prepared or preserved. The metallic salts which have been found in them are those of iron, zinc, copper, and lead. With ferrocyanide of potassium, iron will give a blue color, zinc and lead white precipitates, and copper a rose color followed by chestnut brown. Sulphide of sodium causes with the salts of iron, copper, and lead, a brown discoloration more or less deep, followed by precipitates varying from brown to black; with those of zinc, a white precipitate. The Distilled Waters may be freed from these impurities by animal charcoal, previously well purified. The charcoal should be strongly shaken, eight or ten times in the course of a day, with the impure Water, which should then be allowed to rest, and the next day be filtered. Five grains of the charcoal will be sufficient for a gallon of the Distilled Water. (*Journ. de Pharm.*, Nov. 1862, p. 416.) The volatile oils may be recovered from the Waters containing them, or at least may be transferred to a spirituous menstruum, by mixing olive oil with the water, adding a little solution of potassa so as to form a soap, and a consequent emulsion with the liquid, and then neutralizing by an acid. The fixed oil will rise to the surface,

* Mr. Haselden prefers the process of distillation from the aromatic itself in the instances of dill, caraway, fennel, cinnamon, and pimento, which are not apt to afford to the distilled water such matter as may cause it to become sour; but he prefers trituration for peppermint, spearmint, and pennyroyal waters. He advises, however, that these waters should not be filtered, but prepared in quantity, allowed to settle, and drawn off as wanted. (*P. J. Tr.*, xvi. 14, 15.)

bringing the volatile oil along with it. The latter may then be separated from the former by agitation with alcohol. (T. B. Groves, *P. J. Tr.*, Feb. 1864.)

AQUA. *U. S.*, *Br.* *Water.*

H_2O; 18. (Ā-QUA—ă'kwa.) HO; 9.

"Natural water in its purest attainable state." *U. S.* "Natural water, the purest that can be obtained, cleared, if necessary, by filtration." *Br.*

Aqua communis, *P.G.*; Ὕδωρ, *Gr.*; Eau, *Fr.*; Wasser, *G.*; Acqua, *It.*; Agua, *Sp.*

Water has always been included in the U. S. Pharmacopœia, on account of its great importance as a medical and pharmaceutical agent. It was not admitted into the officinal lists of the British Pharmacopœias until 1839, when it was first recognized by the Edinburgh College. It is more or less concerned in almost all the changes which take place in inorganic matter, and is essential to the growth and existence of living beings, whether animal or vegetable. In treating of a substance of such diversified agency, our limits will allow of a sketch only of its properties and modifications. We shall speak of it under the several heads of *pure water*, *common water*, and *mineral waters*.

PURE WATER. Water, in a pure state, is a transparent liquid, without color, taste, or smell. Its sp. gr. is assumed to be unity, and forms the term of comparison for that of solids and liquids. A cubic inch of it, at the temp. of 15·5° C. (60° F.), weighs very nearly 252·5 grains. In the metric system the weight of 1 C.c. of distilled water taken at 4° C. (39·2° F.) is made equal to 1 gramme, the unit of weight in this system. It is compressible to a small extent, as was proved first by Canton, and afterwards, in an incontestable manner, by Perkins. Reduced in temp. to 0° C. (32° F.), it becomes a solid or ice, with the sp. gr. 0·9175 (Dufour, *Comptes-Rendus*, Juin, 1860); and raised to 100° C. (212° F.), an elastic fluid called steam. In the latter state its bulk is increased nearly 1700 fold, and its sp. gr. so far lessened as not to be much more than half that of atmospheric air. At the temp. of 4° C., or 39·2° F., its density is at the maximum; and consequently, setting out from that point, it is increased in bulk by being either heated or cooled. It has the power of dissolving more or less of all gases, including common air, the constituents of which are always present in natural water. It uniformly exists in the atmosphere, in the form of invisible vapor, even in the driest weather.

Water consists of two atoms of hydrogen 2, and one of oxygen 16 = 18; or, in volumes, of two volumes of hydrogen and one volume of oxygen condensed into two volumes of aqueous vapor or steam. On these data, it is easy to calculate the sp. gr. of steam; which will be 0·0693 (sp. gr. of hydrogen) + 0·5528 (half the sp. gr. of oxygen) = 0·6221.

COMMON WATER. By reason of its extensive solvent powers, water, in its natural state, must be more or less contaminated with foreign matter. Thus, it becomes variously impregnated, according to the nature of the strata through which it percolates. When the foreign substances present are in so small an amount as not materially to alter its taste and other sensible qualities, it constitutes the different varieties of *common water*.

There are almost innumerable shades of difference in common water, as obtained from different localities and sources; but all its varieties may be conveniently arranged under the two heads of soft and hard. A *soft water* is one which contains but inconsiderable impurities, and which, when used in washing, forms a lather with soap. By a *hard water* is understood a variety of water which contains calcareous or magnesian salts, or other impurities, through which it curdles soap, and is unfit for domestic purposes. Tincture of soap is a convenient test for ascertaining the quality of water. In distilled water it produces no effect; in soft water, only a slight opalescence; but in hard water, a milky appearance. The milkiness is due to the formation of an insoluble compound between the fatty acids of the soap and the lime or magnesia of the foreign salt.

The most usual foreign substances in common water, besides oxygen and nitrogen, and matters held in a state of mechanical suspension, are carbonic acid, sulphate and carbonate of calcium, and chloride of sodium (common salt). Carbonic acid is detected by lime-water, which produces a precipitate before the water is boiled, but not afterwards, as ebullition drives off this acid. The presence of sulphate of calcium is shown by precipitates being produced by nitrate of barium, and, after ebullition, by oxalate of ammonium. The former test shows the presence of sulphuric acid, and the latter, after boiling the water, indicates lime not held in solution by carbonic acid. Carbonate of calcium, when held in solution by an excess of carbonic acid, may be detected by boiling the water, which causes it to precipitate; but, even after ebullition and filtration, the water will retain enough carbonate of calcium to give a precipitate with acetate of lead; carbonate of calcium being itself to a minute extent soluble in water. Nitrate of silver will produce a precipitate, if any soluble chloride be present; and, ordinarily, the one present may be assumed to be common salt. Arsenic in minute quantity has been found in water used as drink. At Whitbeck, in Cumberland, England, the inhabitants employ, both as drink and for culinary purposes, a water holding enough arsenic in solution to be quite sensible to tests, without any known injurious consequence. (*Chem. News*, 1860, p. 128.)

Dr. Clark has proposed to purify hard water, when the hardness arises from bicarbonate of calcium, by a process which he calls *liming*. This consists in adding to the water sufficient lime-water to convert the bicarbonate into the very sparingly soluble carbonate. This procedure renders the water soft, and gets rid of all the lime, except that in the minute portion of carbonate dissolved. The merit of this process consists chiefly, not in the removal of lime, but in preventing the formation of organic matters, principally confervæ, the decomposition of which renders the water offensive and unwholesome. Dr. Clark's process has been for some time in successful operation on the water obtained by boring, at the Plumstead water-works, near Woolwich. (*P. J. Tr.*, June, 1856.) River water containing the usual amount of calcareous matter, if allowed to stagnate in open reservoirs, in the summer, will become contaminated with myriads of microscopic plants and animals. This change is prevented, according to Dr. Clark, by his peculiar treatment, which deprives the living organism of the nutriment, derived from loosely combined carbonic acid.

The oxygen and nitrogen present in natural waters are not usually in the same proportion as in atmospheric air; the oxygen in atmospheric air amounting to about 20 per cent. in volume, while the usual gaseous mixture, expelled from fresh water by boiling, contains 32 per cent. (See table on page 222.)

Common water is also divided into varieties according to its source. Thus, we have rain, snow, spring, river, well, lake, and marsh water.

Rain and *snow water* are the purest kinds of natural water. Rain water, to be obtained as pure as possible, must be collected in large vessels in the open fields, at a distance from houses, and some time after the rain has commenced falling; otherwise it will be contaminated with the dust which floats in the atmosphere, and with other impurities derived from roofs. The rain water of large cities contains nitrogenized organic matter, as shown by the odor produced by burning the residue left after the water has been evaporated.

Rain water ordinarily contains atmospheric air, and, according to Liebig, a little nitric acid, the amount of which is increased when the rain descends during a storm. M. Chabrier states as the result of his observations, that rain water contains either nitrous or nitric acid, the one or the other predominating according to the condition of the weather; the nitrous acid being relatively in excess in mild weather, but the nitric when the rain is attended with tempestuous winds. (*Journ. de Pharm.*, Janv. 1872, p. 42.) According to an analysis, made by M. Martin, of rain water which fell at Marseilles during a violent storm, 1000 parts by weight contained 0·004 of chlorine and 0·003 of ammonia. Not a trace of iodine or of nitric acid was discovered. Boussingault has ascertained that the rain which falls in towns contains considerably more ammonia than that which falls in the country. Thus the rain of Paris was found by him to contain three or four parts of ammonia per million; while that collected in a mountainous region, contained about four-fifths of one part only in a million. The average results of Mr. J. B. Lawes and Dr. J. H. Gilbert give one part of ammonia to the million of rain water. Snow water has a peculiar taste, which was supposed to depend on the presence of air more oxygenated than that of the atmosphere; but in point of fact it contains no air, and this accounts for its vapid taste. Rain and snow water is sufficiently pure for most chemical operations.

Spring water (*aqua fontana*) depends entirely for its quality on the strata through which it flows; being purest when it passes through sand or gravel, or where the prevailing rock formation is granitic. On the contrary, where the formation is limestone, the water will, because of the carbonic acid gas dissolved in it, take up the carbonate of lime and become what is called a *hard water*. It almost always contains a trace of common salt, and generally other impurities, which vary according to the locality of the spring.

River water (*aqua fluvialis*) is, generally speaking, less impregnated with saline matter than spring water, because made up in considerable part of rains; while its volume bears a larger proportion to the surface of its bed. It is, however, much more apt to have mechanically suspended in it insoluble matters, of an earthy nature, like clay and silt, which impair its transparency. It is frequently rendered more sightly by being run through porous stone, carbon, or sand filter. The coarse particles are by this filtration removed; but any sewage or other very finely divided organic material is not removed, so that such clean filtered water may be a very deadly poison. Water may be purified for manufacturing purposes by what is termed the alum process,—*i.e.*, by adding 2 grains of alum to a gallon of water, and permitting the impurities to subside for 48 hours. (*Chem. News*, July 23, 1886.)

Well water, like that from springs, is liable to contain various impurities. As a general rule, the purity of the water of a well will be in proportion to its depth and the constancy with which it is used. Well water in large cities always contains a large amount of impurity, both organic and inorganic, the result of sewage contamination. Dr. R. D. Thomson found 147·6 grs., per Imperial gallon, of impurity in a well in London. (*P. J. Tr.*, 1856, p. 27.) The presence of nitrates in water prevents the formation of organic beings, even after it has been long kept. *Artesian* or *overflowing wells*, from their great depth, generally afford a pure water.

Lake water cannot be characterized as having any invariable qualities. The water of most of the lakes in the United States is pure and wholesome.

Marsh water is generally stagnant, and contains vegetable remains undergoing decomposition. It is unwholesome, and ought never to be used internally.

All water which is exposed to the air dissolves a quantity of oxygen and nitrogen, which is determined by the laws of gaseous absorption. It is indeed upon this dissolved oxygen that the life of water-breathing animals depends. In every pure water the proportion between the dissolved nitrogen and oxygen is found to be constant, and it is represented by the following numbers:—oxygen 34·91, and nitrogen 65·09 per cent.: 1000 C.c. of pure water, such as rain water, when saturated dissolves 17·95 C.c. of air. If the water be rendered impure by the introduction of organic matter undergoing oxidation, the proportion between the dissolved oxygen and nitrogen becomes different, owing to the oxygen having been partly or wholly used for the oxidation of this material. This is clearly shown in the following analysis made by Miller of the dissolved gases contained in Thames water collected at various points above and below London.

	Thames water taken at					
	Kingston.	Hammersmith.	Somerset House.	Greenwich.	Woolwich.	Erith.
Total volume of gas per litre..........	C.c. 52·7	C.c.	C.c. 62·9	C.c. 71·25	C.c. 63·05	C.c. 74·3
Carbon dioxide..........................	30·3	......	45·2	55·6	48·3	57·
Oxygen..................................	7·4	4·1	1·5	0·25	0·25	1·8
Nitrogen	15·0	15·1	16·2	15·4	14·5	15·5
Ratio of oxygen to nitrogen............	1:2	1:3·7	1:10·5	1:60	1:52	1:8·1

This table shows that whereas the pure water at Kingston contains the normal quantity of dissolved oxygen, the ratio of nitrogen to oxygen increases in a very rapid rate as the river water becomes contaminated with London sewage, but that this ratio again shows signs of a return to the normal at Erith.

Hence it is clear that an analysis of the gases dissolved in water may prove of much help in ascertaining whether the water is pure or whether it has been contaminated with putrescent organic matter. Indeed, Miller concludes that whenever the proportion between dissolved oxygen and nitrogen rises to more than 1 to 2 the water is unfit for drinking purposes. (Roscoe and Schorlemmer, *Treatise on Chem.*, i. 245.)

The second class of dissolved impurities are inorganic salts, even rain water washing some of these out of the atmosphere. It invariably contains ammoniacal salts, chloride of sodium, and various organic germs. In towns the rain water also contains a larger proportion of nitrates than that falling in the country. It is, however, the spring waters especially which contain the largest amount of mineral matter in solution. The salts which most commonly occur in solution in spring water are: (1) The carbonates of calcium, magnesium, iron, and manganese, dissolved in an excess of carbonic acid. (2) The sulphates of calcium and magnesium; (3) Alkaline carbonates, chlorides, sulphates, nitrates, or silicates.

Spring waters which issue from considerable depths, or which originate in volcanic districts, are always hotter than the mean annual temperature of the locality where they come to the surface.

The term *Aqua*, in the U. S. and Br. Pharmacopœias, may be considered as designating any natural water of good quality which answers well for cooking, and does not curdle soap. Upon the addition of nitrate of barium, nitrate of silver, or oxalate of ammonium, its transparency is but slightly affected; and, upon being evaporated to dryness, it leaves but an inconsiderable residue.

"A colorless, limpid liquid, without odor and taste at ordinary temperatures, and remaining odorless while being heated to boiling, of a perfectly neutral reaction, and containing not more than 1 part of fixed impurities in 10,000 parts.

"The transparency or color of Water should not be affected by hydrosulphuric acid or sulphide of ammonium (abs. of metallic impurities). On heating 100 C.c. of Water, acidulated with 10 C.c. of diluted sulphuric acid, to boiling, and adding enough of a dilute solution of permanganate of potassium (1 in 1000) to impart to the liquid a decided rose-red tint, this tint should not be entirely destroyed by boiling for five minutes (abs. of more than traces of organic or other oxidizable matters)." *U. S.*

The British Pharmacopœia has the following description. "Natural water, the purest that can be obtained, cleared, if necessary, by filtration; free from odor, unusual taste, and visible impurity. To be used whenever 'Water' is ordered in the British Pharmacopœia. In dispensing prescriptions, *aqua* should be understood to mean distilled water." *Br.*

Water should never be kept in leaden cisterns, on account of the risk of its dissolving a small portion of lead. This risk is greater in proportion to the softness and purity of the water; for it is found that the presence of a minute proportion of saline matter, as for example of sulphate of calcium, protects the water from the slightest metallic impregnation. The chlorides are not protective; as they give rise to chloride of lead, which is slightly soluble. The protection has been ascribed to an insoluble film on the surface of the lead, formed by the decomposition of the saline matter. Upon this principle is based a plan of protection by Dr. Schwartz, of Breslau, who proposes to fill leaden pipes through which water is conducted with a strong solution of an alkaline sulphide, which forms a perfectly insoluble coating of sulphide (sulphuret) of lead, said to be quite impermeable by the water afterwards introduced. (*Chem. News*, Sept. 26, 1863, p. 157.) A coating of zinc has been employed for protecting the surface of iron pipes and reservoirs against the action of water, but has failed. Experiment has shown that the water becomes impregnated with the salts of both metals. (*Ibid.*, April 5, 1862, p. 188.)* Mr. A. Wynter Blyth pro-

* Experiments by M. Roux, pharmaceutist of the marine at Rochefort, made by order of the naval authorities, have satisfactorily shown that reservoirs of iron coated with zinc are attacked with great facility by water contained in them, which becomes more or less impregnated with both

poses a new and simple test for lead in drinking water. A solution of cochineal is made by boiling cochineal in water, filtering, and adding a little alcohol to preserve it. A few drops of this solution are added to the water, which, if acid, must be rendered neutral by a trace of alkali; if lead be present, even in the proportion of one-tenth of a grain in a gallon of water, a mauve-blue color will develop, its depth depending upon the quantity of lead in the water. (*Amer. Drugg.*, 1884, p. 93, from *The Analyst.*)

A very important class of dissolved impurities is made up of organic compounds. This organic matter may be derived from a vegetable source, such as leaf-mould and the decomposition products of wood, in which case it is practically harmless, or it may be derived from animal sources, in which case it almost always proves a serious impurity.

The careful observations of students of public health leave no doubt that a number of epidemic diseases, especially cholera and typhoid fever, are often contracted and spread by means of drinking water, contaminated with germs of disease from excreta and general sewage. This impure water may be clear and may have filtered through considerable distances of soil, and yet may contain these poisonous germs. Now nitrogen is one of the characteristic constituents of animal matter as contrasted with vegetable matter, relatively few forms of which contain it, and those are of a character not likely to be found in natural waters. Hence, if water should be impregnated with animal matter, this would be indicated by the presence of nitrogen in solution, either in the form of albumen or albuminous matter, if the animal matter in the water is still unchanged, or, if the animal matter has undergone oxidation, in the form of ammonia or nitrous or nitric acid.

There is, therefore, to be determined in the examination of a water with reference to this presence of organic nitrogenous matter, (1) the ammonia, (2) the unchanged albuminous matter, which, as it is changed into and determined as ammonia, is called "albuminoid ammonia," (3) the nitrates and nitrites present.

The ammonia is first determined by distilling the water made alkaline with carbonate of sodium as long as the distillate carries enough ammonia to be recognized by *Nessler's solution.** For this purpose the distillate is collected successively in volumes of 50 C.c. and the amount of ammonia in each of these separate distillates determined. The smallest quantity of ammonia will produce a yellow color, the tint of which is to be compared with that obtained from the Nessler solution treated with a standard sal ammoniac solution.

After the free ammonia has been distilled off, a solution of caustic soda and permanganate of potash is added and the distillation is continued. Another portion of ammonia now comes off, owing to the action of the permanganate on the nitrogenous organic matter. The amount of ammonia thus obtained is determined and is tabulated as "albuminoid ammonia," because albumen is one of the bodies which is decomposed in this way.

Instead of this method proposed by Wanklyn and Chapman, another process described by Frankland and Armstrong is often used. In this case, the water having been evaporated, the dry residue is submitted to an organic combustion analysis, which gives the "organic nitrogen" and the "organic carbon," and the ratio of these gives an indication as to the presence of albuminous matter rich in nitrogen. If the amount of albuminoid nitrogen indicated by either of these processes exceed 0·15 parts for one million of water, the latter should be rejected as a drinking water. In some large towns, however, the surface well waters have shown albu-

metals in the state of oxides and salts, and especially with those of zinc, to such a degree as to render such vessels improper as recipients of water for drinking. Of the different kinds of water tried, distilled water deprived as far as possible of atmospheric air produced least effect; next in degree of action was spring water; still more energetic was distilled water containing carbonic acid furnished by the earthy bicarbonates of the water submitted to distillation; and more powerful than all was river water containing common salt. (*Journ. de Pharm. et Chim.*, 4e sér., i. 99.)

* This solution is prepared as follows. 35 Gm. of potassium iodide and 13 Gm. of mercuric chloride (corrosive sublimate) are dissolved in about 800 C.c. of hot water, and then a saturated solution of mercuric chloride is gradually added until the precipitate formed ceases to redissolve. 100 Gm. of caustic potash are then dissolved in the liquid, and the cold solution is diluted to one litre and is allowed to deposit any undissolved matter.

minoid nitrogen to the amount of 0·3 to 0·8 parts per million. Such waters are little better than sewage. The free ammonia, moreover, should not exceed 0·08 parts per million, or the water must be considered as containing sewage contamination.

The nitrates and nitrites present can be estimated in another portion of the water by reducing these acids to ammonia by means of the hydrogen evolved from aluminium or zinc-dust in presence of caustic alkalies.

The determination of chlorine is also frequently of great importance, for although mineral waters may be rich in chlorides, ordinary well waters or river waters, which are the chief sources of supply, will not contain much chlorine unless they have been contaminated. Both urine and sewage may contribute this chlorine, as they are highly charged with common salt. As a rule it may be said that water containing more than two grains of chlorine per gallon must be looked upon with suspicion, unless some good reason for the presence of common salt can be assigned.

The following table shows the relative purity of the water-supply of several American cities, as determined by Prof. A. R. Leeds in 1881:

Parts in 100,000.	New York.	Brooklyn.	Jersey City.	Philadelphia.	Boston.	Washington.	Rochester.	Cincinnati.
Free ammonia	0·0027	0·00075	0·00475	0·001	0·01325	0·006	0·0114	0·0115
Albuminoid ammonia	0·027	0·00825	0·0427	0·018	0·0605	0·027	0·023	0·024
Oxygen required	0·81	0·413	0·95	0·46	1·77	0·600	0·790	0·860
Nitrites	None.	None.	None.	None.	None.	None.	None.	None.
Nitrates	0·8325	1·2025	0·9066	0·6845	1·2395	0·8325	0·629	0·740
Chlorine	0·350	0·550	0·235	0·300	0·315	0·270	0·195	0·805
Total hardness	3·300	2·270	3·200	4·400	2·100	4·800	5·500	6·400
Total solids	11·800	6·000	9·300	14·300	8·500	11·500	10·000	16·000
Mineral matter	5·000	5·000	3·400	6·00	2·000	5·500	4·000	9·000
Organic and volatile matter	6·800	1·000	5·900	8·300	6·500	6·000	6·000	7·200

MINERAL WATERS. When natural spring waters are so far impregnated with foreign substances as to have a decided taste, and a peculiar operation on the economy, they are called *mineral waters*. These are conveniently arranged under the heads of *carbonated*, *alkaline*, *sulphuretted*, *saline* (including *magnesian*, *chalybeate*, and *chlorinated*), and *silicious*.

1. *Carbonated waters* are cold, and are characterized by containing an excess of carbonic acid, which gives them a sparkling appearance, and the power of reddening litmus paper. These waters frequently contain the carbonates of calcium, magnesium, and iron, which are held in solution by the excess of carbonic acid. The waters of Seltzer, Spa, Apollinaris, and Pyrmont in Europe, and of the sweet springs in Virginia, belong to this class. For Artificial Carbonic Acid Water, see page 227.)

2. *Alkaline waters* contain a larger quantity of bicarbonate of sodium, as well as common salt and Glauber's salt. These are sometimes warm, such as the springs at Ems and Vichy, but generally cold. The Gettysburg spring water is of this class.

3. *Sulphuretted waters* are such as contain sulphuretted hydrogen, and are distinguished by the peculiar fetid smell of that gas, and by yielding a brown precipitate with the salts of lead or silver. Examples of this kind are the waters of Aix la Chapelle and Harrogate in Europe, and those of the white, red, and salt sulphur springs in Virginia.

4. *Saline waters* are those, the predominant properties of which depend upon saline impregnation. The salts most usually present are the sulphates and carbonates of sodium, calcium, and magnesium, in which latter case the name *magnesian* is given to them; the presence of the chlorides of these alkalies giving the class *chlorinated* waters, which reach their maximum concentration in sea waters; whilst the presence of ferrous salts makes another class, the *chalybeate*. Among magnesian waters may be mentioned those of Friedrichshall, Hunyádi Janos, and Epsom; among chalybeate waters, those of Tunbridge and Brighton in England, of Pyrmont, Wiesbaden, and Spa on the continent, and of Bedford, Pittsburg, and Brandywine in the United States. Potassa is occasionally present, and lithia has been detected by Berzelius in Carlsbad, and other salt springs of Germany, and is also found in some American spring waters. Cæsia and rubidia have also been detected in certain

mineral waters, such as the Dürkheim and Baden-Baden waters, in the former of which these elements were first discovered by Bunsen. Bromine is found in the saline at Theodorshalle, in Germany, as also in the salt wells of Western Pennsylvania, Ohio, and West Virginia. The mineral springs at Saratoga contain a small proportion of iodine and bromine. The principal saline waters are those of Seidlitz in Bohemia, Cheltenham and Bath in England, and Harrodsburg and Saratoga in the United States.

5. *Silicious waters* are those in which the saline contents consist chiefly of alkaline silicates, such as the hot spring waters of Iceland and the geysers of Fire-hole Basin and Gardiner's River, Yellowstone National Park, U. S.

Sea Water. English Channel. In a thousand grains. Water 964·744 grs.; chloride of sodium 27·059; chloride of potassium 0·765; chloride of magnesium 3·667; bromide of magnesium 0·029; sulphate of magnesium 2·296; sulphate of calcium 1·407; carbonate of calcium 0·033. Total 1000 grs. (*Schweitzer.*) The proportion of chloride of sodium is from 36 to 37 parts in 1000 in the ocean, at a distance from land. Its amount is small in the interior of the Baltic. It is perceived that bromine is present in very minute amount; 100 pounds of sea water yielding only 3½ grs. of this element. According to Balard, iodine exists in the water of the Mediterranean; but it has not been detected in the water of the ocean, the bromine being supposed to mask its presence. Beside these ingredients, others are alleged to exist in minute proportion in sea water; as fluorine by Dr. G. Wilson; lead, copper, and silver by MM. Malaguti, Durocher, and Sarzeau; and iron and manganese by M. Usiglio. Anterior to Wilson's researches, Mr. Middleton and Prof. Silliman, jun., had inferred the existence of fluorine in sea water, from its presence in marine animals. The lead and copper above mentioned were found in certain fuci only; the silver in the sea water itself. The presence of silver in sea water has been rendered probable by Mr. F. Field, by a comparative analysis of the same copper sheathing, when new, and after having been on a vessel for many years. The old sheathing was always found to contain more silver than the new (*Chem. Gaz.*, March 2, 1857); and the observations of Mr. Field have been subsequently confirmed by others. Schweitzer's analysis gives a small proportion of carbonate of calcium; but Bibra could not detect any. Dr. John Davy's examinations of sea water show that carbonate of calcium does not exist at a great distance from land, except in very minute proportion, but becomes quite evident at a distance of from fifty to a hundred miles from coasts. Boric acid has been found by Mr. Veatch in the sea water on the coast of California. (See *A. J. P.*, 1860, p. 330.)*

Sea water, filtered, and charged with five times its volume of carbonic acid, forms, according to Pasquier, a gentle purgative, which keeps very well, and is not disagreeable to take. The dose is from half a pint to a pint.

By freezing, sea water is almost entirely freed from saline matter, the ice being nearly pure water. It is obvious that the unfrozen water contains much more than its ordinary proportion of salts; and this is one of the methods of concentrating this and other saline solutions.

Medical Properties of Water. Water is a remedy of great importance. When

* The following analysis of sea water, taken at 2 leagues from Fécamp, on the coast of France, merits special notice from the care with which it was made, and the large quantity operated on. The sp. gr. was 1·026, at 57° F.

Gaseous Contents.	*In one kilog.* litres.	*In one litre.* litres.
Atmospheric air	0·0120	0·0123
Free carbonic acid	traces	traces
" sulphydric acid	traces	traces
Solid Contents.	grs.	grs.
Chloride of potassium	0·09763	0·10019
" sodium	26·09300	26·78913
" lithium	0·00042	0·00043
" ammonium	0·00178	0·00183
" magnesium	3·19300	3·27700
Iodide of sodium	0·00920	0·00944
Bromide of sodium	0·10605	0·10882
" magnesium	0·03084	0·03163
Sulphate of calcium	0·90170	0·92540
" potassium	0·00919	0·00943

Solid Contents.	*In one kilog.* grs.	*In one litre.* grs.
Sulphate of sodium	2·57250	2·64012
" magnesium	0·32736	0·33597
Phosphate of magnesium	0·00046	0·00047
" (ammoniaco-magnesian)	signs	signs
Carbonate of calcium	0·13600	·13959
" magnesium	traces	traces
" iron	0·00021	0·00021
" manganese	signs	signs
Silicic acid	0·01420	0·01457
Organic matter	signs	signs.
Pure water	966·50046	991·91577
Total	1000·00000	1026·3000[illegible]

(*Journ. de Pharm. et de Chim.*, 4e sér., i. 381, 1865.)

taken into the stomach, it acts by its temperature, by its bulk, and by being absorbed. When of the temperature of about 15·5° C. (60° F.), it gives no positive sensation either of heat or cold; between 15·5° C. (60° F.) and 7·2° C. (45° F.), it creates a cool sensation; and below 7·2° C. (45° F.), a decidedly cold one. Between 15·5° C. (60° F.) and 37·7° C. (100° F.), it relaxes the fibres of the stomach, and is apt to produce nausea, particularly if the effect of bulk be added to that of temperature. By its bulk and solvent powers, it allays irritation by diluting the acrid contents of the stomach and bowels, and favoring their final expulsion; and by its absorption, it promotes the secretion of urine and cutaneous transpiration.

Water, externally applied as a bath, is also an important remedy. It may act by its own specific effect as a liquid, or as a means of modifying the heat of the body. It acts in the latter way differently, according to the temperature at which it may be applied. When this is above 36·1° C. (97° F.), it constitutes the vapor or hot bath; when between 36·1° C. (97° F.) and 29·4° C. (85° F.), the warm bath; between 29·4° C. (85° F.) and 18·3° C. (65° F.), the tepid bath; and between 18·3° C. (65° F.) and 0° C. (32° F.), the cold bath.

The general action of the *vapor bath* is to accelerate the circulation, and produce profuse sweating. It acts locally on the skin, by softening and relaxing its texture. In stiffness of the joints, and in various diseases of the skin, it has often proved beneficial.

The *hot bath*, like the vapor bath, is decidedly stimulant. By its use the pulse becomes full and frequent, the veins turgid, the face flushed, the skin red, and the respiration quickened. If the temperature be high, and the constitution peculiar, its use is not without danger; as it is apt to produce a feeling of suffocation, violent throbbing in the temples, and vertigo with tendency to apoplexy. When it acts favorably, it produces profuse perspiration.

The *warm bath*, though below the animal heat, nevertheless produces a sensation of warmth; as its temperature is above that of the surface. It diminishes the frequency of the pulse, renders the respiration slower, lessens the heat of the body, and relaxes the skin. It cannot, therefore, be deemed a stimulant. By relieving certain diseased actions and states, accompanied by morbid irritability, it often acts as a soothing remedy, producing a disposition to sleep. It is proper in febrile exanthematous diseases, in which the pulse is frequent, the skin hot and dry, and the general condition characterized by restlessness. It is contraindicated in diseases of the head and chest.

The *tepid bath* is not calculated to have much modifying influence on the heat of the body. Its peculiar effects are to soften and cleanse the skin, and to promote insensible perspiration.

The *cold bath* acts differently according to its temperature and manner of application, and the condition of the system to which it is applied. When of low temperature and suddenly applied, it acts primarily as a stimulant, by the sudden and rapid manner in which the heat is abstracted; next as a tonic, by condensing the living fibres; and finally as a sedative. It is often useful in diseases of relaxation and debility, when practised by affusion or plunging. But it is essential to its efficacy and safety, that the stock of vitality should be sufficient to create, immediately after its use, those feelings of warmth and invigoration, included under the term reaction. In febrile diseases the use of the cold bath, as advocated by Currie, has been recently viewed with much success. For a discussion of this practice the reader is referred to the last edition of H. C. Wood's Treatise on Therapeutics.

Cold water is frequently applied as a sedative in local inflammations, and as a means of restraining hemorrhage. Its use, however, is scarcely admissible in inflammations of the chest.

Pharm. Uses. Water is used in a vast number of preparations, either as a menstruum, or as a means for promoting chemical action by its solvent power.

Off. Prep. Aqua Destillata.

CARBONIC ACID WATER, or *Soda Water* (so called), (*Aqua acidula simplicior*, F. P.; *Eau gazeuse simple*, Fr.; *Kohlensäure-Wasser*, G.), which was formerly officinal in the U. S. Pharmacopœia, consists of water highly charged with carbonic acid. Water is found to take up its volume of this gas under the pressure of the atmosphere; and Dr. Henry ascertained that precisely the same *volume* of the compressed gas is absorbed under a higher pressure. From this law, the bulk taken up is constant, the quantity being different in proportion as there is more or less driven into a given space. As the space occupied by a gas is inversely as the compressing force, it follows that the quantity of the acid forced into the water will be directly as the pressure. From the principles above laid down it follows that, to saturate water with five times its volume of carbonic acid, as directed in the formula, it must be subjected to a pressure of five atmospheres. Carbonic acid gas compressed into the liquid state is now supplied by the "American Carbonate Co." of New York, and its agencies, in wrought-iron cylinders, which contain either 10 or 20 pounds of compressed gas, equal to 600 or 1200 gallons of gas at normal pressure. This allows of convenient transportation, and guarantees the purity of the gas.

Carbonic acid water is familiarly called in this country "*mineral water*," and "*soda water;*" the latter name, originally applied to the preparation when it contained carbonate of sodium, being from habit continued since the alkali has been omitted.

Carbonic acid water is dispensed in most of the pharmacies in this country. The fountain is usually placed in the cellar, and the tube proceeding from the fountain is made to pass through the floor and counter of the store, and to terminate in a draught tube, by means of which the carbonic acid water may be drawn off at pleasure. In order to have the liquid cool, the tube from the cellar generally terminates in a strong metallic vessel of convenient shape, or a series of block tin pipes called coolers, placed inside the counter apparatus, and surrounded with ice. For some practical suggestions upon the making of carbonic acid water and use of apparatus, see *N. R.*, June, July, August, 1877.

Properties. Carbonic acid water is a sparkling liquid, possessing an agreeable pungent, acidulous taste. It reddens litmus deeply from its state of concentration, and is precipitated by lime-water. Being impregnated with a large quantity of the acid gas under the influence of pressure, it effervesces strongly when freed from restraint. Hence, to preserve its briskness, it should be kept in strong well-corked bottles, placed inverted in a cool place. Several natural waters are of a similar nature; such as those of Seltzer, Spa, Pyrmont, Apollinaris, etc.; but the artificial water has the advantage of a stronger impregnation with the acid gas. Carbonic acid water should be made with every precaution to avoid metallic impurity. Hence the necessity of having the fountain well tinned on the inner surface. Even with this precaution, a slight metallic impregnation is not always avoided, especially in the winter season, when the water is less consumed as a drink, and, therefore, allowed to remain longer in the tubes and stop-cocks. Iron fountains lined with a hard enamel are greatly to be preferred, but the best fountains are now made of cast steel, lined with block tin. When leaden tubes are employed to convey the water, it is liable to be contaminated with this metal, which renders it deleterious. A case of colica pictonum was treated by Dr. Geo. B. Wood, arising from the daily use of the first draught of carbonic acid water from a fountain furnished with tubes of lead. Tubes of pure tin are free from objection, and should be exclusively used.

Copper fountains, well tinned, are liable to the objections that the tin lining wears away by use, and that there is no convenient means of inspecting the interior, owing to the solder joint, which permanently unites the two sections of the fountain. To remove the latter objection, the improvement has been proposed by Dr. R. O. Doremus, of New York, of having the two sections with flanges, securely bolted together, with intervening gutta-percha packing, in order to furnish facilities for examining the interior, to determine whether re-tinning is necessary. Sometimes drops of solder and chips of copper are carelessly left in the fountain, and form an additional source of danger. There can be no doubt that carbonic acid water is not unfrequently rendered poisonous by metallic impregnation. Dr. Doremus has proved, by a chemical examination, that lead and copper are sometimes present. (*A. J. P.*, 1854, p. 422; from the *Am. Med. Monthly.*) Dr. John T. Plummer, of Richmond, Ind., has found lead. The latter metal is detected by sulphuretted hydrogen, which gives with it a black precipitate, and copper by ferrocyanide of potassium, which causes a brown precipitate. In testing for copper, a few drops of the reagent should be added to a glass of the suspected water, placed on a sheet of white paper, when, if even a minute proportion of copper be present, a brownish discoloration will be seen, upon looking down through the liquid.

Medical Properties and Uses. Carbonic acid water is a grateful drink to febrile patients, allaying thirst, lessening nausea and gastric distress, and promoting the secretion of urine. The quantity taken need only be regulated by the reasonable wishes of the patient. It also forms a very convenient vehicle for the administration of magnesia, the carbonated alkalies, sulphate of magnesium, and the saline cathartics generally; rendering these medicines less unpleasant to the palate, and, in irritable states of the stomach, increasing the chances of their being retained. When used for this purpose, six or eight fluidounces (178–236 C.c.) will be sufficient.

AMMONIA. *Ammonia.*

NH_3; 17. (AM-MŌ'NI-A.) NH_3; 17.

All the ammoniacal compounds owe their distinctive properties to the presence of a peculiar gaseous substance, composed of nitrogen and hydrogen, called *ammonia.* This is most easily obtained by the action of lime on chloride of ammonium or sal ammoniac: when the lime unites with the hydrochloric acid, so as to form chloride of calcium and water, and expels the ammonia. It is transparent and colorless, like common air, but possesses an acrid taste, and exceedingly pungent smell. It has a powerful alkaline reaction, and, from this property and its gaseous nature, was called the *volatile alkali* by the earlier chemists. Its sp. gr. is 0·59. It is irrespirable, the glottis closing spasmodically when the attempt is made to breathe it. It consists of one atom of nitrogen 14, and 3 of hydrogen $3 = 17$; or, in volumes, of one volume of nitrogen and three volumes of hydrogen, condensed into two. Its formula is NH_3.

As the gas ammonia exists in the free state, the molecule NH_3 is a definite saturated compound under ordinary conditions. When, however, ammonia gas is mixed with hydrochloric acid gas or its aqueous solution with hydrochloric acid in solution, the two unite to form a new compound, NH_4Cl, which proves to be a definite compound, analogous to potassium or sodium chlorides. Berzelius, therefore, proposed to call this the chloride of *ammonium*, assuming that the monad group $(NH_4)^I$ acted like the monad metal K^I—in forming compounds. And in fact we find that when sulphuric, nitric, carbonic, and other acids are neutralized by *ammonia* gas or solution we get crystallizable salts like $(NH_4)_2SO_4$, NH_4NO_3 and $(NH_4)_2CO_3$, which we therefore call *ammonium* sulphate, nitrate, and carbonate respectively. These are very similar to the corresponding potassium and sodium salts.

The atmosphere contains a minute proportion of ammonia, probably in the state of carbonate. The alkali is sometimes also found in snow. (A. Vogel, *Neues Repert. für Pharm.*, 1872, p. 327.)

Ozonized oxygen oxidizes the elements of ammonia, producing water and nitric acid, which latter, by uniting with undecomposed ammonia, generates nitrate of ammonium. Ordinary oxygen, under the influence of platinum-black, or finely divided copper, likewise oxidizes the elements of ammonia, the nitrogen to the extent only of forming nitrous acid, with the result of producing nitrite of ammonium.

AQUA AMMONIÆ. *U. S.* *Water of Ammonia.*

(Ā'QUA AM-MŌ'NI-Æ.)

"An aqueous solution of Ammonia [NH_3; 17—NH_3; 17], containing 10 per cent., by weight, of the gas." *U. S.* "Ammoniacal gas, NH_3, dissolved in water." *Br.*

Liquor Ammoniæ, *Br.*, Solution of Ammonia; Liquor Ammonii Caustici, *P.G.;* Spiritus Salis Ammoniaci Causticus, Ammonia Aqua Soluta; Ammoniaque liquide, Eau (Solution, Liqueur) d'Ammoniaque, *Fr.;* Salmiakgeist, Aetzammoniak, Ammoniak-Flüssigkeit, *G.*

The U. S. Pharmacopœia of 1880 omits a process for preparing Water of Ammonia. The U. S. P. 1870 contained an excellent process, which is appended.*

* "Take of Chloride of Ammonium, in small pieces, Lime, each, *twelve troyounces;* Water *six pints;* Distilled Water *a sufficient quantity.* Pour a pint of the Water upon the Lime, in a convenient vessel; and, after it has slaked, stir the mixture so as to bring it to the consistence of a smooth paste. Then add the remainder of the Water, and mix the whole thoroughly together.

"Take of Strong Solution of Ammonia *one pint* [Imperial measure]; Distilled Water *two pints* [Imp. meas.]. Mix, and preserve in a stoppered bottle. Sp. gr. 0·959." *Br.*

The title of this preparation was changed, at the revision of the U. S. Pharmacopœia in 1860, from Liquor Ammoniæ to Aqua Ammoniæ, that it might conform in name as well as character with the Waters, among which all the officinal preparations consisting of aqueous solutions of gaseous bodies are included.

The object of the process is to obtain a weak aqueous solution of the alkaline gas ammonia. In the U. S. P. 1870 process, the chloride of ammonium is decomposed by the superior affinity of the lime for its acid, ammonia is disengaged, and the lime, combining with the acid, forms chloride of calcium and water, $2NH_4Cl + Ca2HO = CaCl_2 + 2H_2O + 2NH_3$. The process differs from that of 1850 in introducing the materials into the retort with a large quantity of water, instead of in the dry state. In both cases the gas is driven over by heat, but in the moist plan is accompanied with more watery vapor than in the dry. If the object were to obtain the water of ammonia in the highest possible state of concentration, there might be some advantage in the dry method; but, as a weak solution is contemplated, the wet method is equally efficient, while in all respects it is more convenient, and productive of better results; for, according to Dr. Squibb, the water of ammonia made by the former officinal process has invariably an empyreumatic odor, from which that made by the present process is free. (*Proc. A. P. A.*, 1858, p. 407.) The receiver is intended to retain any water holding in solution undecomposed chloride, or the oily matter sometimes contained in the salt, as well as other impurities, which may be driven over by the heat while the pure gas passes forward into the bottle containing the distilled water, which should not fill it, on account of the increase in the bulk of the water during the absorption of the gas. The tube should extend to near the bottom of the bottle, and pass through a cork, loosely fitting its mouth. To prevent the regurgitation of the water from the bottle into the intermediate vessel, the latter should be furnished with a Welter's safety tube. Very large bottles are improper for keeping the water of ammonia; as, when they are partially empty, the atmospheric air within them may furnish a little carbonic acid to the ammonia.

In preparing solution of ammonia, equal weights of chloride of ammonium and lime are used for generating the gaseous ammonia. This proportion gives a great excess of lime, compared with the quantity required if determined by the molecular weights; but in practice it is found advantageous to have an excess, as well to insure the full decomposition of the chloride of ammonium, as to make up for accidental impurities in the lime.

The British Pharmacopœia gives directions for diluting *Liquor Ammoniæ Fortior*, so as to reduce it to the strength of *Liquor Ammoniæ*. This is effected by mixing one measure of their stronger preparation with two measures of distilled water. The ammonia water of commerce is known as "Aqua Ammoniæ F. F. F.," or "20° ammonia;" it may be diluted by adding 3 parts of water to 2 parts of 20° ammonia water to make officinal water of ammonia. Ammonia water of other strengths may be diluted by consulting the table given on page 231, and applying the rules given in *Remington's Practice of Pharmacy*, p. 82.

Properties. Water of ammonia is "a colorless, transparent liquid, of a very pungent odor, and acrid alkaline taste, and a strongly alkaline reaction. Sp. gr. is 0·959 at 15° C. (59° F.). It is completely volatilized by the heat of a water-bath. On bringing a glass rod dipped into hydrochloric acid near the liquid, dense, white fumes are evolved. On supersaturating Water of Ammonia with diluted sulphuric acid, no empyreumatic odor should be developed. Water of Ammonia

Decant the milky liquid from the gritty sediment into a glass retort, of the capacity of sixteen pints, and add the Chloride of Ammonium. Place the retort on a sand-bath, and adapt to it a receiver, previously connected with a two-pint bottle, by means of a glass tube, reaching nearly to the bottom of the bottle, and containing a pint of Distilled Water. Surround the bottle with ice-cold water; and apply heat, gradually increased, until ammonia ceases to come over. Remove the liquid from the bottle, and add to it sufficient Distilled Water to raise its specific gravity to 0·960. Lastly, keep the liquid in small bottles, well stopped." *U. S.*

should remain clear, or be at most only faintly clouded, when mixed with five times its volume of lime-water (only minute traces of carbonic acid). When supersaturated with nitric acid, the liquid should remain clear on the addition of test-solution of chloride of barium (sulphate) or of nitrate of silver (chloride). Either before or after neutralization with nitric acid, it should not be affected by hydrosulphuric acid (metallic impurities). Test-solution of oxalate of ammonia should produce no cloudiness (calcium). To neutralize 8·5 grammes (or 8·9 C.c.) of Water of Ammonia should require 50 C.c. of the volumetric solution of oxalic acid. Water of Ammonia should be kept in glass-stoppered bottles, in a cool place." *U. S.* Of the British preparation, "85 grains by weight require for neutralization 500 grain-measures of the volumetric solution of oxalic acid, corresponding to 10 per cent. by weight of ammonia, NH_3. One fluidrachm contains 5·2 grains of ammonia." *Br.*

Water of Ammonia is incompatible with acids, and with acidulous and many earthy and metallic salts; but it does not decompose the salts of lime, baryta, or strontia, and only partially decomposes those of magnesia. Commercial solution of ammonia sometimes contains *pyrrol*, *naphthalene*, *aniline*, and *pyridine*. These may be detected by the solution being reddened by nitric acid, and, after having been supersaturated with hydrochloric acid, by its tingeing a slip of fir wood of a rich purple color, characteristic of pyrrol. (*Maclagan.*) The source of these impurities is coal-gas liquor, from which the ammoniacal compounds are largely obtained. Donath (*Dingler's Polytechnisches Journal*, vol. iv. p. 229) tested some ammonia prepared from gas liquor by neutralizing with diluted sulphuric acid, when the liquid assumed a rose color, and a solution of the sulphate emitted the characteristic odor of naphthalene.

Composition. Water is capable of absorbing 670 times its volume of ammoniacal gas at 10° C. (50° F.), and increases in bulk about two-thirds. But the officinal solution of ammonia is by no means a saturated one. Thus, the ammonia contained in the U. S. preparation is about 10 per cent. The following table gives the percentage of ammoniacal gas in aqueous solutions of different densities at the temperature of 14° C. (57·2° F.). (Carius, *Annal. Ch. Pharm.*, xcix. 164.)

Ammonia per cent.	Specific Gravity.	Ammonia per cent.	Specific Gravity.	Ammonia per cent.	Specific Gravity.	Ammonia per cent.	Specific Gravity.
1	0·9959	10	0·9593	19	0·9283	28	0·9026
2	0·9915	11	0·9556	20	0·9251	29	0·9001
3	0·9873	12	0·9520	21	0·9221	30	0·8976
4	0·9831	13	0·9484	22	0·9191	31	0·8953
5	0·9790	14	0·9449	23	0·9162	32	0·8929
6	0·9749	15	0·9414	24	0·9133	33	0·8907
7	0·9709	16	0·9380	25	0·9106	34	0·8885
8	0·9670	17	0·9347	26	0·9078	35	0·8864
9	0·9631	18	0·9314	27	0·9052	36	0·8844

Medical Properties and Uses. When brought into contact with living tissue, ammonia acts as a stimulant, irritant, or caustic, according to the strength of its solution. When applied to the skin it may excite simply burning pain and redness, but in the form even of the present preparation, if the contact be sufficiently maintained, it is capable of destroying the whole dermal tissue; taken internally in a concentrated form it acts as a violent corrosive poison, and may cause rapidly fatal gastro-enteritis, with the destruction of the visceral coats. In some cases it has produced death in a few minutes by entering the larynx and causing œdema, with consequent suffocation. When taken internally in therapeutic doses its action is immediate, and continues but for a few moments. In the stomach it acts as a stimulant antacid, and is often useful in heartburn, sick headache, etc. After absorption it stimulates most powerfully the circulation and respiration, affecting especially the heart and respiratory centres. By full doses the respiratory rate and the arterial pressure are for a few moments enormously increased. Toxic doses are directly paralyzant to the heart muscle, and may cause, if injected into a vein, immediate diastolic arrest of the heart. According to the researches of Bence Jones, ammonia is oxidized in the system with the formation of nitric acid, which is eliminated by the kidneys.

Water of ammonia is a valuable remedy in all forms of sudden syncope. The injection of ammonia into a vein was brought forward by Prof. G. B. Halford, of Melbourne, as a specific against the poison of serpents, and some evidence has been adduced as to its value. As long ago, however, as 1782, Fontana published at Florence a series of experiments showing the uselessness of such injections as a remedy for snake-bite, and recently the subject has been investigated in India by Sir Joseph Fayrer (*Indian Annals Med. Sci.*, 1872), and by a Royal Commission (*Lancet*, Sept. 1874), with the result of completely establishing the truth of the experiments and conclusions of Fontana. In collapse following severe accident, or in sudden cardiac failure from other acute cause, the intravenous injection of aqua ammoniæ has been of the greatest service in arousing the action of the heart. Half a drachm to a drachm diluted in half an ounce to an ounce of water may be slowly thrown directly into a vein. In some cases the drug has been simply used hypodermically, but is almost certain to cause severe local symptoms. On account of its cheapness it is much used as an ingredient in liniments, especially combined with olive or other oil. The internal dose is from ten to thirty drops (0·6–1·9 C.c.), largely diluted.

Off. Prep. and Pharm. Uses. Antimonium Sulphidum Purificatum; Bismuthi et Ammonii Citras; Extractum Glycyrrhizæ Fluidum; Extractum Glycyrrhizæ Purum; Extractum Senegæ Fluidum; Ferri et Ammonii Citras; Ferri et Ammonii Tartras; Ferri et Potassii Tartras; Ferri Oxidum Hydratum; Glycyrrhizinum Ammoniatum; Hydrargyrum Ammoniatum; Linimentum Ammoniæ; Liquor Ferri Acetatis; Liquor Ferri Citratis; Liquor Ferri Nitratis; Spiritus Ammoniæ Aromaticus; Syrupus Calcii Lactophosphatis; Syrupus Senegæ; Sulphur Lotum.

Off. Prep. Br. Linimentum Ammoniæ; Linimentum Hydrargyri; Tinctura Quininæ Ammoniata.

AQUA AMMONIÆ FORTIOR. *U. S.* *Stronger Water of Ammonia.*

(Ā'QUA AM-MŌ'NI-Æ FŎR'TI-ŎR.)

"An aqueous solution of ammonia [NH_3; 17—NH_3; 17], containing 28 per cent., by weight, of the gas." *U. S.* "Ammoniacal gas, NH_3, dissolved in water, and constituting 32·5 per cent. of the solution." *Br.*

Liquor Ammoniæ Fortior, *Br.* Strong Solution of Ammonia. Eau d'Ammoniaque forte, *Fr.*; Starker Salmiakgeist, *G.*

This preparation is too strong for internal exhibition, but forms a convenient ammoniacal solution for reduction, by dilution with one and a half measures of distilled water (two measures British preparation), to the strength of ordinary officinal Water of Ammonia (Aqua Ammoniæ), or for preparing strong rubefacient liniments.

The U. S. Pharmacopœia does not give a process; but in the British, the following formula is given for its preparation.

"Take of Chloride of Ammonium, in coarse powder, *three pounds* [avoirdupois]; Slaked Lime *four pounds* [av.]; Distilled Water *thirty-two fluidounces.* Mix the Lime with the Chloride of Ammonium, and introduce the mixture into an iron bottle, placed in a metal pot surrounded by sand. Connect the iron tube, which screws air-tight into the bottle, in the usual manner, by corks, glass tubes, and caoutchouc collars, with a Woulf's bottle capable of holding a pint [Imp. meas.]; connect this with a second Woulf's bottle of the same size, the second bottle with a flask or other vessel of the capacity of three pints [Imp. meas.], in which twenty-two [fluid]ounces of the Distilled Water are placed, and this vessel, by means of a tube bent twice at right angles, with an ordinary bottle containing the remaining ten [fluid]ounces of Distilled Water. Bottles 1 and 2 are empty, and the latter and the vessel which contains the twenty-two ounces of distilled water are furnished each with a siphon safety tube, charged with a very short column of mercury. The heat of a fire, which should be very gradually raised, is now to be applied to the metal pot, and continued until bubbles of condensible gas cease to escape from the extremity of the glass tube which dips into the water of the flask. The process being terminated, the latter vessel will contain about forty-three fluidounces of the Strong Solution of Ammonia.

"Bottles 1 and 2 will now include, the first about sixteen, the second about ten fluidounces of a colored ammoniacal liquid. Place this in a flask closed by a cork, which should be perforated by a siphon safety tube containing a little mercury, and also by a second tube bent twice at right angles, and made to pass to the bottom of the terminal bottle used in the preceding process. Apply heat to the flask until the colored liquid it contains is reduced to three-fourths of its original bulk. The product now contained in the terminal bottle will be nearly of the strength of Solution of Ammonia, and may be made exactly so by the addition of the proper quantity of Distilled Water, or of Strong Solution of Ammonia." *Br.*

In this process the ammonia is disengaged in the usual manner from chloride of ammonium by the action of lime, as explained under the head of *Aqua Ammoniæ.* But it is perceived, by the details of the process, that the purpose is to obtain both the *stronger* and *ordinary* solution of ammonia at one operation. This is done by connecting the iron bottle containing the materials with a series of four receivers, the first two being empty Woulf's bottles, the third a flask containing twenty-two fluidounces of distilled water, and the fourth an ordinary bottle containing the remainder of the distilled water. In the first two bottles, impurities are condensed with a considerable portion of ammonia; in the flask, the officinal Strong Solution of Ammonia (*Br.*) has been formed by the absorption of the gas; and, in the fourth, a weaker ammoniacal liquid is formed by the absorption of a portion of the gas which has passed through the flask unabsorbed. This last liquid is raised to the strength of the officinal Solution of Ammonia (*Br.*) by forcing into it a portion of ammoniacal gas from the impure contents of the first two bottles. We presume that the receivers are to be kept cool by means of cold water or ice, though no such direction is given in the process. If the solution in the fourth bottle be not of the required officinal strength (sp. gr. 0·959), it may be made so by the addition of stronger solution from the flask, if too weak, or of distilled water, if too strong.

Water of Ammonia is seldom made by the formula of the Pharmacopœia, but is prepared on a large scale, from one of the products of the coal-gas manufacture, by the following more economical process. *Gas liquor* is distilled, and the distillate, which is principally sulphide of ammonium, is converted into sulphate of ammonium by sulphuric acid. The rough sulphate is then gently distilled with milk of lime, the still being connected with a series of glass carboys, arranged like Woulf's bottles, and three-fourths filled with distilled water. In this way solution of ammonia may be obtained of maximum strength.

Properties of Aqueous Ammonia of Maximum Strength. This is a colorless liquid, of an acrid taste, and very pungent smell. It is strongly alkaline, and immediately changes turmeric, when held over its fumes, to reddish brown. Cooled to 40° F. below zero, it concretes into a gelatinous mass, and at 54° C. (130° F.) boils, owing to the rapid disengagement of the gas. Its sp. gr. is 0·875 at 10° C. (50° F.). Anhydrous ammonia is said to dissolve metallic sodium, and the solution is intensely blue. (*Chem. News*, Nov. 4, 1870, p. 217.)

Properties of the Officinal Stronger Water of Ammonia. This has similar properties to those above mentioned. Its sp. gr. is 0·900, *U. S.*, 0·891, *Br.* When of the former density, it contains 28 per cent. of the gas, when of the latter 32·5 per cent. "To neutralize 3·4 Gm. (or 3·9 C.c.) of Stronger Water of Ammonia should require 56 C.c. of the volumetric solution of oxalic acid." *U. S.* "By weight, 52·3 grains require for neutralization 1000 grain-measures of the volumetric solution of oxalic acid. One fluidrachm contains 15·83 grains of Ammonia, NH_3." *Br.* The stronger water of ammonia of commerce usually ranges in density from 0·900 to 0·920. Even when of proper officinal strength at first, it generally becomes weaker by the escape of ammonia. To prevent its deteriorating, it should be kept in closely-stopped bottles in a cool place. If precipitated by lime-water, it contains carbonic acid. After having been saturated with nitric acid, a precipitate by carbonate of ammonium indicates earthy impurity, by nitrate of silver, a chloride, and by chloride of barium, a sulphate. "When diluted with four times its volume of distilled water, it does not give precipitates with solution of lime, oxalate of ammonia, sulphide of ammonium, or ammonio-sulphate of copper" (*Br.*); indicating the absence of carbonates, lime, metals, and sulphides.

When purchasing the Stronger Solution of Ammonia, the apothecary should not trust to its being of the officinal strength; but should ascertain the point by taking its density, either by the specific gravity bottle or the hydrometer. Another method of ascertaining its density is by the *ammonia-meter* of Mr. J. J. Griffin, of London, described and figured in *P. J. Tr.* (x. 413). In reducing it to make Aqua Ammoniæ, the same precaution should be taken; and, if the mixture should not have the sp. gr. 0·959, it should be brought to that density by the addition either of the stronger solution or of distilled water, as the case may require. "Stronger Water of Ammonia should be kept in strong glass-stoppered bottles, not completely filled, in a cool place." *U. S.* *Great care should be exercised in opening these bottles.* It is safer, if the water of ammonia has been kept in a warm room, to cool it with ice before attempting to withdraw the stopper, as the liberated gas, when warm, oftentimes is forced out with extreme violence, and several accidents resulting in injury to the sight of the operator are recorded.

Medical Properties and Uses. This solution is too strong for medical use in its unmixed state. Sufficiently diluted with spirit of camphor and rosemary, it has been much employed as a prompt and powerful rubefacient, vesicatory, or escharotic, in various neuralgic, gouty, rheumatic, spasmodic, and inflammatory affections, in which strong and speedy counter-irritation is indicated. When mere rubefaction is desired, a mixture may be used composed of five fluidounces of the ammoniacal liquid and eight of the diluent liquid; and this will answer even for blistering or cauterizing, unless a very prompt effect is necessary. In the latter case, a lotion may be resorted to consisting of five measures of the ammoniacal to three of the diluent liquid. These mixtures are applied by means of linen folded several times, or a thick piece of flannel saturated with the liniment. A convenient mode is to fill the wooden cover of a large pill or ointment box, an inch or two in diameter, with patent lint, saturate this with the liquid, and press it upon the part. The ammonia is thus prevented from escaping, and a definite boundary given to the inflammation. The application will generally produce rubefaction in from one to eight minutes, vesication in from three to ten minutes, and a caustic effect in a somewhat longer time.

When a solution of ammonia of 25° (sp. gr. 0·905) is mixed with fatty matter, the mixture forms the *vesicating ammoniacal ointment* of Dr. Gondret. The revised formula of this ointment is as follows. Take of lard 32 parts, oil of sweet almonds 2 parts. Melt them together by the *gentle* heat of a candle or lamp, and pour the melted mixture into a bottle with a wide mouth. Then add 17 parts of solution of ammonia of 25°, and mix, with continued agitation, until the whole is cold. The ointment must be preserved in a bottle with a ground stopper, and kept in a cool place. When well prepared, it vesicates in ten minutes. There may be danger of excessive irritation and inflammation of the nostrils, mouth, and air-passages, from the inadvertent inhalation of the gas escaping from a bottle of the stronger water of ammonia, when freshly opened; and serious consequences have occurred from this cause, or the accidental breaking of the bottle. The best antidote, under these circumstances, would be the inhalation of the vapors of vinegar or acetic acid.

Off. Prep. Spiritus Ammoniæ.

Off. Prep. Br. Ammonii Phosphas; Linimentum Camphoræ Compositum; Liquor Ammoniæ; Liquor Ammonii Citratis Fortior; Spiritus Ammoniæ Aromaticus; Spiritus Ammoniæ Fœtidus; Tinctura Opii Ammoniata.

AQUA AMYGDALÆ AMARÆ. *U. S.* *Bitter Almond Water.*

(Ā'QUA A-MY̆G'DA-LÆ A-MĀ'RÆ.)

Aqua Amygdalarum Amararum, *P.G.;* Eau d'Amandes amères, *Fr.;* Bittermandelwasser, *G.*

"Oil of Bitter Almonds, *one part* [or fifteen minims]; Distilled Water, *nine hundred and ninety-nine parts* [or two pints], To make *one thousand parts* [or two pints]. Dissolve the Oil in the Distilled Water, and filter through a well-wetted filter." *U. S.*

Owing to the almost universal employment at this time (1888) of artificial oil of bitter almond (or benzaldehyd), which is free from hydrocyanic acid (such oil being much cheaper than that made from bitter almond), the bitter almond water of pharmacy cannot be relied upon as a medicinal agent, but is used exclusively as a pleasant vehicle. This must be regarded as a fortunate circumstance, because the proportion of hydrocyanic acid was very variable in the former bitter almond water, and doubt and uncertainty about its action always prevailed. Notwithstanding these facts, care must be exercised not to prescribe a larger dose to begin with than two teaspoonfuls (7·5 C.c.), lest the water should have been made from the poisonous oil of bitter almond.* Its principal use in this country is as a vehicle, many physicians prescribing it not for its medicinal virtues, but on account of its agreeable taste and powers of masking the taste of saline substances. Under the same name, a preparation has been much used on the continent of Europe, prepared by distilling bitter almonds with water.† This when fresh is much stronger than the preparation of the U.S. Pharmacopœia, containing, according to an analysis of Geiger, in 1000 parts, 1·2 parts of anhydrous hydrocyanic acid. But, in consequence either of circumstances in the manner of its preparation, or of changes upon being kept, it is of variable and uncertain strength, and cannot be relied on.‡ It has been prescribed with fatal effects; and the greatest caution, therefore, should be observed by the apothecary not to put up the distilled water instead of the officinal.

AQUA ANETHI. *Br.* *Dill Water.*

(Ā'QUĄ Ą-NĒ'THĪ.)

Eau d'Aneth, *Fr.;* Dillwasser, *G.*

"Take of Dill Fruit, bruised, *one pound* [avoirdupois]; Water *two gallons* [Imperial measure]. Distil *one gallon* [Imp. meas.]." *Br.*

This water, which is frequently prescribed in Great Britain, is occasionally used here; it closely resembles caraway water, over which it has no advantages.

AQUA ANISI. *U.S., Br.* *Anise Water.*

(Ā'QUĄ Ą-NĪ'SĪ.)

Eau d'Anis, *Fr.;* Aniswasser, *G.*

"Oil of Anise, *two parts* [or thirty minims]; Cotton, *four parts* [or sixty grains]; Distilled Water, *a sufficient quantity,* To make *one thousand parts* [or two pints]. Add the Oil to the Cotton, in small portions at a time, distributing it thoroughly by picking the Cotton apart after each addition; then pack it firmly in a conical per-

* Under the name of *chloral hydrocyanate* a substance has been introduced (1888) for making cherry laurel and bitter almond water extemporaneously. It occurs in white, translucent rhombic prisms, soluble in water, alcohol, and ether. It has the odor of hydrocyanic acid and chloral, and is said to be a very stable compound. A solution of 6·5 grains of the salt in 1000 grains of Distilled Water corresponds with the officinal bitter almond water of the German Pharmacopœia, which is 1 to 1000. (*Merck's Bulletin.*)

† *Preparation of Bitter Almond Water* (Distilled). H. C. Vielhaber powders ten pounds bitter almonds as finely as possible, separates the fatty oil, which usually amounts to 36 to 38 per cent., by strong pressure, and reduces the almond press-cake to a very fine powder; a quantity of this corresponding to two pounds of almonds is then distilled with water (without alcohol) until about 500 grammes of distillate have been obtained, when the receiver is disconnected, another receiver attached, and the distillation continued as long as the presence of hydrocyanic acid can be recognized by its odor and taste in the distillate; this second distillate is then used in the place of distilled water for distilling another two-pound lot of the almonds, and the operation continued thus, always collecting the first and second distillates separately and utilizing the latter for distilling the next lot, until all the press-cake has been subjected to distillation; the first distillates are mixed, and also the second. The author thus obtained from 10 pounds of almonds about 5 pounds of first and 9 to 10 pounds of second distillate, the former containing a large percentage of volatile almond oil, which is dissolved by adding the officinal (Ph. Germ.) percentage of alcohol (about ¼ of its weight) to the distillate. The percentage of hydrocyanic acid is then determined in the first and second distillates, and sufficient of the latter added to the former to reduce it to the officinal strength (one-tenth of one per cent.). (*Archiv d. Pharm.*, May, 1879, p. 409; *A. J. P.*, July, 1879.) G. A. Zwick prepares distilled bitter almond water by breaking up 12 pounds peach kernels in a mill, then powdering finely, expressing 25 per cent. of fixed oil, powdering the press-cake, introducing this into a still, with water, reserving the first forty fluidounces of distillate, this having been shown by assay to contain the proper amount of hydrocyanic acid, one per mille. (*A. J. P.*, 1881.)

‡ For a method of determining the amount of hydrocyanic acid in bitter almond water, see *Archiv d. Pharm.*, Nov. 1878, p. 408; *A. J. P.*, Feb. 1879.

colator, and gradually pour on Distilled Water, until *one thousand parts* [or two pints] of percolate are obtained." *U. S.*

"Take of Anise fruit, bruised, *one pound* [avoirdupois]; Water *two gallons* [Imperial measure]. Distil one gallon [Imp. meas.]" *Br.*

Anise water is rarely made by distillation, although the product thus secured has a more delicate flavor than the U. S. preparation.

This water is used solely as a vehicle.

AQUA AURANTII FLORUM. *U. S.* *Orange Flower Water.*

(Ă'QUĄ ÂU-RĂN'TĮ-Ī FLŌ'RŬM—âu-răn'shę-ī.)

"The distilled water of the flowers of the Bitter Orange tree, Citrus vulgaris, *Risso* (Citrus Bigaradia, *Duhamel*), *Hist. Nat. des Orang.* plate 30; and of the Sweet Orange tree, Citrus Aurantium, *Risso; Bentl. and Trim. Med. Pl.* vol. i. plate 51. The Orange-Flower Water of commerce is usually three times the strength of that employed in former years." *Br.*

Aqua Aurantii Floris, *Br.;* Orange Flower Water; Aqua Florum Naphæ; Eau (Hydrolat) distillée de Fleurs d'Oranger, Eau de Naphe, *Fr.;* Orangenblüthenwasser, *G.*

"Recent Orange Flowers, *forty parts* [or fifty-four ounces av.]; Water, *two hundred parts* [or sixteen pints], To make *one hundred parts*. Mix them, and, by means of steam, distil *one hundred parts* [or eight pints]. Keep the product in well-stopped bottles, excluded from light." *U. S.*

This preparation is considered by the British Pharmacopœia as an object of importation. According to this authority, it is obtained indiscriminately from the flowers of the bitter and those of the sweet orange tree; and the same is the case with our own officinal standard; though, in Italy and France, where it is largely made, the flowers of the bitter orange are preferred, as yielding the most fragrant product. It may be prepared in the most southern districts of our country from the fresh flowers; and these might be brought to the North for the same purpose, if previously incorporated with one-third or one-quarter of their weight of common salt. The proper method is to arrange the flowers and salt in successive layers in jars of stoneware or glass. They may also be preserved by means of glycerin. Notwithstanding, however, the facility of preparing this Water here, it is generally imported from the south of France, whence it usually comes in cans of tinned copper.

Orange flower water is nearly colorless, though often of a pale yellowish tint. "Orange Flower Water should remain unaffected by hydrosulphuric acid or sulphide of ammonium (metallic impurities), and should not be mucilaginous." *U. S.* From being kept in tinned copper cans, it sometimes contains metallic impurity, which is said to be chiefly carbonate of lead, derived from the lead used as a solder in making the cans. The means of detecting metallic impurity are mentioned under the general observations on distilled waters. Much color, offensive odŏr, or mouldiness indicates impurity derived from the flowers in distillation.

L. Malenfant observed that fresh orange flowers, mixed with cold water, yield, on distillation over the naked fire, a milky water, possessing a somewhat empyreumatic odor and a strong, somewhat acrid taste. Kept for twelve or eighteen months in glass vessels covered with parchment, it loses its empyreuma, and after filtering has an agreeable odor and taste. If the flowers be mixed with boiling water and immediately distilled, the water is limpid, and gradually separates some thick oil of a brownish color; the water has the odor and taste of the flowers, but complicated with a still smell (*goût de feu*), which it loses after long keeping; it seems to alter less rapidly than that obtained by the former process. Distilled by steam a limpid water of a pure odor and taste is at once obtained, free from empyreuma; it may be at once used, and keeps better in the light than when obtained by the two former processes. (*A. J. P.*, June, 1874.) A distilled water of the leaves is also prepared; and sometimes a mixture of the leaves and flowers is employed. But this is a fraud, as the distilled water of the leaves never has the sweet perfume of that of the flowers. (*Journ. de Pharm.*, 4e sér., iii. 249.) Orange flower water is used exclusively on account of its agreeable odor; though it may possess slight powers as a nervous stimulant.

Orange flower water is stored in large glass vessels or carboys in cool cellars by the manufacturers in Grasse, care being taken not to stopper them tightly, but simply to cover the orifice with a piece of paper; this is in direct contradiction of the officinal direction. (See page 236.)

Nitric, sulphuric, or hydrochloric acid produces a red coloration with orange flower water: particularly if the water be shaken with ether to take up the oil and the acid added to the ethereal solution. (*P. J. Tr.*, 1878, p. 248.)

Off. Prep. Syrupus Aurantii Florum.

Off. Prep. Br. Syrupus Aurantii Floris.

AQUA CAMPHORÆ. *U.S., Br.* *Camphor Water.*

(Ă'QUĄ CĂM'PHǪ-RÆ.)

Aqua Camphorata; Eau camphrée, *Fr.*; Kampferwasser, *G.*

"Camphor, *eight parts* [or one hundred and sixteen grains]; Alcohol, *sixteen parts* [half a fluidounce]; Cotton, *sixteen parts* [half an ounce av.]; Distilled Water, *a sufficient quantity*, To make *one thousand parts* [two pints]. Dissolve the Camphor in the Alcohol, and add the solution to the Cotton, in small portions at a time, distributing it thoroughly by picking the Cotton apart after each addition. Expose the Cotton to the air until the Alcohol has nearly evaporated; then pack it firmly in a conical percolator, and gradually pour on Distilled Water, until *one thousand parts* [or two pints] of percolate are obtained." *U. S.*

"Take of Camphor, crushed, *half an ounce* [avoirdupois]; Distilled Water *one gallon* [Imperial measure]. Enclose the camphor in a muslin bag, and attach this to one end of a glass rod, by means of which it may be kept at the bottom of a bottle containing the Distilled Water. Close the mouth of the bottle, macerate for at least two days, and then pour off the solution when it is required." *Br.*

In these processes the object is to effect a solution of the camphor. Water is capable of dissolving but a small proportion of this principle; but the quantity varies with the method employed. The present officinal process is an improvement on former methods, for it undoubtedly secures a saturated solution. The process of U. S. Pharm. 1870, notwithstanding an ordinary amount of care, usually left considerable camphor on the filter not in a finely divided state, and the water passed through not fully saturated. This defect could have been largely overcome by allowing the milky mixture to stand twenty-four hours with occasional agitation before filtering; the present process, however, makes sure of the fine division of the camphor by forming an alcoholic solution, and then securing the distribution of the camphor through the cotton. The present British process is still more inefficient than the old formulas of the different Colleges for their *Mistura Camphoræ*, which has received in the late revision a much more appropriate name. In the present British process no trouble is taken even to comminute the camphor, or to shake it with the water, which is thus allowed to take up what it may be disposed to do by contact with the camphor contained in a bag; though some ingenuity is exhibited in retaining the latter, which is lighter than water, beneath the surface of the liquid by means of a glass rod. The solution thus effected must be extremely feeble, containing probably less than one part in a thousand, which, according to Berzelius, is taken up by water when triturated with camphor. It is besides of uncertain strength, varying with the size of the fragments of camphor. Mr. J. C. Pooley found that 120 grains of camphor, treated according to the officinal directions, gave, when cut into 4 pieces, 6 grains to half a gallon of water, but in 20 pieces gave 20 grains, or about one part to 1750 of water. (*P. J. Tr.*, 2d ser., vii. 162.) The U. S. process is much preferable to the British, as it affords a permanent solution, of sufficient strength to be employed with a view to the influence of the camphor on the system; while the other has little more than the flavor of the narcotic, and is fit only for a vehicle of other medicines. Mr. Wm. B. Addington proposed to add to the camphor just enough alcohol to dissolve it, and triturate the liquor with magnesia, during which process he affirmed that the alcohol evaporated (*A. J. P.*, xlv. 209); and Mr. F. T. Hartzell substituted for alcohol, ether, a few drops of which enabled him to bring the camphor to an impalpable powder. (*Ibid.*, xlvi. 233.) The camphor is separated from its aqueous solution by a solution of pure potassa, and, according to Dr. Paris, by sulphate of magnesium and several other salts. Sir J. Murray proposes a solution of camphor and bicarbonate of magnesium, which contains three grains of the former and six grains of the latter in each fluidounce.

Camphor water has this advantage over camphor in substance, that the latter is with difficulty dissolved by the liquors of the stomach; but it is too feeble a preparation for use when a decided effect is desired. It is usually given in the dose of one or two tablespoonfuls (15–30 C.c.), repeated every hour or two hours.

Off. Prep. Br. Injectio Apomorphinæ Hypodermica; Injectio Ergotini Hypodermica; Liquor Atropinæ Sulphatis.

AQUA CARUI. *Br.* *Caraway Water.*

(Ā′QUĄ CĂR′Ū-Ī.)

Aqua Carvi; Eau distillée de Carvi, *Fr.;* Kümmelwasser, *G.*

"Take of Caraway Fruit, bruised, *one pound* [avoirdupois]; Water, *two gallons* [Imp. meas.]. Distil one gallon [Imp. meas.]." *Br.*

Distilled Caraway Water has the flavor of the fruit or seeds, but is seldom used in the United States. It is usually made from the volatile oil (15 minims in a pint), in the same manner as is cinnamon water.

AQUA CHLORI. *U. S.* *Chlorine Water.*

(Ā′QUĄ CHLŌ′RĪ.)

"An aqueous solution of Chlorine [Cl; 35·4—Cl; 35·4], containing at least 0·4 per cent. of the gas." *U. S.*

Liquor Chlori, *Br.;* Solution of Chlorine; Aqua Chlorata, *P. G.;* Aqua Chlori, Chlorum Solutum, Aqua Oxymuriatica; Eau chlorée, Chlore liquide, *Fr.;* Chlorwasser, *G.;* Aqua Chlorini, *Phar.* 1870.

"Black Oxide of Manganese, *ten parts* [or eighty grains]; Hydrochloric Acid, *forty parts* [or five fluidrachms]; Water, *seventy-five parts* [or ten fluidrachms]; Distilled Water, *four hundred parts* [or seven fluidounces]. Place the Oxide in a flask, add the Acid previously diluted with *twenty-five parts* [or three and a half fluidrachms] of Water, and apply a gentle heat. Conduct the generated Chlorine, by suitable tubes, through the remainder of the Water contained in a small wash-bottle, to the bottom of a bottle having the capacity of *one thousand parts* [or one pint], into which the Distilled Water has been introduced, the neck of which is loosely stopped with cotton, and which is to be kept, during the operation, at a temperature of about 10° C. (50° F.). When the air has been entirely displaced by the gas, disconnect the bottle from the apparatus, and, having inserted the stopper, shake the bottle, loosening the stopper from time to time, until the gas ceases to be absorbed. If necessary, reconnect the bottle with the apparatus, and continue passing the gas and agitating, until the Distilled Water is saturated. Finally, pour the Chlorine Water into dark amber-colored, glass-stoppered bottles, which must be completely filled therewith, and keep them in a dark and cool place." *U. S.*

"Take of Hydrochloric Acid *six fluidounces* [Imperial measure]; Black Oxide of Manganese, in fine powder, *one ounce* [avoirdupois]; Distilled Water *thirty-four fluidounces* [Imp. meas.]. Put the Oxide of Manganese into a gas-bottle, and, having poured upon it the Hydrochloric Acid diluted with two [fluid]ounces of the Water, apply a gentle heat, and, by suitable tubes, cause the gas, as it is developed, to pass through two [fluid]ounces of the Water placed in an intermediate small phial, and thence to the bottom of a three-pint bottle containing the remainder of the water, the mouth of which is loosely plugged with tow. As soon as the chlorine ceases to be developed, let the bottle be disconnected from the apparatus in which the gas has been generated, corked loosely, and shaken until the chlorine is absorbed. Lastly, introduce the solution into a green glass bottle furnished with a well-fitting stopper, and keep it in a cool and dark place." *Br.*

The U. S. and Br. processes are essentially the same. Both are intended to make saturated solutions of chlorine in water. The only material variation in the British formula is the larger proportion of the black oxide of manganese and hydrochloric acid, to the distilled water. The British process differs in directing the disconnection of the apparatus for generating the gas, as soon as it ceases to be produced, instead of after the air in the receiving bottle has been displaced by it. This is a practical improvement which should have been adopted in the U. S. process. Should there be any danger of deficiency of chlorine in the resulting chlorine water, the British process would have the advantage, as it uses not only a larger proportion of the materials for making the gas, but exhausts them.

In both processes, the chlorine gas is extricated from the hydrochloric acid by the black oxide of manganese,* whilst the chloride of manganese and water produced remain in the flask, and the chlorine is passed, through an intermediate vessel containing a little water for purifying it, into the bottle containing the distilled water, loosely stopped, until the vacant part of the bottle is filled with it to the exclusion of the atmospheric air. $MnO_2 + 4HCl = MnCl_2 + Cl_2 + 2H_2O$. The bottle being then corked, is shaken so as to cause the absorption of the gas by the water. Of course the stopper must be from time to time loosened, in order to allow the entrance of air to supply the partial vacuum created by the absorption of the chlorine. The chlorine water is directed to be kept secluded from the light, because otherwise it would be apt to be converted partially into hydrochloric acid, through the union of the chlorine with the hydrogen of the water. In the Br. Pharmacopœia it is ordered to be kept in a green glass bottle, for the purpose, probably, of protecting it from the light; but experiments have shown that it is an orange, and not a green color, which appears to prevent the passage of the chemical rays.†

An extemporaneous chlorine water, containing chloride of potassium and free hydrochloric acid, not more than twenty-four and twelve grains respectively to the pint, may be made as follows. Put in a bottle forty grains of chlorate of potassium, add one-half troyounce of hydrochloric acid. When the bottle begins to be filled with chlorine vapors, add one fluidounce of distilled water. Stopper the bottle, and, when the crystals have dissolved, add distilled water to a pint. (*A. J. P.*, xlii. 208.) The reaction liberates, however, at the same time, the somewhat explosive gas, Cl_2O_4, and may be dangerous at times.

Properties. "A greenish yellow, clear liquid, having the suffocating odor and disagreeable taste of Chlorine, and leaving no residue on evaporation. It instantly decolorizes dilute solutions of litmus and indigo. When shaken with an excess of mercury until the odor of Chlorine has disappeared, the remaining liquid should be at most but faintly acid (limit of hydrochloric acid). On mixing 35·4 Gm. of Chlorine Water with a solution of 0·9 Gm. of iodide of potassium in 20 Gm. of water, the resulting deep red liquid should require for complete decoloration at least 40 C.c. of the volumetric solution of hyposulphite of sodium (corresponding to at least 0·4 per cent. of Chlorine)." *U. S.* Like gaseous chlorine, it destroys vegetable colors. When cooled to about the freezing point, it forms deep yellow crystalline plates, consisting of hydrate of chlorine. It is intended to contain at least twice its volume of the gas. According to MM. Riegel and Walz, chlorine water containing two and a half volumes of the gas at 12·2° C. (54° F.) keeps best. The British solution "immediately discharges the blue color of a dilute solution of indigo. Its sp. gr. is 1·003, and when evaporated it leaves no residue. When 20 grains of iodide of potassium, dissolved in a [fluid]ounce of distilled water, are added to 439 grains by weight (one fluidounce) of this preparation, the mixed solution acquires a deep red color, which requires for its discharge 750 grain-measures of the volumetric solution of the hyposulphite of soda, corresponding to 2·66 grains of chlorine." *Br.* This indicates the quantity of chlorine in the solution, by the amount of the hyposulphite required to decolorise an equivalent quantity of iodine, liberated from the iodide of potassium.

* The oxide of manganese is of course deoxidised. In manufacturing chlorine on the large scale, it is of great importance to reoxidise the manganese, so that it can be used over again. This was first accomplished by Mr. Walter Weldon in 1870, and his "manganese regeneration" process has been universally adopted. It was said that a few years ago there were only two chlorine works in the world that did not regenerate their manganese. (For details, see *Roscoe & Schorlemmer's Chemistry*, vol. ii. part ii. p. 15.

† *Deacon's process.* Mr. Henry Deacon has discovered that chlorine may be made by passing hydrochloric acid vapor and oxygen over sulphate of copper at a temperature from 400° to 700° F., the copper salt coming out unchanged. For details of this process the reader is referred to *Roscoe & Schorlemmer's Chemistry*, vol. i. p. 114.

Chlorine is an elementary gaseous fluid of a greenish-yellow color, and characteristic smell and taste. It is a supporter of combustion. Its specific gravity is 2·47, and its atomic weight 35·4. When the attempt is made to breathe it, even much diluted, it excites cough and a sense of suffocation, and causes a discharge from the mucous membrane of the nostrils and bronchial tubes. Breathed in considerable quantities, it produces spitting of blood, violent pains, and sometimes death.

Medical Properties and Uses. Chlorine water is stimulant and antiseptic. Internally it has been used in typhus, and in chronic affections of the liver; but the diseases in which it has been most extolled are scarlatina, malignant sore throat, and diphtheria. Mr. Wm. M. Dobie found it more effectual in an epidemic of that disease which appeared in Chester, England, in the autumn of 1866, than any other remedy. (*Edin. Med. Journ.*, March, 1867, p. 829.) It is said, also, by Dr. Althaus, to have been used in a late epidemic of the same disease in Germany with highly satisfactory results. (*Med. Times and Gaz.*, July, 1868, p. 56.) Externally it is employed, duly diluted, as a gargle in smallpox, scarlatina, and putrid sore throat, as a wash for ill-conditioned ulcers and cancerous sores, and as a local bath in diseases of the liver. It has been used with advantage as an application to buboes and large abscesses, to promote the absorption of the matter. As it depends upon chlorine for its activity, its medical properties coincide with those of chlorinated lime and chlorinated soda, under which heads they are more particularly given. The dose of chlorine water is from one to four fluidrachms (3·75–15 C.c.), properly diluted. It should not be prescribed in mixtures, almost all organic substances causing a rapid disappearance of the chlorine. Even sugar has this action, and glycerin still more markedly. (*A. J. P.*, xliv. 163.)

Gaseous chlorine has been recommended by Gannal in chronic bronchitis and pulmonary consumption, exhibited by inhalation, in minute quantities, four or six times a day. Its first effect is to produce some dryness of the fauces, with increased expectoration for a time, followed ultimately by diminution of the sputa and amendment. Dr. Christison states that he has repeatedly observed these results in chronic catarrh; and both he and Dr. Elliotson have obtained, in consumption, a more decided improvement of the symptoms from the use of chlorine inhalations than from any other means. The liquid in the inhaler may be formed either of water containing from ten to thirty drops (0·6–1·9 C.c.) of chlorine water, or of chlorinated lime dissolved in forty parts of water, to which a drop or two of sulphuric acid must be added, each time the inhalation is practised. The inhaler should be placed in water heated to about 37·7° C. (100° F.).

AQUA CHLOROFORMI. *Br.* *Chloroform Water.*

(Ā'QUA CHLŌ-RQ-FÖR'MĪ.)

Eau de Chloroforme, *Fr.;* Chloroformwasser, *G.*

"Take of Chloroform *one fluidrachm* [Imp. meas.]; Distilled Water *twenty-five fluidounces* [Imp. meas.]. Put them into a two-pint stoppered bottle, and shake them together until the Chloroform is entirely dissolved in the water." *Br.*

This water contains one-half per cent. of chloroform, and is probably fully saturated. The dose is one-half to two fluidounces (15–60 C.c.).

AQUA CINNAMOMI. *U. S., Br.* *Cinnamon Water.*

(Ā'QUA CĬN-NA-MŌ'MĪ.)

Eau de Cannelle, *Fr.;* Einfaches Zimmtwasser, *G.*

"Oil of Cinnamon, *two parts* [or thirty minims]; Cotton, *four parts* [or sixty grains]; Distilled Water, *a sufficient quantity,* To make *one thousand parts* [or two pints]. Add the Oil to the Cotton, in small portions at a time, distributing it thoroughly by picking the Cotton apart after each addition; then pack it firmly in a conical percolator, and gradually pour on Distilled Water until *one thousand parts* [or two pints] of percolate are obtained." *U. S.*

"Take of Cinnamon Bark, bruised, *twenty ounces* [avoirdupois]; Water *two gallons* [Imperial measure]. Distil a gallon [Imp. meas.]." *Br.*

Of these processes, that of the U. S. Pharmacopœia is the easier, though the second, the British, may yield a sweeter product. On standing, cinnamon water is apt to precipitate, owing to the gradual oxidation and formation of cinnamic acid, which is comparatively insoluble in water; this can be prevented by passing a stream of carbonic acid through the fresh water for a few minutes. (E. Backhaus.) Cinnamon water is much used as a vehicle for other less agreeable medicines, but should be given cautiously in inflammatory affections. For ordinary purposes the U. S. preparation is sufficiently strong when diluted with an equal measure of water. Dr. E. Holmes recommends glycerin as an excellent intermedium between the oil of cinnamon and water. Ten drops of glycerin will effect the solution of a drop of the oil in a fluidounce of water.

Off. Prep. Mistura Cretæ.

Off. Prep. Br. Mistura Cretæ; Mistura Guaiaci; Mistura Spiritus Vini Gallici.

AQUA CREASOTI. *U.S.* *Creasote Water.*

(Ā'QUA CRĒ-A-SŎ'TĪ.)

Eau créosotée, *Fr.;* Kreosotwasser, *G.*

"Creasote, *one part* [or seventy-two minims]; Distilled Water, *ninety-nine parts* [or a sufficient quantity], To make *one hundred parts* [or one pint]. Agitate the Creasote with the Distilled Water until dissolved, and filter through a well-wetted filter." *U.S.*

This preparation contains 4·5 minims of creasote in each fluidounce, and affords a convenient method of administering that medicine. It is about twenty-five per cent. stronger than that formerly officinal. The dose is from one to four fluidrachms (3·75–15 C.c.). It may also be used with advantage as a gargle, lotion, or mixed with cataplasms, to correct fetor, and gently stimulate indolent surfaces.

AQUA DESTILLATA. *U.S., Br.* *Distilled Water.*

H_2O; 18. (Ā'QUA DĔS-TIL-LĀ'TA.) HO; 9.

Eau distillée, Hydrolat simple, *Fr.;* Destillirtes Wasser, *G.*

"Water, *one thousand parts* [or twenty-five pints], To make *eight hundred parts* [or twenty pints]. Distil the Water from a suitable apparatus provided with a block-tin or glass condenser. Collect the first *fifty parts* [or one and a quarter pints] and throw this portion away. Then collect *eight hundred parts* [or twenty pints] and keep the Distilled Water in glass-stoppered bottles." *U.S.*

"Take of Water *ten gallons* [Imperial measure]. Distil from a copper still, connected with a block-tin worm; reject the first half gallon, and preserve the next eight gallons." *Br.*

No natural water is sufficiently pure for certain pharmaceutical purposes; and hence the necessity of the above processes for its distillation. It is best to reject the first portion which comes over, as this may contain carbonic acid and other volatile impurities; and the last portion of the water ought not to be distilled, lest it should pass over with an empyreumatic taste. The distillation is usually performed with the ordinary still and worm; but, to avoid any impurity from the worm or the receiver, the condenser is directed in the U. S. Pharmacopœia to be of block-tin or glass. In the British formula the worm is ordered to be of block-tin; and the same is undoubtedly contemplated in our officinal process; as the ordinary tin-coated sheet-iron, commonly called tin, would be wholly unfit for the purpose. Mr. Brande states that distilled water often derives from the still a foreign flavor, which it is difficult to avoid. He, therefore, recommends that a still and condenser be kept exclusively for distilling water; or, where this cannot be done, that steam be driven through the worm for half an hour, for the purpose of washing it out before it is used, the worm-tub having been previously emptied. J. N. Hurty prefers well water as the source of distilled water, and that it be boiled before collecting the distillate to get rid of ammonia, and to prevent access and growth of spores, that the water be heated to boiling before introducing it into the container, and that it be drawn off by a siphon-tube reaching to the bottom of the vessel, the mouth of which is loosely stopped with cotton. (*Western Druggist*, 1887, p. 4.) Even the use of pure tin, which is generally considered unexceptionable, does not give perfect security against impurity; as water distilled from metallic alembics, with the head and worm of this metal, has a

16

peculiar odor which it retains for some time. Ordinary distilled water invariably contains ammonia, as may be proved by adding a few drops of Nessler's reagent. (See p. 224.) In order to free distilled water from volatile nitrogenous bodies, it is necessary to redistil it after it has been placed in contact with potassium permanganate and caustic potash. After about one-twentieth of the water has come over, the distillate is usually free from ammonia, and leaves no residue on evaporation. If traces of ammonia remain, acid sulphate of potassium is added, and it is redistilled. (*Stas.*)

Properties, etc. Distilled water, as usually obtained, has a vapid and disagreeable taste, and is not perfectly pure; water, to be rendered so, requiring to be distilled in silver vessels. The properties of pure water have already been given under the head of *Aqua*. Distilled water should undergo no change by sulphuretted hydrogen, or on the addition of tincture of soap, subacetate of lead, chloride of barium, oxalate of ammonium, nitrate of silver, or lime-water. "On evaporating 1 litre of Distilled Water, no fixed residue should remain. The transparency or color of Distilled Water should not be affected by hydrosulphuric acid or sulphide of ammonium (abs. of metals), by test-solutions of chloride of barium (sulphate), nitrate of silver (chloride), oxalate of ammonium (calcium), or mercuric chloride, with or without the subsequent addition of carbonate of potassium (ammonium salts or free ammonia). On heating 100 C.c. of Distilled Water acidulated with 10 C.c. of diluted sulphuric acid, to boiling, and adding enough of a dilute solution of permanganate of potassium (1 in 1000) to impart to the liquid a decided rose-red tint, this tint should not be entirely destroyed by boiling for five minutes, nor by subsequently setting the vessel aside, well covered, for ten hours (abs. of organic or other oxidizable matters)." *U.S.* It is uselessly employed in some formulas, but is essential in others. "It gives only a faint yellow coloration when a solution of potassio-mercuric iodide is added to three or four fluidounces." *Br.* As a general rule, when small quantities of active medicines are to be given in solution, and in the preparation of collyria, distilled water should be directed. The following list contains the chief substances which require distilled water as a solvent: tartar emetic, corrosive sublimate, nitrate of silver, the chlorides of barium and calcium, acetate and subacetate of lead, permanganate of potassium, the sulphates of iron and zinc, sulphate of quinine, sulphate, hydrochlorate, and acetate of morphine, and, in general terms, all the alkaloids and their salts. Distilled water is used in preparing the officinal diluted acids, for absorbing gaseous ammonia, and for forming nearly all the officinal aqueous solutions.

AQUA FŒNICULI. *U.S., Br.* *Fennel Water.*

(Ā'QUĄ FŒ-NĬC'Ū-LĪ.)

Eau de Fenouil, *Fr.;* Fenchelwasser, *G.*

"Oil of Fennel, *two parts* [or thirty minims]; Cotton, *four parts* [or sixty grains]; Distilled Water, *a sufficient quantity,* To *make one thousand parts* [or two pints]. Add the Oil to the Cotton, in small portions at a time, distributing it thoroughly by picking the Cotton apart after each addition; then pack it firmly in a conical percolator, and gradually pour on Distilled Water, until *one thousand parts* [or two pints] of percolate are obtained." *U.S.*

"Take of Fennel Fruit, bruised, *one pound* [avoirdupois]; Water *two gallons* [Imperial measure]. Distil one gallon [Imp. meas.]." *Br.*

Fennel water is a pleasant vehicle for other medicines, and useful when a mild aromatic is indicated. The process of the British Pharmacopœia, although more troublesome, furnishes a more delicate and agreeable water.

AQUA LAURO-CERASI. *Br.* *Cherry-Laurel Water.*

(Ā'QUĄ LÂU'RŌ-ÇĔR'Ą SĪ.)

Eau distillée de Laurier-cerise, *Fr.;* Kirschlorbeerwasser, *G.;*

"Take of Fresh Leaves of Cherry Laurel *one pound* [avoirdupois]; Water *two pints and a half* [Imperial measure]. Chop the leaves, crush them in a mortar, introduce them with the water into a retort, and distil one pint of liquid. Shake the product, filter through paper, and adjust the strength of the finished product either by addition of hydrocyanic acid or by diluting the distillate with distilled water, so that 810 grains of it, tested as described in the process for diluted hydrocyanic acid, shall require 150 grain-measures of the volumetric solution of nitrate of silver to be added, before a permanent precipitate begins to form, which corresponds to 0·1 per cent. of real hydrocyanic acid." *Br.*

As the cherry-laurel is little cultivated in the United States, the Water is not officinal; but from experiments by the late Prof. Procter, there is little or no room to doubt that a preparation, identical in its effects, might be made from the leaves of our common wild cherry, *Cerasus serotina.* The imported cherry-laurel water, as found in commerce, is generally impaired by age, and not to be relied on.

A. Ripping, of Rotterdam, proposes to make an artificial cherry-laurel water by adding 6 grammes of oil of cherry-laurel and 4·5 grammes of cyanide of potassium to a half-litre of water, and distilling the mixture in a tubulated retort, a current of carbonic acid gas being passed through it at the same time. The distillate is afterwards diluted with distilled water so as to contain one-tenth per cent. of hydrocyanic acid. (*Archiv d. Pharm.*, 1876, pp. 526–531.)

In a former edition of the Dispensatory it was stated that the best plan of preparing this water is "to thoroughly bruise the leaves, and, having mixed them with at least three times their weight of water, to allow the mixture to stand at a temperature of about 86° F. for at least twelve hours, so that opportunity may be given for those reactions by which the hydrocyanic acid is produced, and then to distil them by means of a current of steam. Without the preliminary maceration the distillation by steam does not afford a satisfactory result; but properly performed, it yields the largest possible product. (*Journ. de Pharm.*, Juillet, 1861, p. 15; and Juin, 1864, p. 523.)" More recent investigations have, however, thrown great doubt upon this statement. Cherry-laurel leaves contain 65 per cent. of water, sufficient to provoke the reactions which result in the formation of a volatile oil and hydrocyanic acid. Water is very prone to hasten the conversion of the volatile oil into benzoic acid by oxidation, and it has been found by Mr. C. Umney (*P. J. Tr.*, x. 467) and by Dr. Moore (*Ibid.*, 604) that the water distilled without previous maceration is somewhat stronger in hydrocyanic acid and decidedly stronger in oil (Umney) than the officinal product. The strength of officinal cherry-laurel water is so uncertain as to render it ineligible. It ought to be a powerful preparation, about one-twentieth the strength of the officinal hydrocyanic acid (Br. Ph.), and yet in commerce it varies as 53 to 100 (Umney). The difference depends upon the age of the preparation, the mode of preparing, and the time of year at which the leaves are gathered. M. Garot (*Annuaire de Thérap.*, 1843, p. 45) has found that the leaves yield only half as much in July as in April. Mr. C. Umney obtained 1·26 grains of acid in 1000 grains in March, in July 1·08 grains, and in November 0·64 gr. (*P. J. Tr.*, x. 468.) Dr. Moore, in an elaborate series of experiments, obtained the largest product in July of one year and in October of the next. Mr. Leger (*Ibid.*, June, 1873) has found the maximum percentage in July, and also that different leaves taken from the same bush on the same day vary enormously; young leaves being much richer than old ones. It is evidently impossible to get a uniform cherry-laurel water, except by following the plan of the French Codex* of testing the product and bringing it to a definite uniform strength; in the French

* The following conclusions, in reference to Cherry-laurel water, were arrived at by a committee of pharmaceutists in Paris, appointed to examine the subject of the distilled waters with a view to the revision of the Codex. 1. The whole of the volatile oil and hydrocyanic acid furnished by cherry-laurel leaves, results from a reaction between two substances analogous to the emulsin and amygdalin of bitter almonds, which can take place only in the presence of water. 2. The quantity of volatile oil furnished by the leaves is always in direct relation to that of hydrocyanic acid. 3. The leaves furnish, by mere contact for twenty-four hours with cold water, only one-third of the quantity which they can be made to yield. 4. The fermentable matter of the leaves is liable to change so that the leaves, after being picked, afford less and less of the acid the longer they are kept; and a moist heat favors change; so that complete decomposition takes place in a few hours. 5. Difference in climate, soil, exposure to the sun, and age of the tree, have but a secondary influence on the productiveness of the leaves. 6. The season of the year, however, has a great influence. The younger the leaf, the greater is its yield; so that, while 0·150 per cent. of the acid was obtained from the forming leaves in spring, those of the autumn yielded only 0·132, those of the winter 0·120, and leaves two years old gave only 0·112. 7. Different plants, under apparently the same

Codex this is 50 milligrammes of acid to a cubic centimetre. The proportion of hydrocyanic acid in the Water diminishes with time. It has been ascertained by M. Deschamps that, if a drop of sulphuric acid be added to a pint of the preparation, it will keep unchanged for at least a year. It is best preserved by the entire exclusion of air and light. M. Lepage found that, preserved in full and perfectly air-tight bottles, both this and bitter-almond water remained unchanged at the end of a year; while if freely exposed to the air, they lost all their hydrocyanic acid and essential oil in two or three months. (*Journ. de Pharm.*, xvi. 346.) In view of the uncertain strength of the Water as obtained from the leaves, it was proposed in France, in reference to the Codex then in preparation, to fix upon a definite proportion of hydrocyanic acid; and the percentage generally adopted was from 0·04 to 0·05. Dr. W. H. Pile proposed an easy volumetric method for estimating the hydrocyanic acid strength of cherry-laurel and bitter-almond waters, as well as of other liquids containing this acid. (See *A. J. P.*, 1862, p. 130.)

Medical Properties. Chérry-laurel water is employed in Europe as a sedative narcotic, identical in its properties with a dilute solution of hydrocyanic acid; but it is of uncertain strength, and should not be allowed to supersede the more definite preparation of the acid now in use. Its fraudulent use in Paris in the preparation of a cordial, in imitation of the genuine cherry cordial, made by fermentation and distillation, and like it called "*kirsch*," has been the subject of no little reprobation. (*Journ. de Pharm. et de Chim.*, 4e sér., i. 33, 1865.) The dose is from thirty minims to a fluidrachm (1·9–3·75 C.c.).

AQUA MENTHÆ PIPERITÆ. *U. S., Br.* *Peppermint Water.*

(Ā'QUA MĔN'THÆ PĬP-ER-Ī'TÆ.)

Eau de Menthe poivrée, *Fr.*; Pfefferminzwasser, *G.*

"Oil of Peppermint, *two parts* [or thirty minims]; Cotton, *four parts* [or sixty grains]; Distilled Water, *a sufficient quantity*, To make *one thousand parts* [or two pints]. Add the Oil to the Cotton, in small portions at a time, distributing it thoroughly by picking the Cotton apart after each addition; then pack it firmly in a conical percolator, and gradually pour on Distilled Water, until *one thousand parts* [or two pints] of percolate are obtained." *U. S.*

"Take of Oil of Peppermint *one fluidrachm and a half;* Water *one gallon and a half* [Imperial measure]. Distil one gallon [Imp. meas.]." *Br.*

Off. Prep. Br. Mistura Ferri Aromatica.

AQUA MENTHÆ VIRIDIS. *U. S., Br.* *Spearmint Water.*

(Ā'QUA MĔN'THÆ VĬR'I-DĬS.)

Eau de Menthe verte, *Fr.*

"Oil of Spearmint, *two parts* [or thirty minims]; Cotton, *four parts* [or sixty grains]; Distilled Water, *a sufficient quantity*, To make *one thousand parts* [or two pints]. Add the Oil to the Cotton, in small portions at a time, distributing it thoroughly by picking the Cotton apart after each addition; then pack it firmly in a conical percolator, and gradually pour on Distilled Water, until *one thousand parts* [or two pints] of percolate are obtained." *U. S.*

"Take of Oil of Spearmint *one fluidrachm and a half;* Water *one gallon and a half* [Imperial measure]. Distil one gallon [Imp. meas.]." *Br.*

The two mint waters are among the most grateful and most employed of this class

circumstances, differ greatly in productiveness, so that 0·176 per cent. was obtained from the most productive, and only 0·092 from the least so. 8. The distillation by steam yields the greatest possible product. The committee, therefore, propose the adoption of this method; the bruised leaves having been previously mixed with at least three times their weight of water, and exposed to a gradually increasing heat, not to exceed 140° F., when all reaction ceases. 9. Bruising is the best method of comminuting the leaves. 10. As it is impossible to obtain a Water always identical from the leaves, the committee propose to fix a definite strength, and state that the proportion generally adopted is from 0·040 per cent. of acid as the minimum, to 0·050, or one-twentieth of one per cent. as the maximum, which is only one-half the strength proposed for bitter-almond water. 11. Though a change rapidly takes place in this and bitter-almond water exposed to the air, yet in bottles full, and perfectly closed by glass stoppers, the change at the end of a year is scarcely perceptible; and this observation applies to the distilled waters in general. (*Journ. de Pharm.*, 1864, p. 520.)

of preparations. Together with cinnamon water, they are used in this country, almost to the exclusion of all others, as the vehicle of medicines given in the form of mixture. They serve not only to conceal or qualify the taste of other medicines, but also to counteract their nauseating properties. Peppermint water is generally thought to have a more agreeable flavor than that of spearmint, but some prefer the latter. Their effects are the same.

AQUA PIMENTÆ. *Br.* *Pimento Water.*

(Ā'QUA PĪ-MĔN'TÆ.)

"Take of Pimento, bruised, 14 ounces [av.]; Water 2 gallons [Imp. meas.]. Distil one gallon [Imp. meas.]" *Br.*

Pimento water is an agreeable aromatic water, used as a vehicle.

AQUA ROSÆ. *U. S., Br.* *Rose Water.*

(Ā'QUA RŌ'ŞÆ.)

Eau distillée de Rose, *Fr.;* Rosenwasser, *G.*

"Recent, Pale Rose, *forty parts* [or forty-eight ounces av.]; Water, *two hundred parts* [or fourteen pints], To make *one hundred parts* [or seven pints]. Mix them, and, by means of steam, distil *one hundred parts* [or seven pints]." *U. S.*

"Take of Fresh Petals of the Hundred-leaved Rose *ten pounds* [avoirdupois] (or an equivalent quantity of the petals preserved while fresh with common salt); Water *five gallons* [Imperial measure]. Distil one gallon [Imp. meas.]." *Br.*

An improvement has been made in this preparation by doubling its strength, experience having shown that the stronger rose water keeps better.

It should be observed that, in the nomenclature of the U. S. Pharmacopœia, the term "Rose" implies only the petals of the flower. These are usually preferred in the recent state; but it is said that, when preserved by being incorporated with one-third of their weight of common salt, they retain their odor, and afford a water equally fragrant with that prepared from the fresh flower. Indeed, Mr. Haselden prefers the salted roses, believing that the water prepared from them is less mucilaginous, less apt to become sour, and keeps its odor better than that prepared from the fresh flowers. (*P. J. Tr.*, xvi. 15.) It is not uncommon to employ the whole flower, including the calyx; but the product is less fragrant than when the petals only are used, as officinally directed.* Rose water is sometimes made by distilling together water and the oil of roses. This is best performed by dropping 10 drops

* A. Monthus states that the petals of the hundred-leaved rose are more odorous the nearer they are to the centre of the flower, and, contrary to what is said in the text, thinks that the calyx should not be rejected in preparing the distilled water. He maintains that so far from injuring the product, it in fact contributes to its preservation, and that the water obtained from the whole flower is less liable to that mucosity, which is the commencement of decomposition. This effect he ascribes to the astringent matter of the calyx, coagulating the mucilaginous matter of the petals, and preventing it from passing over in the distillation. (*Journ. de Pharm.*, 1863, p. 497.)

Milk of Roses. In making this cosmetic it is essential to produce an emulsion which, if it separates after long repose, may be restored by slight agitation. Although other perfumes may be, and are, commonly added to it, the scent of roses should predominate and form its characteristic odor. There are three varieties, the English, French, and German. The latter variety should never be employed as a cosmetic, on account of containing lead.

English. Almonds (blanched) 1½ ounce; Oil of Almonds and White Windsor Soap, of each, 1 drachm; Rose Water ¾ pint. Make an emulsion; to the strained emulsion add a mixture of Essence or Spirit of Roses ½ fluidrachm; Alcohol 2½ fluidounces; and subsequently of Rose Water q. s. to make the whole measure one pint; more alcohol is apt to cause the separation of the ingredients. Some makers add a few drops of oil of bergamot, with two or three drops each of oil of lavender and otto of roses, dissolved in the alcohol.

Or, Oil of Almonds and White Windsor Soap, of each, 1 ounce; Salts of Tartar ½ drachm; Boiling Water ¾ pint. Triturate, and subsequently agitate until perfectly united. When cold, further add Alcohol 2 fluidounces; Spirit of Roses a few drops; Rose Water q. s. to make the whole measure a pint.

French. Tincture of Benzoin (simple) ½ fluidounce; Tincture of Styrax ½ fluidounce; Spirit of Roses 1 to 2 fluidrachms; Alcohol 2½ fluidounces. Mix, and add gradually, with agitation, Rose Water 16½ fluidounces. Augustin recommends the addition of a little carbonate of potassium (say 1 drachm to the pint) when it is intended to be used as a lotion in acne.

Or, Tincture of Benzoin (simple) 1 fluidrachm; Tincture of Balsam of Peru 20 drops; Rose Water ½ pint. The addition of an ounce of alcohol, in lieu of a like quantity of rose water, improves it.

German. Dilute solution of Diacetate of Lead, ½ fluidounce; Lavender Water 2 fluidrachms; Alcohol 2½ fluidounces; Rose Water ¾ of a pint. Mix and agitate.

of oil of rose on a sponge and adjusting it in the upper part of a still in the body of which a gallon of water is placed: the steam from the boiling water will carry over portions of the oil, and the distillate will thus be impregnated.

When properly prepared, it has the delightful perfume of the rose in great perfection. It is most successfully made on a large scale. Like the other distilled waters, it is liable to spoil when kept; and the alcohol which is sometimes added to preserve it is incompatible with some of the purposes to which the water is applied, and is even said to render it sour through acetous fermentation. It is best, therefore, to avoid this addition, and to substitute a second distillation. This distilled water is chiefly employed, on account of its agreeable odor, in collyria and other lotions. It is wholly destitute of irritating properties, unless when it contains alcohol.

Off. Prep. Confectio Rosæ; Mistura Ferri Composita; Unguentum Aquæ Rosæ.
Off. Prep. Br. Mistura Ferri Composita; Trochisci Bismuthi.

AQUA SAMBUCI. *Br.* *Elder-flower Water.*

(Ā'QUA SĂM-BŪ'CĪ.)

"Take of fresh Elder Flowers, separated from the stalks, *ten pounds* [avoirdupois] (or an equivalent quantity of the flowers preserved while fresh with common salt); Water *two gallons* [Imperial measure]. Distil one gallon [Imp. meas.]." *Br.*

Elder flowers yield very little oil upon distillation; and, if the water be needed, it may be best prepared from the flowers. Mr. Haselden prefers the salted flowers to the fresh, for the reason stated under Rose Water. The preparation is little used in this country.

ARGENTUM PURIFICATUM. *Br.* *Refined Silver.*

Ag; 108. (ÄR-ĢĔN'TŲM PŪ-RĮ-FĮ-CĀ'TŬM) Ag; 108.

"Pure metallic silver." *Br.*

Argent raffiné, Argent, *Fr.;* Silber, Raffinirtes Silber, *G.;* Argento, *It.;* Plata, *Sp.*

Silver is occasionally found in the metallic state, sometimes crystallized, at other times combined with gold, antimony, arsenic, or mercury; but usually it occurs in the state of sulphide, either pure or mixed with other sulphides, as those of copper, lead, and antimony. It is sometimes found as a chloride.

The most productive mines of silver are found on this continent, being those of Mexico and Peru, and our own Rocky Mountain territories; the richest in Europe are those of Norway, Hungary, and Transylvania. Mines have been opened and profitably worked in California and Nevada, but at present it is chiefly Colorado and Idaho which furnish the great bulk of the American silver production. Arizona and New Mexico are said also to contain very rich silver deposits which are now being developed. The principal ore is the sulphide. The mineral containing silver, which is most disseminated, is argentiferous galena, which is sulphide of lead, containing a little sulphide of silver. Argentiferous galena exists in several localities in the United States. A mine of silver was opened, about the year 1841, in Davidson County, N. C. The ore is an argentiferous carbonate of lead, yielding about one-third of its weight of lead, from which from 100 to 400 ounces of silver are extracted per ton. (Eckfeldt and Du Bois, *Manual of Coins.*) Native silver is associated, in small quantities, with the native copper of the Lake Superior region; and a little of it has come into the market. The two metals, though more or less mixed, are yet quite distinct, never being alloyed to any considerable extent, showing conclusively that the deposits have not undergone igneous fusion at any time, but that the metals have deposited from solution. The value of the silver produced in the United States for the years 1884, 1885, and 1886, according to the Director of the Mint, was $48,800,000, $51,600,000, and $51,000,000 respectively. The entire production for the world in the year 1885 is stated to be 2,993,805 kilogrammes, valued at $124,422,342.

Extraction. Silver is extracted from its ores by two principal processes, *amalgamation* and *cupellation*. At Freiberg, in Saxony, the ore, which is principally the sulphide, is mixed with a tenth of chloride of sodium, and roasted in a reverberatory furnace. As fast as the sulphide is oxidized to sulphate, this reacts with the sodium chloride, forming silver chloride and sodium sulphate. The roasted mass is then reduced to very fine powder, mixed with half its weight of mercury, one-third of its weight of water, and about a seventeenth of iron in flat pieces, and subjected, for sixteen or eighteen hours, to constant agitation in barrels turned by machinery. The chlorine combines with the iron, and remains in solution as chloride of iron; while the reduced silver forms an amalgam with the mercury. The amalgam is then subjected to pressure in leathern bags, through the pores of which the excess of mercury passes, a solid amalgam being left behind. This is then subjected to heat in a distillatory apparatus, by means of which the mercury is separated from the silver, which is left in a porous mass. In Peru and Mexico the process is similar to that above given, common salt and mercury being used; but slacked lime and sulphide of iron are also employed, with an effect which is not very obvious.

When argentiferous galenas are worked for the silver they contain, they are first reduced, and the argentiferous lead obtained is fused on a large, oval, shallow vessel called a *test*, and exposed to the blast of a bellows, whereby the lead is oxidised, half vitrified, and driven off the test in scales, in the form of *litharge*. The operation being continued on successive portions of argentiferous lead, the whole of the lead is separated, and the silver, not being oxidisable, accumulates on the test as a brilliant fused mass, until its amount is sufficient to be removed. The time required for the separation is much abridged by the process of Mr. Pattinson, of Newcastle, England. This consists in allowing the melted alloy to cool slowly, and separating the crystals which first form, consisting mainly of lead, by means of a perforated ladle. The residue is a very fusible alloy of lead and silver, in which the latter metal is in large proportion, and from which it can be easily separated by cupellation or other means. (*Brande and Taylor.*)

Properties. Silver is a white metal, very brilliant, tenacious, malleable, and ductile. In malleability and ductility, it is inferior only to gold. It is harder than gold, but softer than copper. Its atomic weight is 108, symbol Ag, and sp. gr. from 10·4 to 10·5. It forms but one well-characterised oxide. Exposed to a full red heat, it enters into fusion, and exhibits a brilliant appearance. It is not oxidised in the air, but contracts a superficial tarnish of sulphide of silver by the action of sulphuretted hydrogen in the atmosphere; from which it may be freed by washing it with a strong solution of cyanide of potassium, and, as soon as it becomes bright, washing it with water and drying it. (*Chem. News*, 1866, p. 12.) It is entirely soluble in diluted nitric acid. If any gold be present, it will remain undissolved as a dark-colored powder. From the nitric solution, the whole of the silver may be thrown down by chloride of sodium, as a white precipitate of chloride of silver, characterised by being completely soluble in ammonia. If the remaining solution contain copper or lead, it will be precipitated or discolored by sulphuretted hydrogen. "The solution, deprived of silver by means of chloride of sodium, and filtered, is not colored, *or but slightly so*, and is not precipitated by hydrosulphuric acid." *U. S.* 1870. "If ammonia be added in excess to a solution of the metal in nitric acid, the resulting fluid exhibits neither color nor turbidity" (*Br.*); proving the absence of copper, lead, and other metals.

Off. Prep. Br. Argenti Nitras.

ARGENTI CYANIDUM. *U.S.* *Cyanide of Silver.*

Ag CN; 133·7. (ĂR-ĢĔN'TĪ CȲ-ĂN'Ĭ-DŬM.) Ag C_2 N; 133·7.

Cyanuret of Silver; Argentum Cyanatum; Cyanure d'Argent, *Fr.*; Cyansilber, *G.*

A process for preparing this salt is no longer officinal. Below will be found that of the U. S. P. 1870.*

* "Take of Nitrate of Silver, Ferrocyanide of Potassium, each, *two troyounces*; Sulphuric Acid *a troyounce and a half*; Distilled Water *a sufficient quantity*. Dissolve the Nitrate of Silver in a pint of Distilled Water, and pour the solution into a tubulated glass receiver. Dissolve the Ferrocyanide of Potassium in ten fluidounces of Distilled Water, and pour the solution into a tubulated retort, previously adapted to the receiver. Having mixed the Sulphuric Acid with four fluidounces of Distilled Water, add the mixture to the solution in the retort, and distil, by means of a sand-bath, with a moderate heat, until six fluidounces have passed over, or until the distillate no longer produces a precipitate in the receiver. Lastly, wash the precipitate with Distilled Water, and dry it." *U. S.* 1870.

In the process of 1870 all the silver contained in a given weight of nitrate of silver, placed in a receiver in solution, is converted into cyanide by hydrocyanic acid, produced from ferrocyanide of potassium by the action of sulphuric acid, $AgNO_3 + HCN = HNO_3 + Ag,CN$. The materials in the retort are sufficient to produce a little more hydrocyanic acid than is necessary to convert the whole of the silver in the receiver into cyanide; so that the complete decomposition of the nitrate of silver is insured. Cyanide of silver should be kept in dark amber-colored vials, protected from light.

According to Messrs. Glassford and Napier, the best way of obtaining cyanide of silver is to add cyanide of potassium to a solution of nitrate of silver so long as a precipitate is formed.

Properties. Cyanide of silver is "a white powder, permanent in dry air, but gradually turning brown by exposure to light, odorless and tasteless, and insoluble in water and in alcohol. Insoluble in cold, but soluble in boiling nitric acid, with evolution of hydrocyanic acid; also soluble in water of ammonia and in solution of hyposulphite of sodium. When strongly heated, the salt fuses, gives off cyanogen gas, and, on ignition, metallic silver is left behind." *U. S.*

Its best solvent is cyanide of potassium. It has no medical uses, but is officinal solely for the making of Hydrocyanic Acid.

Off. Prep. Acidum Hydrocyanicum Dilutum.

ARGENTI IODIDUM. *U. S.* *Iodide of Silver.*

Ag I; 234·3. (ÄR-ÇĔN'TĪ Ī-ŎD'Į-DŬM.) Ag I; 234·3.

This is a new officinal salt, which may be readily prepared by adding a solution of iodide of potassium to one of nitrate of silver, and washing and drying the precipitate, which should be kept in dark amber-colored vials, protected from light.

According to the experiments of M. Fizeau, it has the remarkable property of contracting with heat and expanding with cold, differing in this respect from the chlorides and bromides of the same metal, and the iodides of other metals. (*Journ. de Pharm.*, 1867, p. 435.) This appears, however, to be only a partial truth, the iodide having three allotropic forms and a point of maximum density at about 116° C. (240·8° F.). See paper by G. F. Rodwell, in *Chem. News*, xx. 288; xxi. 14. The Pharmacopœia describes it as "a heavy, amorphous, light yellowish powder, unaltered by light if pure, but generally becoming somewhat greenish yellow, without odor and taste, and insoluble in water, alcohol, diluted acids, or in solution of carbonate of ammonium. Soluble in about 2500 parts of stronger water of ammonia. When heated to about 400° C. (752° F.), it melts to a dark red liquid, which, on cooling, congeals to a soft, yellow, slightly translucent mass. When mixed with water of ammonia, it turns white, but regains its yellowish color by washing with water. It is dissolved by an aqueous solution of cyanide of potassium, and the resulting solution yields a black precipitate with hydrosulphuric acid or sulphide of ammonium. If a small quantity of chlorine water be agitated with an excess of the salt, the filtrate acquires a dark blue color on the addition of gelatinized starch. If the salt be boiled with test-solution of carbonate of ammonium previously diluted with an equal volume of water, the resulting filtrate, on being supersaturated with nitric acid, should not be rendered more than faintly opalescent (abs. of chloride)." *U. S.*

Medical Properties. It possesses the general medical properties of nitrate of silver, and Dr. Charles Patterson, of Dublin, states that it may be used without any danger of producing discoloration of the skin, but in this he is probably incorrect. Dr. Patterson found it generally successful in curing the stomach affections of the Irish peasantry, in the treatment of which nitrate of silver had previously proved useful. He succeeded with it in curing several cases of hooping-cough in a short time, and in greatly relieving a case of dysmenorrhœa of three years' standing. Its effects in epilepsy were least satisfactory. The dose is one or two grains (·065–·13 Gm.), three times a day, given in the form of pill; for children, from the eighth to the fourth of a grain (·008–·016 Gm.), according to the age.

ARGENTI NITRAS. *U. S., Br.* *Nitrate of Silver.*

Ag NO₃; 169·7. (ĂR-GĔN'TĪ NĪ'TRĂS.) Ag O, NO₅: 169·7.

Argentum Nitricum Crystallisatum, *P.G.;* Azotas (Nitras) Argenticus; Azotate d'Argent, Nitre lunaire, *Fr.;* Salpetersaures Silberoxyd, Silbersalpeter, *G.*

The U. S. Pharmacopœia does not give a process for making this salt.* The British process is as follows. "Take of Refined Silver *three ounces* [avoirdupois]; Nitric Acid *two and a half fluidounces* [Imperial measure]; Distilled Water *five fluidounces* [Imp. meas.]. Add the Nitric Acid and the Water to the Silver in a flask, and apply a gentle heat till the metal is dissolved. Decant the clear liquor from any black powder which may be present, into a porcelain dish, evaporate, and set aside to crystallize; pour off the clear liquor, and again evaporate and crystallize. Let the crystals drain in a glass funnel, and dry them by exposure to the air, carefully avoiding the contact of all organic substances. To obtain the nitrate in rods, fuse the crystals in a capsule of platinum or thin porcelain, and pour the melted salt into proper moulds. Nitrate of Silver must be preserved in bottles furnished with accurately ground stoppers." *Br.*

The two formulas are essentially the same; but that of the U. S. Pharmacopœia, 1870, is more detailed and precise, with two peculiarities which deserve notice. One of these is the direction to cover the materials in the capsule, during the continuance of the reaction, with a glass funnel. This is in order to economize the nitric acid, a portion of which rises in vapor, and, being condensed on the inner surface of the funnel, falls again into the capsule. The second peculiarity is the fusion of the salt before being dissolved. This would, from the phraseology of the directions, appear to have been intended to get rid of any uncombined nitric acid which might remain in the dry salt. But the effect is to decompose any nitrate of copper that might have been derived from the silver, which, if coin be employed, always contains copper. The heat decomposes the nitrate of copper, and the comparatively insoluble oxide is formed, which remains on the filter when the mass is subsequently dissolved in water and filtered, the nitrate of silver not being decomposed by the heat used.

During the solution of silver in nitric acid, part of the acid is decomposed and nitric oxide is given off, which becomes red by contact with the atmosphere, and the oxygen oxidizes the silver. This is taken up by the remainder of the acid, and produces nitrate of silver in solution, which, by due evaporation, furnishes crystals of the salt. The silver should be pure, and the acid diluted for the purpose of promoting its action. If the silver contain copper, the solution will have a greenish tint, not disappearing on the application of heat; and if a minute portion of gold be present, it will be left undissolved as a black powder. The acid also should be pure. The commercial nitric acid, as it frequently contains both hydrochloric and sulphuric acids, should never be used. The hydrochloric acid gives rise to an insoluble chloride, and the sulphuric, to the sparingly soluble sulphate of silver.† For an account of the manufacture of nitrate of silver on the large scale, see *Druggists' Circular*, 1887, p. 3.

Properties. Nitrate of silver is in "colorless, transparent, tabular, rhombic crys-

* The U. S. Pharmacopœia, 1870, gave the following. "Take of Silver, in small pieces, *two troyounces;* Nitric Acid *two troyounces and a half;* Distilled Water *a sufficient quantity*. Mix the Acid with a fluidounce of Distilled Water in a porcelain capsule, add the Silver to the mixture, cover it with an inverted glass funnel, resting within the edge of the capsule, and apply a gentle heat until the metal is dissolved, and red vapors cease to be produced; then remove the funnel, and, increasing the heat, evaporate the solution to dryness. Melt the dry mass, and continue the heat, stirring constantly with a glass rod, until free nitric acid is entirely dissipated. Dissolve the melted salt, when cold, in six fluidounces of Distilled Water, allow the insoluble matter to subside, and decant the clear solution. Mix the residue with a fluidounce of Distilled Water, filter through paper, and, having added the filtrate to the decanted solution, evaporate the liquid until a pellicle begins to form, and set it aside in a warm place to crystallize. Lastly, drain the crystals in a glass funnel until dry, and preserve them in a well-stopped bottle. By evaporating the mother-water, more crystals may be obtained." *U. S.*

† It is desirable that pure silver, free from copper, should be used in this process. As silver coin always contains copper, it should be purified before being employed. For this purpose, according to the method of M. Lienau, it should be dissolved in nitric acid, and the solution precipitated by chlorine water, which throws down the silver only in the form of chloride. The precipitate is to be well washed with chlorine water, then dissolved in solution of ammonia, and precipitated by clean copper wire. The silver is deposited as a black powder, which, when washed with solution of ammonia, is perfectly pure. (See *A. J. P.*, 1862, p. 368.)

tals, becoming gray or grayish black on exposure to light in presence of organic matter, odorless, having a bitter, caustic and strongly metallic taste and a neutral reaction. Soluble in 0·8 part of water and in 26 parts of alcohol at 15° C. (59° F.), in 0·1 part of boiling water and in 5 parts of boiling alcohol. When heated to about 200° C. (392° F.), the salt fuses to a faintly yellow liquid, which, on cooling, congeals to a purely white, crystalline mass. At a higher temperature the salt is gradually decomposed, with evolution of nitrous vapors. It should be kept in dark amber-colored vials protected from the light." *U. S.* The solution stains the skin of an indelible black color, and is itself discolored by the most minute portion of organic matter, for which it forms a delicate test. The affinity of this salt for animal matter is evinced by its forming definite compounds with albumen and fibrin. The solution also stains linen and muslin in a similar manner; and hence its use in making the so-called indelible ink. To remove these stains, Mr. W. B. Herapath advises to let fall on the moistened spots a few drops of tincture of iodine, which converts the silver into iodide of silver. The iodide is then dissolved by a solution of hyposulphite of sodium, made with half a drachm to a fluidounce of water, or by a moderately dilute solution of caustic potassa, and the spots are washed out with warm water. They are taken out also by a solution of two and a half drachms of cyanide of potassium, and fifteen grains of iodine, in three fluidounces of water. Stains on the skin may be removed by the same reagents. Dr. H. Kraetzer recommends instead of potassium cyanide, a solution of 10 parts sal ammoniac and 10 parts corrosive sublimate in 100 parts of water, with which the stains are said to be removed readily from the hands, and from linen, wool, and cotton without injuring the fabric. (*Archiv d. Pharm.*, 1880, p. 52.) Nitrate of silver is incompatible with almost all spring and river water, on account of a little common salt usually contained in it; with soluble chlorides; with sulphuric, hydrosulphuric, hydrochloric, and tartaric acids, and their salts; with the alkalies and their carbonates; with lime-water; and with astringent infusions. It is sometimes improperly prescribed in pill with tannic acid, by which it is decomposed. Nitrate of silver is an anhydrous salt, consisting of one atom of silver, 108, combined with the monatomic group NO_3, 62, characteristic of nitric acid, = 170.

Impurities and Tests. Hydrochloric acid or a solution of chloride of sodium, added in excess to one of nitrate of silver, should throw down the whole of the silver as a white curdy precipitate darkening on exposure to light, and nothing besides. This precipitate should be entirely soluble in ammonia. If not so, the insoluble part is probably chloride of lead. If the supernatant liquid, after the removal of the precipitate, be discolored or precipitated by sulphuretted hydrogen, the fact shows the presence of metallic matter, which is probably copper or some remains of lead, or both. The solution, after precipitation by hydrochloric acid and filtration, should leave no residue when evaporated. A piece of the salt, heated on charcoal by the blowpipe, melts, deflagrates, and leaves behind a whitish metallic coating. After all, the best sign of the purity of nitrate of silver is the characteristic appearance of the crystals. An aqueous solution of the salt yields with hydrochloric acid a white precipitate of silver chloride, soluble in ammonia. "If all the silver has been precipitated with hydrochloric acid, and the filtrate is evaporated to dryness, no fixed residue should be left (abs. of foreign metallic impurities). 1 Gm. Nitrate of Silver, when completely precipitated by hydrochloric acid, should yield 0·84 Gm. of dry chloride of silver." *U. S.*

Medical Properties and Uses. When nitrate of silver in a pure state is brought in contact with a living tissue, it acts as an escharotic. Owing to the formation of a dense film of coagulated albumen, the depth of its action is very limited; the albuminous coating is at first white, but soon becomes blackish owing to the reduction of the silver. The solution of the salt is, if not too strong, a local stimulant and astringent, and is very largely employed (grs. xx to f℥i) in ordinary angina, or more concentrated (grs. xxx to f℥i) in diphtheria, and is also used in inflammations of the urethral and conjunctival mucous membranes; for the latter purpose the strength should usually not exceed one or two grains to the ounce. As a counter-irritant, stimulant, and alterative, or an escharotic in various external ulcerations, morbid growths, etc., nitrate of silver finds a very wide use. It is largely employed, also, internally in inflammations and ulcerations of the alimentary tract, such as subacute gastritis, pyrosis, ulcer of the stomach, chronic diarrhœa, catarrh of the gall ducts, etc. In all stomachic diseases it should be given half an hour before eating, so as to reach as thoroughly as possible the gastric mucous membrane. Dr. Boudin, of Marseilles, employed it in typhoid fever, and Prof. Wm. Pepper has followed the practice with asserted brilliant results. As it has been found in all the tissues of the body, it is undoubtedly absorbed. It is soluble in peptones, and is probably so taken up, although some believe that it is converted in the stomach into a soluble double chloride with sodium or potassium. It is never used in practical medicine to produce an acute impression on the general system, but for general effects solely as a slowly acting alterative in certain nervous affections, especially epilepsy and chronic spinal inflammation, such as locomotor ataxia, spasmodic tabes, tabes dorsalis, etc. The occasional production of a slate-colored discoloration of the skin is a great drawback to the long-continued use of the nitrate, but it probably never occurs under a course of the remedy of less than two months. It affects also the mucous membrane, and, according to Dr. Branson (confirmed by Dr. Wm. Pepper), an indication of the approach of discoloration is furnished by the occurrence of a dark blue line on the edges of the gums, very similar to that produced by lead, but somewhat darker. When once produced, the discoloration seems to be permanent, although Dr. L. P. Yandell has reported two cases in which the discoloration of the skin disappeared during a course of iodide of potassium for syphilitic disease. (*N. R.*, July, 1873.)

The dose of nitrate of silver (crystals) is the fourth of a grain (0·016 Gm.), gradually increased to half a grain (0·03 Gm.), three times a day. For internal exhibition, the physician should always prescribe the crystals, and never direct the fused nitrate, which may not be pure. Nitrate of silver should always be given in pill, as the solution is decomposed by the liquids of the mouth. In the treatment of epilepsy, Dr. Powell recommends the exhibition at first of grain (0·065 Gm.) doses, to be gradually increased to six grains (0·4 Gm.), three times a day. Its effects vary very much, owing no doubt to the salt being more or less decomposed by the substances used in preparing it in pill, or with which it comes in contact in the stomach. It should not be made up into pill with crumb of bread, as this contains common salt, but with some vegetable powder and mucilage, preferably powdered sugar of milk with an excipient of glucose. But, as all organic substances decompose it more or less, M. Vée proposes the use of inorganic matter, such as nitre, or preferably pure silica obtained by precipitating one of the silicates by an acid, and washing it. The least possible proportion of tragacanth may be used to give adhesiveness to the mass. (*Journ. de Pharm.*, Mai, 1864, p. 408.) In view of the fact that chloride of sodium is used with food, and exists, together with phosphates, in the secretions, and that free hydrochloric acid and albuminous fluids are present in the stomach, it is almost certain that, sooner or later, the whole of the nitrate of silver will be converted into the chloride, phosphate, and albuminate, compounds far less active than the original salt. The experiments of Keller, who analyzed the fæces of patients under the use of this salt, confirm this view. Such being the inevitable result when the nitrate is given, the question arises how far it would be expedient to anticipate the change, and give the silver as a chloride ready formed. Dr. Geo. B. Wood tried the chloride in large doses, in two cases of epilepsy, but without advantage. According to Mialhe, nitrate of silver upon entering the stomach is converted into a soluble and readily absorbable double chloride, by combining with chloride of sodium or of potassium.

When ingested in sufficient dose, nitrate of silver is a violent poison, and has several times caused death. The symptoms are those of toxic gastro-enteritis, with marked constitutional disturbance, especially coma, convulsions, paralysis, and profound alteration of the respiration. The treatment of the poisoning resolves itself into the use of the ordinary antidotes (common salt, soap, alkalies, etc.).

Off Prep. Argenti Nitras Dilutus; Argenti Nitras Fusus.

Off. Prep. Br. Argenti et Potassii Nitras; Argenti Oxidum.

ARGENTI NITRAS DILUTUS. *U.S.* *Diluted Nitrate of Silver.*

(ĂR-ĢĔN'TĪ NĪ'TRĂS DI-LŪ'TŬS.)

"Nitrate of Silver, *fifty parts;* Nitrate of Potassium, *fifty parts,* To make *one hundred parts.* Melt the salts together in a porcelain crucible, at as low a temperature as possible, stirring the melted mass well until it flows smoothly. Then cast it in suitable moulds. Keep the product in dark amber-colored vials, protected from light." *U.S.*

ARGENTI ET POTASSII NITRAS. *Br.* *Nitrate of Silver and Potassium.* [*Mitigated Caustic.*]

(ĂR-ĢĔN'TĪ ĔT PO-TĂS'SI-Ī NĪ'TRĂS.)

"Take of Nitrate of Silver 1 ounce [av.]; Nitrate of Potassium 2 ounces [av.]. Fuse and mix thoroughly together in a capsule of platinum or thin porcelain, and pour the melted mass into proper moulds. Preserve in bottles carefully stoppered." *Br.*

These are new officinal preparations. Their introduction grew out of the frequent demand for a fused nitrate of silver, which would not be so severe in its action as the pure article. The manufacturers have been in the way of furnishing for many years a "*No.* 2 *Lunar Caustic,*" which contains 67 per cent. of pure nitrate of silver; the officinal diluted nitrate contains 50 per cent. of lunar caustic, whilst the British preparation contains but 33 per cent.

Properties. Diluted nitrate of silver is officinally described as "a white, hard solid, generally in form of pencils or cones of a finely granular fracture, becoming gray or grayish black on exposure to light in presence of organic matter, odorless, having a caustic, metallic taste, and a neutral reaction. Each of its constituents retains the solubility in water and in alcohol mentioned respectively under *Argenti Nitras* and *Potassii Nitras.* An aqueous solution of 2 Gm. of Diluted Nitrate of Silver, acidulated with nitric acid, when completely precipitated by hydrochloric acid, should yield not less than 0·84 Gm. of dry chloride of silver. The filtrate, separated from the precipitate, when evaporated to dryness, leaves a residue which is completely soluble in water, and which yields a white, crystalline precipitate with a concentrated solution of bitartrate of sodium." *U.S.*

Medical Properties. This preparation is only used externally. It is similar in its action to the fused nitrate, but less energetic.

ARGENTI NITRAS FUSUS. *U.S.* *Moulded Nitrate of Silver.*

(ĂR-ĢĔN'TĪ NĪ'TRĂS FŪ'SŬS.)

Argenti Nitras, *Br.;* Lunar Caustic; Lapis Infernalis, Argentum Nitricum Fusum, *P.G.;* Azotas (Nitras) Argenticus Fusus; Azotate d'Argent fondu, Pierre infernale, *Fr.;* Höllenstein, Geschmolzenes Salpetersaures Silberoxyd, *G.;* Fused Nitrate of Silver.

"Nitrate of Silver, *one hundred parts* [or one ounce av.]; Hydrochloric Acid, *four parts* [or sixteen minims]. Melt the Nitrate of Silver in a porcelain capsule, at as low a temperature as possible; then add to it, gradually, the Hydrochloric Acid, stir well, and, when nitrous vapors cease to be evolved, pour the melted mass in suitable moulds. Keep the product in dark amber-colored vials, protected from light." *U.S.*

"To obtain the Nitrate in rods, fuse the crystals in a capsule of platinum or thin porcelain, and pour the melted salt into proper moulds. To form Toughened Nitrate of Silver or 'Toughened Caustic,' add 5 parts of nitrate of potassium to 95 parts of the nitrate of silver before fusion. 10 grains of this preparation will yield with hydrochloric acid 8 grains of precipitate, and the filtrate when evaporated will leave a white residue." *Br.*

For most purposes it is desirable to have the nitrate of silver less brittle than in its pure state. Prof. J. L. Smith, of Louisville, Ky., found that this could be effected by adding a little chloride of silver, which rendered the stick tough, without materially impairing its efficiency. Dr. Squibb proposed to accomplish the object by adding 40 grains of hydrochloric acid, with half a fluidounce of distilled water, to two ounces of nitrate of silver, heating the mixture by means of a sand-bath to dryness, and then melting and casting into moulds. (*Proc. A. P. A.*, 1858.)

This process has been adopted in the present U. S. Pharmacopœia. In order to keep the sticks from becoming discolored during the casting process, it is advisable to add a diluted nitric acid (1 in 5) occasionally to the melted nitrate, and carefully prevent the mass from becoming overheated. The British process is merely the continuation of that by which the nitrate is obtained in crystals. As the salt while melting sinks into a common crucible, the fusion is performed in one of porcelain or platinum, the size of which should be sufficient to hold five or six times the quantity of the salt operated on, in order to prevent its overflowing in consequence of the ebullition. Sometimes small portions of the liquid are spirted out, and the operator should be on his guard against this occurrence. When the mass flows like oil, it is completely fused, and ready to be poured into the moulds. These should be warmed, but not greased, as organic matter would thus be furnished, which would partially decompose the fused salt.

Properties. Fused nitrate of silver, as prepared by the above process, is in the form of hard brittle sticks of the size of a goose-quill, at first translucent, but quickly becoming gray or more or less dark under the influence of light, owing to the reduction of the silver, effected probably by organic matter or sulphuretted hydrogen contained in the atmosphere. That the change does not depend on the sole action of light has been proved by Mr. Scanlan, who finds that nitrate of silver in a clean glass tube hermetically sealed undergoes no change by exposure to light. The sticks often become dark-colored and nearly black on the surface, and when broken across, exhibit a crystalline fracture with a radiated surface. Fused nitrate of silver, when pure, is wholly soluble in distilled water; but even fair samples of the fused salt will not totally dissolve, a very scanty black powder being left of reduced silver, arising probably from the salt having been exposed to too high a heat in fusion. Stein (*Schweiz. Wochenschrift für Pharmacie*, 6, 10, 1877) recommends a plan for obtaining sticks of lunar caustic of special diameter or length by taking a glass tube or rod of required outside diameter, and wrapping around it moistened parchment paper, pasting the edges, tying the lower end, and drying. The melted lunar caustic is poured into the paper mould, held upright in a test-tube, and allowed to cool by standing. *Elastic crayons* of nitrate of silver may be made by taking a laminaria tent $\frac{1}{10}$th of an inch (·002 mm.) in diameter, dipping it into thick mucilage, rolling in finely powdered lunar caustic, and drying it. (*Pajot.*) Entirely black lunar caustic is sometimes seen in France, which contains about 2 per cent. of nitrate of potassium and the same quantity of black oxide of manganese. Heller's caustic pencils look like ordinary lead-pencils, and consist of long, thin sticks of lunar caustic, encased in wood; they may be sharpened like lead-pencils, and the point protected by a cap to prevent injury when not in use. "Soluble, with the exception of about 5 per cent. of chloride of silver, in 0·6 part of water and in 25 parts of alcohol at 15° C. (59° F.), in 0·5 part of boiling water, and in 5 parts of boiling alcohol. It is insoluble in ether. Whatever is left undissolved by water is completely soluble in water of ammonia." *U. S.*

Impurities and Tests. Fused nitrate of silver is liable to contain free silver from having been exposed to too high a heat, the nitrates of lead and copper from the impurity of the silver dissolved in the acid, and nitrate of potassium from fraudulent admixture or otherwise. Free silver will be left undissolved as a black powder, after the action of distilled water. A very slight residue of this kind is hardly avoidable; but, if there be much free silver, it will be shown by the surface of a fresh fracture of one of the sticks presenting an unusually dark gray color. (*Christison.*) The mode of detecting lead and copper is explained under nitrate of silver. (See *Argenti Nitras.*) In order to detect nitrate of potassium, a solution of the suspected salt should be treated with hydrochloric acid in excess, to remove silver, and with sulphuretted hydrogen, to throw down other metals if they happen to be present. The filtered liquid, if the salt be pure, will entirely evaporate by heat; if it contain nitrate of potassium, this will be left, easily known by its properties as a nitrate. This impurity sometimes exists in fused nitrate of silver in large amount, varying, according to different statements, from 10 to 75 per cent. According to Dr. Christison, it may be suspected if the sticks present a colorless fracture. Prof.

Pollacci (*Journ. de Pharm.*, 4e sér., xvii. 160) states that if nitrate of silver, after having been heated in a porcelain capsule to redness and cooled, imparts an alkaline reaction to water, it contains nitre. The U. S. Pharmacopœia gives the following quantitative test. "A filtered aqueous solution of 2 Gm. of the salt, acidulated with nitric acid, when completely precipitated by hydrochloric acid, should yield 1·6 Gm. of dry chloride of silver." *U. S.* In the Br. Pharmacopœia the following method is given for testing fused nitrate of silver for impurity, without determining its nature. "Ten grains dissolved in two fluidrachms of distilled water give with hydrochloric acid a precipitate, which, when washed and thoroughly dried, weighs 8·44 grains. The filtrate when evaporated by a water-bath leaves no residue." If the weight of the precipitate be greater or less than here stated, there must be some impurity in the nitrate; and any non-precipitable matter, if solid at the temperature of the water-bath, will be left behind when the filtrate is evaporated.

Medical Properties. Fused nitrate of silver should be restricted to external use. Externally applied, the fused nitrate acts variously as a stimulant, vesicant, and escharotic, and may be employed either dissolved in water, or in the solid state. A drachm of the fused salt, dissolved in a fluidounce of water, forms an escharotic solution, which may often be resorted to with advantage. But fused nitrate of silver is most frequently employed in the solid state; and, as it is not deliquescent nor apt to spread, it forms the most manageable caustic that can be used. When thus employed, it is useful to coat the caustic, as recommended by M. Dumeril, by dipping it into melted engravers' sealing-wax, which strengthens the stick, protects it from change, prevents it from staining the fingers, and affords facilities for limiting the action of the caustic to particular spots. If it is desired, for example, to touch a part of the throat with the caustic, it is prepared by scraping off the sealing-wax with a penknife, to a suitable extent, from one end. Another way to strengthen the stick is to cast it around a platinum wire, as recommended by M. Chassaignac; or around a wick of cotton, according to the plan of M. Blatin. By the latter plan, when the stick is broken, the fragments remain attached. If the fused nitrate be rubbed gently over the moistened skin until this becomes gray, it generally vesicates, causing usually less pain than is produced by cantharides. The fused nitrate is also employed to destroy strictures of the urethra, warts and excrescences, fungous flesh, incipient chancres, and the surface of other ulcers.

It is often of service lightly applied, either in concentrated solution or in stick, to ulcers in expediting their cicatrization. It is very largely employed in the local treatment of inflammations of the mucous membranes, as in cystitis, leucorrhœa, gonorrhœa, conjunctivitis, faucitis, laryngitis, etc. In these cases the strength of the solution must be adapted to the susceptibility and the exact condition of the membrane. In cases of intense and especially specific inflammations, the solution may be a saturated one, the object being to destroy the specific granulations: thus, in gonorrhœal conjunctivitis, and in virulent diphtheritic faucitis, even the solid stick is used by some practitioners, whereas in ordinary conjunctivitis the strength should rarely be above one or two grains to the ounce, and in faucitis twenty to forty grains to the ounce. Strong solutions of nitrate of silver are sometimes used for the aborting of a gonorrhœa, but the treatment is usually considered dangerous, as liable to increase the intensity of the inflammation if unsuccessful. In the advanced stages of gonorrhœa a solution of three to five grains to the ounce may be injected.

Lunar caustic is also frequently used as a topical remedy in various superficial inflammations. The method originated in 1820 by Mr. John Higginbottom of treating erysipelas by the nitrate of silver still finds favor with some of the profession. After thorough washing of the skin with soap and water, and afterwards with pure water, and subsequent drying, a concentrated solution of twenty grains of the nitrate of silver to a drachm of distilled water is applied freely on the inflamed surface and beyond it on the healthy skin by means of a linen mop. In various inflammations of the subcellular tissues nitrate of silver often acts advantageously: thus, applied to the skin in sufficient concentration to blacken the surface, it will sometimes avert a felon or an epididymitis. It has been employed by injection for the radical cure of hydrocele, and in solid stick applied as a fine point to each pustule of smallpox upon the face for the prevention of pitting.

ARGENTI OXIDUM. *U.S., Br.* *Oxide of Silver.*

Ag_2O; 231·4. (ĂR-ǤĔN'TĪ ŎX'Ĭ-DŬM.) AgO; 115·7.

Argentum Oxydatum, Argentic Oxide; Oxyde d'Argent, *Fr.*; Silberoxyd, *G.*

"Take of Nitrate of Silver, in crystals, *half an ounce* [avoirdupois]; Solution of Lime *three pints and a half* [Imperial measure]; Distilled Water *ten fluidounces.* Dissolve the Nitrate of Silver in four [fluid]ounces of the Distilled Water, and, having poured the solution into a bottle containing the Solution of Lime, shake the mixture well, and set it aside to allow the deposit to settle. Draw off the supernatant liquid, collect the deposit on a filter, wash it with the remainder of the Distilled Water, and dry it at a heat not exceeding 212° (100° C.). Keep it in a stoppered bottle." *Br.*

A process for preparing oxide of silver has not been adopted in the present Pharmacopœia: that of the U. S. Pharmacopœia of 1870 is given below.*

Oxide of silver was introduced into the U. S. Pharmacopœia of 1850, and was adopted in the Br. Pharmacopœia from the Dublin. In the processes for making it, nitrate of silver is decomposed by potassa or lime, the oxide being precipitated, and nitrate of potassium or nitrate of calcium, as the case may be, remaining in solution. When thus obtained, the oxide is an olive-brown powder. If the potassa used be not wholly free from carbonic acid, the precipitated oxide will be contaminated with some carbonate of silver. According to Mr. Borland, of London, the carbonate is sometimes sold for the oxide. A third process for obtaining this oxide is that of Gregory, which consists in boiling the moist, recently prepared chloride of silver with a very strong solution of caustic potassa (sp. gr. 1·25 to 1·30), when, by double decomposition, oxide of silver and chloride of potassium are formed. "Oxide of silver should be kept in dark amber-colored vials, protected from the light."

Properties and Tests. "A heavy, dark brownish black powder, liable to reduction by exposure to light, odorless, having a metallic taste and imparting an alkaline reaction to water, in which it is very slightly soluble. It is insoluble in alcohol. When heated, it loses oxygen, and metallic silver is left behind. On adding the Oxide to hydrochloric acid, no effervescence should take place (abs. of carbonate). 1 Gm. of the Oxide, when treated with an excess of hydrochloric acid, should yield 1·236 Gm. of chloride of silver. Oxide of silver should not be triturated with readily oxidizable or combustible substances, and should not be brought in contact with ammonia." *U. S.* When its solution in nitric acid is precipitated by chloride of sodium in excess, the supernatant liquid is not discolored by sulphydrate of ammonium. The non-action of this test shows the absence of most foreign metals, especially copper and lead. It parts with its oxygen with great facility, being decomposed by many organic substances, causing sulphur, amorphous phosphorus, or tannin to take fire when rubbed together with it quite dry, in a mortar.

Medical Properties and Uses. This oxide has been proposed as a substitute for nitrate of silver, as having the general therapeutic virtues of the latter, without its escharotic effect, and objectionable property of discoloring the skin. Experience, however, has shown that it will tint the skin. (*New York Med. Journ.*, June, 1869; *Phila. Med. Times*, vi.) It was first tried as a medicine by Van Mons and Sementini. In 1840 it was employed by Dr. Butler Lane, who considered it to act as a sedative. In 1845 the late Sir James Eyre strongly recommended it in his work on exhausting diseases. Dr. Lane used it with more or less success in nausea, cardialgia, pyrosis, various painful affections of the stomach without organic lesion, dysentery, diarrhœa, night-sweats without other obvious affection, dysmenorrhœa, menorrhagia, leucorrhœa, chronic enlargements of the uterus attended with flooding, etc. The oxide appeared to exert a peculiar control over uterine fluxes. Some of the cases treated required the use of tonics, after the curative influence of the oxide had been exerted. The late Dr. Golding Bird also obtained favorable effects from the use of oxide of silver, and confirmed to a certain extent the results

* "Take of Nitrate of Silver *four troyounces*; Distilled Water *half a pint*; Solution of Potassa *a pint and a half*, or *a sufficient quantity*. Dissolve the Nitrate of Silver in the Water, and to the solution add Solution of Potassa so long as it produces a precipitate. Wash this repeatedly with water until the washings are nearly tasteless. Lastly, dry the precipitate and keep it in a well-stopped bottle, protected from the light." *U. S.* 1870.

of Dr. Lane, especially as to its valuable powers in menorrhagia. In stomach disease characterized by a glairy instead of a watery discharge, Dr. Bird derived not the slightest benefit from the oxide, though he used it in thirty cases. In tænia it has been used successfully in two cases by Mr. Whittel. The dose of oxide of silver is a grain (0·065 Gm.) twice or thrice a day. If pills are ordered, they should not be made with honey, conserve of roses, or other excipient containing glucose; and, indeed, most organic substances, especially in a moist state, deoxidise the oxide, reviving the silver. There would seem to be need of great caution in making these pills. Dr. Jackson has recorded a case in which pills of oxide of silver, muriate of morphia, and extract of gentian exploded violently in the pocket of the patient. (*P. J. Tr.*, xi. 552.) Mr. Ambrose Smith recommends, as among the best excipients, gum arabic, or this with a little syrup. (*Proc. A. P. A.*, 1859, p. 308.) The best method of administering is probably in gelatin capsules, the oxide being introduced in the form of a dry powder. Oxide of silver has been used in an ointment, composed of from five to ten grains to the drachm of lard, as an application to venereal sores, and to the urethral membrane in gonorrhœa, smeared on a bougie.

ARMORACIÆ RADIX. *Br.* *Horse-radish Root.*

(ĂR-MO-RĀ'CI-Æ RĀ'DĬX.)

"The fresh root of Cochlearia Armoracia, *Linn.* From plants cultivated in Britain, and most active in the autumn and early spring before the leaves have appeared." *Br.* (*Nat. Ord:* Cruciferæ, Siliquosæ.)

Armoracia, Br. 1864; Raifort sauvage, Moutarde des Moines, Radis de Cheval, *Fr.;* Meerrettig, *G.;* Rafano rusticano, *It.;* Rabano rusticano, *Sp.*

Gen. Ch. Silicula emarginate, turgid, scabrous with gibbous, obtuse valves. *Willd.*

Cochlearia Armoracia. Willd. *Sp. Plant.* ii. 451; Woodv. *Med. Bot.* p. 400, t. 145. The root of this plant is perennial, sending up numerous very large leaves, from the midst of which a round, smooth, erect, branching stem rises two or three feet in height. The radical leaves are lance-shaped, waved, scolloped on the edges, sometimes pinnatifid, and stand upon strong footstalks. Those of the stem are much smaller, without footstalks, sometimes divided at the edges, sometimes almost entire. The flowers are numerous, white, peduncled, and form thick terminal clusters. The calyx has four ovate, deciduous leaves, and the corolla an equal number of obovate petals, twice as long as the calyx, and inserted by narrow claws. The pod is small, elliptical, crowned with the persistent stigma, and divided into two cells, each containing from four to six seeds.

The horse-radish is a native of western Europe, growing wild on the sides of ditches, and in other moist situations. It is cultivated for culinary purposes in most civilized countries, and is said to have become naturalized in some parts of the United States. Its flowers appear in June.

The root, which is officinal in its fresh state, is long, conical at top, then nearly cylindrical for some inches, at last tapering, whitish externally, very white within, fleshy, of a strong pungent odor when scraped or bruised, and of a hot, biting, somewhat sweetish, and sometimes bitterish taste. Its virtues are imparted to water and alcohol. They depend upon a *volatile oil*, which is dissipated by drying; the root becoming at first sweetish, and ultimately insipid and quite inert. Its acrimony is also destroyed by boiling. The oil may be obtained by distillation with water. It is colorless or pale yellow, heavier than water, very volatile, excessively pungent, acrid, and corrosive, exciting inflammation and even vesication when applied to the skin. Hubatka considers it as identical with the volatile oil of mustard. He combined it with ammonia and obtained crystals of *thiosinamin*, $NH_2.CS.N(C_3H_5)H$, which agreed with that produced from mustard oil. (*Journ. de Pharm.*, 3e sér., v. 42.) According to Gutret, only six parts of it are obtained from 10,000 of the root. Besides this principle, the fresh root contains, according to the same chemist, a bitter resin in minute quantity, sugar, extractive, gum, starch, albumen, acetic acid, acetate and sulphate of calcium, water, and lignin. A. Hilger found in the ashes of the root of horse-radish, lime, magnesia, potassa, a trace of soda and oxide of iron, with sulphuric, hydrochloric, carbonic, phosphoric, and silicic acids in combination. (*Chem. Centralbl.*, p. 597, 1878; *A. J. P.*, 1879,

p. 21.) From observations made by F. L. Winckler, it may be inferred that *myronic acid* exists in the root combined with potassa, and that it is from the reaction between this acid, *myrosine*, also existing in the root, and water, that the volatile oil is produced, in the same manner as oil of mustard from mustard seed. (See *Sinapis*.) Horse-radish, when distilled with alcohol, yields none of the oil. (*Journ. für Prakt. Pharm.*, xviii. 89.) The root may be kept for some time without material injury, if buried in sand in a cool place.

It is said that if to the powder of the dried root, which has become apparently inert, the emulsion of white mustard seed containing myrosine be added, it reacquires its original irritant properties; so that it is the myrosine and not the myronate of potassium which is injured by drying. Hence the powdered root may be added with advantage to mustard in preparing cataplasms, pediluvia, etc. (*Journ. de Pharm. et de Chim.*, xxvii. 268.)*

Medical Properties and Uses. Horse-radish is highly stimulant, exciting the stomach when swallowed, and promoting the secretions, especially that of urine. Externally, it is rubefacient. Its chief use is as a condiment to promote appetite and invigorate digestion; but it is also occasionally employed as a medicine, particularly in dropsy attended with enfeebled digestion and general debility. It has, moreover, been recommended in palsy and chronic rheumatism, both as an internal and an external remedy; and in scorbutic affections is highly esteemed. Cullen found advantage in cases of hoarseness, from the use of a syrup prepared from an infusion of horse-radish and sugar, and slowly swallowed in the quantity of one or two teaspoonfuls, repeated occasionally. The root may be given in the dose of half a drachm (1·95 Gm.) or more, grated or cut into small pieces.

Off. Prep. Br. Spiritus Armoraciæ Compositus.

ARNICÆ FLORES. *U.S.* *Arnica Flowers.*

(ÄR'NI-ÇÆ FLŌ'RĒŞ.)

"The flower heads of Arnica montana. Linné. (*Nat. Ord.* Compositæ.)" *U. S.*

Leopard's Bane; Flores Arnicæ, *P.G.;* Fleurs d'Arnique, *Fr.;* Wohlverleichblüthen, Arnicablüthen, *G.*

ARNICÆ RADIX. *U.S.* *Arnica Root.*

(ÄR'NI-ÇÆ RĀ'DĬX.)

"The rhizome and rootlets of Arnica montana. Linné. (*Nat. Ord.* Compositæ.)" *U. S.* "The dried rhizome and rootlets of Arnica montana." *Br.*

Arnicæ Rhizoma, *Br.;* Racine d'Arnique, *Fr.;* Arnikawurzel, *G.*

Gen. Ch. Calyx with equal leaflets in a double row. *Seed-down* hairy, sessile. *Seeds* of the disk and ray furnished with seed-down. *Receptacle* hairy. *Hayne.*

Arnica montana. Willd. *Sp. Plant.* iii. 2106; *B. & T.* 158. This is a perennial, herbaceous plant, having a woody, brownish, horizontal root, from one to three inches long, and two or three lines thick, ending abruptly, and sending forth numerous slender fibres of the same color. The stem is about a foot high, cylindrical, striated, hairy, and terminating in one, two, or three peduncles, each bearing a flower. The radical leaves are ovate, entire, ciliated, and obtuse; those of the stem, which usually consist of two opposite pairs, are lance-shaped. Both are of a bright green usually consist of two opposite pairs, are lance-shaped. Both are of a bright green color, and somewhat pubescent on their upper surface. The flowers are yellow.

This plant is a native of the mountainous districts of Europe and Siberia, and is found, according to Nuttall, in the northern regions of this continent, west of the Mississippi. It has been introduced into England, and might no doubt be cultivated

* The French Codex contains a formula for a compound *Syrup of Horse-radish* (*Sirop Antiscorbutique*), as follows. Scurvy grass, water cress, horse-radish (root), all fresh, of each, 100 parts, buckbean (marsh trefoil), fresh, 10 parts, bitter orange peel 20 parts, canella 5 parts, white wine 400 parts, sugar 500 parts. Thoroughly contuse and comminute the solid ingredients, macerate for 48 hours with the wine, and distil off 100 parts. Express and strain the residue from the distillation, clarify the liquid with white of egg, and strain; add 300 parts sugar, and make into a syrup of sp. gr. 1·270 whilst boiling; with the rest of the sugar and sufficient water make a thick syrup, mix this with the other syrup, allow to cool, then add the distilled essence. *Iodised Syrup of Horse-radish* may be made by adding one part of tincture of iodine to ninety-nine parts of the compound syrup above.

in this country. The flowers, leaves, and root are employed; but the flowers are usually preferred.

Properties. The whole plant, when fresh, has a strong, disagreeable odor, which is apt to excite sneezing, and is diminished by drying. The taste is acrid, bitterish, and durable. The dried root is cylindrical, contorted, and marked by scars from the insertion of the leaves. Water extracts its virtues. The Pharmacopœia thus describes the flowers and the root.

The flowers are "about one and one-fifth inch (3 cm.) broad, depressed, roundish, consisting of a scaly involucre in two rows, and a small, flat, hairy receptacle, bearing about sixteen yellow, strap-shaped ray-florets, and numerous, yellow, five-toothed, tubular disk-florets; having slender, spindle-shaped achenes, crowned by a hairy pappus. It has a feeble, aromatic odor, and a bitter, acrid taste." *U. S.*

The rhizome is "about two inches (5 cm.) long, and one-eighth or one-sixth of an inch (3 or 4 mm.) thick; externally brown, rough from leaf-scars; internally whitish, with a rather thick bark, containing a circle of resin-cells, surrounding the short wood-wedges, and large, spongy pith. The rootlets numerous, thin, fragile, grayish-brown, with a thick bark containing a circle of resin-cells. Odor somewhat aromatic; taste pungently aromatic and bitter." *U. S.*

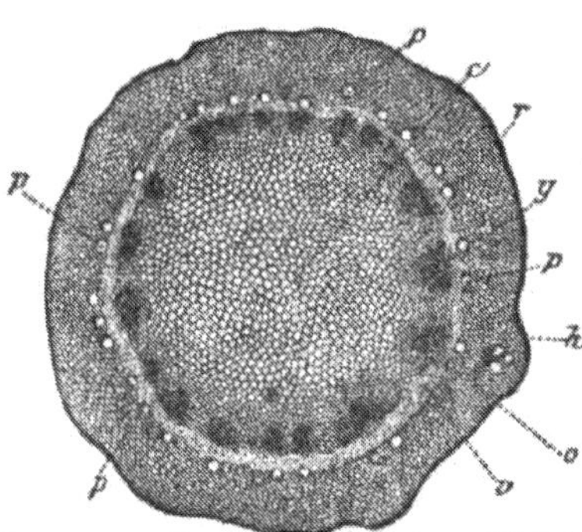

Arnica root. c, pith, marrow; h, outer bark; o, middle bark; p, resin tubes; y, woody bundles.

Bastick (*P. J. Tr.*, x. 389) separated an alkaloid from the flowers, to which he gave the name of *arnicine.*

The *arnicine* of Walz (*N. Jahrb. Pharm.*, 13, p. 175), extracted from both the root and the flowers, is a different substance; it is an amorphous yellow mass of acrid taste, slightly soluble in water, freely in alcohol or ether, and dissolving also in alkaline solutions. It is precipitable from its alcoholic solution by tannic acid or by water. Walz assigns to arnicine the formula $C_{20}H_{30}O_4$; other chemists that of $C_{35}H_{54}O_7$. Arnicine has not yet been proved to be a glucoside, although it is decomposed by dilute acids.

Sigel (1873) obtained from dried arnica root about ½ per cent. of essential oil, and 1 per cent. from the fresh; the oil of the latter had a sp. gr. of 0·999 at 18° C. (64·4° F.). The oil was found to be a mixture of various bodies, the principal being the *dimethyl ether of thymohydroquinone*, $C_{10}H_{12}\left\{\begin{matrix}OCH_3\\OCH_3\end{matrix}\right.$, boiling at about 235° C. (455° F.), and with this, *phloryl isobutyrate* to the extent of one-fifth of the oil, and the *methyl ether* of a *phlorol.* (*Pflanzenstoffe*, 2d ed., p. 1530.) The water from which the oil separates contains *isobutyric acid;* probably also a little *angelic* and *formic acids;* but neither capronic nor caprylic acid, which had been pointed out by Walz. Arnica root contains *inulin*, which Dragendorff extracted from it to the extent of about 10 per cent. (*Pharmacographia*, 2d edition, p. 391.)

Medical Properties and Uses. When taken internally in sufficient dose, arnica acts as an irritant to the stomach and bowels, often producing an emetic and cathartic effect, and is said by Bergius to be diuretic, diaphoretic, and emmenagogue. It is capable of acting as a poison in overdoses, causing burning in the stomach, violent abdominal pains, intense headache, and great nervous disturbance, with, in some cases, marked reduction of the pulse-rate, and finally collapse. A case of tetanic spasm of one side, and ultimate death, under its use, is on record; but there is reason to doubt whether arnica was the real cause of the fatal issue. (*Ann. de Thérap.*, 1854, p. 46.) It is much used by the Germans, who prescribe the flowers and root with advantage in amaurosis, paralysis, and other nervous affections. It is said to prove useful in that disordered condition which succeeds concussion of the brain from falls, blows, etc., and from this circumstance has received the title of *panacea lapsorum.* It has also been recommended in chronic catarrh of the old, intermittent fever and its sequelæ, dysentery, diarrhœa, nephritis, gout, rheumatism, passive hemorrhages, dropsy, chlorosis, amenorrhœa, and various other complaints, in most of which it seems to have been empirically prescribed, and the exact value of the remedy has not been determined. The powdered flowers and leaves are employed as a sternutatory; and the inhabitants of Savoy and the Vosges are said to substitute them for tobacco. They may be given in substance or infusion. The dose of the powder is from five to twenty grains (0·33–1·3 Gm.) frequently repeated. The infusion may be prepared by digesting an ounce of the flowers in a pint of water, of which from half a fluidounce to a fluidounce (15–30 C.c.) may be given every three hours. It should always be strained through linen, in order to separate the fine fibres, which might irritate the throat. A tincture prepared from the flowers is largely used in this country as a domestic remedy in sprains, bruises, etc. It is employed externally. A tincture of the root is now officinal: this would be preferable for internal use. (See *Tinctura Arnicæ Radicis.*)

Off. Prep. of the Flowers. Tinctura Arnicæ Florum.

Off. Prep. of the Root. Extractum Arnicæ Radicis; Extractum Arnicæ Radicis Fluidum; Tinctura Arnicæ Radicis.

Off. Prep. Br. Tinctura Arnicæ.

ARSENIUM. *Arsenic.*

As; 75. (ĂR-SĒ′NĪ-ŬM.) As; 75.

Arsenicum, *U. S.* 1870; Arsenum, Arsenium; Arsenic, *Fr.;* Arsenik, *G.;* Arsenico, *It., Sp.*

This metal was introduced into the U. S. and Dublin Pharmacopœias in 1850, for the purpose of being used to form the iodide of arsenic, and the solution of iodide of arsenic and mercury, at that time two new officinals of those works. It has been rejected by the compilers of the U. S. Pharmacopœia and the British. The Dublin College gave the following formula.

"Take of White Oxide of Arsenic of Commerce two drachms [*Dub. weight*]. Place the Oxide at the sealed end of a hard German glass tube, of about half an inch in diameter and eighteen inches long, and, having covered it with about eight inches of dry and coarsely pulverized charcoal, and raised the portion of the tube containing the charcoal to a red heat, let a few ignited coals be placed beneath the Oxide, so as to effect its slow sublimation. When this has been accomplished, the metallic arsenic will be found attached to the interior of the tube at its distant or cool extremity.

"In conducting this process, the furnace used in the performance of an organic analysis should be employed, and the fuel should be ignited charcoal. It will be proper also to connect the open extremity of the tube with a flue, for the purpose of preventing the possible escape into the apartment of arsenical vapors; and, with the view of keeping it from being plugged by the metal, to introduce occasionally into it, as the sublimation proceeds, an iron wire through a cork, fixed (but not air-tight) in its open extremity."

In the above process, the white oxide (arsenious oxide) is reduced by the agency of ignited charcoal, which attracts the oxygen of the oxide, and revives the metal. On the large scale, metallic arsenic is generally obtained by heating arsenical pyrites ($FeAs,FeS_2$) in earthen tubes; when the metal sublimes, and two mols. of ferrous sulphide, FeS, are left.

Properties. Arsenic is a brittle, crystalline metal, of a steel-gray color, and possessing much brilliancy when recently broken or sublimed. Exposed to the air, its surface becomes dull and blackish. Its texture is granular, and sometimes a little scaly. Rubbed on the hands, it communicates a peculiar odor; but it is devoid of taste. Its sp. gr. is about 5·73 (5·88, *U. S.*). When heated to about 180° C. (356° F.) it sublimes, giving rise to white vapors having a garlicky odor.* Its

* The statement that arsenic on being heated sufficiently passes at once into the state of vapor without fusing was disproved by experiments of Dunnington and Odger, made under the direction of Prof Mallet, of the University of Virginia. They succeeded in fusing arsenic without great difficulty. (*Chem. News*, Aug. 30, 1872.)

atomic weight is 75. It forms two combinations with oxygen, arsenious and arsenic oxides, As_2O_3 and As_2O_5 respectively, to each of which the corresponding acid is known, and three with sulphur, namely, the disulphide or realgar, As_2S_2; the trisulphide or orpiment, As_2S_3, corresponding in composition to arsenious oxide; and the pentasulphide, As_2S_5, corresponding to arsenic oxide. (See *Acidum Arseniosum; also realgar* and *orpiment* in Part II. of this work.) *Arsenic acid* is obtained by distilling off a mixture of twelve parts of nitric and one of hydrochloric acid from four parts of arsenious acid, until the whole acquires the consistence of a thin syrup. The liquid is then poured into a porcelain dish, and evaporated at a moderate heat. Suddenly the arsenic oxide concretes into an opaque white mass, which should be transferred, while warm, to a well-stopped bottle. Arsenic oxide is white, solid, deliquescent, and soluble in six parts of cold and two of boiling water. It forms several acids, corresponding to the several varieties of phosphoric acid, to which it bears a close analogy. With nitrate of silver it gives a brick-red precipitate of arseniate of silver. As a poison it is even more virulent than arsenious oxide. It consists of two atoms of arsenic and five of oxygen (As_2O_5).

Arsenic is much diffused. Besides being present in a great many minerals, it has been detected, in minute proportion, in the earth of graveyards by Orfila; in certain soils and mineral waters by M. Walchner; in the ashes of various plants by M. Stein; and in various kinds of mineral coal, as also in the incrustation formed in the boiler of a sea-going steamer, by M. Daubrée.

ARSENII IODIDUM. *U. S.* *Iodide of Arsenic.*

AsI_3; 454·7. (ĂR'SĒ-NĪ Ī-ŎD'Ĭ-DŬM.) AsI_3; 454·7.

Arsenici Iodidum, *U. S.* 1870; Arsenicum jodatum, Arsenik jodür, *G.*; Iodure d'Arsenic, *Fr.*

"Obtained by the direct combination of iodine and metallic arsenium, or by evaporating to dryness an aqueous mixture of arsenious and hydriodic acids." *Br.*

"Iodide of Arsenic should be kept in glass-stoppered vials, in a cool place." This iodide was introduced into the U. S. Pharmacopœia for the purpose of being used in preparing the solution of iodide of arsenic and mercury. It is made by the direct combination of its constituents, with the aid of a gentle heat.

For U. S. process of 1870 see foot-note.* J. F. Babcock (*Proc. A. P. A.*, 1875, p. 693) proposes to make it by placing a troyounce of iodine in a suitable vessel with 10 or 12 fluidounces of water, and passing sulphuretted hydrogen through until the iodine color is entirely gone; then filtering, heating the filtrate until the odor of sulphuretted hydrogen has been dissipated; then adding a quarter of a troyounce of arsenious acid, heating until dissolved, filtering, and evaporating to dryness. $As_2O_3 + 6HI = 2AsI_3 + 3H_2O$. Nickle's process enables the operator to obtain the salt in a crystalline condition. Arsenic and iodine in equivalent proportions are heated together with carbon disulphide in a flask, to which an upright condenser is attached, until the iodine color disappears. The solution is then evaporated to the crystallizing point.

In the *Berichte d. Deutsch. Chem. Ges.*, 2643, 1881, may be found a process for obtaining this salt chemically pure, by making a hot solution of arsenious acid in hydrochloric acid, and mixing it with a concentrated solution of iodide of potassium, whereupon the teriodide separates as a crystalline powder; this may be washed with hydrochloric acid, sp. gr. 1·120, until a portion of the washings on evaporation ceases to leave a residue of chloride of potassium.

Properties, etc. Iodide of arsenic is an orange red, crystalline solid, soluble in 3·5 parts of water, wholly volatilized by heat, officinally described as in "glossy, orange red, crystalline masses, or shining, orange red, crystalline scales, gradually losing iodine when exposed to the air, having an iodine-like odor and taste, and a

* "Take of Arsenic *sixty grains*; Iodine *three hundred grains*. Rub the Arsenic in a mortar until reduced to a fine powder; then add the Iodine, and rub them together until they are thoroughly mixed. Put the mixture into a small flask or a test-tube, loosely stopped, and heat it very gently until liquefaction occurs. Then incline the vessel in different directions, in order that any portion of the iodine, which may have condensed on its surface, may be returned into the melted mass. Lastly, pour the melted iodide on a porcelain slab, and, when it is cold, break it into pieces, and keep it in a well-stopped bottle." *U. S.* 1870.

neutral reaction. Soluble in 3·5 parts of water and in 10 parts of alcohol at 15° C. (59° F.); also soluble in ether and in disulphide of carbon. It is gradually decomposed by boiling water and by boiling alcohol. By heat the salt is completely volatilized. The aqueous solution has a yellow color, and, on standing, gradually decomposes into arsenious and hydriodic acids. On passing hydrosulphuric acid through the solution, a lemon-yellow precipitate is thrown down. If the salt be heated with diluted nitric acid, vapor of iodine will be given off." *U. S.* It has a great tendency to decompose even at ordinary temperatures, iodine separating and volatilizing, oxygen being absorbed and arsenious acid formed. Iodide of arsenic as found in commerce varies greatly in composition, being usually deficient in arsenic. (See *Ephemeris*, vol. ii. p. 772.) It has been used by Biett as an external application in corroding tubercular skin diseases. By the late Dr. A. T. Thomson it was given internally with alleged advantage in lepra. The ointment used by Biett was composed of three grains of the iodide to an ounce of lard. The dose is an eighth of a grain (0·008 Gm.) three times a day, in pill or solution.

Off. Prep. Liquor Arsenii et Hydrargyri Iodidi.

ASAFŒTIDA. *U.S., Br.* *Asafetida.*

(ĂS-Ą-FŒT'Į-DĄ—ăs-ą-fĕt'į-dą.)

"A gum-resin obtained from the root of Ferula Narthex, Boissier, and of Ferula Scorodosma, Bentham et Hooker. (*Nat. Ord.* Umbelliferæ, Orthospermæ.)" *U. S.* "A gum-resin obtained by incision from the living root of Ferula Narthex, *Boiss.*, and of Ferula Scorodosma, *Benth. and Hook.*, and probably other species." *Br.*

Assafœtida, *Br.;* Asafœtida, *P.G.;* Gummi-resina Asafœtida; Asefétide, Assafœtida, *Fr.;* Stinkasant, Teufelsdreck, *G.;* Assafetida, *It.;* Asafetida, *Sp.;* Ungoozeh, *Pers.;* Hilteet, *Arab.*

Concerning the genus Ferula there has been much dispute by botanists, but at present a much wider range is given to it than formerly. H. Falconer (*Trans. Linn. Soc.*, xx. 285) separated from it the genus *Narthex*, relying chiefly upon the distinctness of the vittæ as characteristic, whilst Bunge separated the genus *Scorodosma* on account of the absence of vittæ. According, however, to Bentham and Hooker, the vittæ in Bunge's type specimens are no more inconspicuous than in various other species of the genus; and, further, the vittæ vary so much that no generic characters can be drawn from them. The genus Ferula is a very difficult one to characterise briefly, and for its description the reader is referred to that of Bentham and Hooker, *Genera Plantarum*, i. 917.

Ferula Narthex. Bois. *Narthex Assafœtida.* Falconer. *Ferula Assafœtida.* Willd. *Sp. Plant.* i. 1413. *B. & T.* This plant was first described from actual observation by H. Falconer, who found it near Kashmir. It has flowered twice in the Edinburgh Botanical Gardens. The root is perennial, fleshy, tapering, simple or divided, a foot or more in length, about three inches thick at top, where it is invested above the soil with numerous small fibres, dark gray and transversely corrugated on the outside, internally white, and abounding in an excessively fetid, opaque, milky juice. The leaves, which spring from the root, are numerous, large and spreading, nearly two feet long, light green above, paler beneath, and of a leathery texture. They are three-parted, with bipinnatifid segments and oblong-lanceolate, obtuse, entire or variously sinuate, decurrent lobes, forming a narrow winged channel on the divisions of the petiole. From the midst of the leaves rises a luxuriant, herbaceous stem, from six to ten feet high, two inches in diameter at the base, simple, erect, round, smooth, striated, solid, and terminating in a large head of compound umbels, with from ten to twenty rays, each surmounted by a roundish partial umbel. It is furnished with numerous branches, springing from the axils of dilated sheathing petioles. The flowers are pale yellow, and the fruit oval, thin, flat, foliaceous, and reddish brown. The plant is said to differ in its leaves and product, in different situations.

It is a native of Persia, Afghanistan, and other neighboring regions; and flourishes abundantly in the mountainous provinces of Laar and Chorassan, where its juice is collected. Burns, in his travels into Bokhara, states that the young plant is eaten with relish by the people, and that sheep crop it greedily.

Ferula Scorodosma. Bentham and Hooker. *Scorodosma fœtidum.* Bunge. *Ferula Assafœtida*, L., of Boissier. *Flora Orientalis*, ii. 994, resembles in its general characters *F. Narthex*, but is not quite so large; has its stem nearly naked with the numerous umbels only at the top, and the few stem leaves lacking the wide sheathing petioles. This plant was first discovered by Lehman in 1844, growing in sandy deserts near the Sea of Aral. About twenty years later it was found by Bunge in Persia.

It is possible that assafetida is obtained from several species of umbelliferous plants, although it seems to be determined that the officinal plants yield the bulk of it. These plants do not agree with the figures given by Engelbert Kaempfer of the plant which he observed in 1687, and to which he gave the name of *Assafœtida Disgunensis*, although Falconer considers the latter plant as identical with his *Narthex assafœtida*, and Borszczon, who studied *F. Scorodosma*, growing wild in the neighborhood of the Caspian Sea, believes this plant the same as that of Kaempfer. It is very likely that the difficulty of identification is due to inaccuracies in the original figure of Kaempfer. *F. Persica* is also said to produce an assafetida-like gum-resin, and was recognized by the Edinburgh Pharmacopœia.

The oldest plants are most productive, and those under four years old are not considered worth cutting, according to the statement of Kaempfer in 1687. At the season when the leaves begin to fade, the earth is removed from about the top of the root, and the leaves and stem, being twisted off near their base, are thrown with other vegetable matters over the root, in order to protect it from the sun. After some time the summit of the root is cut off transversely, and, the juice which exudes having been scraped off, another thin slice is removed, in order to obtain a fresh surface for exudation. This process is repeated at intervals till the root ceases to afford juice, and perishes. During the whole period of collection, which occupies nearly six weeks, the solar heat is as much as possible excluded. The juice collected from numerous plants is put together, and allowed to harden in the sun. Dr. H. W. Bellew visited Kandahar in 1872, and witnessed the collection of the drug; he describes the process essentially as did Kaempfer. The roots varied in size from that of a carrot to the thickness of a man's leg, and their yield from half an ounce to two pounds. The drug, he states, is very much adulterated. The fruit is said to be sent to India, where it is highly esteemed as a medicine. In 1884 Afghanistan was visited by Dr. J. E. T. Aitchison, who found the plains having an altitude of 2000 to 4000 feet, arid and bare in winter, but in the early summer covered with a thick growth of *Ferula fœtida*, *Dorema Ammoniacum*, and *Ferula Galbaniflua.* The great cabbage-like heads of the asafetida plant, representing the primary stage of the flower-heads covered over by the stipules of its leaves, are eaten raw by the natives as a sort of green. In June the asafetida is obtained. The root-stock is first laid bare to the depth of a couple of inches, those plants only which have not reached their flower-bearing stage being selected. A slice is then taken from the top of the root-stock, which is immediately covered with twigs and clay, forming a sort of dome, with an opening towards the north, so that the sun cannot get at the exposed root. About five or six weeks later a thick, gummy, not milky, reddish substance found upon the exposed surface of the root in more or less irregular lumps is scraped off with a piece of iron hoop or removed with a slice of the root and at once placed in a leather bag. The asafetida is then conveyed to Herat, where it is adulterated with a red clay before being sent into commerce.

Assafetida is brought to this country either from India, whither it is conveyed from Bushire, and down the Indus, or by the route of Great Britain. It sometimes comes in mats, but more frequently in cases, the former containing eighty or ninety, the latter from two hundred to four hundred pounds. It is sometimes also imported in casks.

Properties. As found in the shops, assafetida is in irregular masses, softish when not long exposed, of a yellowish or reddish brown color externally, exhibiting when broken an irregular, whitish, somewhat shining surface, which soon becomes red on exposure, and ultimately passes into a dull yellowish brown. This change of color is characteristic of assafetida, and is ascribed to the influence of air and light upon its resinous ingredient. The masses appear as if composed of distinct portions agglutinated together, sometimes of white, almost pearly tears, embedded in a darker, softer, and more fetid paste. Occasionally the *tears* are separate, though rarely in the commerce of this country. They are roundish, oval, or irregular, and generally flattened, from the size of a pea to that of a large almond, sometimes larger, yellowish or brownish externally and white within, and not unlike ammoniac tears, for which they might be mistaken except for their odor, which, however, is weaker than that of the masses. A very fine variety of asafetida is spoken of by Bellew as being procured from the leaf-bud in the centre of the root. It does not come into European commerce, but is the *Kandaharee Hing* of the Indian bazaars. (*P. J. Tr.*, viii. 103.) It occurs in moist flaky pieces and tears, yielding a reddish yellow oil on pressure, and mostly mixed with the remains of leaf-buds.

The odor of asafetida is alliaceous, extremely fetid, and tenacious; the taste, bitter, acrid, and durable. The effect of time and exposure is to render it more hard and brittle, and to diminish the intensity of its smell and taste, particularly the former. Kaempfer assures us that one drachm of the fresh juice diffuses a more powerful odor, through a close room, than one hundred pounds of the drug as usually kept in the stores. The color, which is at first white, becomes pink, and finally the well-known brown, on exposure. Asafetida softens by heat without melting, and is of difficult pulverization. Its sp. gr. is 1·327. (*Berzelius.*) It is inflammable, burning with a clear, lively flame. It yields all its virtues to alcohol, and forms a clear tincture, which becomes milky on the addition of water. "At least 60 per cent. of it should dissolve in alcohol." *U. S.* Macerated in water it produces a turbid red solution, and, triturated with that fluid, gives a white or pink-colored milky emulsion of considerable permanence. Touched with nitric acid (sp. gr. 1·2) the tear becomes of an evanescent green color. When asafetida is dissolved by means of sulphuric acid or ammonia, it exhibits a bluish fluorescence. In 100 parts, Pelletier found 65 parts of resin, 19·44 of gum, 11·66 of bassorin, 3·60 of volatile oil, with traces of acid malate of calcium. The odor of the gum-resin depends on the *volatile oil*, which may be procured by distillation with water or alcohol, and amounts to 6 to 9 per cent., according to Flückiger. It is lighter than water, colorless when first distilled, but becoming yellow with age, of an exceedingly offensive odor, and of a taste at first flat, but afterwards bitter and acrid. It contains, according to Stenhouse, from 15·75 to 23 per cent. of sulphur; but, according to Flückiger, may contain as much as 25 per cent. Hlasiwetz (*Ann. Chem. und Pharm.*, 71, p. 23) considers it a mixture, in variable proportions, of the sulphide and bisulphide of a compound radical, consisting of carbon and hydrogen (C_6H_{11}). A persulphide of allyl, which is sublimed when oil of mustard is heated with persulphide of potassium, is said by Wertheim to have an extremely intense odor of asafetida; a fact which justifies the supposition that it may be identical with the oil of that gum-resin. (*Gmelin*, ix. 377.) The oil boils at about 138° C. (280° F.), but suffers decomposition, yielding sulphuretted hydrogen. When long exposed to the air it becomes slightly acid, and acquires a somewhat different odor. (*Chem. Gaz.*, No. 178, p. 108.)

The resin is, according to Hlasiwetz and Barth (*Ann. Chem. und Pharm.*, 138, p. 61), a mixture containing *ferulaic acid*, $C_{10}H_{10}O_4$, crystallising in iridescent needles, and obtained by precipitating the alcoholic solution with lead acetate, washing the precipitate, and decomposing it with diluted sulphuric acid. Submitted to dry distillation, the resin yields *umbelliferone*, $C_9H_6O_3$, and blue-colored oils. Fused with caustic potash, ferulaic acid yields oxalic acid and carbonic acids, several acids of the fatty series, and proto-catechuic acid. The resin itself treated in like manner, after it has been previously freed from gum, yields resorcin.

Impurities and Adulterations. Asafetida is probably often purposely adulterated; it frequently comes of inferior quality, and mixed with various impurities, such as sand and stones. Portions which are very soft, dark brown, or blackish, with few or no tears, and indisposed to assume a red color when freshly broken, should be rejected. We have been informed that a case seldom comes without more or less of this inferior asafetida, and of many it forms the larger portion. It is sold chiefly for horses. A factitious substance, made of garlic juice and white pitch with a little asafetida, has occurred in commerce. Asafetida is said to be usually mixed with wheat or barley flour, or with earthy matters at the place of its production; the impurities sometimes exceeding 30 per cent. *Hingra* of the Bombay bazaars is a very stony variety, composed largely of earthy matter.

Asafetida is sometimes kept in the powdered state; but this is objectionable, as the drug is thus necessarily weakened by the loss of volatile oil, and is besides rendered more liable to adulteration.

Medical Properties and Uses. The effects of asafetida on the system are those of a moderate stimulant, antispasmodic, efficient expectorant, and feeble laxative. Some consider it also emmenagogue and anthelmintic. Its volatile oil is undoutedly absorbed; as its peculiar odor may be detected in the breath and the secretions. As an antispasmodic simply, it is employed in the treatment of hysteria, hypochondriasis, convulsions of various kinds, spasm of the stomach and bowels unconnected with inflammation, and in numerous other nervous disorders of a merely functional character. From the union of expectorant with antispasmodic powers, it is highly useful in spasmodic pectoral affections, such as hooping-cough and asthma, and in certain infantile coughs and catarrhs, complicated with nervous disorder, or with a disposition of the system to sink. In catarrhal senilis; in the secondary stages of peripneumonia notha, croup, measles, and catarrh; in pulmonary consumption; in fact, in all cases of subacute or chronic disease of the chest in which there is want of due nervous energy, asafetida may be occasionally prescribed with advantage. In the form of enema, it is useful in cases of inordinate accumulation of air in the bowels, and also in the hysteric paroxysm, and other functional convulsions. Its laxative tendency is generally advantageous, but must sometimes be counteracted by opium. It may often be usefully combined with cathartics in flatulent constipation.

It appears to have been known in the East from very early ages, and, notwithstanding its repulsive odor, is at present much used in India and Persia as a condiment. Persons soon habituate themselves to its smell, which they even learn to associate pleasantly with the agreeable effects experienced from its internal use. Children with hooping-cough sometimes become fond of it.

The medium dose is ten grains (0·65 Gm.), which may be given in pill or emulsion. (See *Mistura Asafœtidæ*.) The tincture is officinal, and is much used. When given by injection, the gum-resin should be triturated with warm water. From half a drachm to two drachms (1·95–7·8 Gm.) may be administered at once in this way. It may also sometimes be conveniently given in the form of a suppository. A syrup has been recommended, in which the fetid odor of the drug is obviated by the use of the infusion of wild cherry bark. (See *A. J. P.*, 1871, p. 397.)*

Off. Prep. Emplastrum Asafœtidæ; Mistura Asafœtidæ; Pilulæ Aloes et Asafœtidæ; Pilulæ Asafœtidæ; Pilulæ Galbani Compositæ; Tinctura Asafœtidæ.

Off. Prep. Br. Enema Asafœtidæ; Pilula Aloes et Asafœtidæ; Pilula Asafœtidæ Compositæ; Spiritus Ammoniæ Fœtidus; Tinctura Asafœtidæ.

ASCLEPIAS. *U. S.* *Asclepias.* [*Pleurisy Root.*]

(AS-CLĒ'PI-AS.)

"The root of Asclepias tuberosa. Linné. (*Nat. Ord.* Asclepiadaceæ.)" *U. S.*

Butterfly-Weed; Racine d'Asclépiade tubereuse, *Fr.*; Knollige Schwalbenwurzel, *G.*

Gen. Ch. Calyx small, five-parted. *Corolla* rotate, five-parted, mostly reflexed. *Staminal crown* (or nectary) simple, five-leaved; leaflets opposite the anthers, with a subulate averted process at the base. *Stigmas* with the five angles (corpuscles) opening by longitudinal chinks. *Pollinia* five distinct pairs. *Torrey.*

Several species of Asclepias, besides *A. tuberosa*, have been employed medicinally; and two of these, *A. Syriaca* and *A. incarnata*, were recognized in the Secondary Catalogue of the U. S. Pharm. 1870.

* J. W. Wood prepares syrup of asafetida by dissolving 256 grains of asafetida in two fluidounces of glycerin by the aid of a gentle heat, and straining. He then dissolves 15 drops oil of wintergreen, 5 drops oil of cinnamon, and 1 drop oil of bitter almond, in three fluidrachms of 95 per cent. alcohol, and adds it to the above, together with enough simple syrup to make the whole measure one pint. Each fluidrachm represents two grains of asafetida. (*A. J. P.*, Sept. 1874.)

Asclepias tuberosa. Willd. *Sp. Plant.* i. 1273; Bigelow, *Am. Med. Bot.* ii. 59; Barton, *Med. Bot.* i. 239. The root of the butterfly-weed, or *pleurisy root*, is perennial, and gives origin to numerous stems, which are erect, ascending, or procumbent, round, hairy, of a green or reddish color, branching at the top, and about three feet in height. The leaves are scattered, oblong-lanceolate, very hairy, of a rich, deep green color on their upper surface, paler beneath, and supported usually on short footstalks. They differ, however, somewhat in shape according to the variety of the plant. In the variety with decumbent stems they are almost linear, and in another variety cordate. The beautiful reddish-orange colored flowers occur in terminal or lateral corymbose umbels. The fruit is an erect lanceolate follicle, with flat ovate seeds connected to a longitudinal receptacle by long silky hairs.

This plant differs from other species of Asclepias in not emitting a milky juice when wounded. It is indigenous, growing throughout the United States from Massachusetts to Georgia, and as far west as Texas, and, when in full bloom, in June and July, having a splendid appearance. It is most abundant in the Southern States. The root is the only part used in medicine. It is "large and fusiform, dried in longitudinal or transverse sections; from one to six inches (25 to 150 mm.) long, and about three-quarters of an inch (2 cm.) or more in thickness; the head knotty, and slightly but distinctly annulate, the remainder longitudinally wrinkled; externally orange brown, internally whitish; tough, and having an uneven fracture; bark thin, and in two distinct layers, the inner one whitish; wood yellowish, with large, white, medullary rays; it is inodorous, and has a bitterish, somewhat acrid taste; when long kept it acquires a gray color." *U. S.*

When dried, it is easily pulverized; and its taste is bitter, but not otherwise unpleasant. Mr. E. Rhoads discovered in it a peculiar principle, which he obtained by treating the cold infusion with tannic acid, mixing the precipitate, previously washed and expressed, with litharge, drying the mixture and exhausting it with hot alcohol, and finally decolorizing and evaporating the alcoholic liquor. The product was a yellowish white powder, having the taste of the root, soluble in ether, and much less readily so in water, from which it was precipitated by tannic acid. Mr. Rhoads also found evidence of the existence in the root of tannic and gallic acids, albumen, pectin, gum, starch, a resin soluble and another insoluble in ether, fixed oil, a volatile odorous fatty matter, and various salts, besides from 30 to 35 per cent. of lignin. (*A. J. P.*, xxxiii. 492.)

Medical Properties and Uses. The root of *Asclepias tuberosa* is diaphoretic and expectorant, without being stimulant. In large doses it is often also cathartic. Dr. Pawling, of Norristown, Pa., found it always, when freely given, to diminish the volume and activity of the pulse, while it produced copious diaphoresis (*A. J. P.*, xxxiii. 496); and Dr. Goodbrake, of Clinton, Ill., considers it, from his experience, slightly sedative and astringent. (*Trans. of Illinois State Med. Soc.*, 1857.) In the Southern States it has long been employed by regular practitioners in catarrh, pneumonia, pleurisy, consumption, and other pectoral affections. Its popular name of *pleurisy root* expresses the estimation in which it is held as a remedy in that disease. It has also been useful in diarrhœa, dysentery, and acute and chronic rheumatism. Dr. Lockwood speaks highly of its efficacy in promoting the eruption in exanthematous fevers. (*Buffalo Med. Journ.*, March, 1848.) Much testimony might be advanced in proof of its diaphoretic powers. It is said to be gently tonic, and has been popularly used in pains of the stomach from flatulence and indigestion.

From twenty grains to a drachm (1·3–3·9 Gm.) of the root in powder may be given several times a day; but as a diaphoretic it is best administered in decoction or infusion, made in the proportion of an ounce to a quart of water, and given in the dose of a teacupful every two or three hours till it operates.*

* *Fluid Extract of Asclepias.* Mr. E. Rhoads prepares a *fluid extract* by moistening sixteen ounces of the powdered root with four fluidounces of a menstruum consisting of three pints of alcohol and a pint and a half of water, packing the mixture into a conical glass percolator, pouring on it the remainder of the menstruum, reserving the twelve fluidounces which first pass, evaporating the residue of the filtered liquor by means of a water-bath to four fluidounces, mixing this with the reserved liquor, and filtering at the end of twenty-four hours. This preparation was found effective by Dr. Pawling, in the dose of a fluidrachm (3·75 C.c.) every four hours.

ASPIDIUM. *U. S.* *Aspidium.* [*Male Fern.*]

(AS-PĬD'I-ŬM.)

"The rhizome of Aspidium Filix mas, Swartz, and of Aspidium marginale, Willdenow. (*Nat. Ord.* Filices.)" *U. S.* The dried rhizome with the bases of the footstalks, and portions of the root fibres, of Aspidium Filix mas. *Br.*

Filix Mas, *Br.* and *U. S.* 1870; Rhizoma Filicis, *P.G.;* Radix Filicis maris, Male Shield Fern; Fougère male, *Fr.;* Wurmfarnwurzel, Woldfarnwurzel, Johanniswurzel, *G.;* Félce maschio, *It.;* Helecho, *Sp.*

Gen. Ch. Fruit dots roundish or round, borne on the backs or extremities of free pinnate veins; indusium flat, scarious, orbicular, or round kidney-shaped, covering the sporangia, attached to the receptacle at the centre, or at the sinus opening all round the margin.

Aspidium Filix mas. Willd. *Sp. Plant.* v. 259; Smith, *Flor. Britan.*—*Nephrodium Filix mas.* Lindley, *Flor. Med.* 619.—*Polypodium Filix mas.* Linn.; Woodv. *Med. Bot.* p. 795, t. 267. The male fern has a perennial, horizontal root or rhizome, from which numerous annual fronds or leaves arise, forming tufts from a foot to four feet in height. The stipe, or footstalk, and midrib are thickly beset with brown, tough, transparent scales; the frond itself is oval-lanceolate, acute, pinnate, and of a bright green color. The pinnæ or leaflets are remote below, approach more nearly as they ascend, and run together at the summit of the leaf. They are deeply divided into lobes, which are of an oval shape, crenate at the edges, and gradually diminish from the base of the pinna to the apex. The fructification is in small dots on the back of each lobe, placed in two rows near the base, and distant from the edges. The plant is a native of Europe, Asia, and the north of Africa. It is also said to have been found in some of the Polynesian islands, and grows in Canada, following the Rocky Mountain chain through Mexico, Venezuela, etc., as far south as Peru. In the Eastern United States it is replaced by *A. marginale*, Sw., and *A. Goldianum*, Hook.

A. marginale. Swartz. (*Gray's Manual.*) Frond ovate-oblong in outline (one to two feet long), pale green; pinnæ lanceolate, from a broad almost sessile base; pinnules oblong, obtuse, crowded. This species differs from *A. Filix mas* chiefly in having its fruit dots upon the margins of its evergreen fronds.

The revisers of our Pharmacopœia have perhaps acted prematurely in admitting *Aspidium marginale*, but it is probable that most species of the genus, if not of the natural order, are medicinally active. Mr. J. L. Patterson (*A. J. P.*, 1875) found that the newly recognized *A. marginale* contained all of the active principle of *A. Filix mas*, and Mr. Chas. H. Cressler has demonstrated the activity of its oleoresin. (*Ibid.*, 1878.) On the Pacific slope the indigenous *A. rigidum* is locally used against the tape-worm, and Mr. W. J. Bowman has found in it filicic acid and resin. Popular belief has long ascribed tænicidal virtues to our native *Asplenium Filix fœmina;* and the Kaffirs of South Africa use the rhizome of *Aspidium Athamanticum* under the name of *inkomankomo*, or *uncomocomo*. It is the *pannum* of European commerce. (*P. J. Tr.*, xvi. 447.)

The proper period for collecting the rhizome is during the summer, when, according to M. Peschier, of Geneva, it abounds more in the active principle than at any other season. The same writer informs us that it deteriorates rapidly when kept, and in about two years becomes entirely inert. The rhizomes of other species of fern are frequently substituted for the officinal; and in the dried state it is difficult to distinguish them. The chaff, together with the dead portions of the rhizome and stipes, should be removed, and only such portions as have retained their green color should be used.

Properties, etc. As taken from the ground, the rhizome consists of a long cylindrical caudex, around which are closely arranged, overlapping each other like the shingles of a roof, the remains of the leafstalks or stipes, which are an inch or two in length, from two to four lines thick, somewhat curved and directed upwards, angular, brown, shining, and surrounded near their origin from the rhizome with thin silky scales, of a light brown color. From between these remains of the footstalks emerge numerous small radical fibres. The whole rhizome, thus constituted, presents a somewhat flexible, cylindrical mass, one or two inches thick, and from three inches to a foot or more in length. In this form, however, it is not usually found in our shops. The whole is ordinarily broken up into fragments, consisting of the separated remains of the leafstalks before described, with a small portion of the substance of the rhizome attached to their base, where they are surrounded by the silky scales. These fragments, as seen in the shops, often appear as if long kept, and are probably, in general, much deteriorated by time. The following observations are made by Geiger in relation to the collection and preservation of the rhizome. The inner parts of the fresh rhizome, and of the portions of stalk attached to it, are fleshy and of a light yellowish-green color. In collecting them, all the black discolored portions should be cut away, the fibres and scales separated, and only the sound green parts preserved. These should be immediately but carefully dried, and then pulverized; and the powder should be kept in small well-stopped glass bottles. The powder thus prepared has a pale yellowish color with a greenish tinge.

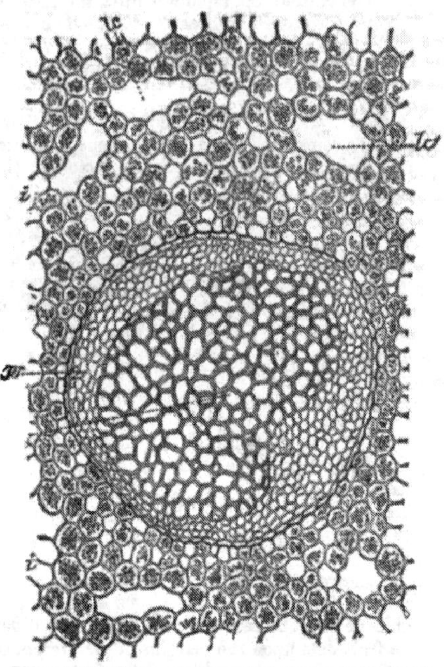

Rhizome of Aspidium. *io*, open interspace; *pr*, prosenchyma; *i*, parenchyma.

The dried rhizome is externally of a brown color, internally yellowish white or reddish, with a peculiar but feeble odor which is most obvious in the powder and decoction, and a sweetish, bitter, astringent, nauseous taste. Microscopic examination shows that it is composed of polyhedral, porous-walled cells and vascular bundles containing scalariform ducts: in *A. Filix mas*, ten of these bundles are larger than the others, and are arranged in a circle near to the surface; whilst in *A. marginale* there are only six bundles in the circle. It has been analyzed by H. Bock, who gives, as its constituents, volatile oil, fixed oil, resin, starch, vegetable jelly, albumen, gum, sugar, tannic and gallic acids, pectin, lignin, and various salts. (See *A. J. P.*, xxiv. 64.) Peschier ascertained that its active properties reside in the ethereal extract, which is the fixed oil in an impure state, containing volatile oil, resin, coloring matter, etc. It is a thick dark liquid, with the odor of the fern, and a nauseous, bitterish, somewhat acrid taste. Dr. E. Luck has found in it a peculiar acid, which he denominates *filicic acid*, and has extracted from the root two others named *tannaspidic* and *pteritannic acids*. (*Chem. Gaz*, ix. 407 and 452.) Luck gave to the filicic acid the formula $C_{13}H_{14}O_4$, but Grabowsky showed that it should be $C_{14}H_{18}O_5$, and that the acid was in reality *dibutyryl phloroglucin*, $C_6H_4(C_4H_7O)_2O_3$. The *aspidin* of Pavesi is not entitled to the name, as, though it may contain, it does not itself constitute the active principle, and is probably little if at all superior to the ethereal extract.

Medical Properties and Uses. Male fern was used by the ancients, and is mentioned as a vermifuge in the works of Dioscorides, Theophrastus, Galen, and Pliny, and was also noticed by some of the earlier modern writers, among whom was Hoffman. But it does not appear to have been generally known till about the year 1775. Madame Nouffer, the widow of a surgeon in Switzerland, had grauually acquired great celebrity in the cure of tape-worm by a secret remedy. Her success was such as to attract the attention of the medical profession at Paris; and some of the most eminent physicians of that city, who were deputed to examine into the subject, having reported favorably of the remedy, the secret was purchased by the King of France, and published by his order. The outlines of her plan were to give a dose of the powdered root of the male fern, and two hours afterwards a powerful cathartic, to be followed, if it should not operate in due time, by some purging salt; and this process was to be repeated, at proper intervals, till the worm should be evacuated. A German physician, named Herrenschwand, had used the male fern in a manner somewhat similar, before Madame Nouffer's secret was known. The oleoresin of Male Fern is certainly a very efficient tænicide, and has entirely superseded the use of the crude drug. In overdoses it is an irritant poison, six drachms having caused death. (*Lancet*, Oct. 14, 1882.) For the expulsion of tape-worm, the patient should live upon milk and a little bread for one day, and the following morning take a full dose (f℥ss to f℥i) of the oleoresin, fasting, and repeating it in two or three hours. At noon the patient may resume the use of food, and in the evening a brisk cathartic should be given. Male fern is said (with doubtful accuracy) to prove more effectual against the tape-worm of the Swiss (*Bothriocephalus latus*) than against the *Tænia solium*, which is more frequent in France and England. (*Bremser.*)

Off. Prep. Oleoresina Aspidii. *Off. Prep. Br.* Extractum Filicis Liquidum.

ATROPINA. *U. S., Br.* *Atropine.*

$C_{17} H_{23} NO_3$; 289. (ĂT-RO-PĪ'NA.) $C_{34} H_{23} NO_6$; 289.

"An alkaloid prepared from Belladonna." *U. S.*

Atropia; Atropinum, *P. G.*; Atropine, *Fr.*; Atropin, *G.*

The U. S. Pharmacopœia has very properly omitted the process for preparing atropine; for process of 1870 see foot-note.* The British process is as follows: "Take of Belladonna Root, recently dried and in coarse powder, *two pounds* [avoirdupois]; Rectified Spirit *ten pints* [Imperial measure]; Slaked Lime *one ounce* [av.]; Diluted Sulphuric Acid, Carbonate of Potassium, of each, *a sufficiency*; Chloroform *three fluidounces*; Purified Animal Charcoal *a sufficiency*; Distilled Water *ten fluidounces*. Macerate the Root in four pints [Imp. meas.] of the Spirit, for twenty-four hours, with frequent stirring. Transfer to a displacement apparatus, and exhaust the root with the remainder of the Spirit by slow percolation. Add the Lime to the tincture placed in a bottle, and shake them occasionally several times. Filter, add the Diluted Sulphuric Acid in very slight excess to the filtrate, and filter again. Distil off three-fourths of the Spirit, add to the residue the Distilled Water, evaporate as rapidly as possible, until the liquor is reduced to one-third of its volume and no longer smells of alcohol; then let it cool. Add very cautiously, with constant stirring, a solution of the Carbonate of Potassium so as nearly to neutralise the acid, care, however, being taken that an excess is not used. Set to rest for six hours, then filter, and add Carbonate of Potassium in such quantity that the liquid shall acquire a decided alkaline reaction. Place it in a bottle with the Chloroform; mix well by frequently repeated brisk agitation, and pour the mixed liquids into a funnel furnished with a glass stop cock. When the Chloroform has subsided, draw it off by the stop-cock, and distil it on a water-bath from a retort connected

* "Take of Belladonna Root, in fine powder, *forty-eight troyounces*; Purified Chloroform *four troyounces and a half*; Diluted Sulphuric Acid, Solution of Potassa, Alcohol, Water, each, *a sufficient quantity*. Mix the powder with a pint of Alcohol, and, having introduced the mixture into a cylindrical percolator, pour alcohol gradually upon it until sixteen pints have passed. From the liquid, thus obtained, distil off twelve pints of Alcohol. To the residue add sufficient Diluted Sulphuric Acid to give it an acid reaction, and, having evaporated the liquid to half a pint, add an equal bulk of Water, and filter through paper. To the filtered liquid add, first a troyounce and a half of the Chloroform, and then Solution of Potassa in slight excess, and shake the whole together at intervals, for half an hour. When the heavier liquid has subsided, separate it, and, having added a troyounce and a half of the Chloroform to the lighter liquid, again shake them together, and separate the heavier from the lighter liquid as before. Add to this lighter liquid the remainder of the Chloroform, and, after agitation, separate the heavier liquid for the third time. Mix the heavier liquids in a capsule, and set the mixture aside until, by spontaneous evaporation, the Atropia is left dry." *U. S.* 1870.

with a condenser. Dissolve the residue in warm Rectified Spirit; digest the solution with a little Animal Charcoal; filter, evaporate, and cool until colorless crystals are obtained." *Br.*

The U. S. process of 1870 is a modification of that of Prof. Procter. (*Proc. A. P. A.*, 1860.) For discussion of this and other processes, see the U. S. Dispensatory, 14th ed.

The British process is a combination of the processes of Mein and Rabourdin (see 14th ed. U. S. Dispensatory), the former being followed until after the addition of carbonate of potassium, and the alkaloid thus liberated being taken up by chloroform as in the latter. The use of lime in the earlier stage of the proceedings is to cause a precipitation of various substances which would otherwise embarrass the subsequent operations. This alkaloid cannot be prepared profitably on the small scale by the pharmacist, and for this reason the Pharmacopœia furnishes several good tests for recognizing its quality, and refrains from giving a process. A new method for preparing atropine is given in *Chem. Centralbl.*, No. 111, 180. (See *Proc. A. P. A.*, 1884, p. 315.)

Properties and Tests. Atropine is in "colorless, or white, acicular crystals, permanent in the air, odorless, having a bitter and acrid taste, and an alkaline reaction. Soluble in 600 parts of water at 15° C. (59° F.), and in 35 parts of boiling water; very soluble in alcohol; also soluble in 3 parts of chloroform and in 60 parts of ether. When heated to 114° C. (237·2° F.), the crystals melt, and, on ignition, are completely dissipated, emitting acrid vapors. Atropine and its salts are decomposed and rendered inert by prolonged contact with potassa or soda, and, if heated with either of them, evolve vapor of ammonia. A solution of Atropine, or of any of its salts, when applied to the eye, strongly dilates the pupil.

"With sulphuric acid Atropine yields a colorless solution, which is neither colored by nitric acid (abs. of and difference from morphine), nor at once by solution of bichromate of potassium (abs. of and difference from strychnine), though the latter reagent, by prolonged contact, causes the solution to turn green. On heating this green solution, diluted with a little water, to boiling, a pleasant odor, recalling that of roses and orange flowers, is developed. The aqueous solution of Atropine, or of any of its salts, is not precipitated by test-solution of platinic chloride (difference from most other alkaloids). With chloride of gold it yields a precipitate which, when recrystallized from boiling water acidulated with hydrochloric acid, is deposited on cooling (rendering the liquid turbid), in minute crystals, forming a dull, lustreless powder on drying (difference from hyoscyamine)." *U. S.*

It is inflammable, giving off an odor like that of benzoic acid, and, when burned in the open air, leaving no residue. By distilling it with bichromate of potassium and sulphuric acid, Dr. E. Pfeiffer succeeded in obtaining crystals of benzoic acid and propylamine. (*A. J. P.*, 1864, p. 226.) Dr. Kraut, by heating it with baryta water, succeeded in obtaining a peculiar acid and peculiar base, the former of which he calls *tropic acid*, $C_9H_{10}O_3$, melting at 117° C., and oxidizable by dilute potassium permanganate to bitter almond oil and benzoic acid, and the latter *tropine*, $C_8H_{15}NO$, melting at 62° C. (*Ibid.*, p. 232.) Ladenburg (*Ber. Chem. Ges.*, 12, 942, and 13, 104) has succeeded in effecting the synthesis of atropine from these two constituents, which when heated over a water-bath in the presence of dilute hydrochloric acid, unite to form the alkaloid. It is said, moreover, that when a little of it, dissolved in a few drops of sulphuric acid, is heated. an odor is given out resembling that of orange flowers. (*A. J. P.*, March, 1864, p. 112.) Hinterberger states that an alcoholic solution of atropine, when cyanogen is passed through it, assumes a blood-red color, and, on spontaneous evaporation, deposits a red, syrupy liquid insoluble in water. (*Gmelin.*) The detection of atropine, in small quantity, is a matter of great difficulty; the best test is the physiological, which consists in placing the suspected liquid in the eye of a cat, or other animal, when, if the alkaloid be present, dilatation of the pupil will occur. According to Brunner, the best chemical test is the aromatic smell, which is produced by adding this alkaloid and a little water to a hot mixture of sulphuric acid and bichromate of potassium or molybdate of ammonium. (*P. J. Tr.*, iv. 385.) For further information see *Belladonna;** also, *A. J. P.*, 1884, p. 206.

Medical Properties and Uses. The local and general effects of atropine on the system are precisely those of belladonna. It is, however, more speedy in its operation, probably in consequence of its easier absorption. Thus, the poisonous action of belladonna is seldom experienced in less than half an hour, while that of atropine shows itself violently in fifteen or twenty minutes. The most prominent effects from small remedial doses are dryness and stricture of the throat, and slight uneasiness of the head, with confusion or giddiness; from somewhat larger doses, dilatation of the pupil, some dimness of vision, frontal headache, hurried respiration, slight delirium, flushed face, and sometimes a scarlet rash. After poisonous doses, the above symptoms occur in a more aggravated form. Two distinct stages of the poisoning can usually be noted. At first there is great dimness or total temporary loss of vision, excessive dilatation of the pupil, headache, delirium, which is always talkative and may be violent, an enormous increase in the frequency of the pulse, which is also small and hard, and an elevation of the bodily temperature, and decided increase of the rate of respiration. Subsequently the second stage develops, and paralytic symptoms set in: the delirium gives way to stupor, restlessness to paralytic weakness, the pulse becomes very feeble, the surface cold, the respirations grow more and more shallow, and death from failure of both respiration and circulation occurs.

In some instances violent convulsions have occurred; nausea and vomiting, and even diarrhœa, are occasionally produced. The atropine is eliminated by the kidneys, and may produce increased diuresis, but usually there is, in cases of poisoning, retention of urine from vesical paralysis. The increase of the heart's action by atropine is chiefly due to its paralyzing the peripheral vagi, the inhibitory nerves of the heart; the final cardiac failure which takes place when poisonous doses have been taken is apparently the result of a direct depressant action on the heart-muscle. Upon the vaso-motor centres atropine in a moderate dose acts as a stimulant, thereby causing a great rise of the arterial pressure. After poisonous doses the primary vaso-motor spasm is followed by dilatation of the vessels, and great fall of the arterial pressure. Upon the spinal cord it acts as a powerful stimulant. Hence the violent convulsions which are sometimes seen in belladonna poisoning. Usually this effect is more or less completely masked by the paralysis of the motor nerves, which is one of the most marked effects of the poison; upon the afferent nerves the poison seems to have but little influence. On all non-striated muscle atropine exerts a very powerful influence, and it is probable, although not certain, that whilst in poisonous amount it lessens and finally paralyzes intestinal movements by a direct action upon the muscular coats, in small doses it increases peristalsis by paralyzing the inhibitory nerves which control this intestinal function. The action of the drug upon the respiratory centres is a very important one, atropine being in moderate doses the most powerful persistent stimulant to the respiratory centre known. The asphyxia of belladonna poisoning is certainly in large measure due to the paralysis of the nerve-trunks, which the poison produces, although it is also probable that the first period of excitation of the respiratory centres is followed by one of depression.

Atropine chiefly depends for its therapeutic powers upon—1st, its sedative action upon the peripheral nerves; 2d, its stimulant action on the respiratory centres; 3d, its influence upon the heart and vaso-motor centres. By virtue of its first-mentioned power it is useful in spasmodic diseases, such as hooping-cough, dysmenorrhœa, local spasms, etc. As the action is upon the nerve-trunks, the remedy is much more effective when it can be applied locally, as by atomization in hooping-cough and asthma, or by hypodermic injection in wry neck. As atropine has some influence upon the afferent nerve, it has some power of relieving pain; but for this action to be marked,

* For the behavior of atropine under the influence of an electric current, see *P. J. Tr.*, 1870, i. 244.

It is stated by H. Bullot that if to an aqueous solution of atropine acidulated with sulphuric acid an aqueous solution of picric acid be added, a precipitate will not form with good English atropine; with that obtained by the method of Simon, there will be a very slight precipitate; with the German alkaloid, an abundant yellow precipitate.

direct application is necessary. On account of its influence upon respiration, it is invaluable in narcotic poisonings and other bodily conditions with failure of the function. In shock and other similar states in which vaso-motor paralysis is an important part of the morbid condition, it is a very useful stimulant. On account of the paralyzing influence which it has upon the inhibitory intestinal nerves, atropine may be used as an adjuvant to more decided laxatives.

On the glandular system atropine exerts a decided influence; its effect upon the salivary and perspiratory glands being at present best understood. The remarkable action which it has in checking the functional activity of these glands is probably exerted through the nervous system, for in Keuchel's experiments it was distinctly proved that the chorda tympani nerve, excitation of which normally provokes salivation in atropine poisoning, is paralyzed. In a case recorded by Dr. James Andrew two-thirds of a grain of atropine occasioned the most alarming symptoms, which continued for several days (*Ed. Month. Journ. of Med. Sci*, xiv. 34); and a lady, under the care of M. Roux, of Brignolles, took somewhat more than a grain, with the same alarming symptoms (*Ann. de Thérap.*, 1861, p. 14); though, in both cases, recovery took place under treatment. In a child three years old less than half a grain was followed by similar dangerous symptoms, and the same favorable result. (*Med. Times and Gaz.*, Dec. 1850, p. 601.) A solution of atropia dropped into the eye produces dilatation of the pupil after ten or fifteen minutes, without causing congestion or inflammation; and the dilatation will usually continue for three or four days. Sometimes it is said that the dilatation is followed by contraction of the pupil, especially when the dose is large. The alkaloid also produces its characteristic constitutional effects when applied to the skin denuded of the epidermis, or to a mucous membrane, as of the rectum, vagina, etc., and especially when injected into the subcutaneous areolar tissue. The remedies for its poisonous operation are the same as those for belladonna; the most prominent being evacuation of the stomach, cold applications to the head, the preparations of opium internally, and stimulants when the strength is failing. As the value of atropine in opium poisoning, which seems unquestionable, is due to its influence on the respiratory centres, it is far from certain that opium is of at all proportionate advantage in poisoning by belladonna, etc. The officinal compound solution of iodine has been given as a chemical antidote to atropine, and with asserted advantage. It acts by forming an insoluble compound with the alkaloid. (See *Belladonna.*)

Atropine may be used internally for all the purposes for which belladonna is given; and it is very largely used as a local remedy, for application to the eye, or to the surface of the body, or for subcutaneous injection; and for these purposes it has the advantage over the ordinary preparations of belladonna, of greater precision of dose, quicker action, and greater neatness and cleanness. In ptyalism and in colliquative sweats the most prompt effects can be obtained from the hypodermic use of atropine. The hypodermic dose of atropine may be set down as the one-hundredth of a grain, the dose by the mouth as the one-seventy-fifth of a grain, although in serious cases these amounts may be much exceeded. Thus, in some cases of opium poisoning, one-twentieth of a grain (0·003 Gm.) may be exhibited at once. On the other hand, in susceptible persons, one-hundredth of a grain (0·0006 Gm.) will produce decided dryness of the throat, and the one-fiftieth of a grain (0·0012 Gm.) is alleged to have caused toxic symptoms. As the atropine itself is insoluble, the sulphate should always be preferred. For application to the sound skin, the form of ointment is most convenient. This may be made by rubbing a grain of the alkaloid first with four minims of alcohol, and then with a drachm of lard. Glycerin and olein also have been recommended as vehicles of atropine for external use, and may be incorporated with it in the same proportion.

When solution of sulphate of atropine is used for dilating the pupil, it may be either dropped into the eye within the lower lid, or may be introduced on small slips of paper previously saturated with the solution and dried, or, what is still more convenient, by means of minute circular disks of gelatin, made by mixing the solution with gelatin and evaporating so as to procure a thin film, which is to be cut into circular pieces. These have the advantage over paper that they do not require to be subsequently removed from the eye.

The external use of atropine is not without danger, unless great caution be observed. A case is on record in which an ointment composed of three grains of the sulphate and two drachms of lard, applied upon a vesicated surface on the neck, produced in a few minutes the most violent symptoms of belladonna poisoning, ending in death in two hours. (*Ann. de Thérap.*, 1867, p. 9.) The solution of atropine or its salts is very apt to have developed in it a fungous growth with consequent decomposition of the alkaloid.

The physiological action of *tropine hydrochlorate* has been partially investigated by Dr. H. G. Beyer. (*Med. News*, Aug. 27, 1887.) He concludes that it gives rise to vaso-motor constriction by exciting the vaso-motor constrictors, and that some terebene causes vaso-motor dilatation by exciting vaso-motor dilator nervous elements.

Off. Prep. Br. Atropinæ Sulphas; Unguentum Atropinæ.

ATROPINÆ SULPHAS. *U. S., Br.* *Sulphate of Atropine.**

(ĂT-RO-PĪ'NÆ SŬL'PHĂS.)

$(C_{17}H_{23}NO_3)_2, H_2SO_4$; 676. $C_{34}H_{23}N_2O_6, HOSO_3$; 338.

Sulphate of Atropia; Atropinum Sulfuricum, *P. G.*; Sulfate d'Atropine, *Fr.*; Schwefelsaures Atropin, *G.*

"Take of Atropine *one hundred and twenty grains*; Distilled Water *four fluid-drachms*; Diluted Sulphuric Acid *a sufficiency*. Mix the Atropine with the Water and add the Acid gradually, stirring them together until the alkaloid is dissolved, and the solution is neutral. Evaporate it to dryness at a temperature not exceeding 100° (37.8° C.)." *Br.*

The U. S. Pharmacopœia gives no process for preparing this salt. The officinal formula of 1870 is essentially the process of M. Ch. Maitre.† Atropine being soluble in ether while its sulphate is insoluble in that fluid, a convenient method is afforded for preparing the sulphate with little evaporation. By adding the mixed acid and alcohol to the ethereal solution, the sulphate is formed, and, being insoluble in the ether, is deposited; while the little left dissolved in the alcohol is obtained by spontaneous evaporation. The quantity of acid added, is intended to saturate the alkaloid; but if the saturation should not be exact, it would be easy to render it so by the addition of a little more alkaloid or a little more acid, as the case might be.

From the great facility with which atropine undergoes change, much caution is necessary in preparing its salts; and the process was arranged in reference to this caution. Upon the addition of the mixed acid and alcohol to the ethereal solution, the liquid becomes milky, and deposits on the sides of the vessel a copious precipitate, of a viscid appearance, which soon dries upon the decantation of the ether, and the placing of the vessel in a drying room. To succeed with this process, it is necessary that the liquids employed should be carefully freed from water, the sulphuric acid being monohydrated, and that the temperature should be kept as low as possible. There should be no excess of acid; and, if such an excess should be found upon applying the test of litmus paper, the solution should be neutralised by a portion of reserved solution of atropine. (*A. J. P.*, xxviii. 361; from *Répert. de Pharm.*)

* *Atropine Salicylate.* This salt is alleged to have advantages over the sulphate, mainly because of its more rapid and efficient action, provided it be pure and perfectly neutral. It may be prepared by Frederici's process, which is to dissolve 23 parts of atropine in pure alcohol by a gentle heat, and to add enough salicylic acid (about 18 parts) to render the solution neutral, which is determined by the use of litmus paper. The solution is carefully evaporated, and finally dried in a drying oven. It is deliquescent, and should be kept in securely-stopped vials. The dose is the same as that of the sulphate.

Atropinum Santonicum, a compound of atropine and santonic acid, is described by Herr Bombelon (*Pharm. Zeitung*, April, 1886) as an amorphous non-hygroscopic powder, readily soluble in water, which presents advantages over all other atropine salts in being non-irritating, and also affording a solution which is stable if kept in yellow glass bottles to avoid the formation of photo-santonic acid. One drop of a solution of 0·01 Gm. in 20 Gm. of water is sufficient to dilate the pupil, the dilatation disappearing in from twelve to twenty-four hours.

† "Take of Atropia *sixty grains*; Stronger Ether *four fluidounces and a half*; Sulphuric Acid *six grains*; Stronger Alcohol *a fluidrachm*. Dissolve the Atropia in the Ether; then mix the Acid and Alcohol, and add the mixture, drop by drop, to the ethereal solution until the Atropia is saturated. Allow the liquid to stand until the precipitate formed is deposited. Then decant the ether, and expose the residue to spontaneous evaporation until the salt is dry." *U. S.* 1870.

In the British process the same object of avoiding decomposition by heat is attained by the low temperature at which the evaporation is effected.

Properties. "A white, indistinctly crystalline powder, permanent in the air, odorless, having a very bitter, nauseating taste, and a neutral reaction. Soluble in 0·4 part of water and 6·5 parts of alcohol at 15° C. (59° F.), very soluble in boiling water and in boiling alcohol; also soluble in 0·3 part of absolute alcohol. When heated on platinum foil, the salt is decomposed and wholly dissipated, emitting acrid vapors. On adding test-solution of carbonate of sodium to a concentrated aqueous solution of the salt, a white precipitate is obtained, which answers to the reactions of atropine. (See *Atropina.*) The salt, or its solution, when applied to the eye strongly dilates the pupil. An aqueous solution of the salt yields, with test-solution of chloride of barium, a white precipitate insoluble in hydrochloric acid." *U. S.*

If it be required to procure the sulphate in the form of crystals, which may sometimes be desirable, to avoid adulteration, the process of M. Laneau may be employed. A solution of crystallized atropine in absolute alcohol, in the proportion of 2·89 parts of the former to 4 parts of the latter by weight, having been made with the assistance of a gentle heat, 0·4 part of sulphuric acid of the sp. gr. 1·85, diluted with 3 parts of absolute alcohol, is to be gradually added, and stirred with a glass rod, until saturation, as shown by test-paper, is effected. The solution is then allowed to evaporate spontaneously, and the thinner the stratum the sooner will the process be completed. The crystals are in colorless needles more or less interlaced. (See *A. J. P.*, 1863, p. 315.)

The effects of the salt on the system are precisely the same as those of atropine, and it may be used in the same dose. Its great advantage over the alkaloid is its solubility in water. A solution of the salt in the proportion of one part to one hundred of the solvent has been found instantaneously efficacious in the relief of toothache, applied in the quantity of a drop or two (0·06–0·12 C.c.) to the denuded dental pulp; and it is said, in the same quantity, to produce complete insensibility of the dental nerves, in cases in which an artificial tooth is inserted in a living root. (*Ann. de Thérap.*, 1861, p. 19.)

AURANTII AMARI CORTEX. *U. S.* *Bitter Orange Peel.*

(ÂU-RĂN'TI-Ī A-MĀ'RĪ CÔR'TĔX—âu-răn'she-ī.)

"The rind of the fruit of Citrus vulgaris. Risso. (*Nat. Ord.* Aurantiaceæ.)" *U. S.*

AURANTII CORTEX. *Bitter Orange Peel.* "The dried outer part of the rind or pericarp of Citrus vulgaris, *Risso* (Citrus Bigaradia, *Duhamel*)." *Br.*

Aurantii pericarpium; Cortex Fructus Aurantii, *P.G.;* Cortex Aurantiorum, Cortex Pomorum Aurantii; Écorce (Zestes) d'Oranges amères, Écorce de Bigarade, *Fr.;* Pomeranzenschale, *G.*

AURANTII DULCIS CORTEX. *U. S.* *Sweet Orange Peel.*

(ÂU-RĂN'TI-Ī DŬL'CIS CÔR'TĔX—âu-răn'she-ī.)

"The rind of the fruit of Citrus Aurantium. Risso. (*Nat. Ord.* Aurantiaceæ.)" *U. S.*

Cortex Aurantiorum Dulcium; Écorce (Zestes) d'Oranges douces, *Fr.;* Apfelsinenschalen, *G.;* Scorza del Frutto dell' Arancio, *It.;* Corteza de Naranja, *Sp.*

AURANTII FLORES. *U. S.* *Orange Flowers.*

(ÂU-RĂN'TI-Ī FLŌ'RĒŞ—âu-răn'she-ī.)

"The partly expanded, fresh flowers of Citrus vulgaris and Citrus Aurantium. Risso. (*Nat. Ord.* Aurantiaceæ.)" *U. S.*

Flores Naphæ; Fleurs d'Oranger, *Fr.;* Orangenblüthen, Pomeranzenblüthen, *G.*

AURANTII FRUCTUS. *Br.* *Bitter Orange.*

(ÂU-RĂN'TI-Ī FRŬC'TŬS—âu-răn'she-ī.)

"The ripe fruit of Citrus vulgaris, *Risso* (Citrus Bigaradia, *Duhamel*)." *Br.*

Gen. Ch. Calyx five-cleft. *Petals* five, oblong. *Anthers* twenty, the filaments united into different parcels. *Berry* nine-celled. *Willd.*

This very interesting genus is composed of small evergreen trees, with ovate or oval-lanceolate and shining leaves, odoriferous flowers, and fruits which usually combine beauty of color with a fragrant odor and grateful taste. They are all natives of warm climates. Though the species are not numerous, great diversity exists in the character of the fruit; and many varieties, founded upon this circumstance, are noticed by writers. In the splendid work on the natural history of the *Citrus* by Risso and Poiteau, 169 varieties are described under the eight following heads:—1, sweet oranges, 2, bitter and sour oranges, 3, bergamots, 4, limes, 5, shaddocks, 6, lumes, 7, lemons, and 8, citrons. Of these it is difficult to decide which have just claims to the rank of distinct species, and which must be considered merely as varieties. Those employed in medicine may be arranged in two sets, of which the orange, *C. Aurantium*, and the lemon, *C. medica*, are respectively the types; the former characterized by a winged, the latter by a naked or nearly naked petiole. The form and character of the fruit, though not entirely constant, serve as the basis of subdivisions. *C. decumana*, which yields the *shaddock*, agrees with *C. Aurantium* in the form of its petiole.

Citrus Aurantium. Willd. *Sp. Plant.* iii. 1427; *B. & T.* 51. The orange-tree grows to the height of about fifteen feet. Its stem is rounded, much branched, and covered with a smooth, shining, greenish brown bark. In the wild state, and before inoculation, it is often furnished with axillary spines. The leaves are ovate, pointed, entire, smooth, and of a shining pale green color. When held between the eye and the light, they exhibit numerous small transparent vesicles, filled with volatile oil; and, when rubbed between the fingers, are highly fragrant. Their footstalks are about an inch long, and have wings or lateral appendages. The flowers, which have a delightful odor, are large, white, and attached by short peduncles, singly, or in clusters, to the smallest branches. The calyx is saucer-shaped, with pointed teeth. The petals are oblong, concave, white, and beset with numerous small glands. The filaments are united at their base in three or more distinct portions, and support yellow anthers. The germen is roundish, and bears a cylindrical style, terminated by a globular stigma. The fruit is a spherical berry, often somewhat flattened at its base and apex, rough, of a yellow or orange color, and divided internally into nine vertical cells, each containing from two to four seeds, surrounded by a pulpy matter. The rind of the fruit consists of a thin exterior layer, abounding in vesicles filled with a fragrant volatile oil, and of an interior one, which is thick, white, fungous, insipid, and inodorous. There are two varieties of *C. Aurantium*, considered by some as distinct species. They differ chiefly in the fruit, which in one is sweet, in the other sour and bitterish, and has a darker and rougher rind. The first retains the original title, the second is called *Citrus vulgaris* by De Candolle, and *C. Bigaradia* by Risso. The Seville orange is the product of the latter.*

This beautiful evergreen, in which the fruit is mingled, in every stage of its growth, with the blossoms and foliage, has been applied to numerous purposes of utility and ornament. A native of China and India, it was introduced into Europe at a very early period, was transplanted to America soon after its first settlement, and is now found in every civilized country where the climate is favorable. The fruit is brought to us chiefly from Florida, the south of Europe, and the West Indies. The Florida and Havana oranges have the sweetest and most agreeable flavor.

Various parts of the plant are used in medicine. The leaves, which are bitter and aromatic, are employed in some places in the form of infusion as a gently stimulant diaphoretic. They yield by distillation with water a volatile oil, which is said to be often mixed by the distillers with the oils obtained from the flowers and unripe fruit. In regard to polarized light, it has a rotatory power to the left, which is considerably weakened by the prolonged action of heat. (Chautard, *Journ. de Pharm.*, 3e sér., xliv. 28.) The fresh flowers may be kept for some time by mixing them well with

* A variety of the orange, called the *Mandarin Orange* (*Citrus Bigaradia Sinensis* or *C. Bigaradia myrtifolia*), which is probably a native of China, but cultivated in Sicily, the south of Italy, and Florida, bears a fruit much smaller than the common orange, round but flattened above and below, with a smooth, thin, delicate rind, and a very sweet delicious pulp. A volatile oil is obtained from the rind by expression, of a yellow color, a very bland agreeable odor, different from that of the orange or lemon, and a not unpleasant taste, like that of the rind. When freed from coloring matter by distillation, it was found by M. S. de Luca to be a pure hydrocarbon, with the formula $C_{20}H_{16}$. (*Journ. de Pharm.*, 3e sér., xxxiii. 52.)

half their weight of chloride of sodium, pressing the mixture in a suitable jar, and keeping it well closed in a cool place. They are officinally described as follows. "About half an inch (12 mm. long; calyx small, cup-shaped, five-toothed; petals five, oblong, obtuse, rather fleshy, white and glandular-punctate; stamens numerous, in about three sets; ovary globular, upon a small disk, with a cylindrical style, and a globular stigma; odor very fragrant; taste aromatic and somewhat bitter." *U. S.* The dried flowers are used on the continent of Europe as a gentle nervous stimulant, in the form of infusion, which may be made in the proportion of two drachms to the pint of boiling water, and taken in the dose of a teacupful. The flowers should be dried in the shade, at a temperature between 24° C. (75° F.) and 35° C. (95° F.). (*Annuaire de Thérap.*, 1861, p. 59.)

An oil is obtained also from the flowers by distillation, which is called *neroli* in France, and is much used in perfumery, and in the composition of *liqueurs*. (See *Oleum Aurantii Florum.*) It is an ingredient of the famous Cologne water. That obtained from the flowers of the Seville or bitter orange (*C. vulgaris*) is deemed the sweetest. It was introduced into the Edinburgh Pharmacopœia, with the title of *Aurantii Oleum*, to serve for the preparation of orange-flower water. Soubeiran considers this oil rather as a product of the distillation than as pre-existing in the flowers. The fact may thus be explained, that orange-flower water, made by dissolving even the finest neroli in water, has not the precise odor of that procured by distillation from the flowers. Pure neroli has a rotating power to the right, in this respect differing from the oil of the leaves. (*Chautard.*)

The fruit is applied to several purposes. Small unripe oranges, about the size of a cherry or less, previously dried, and rendered smooth by a turning-lathe, are sometimes employed to maintain the discharge from issues. They are preferred to peas on account of their agreeable odor, and by some are thought to swell less with the moisture; but this is denied by others, and it is asserted that they require to be renewed at the end of twenty-four hours. These fruits are sometimes found in commerce under the name of *orange berries*. They are of a grayish or greenish brown color, fragrant odor, and bitter taste, and are said to be used for flavoring cordials. A volatile oil is obtained from them by distillation, known to the French by the name of *essence de petit grain*, and employed for similar purposes with that of the flowers. The oil, however, which now goes by this name, is said to be distilled from the leaves, and those of the bitter orange yield the best. The oils from the unripe and the ripe fruit have a rotating power to the right, the latter much greater than the former; and this property might serve to distinguish them from the oil of the leaves. Several of the oils from the Aurantiaceæ deposit a crystalline substance, differing from camphor. (*Chautard.*) The juice of the Seville orange is sour and bitterish, and forms with water a refreshing and grateful drink in febrile diseases. It is employed in the same manner as lemon-juice, which it resembles in containing citric acid, though in much smaller proportion. The sweet orange is more pleasant to the taste, and is extensively used as a light refrigerant article of diet in inflammatory diseases, care being taken to reject the membranous portion. The rind both of the sweet and bitter varieties is directed by the U. S. Pharmacopœia, the bitter only by the British. With the latter the outer portion is that considered officinal; as the inner is destitute of activity, and by its affinity for moisture renders the peel liable to become mouldy. The best mode of separating the outer rind when its desiccation and preservation are desired, is to pare it from the orange in narrow strips with a sharp knife, as we pare an apple. When the object is to use the fresh rind for certain pharmaceutical purposes, as for the preparation of the *confection of orange peel*, it is best separated by a grater. The dried peel, sold in the shops, is usually that of the Seville orange, and is brought chiefly from the Mediterranean.

Properties. Orange peel has a grateful aromatic odor, and a warm bitter taste, which depend upon the volatile oil contained in its vesicles. "Bitter orange peel is in narrow, thin bands or in quarters; epidermis of a dark brownish green color, glandular, and with very little of the spongy, white, inner layer adhering to it." *U. S.* The sweet peel is orange yellow and less bitter. Both yield their sensible properties to water and alcohol. The bitter principle, *hesperidin*, $C_{22}H_{26}O_{12}$, was discovered by

Lebreton in 1828, but its character as a glucoside was established first by Hilger and Hoffmann. (*Ber. der Chem. Ges.*, 9, 26, 685.) Treated with dilute acids it yields *hesperetin*, $C_{16}H_{14}O_6$, and glucose. It is crystalline (fusing point 250°–251° C.), and may be prepared by Paterno and Briosi's process, as follows. The cut and bruised oranges are covered with diluted alcohol, potassa solution added in excess, the liquor filtered after two days, and impure hesperidin precipitated by hydrochloric acid; the precipitate is boiled with acetic acid for ten minutes, and, after cooling, filtered from the resinous mass left. The hesperidin gradually separates from the filtrate upon standing, in white fine needles. From 4000 oranges about 6 ounces av. of the principle were obtained. (*Berichte d. Chem. Ges.*, 1876, pp. 250–252.) Tanret found in the rind of the bitter orange, 1. A crystalline acid, $C_{44}H_{28}O_{14}$; 2. a non-crystalline resinous body; 3. *hesperidin*; 4. *isohesperidin*, a crystalline glucoside isomeric with hesperidin; 5. *aurantianarin*, a new glucoside, to which the bitterness of the peel is due. (*P. J. Tr.*, 1886, p. 839.) The oil may be obtained by expression from the fresh grated rind, or by distillation with water. It is imported into the United States in tinned copper cans. It has properties resembling those of the oil of lemons, but spoils more rapidly on exposure to the air, acquiring a terebinthinate odor. The perfumers use it in the preparation of Cologne water, and for other purposes; and it is also employed by the confectioners. According to Dr. Imbert-Gourbeyre, they who are much exposed to the inhalation of the oil of bitter oranges are apt to be affected with cutaneous eruptions, and various nervous disorders; as headache, tinnitus aurium, oppression of the chest, gastralgia, want of sleep, and even muscular spasm. He thinks that the oils of the Aurantiaceæ have much resemblance to camphor in their effects. (*Pharm. Centralblatt*, Feb. 1854, p. 128.)

Medical Properties and Uses. Bitter orange peel is a mild tonic, carminative, and stomachic; the sweet is simply aromatic; but neither is much used alone. They are chiefly employed to communicate a pleasant flavor to other medicines, to correct their nauseating properties, and to assist their stimulant impression upon the stomach. They are a frequent and useful addition to bitter infusions and decoctions, as those of gentian, quassia, columbo, and especially Peruvian bark. It is obviously improper to subject orange peel to long boiling; as the volatile oil, on which its virtues chiefly depend, is thus driven off. The dose in substance is from half a drachm to a drachm (1·95–3·9 Gm.) three times a day. Large quantities are sometimes productive of mischief, especially in children, in whom violent colic and even convulsions are sometimes induced by it. We have known the case of a child, in which death resulted from eating the rind of an orange.

When orange peel is used simply for its agreeable flavor, the rind of the sweet orange is preferable; as a tonic, that of the Seville orange.

Off. Prep. of Bitter Orange Peel. Extractum Aurantii Amari Fluidum; Tinctura Aurantii Amari; Tinctura Cinchonæ Composita; Tinctura Gentianæ Composita.

Off. Prep. Br. Infusum Aurantii; Infusum Aurantii Compositum; Infusum Gentianæ Compositum; Spiritus Armoraciæ Compositus; Tinctura Aurantii; Tinctura Cinchonæ Composita; Tinctura Gentianæ Composita.

Off. Prep. of Sweet Orange Peel. Syrupus Aurantii; Tinctura Aurantii Dulcis.

Off. Prep. of the Flowers. Aqua Aurantii Florum.

Off. Prep. of the Fruit. Br. Tinctura Aurantii Recentis; Vinum Aurantii.

AURI ET SODII CHLORIDUM. *U.S. Chloride of Gold and Sodium.*

(ÂU'RĪ ĔT SŌ'DI-Ī CHLŌ'RI-DŬM.)

"A mixture composed of equal parts of dry Chloride of Gold [**$AuCl_3$; 302·4.** — $AuCl_3$; 302·4], and Chloride of Sodium [**NaCl; 58·4.** — NaCl; 58·4]." *U.S.*

This new officinal is the first preparation of gold to enter the U.S. Pharmacopœia. It may be prepared by dissolving gold in nitro-hydrochloric acid, evaporating the solution to dryness, weighing, and dissolving the dry mass in eight times its weight of distilled water. To this solution a weight of pure decrepitated common salt equalling that of the dry chloride of gold is added, previously dissolved in four parts of water. The mixed solution is then evaporated to dryness, being in the mean time constantly stirred with a glass rod. A process for making this salt from gold coin without requiring the preliminary purification necessary in the above process may be found in *Proc. A. P. A.*, 1882, p. 311.

Properties. The salt is of a golden yellow color, and, when crystallized, is in the form of long prismatic crystals, unalterable in the air. The Pharmacopœia describes it as "an orange yellow powder, slightly deliquescent in damp air, odorless, having a saline and metallic taste, and a slightly acid reaction. The compound is very soluble in water; at least one-half of it should be soluble in cold alcohol. When exposed to a red heat, it is decomposed and metallic gold is separated. A fragment of the compound imparts an intense, persistent, yellow color to a non-luminous flame. Its aqueous solution yields, with test-solution of nitrate of silver, a white precipitate insoluble in nitric acid, but soluble in ammonia. On bringing a glass rod dipped into water of ammonia close to a portion of the compound, no white fumes should make their appearance (abs. of free acid). If 0·5 Gm. of Chloride of Gold and Sodium be dissolved in 20 C.c. of water, and treated with a clear solution of 2 Gm. of ferrous sulphate in 20 C.c. of water acidulated with a few drops of sulphuric acid, a brown precipitate of metallic gold will be thrown down. If, after at least two hours, this precipitate be separated, well washed, dried and ignited, the residue of metallic gold should weigh not less than 0·162 Gm. (corresponding to 32·4 per cent. of metallic gold)." *U. S.*

Medical Properties. The precise action of this salt upon the system is not known, but there is reason for believing that it exerts some influence upon the general nutrition, and is therefore alterative. By many gynæcologists it is believed to have a specific direction to the genital organs, and it is much used in hysteria, ovarian irritation and neuralgia, chronic ovaritis, and even chronic uterine inflammation. For frictions on the gums and tongue, Chrestien recommends the following formula. Crystallized chloride of gold and sodium, one grain; powdered orris root, deprived of its soluble parts by alcohol and water, and dried, two grains. Mix. At first the fifteenth part of this powder is used daily by frictions; afterwards the fourteenth, the thirteenth, etc., until, increasing gradually, the tenth or eighth part is employed. The use of four grains of the salt in this way is said commonly to cure bad cases of recent syphilis; such, for example, as are characterized by the coexistence of chancres, warts, and buboes; it is also affirmed to have resolved chronic glandular tumors in the neck. The patient should swallow his saliva while the frictions are practised. (*B. and F. Medico-Chir. Rev.*, Am. ed., July, 1857, p. 172.) It may be given in lozenges, each containing the twelfth of a grain (0·005 Gm.), by mixing immediately five grains of the salt with an ounce of powdered sugar, and making the whole with mucilage of tragacanth into a proper mass, to be divided into sixty lozenges. Pills, containing the same dose, may be formed by dissolving ten grains of the dried salt in a drachm of distilled water, and forming the solution into a pilular mass with a mixture of four drachms of potato starch and one drachm of gum arabic, to be divided into one hundred and twenty pills. (*Journ. de Pharm.*, xx. 648.)

AZEDARACH. *U.S.* *Azedarach.*

(Ą-ZĔD'Ą-RĂCH.)

"The bark of the root of Melia Azedarach. Linné. (*Nat. Ord.* Meliaceæ.)" *U. S.*

Pride of India, Pride of China, Common Bead Tree; Écorce d'Azédarach, Écorce de Margousier, *Fr.*; Zedrachrinde, *G.*

Gen. Ch. *Calyx* five-toothed. *Petals* five. *Nectary* cylindrical, toothed, bearing the *anthers* in the throat. *Drupe* with a five-celled nut. *Willd.*

Melia Azedarach. Willd. *Sp. Plant.* ii. 558; Michaux, *N. Am. Sylv.* iii. 4. *M. Azadirachta*, *B. & T.* 62. This is a beautiful tree, thirty or forty feet high, with a trunk fifteen or twenty inches in diameter. When alone, it attains less elevation, and spreads out into a capacious summit. Its leaves are large and doubly pinnate, consisting of smooth, acuminate, denticulate, dark green leaflets, disposed in pairs with an odd one at the end. The flowers are of a lilac color, delightfully fragrant, and in beautiful axillary clusters near the ends of the branches. The fruit is a round drupe, about as large as a cherry, and yellowish when ripe.

This species of Melia is a native of Syria, Persia, and the north of India, and is cultivated as an ornament in different parts of the world. It is abundant in our Southern States, and has even become naturalized. North of Virginia it does not flourish, though small trees may sometimes be seen in sheltered situations. It flowers early in the spring.

Properties. "The bark is in curved pieces or quills of variable size and thickness; outer surface red-brown, with irregular, blackish, longitudinal ridges; inner surface whitish or brownish, longitudinally striate; fracture more or less fibrous; upon transverse section tangentially striate, with yellowish bast-fibres; inodorous, sweetish, afterward bitter and nauseous. If collected from old roots, the bark should be freed from the thick, rust-brown, nearly tasteless, corky layer." *U. S.*

Jacobs (*A. J. P.*, 1879, p. 444) believes that the active principle is a yellowish white resin, and that the activity of the bark resides in the liber. Hanausek (1878) states that two kinds of oil of azedarach are used in Eastern Asia,—one from the fruit and the other from the seeds; the former is used medicinally, the latter only for burning. The closely related *Azadirachta Indica*, according to Broughton (*P. J. Tr.*, 1873, p. 992), contains a bitter amorphous resin, $C_{36}H_{50}O_{11}$, which fuses at 92° C. (197·6° F.), and a crystallized principle, melting at 175° C. (347° F.). Cornish (*Indian Annals of Med. Sc.*, 4, p. 104) had previously announced the presence of a bitter alkaloid, to which he gave the name *margosine*, from the Portuguese name for the tree, Margosa.

Medical Properties and Uses. The decoction of this bark is cathartic and emetic, and in large doses is said to produce narcotic effects similar to those of spigelia, especially if gathered at the season when the sap is mounting; but in a number of experiments made by Dr. H. C. Wood with extracts from the dried bark and fruit, it was found impossible to produce toxic symptoms in frogs or rabbits. Robins eating of the sweetish fruit, of which they are very fond, are often rendered so far insensible as to be picked up under the tree; though they usually recover in a few hours. It has been suggested that sufficient alcohol is produced by the spontaneous fermentation of the berries to cause intoxication. Children are said to eat the fruit without inconvenience, and possibly the robins simply choke themselves with the large berries. The bark is considered in the Southern States an efficient anthelmintic, and appears to enjoy, in some places, an equal degree of confidence with the pinkroot. The form of decoction is usually preferred. A quart of water is boiled with four ounces of the fresh bark to a pint, of which the dose for a child is a tablespoonful every two or three hours, till it affects the stomach or bowels. Another plan is to give a dose morning and evening for several successive days, and then to administer an active cathartic. The *fresh* bark and the fruit are said to be superior as vermifuges, but are not to be found in our Northern drug stores. A fluid extract and syrup of azedarach are proposed by J. J. Miles (*A. J. P.*, Aug. 1874), the former made in the usual way with diluted alcohol, except that 6 troyounces of white sugar are added. The syrup is made by taking 4 fluidounces of the fluid extract, 8 fluidounces of vanilla syrup, and sufficient simple syrup to make a pint.

BALSAMUM PERUVIANUM. *Balsam of Peru.*

(BĂL'SĄ-MŬM PĘ-RÛ-VĮ-Ā'NŬM.)

"A balsam obtained from Myroxylon Pereiræ. Klotzsch. (*Nat. Ord.* Leguminosæ, Papilionaceæ.)" *U. S.* "A balsam exuded from the trunk of Myroxylon Pereiræ, *Klotzsch* (Toluifera Balsamum, var. *Baill.*), after the bark has been beaten, scorched, and removed." *Br.*

Balsamum Peruvianum Nigrum, Balsamum Indicum; Baume des Indes, Baume de Pérou, *Fr.*; Peruvianischer Balsam, *G.*; Balsamo del Peru, *It.*; Balsamo negro, *Sp.*

Gen. Ch. *Calyx* subincurved, irregularly dentate. *Vexillum* broadly orbiculate; four inferior *petals* sub-equal, free, narrow. *Stamens* deciduous with the petals, free or at their extreme base very shortly connate. *Ovaries* long, stipitate, near the apex two ovulate. *Styles* short incurved, with a minute terminal stigma. *Legume* stipitate, compressed, indehiscent, with the apex indurated, and one-seeded. *Seed* one, subreniform, with a thin testa. *Cotyledons* plano-convex. *Radicle* very short, incurved. (Bentham and Hooker, *Genera Plantarum*, ii. 559.)

De Candolle and other botanists considered that the genera Myroxylon and Toluifera of Linnæus are not distinct from Myrospermum of Jacquin, but it is now generally recognized that the two Linnean genera are, taken together, entitled to rank as a single genus. To this the title of Myroxylon is now generally applied, although according to the strict rules of botanical nomenclature it should be called Toluifera. In regard to the species now under consideration there has been much discussion, and although the plant is now well known botanically, botanists are not agreed as to its specific distinctness; Ruiz (*Flora Peruviana*), Carson (*A. J. P.*, 1860, p. 297), Baillon, and others believing it to be identical with the tree which yields balsam of Tolu. Flückiger and Hanbury (*Pharmacographia*, 2d ed., 205) give the following points of difference: in *M. Pereiræ* the branches come off near the ground, the calyx is widely cup-shaped, and shallow, the racemes loose, 6 to 8 inches long, and the legume much narrowed at its base; whilst in *M. Toluifera* the trunk does not branch for 30 or 40 feet, the calyx is rather tubular, the racemes dense and 3 to 4½ inches long, the legume scarcely narrowed at the base. Besides the officinal species, there are others of the genus which possess medical virtues, and have been more or less employed.* The pod of *M. frutescens* (Jacq.), growing in Trinidad, is popularly used in that island as a carminative, and externally, in the form of tincture, as a lotion in rheumatic pains; and by incisions in the stem a small quantity of balsamic juice is obtained not distinguishable from balsam of Tolu.† (*P. J. Tr.*, Sept. 1862, p. 108.) Another species is known in Paraguay under the name of *quinoquino*, the bark of which is used, in powder and decoction, as a remedy in wounds and ulcers; and from the trunk of which a juice is obtained, which in its concrete state closely resembles dried balsam of Peru. (*Ibid.*, Oct. 1862, p. 183.)‡

Myroxylon Pereiræ, Klotzsch; *Myrospermum Pereiræ*, Royle et Auctores; "*Myrospermum of Sonsonate*," Pereira; is a handsome tree, with a straight, round, lofty stem, a smooth ash-colored bark, and spreading branches at the top. The leaves are alternate, petiolate, and unequally pinnate. The leaflets are from five to eleven, shortly petiolate, oblong, oval-oblong, or ovate, about three inches long by somewhat less than an inch and a half in breadth, rounded at the base, and contracting abruptly at top into an emarginate point. When held up to the light, they exhibit, in lines parallel with the primary veins, beautiful rounded and linear pellucid spots. The common and partial petioles and midribs are smooth to the naked eye, but, when examined with a microscope, are found to be furnished with short hairs. The fruit, including the winged footstalks, varies from two to four inches in length. At its peduncular extremity it is rounded or slightly tapering; at the top enlarged, rounded, and swollen, with a small point at the side. The mesocarp, or main investment of the fruit, is fibrous, and contains in distinct receptacles a balsamic juice, which is most abundant in two long receptacles or vittæ, one upon each side. The yellowish-white beans yielded to Mr. Rother (*P. J. Tr.*, xv. 244) two per cent. of coumarin; the husks, a brown, extremely bitter, somewhat acrid resin. A gum-resin exudes in small quantities from the trunk of the tree, which, though containing, besides gum and resin, a small proportion of volatile oil, is distinct from the proper balsam, and yields no cinnamic acid. (Attfield, *P. J. Tr.*, Dec. 1863.)

* For an account of the various imperfectly described species related to this plant, see 14th Ed. U. S. D.

† The name *Brasilian Balsam* has been proposed for the product of *M. Peruiferum*. It differs from balsam of Peru in odor, and in having a slightly pungent, but not warm, aromatic taste; in being permanently soluble in 90 per cent. alcohol in all proportions; also in mixing with castor oil in all proportions, forming with bisulphide of carbon a clear light brown solution with residue, and in the deposit, by its chloroform solution, of a powdery precipitate upon standing. At 17° C. its specific gravity is 1·031. Its general constitution is very similar to that of balsam of Peru, containing volatile oil, myroxylin, cinnamic and tannic acids, and resin. (*P. J. Tr.*, 3d ser., xi. 818.)

‡ A substance which is sometimes offered for sale as the genuine Peru Balsam is that yielded by the *Myroxylon Peruiferum*, and known as *Oleo-Balsam*. This in bulk is of a dark brown color, but in thin layers is dark red. Its odor is smoky, feebly fragrant; its taste slightly pungent, leaving a choking, disagreeable, persistent feeling. It is entirely soluble in ether and in rectified spirits. It is especially to be distinguished from Peru Balsam by its behavior with sulphuric acid. When Peru Balsam is treated with sulphuric acid, and cold water poured upon it, a beautiful violet is imparted to the surface, and the whole mass has a bright shade. The same procedure yields with the Oleo-Balsam a gray mass. For further information see *P. J. Tr.*, xv. 771.

This tree grows in Central America, in the State of San Salvador, upon the Pacific coast. It is found in the wild forests, singly or in groups, but the trees are owned by individuals. Dr. Charles Dorat states that it is never found at a greater height on the mountains than one thousand feet, that it begins to be productive after five years, and continues to yield for thirty years or more, and that the aroma of its flowers is perceived at the distance of one hundred yards. (*A. J. P.*, xxxii. 303.) In 1861 the tree was introduced in Ceylon with complete success. The balsam is collected from it exclusively by the aborigines, on lands reserved to them, within a small district denominated the Balsam Coast, extending from Acajutla to Port Libertad. Early in November or December the bark is beaten on four sides of the trunk, so as to separate it from the wood without breaking it; intermediate strips being left sound, in order not to destroy the life of the tree. The bruised bark soon splits, or cuts are made in it. Five or six days after the beating the injured surface is set on fire, and about a week later the bark, if it has not fallen off spontaneously, is removed. The juice now begins to exude freely from the exposed wood, which the natives cover with rags. The latter, when saturated, are boiled in water in large jars, and the liquid allowed to stand; whereupon the water rises to the top, and is poured off, leaving the balsam, which is put into calabashes or bladders. It is then taken for sale to the neighboring towns, where it is purified by subsidence and straining, and put into jars or metallic drums for exportation. The destroyed bark is said to renew itself in two years, so that by care a tree can be long worked; two pounds is stated to be the average yearly yield. The export from San Salvador in 1876 was over $78,000 in value.

A substance called *white balsam* (*Balsamo blanco*) is procured from the fruit by expression. This has been confounded with the balsam of Tolu, but is wholly distinct. It is of a semi-fluid or soft-solid consistence, somewhat granular, and, on standing, separates into a white resinous crystalline deposit, and a superior translucent more fluid portion. The smell, though quite distinct from that of the balsam of Tolu and Peru, is not disagreeable. Dr. Stenhouse has obtained from it a peculiar resinous body, readily crystallizable, and remarkably indifferent in its chemical affinities, which he denominates *myroxocarpin*. (*P. J. Tr.*, x. 290.) Dr. Dorat, however, denies that the white balsam is produced by the same tree, or in the same vicinity.

Another substance obtained from the same tree, and much used in Central America, is a tincture of the fruit, made by digesting it in rum. It is called *balsamito* by the inhabitants, and is said to be stimulant, anthelmintic, and diuretic. It is also used as an external application to gangrenous or indolent ulcers, and as a wash to the face to remove freckles. According to Dr. Dorat, the balsamito is not the tincture, but an alcoholic extract of the young fruit. Neither this nor the white balsam reaches the markets of this country.

The balsam of Peru was named from its place of exportation; and it was long thought to be a product of Peru. It is now shipped partly from the Pacific coast, and partly from the Balize or other Atlantic ports, whither it is brought across the country. It was Guibourt who first made known the fact of its exclusive production in Central America. As imported, it is usually in tin canisters, with a whitish scum on its surface, and more or less deposit, which is dissolved with the aid of heat.

Properties. Balsam of Peru is viscid like syrup or honey, of a dark reddish brown color, a fragrant odor, and a warm bitterish taste, leaving when swallowed a burning or prickling sensation in the throat. When exposed to flame it takes fire, diffusing a white smoke and fragrant odor. Containing resin, volatile oil, and both benzoic and cinnamic acids, it is properly considered a balsam, though probably somewhat altered by heat. Alcohol entirely dissolves it, taking up one part in five. (*Br.*) "A thick liquid, brownish black in bulk, reddish brown and transparent in thin layers, having a syrupy consistence, a somewhat smoky, but agreeable and balsamic odor, and a warm, bitter, afterward acrid taste. Sp. gr. 1·135 to 1·150." *U. S.* Boiling water extracts the acid. The oily liquid which separates on agitating Peru balsam with caustic potash or soda, called *Peru balsam oil* by Stolze, *cinnamein* by Frémy, may be separated by fractional distillation into three portions, viz.:—*benzyl alcohol*, C_7H_8O, passing over at about 200° C. (392° F.); *benzylic benzoate*,

$C_7H_5O_2,C_7H_7$, the principal portion, boiling at 303°–304° C. (577·5°–579° F.); and *benzylic cinnamate*, $C_9H_7O_2,C_7H_7$, passing over at about the boiling point of mercury. The crude oil likewise contains small quantities of free cinnamic and benzoic acids, resulting from the decomposition of the benzylic ether by the alkali used in separating it, and equivalent to the free benzylic alcohol also contained in it. According to Kraut (*Am. Ch. Pharm.*, 153, p. 129), the benzylic cinnamate constitutes nearly 60 per cent. of the balsam.

Peru balsam appears to contain only a single resin, yielding, by analysis, 66·3 to 67·25 per cent. of carbon, and 6·22 to 6·32 per cent. of hydrogen (Kraut, *loc. cit.*). This resin separated from the alkaline solution of the balsam by hydrochloric acid is brown, has a faint odor of vanilla, and when fused with potash yields protocatechuic acid, together with a little benzoic acid. The resin yielded about two-thirds its weight of protocatechuic acid. (Kachler, *Zeitsch. für Ch.*, [2] 6, 59.) The tree also exudes a gum-resin, which, according to Attfield (*P. J. Tr.*, 1864, p. 248) contains 77·4 per cent. of a resin, non-aromatic, and devoid of cinnamic acid, and therefore entirely distinct from balsam of Peru. The leaves of the tree contain a fragrant oil.

The balsam is said to be adulterated in Europe (especially at Bremen) with castor oil, copaiba, Canada turpentine, etc. (*P. J. Tr.*, xii. 549); and a factitious substance has been sold in this country for the genuine balsam, prepared by dissolving balsam of Tolu in alcohol. This may be distinguished by taking fire readily, and burning with a blue flame. (*N. Y. Journ. of Pharm.*, i. 133.) It would, moreover, undergo diminution in volume when mixed with water, which is not the case with the genuine balsam. (*Br.*) A method of detecting castor oil, proposed by Dr. Wagner, is to expose a small portion of the suspected balsam to distillation until somewhat more than one-half has passed, to shake the distillate with baryta water, to remove by means of a pipette the layer of oil floating on the surface, and to shake this with a concentrated solution of bisulphite of sodium. If castor oil be present, the liquid will immediately become a crystalline mass. (*A. J. P.*, xxx. 570.) The officinal tests of purity are as follows. "It is entirely soluble in 5 parts of alcohol, and should not diminish in volume, when agitated with an equal bulk of benzin, or water (abs. of fixed oils and alcohol). It is readily miscible with absolute alcohol, chloroform, or glacial acetic acid. If 1 volume of the Balsam be triturated with 2 volumes of sulphuric acid, a tough, homogeneous, cherry-red mixture should result. If this be washed, after a few minutes, with cold water, it should be converted into a resinous mass which is brittle, when cold. A mixture of 3 parts of the Balsam with 1 part of disulphide of carbon remains clear; but a mixture of 1 part of the Balsam with 3 parts of disulphide of carbon separates from the Balsam about 40 per cent. of resin. The liquid poured off from the latter should be transparent, should not have a deeper color than light brownish, and should not exhibit more than a faint fluorescence (abs. of gurjun balsam). When distilled with 200 times its weight of water, no volatile oil should pass over." *U. S.* Prof. Flückiger relies upon the specific gravity, which should be between 1·140 and 1·145, and the *lime test*, in which 10 drops of the balsam are shaken with 6 grains (0·4 Gm.) of slaked lime, forming, if there be no adulteration, a soft mixture, which does not harden. *Grote's test* consists in shaking 3 drops of balsam with 2 C.c. of officinal ammonia water; if, after standing, the mixture solidifies, colophony or other adulterant is present: benzoin, storax, and certain other substances cannot be detected by this test. (*A. J. P.*, 1881, pp. 302, 361.)

Medical Properties and Uses. This balsam is a warm stimulating stomachic and expectorant, and has been recommended in chronic catarrhs, certain forms of asthma, phthisis, and other pectoral complaints attended with debility. It has also been used in gonorrhœa, leucorrhœa, amenorrhœa, chronic rheumatism, and palsy. At present, however, it is little employed by American physicians. As an external application it has been found beneficial in chronic indolent ulcers. The dose is half a fluidrachm (1·9 C.c.). It is best administered diffused in water with sugar and the yolk of eggs or gum arabic, or in smaller doses dropped on a lump of sugar. When prescribed as an addition to expectorant mixtures, sufficient mucilage of acacia should be ordered with it to suspend it properly.

BALSAMUM TOLUTANUM. *U. S., Br.* *Balsam of Tolu.*

(BĂL'SA-MŬM TŌ-LŪ-TĀ'NŬM.)

"A balsam obtained from Myroxylon toluifera. Kunth. (*Nat. Ord.* Leguminosæ, Papilionaceæ.)" *U. S.* "A balsam which exudes from the trunk of Myroxylon Toluifera after incisions have been made in the bark." *Br.*

Baume de Tolu, Baume de Carthagène, *Fr.;* Tolubalsam, *G.;* Balsamo del Tolu, *It.;* Balsamo de Tolu, *Sp.*

For a long time the tree from which this balsam is derived retained the name of *Toluifera Balsamum*, given to it by Linnæus. Ruiz, one of the authors of the Flora Peruviana, considered it identical with *Myroxylon Peruiferum;* but M. Achille Richard determined that it was a distinct species, and gave it the appropriate specific name of *Toluiferum*, which is now recognized by the Pharmacopœias.

The balsam is procured by making V-shaped incisions in the trunk quite through the bark. The juice is received in small calabash cups, which are inserted in slight excavations beneath the point of the two vertical incisions meeting at the lower end; and Mr. Weir has seen as many as twenty cups at a time on one tree. The collectors go from tree to tree, emptying the cups into flasks of raw hide. In these skin vessels the juice is taken to the different ports on the river, where it is transferred to tin cans. (Weir, *Ibid.*) It is brought from Carthagena in calabashes or baked earthen jars, or in tin or glass vessels.

Properties. As first imported, balsam of Tolu has a soft tenacious consistence, which varies considerably with the temperature. By age it becomes hard and brittle like resin. It is shining, translucent, of a reddish or yellowish brown color, a highly fragrant odor, and a warm, somewhat sweetish and pungent, but not disagreeable taste. Exposed to heat, it melts, inflames, and diffuses an agreeable odor while burning. It is entirely soluble in volatile oils. The officinal description of it is as follows. "A yellowish or brownish yellow, semi-fluid or nearly solid mass, transparent in thin layers, brittle when cold, having an agreeable, balsamic odor, and a mild, aromatic taste. It is entirely soluble in alcohol, and the solution shows an acid reaction with test-paper. It is almost insoluble in water and in benzin. Warm disulphide of carbon removes from the Balsam scarcely anything but cinnamic and benzoic acids. On evaporating the disulphide, no substance having the properties of resin should be left behind." *U. S.* Boiling water extracts its acid. Distilled with water it affords a small proportion of volatile oil; and, if the heat be continued, an acid matter sublimes. Mr. Hatchett states that, when dissolved in the smallest quantity of solution of potassa, it loses its own characteristic odor, and acquires that of the clove pink. G. L. Ulex gives as a test of the purity of the balsam, that, if heated in sulphuric acid, it dissolves without disengagement of sulphurous acid, and yields a cherry-red liquid. (*Archiv der Pharm.*, Jan. 1853.) The balsam is a mixture of volatile oil, free acid, and resin. The volatile oil is obtained by distilling the balsam with water, and may amount to a little over 1 per cent. This oil is chiefly *tolene*, $C_{10}H_{16}$, boiling at 170° C. (338° F.), and rapidly hardening by absorption of oxygen from the air. The free acid, according to Deville and Scharling, consists of benzoic and cinnamic acids, which statement has been recently confirmed by Flückiger. (*Pharmacographia*, 2d ed., p. 204.) Busse (*Ber. Chem. Ges.*, 1876, p. 833) has shown, moreover, that the benzylic ethers of both cinnamic and benzoic acids are present in the balsam, the benzyl cinnamate in larger amount.

According to Kopp, there are two resins in Tolu balsam, one easily soluble in alcohol, $C_{18}H_{18}O_4$, and another sparingly soluble, $C_{18}H_{20}O_5$. According to Deville, however, there is only one resin, that to which the second formula belongs. Trommsdorff obtained 88 per cent. of resin, 12 of acid, and only 0·2 of volatile oil. According to Mr. Heaver, the balsam yields by distillation about one-eighth of its weight of pure cinnamic acid. The acid distils over in the form of a heavy oil, which condenses into a white crystalline mass. It may be freed from empyreumatic oil by pressure in bibulous paper, and subsequent solution in boiling water, which deposits it in minute colorless crystals, upon cooling. (*A. J. P.*, xv. 77.) A factitious balsam of Tolu is described by Dr. R. V. Mattison (*A. J. P.*, 1876, p. 51), which contained 63 per cent. of storax.

Medical Properties and Uses. Balsam of Tolu is a stimulant stomachic, with a peculiar tendency to the pulmonary organs. It is given with some advantage in chronic catarrh and other pectoral complaints, in which a gently stimulating expectorant is demanded; but should not be prescribed until after the reduction of inflammatory action. Independently of its medical virtues, its agreeable flavor renders it a popular ingredient in expectorant mixtures. Old and obstinate coughs are said to be sometimes greatly relieved by the inhalation of the vapor proceeding from an ethereal solution of this balsam. From ten to thirty grains (0·65–1·95 Gm.) may be given at a dose, and frequently repeated. The best form of administration is that of emulsion, made by triturating the balsam with mucilage and loaf sugar, and afterwards with water.

Off. Prep. and Pharm. Uses. Syrupus Tolutanus; Tinctura Benzoini Composita; Tinctura Tolutana; Pilula Ferri Iodidi; Pilula Phosphori.

BARIUM. *Barium.*

Ba; 136·8. (BĀ'RĮ-ŬM.) Ba; 136·8.

This is the metal present in the earth baryta. It was first obtained in 1808 by Sir H. Davy, who describes it as a difficultly fusible metal, of a silvery gray color, decomposing water readily, and considerably heavier than sulphuric acid. When exposed to the air, it instantly becomes covered with a crust of baryta, and when gently heated, burns with a deep red light (or greenish light according to Clarke). The compounds of barium formerly officinal are the chloride and the carbonate.

Baryta (or barium oxide) may be obtained from the native carbonate by intense ignition with carbonaceous matter; or from the native sulphate, by ignition with charcoal, which converts it into sulphide of barium, subsequent solution of the sulphide in nitric acid, and strong ignition of the nitrate formed to dissipate the acid. As thus obtained, it is an anhydrous solid, caustic, alkaline, difficultly fusible, and of a grayish white color. Its sp. gr. is about 4. It acts on the animal economy as a poison. When sprinkled with water it slakes like lime, becomes hot, and is reduced to the state of a white pulverulent hydrate. The same hydrate is formed in mass, when the anhydrous earth is made into a paste with water, and exposed to a red heat in a platinum crucible. The excess of water is expelled, and the hydrate, undergoing fusion, may be poured out and allowed to congeal. Barium hydrate dissolves in water, and forms the reagent called *baryta-water*. A boiling saturated solution, as it cools, yields crystals of barium hydrate containing eight molecules of water of crystallization.

An economical process for obtaining barium hydrate in crystals has been published by Dr. Mohr, of Coblentz. It consists in adding to a boiling solution of caustic soda an equivalent quantity of chloride of barium and nitrate of barium. In consequence of the usual impurities in caustic soda, a precipitate is formed of some carbonate and sulphate of barium, which is easily separated by subsidence from the solution of barium hydrate, kept hot. This, when clear, is drawn off by a siphon, and put in a suitable covered vessel to cool and crystallize; when the whole liquid is often converted into a mass of acicular crystals. (*P. J. Tr.*, Dec. 1856.) Baryta consists of one atom of barium 136·8, and one of oxygen 16 = 152·8. Its chemical formula is, therefore, BaO. *Carbonate of barium*, $BaCO_3$; mol. wt. 196·8, is the native carbonate, a rare mineral, discovered in 1783 by Dr. Withering, in honor of whom it is called *Witherite*. It is found in Sweden and Scotland, but most abundantly in the lead mines of the north of England. It occurs usually in grayish, or pale yellowish gray, fibrous masses, but sometimes crystallized. Its sp. gr. varies from 4·2 to 4·4. It is generally translucent, but sometimes opaque. It effervesces with acids, and, before the blowpipe, melts into a white enamel without losing its carbonic acid. It is distinguished from the carbonate of strontium, with which it is most liable to be confounded, by its greater specific gravity, and by its yielding a light greenish rather than a reddish flame upon the burning of alcohol impregnated with its solution in hydrochloric acid. If strontia be present, the reddish flame will show it.

When pure, carbonate of barium is entirely soluble in hydrochloric acid. Any sulphate of barium present is left undissolved. If neither ammonia nor sulphuretted hydrogen produces discoloration or a precipitate in the hydrochloric acid solution, the absence of alumina, iron, copper, and lead is shown. Lime may be detected by adding an excess of sulphuric acid, which will throw down the baryta as a sulphate, and afterwards testing the clear liquid with carbonate of sodium, which, if lime be present, will produce a precipitate of carbonate of calcium.

Carbonate of barium acts as a poison on the animal economy. Its only pharmaceutical use is to prepare chloride of barium. (For *Chloride* and *Sulphate of Barium*, see Part II.)

BEBERINÆ SULPHAS. *Br.* *Sulphate of Beberine.*

(BĔ-BE̥-RĪ′NÆ SŬL′PHĂS.)

Beberiæ Sulphas; Sulphate of Bibirine; Sulfate de Bébéerine, *Fr.;* Schwefelsaures Bebirin, *G.*

"Prepared from Nectandra or Bebeeru bark. It is probably a mixture of sulphates of beberine, $C_{36}H_{42}N_2O_6$, nectandrine, $C_{40}H_{46}N_2O_8$, and other alkaloids." *Br.*

"Take of Bebeeru Bark [Nectandra, *U. S.*], in coarse powder, *one pound* [avoirdupois]; Sulphuric Acid *half a fluidounce* [Imperial measure]; Slaked Lime *three-quarters of an ounce*, or *a sufficiency;* Solution of Ammonia *a sufficiency;* Rectified Spirit *sixteen fluidounces*, or *a sufficiency;* Diluted Sulphuric Acid *a sufficiency;* Water *one gallon* [Imp. meas.]; Distilled Water *a sufficiency*. Add the Sulphuric Acid to the Water; pour upon the Bebeeru Bark enough of this mixture to moisten it thoroughly; let it macerate for twenty-four hours, place it in a percolator, and pass through it the remainder of the acidulated water. Concentrate the acid liquor to the bulk of one pint, cool, and add gradually the Lime in the form of milk of lime, agitating well, and taking care that the fluid still retains a distinct acid reaction. Let it rest for two hours; filter through calico; wash the precipitate with a little cold Distilled Water, and to the filtrate add Solution of Ammonia until the fluid has a faint ammoniacal odor. Collect the precipitate on a cloth, wash it twice with ten ounces of cold water, squeeze it gently with the hand, and dry it by the heat of a water-bath. Pulverize the dry precipitate, put it into a flask with six ounces of the Rectified Spirit, boil, let it rest for a few minutes, and pour off the spirit. Treat the undissolved portion in a similar manner with fresh spirit until it is exhausted. Unite the spirituous solutions, add to them four ounces of Distilled Water, and distil so as to recover the greater part of the spirit. To the residue of the distillation add by degrees, and with constant stirring, Diluted Sulphuric Acid till the fluid has a slight acid reaction. Evaporate the whole to complete dryness on the water-bath, pulverize the dry product, pour on it gradually one pint [Imp. meas.] of cold Distilled Water, stirring diligently; filter through paper; evaporate the filtrate to the consistence of syrup, spread it in thin layers on flat porcelain or glass plates, and dry it at a temperature not exceeding 140° F. (60° C.). Preserve the product in stoppered bottles." *Br.*

In the above process the bark is exhausted by water acidulated with sulphuric acid; lime is added to separate various inert matters, still leaving the acid in excess, as otherwise it might precipitate the beberine itself; the filtered liquor is treated with ammonia which throws down the beberine; the precipitate is exhausted by alcohol which dissolves the alkaloid; and the solution, having been concentrated, is treated with sulphuric acid so as to form the sulphate, which is obtained by evaporation to dryness. It is obvious that the salt of beberine thus obtained must be very impure, and among other substances probably contains a portion of *sipirine*, another alkaloid of the bark. Indeed, Prof. Flückiger has found the commercial article to yield a very trifling amount, less than 25 per cent., of the pure alkaloid. It is in dark brown translucent scales, yellow when reduced to powder, of a strongly bitter taste, and soluble in water and alcohol. According to the Br. Pharmacopœia, "its watery solution gives with chloride of barium a white precipitate, and with caustic soda a yellowish-white precipitate, which is dissolved by agitating the mixture with twice its volume of ether; and the ethereal solution, separated by a pipette, and evaporated, leaves a yellow translucent residue, entirely soluble in diluted acids. If the whole of the precipitate produced is dissolved by ether, it cannot contain sipirine, which is insoluble in that menstruum. It is "entirely destructible by heat, and water forms with it a clear brown solution." According to Dr. Flückiger (*P. J. Tr.*, xi. 193, 1869), pure beberine is a white, amorphous powder, whose concentrated watery solution is not precipitated by tartar emetic, but affords abundant white precipitates with phosphate of sodium, nitrate, iodide, or iodohydrargyrate of potassium, perchloride of mercury, platinocyanide of potassium, and nitric or iodic acid. Its acetate yields yellow amorphous precipitates with red or yellow prussiate of potassium, chromate or bichromate of potassium, or bichloride of platinum. Mr. D. B. Dott has confirmed the results of Prof. Flückiger's examination, although he found a larger percentage of alkaloids than the latter did. Owing to the difficulty of obtaining the alkaloids in crystals, it was almost impossible to ascertain the quantity present. (*Year-Book of Pharmacy*, 1881, p. 442; 1885, p. 420.) Beberine was shown by Walz in 1860 to be identical with *buxine*, obtained from *Buxus sempervirens.* This statement was confirmed by Flückiger, who proved that *pelosine* was identical with both of the above principles. (*P. J. Tr.*, xi., 1870, p. 192.) The alkaloid dried at 100° C. has the formula $C_{18}H_{21}NO_3$.

Sulphate of beberine is a tonic, supposed to possess antiperiodic powers, and has been given in intermittent fever and other periodical diseases. It is thought to be useful also in various uterine diseases, as dysmenorrhœa, menorrhagia, and leucorrhœa; and has been recommended in blennorrhœal discharges, and in atony of the kidneys and bladder. (Dr. A. P. Merrill, *Half-Yearly Abstract of Med. Sci.*, xlv. 249.) The dose is from two to five grains (0·13–0·33 Gm.) (See *Nectandra.*)

BELÆ FRUCTUS. *Br.* *Bael Fruit.*

(BĒ'LÆ FRŬC'TŪS.)

"The dried half-ripe fruit of Ægle Marmelos." *Br.*

Indian Bael, Bengal Quince, *E.;* Bael, Coing du Bengale, *Fr.;* Baelfrucht, Bengalische Quitte, *G.*

This is a newly introduced officinal of the British Pharmacopœia, known to some extent in Great Britain, but scarcely at all in the United States; and probably sanctioned by the British Council out of compliment to practitioners in the East Indies, who are said to have used it with advantage. It is the unripe fruit of the *Ægle Marmelos* of De Candolle, belonging to the Aurantiaceæ, and with the following generic character. "*Flowers* bi-sexual. *Petals* 4-5 patent. *Stamens* 30-40, with distinct filaments, and linear-oblong anthers. *Ovary* 8-15 celled, with numerous ovules in each cell. *Style* very short and thick. *Stigma* capitate. *Fruit* baccate, with a hard rind, 8-15 celled, the cells 6-10 seeded. *Seed* with a woolly coat, covered with a slimy liquid." (*Wight & Arnott.*)

This species of Ægle, sometimes called the *Bengal quince*, is a rather large tree, with an erect stem, and few and irregular branches, covered with an ash-colored bark, and furnished in general with strong, very sharp, axillary thorns, single or in pairs. The leaves are ternate, with oblong-lanceolate, crenulated, slightly dotted leaflets, of which the terminal is largest. The flowers are large, white, and in small terminal or axillary panicles. The fruit is a berry, of about the size of a large orange, somewhat spherical, but flattened at the base, and depressed at the insertion of the stem, with a hard smooth shell, and from 10 to 15 cells, containing besides the seeds a large quantity of exceedingly tenacious mucilage, which, when dried, is hard and transparent. The tree is a native of Hindostan and of Farther India. It is figured in *P. J. Tr.*, Oct. 1850, p. 166.

Several parts of the tree are used in India. The ripe fruit is described as fragrant, and of a delicious flavor; and a sort of sherbet prepared from it is deemed useful in febrile affections. The mucilage about the seeds is applied to various purposes in the arts, in connection with its viscid properties. The rind is used in dyeing. The flowers are deemed refrigerant by the native physicians. The fresh leaves yield by expression a bitterish and somewhat pungent juice, which, diluted with water, is occasionally used in the early stage of catarrhal and other fevers. The bark of the stem and root is thought to possess febrifuge properties. But it is the unripe or half-ripe fruit that is chiefly employed, and is the part recognized by the Br. Pharmacopœia.

Properties. The dried fruit is imported into England in vertical slices, or in broken pieces consisting of a part of the rind with the adherent pulp and seeds. The "rind is about a line and a half thick, covered with a smooth pale brown or grayish epidermis, and internally, as well as the dried pulp, brownish orange, or cherry-red" (*Br.*) When moistened, the pulp becomes mucilaginous. The fruit is astringent to the taste, and yields its virtues to water by maceration or decoction. Mr. Pollock found in it tannic acid, a concrete essential oil, and a vegetable acid (*Med. Times and Gaz.*, Feb. 1864, p. 199), but Prof. Flückiger states that neither a ferric nor a ferrous salt shows the infusion to contain any appreciable quantity of tannin, nor is the drug in any sense possessed of astringent properties. (*Pharmacographia*, 2d ed., p. 131.)

The difficulty of obtaining bael in England is said to have led to the substitution for it of mangosteen, the fruit of *Garcinia Mangostana*. This is in irregular fragments of the rind, without any adhering pulp. The pieces are convex, three or four lines or more in thickness, externally covered with a smooth, deep reddish brown, easily separable coating, and internally pale reddish brown or reddish yellow, smooth, with projecting vertical lines. (Prof. Bentley, *P. J. Tr.*, May, 1867, p. 654.)

Medical Properties and Uses. Bael, as the medicine is called in India, is said to possess astringent properties which render it useful in diarrhœa, dysentery with debility of the mucous membrane, and other diseases of the bowels with relaxation, which it relieves without inducing constipation. It is much used by some practitioners in India, generally in the form of decoction, made by slowly boiling down a pint of water with two ounces of the dried fruit to four fluidounces. Of this one or two fluidounces (30–60 C.c.) are given in acute cases every two or three hours, in chronic cases two or three times a day. A liquid extract is directed in the Br. Pharmacopœia, the dose of which may be one or two fluidrachms (3·75–7·5 C.c.). Mr. Waring, of the East India medical service, recommends an extract in the dose of half a drachm or a drachm (1·95–3·9 Gm.).

Off. Prep. Br. Extractum Belæ Liquidum.

BELLADONNÆ FOLIA. *U.S., Br.* *Belladonna Leaves.*

(BĔL-LA-DŎN'NÆ FŎ'LI-A.)

"The leaves of Atropa Belladonna. Linné. (*Nat. Ord.* Solanaceæ.)" *U. S.* "The fresh leaves, with the branches to which they are attached, of Deadly Nightshade, Atropa Belladonna; also the leaves separated from the branches and carefully dried; gathered, when the fruit has begun to form, from plants growing wild or cultivated in Britain." *Br.*

Folia (s. Herba) Belladonnæ; Feuilles de Belladone, *Fr.;* Tollkirschen-Blätter, Wolfskirschen-Blätter, Tollkraut, *G.*

BELLADONNÆ RADIX. *U.S., Br.* *Belladonna Root.*

(BĔL-LA-DŎN'NÆ RA'DĬX.)

"The root of Atropa Belladonna. Linné. (*Nat. Ord.* Solanaceæ.)" *U. S.* "The root of Atropa Belladonna, *Linn.*, from plants growing wild or cultivated in Britain and carefully dried; or imported in a dried state from Germany." *Br.*

Racine de Belladone, Belladone, *Fr.;* Gemeine Tollkirsche, Wolfskirsche, Tollkirschen-Wurzel, Wolfskirschen-Wurzel, *G.;* Belladonna, *It.;* Belladona, Belladama, *Sp.*

Gen. Ch. Corolla bell-shaped. *Stamens* distant. *Berry* globular, two-celled. *Willd.*

Atropa Belladonna. Willd. *Sp. Plant.* i. 1017; Carson, *Illust. of Med. Bot.* ii. 19, pl. lxv.; *B. & T.* 193. The belladonna, or *deadly nightshade*, is an herbaceous perennial, with a fleshy, creeping root, from which rise several erect, round, purplish, branching stems, to the height of about three feet. The leaves, which are attached by short footstalks to the stem, are in pairs of unequal size, oval, pointed, entire, of a dusky green on their upper surface, and paler beneath. The flowers are large, bell-shaped, pendent, of a dull reddish color, with solitary peduncles, rising from the axils of the leaves. The fruit is a roundish berry with a longitudinal furrow on each side, at first green, afterwards red, ultimately deep purple, slightly resembling a cherry, and containing, in two distinct cells, numerous seeds, and a sweetish violet-colored juice. The calyx adheres to the base of the fruit.

The plant is a native of Europe, where it grows in shady places, along walls, and amidst rubbish, flowering in June and July, and ripening its fruit in September

It grows vigorously under cultivation in this country, and retains all its activity, as shown by the observations of Mr. Alfred Jones. (*A. J. P.*, xxiv. 106.) All parts of it are active. The leaves and roots are directed by the United States and British

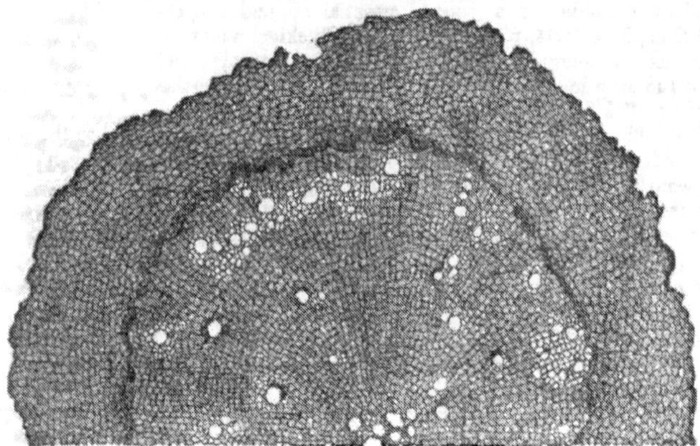

Transverse Section of Belladonna Root.

Pharmacopœias; the latter including the young branches, which are probably not less efficient. The leaves should be collected in June or July, when the plant is in flower, the roots in the autumn or early in the spring, and from plants three years old or more. Leaves which have been kept long should not be used, as they undergo change through absorption of atmospheric moisture, emitting ammonia, and probably losing a portion of their active nitrogenous matter. It has been affirmed that the finest-looking leaves are to be rejected, as probably being those of cultivated plants, and inferior in strength to the smaller and less sightly leaves of the wild plant. (*A. J. P.*, xxvii. 455.) This is, however, probably an error, as the analyses made by Mr. A. W. Gerrard (*P. J. Tr.*, xv. 153) show that while the wild belladonna plant contains a little more alkaloid than the cultivated, the difference is not sufficient to be of material consequence. The same investigator found that the leaf yields the alkaloid most abundantly, the root, fruit, and stem being the next in order, and that the period of flowering, between two and four years of age, is the best time for collecting the plant. The dried leaves as they occur in the American market appear to vary remarkably in the percentage of alkaloid; the best are fully equal to the finest English leaves. Specimens which contain much stem or are musty should always be rejected as weak in active principle. (See paper by Prof. V. Coblentz, *American Druggist*, July, 1885.) Mr. Holmes has found in the English market the root of *Medicago sativa* used as an adulterant. (*P. J. Tr.*, 1882.)

Properties. The "leaves are from four to six inches (10 to 15 cm.) long, broadly ovate, narrowed into a petiole, tapering at the apex, entire on the margin, smooth, thin, the upper surface brownish green, the lower surface grayish green, having a slight odor, and a bitterish, disagreeable taste." *U. S.* The root occurs "in cylindrical, somewhat tapering, longitudinally wrinkled pieces, from half an inch to an inch (12 to 25 mm.) or more in thickness; externally brownish gray, internally whitish; nearly inodorous, having a sweetish, afterward bitterish and strongly acrid taste, and breaking with a nearly smooth and mealy fracture. Roots which are tough and woody, breaking with a splintery fracture, should be rejected."* *U. S.*

* *Japanese Belladonna.* There have recently appeared in European commerce certain rhizomes from two to six inches long, about one-half inch in diameter, rarely branched, cylindrical or slightly compressed, knotty, bent, with circular disk-like scars, of a pale brown color, not whitish when abraded, with a slightly mousy, narcotic odor, and a taste nearly free from bitterness. Mr. E. M. Holmes believes this Japanese belladonna to be derived from *Scopolia Japonica*, Max. Dr. A. Langgaard has found in it two alkaloids, one in very small amount, *scopolenine*, and one which is very closely allied to, if not identical with, atropine. (*A. J. P.*, 1880, pp. 356, 456; 1881, p. 450.)

As to the relative strength of these two parts, M. Hirtz, of Strasburg, has inferred from his experiments that the root yields an extract five times stronger than that obtained from the leaves, but did not determine the relative yield of extract; whilst Lefort obtained from young roots 0·6, old roots 0·25, dried leaves 0·44 per cent. of atropine; and Dragendorff obtained 0·66 from dried leaves, and 0·4 per cent. from the roots. (*Jahresb.*, 1874, p. 96.) Both the leaves and root, as well as all other parts of the plant, impart their active properties to water and alcohol. Brandes rendered it probable that these properties reside in a peculiar alkaline principle, which he supposed to exist in the plant combined with an excess of malic acid, and appropriately named *atropine.* Besides malate of atropine, Brandes found in the dried herb two principles, a green resin (chlorophyll), wax, gum, starch, albumen, lignin, and various salts. The alkaloid principle was first, however, procured in a state of purity by Mein, a German apothecary, who extracted it from the root. Ladenburg (1879–1884) has exhaustively studied the several sources of atropine and the allied alkaloids that exert a mydriatic action, and found that there are three alkaloids, *atropine*, *hyoscyamine*, and *hyoscine*, which possess the common formula $C_{17}H_{23}NO_3$, and in belladonna root, *belladonine*, $C_{17}H_{23}NO_4$. Of these, atropine occurs in the *Atropa belladonna* and in *Datura stramonium*, hyoscyamine in these plants and also in *Hyoscyamus niger* and *Duboisia myoporoides:* hyoscine is found in *Hyoscyamus niger* alone, and belladonine in belladonna root alone. The first of the alkaloids, of the formula $C_{17}H_{23}NO_3$, *atropine*, fuses at 114° C.–115° C. (237·2° F.–239° F.) and forms a double gold chloride, fusing at 135° C.–137° C. (275° F.–278·6° F.); the second, the alkaloid known under the several names of *hyoscyamine*, *daturine*, and *duboisine*,* fuses at 107° C. (224·6° F.), and yields a gold salt, fusing at 159° C. (318·2° F.); and the third, *hyoscine*, only obtained as yet in the form of a syrup, but forming a crystalline gold salt, which fuses at 196° C.–198° C. (384·8° F.–388·4° F.), and is less soluble than the hyos-

Scopolenine is said by Dr. Waring to be equal if not superior in mydriatic properties to belladonna (*Brit. Med. Journ.*, June 6, p. 1145); this is confirmed by Pierd Houy, who also noted as characteristic a return of the maximum dilatation some hours after it had been previously reached. (*Nouv. Remèdes*, 1886, No. 3, p. 282.)

* *Medical Properties and Uses of Duboisine.* When about $\frac{1}{60}$th of a grain (0·001 Gm.) of duboisine is injected hypodermically in man, in the course of five or ten minutes, dryness of the mouth, thirst, acceleration of the pulse, and dryness and redness of the skin begin successively to appear. As these symptoms are accompanied by dilatation of the pupil and disorder of vision, the subject of them appears to be suffering from atropine poisoning. Even from the amount named, symptoms more severe are sometimes produced, such as vertigo, great muscular weakness, and, in several instances, a sudden very pronounced fall of the pulse, with great abatement of the force. In a case (*Detroit Lancet*, Feb. 1881, p. 369) in which an eighth of a grain is said to have been taken, at the end of three-quarters of an hour the patient could scarcely stand; he shortly afterwards passed into a state of complete unconsciousness, not preceded by delirium, and accompanied, it is stated, with natural breathing. In the absence of delirium and in the natural respiratory movements (if correctly reported), this case separates itself from one of atropine poisoning; whilst in the slowing of the pulse, after large doses of duboisine, first pointed out by Gubler (*Bull. Thérap.*, vol. xciv., p. 426), we have another point of difference.

The effect of the new alkaloid upon the lower mammals is similar to that which it exerts upon man. It has been studied physiologically by Ringer and Tweedy (*Lancet*, 1878, vol. i.), by N. Epifanon (*Hoffmann und Schwalbe's Jahresberichte*, ix. 206), and by G. Tiger (*Ibid.*), with results which want of space forbids us fully to discuss. The likeness in its action to that of atropine is maintained, excepting that the new alkaloid is much more powerful, and, according to Tiger, does not stimulate the respiratory centre, though this latter assertion needs confirmation.

When placed upon the conjunctiva, duboisine acts as a mydriatic more rapidly than does atropine, full dilatation being obtained with it in 10 to 15 minutes, soon followed by complete paralysis of accommodation. These effects pass off much more quickly than after the belladonna alkaloid, but it is so prone, when applied to the eye, to produce slight toxic symptoms, that its usefulness is much curtailed. Dr. Wm. F. Norris has found it less irritant to the eyes than the atropine, and therefore especially adapted to the treatment of inflammatory affections. Duboisine has been employed scarcely at all in internal medicine. As a substitute for atropine it has been used for the purpose of arresting the night-sweats of phthisis, but Fraentzel states that it is inferior to the older alkaloid. Dujardin-Beaumets and Desnos (*Bull. Gén. Thérap.*, 1880) have employed it with alleged advantage in the treatment of Basedow's disease, given subcutaneously in the dose of one-fourth to one milligramme a day.

Mr. C. M. Chadwick (*Brit. Med. Journ.*, Feb. 1887) reports a case in which severe poisoning followed the placing of two disks which were supposed to contain one-hundredth of a grain of the sulphate of duboisine in the eyes. There was great thickness and indistinctness of speech, with irregularity of gait, ending in almost complete paralysis of the legs, visional hallucinations, and delirium, resembling that of belladonna poisoning. The pulse, however, was slow.

cyamine gold salt. In *Duboisia myoporoides* (see Part II.) the only alkaloid present seems to be the second of these, and the complete identity of it with the purified alkaloid of *hyoscyamus* has been established by Ladenburg, both by analysis of the free alkaloid and its salts, and by study of the action of different reagents upon it.* Hyoscyamine is more soluble in water and dilute alcohol than atropine, and, as already stated, forms a gold salt of different fusing point. Its decomposition products under the influence of caustic baryta, or hydrochloric acid, are the same as those of atropine, viz., *tropine* and *tropic acid.* Regnauld and Valmont have confirmed Ladenburg's results as far as atropine and hyoscyamine are concerned. (*A. J. P.*, Dec. 1881, p. 610.) Hübschmann (*Schweiz. Zeits. Pharm.*, 1858, p. 123) and Kraut (*Ann. der Ch. und Pharm.*, 148, p. 236) both described, under the name of *belladonine*, a second alkaloid extracted from belladonna. Ladenburg (1884) finds that *belladonine* is probably the tropate of oxytropine, $C_8H_{15}NO_2$, which uniting with tropic acid, $C_9H_{10}O_3$, with elimination of water, gives $C_{17}H_2N_2O_4$, so that it may be called an oxy-atropine. For the mode of preparing atropine and its properties, see the article *Atropina.* Dunstan and Ransom have devised processes for isolating the alkaloids from the root and leaves which they assert are simple and accurate. (See *A. J. P.*, 1884, p. 277; *Proc. A. P. A.*, 1886, p. 392.)†

The imported belladonna, especially that from Germany, is occasionally adulterated. (See 15th edition U. S. D., page 284.) W. Will published, in 1888, the results of an investigation undertaken at the request of the Schering manufactory to determine why the proportion of hyoscyamine and atropine in a root seems to vary with the method of working, and reached the surprising conclusion that hyoscyamine can be changed into atropine under a variety of circumstances, such as fusion, action of weak soda solution (even at ordinary temperatures), and of ammonia.

The change of the optical activity of the hyoscyamine into the inactive atropine, the alteration of fusing point in the two alkaloids, and of their double gold chloride salts, all confirm the results of the investigation. (*Ber. der Chem. Ges.*, 1888, p. 1717.)

Medical Properties and Uses. The action of belladonna upon the system is that of atropine. (See p. 265.) All parts of the plant are poisonous. It is not uncommon, in countries where it grows wild, for children to pick and eat the berries, allured by their fine color and sweet taste. Soon after the poison has been swallowed, its peculiar influence is experienced in dryness of the mouth and fauces, burning in the throat and stomach, great thirst, difficult deglutition, nausea and ineffectual retching, loss of vision, vertigo, and intoxication or delirium, with violent gestures and sometimes fits of laughter, and followed by coma. A feeble pulse, cold extrem-

* Ladenburg has collected additional facts and embodied them in a valuable historical sketch of these researches in the *Annalen.* (See *A. J. P.*, 1883, p. 463; also, *Ibid.*, 1884, p. 206.)

† *Homatropine. Homatropia. Oxytoluyl-tropeïne.* ($C_{16}H_{21}NO_3$.) This alkaloid is one of the derivatives of *tropeïne*, produced by heating *tropine* gently in contact with organic acids and diluted hydrochloric acid. The most important of this group from a therapeutic point of view is homatropine; it is prepared from tropine, amygdalic (phenyl-glycolic, or benzo-glycolic) acid, and diluted hydrochloric acid. Merck has succeeded in crystallizing it in transparent colorless prisms by recrystallization from its ethereal solution. It is not easily soluble in water, although it is *hygroscopic and very deliquescent*; the crystals melt at 95·5° C. to 98·5° C. (203·9° F. to 208·9° F.). (*Ber. d. Deutsch. Chem. Ges.*, 1880, p. 340.) The most useful salt has been shown to be the *hydrobromate of homatropine*, $C_{16}H_{21}NO_3.HBr$, which is crystallizable and not hygroscopic, soluble in 10 parts of water, making a solution which is reasonably permanent. When taken internally, homatropine produces symptoms which are mostly similar to those caused by atropine, except that the pulse-frequency is lessened instead of being increased. There is also fall of the arterial pressure, which, with the slowing of the pulse, is probably caused by a direct action of the alkaloid upon the heart-muscle or its contained ganglia. In overdose, homatropine produces death by paralyzing the respiratory centres, but no case of serious poisoning by it has occurred in man. In practical medicine the only use which has been made of it is as a mydriatic. Its action on the eye is practically identical with that of atropine, except that it is somewhat more feeble and much more temporary. The pupil begins to dilate in from fifteen to twenty minutes after the instillation of a solution of the hydrobromate, four grains to the ounce of water, and accommodation fails in from forty to ninety minutes, recovery being complete in from one to twelve hours. It is less irritating to the conjunctiva, and much less prone to produce serious systemic disturbance, when used as a mydriatic, than is atropine. When it is only desired to examine the fundus oculi, a solution of the strength of three grains to the ounce suffices, but to paralyze the accommodation, repeated instillations of a stronger solution are required.

ities, subsultus tendinum, deep coma or delirium, and sometimes convulsions, precede death. To obviate the poisonous influence of the belladonna, the most effectual method is to evacuate the stomach as speedily as possible, by means of emetics or the stomach-pump, and afterwards to cleanse the bowels by purgatives and enemata. The infusion of galls may be serviceable as an antidote. Bouchardat recommends the ioduretted solution of iodide of potassium; and a case is recorded in which it seems to have been useful. (*Ann. de Thérap.*, 1854, p. 14.)

Belladonna has been used as a medicine from early times. The leaves were first employed externally to discuss scirrhous tumors, and heal cancerous and other ill-conditioned ulcers; and were afterwards administered internally for the same purpose. Much evidence of their usefulness in these affections is on record, and even Dr. Cullen spoke in their favor; but this application of the medicine has fallen into disuse. It is now more esteemed in nervous diseases; for an account of its use in these and other disorders the reader is referred to the article on atropine. Belladonna has acquired considerable credit as a preventive of scarlatina; an application of the remedy first suggested by the author of the *homœopathic* doctrine; but it is absolutely devoid of any such power.

The extract is much used locally. Rubbed upon the areola of the breast, it has been found to arrest the secretion of milk; and upon the abdomen, to relieve the vomiting of pregnancy, and other irritations sympathetic with the gravid uterus. Applied, in the form of a large plaster, above the pubes, it has been found very useful in relieving dysenteric tenesmus, and, as a dressing to a blistered surface over the abdomen, has been asserted to effect a cure in epidemic cholera. (*Ann. de Thérap.*, 1860, p. 49.) In cardiac diseases the plaster is often applied with advantage over the heart. The decoction or extract, applied to the neck of the uterus, is asserted to have hastened tedious labor dependent on rigidity of the os tincæ; and spasmodic stricture of the urethra, neck of the bladder, and sphincter ani, anal fissures, and painful uterine affections, have been relieved by the local use of the extract, either smeared upon bougies, or administered by injection. In the latter mode it has relieved strangulated hernia. It is asserted also to be useful in paraphimosis. The inhalation of the vapor from a decoction of the leaves or extract has been recommended in spasmodic asthma. For this purpose, two drachms of the leaves, or fifteen grains of the aqueous extract, are employed to the pint of water. A much better plan is to smoke the dried leaves, either in the form of a cigarette or in a pipe. Relief is said to have been obtained in phthisis by smoking the leaves, infused when fresh in a strong solution of opium, and then dried.

Belladonna may be given in substance, but is very rarely used except in extract. The dose of the powdered leaves is for children from the eighth to the fourth of a grain (0·008–0·016 Gm.), for adults one or two grains (0·065–0·13 Gm.), repeated daily, or twice a day, and gradually increased till the characteristic effects are experienced.

From its quicker action, more uniform strength, and greater cleanliness, *atropine* has been largely substituted for extract of belladonna for local use. (See *Atropine.*)

Off. Prep. of the Leaves. Extractum Belladonnæ Alcoholicum; Tinctura Belladonnæ.

Off. Prep. Br. Extractum Belladonnæ; Succus Belladonnæ; Tinctura Belladonnæ.

Off. Prep. of the Root. Abstractum Belladonnæ; Emplastrum Belladonnæ; Extractum Belladonnæ Fluidum.

Off. Prep. Br. Atropina; Extractum Belladonnæ Alcoholicum; Linimentum Belladonnæ.

BENZINUM. *U.S.* *Benzin.*

(BĔN-ZĪ'NŬM.)

"A purified distillate from American Petroleum, consisting of hydrocarbons, chiefly of the marsh-gas series [C_5H_{12}; C_6H_{14}—$C_{10}H_{22}$; $C_{12}H_{26}$] and homologous compounds, having a sp. gr. from 0·670 to 0·675, and boiling at 50° to 60° C. (122° to 140° F.).

"Benzin should be carefully kept in well-stopped bottles or cans, in a cool place, remote from lights or fire." *U. S.*

Petroleum Benzin, Petroleum Ether.

This useful product of petroleum is officinal for the first time; it is obtained in the process of purifying petroleum by fractional distillation (see *Petroleum*, Part II.), and it is defined in the Pharmacopœia as "a transparent, colorless, diffusive liquid, of a strong, characteristic odor, slightly resembling that of petroleum, but much less disagreeable; neutral in reaction; insoluble in water, soluble in about 6 parts of alcohol, and readily so in ether, chloroform, benzol, and fixed and volatile oils. It is highly inflammable, and its vapor, when mixed with air and ignited, explodes violently. Benzin, when evaporated upon the hand, should leave no odor, and, when evaporated in a warmed dish, should leave no residue (abs. of heavy hydrocarbons). When boiled a few minutes with one-fourth its volume of spirit of ammonia and a few drops of test-solution of nitrate of silver, the ammoniacal liquid should not turn brown (abs. of pyrogenous products, and sulphur compounds); and it should require 6 parts of officinal alcohol to dissolve it (difference from benzol). If 5 drops are added to a mixture of 40 drops of sulphuric acid with 10 drops of nitric acid, in a test-tube, the liquid warmed and set aside for half an hour, and then diluted, in a shallow dish, with twice its volume of water, it should not have the bitter-almond-like odor of nitro-benzol (abs. of benzol)." *U. S.* Petroleum benzin must be carefully distinguished from benzol (called benzene by English chemists), a product derived from coal tar (see *Benzol*, Part II.). Although the Pharmacopœia gives a test to distinguish an admixture with benzol, this adulteration of benzin is hardly likely to take place here in the near future because of the great difference in price. The principal consumption of benzin at present is in the arts as a solvent, and as a substitute for oil of turpentine, which it resembles very much in its solvent properties. In pharmacy it has been used to deprive powdered drugs of their fixed oil by percolation (see *Charta Sinapis*), to obtain volatile oils by percolating the oily drug with the benzin, and subsequently evaporating the mixture spontaneously, as a substitute for ether in making oleoresins, and for many other purposes to which it is adapted on account of its powers as a solvent. Benzin is a good solvent for fats, resins, caoutchouc, and some of the alkaloids.

BENZOINUM. *U.S., Br.* *Benzoin.*

(BĔN-ZO-Ī'NŬM.)

"A balsamic resin obtained from Styrax Benzoin. Dryander. (*Nat. Ord.* Styraceæ.)" *U. S.* "A balsamic resin obtained from Styrax Benzoin, *Dry.*; and probably from one or more other species of Styrax, *Linn.* It is generally procured by making deep incisions in the bark of the trees, and allowing the liquid that exudes to concrete by exposure to the air." *Br.*

Benzoe, *P.G.*; Resina Benzoe, Asa Dulcis; Gum Benjamin; Benjoin, *Fr.*; Benzöe, *G.*; Belzoino, *It.*; Benjui, *Sp.*

The botanical source of benzoin was long uncertain. At one time it was generally supposed in Europe to be derived from the *Laurus Benzoin* of this country. This error was corrected by Linnæus, who, however, committed another, in ascribing the drug to *Croton Benzoë*, a shrub which he afterwards described under the name of *Terminalia Benzoin.* Mr. Dryander was the first who ascertained the true benzoin-tree to be a *Styrax;* and his description, published in the 77th vol. of the London Philosophical Transactions, has been copied by most subsequent writers.

Gen. Ch. Calyx inferior. *Corolla* funnel-shaped. *Drupe* two-seeded. *Willd.*

Styrax Benzoin. Willd. *Sp. Plant.* ii. 623. (*B. & T.*, 169.) This is a tall tree of quick growth, sending off many strong round branches, covered with a whitish downy bark. Its leaves are alternate, entire, oblong, pointed, smooth above, and downy beneath. The flowers are in compound, axillary clusters, nearly as long as the leaves, and usually hang, all on the same side, upon short slender pedicels.

The benzoin, or *benjamin-tree*, is a native of Sumatra, Java, Borneo, Laos, and Siam. By wounding the bark near the origin of the lower branches, a juice exudes, which hardens upon exposure, and forms the *benzoin* of commerce. The trees, which are either wild or cultivated, are deemed of a proper age to be wounded at six years, when the trunks are usually about seven or eight inches in diameter. The operation is performed annually, and the product on each occasion from one tree never exceeds three pounds. The juice which first flows is the purest, and affords the whitest and most fragrant benzoin. It is exported chiefly from Bangkok in Siam, and Acheen in Sumatra. *Siam benzoin* is usually imported in cubic blocks, which take their form from the wooden boxes in which the soft resin has been packed. It is brittle, with a peculiar, vanilla-like fragrance, but bitter taste. It may be a compact mass, containing more or less numerous opaque white tears imbedded in a rich amber-colored translucent resin, mixed to a greater or less extent with bits of bark, wood, etc. In some specimens these tears are exceedingly small, in others almost wanting. The finest variety is composed almost entirely of these tears, loosely agglutinated together. According to Mr. E. M. Holmes, Siam benzoin is produced by a tree whose leaves are rather thinner and have a less marked venation than the leaves of the *Styrax Benzoin*. *Sumatra benzoin* differs from the Siam in having a much grayer color; the resin is grayish brown, the tears usually fewer than in the finer variety, and the bits of wood, etc., more abundant. The odor differs from, and is less agreeable than, that of Siam benzoin. *Palembang benzoin* resembles Sumatra benzoin, but is somewhat more transparent, and is stated to yield a larger percentage of benzoic acid. It is also asserted that it can be distinguished by its tincture when dropped into water, not producing milkiness, but a flocculent deposit.* *Penang benzoin* also resembles Sumatra benzoin, but has an odor which is more like that of storax, and it is probably not yielded by the *Styrax Benzoin*; possibly it is the product of *S. subdenticulata*.

Properties. Benzoin has a fragrant odor, with very little taste; but, when chewed for some time, leaves a sense of irritation in the mouth and fauces. It breaks with a resinous fracture, and presents a mottled surface of white and brown or reddish brown; the white spots being smooth and shining, while the remainder, though sometimes shining and even translucent, is usually more or less rough and porous, and often exhibits impurities. In the inferior kinds, the white spots are very few, or entirely wanting. Benzoin is easily pulverized, and, in the process of being powdered, is apt to excite sneezing. Its sp. gr. is from 1·063 to 1·092. "In lumps consisting of agglutinated, yellowish brown tears, which are internally milk white, or in the form of a reddish brown mass, more or less mottled from whitish tears imbedded in it. It is almost wholly soluble in 5 parts of moderately warm alcohol, and in solution of potassa. When Benzoin is boiled with milk of lime, the hot filtrate should not give off the odor of oil of bitter almond on the addition of test-solution of permanganate of potassium (abs. of cinnamic acid)." *U. S.* When heated it melts, and emits thick, white, pungent fumes, which excite cough when inhaled, and consist chiefly of benzoic acid. It is wholly soluble, with the exception of impurities, in alcohol, and is precipitated by water from the solution, rendering the liquor milky. It imparts to boiling water a notable proportion of benzoic acid. Lime-water and the alkaline solutions partially dissolve it, forming benzoates, from which the acid may be precipitated by the addition of other acids. Its chief constituents are resin and benzoic acid; and it therefore belongs to the balsams. The white tears and the brownish connecting medium are said by Stolze to contain nearly the same proportion of acid, which, according to Bucholz, is 12·5 per cent., to Stolze, 19·8 per cent. In a more recent examination by Kopp, the white tears were found to contain from 8 to 10 per cent. of acid, and the brown 15 per cent. (*Journ. de Pharm.*, 3e sér., iv. 46.) The resin is of three kinds, one extracted with the benzoic acid by a boiling solution of carbonate of potassium in excess, another dissolved by ether from the residue, and the third affected by neither of these solvents. Besides benzoic acid and resin, the balsam contains a little extractive, and traces of volatile oil. Benzoin retards the oxidation of fatty matters, and thus tends to prevent rancidity.

It appears from recent researches that benzoin, besides its own characteristic acid, often contains also cinnamic acid, which is found more especially in the white tears. Indeed, Hermann Aschoff obtained from some benzoin of Sumatra a pure cinnamic

* A factitious substance has been sold in our markets for benzoin, consisting of chips of wood agglutinated by a resinous substance, with no benzoic acid, and only a trace of cinnamic. (J. M. Maisch, *A. J. P.*, xxxv. 494.)

acid, without any benzoic; and Messrs. Kolbe and Lautermann, upon examining a specimen of the tears, discovered what they at first supposed to be a peculiar acid, but which, on further investigation, proved to be a mixture of the cinnamic and benzoic acids. Aschoff recommends the following method of detecting *cinnamic acid*. Boil the benzoin with milk of lime, filter, decompose with hydrochloric acid, and add either bichromate of potassium with sulphuric acid, or permanganate of potassium, when, if cinnamic acid be present, the odor of oil of bitter almonds will be perceived. The two acids, which, when they occur together in benzoin, are said to be always mixed in the same proportion, may be at least partially separated by simple crystallization; their melting points being very different, that of benzoic acid 121° C. (249° F.), and that of the mixed acid, consisting of one part of the cinnamic and two of the benzoic, only 25·5° C. (78° F.). (*P. J. Tr.*, 1863, p. 77.) According to Mr. A. C. Curtis, *cinnamein* may be obtained by boiling benzoin with twice its bulk of lime in forty parts of water for fifteen or twenty minutes, filtering, cooling, adding hydrochloric acid, washing the precipitate, and recrystallizing from water acidulated with hydrochloric acid. (*A. J. P.*, 1872, p. 486.)

Rump (1878) treated Siam benzoin with caustic lime, precipitated the benzoic acid with hydrochloric acid, and agitated the liquid with ether. The latter on evaporating afforded a mixture of benzoic acid and *vanillin*, $C_8H_8O_3$. Subjected to dry distillation, benzoin affords as chief product benzoic acid, together with empyreumatic products, among which Berthelot has proved the presence (in Siam benzoin) of *styrol*, C_8H_8. The latter was also obtained in 1874 by Theegarten from Sumatra benzoin by distilling it with water. (*Ber. Chem. Ges.*, 1874, p. 727.)

Medical Properties and Uses. Benzoin is stimulant and expectorant, and was formerly employed in pectoral affections; but, except as an ingredient of the compound tincture of benzoin, it has fallen into disuse. Trousseau and Pidoux recommend strongly its inhalation in chronic laryngitis. Either the air of the chamber may be impregnated with its vapor by placing a small portion upon some live coals, or the patient may inhale the vapor of boiling water to which the balsam has been added. It is employed in pharmacy for the preparation of benzoic acid (see *Acidum Benzoicum*); and the milky liquor resulting from the addition of water to its alcoholic solution is sometimes used as a cosmetic, under the impression that it renders the skin soft. A tincture has been strongly recommended in anal fissure. In the East Indies, the balsam is burnt by the Hindoos as a perfume in their temples.*

Off. Prep. Adeps Benzoinatus; Tinctura Benzoini; Tinctura Benzoini Composita.

Off. Prep. Br. Acidum Benzoicum; Adeps Benzoatus; Tinctura Benzoini Composita; Unguentum Cetacei.

BISMUTHI CITRAS. *U. S., Br.* *Citrate of Bismuth*

$BiC_6H_5O_7$; 399. (BĬS-MŪ'THĪ CĪ'TRĂS.) $BiO_3, C_{12}H_5O_{11}$; 399.

Bismuthum Citricum, Citrate de Bismuth, *Fr.*; Citronensaures Wismuth, *G.*

"Subnitrate of Bismuth, *ten parts*; Citric Acid, *seven parts*; Distilled Water, *a sufficient quantity*. Boil the Subnitrate of Bismuth and the Citric Acid with *forty*

* A styptic liquid, prepared by a Roman pharmaceutist named *Pagliari*, and kept secret for a time, has acquired some reputation among the French army surgeons. It is made by boiling, for six hours, eight ounces of tincture of benzoin (containing about two ounces of the balsam), a pound of alum, and ten pounds of water, in a glazed earthen vessel, stirring constantly, and supplying the loss with hot water. The liquor is then strained and kept in stopped bottles. It is limpid, styptic, of an aromatic smell, and said to have the property of causing an instantaneous coagulation of the blood. (See *Am. Journ. of Med. Sci.*, N. S., xxv. 199.)

M. Meyer, believing that the long boiling in the foregoing process is injurious, if in no other way, by dissipating the benzoic acid, proposes to dispense with it, and has substituted the following formula, which furnishes a product always identical. Take tears of benzoin, 6 grammes (about ℥iss), alcohol at 90° C. 15 grammes; dissolve and add of water 300 grammes, alum 30 grammes; mix and boil till the liquid becomes clear. The liquid should mark 6° on the hydrometer. (*Journ. de Pharm. et de Chim.*, 4e sér., v. 123.)

Fumigating pastiles are made from 16 parts of benzoin, 4 of balsam of Tolu, 4 of yellow saunders, 1 of labdanum, 48 of charcoal, 2 of nitre, 1 of tragacanth, 2 of gum arabic, and 12 of cinnamon-water, by reducing the solid ingredients to powder, and mixing the whole into a plastic mass, which is to be formed into cones, flattened at the base, and dried first in the air, and then in a stove (Soubeiran, *Trait. de Pharm.*, 3e ed., i. 463.)

parts of Distilled Water, until a drop of the mixture yields a clear solution with water of ammonia. Then add *five hundred parts* of Distilled Water, allow the suspended matter to deposit, wash the precipitate (first by decantation, and afterward on a strainer), with Distilled Water, until the washings are tasteless, and dry the residue at a gentle heat." *U. S.*

"Take of Subnitrate of Bismuth 5½ ounces [av.]; Nitric Acid 11 fluidounces [Imp. meas.] or a sufficiency; Citric Acid 4 ounces [av.]; Bicarbonate of Sodium 8 ounces [av.]; Distilled Water a sufficiency. Heat the Subnitrate of Bismuth with the Nitric Acid until the salt is dissolved. Pour in some water, with constant stirring, until the cloudiness produced by the water no longer rapidly disappears. Dissolve the Bicarbonate of Sodium in Distilled Water, add the Citric Acid, boil until all gas is expelled, and then add the liquid to the clear or only faintly opalescent solution of bismuth until no further precipitate is produced. Heat to boiling, occasionally stirring. Set the whole aside to cool. When cold, filter, and wash the precipitate of citrate of bismuth until no free nitric acid remains. Dry the product over a water-bath." *Br.*

Properties. "A white amorphous powder, permanent in the air, odorless and tasteless, insoluble in water or alcohol, but soluble in water of ammonia. When strongly heated, the salt chars, and, on ignition, leaves a more or less blackened residue with a yellow surface, which is dissolved by warm nitric acid. This solution, on being dropped into water, occasions a white turbidity. The ammoniacal solution, when treated with hydrosulphuric acid in excess, yields a black precipitate. The filtrate deprived, by heat, of the excess of hydrosulphuric acid and cooled, when boiled with lime-water, produces a white precipitate, and when a portion of it is mixed with an equal volume of concentrated sulphuric acid and cooled, a brown or brownish black zone should not appear around a crystal of ferrous sulphate dropped into the liquid (abs. of nitrate)." *U. S.*

Composition. As citric acid ($H_3C_6H_5O_7$) is tribasic, one atom of bismuth, being trivalent, will exactly replace the three hydrogen atoms of the citric acid and form a neutral citrate of bismuth. When subnitrate of bismuth is boiled with a solution of citric acid it is decomposed, the nitric acid is replaced by the citric acid, and the insoluble citrate of bismuth is formed; the completion of the process is known by the mixture yielding a clear solution with water of ammonia.

Medical Properties. This salt is not used itself in medicine, but has been made officinal for pharmaceutical purposes.

Off. Prep. Bismuthi et Ammonii Citras.

BISMUTHI ET AMMONII CITRAS. *U. S., Br.* *Citrate of Bismuth and Ammonium.*

(BĬŞ-MŪ'THĪ ĔT ĂM-MŌ'NĮ-Ī CĬ'TRĂS.)

Citrate de Bismuth et d'Ammoniaque, *Fr.;* Citronensaures Wismuthoxyd-Ammonium, *G.*

"Citrate of Bismuth, *ten parts;* Water of Ammonia, Distilled Water, each, *a sufficient quantity.* Mix the Citrate of Bismuth with *twenty* (20) *parts* of Distilled Water to a smooth paste, and gradually add Water of Ammonia until the salt is dissolved, and the liquid has a neutral or only faintly alkaline reaction. Then filter the solution, evaporate it to a syrupy consistence, and spread it on plates of glass, so that, on drying, the salt may be obtained in scales. Keep the product in small, well-stopped vials, protected from light." *U. S.*

"Take of Solution of Citrate of Bismuth and Ammonium *one pint* [Imp. meas.] or a sufficiency. Evaporate the solution over a water-bath to the consistence of a syrup. Spread the resulting fluid in thin layers on glass or porcelain plates, and dry at a temperature not exceeding 100° F. (37·8° C.). Remove the scales and preserve them in a stoppered bottle." *Br.*

This salt is officinal for the first time, although it has been used quite extensively during the last ten years, principally for preparing extemporaneously the London Liquor Bismuthi originally suggested by Schacht. (See *Liquor Bismuthi et Ammoniæ Citratis.*)

Properties. "Small, shining, pearly or translucent scales, becoming opaque on exposure to air, odorless, having a slightly acidulous and metallic taste, and a neutral or faintly alkaline reaction. Very soluble in water and but sparingly soluble in alcohol. When strongly heated, the salt melts, then chars, and finally leaves a more or less blackened residue with a yellow surface, which is dissolved by warm nitric acid. This solution, on being dropped into water, occasions a white turbidity. The aqueous solution of the salt, when boiled with solution of potassa, evolves vapor of ammonia; and, when treated with hydrosulphuric acid, yields a black precipitate. If the filtrate be deprived, by heat, of the excess of hydrosulphuric acid and cooled, a portion of it, boiled with lime-water, produces a white precipitate. Another portion, after being mixed with an equal volume of concentrated sulphuric acid and cooled, should not produce a brown or brownish black zone around a crystal of ferrous sulphate dropped into the liquid (abs. of nitrate)." *U. S.* As frequently seen in commerce it is not entirely soluble in water: this is due to the loss of ammonia through exposure, and a few drops of water of ammonia, added to the turbid solution, are generally sufficient to restore its transparency. The Committee of Revision very properly omitted to give its chemical formula, as it is by no means proved that it has a definite composition. It is believed by some to be a true double citrate, $Bi,C_6H_5O_7(NH_4)_2C_6H_5O_7$. On the other hand, Bartlett (*Zeitsch. für Chem.*, 1865, p. 350) obtained on evaporation of the ammoniacal solution $BiC_6H_5O_7,NH_3+3H_2O$, and Rother (*Jahresbericht*, 1876, p. 564) obtained on crystallizing from warm ammonia $Bi,C_6H_5O_7$, $3NH_3+3H_2O$. "Ten grains dissolved in water, and treated with sulphuretted hydrogen in excess, yield a precipitate which, when washed and dried, weighs about six and a half grains." *Br.*

Medical Properties. This salt differs from the older preparations of bismuth in its solubility, and for this reason probably is more rapid, more astringent, and more irritant in its action. In cases of irritation or inflammation of the gastro-intestinal mucous membrane it is very much inferior to the insoluble preparations, but when there is relaxation with excessive discharges it may usefully be employed. The dose is from one to three grains (·065–·20 Gm.).

BISMUTHI ÓXIDUM. *Br.* *Oxide of Bismuth.*

Bi_2O_3; 468. (BĬṢ-MŪ′THĪ ŎX′Ị-DŬM.) Bi_2O_3; 468.

Oxyde de Bismuth, *Fr.*; Bismuthum Oxydatum, Oxydum Bismuthicum; Wismuthoxyd, *G.*

"Take of Subnitrate of Bismuth *one pound* [avoirdupois]; Solution of Soda *four pints* [Imp. meas.]. Mix and boil for five minutes; then having allowed the mixture to cool and the oxide to subside, decant the supernatant liquid, wash the precipitate thoroughly with distilled water, and finally dry the oxide by the heat of a water-bath." *Br.*

The subnitrate of bismuth is decomposed by the solution of soda in this process, hydrate of bismuth being formed, which is precipitated, whilst nitrate of sodium remains in solution. $2(BiNO_4,H_2O)+2NaHO=Bi_26HO$ (or $Bi_2O_3,3H_2O$) + $2NaNO_3$. At the temperature of 100° C. (212° F.) the hydrate of bismuth is decomposed, water is liberated, and the anhydrous oxide is left.

Properties. Oxide of bismuth is a powder of a dull lemon yellow color, insoluble in water, but soluble in nitric acid mixed with half its volume of water without effervescence.

Medical Properties. The oxide of bismuth resembles the subnitrate in its medical properties, and may be administered in similar doses.

BISMUTHI SUBCARBONAS. *U.S.*, *Br.* *Subcarbonate of Bismuth.*

(BĬṢ-MŪ′THĪ SŬB-CĀR-BŌ′NĂS.)

$(BiO)_2CO_3,H_2O$; 530. BiO_3,CO_2HO; 265.

Bismuthi Carbonas, *Br.*; Carbonate of Bismuth; Bismuthum Subcarbonicum, Subcarbonas Bismuthicus; Sous-carbonate de Bismuth, *Fr.*; Basisches Kohlensaures Wismuthoxyd, *G.*

A process for this salt is no longer officinal; that of the Pharm. 1870 will be found in the foot-note below.*

* "Take of Bismuth, in pieces, *two troyounces*; Nitric Acid *eight troyounces and a half*; Water of Ammonia *five fluidounces*; Carbonate of Sodium *ten troyounces*; Distilled Water *a sufficient quan-*

"Take of Purified Bismuth, in small pieces, *two ounces* [avoirdupois]; Nitric Acid *four fluidounces* [Imperial measure]; Carbonate of Ammonium *six ounces* [avoird.]; Distilled Water *a sufficiency*. Mix the Nitric Acid with three [fluid]ounces [Imp. meas.] of Distilled Water, and add the Bismuth in successive portions. When effervescence has ceased, apply for ten minutes a temperature approaching that of ebullition, and afterwards decant the solution from any insoluble matter that may be present. Evaporate the solution until it is reduced to two fluidounces [Imp. meas.], and add this in small quantities at a time to a cold filtered solution of the Carbonate of Ammonium in two pints [Imp. meas.] of Distilled Water, constantly stirring during admixture. Collect the precipitate on a calico filter, and wash it with Distilled Water until the washings pass tasteless. Remove now as much of the adhering water as can be separated from the precipitate by slight pressure with the hands, and finally dry the product at a temperature not exceeding 150° F. (65·5° C.)." *Br.*

This preparation was first made officinal in the 1860 edition of the U. S. Pharmacopœia. As metallic bismuth generally contains arsenic, it is very important to provide that this should be left behind, in the processes for making its medicinal preparations. It is on this account that the formula of U. S. Pharm. 1870 was so elaborate. The bismuth is first dissolved in nitric acid, a portion of which oxidizes the metal, with the evolution of nitrous vapors, while another portion combines with the oxide produced to form nitrate of bismuth. At the same time the arsenic is also oxidized at the expense of the nitric acid, and unites with a portion of the oxidized metal so as to produce the arseniate of bismuth. Both of these salts, therefore, are contained in the solution, which is very concentrated. Both have the property, when their solution is diluted with water, of separating into two salts, one an insoluble subsalt which is deposited, and the other a soluble acid salt which is held in solution. But the arseniate is more disposed to the change than the nitrate, and requires for the purpose a smaller amount of water of dilution. Hence, the first direction, after the metal has been dissolved, is to add a moderate quantity of distilled water, insufficient to cause the decomposition of the nitrate. From this diluted solution the insoluble subarseniate is slowly deposited, so as, in the course of twenty-four hours, to free it almost if not entirely from the poisonous metal. This is separated by filtration, and the solution is now diluted with a much larger quantity of distilled water, which causes a copious deposition of subnitrate of bismuth. But, in order not to waste the acid nitrate remaining in solution, this is decomposed by ammonia, which takes most of the nitric acid, and precipitates the bismuth combined with the remainder, in the form of subnitrate. The whole of the precipitated subnitrate, thus freed from arsenic, is redissolved in nitric acid, and the solution of the nitrate now obtained, being diluted with just so much water as to produce a commencing precipitation of subnitrate, is freed by filtering from the small quantity formed, and slowly added to a solution of carbonate of sodium. An interchange of principles takes place; nitrate of sodium and carbonate of bismuth are formed, the former of which remains in solution, and the latter is deposited. This part of the process tends still further to get rid of the arsenic; for if any of the arsenic acid or arseniate of bismuth exist in the solution, the poisonous acid would combine with the soda, and, thus forming a soluble salt, would be retained by the water. Nothing now remains but to wash, dry, and powder the precipitate.

tity. Mix four troyounces and a half of the Nitric Acid with four fluidounces of Distilled Water in a capacious glass vessel, and, having added the Bismuth, set the whole aside for twenty-four hours. Dilute the resulting solution with ten fluidounces of Distilled Water, stir it thoroughly, and, after twenty-four hours, filter through paper. To the filtered liquid, previously diluted with unequal measure of Distilled Water, slowly add the Water of Ammonia, constantly stirring. Transfer the whole to a strainer, and after the precipitate has been drained, wash it with two pints of Distilled Water, and drain it again. Then place the precipitate in a proper vessel, add the remainder of the Nitric Acid, and afterwards four fluidounces of Distilled Water, and set the solution aside. At the end of twenty-four hours, filter through paper. Dissolve the Carbonate of Sodium in twelve fluidounces of Distilled Water, with the aid of heat, and filter the solution through paper. To this, when cold, slowly add the solution of nitrate of bismuth, with constant stirring. Transfer the whole to a strainer, and after the precipitate has been drained, wash it with Distilled Water until the washings pass tasteless. Lastly, press, dry it on bibulous paper with a gentle heat, and rub it into powder." *U. S.* 1870.

The British process is more simple, because, using bismuth already purified, it is without the preliminary measures taken in the U. S. process to separate the arsenic.

Properties. Subcarbonate of bismuth is "a white, or pale yellowish white powder, permanent in the air, odorless and tasteless, and insoluble in water or alcohol. When heated to redness, the salt loses moisture and carbonic acid gas, and leaves a yellow residue which is soluble in nitric or in hydrochloric acid, and which is blackened by hydrosulphuric acid." *U. S.* Its sp. gr. is about 4. It effervesces with acids, and, when exposed to heat, loses 9·5 per cent. of its weight (*U. S.* 1870) in consequence of the escape of carbonic acid, and is converted into the anhydrous teroxide, of a light yellow color. When mixed with sulphuric acid, and subjected to Marsh's test, it should yield no arsenic, or merely a trace.

Tests. "On dissolving 1 part of the salt in 6 parts of warm nitric acid (sp. gr. 1·200), a copious effervescence takes place, and no residue should be left (abs. of insoluble foreign salts). On pouring this solution into 50 parts of water, a white precipitate is produced, and, on filtering and concentrating the filtrate to 6 parts, a portion of this, mixed with 5 times its volume of diluted sulphuric acid, should not become cloudy (abs. of lead). If another portion be precipitated with an excess of water of ammonia, the supernatant liquid should not exhibit a blue tint (copper). On diluting a third portion with 5 volumes of distilled water, the filtrate should not be affected by test-solution of nitrate of silver (chloride), or of nitrate of barium (sulphate); nor by hydrochloric acid (silver). If the salt be boiled with acetic acid diluted with an equal volume of water, and the cold filtrate freed from Bismuth by hydrosulphuric acid, the new filtrate should leave no fixed residue on evaporation (alkalies and alkaline earths). On boiling 1 Gm. of the salt with 10 C.c. of solution of soda (sp. gr. 1·260), and holding a glass rod dipped in acetic acid over the test tube, not more than a faint, white cloud, but no heavy, white fumes, should appear (only traces of ammonia). If the preceding mixture, after thorough boiling, be diluted with water to 50 C.c. and filtered, the filtrate, when supersaturated with hydrochloric acid, and treated with hydrosulphuric acid, should not deposit more than a trace of a precipitate, which should not have a yellow or orange color (only traces of antimony, arsenic, tin). On boiling 1 Gm. of the salt with 10 C.c. of strong solution of soda, decanting the liquid from the precipitated oxide of bismuth into a long test-tube, and adding about 0·5 Gm. of aluminium wire cut into small pieces (a loose plug of cotton being pushed a short distance down the tube) the generated gas should not impart any color or tint to paper wet with test-solution of nitrate of silver and kept over the mouth of the test-tube for half an hour (abs. of more than traces of arsenic)." *U. S.* "The nitric acid solution gives no precipitate with diluted sulphuric acid or with solution of nitrate of silver. If to nitric acid mixed with half its volume of distilled water as much carbonate of bismuth be added as the acid will dissolve, one volume of this solution poured into twenty volumes of water will yield a white precipitate." *Br.* If arsenic were present, a precipitate would take place with a much smaller proportion of water.

Medical Properties and Uses. This salt was brought into notice by M. Hannon, of Brussels (*Ann. de Thérap.*, 1857, p. 214), who, conceiving that it was more tonic than the subnitrate, recommended it as a substitute. It is, however, therapeutically equivalent to the older preparation, having the same range of application to the treatment of disease and the same dose.

BISMUTHI SUBNITRAS. *U.S., Br.* *Subnitrate of Bismuth.*

$BiO\,NO_3.\,H_2O$; 306. (BĬȘ-MŪ'THĪ SŬB-NĪ'TRĂS.) $BiO_3, NO_5.\,2HO$; 306.

Bismuthum Album, *Br.;* White Bismuth; Bismuthum Subnitricum, *P.G.;* Bismuthum Hydrico-nitricum, Magisterium Bismuthi, Subazotas (s. Subnitras) Bismuthicus; Sous-azotate de Bismuth, *Fr.;* Basisches Salpetersaures Wismuthoxyd, *G.;* Oxynitrate of Bismuth.

A process for subnitrate of bismuth is no longer officinal. The process of U. S. P. 1870 is given in the foot-note.*

* Take of Bismuth, in pieces, *two troyounces;* Nitric Acid *eight troyounces and a half;* Carbonate of Sodium *ten troyounces;* Water of Ammonia *five fluidounces;* Distilled Water *a sufficient quantity.* Mix four troyounces and a half of the Nitric Acid with four fluidounces of Distilled

"Take of purified Bismuth, in small pieces, *two ounces* [avoirdupois]; Nitric Acid *four fluidounces* [Imperial measure]; Distilled Water *a sufficiency*. Mix the Nitric Acid with three [fluid]ounces of Distilled Water, and add the Bismuth in successive portions. When effervescence has ceased, apply for ten minutes a heat approaching that of ebullition, and decant the solution from any insoluble matter that may be present. Evaporate the solution until it is reduced to two fluidounces, and pour it into half a gallon of Distilled Water. When the precipitate which forms has subsided, decant the supernatant liquid, add half a gallon [Imp. meas.] of Distilled Water to the precipitate, stir them well together, and, after two hours, decant off the liquid, collect the precipitate on a calico filter and fold it with the calico and press it with the hands, and dry it at a temperature not exceeding 150° F. (65 5° C)." *Br.*

The alterations from the old process, in the U. S. P. formula of 1870, were based upon the wish to get rid of any arsenic that might be present in the bismuth used. This is accomplished by first preparing the carbonate, by adding the nitric acid solution of bismuth to a solution of carbonate of sodium in excess, whereby most of the arsenic is retained in the solution, probably as arseniate of sodium, while the insoluble carbonate is precipitated. This is dissolved, with the aid of heat, in nitric acid, so as to make a very concentrated solution of the nitrate, to which, when cold, just so much water is added as to begin to produce a permanent turbidness. The object of this is to allow any arsenic that may be still present to be deposited, which happens for reasons stated in explaining the process for procuring the subcarbonate. (See page 291.) The deposited matter having been precipitated, only the pure nitrate remains in solution, which is made to yield the subnitrate by large dilution with water, and still more completely by the addition of ammonia.

In the British formula, the old method is pursued of simply dissolving the bismuth, which has been previously purified, in nitric acid somewhat diluted, concentrating the solution, and precipitating by adding it to a large quantity of water. When bismuth is added to dilute nitric acid, red fumes are copiously given off, and the metal, oxidized by the decomposition of part of the nitric acid, is dissolved by the remainder so as to form a solution of the ternitrate of bismuth. It is unnecessary to have the metal in powder; as it dissolves with great facility when added to the acid in fragments. When the solution is completed, the liquor should be added to the water, and not the water to the solution. In order to have a smooth light powder, which is most esteemed, the precipitate should be well washed to remove every trace of free nitric acid, and dried as speedily as possible. In the use of this formula it is taken for granted that the bismuth has been ascertained to be free from arsenic; and, if it prove upon the application of Marsh's test to be otherwise, means should certainly be employed to purify it before using it. Measures for this purpose are mentioned under *Bismuthum Purificatum.* Should the subnitrate or subcarbonate be ascertained to contain arsenic, it may, as suggested by Dr. Herapath, be purified by boiling it with solution of caustic soda or potassa, twice successively, then thoroughly washing the residue, which will be yellow oxide of bismuth, dissolving it again in nitric acid, and precipitating by water as before. (*Chem. News*, 1863, p. 77.) In the washing of subnitrate of bismuth, the salt is asserted to lose a portion of its nitric acid; and the change may be considerable, if the washing be continued so long as the liquid comes away in any degree acid-

Water, in a capacious glass vessel, and, having added the Bismuth, set the whole aside for twenty-four hours. Dilute the resulting solution with ten fluidounces of Distilled Water, stir it thoroughly, and, after twenty-four hours, filter through paper. Dissolve the Carbonate of Sodium in twenty fluidounces of Distilled Water with the aid of heat, and filter the solution through paper. To this, when cold, slowly add the solution of nitrate of bismuth, with constant stirring. Transfer the whole to a strainer, and, after the precipitate has been drained, wash it with Distilled Water until the washings pass tasteless, and drain again as completely as possible. Then place the moist precipitate in a capacious vessel, gradually add the remainder of the Nitric Acid, and afterwards four fluidounces of Distilled Water, and set the solution aside. At the end of twenty-four hours, filter through paper, and to the filtered liquid, previously diluted with four pints of Distilled Water, slowly add the Water of Ammonia, with constant stirring. Transfer the whole to a strainer, and, after the precipitate has been drained, wash it with two pints of Distilled Water, drain it again, and press out as much of the liquid as possible. Lastly, dry it upon bibulous paper with a gentle heat, and rub it into powder." *U. S.* 1870.

ulous. It has been ascertained by Julius Löwe that this effect may be avoided by washing with a very dilute solution of nitrate of ammonium, containing one part in 500 parts of water. (*Chem. Gaz.*, March 15, 1859, p. 119.)* *Bismuthous nitrate*, a crystalline salt ($Bi3NO_3,5H_2O$), is deposited from a solution of bismuth in nitric acid. This has been used by Dr. Balmanno Squire dissolved in glycerin, under the name of *Glycerole of Nitrate of Bismuth.* (*P. J. Tr.*, Nov. 11, 1876.) W. W. Moorhead prepares it by taking two troyounces of crystalline nitrate of bismuth and dissolving in sufficient glycerin to make eight fluidounces. No heat should be used. This preparation can be diluted with an equal bulk or less of water, or one part can be added to forty-eight of water without ready precipitation, but one part to twelve, eight, or six of water soon precipitates. (*A. J. P.*, 1877, p. 98; also pp. 23 and 89.)

Properties. Subnitrate of bismuth is "a heavy, white powder, permanent in the air, odorless and almost tasteless, showing a slightly acid reaction when moistened on litmus paper, and insoluble in water or alcohol. When heated to redness, the salt gives off moisture, and afterward nitrous vapors, leaving a yellow residue which is soluble in nitric or in hydrochloric acid, and which is blackened by hydrosulphuric acid. On dissolving 1 part of the salt in 5 parts of warm nitric acid (sp. gr. 1·200), no effervescence should occur (abs. of carbonate), and no residue should be left (abs. of insoluble foreign salts). The reactions, for purity, of this solution, as well as those of the original salt, should be the same as those mentioned under *Bismuthi Subcarbonas.*" *U. S.* It is readily soluble in the strong acids, from which it is precipitated by water. The fixed alkalies dissolve it sparingly, and ammonia more readily. It is darkened by hydrogen sulphide gas, but not by exposure to light, unless it contains a little silver, or is subjected to the influence of organic matter. If the nitric solution is not precipitated by dilute sulphuric acid, it is free from lead. It sometimes contains arsenic, which may be detected by acting on it with pure sulphuric acid, evaporating to dryness, dissolving in hot distilled water, and testing a part of the solution by Marsh's apparatus. By this method M. Lassaigne detected one-sixth of 1 per cent. of arsenic in a sample of subnitrate sold in Paris. M. Glénard proposes two new methods of searching for arsenic in the subnitrate; one merely qualitative, the other quantitative. The first consists in strongly heating a mixture of the suspected salt with acetate of potassium. The least trace of arsenic will be detected by the strong and offensive odor produced, owing to the formation of cacodyl. In the second, the subnitrate of bismuth is heated with pure hydrochloric acid. If arsenic be present it will rise in vapors in the form of chloride. These should be carefully collected and condensed, and then treated with an excess of sulphuretted hydrogen. The sulphide of arsenic precipitated will be the measure of the metal. (*Ann. de Thérap.*, 1868, p. 176.) M. Lassaigne has found as much as 27 per cent. of chloride of bismuth in this preparation, when obtained by precipitating, with water, a solution of bismuth in a mixture of nitric and hydrochloric acids. The same impurity is introduced, to a small extent, by using common water containing chlorides; and subsulphate of bismuth renders the preparation impure, when the water used contains sulphate of calcium. (*Journ. de Chim. & Méd.*, 1855, p. 276.) These facts show the necessity of using distilled water. As regards the origin of the chlorine sometimes existing in commercial subnitrate of bismuth, it is asserted by Mr.

* In order to avoid the handling of large volumes of liquid, as well as the loss of bismuth by the production of soluble salts, A. Lalieu proposes the following process, which, he says, yields a much larger, purer, and denser product: 200 grammes of bismuth are dissolved in a sufficient quantity of nitric acid; the clear solution is decanted and poured into about 8 litres of water containing 500 grammes of water of ammonia. The precipitate is washed, transferred to a capsule, and 50 to 60 grammes of caustic soda, dissolved in a little water, are added to it. The capsule is then exposed for 15 to 20 minutes to the heat of a water-bath, and the contents stirred up several times. After having again become cold, the supernatant liquor is poured off, the precipitate is thoroughly washed, and a quantity of nitric acid, representing 48·5 grammes of anhydrous nitric acid (to be determined from the sp. gr., etc.), is added to it in small portions at a time, and under constant stirring. If, during this addition, the mass should become too thick, a little water may be added, but not enough to destroy the pasty consistence of the mass. The capsule is then replaced for a few minutes on the water-bath, and the mass well stirred. The latter, which had been yellow, becomes soon perfectly white, and somewhat more liquid. It is then diluted with a little water, the precipitate collected on a filter placed on a muslin strainer, washed, drained, pressed, and dried. The product amounts to about 265 grammes. (*L'Union Pharmaceutique*, No. 8; *N. R.*, Nov. 1878.)

R. C. Tichborne to be a common practice with the manufacturer, in order to save the bismuth existing in the mother-liquor, after the deposition of the subnitrate, to precipitate it with chloride of sodium, thus obtaining an insoluble oxychloride of bismuth, which is then added to the previous product. (*P. J. Tr.*, 1860, p. 413.) For the modes of detecting and separating it, the reader is referred to the *Chemical News* (1863, p. 109). The metal thallium is said to be present in most specimens of the pharmaceutical preparations of bismuth, whilst the fetid odor of the breath so often produced when the subnitrate is administered is believed to be due to traces of tellurium. (Brownen, *P. J. Tr.*, Oct. 16, 1875.) It has also been said that the arsenic usually present in minute quantities is the cause of the garlicky odor of the breath. Dr. E. R. Squibb (*Ephemeris*, Sept. 1882) states, however, that the "bismuth breath" has been noticed in patients who were taking a preparation of bismuth in which the absence of both tellurium and arsenic was conclusively shown. The cause of the peculiar odor is, therefore, at present doubtful. Phosphate of calcium has been ascertained to be an occasional adulteration of the subnitrate. A ready method of detecting it, suggested by M. Roussin, has proved to be fallacious, and may lead to false decisions as to the presence of the phosphate. There can be no difficulty in detecting the adulteration by the U. S. P. tests. Subnitrate of bismuth was called, by the earlier chemists, *magistery of bismuth*. It is incompatible with iodide of potassium (slowly forming a brick-red iodide of bismuth), and with alkaline bicarbonates.

Medical Properties. Owing to the difficulty of dissolving it, the subnitrate of bismuth has been thought not to be absorbed at all when ingested. The peculiar garlicky odor which it often imparts to the breath of those taking it, unless it be really due to the presence of tellurium in the bismuth, shows, however, that this is a mistake, and the French chemists MM. Bergeret and Mayençon affirm that they have found bismuth in the urine of those taking it. Its solution and absorption in the stomach must, however, be exceedingly slow, and it does not have the power of impressing the general system. First introduced as a medicine by Dr. Odier, of Geneva, it has come into very extensive use for its local effects upon irritated mucous membrane, to which it seems to be sedative, feebly astringent, and very soothing. It is one of our most useful remedies in subacute gastritis, gastralgia, pyrosis, gastric ulcers, and similar stomachic diseases. Owing to its great insolubility when taken into the stomach, it escapes into the intestine and there exerts its specific influence; it is, therefore, very useful in diarrhœas of irritation, and even in dysentery. In diarrhœas of relaxation it is of little service. Subnitrate of bismuth is also a very useful topical application in various mucous inflammations, other than gastro-intestinal; thus it is used with advantage by injection (gr. v–xx to f℥i of mucilage) in the first stage of gonorrhœa, in leucorrhœa, and in rectal irritation, by snuffing in coryza, etc. M. Trousseau has successfully employed subnitrate of bismuth in the diarrhœa of children in the form of enema, in the dose of two scruples, mixed with thick flaxseed tea. Its use always blackens the stools. The dose of subnitrate of bismuth, usually prescribed, is five to ten grains (0·33–0·65 Gm.) twice or thrice a day, given in powder or suspended in a thick mucilage. It may, however, be advantageously employed in much larger doses. M. Monneret, who was the first to recommend it in diarrhœa, used from half an ounce to an ounce (15·5–31·1 Gm.) daily, in divided doses, in the diarrhœa of adults; from half a drachm to a drachm (1·95–3·9 Gm.) in that of infants; and from a drachm to two drachms (3·9–7·8 Gm.) in painful affections of the stomach. In these large doses the medicine is perfectly safe; and yet Orfila mentions, as resulting from an overdose, gastric distress, nausea, vomiting, diarrhœa or constipation, colic, heat in the breast, slight rigors, vertigo, and drowsiness, results which were undoubtedly due to the presence of irritant impurities. In gastric inflammations the subnitrate, administered before meals, comes immediately in contact with the diseased surface; but when it is desired to reach the intestinal mucous membrane, the remedy should be given about two hours after eating, when the contents of the stomach are passing into the intestines. M. Rodolfi, of Breccia, has found the use of the subnitrate, associated with bicarbonate of sodium and sulphur, to be very efficient in controlling the night-sweats of phthisis.

As has been shown by Theodore Kocher, even the insoluble preparations of bismuth are active antiseptics, and they were for a time much used in Germany in the treatment of wounds. It was claimed for them that they acted like iodoform and were not capable of producing poisonous symptoms. Further experience has shown, however, that this is incorrect; that when applied in large quantities to extensive wounded surfaces they are capable of yielding so much bismuth to absorption as to produce a poisoning, which is characterized by acute stomatitis, with a peculiar black discoloration of the mucous membrane, usually beginning upon the borders of the teeth, but spreading over the whole mouth, followed by an intestinal catarrh, with pain and diarrhœa: in severe cases desquamative nephritis, as shown by albuminous urine and epithelial tube-casts, may also occur.

Off. Prep. Br. Trochisci Bismuthi.

BISMUTHUM. *Br.* *Bismuth.*

Bi; 210. (BĬṢ-MŪ'THŬM.) Bi; 210.

"A crystalline metal. In its crude state it is impure." *Br.*

Etain de Glace, Bismuth, *Fr.;* Wismuth, *G.;* Bismutte, *It.;* Bismut, *Sp.*

Bismuth occurs usually in the metallic state, occasionally as a sulphide or telluride, and rarely as an oxide. It is found principally in Saxony. It occurs also in Cornwall, and has been found at Monroe, in Connecticut, in Archer County, Texas (*A. J. P.*, 1871, p. 228), and in Colorado with gold and silver ores. It has also been discovered largely in South Australia, whence a quantity of it has been sent into commerce. (*P. J. Tr.*, Aug. 1867, p. 95.) It is obtained almost entirely from native bismuth, which is heated by means of wood or charcoal, whereby the metal is fused and separated from its gangue. Most of the bismuth of commerce comes from Saxony, although it is now (1881) also largely obtained from Bolivia. The bismuth from South America is said to be naturally free from arsenic, and to be therefore preferable for pharmaceutical purposes.

Bismuth was first recognized as a metal by Agricola in 1520. Before that period it was confounded with lead. It is a brittle, pulverizable, brilliant metal, of a crystalline texture, and of a white color with a slight reddish tint. Its crystals are rhombohedral, but with an angle of 87° 40′, which makes it difficult to distinguish them from cubes, in which the angle would be 90°. Indeed, many books still speak of it as cubical in form. It undergoes but a slight tarnish in the air. Its sp. gr. is 9·8, 9·83, *Br.* (purified), melting point 264° C. (507° F.). When impure bismuth solidifies after fusion, globules of the metal, nearly pure, are thrown up from the mass. This takes place when the metal contains as much as 50 per cent. of impurity. The same phenomenon does not occur when pure bismuth is melted. (*R. Schneider.*) At a high temperature, in close vessels, bismuth volatilizes, and may be distilled over. When heated in the open air to a full red heat, it takes fire, and burns with a faint blue flame, forming an oxide of a yellow color. This is the *teroxide*, and consists of two atoms of bismuth 420, and three of oxygen 48 = 468. There is another compound of bismuth and oxygen, consisting of two atoms of the former and five atoms of the latter, which is called *bismuthic oxide*, Bi_2O_5. It is obtained in the form of a hydrate by boiling nitrate of bismuth in solution of potassa, washing the precipitate, and mixing it while moist with solution of potassa into which chlorine is passed. A mixture of bismuthous and bismuthic oxides is precipitated, from which the former is separated by digestion with nitric acid. The hydrated oxide remaining, when washed and dried, is in the form of a red powder, which gives up its water at 130° C. (266° F.), and at a higher heat loses oxygen. Bismuth is acted on feebly by hydrochloric acid, but violently by nitric acid, which dissolves it with a copious liberation of red fumes. Sulphuric acid, when cold, has no action on it, but at a boiling heat effects its solution with the liberation of sulphurous acid. As it occurs in commerce, it is generally contaminated with other metals, among which are arsenic in minute quantity, traces of silver, cadmium, nickel, and iron, and sometimes a very small proportion of thallium. It may be purified from all contaminating metals by dissolving the bismuth of commerce in diluted nitric acid, precipitating the clear solution by adding it to water, and reducing the white powder thus obtained with black flux. The same precipitate is obtained by adding ammonia to the nitric solution; if the supernatant liquor is blue, the presence of copper is indicated; if the precipitate is yellowish, iron is present.

Pharm. Uses, etc. Bismuth is not used in medicine in an uncombined state, but is employed pharmaceutically to obtain the subcarbonate and subnitrate of bismuth, the only medicinal preparations formed from this metal. In the arts it is used to form a white paint for the complexion, called *pearl white;* and as an ingredient of the best pewter.

Off. Prep. Br. Bismuthum Purificatum.

BISMUTHUM PURIFICATUM. *Br.* *Purified Bismuth.*

(BĬŞ-MŪ′THŬM PŪ-RĮ-FĮ-CĀ′TŬM.)

Bismuth purifié, *Fr.;* Gereinigtes Wismuth, *G.*

"Take of Bismuth 10 ounces [av.]; Cyanide of Potassium ½ ounce [av.]; Sulphur 80 grains; Carbonate of Potassium, recently ignited, Carbonate of Sodium, recently ignited, of each a sufficiency. Melt the Bismuth in a crucible. Add the Cyanide of Potassium and Sulphur, previously mixed. Heat the whole to low redness for about fifteen minutes, constantly stirring. Remove the crucible from the fire, and let it cool until the flux has solidified to a crust. Pierce two holes in the crust, and pour the still fluid bismuth into another crucible. Remelt this partially purified bismuth with about five per cent. of a mixture of equal parts of the dried Carbonates of Potassium and Sodium, heating to bright redness and constantly stirring. Remove the crucible from the fire, cool, and pour out the bismuth into suitable moulds." *Br.*

The object of the above process is to separate contaminations of copper, arsenic, and other impurities found in commercial bismuth. The first part of the process is a modification of Hugo Tamm's method for separating the copper, whereby the melted metal is brought into contact with potassium sulphocyanate, which, acting as a flux, forms a compound with the copper, which separates as a crust. The partially purified bismuth is then remelted in contact with a small quantity of dried carbonates of potassium and sodium, which separates iron, cooled, and poured into moulds.

A mode of purifying bismuth is given in the U. S. Pharmacopœia of 1870 in the process for preparing the subnitrate. That of the former British Pharmacopœia was different; consisting in the oxidation of the arsenic and other contaminating metals that may be present, by means of the nitric acid of the nitre, and their consequent separation from the bismuth, the great mass of which remains behind unaffected. This method was referred to in the twelfth edition of the Dispensatory (p. 1025); where also the plan of M. W. Pierre is mentioned, consisting in the addition of from 2·5 to 5 per cent. of zinc to the bismuth, and strongly heating the mixture in a crucible, with a piece of charcoal to prevent the oxidation of the zinc. Both the arsenic and zinc are driven off. (*Chem. News*, Jan. 16, 1861.) According to Mr. Tilden, the British officinal process was both wasteful of the bismuth and incapable of removing the impurities. (*P. J. Tr.*, ser. 3, i. 505.) For other methods of purification, see *Schweiz. Woch. f. Ph.*, No. 5; *A. J. P.*, Sept. 1877.

"Dissolved in a mixture of equal volumes of nitric acid and distilled water, it forms a solution which by evaporation yields colorless crystals, that are decomposed on the addition of water, giving a white precipitate. If the mother liquor from which the crystals have been separated be evaporated with hydrochloric acid until all the nitric acid is dissipated, a little of the product yields no evidence of arsenium on being examined by the hydrogen test commonly known as Marsh's Test; no blue coloration on adding water and excess of ammonia, and no precipitate on filtering and saturating the ammoniacal filtrate with nitric acid; no white precipitate with diluted sulphuric acid; no red or black precipitate with sulphide of sodium; and no blue precipitate with ferrocyanide of potassium." *Br.*

Off. Prep. Br. Bismuthi Carbonas; Bismuthi Citras; Bismuthi et Ammonii Citras; Bismuthi Oxidum; Bismuthi Subnitras; Liquor Bismuthi et Ammonii Citratis; Trochisci Bismuthi.

BRAYERA. *U. S., Br.* *Brayera.*

(BRĀY-Ē'RĄ.)

"The female inflorescence of Brayera anthelmintica. Kunth. (*Nat. Ord.* Rosaceæ, Roseæ.)" *U. S.* "The dried panicles (chiefly of the female flowers) of Hagenia Abyssinica, *Willd.* (Brayera anthelmintica, *Kunth.*)" *Br.*

Cusso, *Br.*; Kousso: Koosso; Flores Kosso, *P.G.*; Kusso, *E.*; Cousso, Kousso, *Fr.*; Kosso, Kusso, Cusso, *G.*

Gen. Ch. "*Calyx* with the tube bibracteolate at the base, turbinate; throat internally constricted by a membranous ring; the limb with two series of segments, each five in number, the outer much larger. *Petals* five, inserted in the throat of the calyx, small, linear. *Stamens* from 15 to 20, inserted with the petals. *Filaments* free, unequal. *Anthers* bilocular, dehiscing longitudinally. *Carpels* two at the bottom of the calyx, free, unilocular, containing one or two pendulous ovules. *Styles* terminal, exserted from the throat of the calyx, thickened upward. *Stigmas* subpeltate, dilated, crenate, oblong." The flowers are said to be diœcious; though the male have well-developed carpels.

Brayera anthelmintica. Kunth; De Cand. *Prodrom.* ii. 580; Pereira, *Mat. Med.*, 3d ed., ii. 1818.—*Hagenia Abyssinica.* Lamarck.—*B. & T.*, 102.—*Bancksia Abyssinica.* Bruce. This is a tree about twenty feet high, growing on the table-land of Abyssinia, at an elevation of from three thousand to eight thousand feet. The branches exhibit circular cicatrices, left by the fallen leaves. These are crowded near the ends of the branches, large, pinnate, sheathing at the base, with opposite, lanceolate, serrate leaflets, villose at the margin, and nerved beneath. The unisexual flowers are tinged with purple, pedicelled, with an involucre of four roundish, oblong, obtuse, membranous bracts, and are arranged in fours, upon hairy, flexuous, bractate peduncles, with alternate branches. They are small and of a greenish color, becoming purple. These and the unripe fruit are the parts of the plant employed. The petals are apt to be wanting in the dried flowers. They are brought from Abyssinia packed in boxes, reaching Europe chiefly by way of Aden and Bombay. The Abyssinian name of the medicine has been variously spelled by European writers kosso, kousso, cusso, cosso, etc.; but koosso is deemed the most appropriate English title, as it indicates the proper pronunciation of the word. The fruit of the tree is said to be used as an anthelmintic in Abyssinia, but Dragendorff failed to detect any active principle in it.

Properties. The dried flowers are in unbroken though compressed clusters. The male flowers are usually collected, so that ordinarily the general color of the mass is greenish yellow or light brown; sometimes the female flowers constitute the bulk of the drug, which then has a distinct reddish tint, and is often known in commerce as *Red Koosso.* In accordance with our Pharmacopœia this commercial variety should alone be used. The officinal description is as follows. "In bundles or rolls, or compressed clusters, consisting of panicles about ten inches (25 cm.) long, with a sheathing bract at the base of each branch; the two roundish bracts at the base of each flower, and the four or five obovate, outer sepals, are of a reddish color, membranous and veiny; calyx top-shaped, hairy, enclosing two carpels or nutlets. Its odor is slight, fragrant, and tea-like, and its taste bitter and nauseous." As the medicine, from its high price, is apt to be adulterated, it should be procured in the unpowdered state, in which the botanical characters of the flower will sufficiently test its genuineness. It has a fragrant balsamic odor; and the taste, slightly perceptible at first, becomes in a short time somewhat acrid and disagreeable. Analyzed by Wittstein, it was found to contain in 100 parts, 1·44 of fatty matter and chlorophyll, 2·02 of wax, 6·25 of bitter acrid resin, 0·77 of tasteless resin, 1·08 of sugar, 7·22 of gum, 24·40 of tannic acid, 40·97 of lignin, 15·71 of ashes, with 0·14 part of loss. To Clemens Willing it yielded a small quantity of volatile oil, having the odor of the flowers, much extractive, tannic acid coloring iron green, a crystallizable acid, and a resin with a bitter and astringent taste and the odor of the oil. (*Chem. Centralblatt*, 1855, p. 224.) In which of these constituents the virtues of the medicine reside, is not positively determined, but *koossin* or *kosin* of Signor Pavesi is probably the active principle.

The composition of koosso has been since investigated by Dr. C. Bedall, of Munich, who determined that the kosin or tæniin of Pavesi is identical with the bitter acrid resin of Wittstein. It may be obtained by treating koosso repeatedly with alcohol to which hydrate of lime has been added; the residue is boiled with water; the liquids are mixed, filtered, and distilled; and the residue treated with acetic acid, which precipitates the kosin in a white flocculent form, soon becoming denser and resin-like, and, on drying, yellowish, or, at a higher temperature, brown. The product is 3 per cent. In bulk, kosin has an odor like that of Russian leather, a persistent bitter and acrid taste, a yellowish or yellowish white color, and an indistinct crystalline appearance under the microscope. It is very sparingly soluble in water, but freely so in alcohol, ether, and alkaline solutions. (*A. J. P.*, 1872, p. 394.) Its formula, according to Flückiger, is $C_{31}H_{38}O_{10}$. It fuses at 142° C. (287·6° F.), and remains after cooling an amorphous yellow mass, but if touched with alcohol it immediately assumes the form of stellate tufts of crystals. This may be repeated at pleasure, kosin not being altered by cautious fusion. (*Pharmacog.*, 2d ed., p. 258.) Kosin is not decomposed by boiling dilute acids. It dissolves in strong sulphuric acid, giving a yellow solution, which becomes turbid by addition of water, white amorphous kosin being thrown down. From the fact that at the same time an odor of isobutyric acid is evolved, Flückiger considers that it may be a compound ether of that acid.

Koossinate of Sodium has been recommended by Pavesi as a very eligible preparation for obtaining the virtues of koossin; a process is given in *Amer. Drug.*, 1884, p. 96; *A. J. P*, 1885, p. 239.

Medical Properties. Koosso is highly valued in Abyssinia as a vermifuge. Bruce speaks of it in his travels, and gives a figure of the plant. Dr. Brayer, a French physician, practising in Constantinople, employed the medicine effectively, and published a treatise on it at Paris, so long ago as 1823. It was in his honor that Kunth adopted the generic title of the plant. Much attention has recently been attracted to this medicine; and trials made with it have proved that it has extraordinary efficacy in the destruction and expulsion of the tape-worm. Its effects, when taken internally, are not very striking. In the ordinary dose it sometimes produces heat of stomach, nausea, and even vomiting, and shows a tendency to act on the bowels, though this effect is not always produced. It appears to act exclusively as a poison to the worms; and has been found equally effectual in both kinds of tape-worm. The medicine is taken in the morning upon an empty stomach, a light meal having been made the preceding evening. A previous evacuation of the bowels is also recommended. The flowers are given in the form of powder, mixed with half a pint of warm water; the mixture being allowed to stand for fifteen minutes, then stirred up, and taken in two or three draughts at short intervals. The medicine may be preceded and followed by lemonade. The medium dose for an adult is half an ounce (15·5 Gm.), which may be diminished one-third for a child of 12 years, one-half for one of 6, and two-thirds for one of 3. Should the medicine not act on the bowels in three or four hours, a brisk cathartic should be administered. One dose is said to be sufficient to destroy the worm. Should the quantity mentioned not prove effectual, it may be increased to an ounce (31·1 Gm.).

The principle kosin has been considerably used in Germany, and Dr. Bedall recommends it as one of the best tæniafuges; two scruples (2·6 Gm.) being sufficient to discharge the worm; and, taken in 2 or 4 powders, it usually agrees with the patient; only exceptionally causing transient nausea and vomiting; but Buchheim found *pure* kosin less powerful as an anthelmintic than that which was not pure, whilst Arena (*Pharm. Zeitschr. f. Russl.*, 1879, p. 655) believes that kosin is not the active principle at all, but that the activity of koosso resides exclusively in the green slightly bitter resin, which is soluble in alcohol and ether. If this view be correct it explains the greater efficacy of freshly-powdered koosso, for the green resin turns yellow by age and loses its power.

Off. Prep. Extractum Brayeræ Fluidum; Infusum Brayeræ.

Off. Prep. Br. Infusum Cusso.

BROMUM. *U.S., Br.* *Bromine.*

Br; 79·8. (BRŌ'MŬM.) Br; 79·8.

"A liquid non-metallic element, obtained from sea-water, and from some saline springs." *Br.*

Brominium, *U. S.*, 1870; Bromum, *P. G.;* Brome, *Fr.;* Brom, *G.;* Bromo, *It.*

Bromine is an elementary body, possessing many analogies to chlorine and iodine. It was discovered in 1826 by M. Balard, of Montpellier, in the bittern of sea-salt works, in which it exists as a bromide of magnesium. Since then it has been found in the waters of the ocean, in certain marine animals and vegetables, in various aquatic plants, as the water-cress, in numerous salt springs, and in the mineral kingdom. It has also been detected by M. Mène in the coal-gas liquor of the Paris gas works. In the United States it was first obtained by Professor Silliman, who found it in the bittern of the salt works at Salina, in the State of New York. It was discovered in the salt wells, near Freeport, Pa., by Dr. David Alter, but is now obtained in largest amount from the brines of West Virginia. The chief works are located at Parkersburg and Mason City, W. Va., and Pomeroy, Ohio. The annual production of bromine in the United States for five years was as follows: 1882, 250,000 lbs.; 1883, 301,100 lbs.; 1884, 281,100 lbs.; 1885, 310,000 lbs.; 1886, 428,334 lbs. The notable increase in 1886 was mainly due to the Michigan production, which now equals that of West Virginia. (*U. S. Geol. Survey*, 1886.)

Preparation. The original salt-liquor or brine is pumped out of the ground at 9° B., evaporated to about 15° in large iron pans, then allowed to settle, and is further evaporated in wooden tanks heated by steam pipes to the point of crystallization. These tanks, five in number, are placed at different elevations, one above the other. Each day the liquor is run off from No. 1, the highest, to No. 2; next day to No. 3, and so on until it reaches No. 5, the crystallized salt being removed from each tank after draining off the liquor. The brine which reaches No. 5 is bittern, and consists chiefly of chlorides of calcium, magnesium, sodium, and some aluminium, with varying percentages of bromides of sodium and calcium.

The bittern marking 30° to 38° B. is evaporated to about 45° B. By this further evaporation an additional percentage of impure salt is removed, the liquor is then run into stone stills, materials for generation of chlorine added, and heat applied by means of steam until the bromine has been all eliminated and vaporized. It is condensed and collected in cooled receivers. (*Proc. A. P. A.*, 1877, p. 448.) An improved bromine still is figured in *N. R.*, April, 1877; see, also, *N. R.*, 1883, p. 108; *Amer. Drug.*, 1884, p. 121.

The bittern of the salt works of Schoenbeck, in Germany, which contains only seven-tenths of one part of bromine in 1000 parts, is subjected to several successive operations, whereby the solution is reduced in bulk, and so far purified as to contain chiefly the bromide and chloride of magnesium. The chlorine is separated in the form of hydrochloric acid gas, by heating the liquid with sulphuric acid, at a temperature not exceeding 259° F.; the sulphates are crystallized out; and the bromine is evolved in the usual manner by sulphuric acid and manganese dioxide. The last operation, occupying six hours, is performed in a leaden still, of sufficient capacity to contain a charge of 84 pounds of the concentrated bittern, 60 or 70 pounds of weak sulphuric acid from the leaden chambers, and 40 pounds of manganese dioxide. The product is 4 pounds of bromine. (Moritz Hermann, *Journ. de Pharm.*, Janv. 1854.)

Bromine has also been obtained from sea-weeds by carbonizing them, lixiviating the carbonaceous residue, and then separating the ingredients, among which are iodine and bromine. For details, see *Chem. News* (July 6, 1866, p. 2). More than two-thirds of the bromine is used for the manufacture of potassium and sodium bromides for medicinal use, and for photography; the remainder is used for aniline colors.

Properties. Bromine is a volatile liquid, of a dark red color when viewed in mass, but hyacinth-red in thin layers. Its taste is very caustic, and its smell strong and disagreeable, having some resemblance to that of chlorine.* Its sp. gr. is very

* Inhaled in the form of vapor it produces intense irritation, and endangers asphyxia through spasm of the glottis. A case which had nearly proved fatal, was apparently saved by throwing steam sufficiently cooled into the larynx. (G. P. Duffield, *A. J. P.*, 1868, p. 288.)

nearly 3 (2·99, *U. S.*, 2·97 to 3·14, *Br.*). At —24·5° C. (—12° F., *Baumhauer*,* —7·2° C., *Philipp*) it becomes a hard, brittle, crystalline solid, having a dark leaden color, and a lustre nearly metallic. It boils at about 63° C. (145·4° F.), forming a reddish vapor resembling that of nitrous acid, and of the sp. gr. 5·54. It evaporates readily, a single drop being sufficient to fill a large flask with its peculiar vapor. "Agitated with solution of soda in such proportion that the fluid remains very slightly alkaline, it forms a colorless liquid, which, if colored by the further addition of a small quantity of the bromine, does not become blue on the subsequent addition of a cold solution of starch" (*Br.*); thus showing the absence of iodine.

Bromine is sparingly soluble in water (in 33 parts at 15° C. (59° F.), *U. S.*), to which it communicates an orange color, more soluble in alcohol, and still more so in ether, chloroform, and carbon bisulphide. By the aid, however, of bromide of potassium, it may be dissolved to any desirable extent in water. Its alcoholic and ethereal solutions lose their color in a few days, and become acid from the generation of hydrobromic acid. It bleaches vegetable substances like chlorine, destroys the color of sulphate of indigo, and decomposes organic matters. Its combination with starch has a yellow color. It corrodes the skin and gives it a deep yellow stain. Bromine is intermediate in its affinities between chlorine and iodine; since its combinations are decomposed by chlorine, while, in its turn, it decomposes those of iodine. It forms acids which are analogous in properties and composition to the corresponding acids of chlorine and iodine. It combines also with chlorine, forming chloride of bromine, which probably has the formula $BrCl_5$. This is prepared by passing chlorine through bromine, and condensing the vapors at a low temperature. It is a reddish yellow liquid, very volatile, soluble in water, with a penetrating odor and disagreeable taste.

Commercial bromine sometimes contains as much as 6 or 8 per cent. of *carbon tetrabromide*, as ascertained by M. Poselger. He discovered the impurity by submitting some bromine to distillation, during the progress of which the boiling point rose to 120° C. (248° F.). The residuary liquid at this temperature was colorless, and when freed from a little bromine, proved to be bromide of carbon, as an oily, aromatic liquid.† Chlorine and iodine are also frequently found in bromine, the former impurity being more common in the American and the latter in the German bromine.

The U. S. P. gives the following tests for determining the purity of bromine. "If 3 Gm. of Bromine be mixed with 30 C.c. of water and enough water of ammonia to render the solution colorless, the liquid then digested with carbonate of barium, filtered, evaporated to dryness, and the residue gently ignited, the latter should be soluble in absolute alcohol without leaving more than 0·26 Gm. of residue (abs. of more than 3 per cent. of chlorine). If an aqueous solution of Bromine be poured upon reduced iron and shaken with the latter until it has become nearly colorless, then filtered, mixed with gelatinized starch, and a few drops of bromine solution be now carefully poured on top, not more than a very faint blue zone should appear at the line of contact of the two liquids (limit of iodine)." *U. S.*

In testing for bromine in mineral or saline waters, the water is evaporated in order to crystallize most of the salts. The solution, after having been filtered, is placed in a narrow tube, and a few drops of strong chlorine-water are added. If this addition produces an orange color, bromine is present. The water examined, in order that the test may succeed, must be free from organic matter, and the chlorine not be added in excess. Bromine may be detected in marine vegetables by carbonizing them in a covered crucible, exhausting the charcoal, previously pulverized, with boil-

* See *A. J. P.*, Oct. 1872, p. 452. The higher degree usually given in chemical works is ascribed by Baumhauer to the presence of water in the bromine examined.

† It is stated by T. L. Phipson, that he has found in commercial bromine, accounted pure, a notable amount of cyanogen, and that it may be detected as follows. Take of iron filings and bromine, of each half an ounce; add to the filings 2 or 2·5 ounces of water; introduce the bromine very gradually, stirring steadily; filter rapidly while warm from the reaction; and put the filtered liquid in a partially closed bottle. In the course of some hours a deposit of ferricyanide of iron (Berlin blue) will have formed, and may be collected on a filter. In the course of two days, the whole of the cyanogen will be deposited. In the samples of bromine thus examined he had found from 0·5 to 1 per cent. of cyanogen. (*Chem. News*, 1873, p. 51.)

ing distilled water, precipitating any alkaline sulphide present in the solution by sulphate of zinc, and then adding successively a few drops of nitric acid and a portion of ether, shaking the whole together. If bromine be present, it will be set free and dissolve in the ether, to which it will communicate an orange color. (*Dupasquier.*) According to Reynoso, a more delicate test is furnished by hydrogen peroxide (ozonized water), which liberates bromine from its compounds, without reacting on it when free. The mode of proceeding is as follows. Put a piece of barium peroxide in a test-tube, and add successively distilled water, pure hydrochloric acid, and ether. The materials are here present for generating hydrogen peroxide; and so soon as bubbles are seen to rise to the surface, the substance suspected to contain bromine is added, and the whole shaken together. If a bromide be present, the hydrochloric acid will give rise to hydrobromic acid; and the hydrogen peroxide, acting on this will set free the bromine, which will dissolve in the ether, and give it a yellow tint and the odor of bromine.

Medical Properties. Bromine, from its analogy to iodine, was early tried as a remedy, and the result has demonstrated its value as a therapeutic agent. It acts like iodine as an alterative, and probably also as a stimulant to the lymphatic system, thereby promoting absorption. It has been employed in bronchocele, scrofulous tumors and ulcers, secondary and tertiary syphilis, amenorrhœa, diphtheritic affections, chronic diseases of the skin, and hypertrophy of the ventricles. Magendie recommends it in cases in which iodine does not operate with sufficient activity, or has lost its effect by habit. The form in which it is employed is aqueous solution, the dose of which, containing one part of bromine to forty of distilled water, is about six drops (0·36 C.c.) taken several times a day in water. Locally in its concentrated state it is a very powerful and deep caustic. When used as a wash for ulcers, from ten to forty minims may be added to a pint of water. The use of bromine as a caustic in hospital gangrene was proposed by Dr. Goldsmith during the war of the rebellion, and became universal in the army hospitals. Applied pure by means of a glass rod, it destroyed the diseased tissues more rapidly and thoroughly than did even strong nitric acid. Of the compounds of bromine, the bromides of potassium, ammonium, iron, and mercury have been chiefly used. Some of them have been found to exercise a remarkable influence in allaying nervous irritation, and are now much employed for that purpose. See these titles respectively in the different parts of this work.* The *chloride of bromine* has been used in cancer by Landolfi, of Naples, both externally as a caustic and internally. But a committee of the French Academy reported decidedly against it, not only as inefficacious, but as sometimes positively injurious. (*Gaz. Hebdom. de Méd. et Chir.*, Mai 9, 1856.)

Dr. J. Lawrence Smith, of Louisville, Ky., proposes the following as a convenient formula for a solution of bromine. Dissolve 160 grains of bromide of potassium in two fluidounces of water, add one troyounce of bromine, and, stirring diligently, pour in sufficient water to make the solution measure four fluidounces. The solution should be kept in accurately stopped bottles. This is a suitable preparation for application to hospital gangrene, and may be diluted to any desirable extent with water. (*A. J. P.*, 1863, p. 202.)

Bromine, in an overdose, acts as a corrosive poison. The best antidote, according to Mr. Alfred Smee, is ammonia. A case of poisoning by this substance, which proved fatal in seven hours and a half, is related by Dr. J. R. Snell. The amount swallowed was about an ounce, and the symptoms generally were those produced by the irritant poisons: such as violent inflammation of the lips, mouth, tongue, and œsophagus, with incessant burning pain, followed, in two hours and a half, by prostration, ending in death. (*New York Journ. of Med.*, Sept. 1850.) The ammonia should, of course, be given largely diluted and mixed with sweet oil.

Bromine is extensively used in photography and in the manufacture of coal-tar colors.

* *Bromide of Iodine* in aqueous solution is sometimes employed, which is made by rubbing 10 parts of iodine with 40 parts distilled water, introducing into a flask, adding 20 parts of bromine, and shaking until the iodine is dissolved. 530 parts of distilled water is added, and the whole filtered. 20 parts contain 1 part of terbromide of iodine. A solution containing 15 per cent. is sometimes found in commerce.

BRYONIA. *U. S.* *Bryonia.* [*Bryony.*]

(BRȲ-Ō'NĬ-Ȧ.)

"The root of Bryonia alba, and of Bryonia dioica. Linné. (*Nat. Ord.* Cucurbitaceæ.)" *U. S.*

Bryone couleuvrée, *Fr.;* Zaunrübe, Giehtrübe, *G.*

Bryonia alba, or white bryony, is a perennial, climbing, herbaceous plant, growing in thickets and hedges in different parts of Europe. It bears rough, heart-shaped, five-lobed leaves, small yellow monœcious flowers, arranged in racemes, and roundish black berries about the size of a pea. Another species, called *B. dioica*, with diœcious flowers and red berries, bears so close a resemblance in character and properties to the preceding, that it is considered by some botanists merely a variety. The roots of both plants are gathered for use. When fresh they are spindle-shaped, sometimes branched, a foot or two in length, as thick as the arm, or even thicker, externally yellowish gray and circularly wrinkled, within white, succulent, and fleshy, of a nauseous odor, which is lost in great measure by drying, and of a bitter, acrid, very disagreeable taste. The peasants are said sometimes to hollow out the top of the root, and to employ the juice which collects in the cavity as a drastic purge. (*Mérat and De Lens.*) The berries are also purgative, and are used in dyeing. *B. Americana*, Lam., and *B. Africana*, Thunb., are respectively used in the West Indies and Africa as hydragogue cathartics in dropsy. The berries of the European *Black Bryony*, *Tamus communis*, are said to be an irritant poison, and M. Coutagne has found that their tincture causes in animals paralysis and convulsions. (*Rép. de Pharm.*, Nov. 1884.)

Properties. As kept in the shops, the root is in circular transverse slices, externally yellowish gray and longitudinally wrinkled, internally of a whitish color, becoming darker by age, concentrically striated, light, brittle, and readily pulverizable, yielding a whitish powder. It is officinally described as follows. "In transverse sections about two inches (5 cm.) in diameter, the bark gray-brown, rough, thin, the central portion whitish or grayish, with numerous small wood-bundles arranged in circles and projecting, radiating lines; inodorous, taste disagreeably bitter." Besides a peculiar bitter principle called *bryonin*, the root contains starch in considerable proportion, gum, resin, sugar, a concrete oil, albumen, and various salts. It yields its active properties to water. *Bryonin*, $C_{48}H_{80}O_{19}$, may be obtained by mixing the powdered root with one-sixth of its weight of purified animal charcoal, in fine powder, putting the mixture into a percolator, already containing a quantity of animal charcoal equal to that mixed with the bryony, and then percolating successively with strong alcohol, diluted alcohol, and sufficient water to displace the alcoholic liquid. The tincture thus obtained yields the bryonin by spontaneous evaporation. This is extremely bitter, soluble in water and alcohol, insoluble in ether, unaltered by the alkalies, and dissolved by sulphuric acid, with the production of a blue color. It purges actively in the dose of two grains. (*A. J. P.*, xxviii. 166.) When treated with acids bryonin is resolved into sugar and two peculiar substances, one soluble in ether, called *bryoretin*, $C_{21}H_{35}O_7$, the other insoluble in that liquid, and named *hydrobryoretin*, $C_{21}H_{37}O_8$. It is, therefore, a glucoside. (G. F. Waltz. See *A. J. P.*, 1859, p. 251; see, also, report of investigation by C. F. Heller, *A. J. P.*, 1887, p. 68.)

Medical Properties. Bryony is an active hydragogue cathartic, in large doses sometimes emetic, and disposed, if too largely administered, to occasion inflammation of the alimentary mucous membrane. It appears also to have direct relations with the nervous system, and it has in a number of cases produced serious or even fatal poisoning. Vomiting and purging have been commonly present, but in some cases there has been no diarrhœa. Giddiness, delirium, and dilated pupils, coupled with fall of the bodily temperature, imperceptible pulse, cold perspiration, and other manifestations of collapse, are the usual symptoms. Eighty minims of the homœopathic tincture caused very serious but not fatal poisoning. (For cases see *P. J. Tr.*, 1858, p. 542; *Lancet*, May 9, 1868; *Brit. Med. Jour.*, 1883, ii. 1067; *Ther. Gaz.*, ii. 35; also *Woodman and Tidy.*) The recent root is highly irritant, and is said, when bruised and applied to the skin, to be capable of producing vesication. The medicine was well known to the ancients, and has been employed by modern physicians as a hydragogue cathartic in dropsy; but is now superseded by jalap. The dose of the powdered root is from a scruple to a drachm (1·3–3·9 Gm.).

Off. Prep. Tinctura Bryoniæ.

BUCHU. *U. S.* *Buchu.*

(BŪ'SHŪ.)

"The leaves of Barosma betulina, Bartling, Barosma crenulata, Hooker, and Barosma serratifolia, Willdenow. (*Nat. Ord.* Rutaceæ, Diosmeæ.)" *U. S.* "The dried leaves of Barosma betulina, *Bart. and Wendl.*, Barosma crenulata, *Hook.*, and Barosma serratifolia, *Willd.*" *Br.*

Buchu Folia, *Br.;* Folia Bucco, Folia Diosmæ, s. Barosmæ; Feuilles de Bucco (Booko, Buchu), *Fr.;* Buckublätter, Buccoblätter, *G.*

The leaves of the officinal and other Barosmas (so named from βαρος, and οσμη strong odor), and of some *Agathosmas*, are collected by the Hottentots, who value them on account of their odor, and, under the name of *bookoo* or *buchu*, rub them, in the state of powder, upon their greasy bodies.

Gen Ch. Calyx five-cleft or five-parted. Disk lining the bottom of the calyx, generally with a short scarcely prominent rim. *Petals* five, with short claws. *Filaments* ten; the five opposite the petals sterile, petaloid; the other five longer, subulate. *Style* as long as the petals. *Stigma* minute, five-lobed. *Fruit* composed of five cocci, covered with granular dots at the back. These plants are small shrubs, with opposite leaves and peduncled flowers. *Lindley.*

The officinal species are all erect, slender shrubs with opposite leaves, dotted with conspicuous pellucid oil glands, smooth, angular, purplish branches, often of a purplish color, white flowers, and a fruit of five erect carpels. They are chiefly distinguished by their leaves.

Barosma crenata. Lindley, *Flor. Med.* p. 213.—*Diosma crenata.* De Cand. *Prodrom.* i. 714.—*Barosma crenulata.* Hooker. *B. & T.* 46. The leaves are opposite, ovate or obovate, acute, serrated and glandular at the edge, coriaceous, and full of small pellucid dots on the under surface. The flowers are white or of a reddish tint, and stand solitarily at the end of short, lateral leafy shoots.

B. serratifolia. Willd. *Sp. Plant.* p. 257; Lind. *Flora Med.* p. 213; *B. & T.* 47. The leaves are linear lanceolate, equally narrowed towards either end, three-nerved, with a truncate apex, which is always furnished with an oil cell, and a sharply serrulate margin. Their length is from an inch to an inch and a half; their width one-fifth of an inch.

B. betulina. Bartling. The leaves of this species are cuneate-obovate, apex recurved, with their margin sharply denticulate by spreading teeth. They are from one-half to three-quarters of an inch long, by three-tenths to five-tenths of an inch wide.

Properties. Buchu leaves are officinally described as follows. "About three-fifths of an inch (15 mm.) long, roundish-obovate with a rather wedge-shaped base, or varying between oval and obovate, obtuse, crenate or serrate, with a gland at the base of each tooth, pale green, thickish, pellucid-punctate; strongly aromatic, somewhat mint-like, pungent and bitterish. The leaves of *Barosma serratifolia* are about one inch (25 mm.) long, linear-lanceolate, thinner than, but otherwise like the preceding." *U. S.* The leaves of *B. crenata* constitute the *short buchu* or *round buchu*, whilst those of *B. serratifolia* are the *long buchu* of commerce. It is said that the leaves of *B. crenulata* are at present comparatively infrequent in commerce, the parcels usually consisting of those of one of the other species almost unmixed. The species can be recognized by the characters already given. Mixed with buchu leaves, or sometimes constituting the bulk of the parcel, the leaves of the *Empleurum serrulatum* sometimes occur. They are to be distinguished by being longer and narrower than any buchu leaf, with a sharp-pointed apex, parallel sides, and coarse denticulation.

Flückiger obtained from *B. betulina* 1·56 per cent. of volatile oil, which had the odor of peppermint rather than of buchu, and deviated the plane of polarization considerably to the left. On exposure to cold it furnished a camphor, which, after re-solution in alcohol, crystallized in needle-shaped forms. After repeated purification in this manner, the crystals of *Barosma camphor*, or *diosphenol*, have a peppermint odor; they fuse at 85° C. and begin to sublime at 110° C. After fusion they again solidify only at 50° C. Submitted to elementary analysis, the crystals yielded 74·08 per cent. of carbon and from 9 to 10 per cent. of hydrogen. Barosma camphor is abundantly soluble in bisulphide of carbon. The crude oil from which the camphor had been separated had a boiling point of about 200° C., quickly rising to 210° C. or even higher. The oil which distilled between these temperatures, rectified over sodium, gave approximately the formula $C_{10}H_{18}O$. (*Pharmacographia*, 2d ed., p. 109.) Prof. Spica examined *B. crenata* and found the volatile oil to differ from that obtained by Prof. Flückiger from *B. betulina*; the stearopten was similar to diosphenol, but upon analysis gave the figures $C_{10}H_{16}O_2$, and hence is regarded by Prof. Spica as an oxycamphor. The elæopten was a greenish-yellow oil, having a pleasant odor and a pungent, peppermint-like taste; by fractioning, it was separated into a portion isomeric with borneol, resembling thymol in smell and taste, and having the composition $C_8H_{12}O$, to which the name of *dioscamphor* was given. A substance extracted by alcohol from the residue after the removal of the oil Prof. Spica named *diosmin*. (*P. J. Tr.*, 1885, p. 106.) Wayne's experiments (*A. J. P.*, 1876, p. 19) appear to indicate that the oil also contains a substance capable of being converted into salicylic acid. Prof. J. M. Maisch believes that buchu leaves do not contain salicylic acid, although the stearopten of the oil gives a blackish color with ferric chloride. (*A. J. P.*, July, 1881.) The yield of ash varies, according to the researches of H. W. Jones (*P. J. Tr.*, ix. 673), from 4·69 to 4·40 in *B. betulina*, 4·32 to 5·39 in *B. crenulata*, 5·03 to 5·22 in *B. serratifolia*; the ash itself was remarkable as containing a great deal of manganese. The short-leaved buchu was found by Mr. P. W. Bedford to yield an average of 1·21 per cent. of volatile oil; while the long-leaved, though more highly valued in the market, gave only 0·66 per cent., showing its great inferiority in strength. (*Proc. A. P. A.*, 1863, p. 211.)

Medical Properties. The Hottentots have long used buchu in a variety of diseases. From these rude practitioners the remedy was borrowed by the resident English and Dutch physicians, by whose recommendation it was employed in Europe, and has come into general use. Its activity depends upon the volatile oil which is eliminated by the kidneys. Under its action there is no marked increase in the amount of the urine, hence the remedy is of no value in dropsies; but the oil affects very decidedly the mucous membrane of the genito-urinary tract. The remedy is very useful in diseases of the urinary organs, such as gravel, chronic catarrh of the bladder, morbid irritation of the bladder and urethra, diseases of the prostate, and retention or incontinence of urine from a loss of tone in the parts concerned in its evacuation. It should be given when the inflammation is not severe, but not when it is in that condition of chronicity requiring oil of turpentine, tincture of cantharides, or other more stimulant diuretics. The best preparation for use is the fluid extract, of which the dose is a fluidrachm (3·75 C.c.) repeated three or four times a day.

Off. Prep. Extractum Buchu Fluidum.

Off. Prep. Br. Infusum Buchu; Tinctura Buchu.

BUTYL-CHLORAL HYDRAS. *Br.* *Hydrate of Butyl-Chloral.*

$C_4H_5Cl_3O, H_2O$. (BŪ′TȲL-ÇHLŌ′RĂL HȲ′DRĂS.)

Chloral butylicum; Butyl chloralhydrate; Hydrate de chloral butylique, *Fr.*; Butylchloralhydrat, *G.*

"Butyl-chloral, produced by the action of dry chlorine gas on aldehyd cooled to a temperature of 14° F. (—10° C.), separated by fractional distillation, and converted into the solid hydrous butyl-chloral by the addition of water." *Br.*

This substance was discovered by Krämer and Pinner, of Berlin, during an examination of the accumulated by-products of the chloral factory of Schering. It was named croton-chloral hydrate because it was believed to bear a relationship to crotonic acid, the peculiar acid of croton oil; this was subsequently disproved by Pinner, who showed that it belonged to the butyl series. (*Ber. d. Chem. Ges.*

vii. 1321, 1561.) It is made by passing dry chlorine through aldehyd cooled to —10° C. (14° F.), in an apparatus similar to that used in making chloral. Fractional distillation is resorted to, and the product boiling between 163° C. (325·4° F.) and 165° C. (329° F.) is reserved; this is butyl-chloral, a colorless oily liquid. The necessary amount of water is added, and butyl-chloral hydrate is obtained.

Properties. Butyl-chloral hydrate occurs in the form of crystalline, micaceous scales of a pungent odor, sparingly soluble in water, freely soluble in alcohol, hot water, and glycerin, but insoluble, or nearly so, in chloroform, a property which may be employed to separate it from ordinary chloral hydrate. When treated with caustic alkalies it is converted into formic acid, potassium chloride, and allylene dichloride, $C_3H_4Cl_2$. "It fuses at about 172° F. (77°·8 C.) to a transparent liquid, which, in cooling, commences to solidify at about 160° F. (71°·1 C.) Soluble in about fifty parts of water, in its own weight of glycerine and of rectified spirit, and nearly insoluble in chloroform. The aqueous solution is neutral or but slightly acid to litmus paper. It does not yield chloroform when heated with solutions of potash or soda or with milk of lime." *Br.*

Medical Properties and Uses. Butyl-chloral was proposed by Liebreich, in 1870, as a remedy for the treatment of trigeminal neuralgia. He states that a drachm of it causes deep sleep, accompanied by anæsthesia of the head, with complete loss of irritability of the eyeball and of the trigeminal nerve, the circulation being kept up with great tenacity, and death, if the dose has been large enough, resulting from the arrest of respiration. These statements of Liebreich were contradicted by the research of J. von Mering and of H. W. Schmidt, who found that no anæsthesia was produced unless sufficient doses were given to cause complete narcosis, and that the general course of the symptoms caused by the croton-chloral were exactly parallel to those produced by the chloral hydrate. Nevertheless a number of observers have used croton-chloral with asserted good results in the treatment of tic-douleureux. The relief obtained is, unfortunately, only temporary and palliative. The drug has been commonly administered in doses of from 5 to 20 grains, in syrup. The safer plan is to give 5 grains every half-hour until 30 grains have been taken or relief afforded. The original formula of Liebreich was—Butyl Chloral 5 to 10 parts; Glycerin 20 parts; Distilled Water 130 parts. Dose, half a fluidounce, followed in five minutes by a second dose, ten minutes later by a third dose, unless relief is afforded. It is not sure that such medication would be safe. The dose given by the British Pharmacopœia is 5 to 15 grains.

CAFFEA. *Coffee.*

(CAF'FE-A.)

"The seed of Coffea Arabica." *U. S.* 1870. (*Nat. Ord.* Rubiaceæ.)

Semen Caffeæ; Café, *Fr.;* Kaffee, *G.;* Caffè, *It.;* Café, *Sp.;* Bun, *Ar.;* Copi cotta, *Cingalese;* Kaeva, *Malay.*

Although this substance was omitted in the Pharmacopœia of 1880, its great importance as a dietetic and its use as a medicine require a notice here.

Gen. Ch. "*Calyx* with a small, 4-5 toothed limb. *Corolla* tubular, funnel-shaped, with a 4-5 parted spreading limb. *Stamens* 4-5, inserted in the middle of the upper part of the tube, exserted or enclosed. *Style* bifid at the apex. *Berry* umbilicate, naked or crowned with the calyx, containing two seeds enclosed in a parchment-like putamen." *Lindley.*

Coffea Arabica. Linn. *Sp. Plant.* 245; *Bot. Mag.* t. 1303; *B. & T.* 144. The coffee plant is a small tree, from fifteen to thirty feet in height. The branches are opposite, the lower spreading, the upper somewhat declining, and gradually diminishing in length, as they ascend, so as to form a pyramidal summit, which is covered with green foliage throughout the year. The leaves are opposite, upon short footstalks, oblong-ovate, acuminate, entire, wavy, four or five inches long, smooth and shining, of a dark green color on their upper surface, paler beneath, and accompanied with a pair of small pointed stipules. The flowers are white, with an odor not unlike that of the jasmine, and stand in groups in the axils of the upper leaves. The calyx is very small, the corolla salver-form, with a nearly cylindrical tube, and a flat border divided into five lanceolate, pointed segments. The stamens project above the tube. The fruit, which is inferior, is a roundish berry, umbilicate at top, at first green, then red, and ultimately dark purple. It is about as large as a cherry, and contains two seeds surrounded by a paper-like membrane, and enclosed in a yellowish purple matter. These seeds, divested of their coverings, constitute coffee.

This tree is a native of Southern Arabia and Abyssinia, and probably pervades Africa about the same parallel of latitude, as it is found growing wild in Liberia, on the western coast of the continent. It is cultivated in various parts of the world where the temperature is sufficiently elevated and uniform. Considerable attention has long been paid to its culture in its native country, particularly in Yemen, in the vicinity of Mocha, from which the demands of commerce were at first almost exclusively supplied. About the year 1690, it was introduced by the Dutch into Java, and in 1718, into their colony of Surinam. Soon after this latter period, the French succeeded in introducing it into their West India Islands, Cayenne, and the Isles of France and Bourbon; and it has subsequently made its way into the other West India Islands, various parts of tropical America, Hindostan, and Ceylon.

The tree is raised from the seeds, which are sown in a soil properly prepared, and, germinating in less than a month, produce plants which, at the end of the year, are large enough to be transplanted. These are then set out in rows at suitable distances, and in three or four years begin to bear fruit. It is customary to top the trees at this age, in order to prevent their attaining an inconvenient height, and to increase the number of the fruit-bearing branches. It is said that they continue productive for 30 or 40 years. Though almost always covered with flowers and fruit, they yield most largely at two seasons, and thus afford two harvests during the year. Various methods are employed for freeing the seeds from their coverings; but that considered the best is, by means of machinery, to remove the fleshy portion of the fruit, leaving the seeds surrounded only by their papyraceous envelope, from which they are, after drying, separated by peeling and winnowing mills.

The character of coffee varies considerably with the climate and mode of culture. Consequently, several varieties exist in commerce, named usually from the sources from which they are derived. The *Mocha Coffee*, which is in small roundish grains, takes precedence of all others. The *Java Coffee* is highly esteemed in this country; but our chief supplies are derived from the West Indies and South America. Some good coffee has been brought from Liberia. Coffee improves by age, losing a portion of its strength, and acquiring a more agreeable flavor. It is said to be much better when allowed to ripen perfectly on the tree, than as usually collected. The grains should be hard, and should readily sink in water. When soft, light, black or dark colored, or musty, they are inferior.

Properties. Coffee has a faint, peculiar odor, and a slightly sweetish, somewhat austere taste. An analysis by M. Payen gives for its constituents, in 100 parts, 34 of cellulose, 12 of hygroscopic water, 10 to 13 of fatty matter, 15·5 of glucose, with dextrin and a vegetable acid, 10 of legumin, 3·5 of *chlorogenate of potassium and caffeine*, 3 of a nitrogenous body, 0·8 of free caffeine (see article *Caffeina*) 0·001 of concrete volatile oil, 0·002 of fluid volatile oil, and 6·697 of mineral substances. (*Journ. de Pharm.*, 3e sér., x. 266.) Pfaff recognized, in the precipitate produced by acetate of lead with the decoction of coffee, two peculiar principles, one resembling tannin, called *caffeo-tannic acid*, and the other an acid, called by him *caffeic acid*. The latter is thought to be identical with the *chlorogenic acid* of Payen. When strongly heated, it emits the odor of roasted coffee, and it is supposed to be the principle to which the flavor of coffee as a drink is owing. A remarkable property of caffeic acid is that, when acted on by sulphuric acid and manganese dioxide, it is converted into quinone, being in this respect analogous to quinic acid. The *sugar* of coffee is probably neither glucose as supposed by Payen, nor cane-sugar as stated by Rochleder, but peculiar; for, when the coffee is roasted, it does not answer to Trommer's test for glucose. Caffeo-tannic acid has been ascertained by Hlasiwetz to be a glucoside with the formula $C_{14}H_8O_7$, and resolvable into glucose and a peculiar crystallizable acid, $C_9H_8O_4$, named by him caffeic acid (*Journ.*

de Pharm., 1867, p. 307), and which may be obtained from coffee, by boiling a solution of the extract with caustic potassa, treating the resulting liquid with sulphuric acid in excess, and extracting the caffeic acid with ether, which yields it somewhat impure by evaporation. (*Ibid.*, January, 1868, p. 75.) The coffee fat, which ranges in different varieties from 14 to 21 per cent., is, when purified, white, without odor, of a buttery consistence, melting at 37·5° C., and becomes rancid on exposure to the air. According to Rochleder (*Wien. Akad. Ber.*, xxiv. 40), it contains the glyceride of palmitic acid and of an acid of the composition $C_{12}H_{24}O_2$.

Coffee undergoes considerable change during the roasting process. It swells up very much, acquiring almost double its original volume, while it loses from 15 to 30 per cent. of its weight. (*Pharm. Centralblatt*, 1850, p. 687.) It acquires, at the same time, a peculiar odor entirely different from that of the unroasted grains, and a decidedly bitter taste. An active empyreumatic oil is developed during the process, probably at the expense of a portion of the caffeine. Much of the alkaloid, however, escapes change, and a portion of it is volatilized. The excellence of the flavor of roasted coffee depends much upon the manner in which the process is conducted, and the extent to which it is carried. It should be performed in a covered vessel, over a moderate fire, and the grains should be kept in constant motion. When they have acquired a chestnut brown color, the process should cease. If too long continued, it renders the coffee bitter and acrid, or, by reducing it to charcoal, deprives it entirely of flavor. During a severe roasting it loses a portion of caffeine, which sublimes; while in a slight roasting it loses none: yet ordinary coffee for drinking, prepared by percolation, contains rather more caffeine when prepared from strongly roasted than from slightly roasted coffee, because the caffeine is more easily extracted from the former. (Herman Aubert. See *A. J. P.*, 1873, p. 121.) The coffee should not be roasted long before it is used, and should not be kept in the ground state. Paul and Cownley found in preparing "low and medium roasted" coffee no perceptible loss of alkaloid, whilst in "over-roasted" coffee the loss amounted to one-third. The average amount of caffeine in moderately roasted coffee they fix at 1·3 per cent. (*P. J. Tr.*, 1887, p. 822.)

Medical and Economical Uses. More attention has been paid to the effects of coffee on the system in the roasted than in the crude state. Unroasted coffee has been employed in intermittent fever; but it is much inferior to quinine. It has been given in powder, in the dose of a scruple every hour; in decoction, prepared by boiling an ounce with eighteen ounces of water down to six; or in extract, in the dose of from four to eight grains.

The action of coffee is directed chiefly to the nervous system. When swallowed it produces a warming cordial impression on the stomach, quickly followed by a diffused agreeable nervous excitement, which extends itself to the cerebral functions, giving rise to increased vigor of imagination and intellect, without any subsequent confusion or stupor such as characterizes the action of narcotic medicines. Indeed, one of its most extraordinary effects is a disposition to wakefulness, which continues for several hours after it has been taken. It is even capable of resisting, to a certain extent, the intoxicating and soporific influence of alcohol and opium, and may sometimes be advantageously employed for this purpose. It also moderately excites the circulatory system, and stimulates the digestive function. A cup of coffee, taken after a hearty meal, will often relieve the sense of oppression so apt to be experienced, and enable the stomach to perform its office with comparative facility. The exhilarating effects of coffee, united with its delicious flavor when suitably qualified by cream and sugar, have given rise to its habitual employment as an article of diet. Its use for this purpose has prevailed from time immemorial in Persia and Arabia. In 1517 it was introduced by the Turks into Constantinople, whence it was carried to France and England about the middle of the succeeding century, and has since gradually made its way into almost universal use. It cannot be supposed that a substance, capable of acting so energetically upon the system, should be entirely destitute of deleterious properties. Accordingly, if taken in large quantities, it leaves, after its first effects, a degree of nervous derangement or depression equivalent to the previous excitement; and its habitual immoderate employment is well known very greatly to injure the tone of the stomach, and frequently to occasion troublesome dyspeptic and nervous affections. This result is peculiarly apt to take place in individuals of susceptible nervous systems, and in those of sedentary habits. We have repeatedly known patients, who have long suffered with headache and vertigo, to get rid of them by abstaining from coffee.

In the treatment of disease, coffee has been less employed than might have been expected from its effect upon the system. There can be no doubt that it may be advantageously used in various nervous disorders. In a tendency to stupor or lethargy dependent on deficient energy of the brain, without congestion or inflammation, it would be found useful by stimulating the cerebral functions. In light nervous headaches, and even in sick headache not caused by the presence of offending matter in the stomach, it often proves temporarily useful. It has acquired much reputation as a palliative in the paroxysms of spasmodic asthma, and has been recommended in hooping-cough, and in hysterical affections. The Egyptians are said to have formerly employed it as a remedy in amenorrhœa. Hayne informs us that in a case of violent spasmodic disease, attended with short breath, palpitation of the heart, and a pulse so much increased in frequency that it could scarcely be counted, immediate relief was obtained from a cup of coffee, after the most powerful antispasmodics had been used in vain for several hours. By the late Dr. Dewees it was highly recommended in cholera infantum, and it has even been used with asserted advantage in cholera. It is said also to have been used successfully in obstinate chronic diarrhœa, and the late Dr. Chapman, of Philadelphia, found it highly useful in calculous nephritis. Under the impression of its diuretic powers, it has been recommended in dropsy. A very concentrated infusion of coffee is serviceable in opium poisoning, but the alkaloid caffeine is probably preferable.

Roasted coffee is said to have the effect of destroying offensive and noxious effluvia from decomposing animal and vegetable substances, and therefore to be capable of beneficial application as a disinfecting and deodorizing agent. The powder of the grains should be roasted until it becomes dark brown, and then sprinkled, or placed in plates, in the infected place.

Coffee is usually prepared in this country by boiling the roasted grains, previously ground into a coarse powder, in water for a short time, and then clarifying by the white of an egg. Some prefer the infusion, made by a process similar to that of percolation. It has more of the aroma of the coffee than the decoction, with less of its bitterness. The proper proportion for forming the infusion for medical use is an ounce to a pint of boiling water, of which a cupful may be given warm for a dose, and repeated, if necessary. A *syrup of coffee* is prepared by Dorvault in the following manner. Treat a pound of ground roasted coffee by percolation with boiling water until two pints have passed. Evaporate eight pounds of simple syrup to six, add the infusion, and strain. Two tablespoonfuls of this syrup may be added to a cup of hot water or milk. It is also used with carbonic acid water. For processes for preparing fluid extracts of green or roasted coffee see Part II.

Coffee depends for its physiological activity upon caffeine and the empyreumatic oil formed during the roasting, probably at the expense of the caffeine. There is much reason for believing that coffee and tea when taken internally lessen the waste of tissue and the elimination of urea. The experiments of Prof. Lehmann seem to show that in this action the empyreumatic oil is at least as active as is caffeine.

The *leaves* of the coffee plant possess properties analogous to those of the fruit, and are extensively used by the Malays. Dr. Stenhouse found them to contain caffeine in larger proportion than the coffee-bean, and also caffeic acid. The leaves are prepared for use by drying over a clear fire and then powdering by rubbing in the hands. The powder is made into an infusion like common tea. The taste is said to be like that of tea and coffee combined. (*P. J. Tr.*, xii. 443, xiii. 207 and 382, and xvi. 1067.)

CAFFEINA. *U.S., Br.* *Caffeine.*

$C_8 H_{10} N_4 O_2 . H_2 O$; 212. (CAF-FE-Ī'NA.) $C_{16} H_{10} N_4 O_4 . 2HO$; 212.

Caffeia, Theina, Guarina.

"A proximate principle of feebly alkaloidal power, generally prepared from the dried leaves of Camellia Thea, Link (*Nat. Ord.* Ternstrœmiaceæ), or from the dried seeds of Coffea Arabica, Linné (*Nat. Ord.* Rubiaceæ); or from Guarana, and occurring also in other plants."* *U.S.* "An alkaloid usually obtained from the dried leaves of Camellia Thea, *Link;* or the dried seeds of Coffea Arabica, *Linn.*, by evaporating aqueous infusions from which astringent and coloring matters have been removed." *Br.*

Caffeine (*Caffeia*) was first discovered by Runge, and afterwards by Robiquet. Strecker first proved it to be methyl-theobromine by making it from theobromine synthetically.† (*Ann. Chem. Pharm.*, 118, 170.) It may be obtained in the following manner. Exhaust bruised coffee by two successive portions of boiling water, unite the infusions, add acetate of lead in order to precipitate various principles accompanying the caffeine, filter, decompose the excess of acetate of lead in the filtered liquor by sulphuretted hydrogen, concentrate by evaporation, and neutralise with ammonia. The caffeine is deposited in crystals upon cooling, and may be purified by redissolving in water, treating with animal charcoal, and evaporating. H. J. Versmann, of Lubeck, recommends the following process as more economical. Powdered coffee, mixed with one-fifth of its weight of slaked lime, is exhausted, by means of percolation, with alcohol of 0·863; the tincture is distilled to separate the alcohol; the residue is rinsed out of the still with warm water, and the supernatant oil separated; the liquid is evaporated so as to solidify on cooling; and the crystalline mass thus obtained, having been expressed and dried by pressure in bibulous paper, is purified by solution in water with animal charcoal, and recrystallization. (*Chem. Gaz.*, 1852, p. 67.) H. Leuchsenring obtains caffeine by availing himself of its property of subliming unchanged by heat. He precipitates a concentrated decoction of coffee by a weak solution of acetate of lead, filters, evaporates to dryness, mixes the residue with sand, and sublimes as in Mohr's process for procuring benzoic acid. (*A. J. P.*, xxxii. 25.) Still another method, proposed by Vogel, is to treat coffee, ground to powder, with benzin, which dissolves the caffeine and an oily substance, to separate the benzin by distillation, to treat the residue with boiling water, which dissolves the caffeine, and deposits it in a crystalline form, after filtration and concentration. (*Journ. de Pharm.*, 3e sér., xxxv. 436.) Paul and Cownley's process for estimating the caffeine in coffee is to mix finely powdered coffee with moist lime, and exhaust with alcohol by hot repercolation. The alcohol is evaporated off, and the residue mixed with water and a few drops of diluted sulphuric

* The United States Pharmacopœia allows caffeine to be prepared from either one of the ordinary commercial sources, but because tea leaves contain a much larger percentage of the alkaloid than does the coffee berry, and are frequently thrown into commerce in a damaged condition, unfit for use as a beverage, commercial caffeine is almost always prepared from them. If the assertion of Dr. Thomas J. Mays, that theine, though chemically identical with caffeine, is physiologically different, be confirmed, it will become necessary to recognise theine as an officinal alkaloid, and direct that caffeine be prepared from coffee. The argument that tea and coffee differ in their gross effects on the human body, and that therefore the alkaloids cannot be identical, has no force, because coffee contains an active empyreumatic oil, developed during the process of roasting. How far the conclusions arrived at by Dr. Mays by experiments upon frogs must be accepted still remains a matter of opinion. We think, however, that further physiological studies of the three alkaloids, theine, caffeine, and guaranine, are necessary before their physiological diversity can be considered established. The clinical results obtained by Dr. Mays (*Med. News*, vol. xlviii.) are sufficient to warrant the trial of theine as a local anæsthetic injected in a dose of a third of a grain over painful nerves.

† In an examination of 25 varieties of coffee, Prof. Dragendorff found a variation in the amount of caffeine of 0·6 to 2·2 per cent. The most important varieties were as follows:

Brown Preang	0·71 per cent.	First native Ceylon	0·87 per cent.
Finest Mocha	0·64 "	Second " "	1·54 "
Yellow Menado	1·22 "	Third " "	1·59 "
Finest plantation Jamaica	1·43 "	Costa Rica	1·18 "
First Surinam	1·78 "	West Indian	1·22 "
Pearl plantation Ceylon	0·78 "	Rio	1·14 "
Yellow Java	0·88 "	Jamaica	0·67 "
Gray Java	2·21 "	Santos	1·46 "

acid; the mixture is filtered, and the filtrate and washings, when cool, treated with chloroform to wash out the alkaloid; the chloroformic solution is evaporated in a tared capsule, and the residue weighed as caffeine. (*P. J. Tr.*, 1887, p. 565. For another method, by E. D. Smith, see *Pharm. Era*, 1887, p. 17.)

Properties. Caffeine is in "colorless, soft and flexible crystals, generally quite long, and of a silky lustre, permanent in the air, odorless, having a bitter taste and a neutral reaction. Soluble in 75 parts of water and in 35 parts of alcohol at 15° C (59° F.); in 9·5 parts of boiling water and very soluble in boiling alcohol; also soluble in about 6 parts of chloroform, but very slightly soluble in ether or in disulphide of carbon. When heated to 100° C. (212° F.), the crystals lose 8·49 per cent. in weight (of water of crystallization); and when heated on platinum foil, they are completely volatilized without carbonizing. On heating Caffeine with chlorine water, or treating it with concentrated nitric acid, it is decomposed; on evaporating afterward at a gentle heat, a yellow mass is left, which, when moistened with water of ammonia, assumes a purplish color. Sulphuric or nitric acid should dissolve it without color, and its aqueous solution should not be precipitated by test-solution of iodide of mercury and potassium (abs. of other alkaloids)." *U. S.* It is precipitated from its aqueous solution by no reagent except tannic acid and solution of iodide of potassium and mercury. When this solution, made by saturating iodide of potassium with red oxide of mercury, is added to a solution of caffeine, a precipitate is produced, which soon takes the form of white, shining, acicular crystals. This reaction is proposed as a test of caffeine by Prof. Dellfs; for, though the same solution will precipitate the other alkaloids, the product is always amorphous. (*Chem. Gaz.*, Feb. 15, 1855.) Caffeine is remarkable for containing a larger proportion of nitrogen than almost any other proximate vegetable principle, in this respect equalling some of the most highly animalized products.

Medical Properties. The alkaloid caffeine,* given in large dose to the lower animals, produces hurried respiration, restlessness, slightly lowered followed by markedly elevated temperature, tetanic and clonic convulsions, progressive paralysis, and finally death from paralytic arrest of respiration. The cause of the convulsions in mammals is not determined, but in the frog they are of spinal origin, for both Pratt and Le Blond have found that section of the cord does not arrest them below the point of section, whilst destruction of the cord (Pratt and Leven) prevents their development. The alkaloid certainly acts upon the muscles of the frog, as is readily demonstrated by throwing an isolated piece of the gastrocnemius into a 1 per cent. or even a weaker solution of the citrate of caffeine; in from two to three minutes the muscle will become contracted, swollen, stiff, and unable to respond to the galvanic current. Both Leven and Binz have found that caffeine has a very distinct effect in elevating arterial pressure when given in a moderate dose, but toxic doses act upon the heart-muscle as a depressant and paralysant, producing first fall of the arterial pressure and finally cardiac arrest. In the experiments of Leven, isolation of the heart from the nerve-centres did not prevent the increase, caused by moderate doses, of the cardiac pressure and the pulse-rate, proof that the stimulant action is upon the heart itself or upon the vaso-motor system.

There have been a few cases of poisoning by caffeine; a drachm of the citrate swallowed by an adult was followed by burning at the throat, giddiness, faintness, nausea, tremor of the extremities, abdominal pain, mental distress, great cardiac oppression, and finally collapse. Consciousness was not impaired, and there was no headache until the patient began to recover. A decoction of 8 ounces of freshly roasted coffee, taken for the purpose of producing abortion, caused pronounced choreic tremors, great restlessness, quickened respiration, and rapid pulse, with very strong, even violent, heart-beats. In doses of 3 to 5 grains caffeine produces in the healthy individual a peculiar wakefulness, with stimulation of the cerebrum, and some increase of the urinary secretion and force of the pulse. There is usually marked increase of

* Professor W. Filehne (*Archiv für Anatomie und Physiologie* (*Physiol. Abtheil.*), 1886, Nos. 1, 2) has made an investigation of the physiological action of certain derivatives and decomposition products of caffeine, namely, hydroxy-caffeine, diethoxy-hydroxy-caffeine, ethoxy-caffeine, caffeidine, caffuric acid, hypo-caffeine, caffoline, guanineine, uric acid. An abstract of the original paper will be found in the *Therapeutic Gazette*, 1886, page 628.

the mental activity and of the capability for sustaining mental work. About two hours after the ingestion of 12 grains by Dr. Pratt, there was intense physical restlessness and mental anxiety, with obstinate sleeplessness, active and persistent thinking, general muscular tremulousness, and frequent urination.

In doses of 3 to 5 grains caffeine has been used of late years as a cerebral stimulant, as a cardiac stimulant, and as a diuretic. It is certainly a valuable remedy in some cases of nervous headaches. Either in the form of the alkaloid or its salts, or in that of a strong decoction of coffee, it has long been a standard remedy in opium-poisoning, in which it seems to act partly by promoting wakefulness, partly by a direct stimulating influence upon the respiratory centres. In a series of experiments Dr. J. Hughes Bennett found that within narrow limits there was a direct physiological antagonism between caffeine and morphine. The power of caffeine in opium-poisoning does not, however, compare with that of atropine, and in Bennett's experiments on cats, if a little too much of the narcotic was given the caffeine was without pronounced influence. Caffeine, originally recommended by Prof. Riegel as a substitute for digitalis in cardiac doses, has been used by large numbers of practitioners often with excellent results. It is to be employed in the same class of cases as is digitalis, namely, where the working power of the heart-muscle is less than the work required of the heart. Its action differs from that of digitalis in being much more prompt, less persistent, and not cumulative. Dr. Böcker gives from 8 to 30 grains of the powdered citrate in divided doses in twenty-four hours, beginning with smaller quantity and rapidly increasing until the result is achieved. Dr. H. C. Wood has frequently used it for the relief of cardiac failure in doses of 8 to 15 grains a day, often with an excellent result. It is, perhaps, less certain than digitalis, but is not only more prompt, but also much less apt to derange the stomach. On account of its distinct diuretic action it is a very valuable remedy in the treatment of cardiac dropsy, and is also often useful in chronic Bright's disease when there is no tendency to irritation of the kidneys. It would probably prove a useful drug in cases of sudden collapse from various causes. The ordinary salts of it are, however, not available for hypodermic use, because they are decomposed in the presence of water. The double benzoinate of sodium and caffeine has been proposed as moderately stable and free from irritant properties; the following formula has been commended by M. Tanret for hypodermic use: Sodii salicyl., 31 gr.; Caffeinæ, 40 gr.; Aquæ destillat., 60 gr. For internal administration the soluble preparation known as the citrate of caffeine is usually preferred. Dose, from 3 to 6 grains.

Off. Prep. Br. Caffeinæ Citras.

CAFFEINÆ CITRAS. *Br.* *Citrate of Caffeine.*

$C_8H_{10}N_4O_2, H_3C_6H_5O_7$. (CĂF-FE-Ī'NÆ CĪ'TRĂS.)

"A weak compound of caffeine and citric acid." *Br.*

"Take of Caffeine 1 ounce [av.]; Citric Acid 1 ounce [av.]; Distilled Water 2 ounces [Imp. meas.]. Dissolve the Citric Acid in the Water, and stir the Caffeine into the heated solution. Evaporate to dryness on a water-bath, constantly stirring towards the end of the operation. Reduce to a fine powder." *Br.*

This is a new officinal of the British Pharmacopœia; although defined as a weak compound of caffeine and citric acid, it is not regarded by chemists as a chemical salt, but as a mechanical mixture of the two substances composing it. It is officinally described as "a white inodorous powder with an acid and faintly bitter taste and an acid reaction on litmus. It is soluble in a mixture of two parts of chloroform and one part of rectified spirit. With a little water it forms a clear syrupy solution, which on dilution yields a white precipitate of caffeine that redissolves when ten parts of water have been added. Heated in the air, the salt chars and burns, leaving a mere trace of ash. From a boiling aqueous solution excess of lime water gives a white precipitate. Tannic acid yields a white precipitate soluble in excess of the reagent. If to a little of the salt a crystal of chlorate of potassium be added, and a few drops of hydrochloric acid, and the mixture be evaporated to dryness in a porcelain dish, a reddish residue results, which becomes purple when moistened with solution of ammonia." *Br.*

Medical Properties and Uses. The citrate of caffeine is possessed of the physiological and therapeutical properties of caffeine. The dose is from 3 to 8 grains.

CALAMINA PRÆPARATA. *Br.* *Prepared Calamine.*

(CĂL-Ą-MĪ'NĄ PRÆ-PĄ-RĀ'TĄ.)

Lapis Calaminaris Præparata.

"Native carbonate of zinc, calcined in a covered earthen crucible at a moderate temperature, powdered, and freed from gritty particles by elutriation." *Br.*

Calamine is found in the United States, but more abundantly in Germany and England. It usually occurs in compact or earthy masses, or concretions, of a dull appearance, readily scratched by the knife, and breaking with an earthy fracture; but sometimes it is found crystallized. Its color is very variable; being, in different specimens, grayish, grayish yellow, reddish yellow, and, when very impure, brown or brownish yellow. Its sp. gr. varies from 3·4 to 4·4. Before the blowpipe it does not melt, but becomes yellow and sublimes. When of good quality, it is almost entirely soluble in the dilute mineral acids; and, unless it has been previously calcined, emits a few bubbles of carbonic acid. If soluble in sulphuric acid, it can contain but little carbonate of calcium, and no sulphate of barium.

Calamine must be impalpable before being used in medicine. The following is the U. S. formula of 1850. "Take of Calamine a convenient quantity. Heat it to redness, and afterwards pulverize it; then reduce it to a very fine powder in the manner directed for Prepared Chalk." The object of this process is to bring the native carbonate of zinc, or calamine, to the state of an impalpable powder. Calamine, as sold in England and the United States, was formerly almost always spurious, consisting wholly or principally of sulphate of barium, colored with sesquioxide of iron. Of six samples analyzed by Mr. F. Bringhurst, of Wilmington, Del., five were totally devoid of zinc, and the sixth contained only 2 per cent. of the oxide. (*A. J. P.*, July, 1857.) But more recently (*P. J. Tr.*, 1886), Mr. R. H. Davis has found that most of the calamine sold as such in Great Britain is genuine. Prepared calamine is in the form of a pinkish or flesh-colored powder, of an earthy appearance. Sometimes it is made up into small masses. It is used only as an external application, being employed as a mild astringent and exsiccant in excoriations and superficial ulcerations. For this purpose it is usually dusted on the part, and hence the necessity for its being in very fine powder. It is often employed in the form of cerate.

The British Pharmacopœia describes it as "a pale pinkish-brown powder, without grittiness; almost entirely soluble, with effervescence, in acids."

Off. Prep. Br. Unguentum Calaminæ.

CALAMUS. *U. S.* *Calamus.* [*Sweet Flag.*]

(CĂL'Ą-MŬS.)

"The rhizome of Acorus Calamus. Linné. (*Nat. Ord.* Araceæ.)" *U. S.*

Rhizoma Calami, *P.G.;* Radix Calami Aromatici, Radix Acori; Acore vrai, Acore odorant, *Fr.;* Kalmuswurzel, *G.;* Calamo Aromatico, *It.*, *Sp.*

Gen. Ch. *Spadix* cylindrical, covered with florets. *Corolla* six-petalled, naked. *Style* none. *Capsule* three-celled. *Willd.*

Acorus Calamus. Willd. *Sp. Plant.* ii. 199; Barton, *Med. Bot.* ii. 63; *B. and T.* 279. The sweet flag, or calamus, has a perennial, horizontal, jointed, somewhat compressed root (rhizome), from half an inch to an inch thick, sometimes several feet in length, sending off numerous round and yellowish or whitish radicles from its base, and bunches of brown fibres resembling coarse hair from its joints, internally white and spongy, externally whitish with a tinge of green, variegated with triangular stains of light brown and rose color. The leaves are all radical, sheathing at the base, long, sword-shaped, smooth, green above, but, near their origin from the root, of a red color variegated with green and white. The scape or flower-stem resembles the leaves, but is longer, and from one side, near the middle of its length, sends out a cylindrical spadix, tapering at each end, about two inches in length, and crowded with greenish yellow flowers. These are without calyx, and have six small, concave, membranous, truncated petals. The fruit is an oblong capsule, divided into three cells, and containing numerous oval seeds.

This is an indigenous plant, growing throughout the United States, in low, wet, swampy places, and along the sides of ditches and streams, and flowering in May and June. It is also a native of Europe and Western Asia; and a variety is found in India. The European plant differs slightly from the American. The leaves as well as the root have an aromatic odor; but the latter only is employed. It should be collected late in the autumn, or in the spring. After removal from the ground, the rhizomes are washed, freed from their fibres, and dried with a moderate heat. By drying they lose nearly one-half their diameter, but are improved in odor and taste.

Properties. The roots, as kept in the shops, are "in sections of various lengths, unpeeled, about three-quarters of an inch (2 cm.) broad, subcylindrical, longitudinally wrinkled; on the lower surface marked with the circular scars of the rootlets in wavy lines, externally reddish brown, somewhat annulate from remnants of leaf-sheaths; internally whitish, of a spongy texture, breaking with a short, corky fracture, showing numerous oil-cells and scattered wood-bundles, the latter crowded within the subcircular nucleus-sheath. It has an aromatic odor, and a strongly pungent taste." *U. S.* Their texture is light and spongy, their color internally whitish or yellowish white, and their fracture short and rough. A variety imported from Germany consists exclusively of the interior portion of the root. The pieces are usually long, slender, irregularly quadrangular, and of a grayish white color.

The odor of calamus is strong and fragrant; its taste warm, bitterish, pungent, and aromatic. Its active principles are taken up by boiling water. From 100 parts of the fresh root of the European plant, Trommsdorff obtained 0·1 of volatile oil, 2·3 of soft resin, 3·3 of extractive with a little chloride of potassium, 5·5 of gum with some phosphate of potassium, 1·6 of starch analogous to inulin, 21·5 of lignin, and 65·7 of water. Sixteen ounces of the dried root afforded to Neumann about two scruples of volatile oil. The oil is at first yellow, but ultimately becomes red, and has the smell and taste of calamus. Kurbatow (*Annal. d. Chemie*, vol. 173, p. 4) examined oil of calamus, and found that the portion boiling below 170° C. (338° F.) yielded after treatment with sodium a terpene, $C_{10}H_{16}$, having sp. gr. ·8793 at 0° C. (32° F.); and having a boiling point of 158° C. (316·4° F.). The extractive matter has an acrid and sweetish taste. H. Thoms obtained from calamus rhizomes a bitter principle, which he named *acorin*, in the form of a clear, thick, yellow liquid, having a neutral reaction, aromatic odor, and bitter, aromatic taste. It is a glucoside, having the formula $C_{36}H_{60}O_6$, splitting into oil of calamus and sugar; insoluble in water, but readily soluble in absolute alcohol, methylic alcohol, and chloroform. By oxidation *acoretin*, a neutral resin, is formed, and from the extract remaining after the acorin is removed he obtained an alkaloid which he named *calamine;* this is crystalline, insoluble in water and ether, but soluble in alcohol, chloroform, and acetone. (*Archiv d. Pharm.*, 1886, p. 465; *P. J. Tr.*, 1886, p. 1085.) The root is sometimes attacked by worms, and deteriorates by keeping. The India variety is more slender than the European, and has a stronger and more pleasant flavor.

Medical Properties and Uses. Calamus is a feeble aromatic, which may be used with advantage in pain or uneasiness of the stomach or bowels arising from flatulence, and as an adjuvant to tonic or purgative medicines. It was probably known to the ancients, and is supposed to have been the *ἄκορον* of the Greeks; but the *calamus aromaticus* of Dioscorides was a different product, having been derived, according to Dr. Royle, from a species of *Andropogon.* The medicine is at present not much used. The dose in substance is from a scruple to a drachm (1·3–3·9 Gm.). An infusion, made in the proportion of an ounce of the root to a pint of boiling water, is sometimes given in the dose of a wineglassful (60 C.c.) or more.

Off. Prep. Extractum Calami Fluidum.

CALCIUM. *Calcium.*

Ca; 40. (CĂL'CI-ŬM.) Ca; 40.

This is the metal characteristic of lime, and consequently of all calcareous substances. It was obtained by Dr. Matthiessen, in 1855, in masses of the size of a pea, by the electrolysis of chloride of calcium with a Bunsen battery. It is a pale yellow metal, remarkably glittering when freshly filed. Its fracture is jagged, becoming granular. It is malleable and very ductile. In a dry air it remains unaltered; but it soon tarnishes in a moist one. It melts at a red heat, and afterwards burns with splendor, forming lime, or calcium oxide. (*Chem. Gaz.*, June 15, 1855.)

Calcium is a very abundant element in nature, existing in the mineral kingdom chiefly as a carbonate, in the form of limestone, marble, chalk, and calcareous spar; and as a phosphate and carbonate in the bones and shells of animals.

CALCII BROMIDUM. *U. S.* *Bromide of Calcium.*

Ca Br₂; 199·6. (CĂL'CI-Ī BRO-MĪ'DŬM.) Ca Br; 99·8.

Calcium Bromatum, Bromure de Calcium, Bromure de Chaux, *Fr.;* Brom calcium, *G.*

"Bromide of Calcium should be preserved in well-stopped bottles." *U.S.* Although this salt has been largely used, it has never been officinal until the present revision. It is prepared by M. Boedecker by first forming a bromide of sulphur, by the addition of 20 parts of the flowers of sulphur to 240 parts of bromine; this is added to a milk of lime containing 140 parts of fresh lime. The sulphate and bromide of calcium are formed and are readily separated. (*Journ. de Pharm.*, 4e sér., viii. 463.) Mr. Jas. R. Mercein puts five ounces of bromine and two and a half pints of water in a half gallon specie jar, passes a stream of sulphuretted hydrogen through the bromine until it is all taken up, filters, drives off excess of sulphuretted hydrogen by heat, distils the solution of hydrobromic acid thus obtained until four-fifths have passed over, saturates this with excess of precipitated carbonate of calcium, filters and evaporates. (*A. J. P.*, xliv. 100.) Mr. Macdonald (*Ibid.*, 1873) employs the following method. Dissolve 4 ounces of bromide of ammonium in a pint of water. Put in a flask and bring to the boiling point. Keep boiling, and add milk of lime (made from *pure* calcined lime) in small quantities, until ammoniacal vapors cease to be evolved. The operator can easily tell when this point has been reached, by the sense of smell. Filter the solution, evaporate to a syrupy consistency, remove from the fire, and stir until cold.

Properties. "A white, granular salt, very deliquescent, odorless, having a pungent, saline and bitter taste and a neutral reaction. Soluble in 0·7 part of water and in 1 part of alcohol at 15° C. (59° F.); very soluble in boiling water and in boiling alcohol. At a dull red heat the salt fuses without losing anything but moisture. At a higher temperature it is partially decomposed. An aqueous solution of the salt yields, with test-solution of oxalate of ammonium, a white precipitate soluble in hydrochloric, but insoluble in acetic acid. If disulphide of carbon be poured into a solution of the salt, then chlorine water added drop by drop, and the whole agitated, the disulphide will acquire a yellow or yellowish brown color without a violet tint." *U. S.*

Tests. "If diluted sulphuric acid be dropped upon the salt, the latter should not at once assume a yellow color (abs. of bromate). If 1 Gm. of the salt be dissolved in 10 C.c. of water, some gelatinized starch added and then a few drops of chlorine water carefully poured on top, no blue zone should make its appearance at the line of contact of the two liquids (iodide). On adding to 1 Gm. of the salt dissolved in 20 C.c. of water, 5 or 6 drops of test-solution of nitrate of barium, no immediate cloudiness or precipitate should make its appearance (sulphate). If a solution of the salt be precipitated with an excess of nitrate of silver, the washed precipitate for some time shaken with a cold, saturated solution of carbonate of ammonium, and the decanted and filtered liquid supersaturated with nitric acid, not more than a faint cloudiness, insufficient to produce a precipitate, should appear (limit of chloride). On adding to the aqueous solution, first, chloride of ammonium, then test-solution of carbonate of ammonium and water of ammonia in slight excess, and gently warming, the filtrate separated from the resulting precipitate should not be rendered more than faintly turbid by test-solution of phosphate of sodium (limit of magnesium). 1 Gm. of the dry salt, when completely precipitated by nitrate of silver, yields, if perfectly pure, 1·878 Gm. of dry bromide of silver." *U. S.*

Medical Properties and Uses. Bromide of calcium was proposed by Dr. Hammond, in 1871, as a substitute for the corresponding salt of potash. It has failed to gain much support from the medical profession, but is sometimes employed as an adjuvant in epilepsy and hysteria. Its action upon the lower animals has been partially investigated by Guttmann (*Phila. Med. Times*, iv. 361), who finds that it acts as a sedative to the nerve-centres, but lacks the depressant cardiac action of the bromide of potassium. The dose is half to two drachms (0·95–7·8 Gm.).

CALCII CARBONAS PRÆCIPITATUS. *U. S. Precipitated Carbonate of Calcium.*

Ca CO_3; 100. (CĂL′CI̦-Ī CĂR-BŌ′NAS PRÆ-CĬP-I̦-TĀ′TŬS.) Ca O, CO_2; 50.

Calcis Carbonas Præcipitata, *Br.;* Calcaria Carbonica Præcipitata, *P. G.;* Carbonas Calcicus Præcipitatus, Creta Præcipitata; Carbonate de Chaux précipité, Craie précipitée, *Fr.;* Präcipitirter kohlensauer Kalk, *G.*

A formula for this preparation is found in the Pharmacopœia of 1870.*

"Take of Chloride of Calcium *five ounces* [avoirdupois]; Carbonate of Sodium *thirteen ounces* [avoird.]; Boiling Distilled Water *a sufficiency*. Dissolve the Chloride of Calcium and the Carbonate of Sodium each in two pints [Imperial measure] of the Water; well mix the two solutions; and allow the precipitate to subside. Collect this on a calico filter, wash it with boiling Distilled Water until the washings cease to give a precipitate with nitrate of silver, and dry the product at the temperature of 212° F. (100° C.)." *Br.*

The processes do not essentially differ. In each a mutual interchange of principles takes place, resulting in the production of chloride of sodium which remains in solution, and carbonate of calcium which is deposited, $CaCl_2 + Na_2CO_3 = CaCO_3 + 2NaCl$. Any peculiar advantage of the preparation must depend on the minute division of its particles. According to Dr. Bridges, this effect is best obtained by employing the solutions at the boiling temperature, a precaution which is observed in most processes now. (*A. J. P.*, xvi. 163.) When properly made, it is "a very fine, white, impalpable powder, permanent in the air, odorless and tasteless, and insoluble in water or alcohol. Wholly soluble in hydrochloric, nitric, or acetic acid with copious effervescence. By exposure to a red heat the salt loses carbonic acid gas, and the residue has an alkaline reaction. A neutral solution of the salt in acetic acid yields, with test-solution of oxalate of ammonium, a white precipitate soluble in hydrochloric, but insoluble in acetic acid. On adding to another portion of the same solution, first, chloride of ammonium, then test-solution of carbonate of ammonium and water of ammonia in slight excess, and gently warming, the filtrate separated from the resulting precipitate should not be rendered more than faintly turbid by test-solution of phosphate of sodium (limit of magnesium). A solution of the salt in hydrochloric acid, freed from carbonic acid gas by heat, should not be rendered turbid, when supersaturated with water of ammonia (abs. of aluminium, iron, or phosphate)." *U. S.*

Medical Properties and Uses. For ordinary use, it probably has no such superiority over prepared chalk as to counterbalance its greater expensiveness, but it is preferred by some in the preparation of tooth-powders. The dose is from 10 to 40 grains (0·65–2 6 Gm.) or more.

Off. Prep. Br. Trochisci Bismuthi.

CALCII CHLORIDUM. *U. S., Br. Chloride of Calcium.*

Ca Cl_2; 110·8. (CĂL′CI̦-Ī CHLŌ′RI̦-DŬM.) Ca Cl; 55·4.

"Chloride of Calcium, deprived of its water by fusion at a low red heat. It should be preserved in well-stopped bottles." *U. S.*

Calcaria Muriatica, Chloridum Calcicum; Muriate of Lime, Hydrochlorate of Lime; Chlorure de Calcium, Hydrochlorate de Chaux, *Fr.;* Chlorcalcium, Salzsaures Kalk, *G.*

Chloride of calcium consists of chlorine, united with calcium, the metallic radical

* "Take of Solution of Chloride of Calcium *five pints and a half;* Carbonate of Sodium *seventy-two troyounces;* Distilled Water *a sufficient quantity*. Dissolve the Carbonate of Sodium in six pints of Distilled Water. Heat this solution and the Solution of Chloride of Calcium, separately, to the boiling point, and mix them. After the precipitate has subsided, separate it from the supernatant liquid by decantation, and wash it with boiling Distilled Water until the washings cease to be affected by a solution of nitrate of silver. Lastly, dry the precipitate on bibulous paper." *U. S.* 1870.

of lime. It may be readily formed by saturating hydrochloric acid with chalk or marble, evaporating to dryness, and heating to redness. The hydrochloric acid, by reacting with the lime, forms chloride of calcium and water, the latter of which is dissipated at a red heat, $CaCO_3 + 2HCl = CaCl_2 + CO_2 + H_2O$. The Br. Pharmacopœia, after neutralizing the acid with carbonate of calcium, adds a little solution of chlorinated lime and slaked lime, filters, evaporates till the chloride becomes solid, and, instead of igniting the residue, dries it at about 204·4° C. (400° F.). Its composition is $CaCl_2,2H_2O$.

Properties. Chloride of calcium is in "colorless, slightly translucent, hard and friable masses, very deliquescent, odorless, having a hot, sharp, saline taste, and a neutral or faintly alkaline reaction. Soluble in 1·5 parts of water and 8 parts of alcohol at 15° C. (59° F.); very soluble in boiling water, and soluble in 1·5 parts of boiling alcohol. At a low red heat the salt fuses to an oily liquid which, on cooling, solidifies to a mass of the original appearance, entirely soluble in water. The aqueous solution yields, with test-solution of oxalate of ammonium, a white precipitate, soluble in hydrochloric but insoluble in acetic acid. With test-solution of nitrate of silver, it yields a white precipitate soluble in ammonia. The dilute aqueous solution should not be precipitated by water of ammonia (aluminium, iron, etc.), nor by test-solution of chloride of barium (sulphate). On adding to the aqueous solution, first, chloride of ammonium, then test-solution of carbonate of ammonium and water of ammonia in slight excess, and gently warming, the filtrate separated from the resulting precipitate should not be rendered more than faintly turbid by test-solution of phosphate of sodium (limit of magnesium)." *U. S.* On account of its avidity for water, the fused salt is used for drying gases. The crystallized salt is also very deliquescent, and has the form of colorless, transparent, striated, six-sided prisms. The crystals, on exposure to heat, first dissolve in their water of crystallization, and after this has evaporated, undergo the igneous fusion. With ice or snow they form a powerful frigorific mixture. "The salt evolves no chlorine or hypochlorous acid on the addition of hydrochloric acid, is entirely soluble in twice its weight of water, and is not precipitated by lime-water." *Br.* Chloride of calcium exists in the water of the ocean and of many springs. It is usually associated with common salt and chloride of magnesium, from which it is separated with difficulty. When crystallized it contains six molecules of water.

Chloride of calcium is used medicinally in solution only.*

CALCII HYDRAS. *Br.* *Hydrate of Calcium.*

(CĂL'CI̦-Ī HȲ'DRĂS.)

Calcis Hydras; Hydrate of Lime; Slaked Lime.

"Hydrate of calcium, $Ca(HO)_2$, with some impurities." *Br.*

"Take of Lime 2 pounds [av.]; Distilled Water 1 pint [Imp. meas.]. Place the lime in a metal pot, pour the water upon it, and when vapor ceases to be disengaged cover the pot with its lid and set it aside to cool. When the temperature has fallen to that of the atmosphere, put the slaked lime on an iron-wire sieve, and by gentle agitation cause the fine powder to pass through the sieve, rejecting what is left. Put the powder into a well-stoppered bottle, and keep it excluded as much as possible from the air. Slaked lime should be recently prepared." *Br.*

For an account of the physical and medical properties of this slaked lime, see *Calx.*

Off. Prep. Br. Liquor Calcis; Liquor Calcis Saccharatus.

CALCII HYPOPHOSPHIS. *U. S.* *Hypophosphite of Calcium.*

$Ca\,H_4\,(PO_2)_2$; 170. (CĂL'CI̦-Ī HȲ-PO̦-PHŎS'PHI̦S.) CaO, 2HO, PO; 85.

Calcis Hypophosphis; Hypophosphite of Lime; Calcaria Hypophosphorosa, Hypophosphis Calcicus; Hypophosphite de Chaux, *Fr.*; Unterphosphorigsaurer Kalk, *G.*

Attention has been called to the hypophosphites as a class of salts, in consequence of their recommendation by Dr. Churchill, of Paris, in the treatment of phthisis, in

* *Liquor Calcii Chloridi* was officinal in Pharm. 1870. A convenient method of making this preparation is to dissolve 228 grains of fused chloride of calcium in 1 fluidounce of distilled water and filter if necessary.

which they are thought to be useful by furnishing phosphorus to the tissues. One of the first papers on their mode of preparation and qualities was communicated by Prof. Procter. (See *A. J. P.*, xxx. 118.) Hypophosphorous acid consists of one atom of phosphorus, two of oxygen, and three of hydrogen, of which latter, however, only one is replaceable by metal. It is, therefore, a monobasic acid. It has a strong affinity for oxygen, and acts as a powerful deoxidizing or reducing agent, which property it is supposed to owe to the presence of the unreplaceable hydrogen atoms, sometimes termed "aldehydic" hydrogen. When heated, it is resolved into phosphuretted hydrogen and phosphoric acid. Its salts are generally soluble in water and deliquescent, and many of them are soluble in alcohol. They are converted into phosphates by heat, with the escape of phosphuretted hydrogen; and some of them are explosive.

Hypophosphite of calcium has attracted most attention, and would meet the views of those who wish to supply phosphate of calcium to the system, as the hypophosphorous acid is converted into the phosphoric by its deoxidizing power. To prepare it Prof. Procter gave the following formula. Slake 4 lbs. avoird. of lime with a gallon of water, add it, in a deep boiler, to 4 gallons of boiling water, and mix thoroughly. To the mixture add a pound (avoird.) of phosphorus, and continue the boiling, adding hot water from time to time to keep up the measure, until the combination is complete, and phosphuretted hydrogen is no longer evolved. It is necessary that provision should be made for the escape of the gas, which takes fire spontaneously in contact with the air. There are formed in the liquid, phosphate and hypophosphite of calcium, the phosphorus having become oxidized at the expense of the water, the hydrogen of which has escaped in combination with another portion of phosphorus, which is therefore lost. The liquid is filtered to separate the insoluble phosphate and residuary lime, then concentrated, and refiltered to separate the carbonate of calcium formed by the action of the air on a little lime held in solution, and lastly evaporated till a pellicle appears; after which the salt may be allowed to crystallize by setting the liquid aside, or may be obtained in the granular form by continuing the heat, and stirring. The salt should be introduced into bottles. The British Pharmacopœia has practically adopted this process, but any uncombined lime remaining in the solution is separated by passing carbonic acid gas through it.

Hypophosphite of calcium is "in colorless or white, six-sided prisms, or thin, flexible scales, of a pearly lustre, permanent in dry air, odorless, having a nauseous, bitter taste and a neutral reaction. Soluble in 6·8 parts of water at 15° C. (59° F.), and in 6 parts of boiling water; insoluble in alcohol. When heated in a dry test-tube, the salt decrepitates, gives off water, then evolves spontaneously-inflammable phosphoretted hydrogen, leaving a reddish residue which amounts to about 80 per cent. The aqueous solution yields, with test-solution of oxalate of ammonium, a white precipitate soluble in hydrochloric, but insoluble in acetic acid. Acidified with hydrochloric acid and added to excess of test-solution of mercuric chloride, it produces a white precipitate of mercurous chloride, and, on further addition, metallic mercury separates.

"When dissolved in water, the salt should leave no insoluble residue (insoluble salts of calcium). The aqueous solution should yield no precipitate with test-solution of acetate of lead (soluble phosphate), nor, after being acidulated with nitric acid, with test-solution of chloride of barium (soluble sulphate). On adding to the aqueous solution, first, chloride of ammonium, then test-solution of carbonate of ammonium and water of ammonia in slight excess, and gently warming, the filtrate separated from the resulting precipitate should not be rendered more than faintly turbid by test-solution of phosphate of sodium (limit of magnesium)." *U. S.* "Five grains boiled for ten minutes with a solution of twelve grains of permanganate of potassium yields, on filtration, a nearly colorless solution." *Br.*

The solubility of hypophosphite of calcium is increased by the addition of hypophosphorous acid. For a method of purifying alkaline hypophosphites, see *Journ. de Ph. d'Anvers*, 1879, p. 57; *N. R.*, 1879, p. 142.

As the soluble salts of mercury, copper, and silver are reduced by the hypophosphites, they are of course incompatible with it in prescriptions. With the hypophosphite of calcium, all the soluble sulphates and carbonates produce precipitates. As the hypophosphites are insoluble in cod-liver oil, they should be dissolved in syrup before being added to the oil. (See *Syrupus Calcii Hypophosphitis.*)

Medical Properties and Uses. The hypophosphite of calcium has been with the other hypophosphites strongly recommended in chronic phthisis, and is still much used; but the weight of testimony appears to be opposed to the first favorable impressions; and, though some cases may have seemed to be benefited, yet great care must be taken not to allow a reliance on the hypophosphites to interfere with the use of remedies known to be efficient, as cod-liver oil, and supporting measures generally. The remedy has also been highly commended in scrofulous diseases and in cases of defective nutrition of the nerve centres; but in most of these latter cases some direct preparation of phosphorus is probably superior, as it is not proven and not probable that the hypophosphites can yield up their phosphorus to the nerve centres. The dose of either of the hypophosphites is from ten to thirty grains (0·65–1·95 Gm.), three times a day.

Off. Prep. Syrupus Hypophosphitum.

CALCII PHOSPHAS PRÆCIPITATUS. *U.S.* *Precipitated Phosphate of Calcium.*

$Ca_3(PO_4)_2$; 310. (CĂL'CI-Ī PHŎS'PHĂS PRÆ-CĬP-I-TĀ'TŬS.) $3CaO, PO_5$; 155.

Calcis Phosphas, *Br.;* Phosphate of Calcium; Calcaria Phosphorica, *P. G.;* Phosphas Calcicus Præcipitatus; Précipitated Phosphate of Lime, Phosphate de Chaux hydraté, *Fr.;* Phosphorsaure Kalkerde, *G.*

A formula for this preparation was given in the U. S. Pharmacopœia of 1870.*

"Take of Bone Ash *four ounces* [avoirdupois]; Hydrochloric Acid *six fluidounces* [Imperial measure]; Water *two pints* [Imp. meas.]; Solution of Ammonia *twelve fluidounces* or *a sufficiency;* Distilled Water *a sufficiency.* Digest the Bone Ash in the Hydrochloric Acid diluted with a pint of Water, until it is dissolved. Boil for a few minutes; filter; add the remainder of the Water, and afterwards the Solution of Ammonia, until the mixture acquires an alkaline reaction; and, having collected the precipitate on a calico filter, wash it with boiling Distilled Water as long as the liquid which passes through occasions a precipitate, when dropped into solution of nitrate of silver acidulated with nitric acid. Dry the washed product at a temperature not exceeding 212° F. (100° C.)." *Br.*†

This preparation, whatever opinion may be entertained of its real powers, has been very properly retained in the U. S. Pharmacopœia, as it is considerably used, and is by some much esteemed. One of its more recent uses was to replace carbonate of magnesium in the process for medicated waters. Experience has shown, however, that its insolubility is not as great as supposed, and cotton has been substituted.

The hydrochloric acid dissolves the phosphate of calcium of the bones, and lets it fall, on the addition of ammonia, in a state of minute division. The ablution is intended to free it from adhering chloride of ammonium. The salt thus obtained is, for the sake of distinction, called *bone phosphate of calcium.* It is "a light, white, amorphous powder, permanent in the air, odorless, tasteless, and insoluble in water or alcohol. Wholly soluble in nitric or in hydrochloric acid without effervescence (abs. of carbonate). At an intense heat it is fusible without decomposition. A solution of the salt in diluted nitric acid, after being mixed with an excess of acetate of sodium, yields a white precipitate with test-solution of oxalate of ammo-

* "Take of Bone, calcined to whiteness, and in fine powder, *four troyounces;* Muriatic Acid *eight troyounces;* Water of Ammonia *twelve fluidounces,* or *a sufficient quantity;* Distilled Water *a sufficient quantity.* Macerate the Bone in the Acid, diluted with a pint of Distilled Water, until it is dissolved, and filter the solution. Add another pint of Distilled Water, and then, gradually, Water of Ammonia, until the liquid acquires an alkaline reaction. Mix the precipitate obtained, while yet in the state of magma, with twice its bulk of boiling Distilled Water, and pour the whole upon a strainer. Wash the precipitate with boiling Distilled Water until the washings cease to be affected by a solution of nitrate of silver, acidulated with nitric acid. Lastly, dry the precipitate with a gentle heat." *U. S.*

† For an apparatus for preparing *phosphate of calcium* on a large scale, see *Journ. de Pharm.,* Sept. 1, 1876, p. 193.

nium, and a lemon yellow precipitate with test-solution of ammonio-nitrate of silver. On dissolving 1 Gm. of the salt in hydrochloric acid, and subsequently adding water of ammonia, the salt is precipitated unaltered. The precipitate should yield nothing to a boiling solution of potassa (abs. of aluminium), and, when washed and dried, should weigh 1 Gm." *U. S.*

"Ten grains dissolve perfectly and without effervescence in diluted hydrochloric acid, and the solution yields with ammonia a white precipitate, insoluble in boiling solution of potash, and weighing nearly ten grains when washed and dried." *Br.*

Medical Uses. In the form of burnt hartshorn, phosphate of calcium formerly enjoyed a brief popularity in the treatment of rickets and mollities ossium, in which its use seemed to be indicated upon obvious chemical grounds. In 1851, Benecke suggested that, as it is essential in animals as well as plants to the formation of cells, it might be found useful in certain pathological states of the system characterized by defective nutrition, such as the scrofulous affections, and from that time its use has gradually become more frequent, and, in connection with other phosphates, as those of iron, sodium, and potassium, it has acquired no little reputation in different forms of scrofula, mollities ossium, rickets, and even chronic phthisis. It is also thought to have proved useful by hastening the union of fractured bones; and M. Alphonse Milne-Edwards is said to have shown, by experiments upon dogs and rabbits, that, in these animals, the callus in fractured bones forms more quickly under its use than without it. (*Med. Times and Gaz.*, May, 1856, p. 489.) Though insoluble in water, it is probably in general dissolved by the gastric liquids, in consequence of the acid present in them; but it is best administered in acid solution, and is at present very extensively used dissolved in lactic acid and emulsified with cod-liver oil. The dose is from ten to thirty grains (0·65–1·95 Gm.).

Off. Prep. Syrupus Calcii Lactophosphatis.

Off. Prep. Br. Pulvis Antimonialis.

CALCII SULPHAS. *Br. Sulphate of Calcium.*

(CĂL'CI-Ī SŬL'PHĂS.)

Calcis Sulphas; Sulphate of Lime; Gypsum; Plaster of Paris.

"Native sulphate of calcium ($CaSO_4,2H_2O$) rendered nearly anhydrous by heat." *Br.*

The native sulphate is known as *gypsum*, and in its massive variety as *alabaster*. When powdered gypsum is carefully heated to 110°–120° C. it loses its water of crystallization and becomes *plaster of Paris*. This is capable of uniting with water again and solidifying, a property largely applied in practice, as in making plaster casts or models, and somewhat in surgery.

Medical Properties and Uses. Gypsum is used by surgeons for mechanical purposes, and not at all in internal medicine. It is so slightly soluble in water that it may be considered for ordinary purposes insoluble. According to Bucholz, it is soluble in 460 parts of water cold or hot, according to Giese, in 380 parts of cold and 388 of boiling water. Notwithstanding the statement of Bucholz, the fact has been well established that its solubility varies with the temperature, but, like that of sulphate of sodium, very unequally. Thus, according to M. Poggiale, it is greatest at 35° C. (95° F.), and above or below that temperature gradually diminishes, so that at 100° C. (212° F.), or the boiling point of water, it is very nearly the same as at 5° (41° F.), not far from the freezing point. (*Journ. de Pharm.*, 4e sér., v. 86.) The other point is that, when deprived of its water by heat, and reduced to the state of a white powder, it rapidly absorbs water added to it, and from the state of semi-liquid paste into which it is brought with that fluid, quickly hardens without change of bulk. It is this property which fits plaster of Paris so well for all kinds of moulding; and to this also it owes its peculiar adaptability to the purpose of a splint. To prepare it for use, the gypsum must first be deprived of the greater part of its water by exposure to a heat of 100° C. (212° F.), or from that to 121·1° C. (250° F.). It loses both its molecules of water of crystallization at a temperature of from 110°–120° C. (230°–248° F.), and is then known as *burnt gypsum*. If heated above 205° C. (401° F.) it becomes *dead-burnt*, and does not take up water readily and does not harden. When dehydrated, it is reduced to fine powder, and kept in air-tight vessels for use. As thus prepared, if mixed with two parts of water, it forms a semi-liquid cream-like mass, which becomes solid and hard in fifteen or twenty minutes, the temperature rising during the process, as in the slaking of lime. The hydrated gypsum expands in solidifying, hence its advantages in preparing casts,—the expansion causes it to fill accurately all interstices. According to Mr. T. E. Stark, a medical officer in the British army, flannel is the best material for bandages to be used with gypsum. It should be cut into strips an inch and a half broad and two or three yards long, which should first be spread on a table and rubbed well with the powdered gypsum on both sides, and always in the direction of the thread. The bandages should then be rolled up loosely, and kept for use in air-tight cases. Thus applied, the bandages, first thoroughly wetted, should be rolled round the limb, overlapping at the edges, so as to make a uniform covering. After application, it should be left to harden, which generally happens in fifteen or twenty minutes. A simpler method of using the gypsum for this purpose is, after the application of the bandages, to paint the whole thoroughly and carefully with the milk of gypsum, which will solidify, and enclose the part in a firm case.

Off. Prep. Br. Calx Sulphurata.

CALENDULA. *U. S.* *Calendula.* [*Marigold.*]

(CĄ-LĔN'DŪ-LĄ.)

"The fresh, flowering herb of Calendula officinalis. Linné. (*Nat. Ord.* Compositæ.)" *U. S.*

Fleurs de Tous les mois, Souci, *Fr.;* Ringelblume, *G.*

Gen. Ch. Flower-head heterogamous, rayed, with the female flowers of the ray fertile, in one or two rows, the hermaphrodite of the disk sterile. *Involucre* broad, with linear, acuminate, subequal, often scarious bracts in one or two rows. *Receptacle* flat, naked. *Corolla* of female flowers ligulate, with the lamina entire or three dentate. Hermaphrodite flowers, regular, tubular, with an enlarged limb shortly five cut at the apex. *Anthers* sagittate, with the auricles setaceous-mucronate or caudate. *Style* of the hermaphrodite flower undivided. *Achenia* bare; those of the ray incurved, 2-3 serrate, heteromorphous usually upon the back, or everywhere muricate; the outer often elongate, linear, sometimes empty; the intermediate broader, often alate; the interior shorter, more incurved; those of the disk thin, smooth, empty. (Bentham & Hooker, *Genera Plantarum*, ii. 454.)

Calendula officinalis. L. The common marigold of the gardens is too well known to need description, other than that of the Pharmacopœia.

Properties. "Stem somewhat angular, rough; leaves alternate, thickish, hairy, spatulate or oblanceolate, slightly toothed, the upper ones sessile; flower-heads nearly two inches (5 cm.) broad, the yellow strap-shaped ray-florets in one or several rows, fertile, the achenes incurved and muricate; odor slightly narcotic; taste bitter and saline." *U. S.* The odor is much stronger in the fresh than in the dry herb, and, on exposure to the sun, the yellow color fades into whitish. Among its constituents is a peculiar principle, called *calendulin*, discovered by Geiger most abundantly in the flowers, and considered by Berzelius as analogous to bassorin, though soluble in alcohol. *French* or *African Marigold*, so called, is very frequently substituted for the officinal drug. It is the *Tagetes patula L.* and *T. erecta*, Lin., both of Mexico. The flowers are readily distinguished by the scales of the involucre being united to form a tube, and by the slender, flattish achenes being crowned with a few chaffy or awned scales. The broadly strap-shaped ray-florets are toothed, and light or deep orange color sometimes striped with red.

Medical Properties and Uses. The medical properties of this new officinal are probably very feeble, if indeed they be not altogether apocryphal. In the days of therapeutic darkness the plant was thought to be antispasmodic, sudorific, deobstruent, and emmenagogue, and was given in low forms of fever, scrofula, jaundice, amenorrhœa, etc. Both the leaves and flowers were used; but the latter were preferred, and were usually administered in the recent state in the form of tea. An extract was also prepared, and employed in cancerous and other ulcers, sick stomach, etc. The tincture has been used to a considerable extent as an embrocation in sprains, bruises, etc., and probably is of as much value as simple alcohol.

Off. Prep. Tinctura Calendulæ.

CALUMBA. *U. S.* *Calumba.* [*Columbo.*]

(CĄ-LŬM'BĄ.)

"The root of Jateorrhiza Calumba. Miers. (*Nat. Ord.* Menispermaceæ.)" *U. S.* "The dried transversely cut slices of the root of Jateorrhiza Calumba, *Miers; Cocculus palmatus, D. C.*" *Br.*

Calumbæ Radix, *Br.;* Radix Colombo, *P. G.;* Radix Columbo; Colomba, *U. S.* 1850; Colombo, *Fr.;* Columbowursel, *G.;* Columba, *It.;* Raiz de Columbo, *Sp.;* Kalumbo, *Port.;* Calumb, *Mozambique.*

The columbo plant was long but imperfectly known. Flowering specimens of a plant gathered by Commerson, about the year 1770, in the garden of M. Poivre in the Isle of France, and sent to Europe with that botanist's collection, were examined by Lamarck, and described under the name of *Menispermum palmatum.* But its original locality was unknown, and it was only conjectured to be the source of columbo. In the year 1805, M. Forten, while engaged in purchasing the drug in Mozambique, obtained possession of a living offset of the root, which, being taken to Madras, and planted in the garden of Dr. Anderson, produced a male plant, which was figured and described by Dr. Berry. From the drawing thus made, the plant was referred to the natural family of the Menispermaceæ; but, as the female flowers were wanting, some difficulty was experienced in fixing its precise botanical position. De Candolle, who probably had the opportunity of examining Commerson's specimens, gave its generic and specific character; but confessed that he was not acquainted with the structure of the female flower and fruit. This desideratum, however, was supplied by ample drawings sent to England by Mr. Telfair, of Mauritius, made from plants which were propagated from roots obtained by Captain Owen in 1825, while prosecuting his survey of the eastern coast of Africa. The plant was first placed in the genus Cocculus, which was separated by De Candolle from Menispermum. Subsequently, Mr. J. Miers established a new genus, which has been received by botanists, giving to it the name of Jateorrhiza. M. Miers also separated his plant specifically from *C. palmatus* of De Candolle, describing it under the name of *Jateorrhiza Calumba.* This species is now recognized by both the U. S. and Br. Pharmacopœias. But the very careful researches of Mr. Hanbury (*Pharmacographia*, 2d ed., p. 23) have led him to consider the specific differences as unimportant and inconstant. These differences are that in *J. palmata* "the lobes at the base of the leaf overlap, and the male inflorescence is nearly glabrous; while in *J. Calumba* the basal lobes are rounded, but do not overlap, and the male inflorescence is setose-hispid." The plants are probably only varieties of one species, and it is almost certain that columbo is derived from each of them.

Gen. Ch. *Sepals* 6, in two rows, somewhat unequal, thin. *Petals* 6, shorter than the sepals. Male flowers: *Stamens* 6, free, with the apex recurved-clavate. *Anthers* unilocular with the apex extrorse, dehiscent by a transverse cleft. Female flowers: *Carpels* 3, with lacerate, reflex stigmata. *Drupe* ovoid with a subterminal cicatrix of the style. *Putamen* somewhat concave in its inner face. *Seed* meniscoid; albumen fleshy, ruminate; embryo somewhat curved. *Cotyledons* laterally bivaricate." (Bentham and Hooker, *Genera Plantarum*, i. 34.)

"The plants of this genus, natives of intertropical Africa, are all climbers, distinguished by a very peculiar habit, having very large deeply-lobed leaves, upon very long petioles, and clothed with long strigose hairs; their inflorescence is in long slender racemes; the fruit is a drupe containing a putamen covered with a dense hairy coating imbedded in the fleshy mesoderm." (*Ann. Mag. Nat. Hist.*, Feb. 1864.)

Cocculus palmatus. De Cand. *Syst. Veg.* i. 523; Woodv. *Med. Bot.* 3d ed., v. 21; Hooker, *Curtis's Bot. Mag.*, Nos. 2970, 2971. *Jateorrhiza palmata.* Miers, *Annals and Mag. of Nat. Hist.*, Feb. 1864, p. 183. *B. & T.* 13. This is a climbing plant, with a perennial root, consisting of several fasciculated, fusiform, somewhat curved, and descending tubers, as thick as an infant's arm. The stems, of which one or two proceed from the same root, are twining, simple in the male plant, branched in the female, round, hairy, and about as thick as the little finger. The leaves, which stand on rounded, glandular hairy footstalks, are alternate, distant, cordate, with three, five, or seven entire, acuminate, wavy, somewhat hairy lobes, and as many nerves, each running into one of the lobes. The flowers are small and inconspicuous, and arranged in solitary axillary racemes, which, in the male plant, are compound, in the female, simple, and in both, shorter than the leaves.

Jateorrhiza Calumba. Miers. Br. Pharm.—*Cocculus palmatus.* Wallich, non De Cand.—*Menispermum Columba.* Roxb. *Flor. Ind.* This species is characterized by "rounded, angularly striate, roughly pilose branches; broadly orbicular, sinuously lobed leaves, with rounded sinuses; the lobes being 5 in number, broadly ovate, acute, mucronately acuminate; the basal deeply divaricate and hence broadly cordate; 7 to 9 nerved, opaque above, on both sides furnished with short, adpressed, somewhat curved, reddish hairs, beneath, pale, strongly reticulate with prominent nerves and veins; the petiole somewhat slender, striate, tortuous, and roughly glandular; the racemes axillary, solitary or many; the rachis greatly elongated, striate, bristly, with elongated, smooth, divaricate, almost capillary, subflexuous, few-flowered branches; the flowers sessile, and almost without bracts." (*Miers.*)

Both of these so-called species are natives of Mozambique, on the south-eastern coast of Africa, where they grow wild in great abundance in the thick forests extending from the sea many miles into the interior. They are not cultivated. The root is dug up in March, when dry weather prevails. From the base of the root numerous fusiform offsets proceed, less fibrous and woody than the parent stock. These offsets are separated and cut into transverse slices, which are dried in the shade. The old root is rejected.

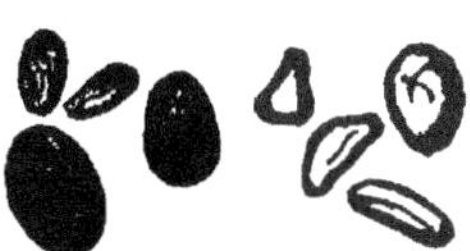
Magnified starch granules of calumba root.

Columbo is a staple export of the Portuguese from their dominions in the south-east of Africa. It is taken to India, and thence distributed. It was formerly supposed to be a product of Ceylon, and to have derived its name from Colombo, a city of that island, from which it was thought to be exported. It is possible that, when the Portuguese were in possession of Ceylon, Colombo may have been the entrepot for the drug brought from Africa, and thus have given origin to its name. Some, however, consider a more probable derivation to be from the word *calumb*, which is said to be the Mozambique name for the root. Dr. Christison has been misinformed in relation to the cultivation of the true columbo plant in this country. (*Dispensatory*, Am. ed., p. 304.)

Properties. "In nearly circular disks, one and one-fifth to two and two-fifths inches (3 to 6 cm.) in diameter, yellowish gray, depressed in the centre, with two or three interrupted circles of projecting wood-bundles, distinctly radiate in the outer portion; fracture short, mealy; odor slight; taste mucilaginous, slightly aromatic, persistently bitter." *U. S.* Along with the disks are sometimes a few cylindrical pieces an inch or two in length. The cortical portion is thick, of a bright yellow, slightly greenish color internally, but covered with a brownish, wrinkled epidermis. The interior or medullary portion, which is readily distinguishable from the cortical, is light, spongy, yellowish, usually more or less shrunk, so that the pieces are thinnest in the centre; and is often marked with concentric circles and radiating lines. Those pieces are to be preferred which have the brightest color, are most compact and uniform, and least worm-eaten. The odor of columbo is slightly aromatic. The taste is very bitter, that of the cortical much more so than that of the central portion, which is somewhat mucilaginous. The root is easily pulverized. The powder is greenish, becoming browner with age, and deepening when moistened. As it attracts moisture from the air, and is apt to undergo decomposition, it should be prepared in small quantities.

M. Planche analyzed columbo in 1811, and found it to contain a nitrogenous substance, probably albumen, in large quantity, a bitter yellow substance not precipitated by metallic salts, and one-third of its weight of starch. He obtained also a small proportion of volatile oil, salts of lime and potassa, oxide of iron, and silica. Wittstock, of Berlin, afterwards isolated a principle, which he called *colombin.* This crystallizes in beautiful transparent quadrilateral prisms of the formula $C_{21}H_{22}O_7$, is without smell, and is extremely bitter. It is but very slightly soluble in water, alcohol, or ether, at ordinary temperatures, and yet imparts to these fluids a strongly bitter taste. It is more soluble in boiling alcohol, which deposits it upon cooling. The best solvent is dilute acetic acid. It is taken up by alkaline solutions, from which it is precipitated by acids. It has neither acid nor alkaline properties, and its alcoholic and acetic solutions are not affected by the metallic salts, or the infusion of galls. It is obtained by exhausting columbo by means of alcohol of the sp. gr. 0·835, distilling off three-quarters of the alcohol, allowing the residue to stand for some days till crystals are deposited, and lastly treating these crystals with alcohol and animal charcoal. The mother-waters still contain a considerable quantity of colombin, which may be separated by evaporating with coarsely powdered glass to dryness, exhausting the residue with ether, distilling off the ether, treating the residue with boiling acetic acid, and evaporating the solution to crystallization.

P. E. Alessandri isolated *calumbine*, which he considers an alkaloid, by the following process. An infusion of columbo is made with a 3 per cent. solution of oxalic acid; the yellow bitter liquid is neutralized with ammonia and evaporated to one-third its bulk; it is, when cooled, treated with ether, separated, and the ethereal solution on evaporation yields pure white calumbine. (*L'Orosi*, v. 1; *P. J. Tr.*, 1882, p. 995.)

From the researches of Dr. Bödeker it appears that another bitter principle exists in columbo, which corresponds in composition and chemical relations with *berberine*, the active principle of *Berberis vulgaris*, and is assumed to be identical with that substance. It was obtained by exhausting columbo with alcohol of 0·889, distilling off the alcohol, allowing the residual liquor to stand for three days so as to deposit the columbin, evaporating the supernatant liquid together with the aqueous washings of the colombin to dryness, exhausting the residue with boiling alcohol of 0·863, treating the solution thus obtained as the former one, submitting the residue to the action of the boiling water, filtering and adding hydrochloric acid, collecting the precipitate thus formed on a filter, drying it with bibulous paper, and finally, in order to separate adhering acid, dissolving it in alcohol, and precipitating with ether. The result was an imperfectly crystalline, bright yellow powder, of a disagreeable, bitter taste, supposed to be *berberine hydrochlorate.* It is stated that berberine is present in columbo in much larger proportion than columbin, and being freely soluble in hot water and alcohol, while columbin is but slightly so, is probably more largely extracted in the ordinary liquid preparations of the root. (*A. J. P.*, xx. 322.) A third constituent, *columbic acid*, was also discovered by Bödeker. It is yellow, amorphous, nearly insoluble in cold water, but dissolving in alcohol and in alkaline solutions. It tastes somewhat less bitter than *columbin.* Bödeker surmises that it may exist in combination with the berberine, and has pointed out a connection between the three bitter principles of columbo. If we suppose a molecule of ammonia, NH_3, to be added to two molecules of *columbin*, $C_{21}H_{22}O_7$, the complex molecule thence resulting will contain the elements of *berberine*, $C_{20}H_{17}NO_4$, *columbic acid*, $C_{22}H_{24}O_7$, and water, $3H_2O$. (*Pharmacographia*, p. 25.) Alessandri obtains *berberine* from columbo by neutralizing a cold infusion, made with diluted oxalic acid (3 per cent.), with baryta; the precipitate which is produced is separated. The liquid is heated, allowed to stand for twenty-four hours to allow the barium oxalate to deposit, filtered, and then a current of carbonic acid is passed through to remove baryta. It is then treated by shaking the ammoniacal liquid with ether as in Alessandri's process for calumbine (see above), and, after the ethereal layer is separated, the aqueous liquid is evaporated to dryness. Berberine is obtained from the extract by treating the latter with alcohol, the berberine being purified by washing with ether. *Calumbic acid* may be obtained from the precipitate produced by the addition of baryta to the oxalic acid infusion. (*L'Orosi*, v. 1; *P. J. Tr.*, 1882, p. 995.)

There can be little doubt that both columbin and berberine contribute to the remedial effects of columbo. The virtues of the root are extracted by boiling water and by alcohol. Precipitates are produced with the infusion and tincture by infusion of galls, and solutions of acetate and subacetate of lead; but the bitterness is not affected.

Adulterations. It is said that the root of *white bryony*, tinged yellow with the tincture of columbo, has sometimes been fraudulently substituted for the genuine root; but the adulteration is too gross to deceive those acquainted with the characters of either of these drugs. American columbo, which is the root of *Frasera Walteri*, is said to have been sold in some parts of Europe for the genuine. Independently of the sensible differences between the two roots (see *Frasera*), M. Stolze, of Halle, states that, while the tincture of columbo remains unaffected by the sulphate or sesquichloride of iron, and gives a dirty-gray precipitate with tincture of galls, the tincture of frasera acquires a dark green color with the former reagent, and is not affected by the latter. (*Duncan.*) Under the name of *columbo wood*, or *false columbo*, the wood of *Coscinium fenestratum*, a plant of the family of Menispermaceæ, growing in Ceylon, has been imported into England, and offered for sale in the drug market. (*P. J. Tr.*, x. 321, and xii. 185.)

Medical Properties and Uses. Columbo is among the most useful of the mild tonics. Without astringency, with very little stimulating power, and generally acceptable to the stomach, it answers admirably as a remedy in simple dyspepsia, and in the debility of convalescence, especially when the alimentary canal is left enfeebled. Hence, it is often prescribed in the declining stages of remittent fever, dysentery, diarrhœa, cholera morbus, and cholera infantum. The absence of irritating properties renders it also an appropriate tonic in the hectic fever of phthisis, and kindred affections. It has been highly recommended in vomiting, unconnected with inflammation of the stomach, as in the sickness of pregnant women. It is frequently administered in combination with other tonics, aromatics, mild cathartics, and antacids. A favorite remedy of Dr. Geo. B. Wood for the permanent cure of a disposition to the accumulation of flatus in the bowels, was an infusion made with half an ounce of columbo, half an ounce of ginger, a drachm of senna, and a pint of boiling water, and given in the dose of a wineglassful three times a day. Columbo is much used by the natives of Mozambique in dysentery and other diseases. (*Berry.*) It was first introduced to the notice of the profession in Europe by François Redi, in the year 1685. It is most commonly prescribed in the state of infusion. (See *Infusum Calumbæ.*) The dose of the powder is from ten to thirty grains (0·65–1·95 Gm.), and may be repeated three or four times a day. It is frequently combined with powdered ginger, subcarbonate of iron, and rhubarb.

Off. Prep. Extractum Calumbæ Fluidum; Tinctura Calumbæ.

Off. Prep. Br. Extractum Calumbæ; Infusum Calumbæ; Mistura Ferri Aromatica; Tinctura Calumbæ.

CALX. *U. S., Br.* *Lime.*

Ca O; 56. (CALX.) Ca, O; 28.

"An alkaline earth, oxide of calcium, CaO, with some impurities, obtained by calcining chalk or limestone so as to expel carbonic acid." *Br.*

Calcaria Usta, *P.G.;* Calcaria, Calx Viva, Calx Usta, Oxydum Calcicum; Burned Lime; Quicklime; Chaux, Chaux vive, *Fr.;* Kalk, Gebrannter Kalk, *G.;* Calce, *It.;* Calvira, *Sp.*

Lime, which is ranked among the alkaline earths, is a very important pharmaceutical agent, and forms the principal ingredient in several standard preparations. It is a very abundant natural production. It is never found free, but mostly combined with acids; as with carbonic acid in chalk, marble, calcareous spar, limestone, and shells; with sulphuric acid in the different kinds of gypsum, with phosphoric acid in the bones of animals; and with silica in a great variety of minerals.

Preparation. Lime is prepared by calcining, by a strong heat, some form of the native carbonate. The carbonic acid is thus expelled, and the lime remains. When the lime is intended for nice chemical operations, it should be obtained from pure white marble or oyster shells. For the purpose of the arts it is procured from common limestone, by calcining it in kilns of peculiar construction. When obtained in this way it is generally impure, being of a grayish color, and containing alumina, silica, sesquioxide of iron, and occasionally a little magnesia and oxide of manganese.

The officinal lime of the United States and British Pharmacopœias is the lime of commerce, and therefore impure. It may be obtained purer by exposing pure white marble, broken into small fragments, in a covered crucible, to a full red heat for three hours, or till the residuum, when slaked and suspended in water, no longer effervesces on the addition of hydrochloric acid.

Properties. Lime is in "hard, white or grayish white masses, gradually attracting moisture and carbonic acid gas on exposure to air and falling to a white powder, odorless, having a sharp, caustic taste and an alkaline reaction. Soluble in 750 parts of water at 15° C. (59° F.) and in 1300 parts of boiling water; insoluble in alcohol. When heated to a white heat, lime is neither fused nor altered. Brought in contact with about half its weight of water, it absorbs the latter, becomes heated and is gradually converted into a white powder (slaked lime). Lime mixed with water to a thin milk, should be dissolved by nitric acid with but little effervescence (limit of carbonate), and without leaving more than a slight residue of insoluble matter. Lime should be preserved in well-closed vessels, in a dry place. Distilled water agitated with slaked lime should give the reactions mentioned under *Liquor Calcis.*" *U.S.*

Lime is the oxide of calcium, and consists of one atom of calcium 40, and one of oxygen 16. Its sp. gr. is 3·08, whilst the hydrate has the sp. gr. 2·078. (*Filhol.*) Its solubility in water is greatly increased by the addition of sugar or glycerin. (See *Syrupus Calcis.*) It is distinguished from the other alkaline earths by forming a very deliquescent salt (*chloride of calcium*) by reaction with hydrochloric acid, and a sparingly soluble one with sulphuric acid. All acids, acidulous, ammoniacal, and metallic salts, borates, alkaline carbonates, and astringent vegetable infusions are incompatible with it.

Medical Properties. Lime acts externally as an escharotic, and was formerly applied to ill-conditioned ulcers. The *lime ointment* of Spender is made by incorporating four parts of washed slaked lime with one part of fresh lard and three parts of olive oil, previously warmed together. Mixed with potassa, lime forms an officinal caustic. (See *Potassa cum Calce.*) As an internal remedy, it is always administered in solution. (See *Liquor Calcis.*)

Off. Prep. and Pharm. Uses. Liquor Calcis; Syrupus Calcis; Potassa cum Calce; Calx Sulphurata; Chloroformum Purificatum; Liquor Potassæ; Liquor Sodæ; Sulphur Præcipitata.

Off. Prep. Br. Calcii Hydras.

CALX CHLORATA. *U.S.* *Chlorinated Lime.*

(CĂLX CHLO-RĀ'TA.)

Calx Chlorinata, *Pharm.* 1870. *Br.* Chloride of Lime. "A compound resulting from the action of Chlorine upon Hydrate of Calcium, and containing at least 25 per cent. of available Chlorine." *U.S.* "A product obtained by exposing slaked lime to the action of chlorine gas so long as the latter is absorbed." *Br.*

"Chloride of Lime should be preserved in well-closed vessels, in a cool and dry place." *U.S.*

Hypochlorite of Lime or Calcium, Oxymuriate of Lime or Calcium, Bleaching Powder; Calcaria Chlorata, *P.G.;* Chloris Calcicus, Chloruretum Calcis, Calcis Chloridum, Calcii Hypochloris, *Lat.;* Chlorure de Chaux, Poudre de Tennant ou de Knox, *Fr.;* Chlorkalk, Bleichkalk, *G.;* Cloruro di Calce, *It.*

This compound was originally prepared and brought into notice as a bleaching agent, in 1798, by Tennant, of Glasgow. Subsequently it was found to have valuable properties as a medicine and disinfectant; and, accordingly, it has been introduced into the United States and British Pharmacopœias.

The following is an outline of the process for preparing chlorinated lime on the large scale. A rectangular chamber is constructed, generally of silicious sandstone, the joints being secured by a cement of pitch, rosin, and dry gypsum. At one end it is furnished with an air-tight door, and on each side with a glass window, to enable the operator to inspect the process during its progress. The slaked or hydrated lime is sifted, and placed on wooden trays eight or ten feet long, two broad, and one inch deep. These are piled within the chamber to a height of five or six feet on cross-bars, by which they are kept about an inch asunder, in order to favor the circulation of the gas over the lime. The chlorine is generated in a leaden vessel nearly spherical, the lower portion of which is surrounded with an iron case, leaving an interstice two inches wide, intended to receive the steam for the purpose of producing the requisite heat. In the leaden vessel are five apertures. The first is in the centre of the top, and receives a tube which descends nearly to the bottom, and through which a vertical stirrer passes, intended to mix the materials, and furnished, at the lower end, with horizontal cross-bars of iron, or of wood sheathed with lead. The second is for the introduction of the common salt and manganese. The third admits a siphon-shaped funnel, through which the sulphuric acid is introduced. The fourth is connected with a pipe to lead off the chlorine. The fifth, which is near the bottom, receives a discharge-pipe, passing through the iron case, and intended for drawing off the residuum of the operation. The pipe leading off the chlorine terminates, under water, in a leaden chest or cylinder, where the gas is washed from hydrochloric acid. From this intermediate vessel the chlorine finally passes, by means of a pretty large leaden pipe, through the ceiling of the chamber containing the lime. The process of impregnation generally lasts four days, this time being necessary to form a good bleaching powder. If it be hastened, heat will be generated, which will favor the production of chloride of calcium, with a proportional diminution of chloride of lime.

The proportions of the materials generally adopted are 10 cwt. of common salt, mixed with from 10 to 14 cwt. of manganese dioxide: to which are added, in successive portions, from 12 to 14 cwt. of strong sulphuric acid, diluted before being used until its sp. gr. is about 1·65, which is accomplished by adding about one-third of its weight of water. In factories in which sulphuric acid is also made, the acid intended for this process is brought to the sp. gr. 1·65 only, whereby the expense of further concentration is saved.

The importation of "bleaching powder" into the United States for the year 1887 was 103,087,827 lbs.

Properties. Chlorinated lime is "a white or grayish white, dry, or but slightly damp powder, or friable lumps, becoming moist and gradually decomposing on exposure to air, having a feeble, chlorine-like odor, and a disagreeable, saline taste. It is partially soluble in water and in alcohol. On dissolving Chlorinated Lime in diluted hydrochloric acid, chlorine gas is given off, and there should not remain more than a trifling amount of insoluble matter. Its solution in diluted acetic acid yields, with test-solution of oxalate of ammonium, a white precipitate soluble in hydrochloric acid. The aqueous solution quickly destroys the color of a dilute solution of litmus or of indigo." *U. S.* When perfectly saturated with chlorine it dissolves almost entirely in water. When exposed to heat, it gives off oxygen, and some chlorine, and is converted into chloride of calcium. It is incompatible with the mineral acids, carbonic acids, and the alkaline carbonates. The acids evolve chlorine copiously, and the alkaline carbonates cause a precipitate of carbonate of calcium. (See *Liquor Sodæ Chlorinatæ.*)*

Chlorinated lime is an oxidizing agent, the oxygen being derived from water, the hydrogen of which unites with the chlorine to form hydrochloric acid. It has a

* Chlorinated lime is constantly becoming weaker on exposure, giving off chlorine or hypochlorous acid, probably through the influence of the atmospheric carbonic acid, which sets them free by combining with the lime. But it would seem that, even when closely confined, it sometimes at least gives off gaseous matter, as we have an account of a well-stopped bottle containing it having been broken by a violent explosion, without any peculiar exposure to heat. (See *A. J. P.*, 1861, p. 72.) M. Barreswil has found that the subjection of chlorinated lime to strong pressure greatly diminishes the tendency to decomposition. It is rendered in this way as hard as a stone, and may be kept long without undergoing change. (*Chem. News*, No. 58, p. 33.)

powerful action on organic matter, converting sugar, starch, cotton, linen, and similar substances into formic acid, which unites with the lime. (*W. Bastick.*) It also acts energetically on the volatile oils, including oil of turpentine, producing chloroform. (J. Chautart, *Journ. de Pharm.*, Mars, 1855.)

Composition. The composition of bleaching powder is represented by the formula $CaOCl_2$, and it was formerly supposed to be a direct compound of lime with chlorine. This view, however, is not consistent with its reactions, for when distilled with dilute nitric acid it readily yields a distillate of aqueous hypochlorous acid, and when treated with water it is resolved into chloride and hypochlorite of calcium, the latter of which may be separated in crystals by exposing the filtered solution to a freezing mixture, or by evaporating it in a vacuum over oil of vitriol, and leaving the dense frozen mass to thaw upon a filter. A solution of calcium chloride mixed with hypochlorite then passes through, and feathery crystals remain on the filter, very unstable, but consisting, when recently prepared, of hydrated calcium hypochlorite, $Ca(OCl)_2 4H_2O$. These results seem at first sight to show that the bleaching powder is a mixture of chloride and hypochlorite of calcium, formed according to the equation $2CaO + Cl_4 = CaCl_2 + Ca(ClO)_2$; but if this were its true constitution, the powder when digested with alcohol ought to yield a solution of calcium chloride containing half the chlorine of the original compound, which is not the case. Its constitution is, therefore, better represented by the formula $Ca\left\{\begin{matrix}Cl\\OCl\end{matrix}\right.$, suggested by Dr. Odling, this molecule being decomposed by water into chloride and hypochlorite in the manner just explained, and yielding with dilute nitric acid or sulphuric acid a distillate containing hydrochloric and hypochlorous acids, $CaCl(OCl) + 2HNO_3 = Ca(NO_3)_2 + HCl + HClO$. (Lunge and Schaeppi, *A. J. P.*, Dec. 1881, p. 608, and Lunge and Naef, *Ber. der Chem. Ges.*, 1883, p. 840.)*

Impurities and Tests. Chlorinated lime may contain a great excess of lime, from imperfect impregnation with the gas. This defect will be shown by the large proportion insoluble in water. If it contain much chloride of calcium, it will be quite moist, which is always a sign of inferior quality. When long and insecurely kept, it deteriorates from the gradual formation of chloride of calcium and carbonate of calcium. Several methods have been proposed for determining its bleaching power, which depends solely on the proportion of loosely combined chlorine. Walter proposed to add a solution of the bleaching powder to a standard solution of sulphate of indigo, in order to ascertain its decolorizing power; but the objection to this test is that the indigo of commerce is very variable in its amount of coloring matter. The oxidation of an arsenious acid solution is largely used in practice. Lunge (*Ber. der Chem. Ges.*, 1886, p. 869) has also proposed to use hydrogen peroxide (H_2O_2) solution for the valuation of bleaching powder. The two solutions both liberate oxygen in exactly equal amount. This is measured in a nitrometer. According to Wittstein and Claude, the test of sulphate of iron, which was formerly officinal, is not reliable. The present volumetric method, which is based upon that of the British Pharmacopœia, is preferred. "If 0·71 Gm. of Chlorinated Lime be mixed with a solution of 1·25 Gm. of iodide of potassium in 120 C.c. of water, and 9 Gm. of diluted hydrochloric acid be then added, the red-brown liquid should require for complete decoloration not less than 50 C.c. of the volumetric solution of hyposulphite of sodium." *U. S.*

The following is the test given in the British Pharmacopœia. "When fresh, five grains mixed with fifteen grains of iodide of potassium, and dissolved in four fluidounces of water, produces, when acidulated with one fluidrachm of hydrochloric acid, a reddish solution, which requires for the discharge of its color at least 467 grain-measures of the volumetric solution of hyposulphite of sodium, corresponding

* According to Lunge's investigations, the best temperature for the absorption of chlorine by the calcium hydrate is 40°–45° C.; from pure calcium hydrate a bleaching powder of 43 per cent. active chlorine can be gotten, in which case allowance for 4 per cent. of moisture in the hydrate is made; strong mineral acids, when not used in excess, liberate only hypochlorous acid; dry carbon dioxide at normal temperature does not set free any chlorine, but at moderately elevated temperature drives off almost all the chlorine.

to 33 per cent. of available chlorine." In this process iodine is separated by the chlorine in equivalent quantity, and imparts color to the liquid, which is removed by the hyposulphite of sodium, by forming colorless compounds with the iodine; and the quantity required for this purpose measures the quantity of iodine, and consequently that of the chlorine present in the chlorinated solution. (See *Sodii Hyposulphis.*)

Medical Properties and Uses. Chlorinated lime, externally applied, is a desiccant and disinfectant, and has been used with advantage in solution, as an application to ill-conditioned ulcers, burns, chilblains, and cutaneous eruptions, especially itch; as a gargle in putrid sore throat; and as a wash for the mouth to disinfect the breath, and for ulcerated gums. Internally, it is stimulant and alterative. It has been used to some extent internally, in adynamic dysentery, typhus fever, and various other low diseases: it may be considered as therapeutically equivalent to chlorine. The dose internally is from three to six grains (0·2–0·4 Gm.), dissolved in one or two fluidounces (30–60 C.c.) of water, filtered and sweetened with syrup. It should never be given in pills. As it occurs of variable quality, and must be used in solution more or less dilute, according to the particular purpose to which it is to be applied, it is impossible to give any very precise directions for its strength as an external remedy. From one to four drachms of the powder added to a pint of water, and the solution filtered, will form a liquid within the limits of strength ordinarily required. For the cure of itch, M. Derheims has recommended a much stronger solution—three ounces of the chloride to a pint of water, the solution being filtered, and applied several times a day as a lotion, or constantly by wet cloths. When applied to ulcers, their surface may be covered with lint dipped in the solution. When used as an ointment, to be rubbed upon scrofulous enlargements of the lymphatic glands, this may be made of a drachm of the chloride to an ounce of lard. Chlorinated lime is less eligible for some purposes than the solution of chlorinated soda. (See *Liquor Sodæ Chloratæ.*)

Chlorine gas is a very active germicide, and as chlorinated lime affords the best practical method of using it for ordinary disinfecting purposes, it seems proper to discuss the subject at this place. It has been proved by the concurrent results of numerous experimenters that chlorine, if present in the proportion of one part in one hundred in the atmosphere of a room, is able to destroy disease-germs, provided that the air and the objects are moist, and that the exposure continues for upward of one hour. In the case of any infected room or confined space, as the hold of a ship, it seems to us, however, that the endeavor should be to have a larger proportion of the chlorine gas present for several hours, and, if it can be readily accomplished, steam should also be allowed to enter with the gas, so as to make sure that all parts shall be thoroughly moistened. The importance of this is shown by the experiments of Fischer and Proskauer, who find that dry anthrax spores maintained their integrity for one hour when exposed to the action of a dry chlorine atmosphere containing about forty-five per cent. of chlorine, whereas moistened spores were killed by an hour's exposure to a moist atmosphere containing four per cent. of chlorine. Dr. Sternberg found that six hours' exposure of vaccine lint upon ivory points to a moist atmosphere containing one part of chlorine in one hundred was sufficient to destroy the infective power of the lint. Chlorine is not only germicidal, but it also has the power of decomposing sulphuretted hydrogen compounds, and thereby deodorizing. In all these employments of chlorine it must be remembered that it is not possible for human beings to breathe a chlorinated air, and that the apartment must be, therefore, empty, and also as hermetically sealed as possible to prevent the escape of the gas. The experiments of Dr. Duggan show that the hypochlorites as derived from chlorinated lime are very active germicides, one part to four hundred being capable of destroying moist germs in two minutes, and six parts to ten thousand killing the spores of the anthrax-bacillus in six hours. A half of one per cent. of the hypochlorites in solution is said to be sufficient to destroy spores almost instantly. Ordinary bleaching powder contains from twenty-five to forty per cent. of available chlorine; one part of the powder to one hundred of water is strong enough for ordinary purposes. The odor and taste of this solution are such that it can scarcely be considered a dangerous poison, and it has been affirmed, although with doubtful correctness, that such solution will not injure clothing, bedding, etc. The cost of bleaching powder for use in small quantities is so small that even a saturated solution may be prepared for use in the sick-room at a nominal cost. *For the destruction of disease-germs in urine, fecal discharges, sputa, etc., such saturated solution of bleaching powder appears to be in all respects the best disinfectant known.* As it is important to destroy the germs as soon as possible, this solution should be put into the receptacle to be used by the patient *before* the discharges are ejected into them. As the chlorinated solution attacks metals, it is essential that the spit-cups, etc., be made of china.

In consequence of its powers as a disinfectant, chlorinated lime is a very important compound in its application to medical police. It may be used with advantage for preserving bodies from exhaling an unpleasant odor, before interment, in the summer season. In juridical exhumations its use is indispensable; as it effectually removes the disgusting and insupportable fetor of the corpse. The mode in which it is applied, in these cases, is to envelop the body with a sheet completely wet with a solution, made by adding about a pound of the chloride to a bucketful of water. This solution may also be employed for disinfecting dissecting rooms, privies, common sewers, docks, and other places with offensive effluvia.

Chlorinated lime acts exclusively by its chlorine, which, being loosely combined, is disengaged by the slightest affinities. It should, therefore, be carefully kept from contact with the air and organic substances, which cause rapid loss of chlorine, and the modern method of putting it up for ordinary use in hermetically sealed pasteboard boxes is a great convenience. Mr. R. C. Bicknell examined commercial chlorinated lime put up in these boxes for available chlorine; he found the top layers usually deficient in strength, but in the interior from 30 to 35 per cent. of chlorine. Some of the packages assaying 30 per cent. of chlorine were more than a year old. (*A. J. P.*, 1886, p. 593.) All acids, even the carbonic, disengage it; and, as this acid is a product of animal and vegetable decomposition, noxious effluvia furnish the means, to a certain extent, of their own disinfection. But the stronger acids disengage the chlorine far more readily, and among these, sulphuric acid is the most convenient. Accordingly, the powder may be dissolved in a very dilute solution of this acid; or a small quantity of the acid may be added to an aqueous solution ready formed, if a more copious evolution of chlorine be desired than that which takes place from the mere action of the carbonic acid of the atmosphere.

Chlorinated lime may be advantageously applied to the purpose of purifying offensive water, a property which makes it invaluable on long voyages. When used for this purpose, from one to two ounces of the chloride may be mixed with about sixty-five gallons of the water. The water must afterwards be exposed for some time to the air, and allowed to settle, before it is fit to drink.

Strong insecticide properties have been ascribed to chlorinated lime. Hence it is recommended to sprinkle it on vegetables, flowers, fruit-trees, etc., which are apt to be attacked by worms and insects.

Off. Prep. Liquor Sodæ Chloratæ.

Off. Prep. Br. Liquor Calcis Chlorinatæ.

CALX SULPHURATA. *U.S., Br.* *Sulphurated Lime.*

(CĂLX SŬL-PHŪ-RĀ´TĄ.)

"A mixture (commonly misnamed Sulphide of Calcium) consisting chiefly of Sulphide of Calcium [**CaS**; **72.**—CaS; 36] and Sulphate of Calcium [$\mathbf{CaSO_4}$; **136.**—CaO,SO_3; 68], in varying proportions, but containing not less than 36 per cent. of absolute Sulphide of Calcium." *U.S.* "A mixture containing not less than 50 per cent. of sulphide of calcium (CaS)." *Br.*

"Lime, in very fine powder, *one hundred parts;* Precipitated Sulphur, *ninety parts.* Mix the Lime and Sulphur intimately, pack the mixture with gentle pressure in a crucible so as to nearly fill it, and having luted down the cover, expose the crucible for one hour to a low red heat, by means of a charcoal fire so arranged that the upper part of the crucible shall be heated first. Then remove the crucible, allow it to cool, rub its contents to powder, and at once transfer the latter to small, glass-stoppered vials." *U. S.*

"Take of Sulphate of Calcium, in fine powder, 7 ounces [av.]; Wood Charcoal, in fine powder, 1 ounce [av.]. Mix thoroughly. Heat to redness in an earthen crucible until the black color has disappeared. Cool, and at once place the whitish residue in a stoppered bottle." *Br.*

By the latter method, by decomposing a mixture of seven parts of sulphate of calcium and one part of charcoal, heated in a crucible to a red heat, carbonic oxide is formed, which combines with the oxygen of calcium sulphate, and calcium sulphide is produced, $CaSO_4 + 4CO = CaS + 4CO_2$. A less convenient method is to pass sulphuretted hydrogen over red-hot lime, although if the lime be pure a better product is insured. This preparation, which was introduced into both Pharmacopœias at the last revision, is of doubtful utility, particularly in the form in which it is produced when made by the officinal process. The amount of sulphide of calcium present must vary considerably according to circumstances. The medicinal activity is alone measured by the quantity of sulphide in the finished preparation, sulphate of calcium, the other constituent, being inert. It is to be regretted that a method of purification was not appended.

Properties. Sulphurated lime is "a grayish white or yellowish white powder, gradually altered by exposure to air, exhaling a faint odor of hydrosulphuric acid, having an offensive, alkaline taste and an alkaline reaction. Very slightly soluble in water and insoluble in alcohol. On dissolving Sulphurated Lime with the aid of acetic acid, hydrosulphuric acid is abundantly given off, and a white precipitate (sulphate of calcium) is thrown down. The filtrate yields, with test-solution of oxalate of ammonium, a white precipitate soluble in hydrochloric, but insoluble in acetic acid." *U. S.*

Test. "If 1 Gm. of Sulphurated Lime be gradually added to a boiling solution of 1·25 Gm. of sulphate of copper in 50 C.c. of water, the mixture digested on a water-bath for fifteen minutes, and filtered when cold, no color should be imparted to the filtrate by 1 drop of test-solution of ferrocyanide of potassium (presence of at least 36 per cent. of real sulphide of calcium)." *U. S.* "If eight grains be added to a cold solution of fourteen grains of sulphate of copper in an ounce of water, a little hydrochloric acid be added, and the mixture be then well stirred and heated to a temperature approaching that of ebullition until all action has ceased, the filtered liquid should give no red color with ferrocyanide of potassium." *Br.*

Sulphydrate of calcium is formed when sulphuretted hydrogen is passed into milk of lime as long as it is absorbed. It is in the form of a paste of a greenish gray color, and exhales a strong odor of sulphuretted hydrogen.

Medical Properties. It is used as a *depilatory*, and is applied in a layer on the part which is to be deprived of hair. At the end of fifteen minutes it is removed with a wet sponge, which at the same time detaches the hairs. On account of this preparation giving out sulphuretted hydrogen, it should not be applied near the mouth or nose. An impure aqueous solution of sulphide of calcium, necessarily containing hyposulphite of calcium from the manner of its preparation, is used with great success, in Belgium, in itch, the cure of which it effects in a few hours. It is made by boiling together one part of sublimed sulphur, two of lime, and ten of water. The liquid is allowed to cool, and the clear part poured off, and kept in well-stopped bottles. For an explanation of the reaction which takes place, see *Sulphur Præcipitatum*. The patient, after having been well washed with soap and tepid water in a bath, is rubbed over with the liquid, which is allowed to dry on the skin for a quarter of an hour. A second bath is then taken, which completes the cure. The preparation, when it dries, leaves on the skin a thin layer of the sulphur compound, which destroys the itch insect and its eggs.

Sulphide of calcium has been strongly recommended by Ringer, Duhring, and other authorities as a remedy for furuncular eruptions, and it has also been used successfully in acne. It is given in doses of from one-tenth to one-half grain (0·00648–0·0324 Gm.).

CAMBOGIA. *U.S., Br.* *Gamboge.*

(CĂM-BŌ'ĢI-Ą.)

"A gum-resin obtained from Garcinia Hanburii. Hooker filius. (*Nat. Ord.* Guttiferæ.)" *U.S.* "A gum-resin obtained from Garcinia Hanburii, Hook. fil. (Garcinia Morella, *var.* pedicellata, Hanbury)." *Br.*

Gambogia, *Pharm.* 1870; Gomme gutte, *Fr.;* Gummigutt, *G.;* Gomma-gotta, *It.;* Gutta gamba, *Sp.*

Several plants belonging to the natural family of Guttiferæ, growing in the equatorial regions, yield on incision a yellow opaque juice, which hardens on exposure, and bears a close resemblance to gamboge; but it is only from a particular tree, growing in Siam, that the officinal gum-resin is procured.* Formerly the United States and all the British Pharmacopœias ascribed it to *Stalagmitis Cambogioides.* Both the genus and species were established by Murray, of Göttingen, in 1788, from dried specimens belonging to König, procured in Ceylon; and, from information derived from the same source, it was conjectured by Murray that the tree yielded not only the gamboge of Ceylon, but that also collected in Siam. On this authority the British Colleges made the references alluded to. But it was ascertained by Dr. Graham, of Edinburgh, that there is no such plant as *Stalagmitis Cambogioides;* the description of Murray having been drawn up from accidentally conjoined specimens of two trees belonging to different genera; one being the *Xanthochymus ovalifolius* of Roxburgh, and the other, the *Hebradendron Cambogioides* of Graham. By several botanists the gum-resin has been ascribed to *Garcinia Cambogia,* also a tree of Ceylon belonging to the Guttiferæ, and yielding a yellowish concrete juice; but a specimen of this juice, sent to Edinburgh, was found by Dr. Christison to differ from gamboge both in composition and appearance, being of a pale lemon-yellow color. Thus it appears that neither of these references is correct; and, besides, the fact seems to have been overlooked that commercial gamboge is never obtained from Ceylon, but exclusively from Siam and Cochin-China. A gum-resin from Ceylon having been found similar in composition to the gamboge of commerce, and the tree which produced it having been referred by Dr. Graham to a new genus, and named by him *Hebradendron Cambogioides,* the Edinburgh College, in the last edition of its Pharmacopœia, was induced to adopt this Ceylon gamboge as officinal, and to recognize the name proposed by Dr. Graham for the tree producing it. But, as this variety is never found in western commerce, and exists only in cabinets, or the bazaars of India, it scarcely merited a place in an officinal catalogue; moreover the genus Hebradendron is not acknowledged by botanists. The *H. Cambogioides* is the *Garcinia pictoria* of Roxburgh (*Flor. Ind.,* ii. 627), which Sir Joseph Hooker considers to be a variety of the *G. Morella* (Desrous.); though Beddome keeps it distinct on account of its having the fertile flower bearing "the staminodes in bundles, and the stigma very small and 4-lobed." Several years since, Dr. Christison received from Singapore specimens of the gamboge plant cultivated in that island, and derived from Siam, which proved to be a Garcinia, differing from the *G. elliptica* of Wallich chiefly in having its male flower upon pedicels. More recently Mr. Hanbury obtained from the same source numerous specimens of the same plant, and was enabled to confirm the statement of Dr. Christison; but he also found that the plant approached very near to the *Garcinia Morella* of Desrousseaux, from which it could be distinguished only by its pedicellate flowers. These specimens were afterwards submitted to the inspection of Mr. Thwaites in Ceylon, who is perfectly familiar with the Garcinias of that island, and were pronounced by him to belong to a variety of *G. Morella,* scarcely differing from the Ceylon plant, except in having pedicelled instead of sessile flowers; for these two varieties the names of *G. Morella,* var. *sessile,* and *G. Morella,* var. *pedicellata,* were proposed. Sir Joseph Hooker, however, determined (*Journ. Linn. Soc.,* xiv. 485) that the var. *pedicellata* is a distinct species, differing from *G. Morella* in having not only its flowers pedicellate, but also its leaves more ovate and much larger, and its fruit larger: he very properly gave it the specific name

* According to observations of Messrs. Baildon and Jamie, gamboge is obtained exclusively from the province of Cambodia; the plant being found in no other part of Siam or in Cochin-China. (*Journ. de Pharm.,* Juillet, 1874, p. 65.)

of Hanburii to commemorate the contributions of the late Mr. Hanbury to pharmaceutical science, and his connection with the history of the present plant.

Gamboge is said to be procured in Siam by breaking off the leaves and shoots of the tree, the juice, which is contained in ducts or latex vessels in the bark, issuing in drops, and, being received in suitable vessels, it gradually thickens, and at length becomes solid. Dr. Jamie, of Singapore, states that incising the trunk and larger branches is often practised. The juice is frequently received into the hollow joints of the bamboo, and the water expelled by mild continuous heat. In this way the so-called pipe gamboge is formed, the contraction during drying causing the cylinders to be hollow. The name *gummi gutta*, by which it is generally known on the continent of Europe, probably originated from the circumstance that the juice escapes from the plant by drops. The officinal title was undoubtedly derived from the province of Cambodia, in which the gum-resin is collected. It was first brought to Europe by the Dutch about the middle of the seventeenth century. We import gamboge from Canton and Calcutta, whither it is carried by the native or resident merchants. There is no difference in the appearance or character of the drug as brought from these two ports; an evidence that it is originally derived from the same place.

Varieties. The best gamboge is in cylindrical rolls, from one to three inches in diameter, sometimes hollow in the centre, sometimes flattened, often folded double, or agglutinated in masses so that the original form is not always easily distinguishable. The pieces sometimes appear as if rolled, but are in general striated longitudinally from the impression made by the inner surface of the bamboo. They are externally of a dull orange color, which is occasionally displaced by greenish stains, or concealed by the bright yellow powder of the drug, slightly adhering to the surface. In this form the drug is sometimes called *pipe gamboge*. Another variety is imported under the name of *cake* or *lump gamboge*. It is in irregular masses of two or three pounds or more, often mixed with sticks and other impurities, containing many air cells, less dense, less uniform in texture, and less brittle than the former variety, and breaking with a dull and splintery instead of a shining and conchoidal fracture. The worst specimens of this variety, as well as of the cylindrical, are sometimes called by the druggists *coarse gamboge*. They differ, however, from the preceding, only in containing a greater amount of impurities. Indeed, it would appear, from the experiments of Christison, that all the commercial varieties of this drug have a common origin, and that cake or lump gamboge differs from the cylindrical, only in the circumstance that the latter is the pure concrete juice; while to the former, farinaceous matter and other impurities have been added for the purpose of adulteration. The inferior kinds of gamboge may be known by their greater hardness and coarser fracture; by the brownish or grayish color of their broken surface, which is often marked with black spots; by their obvious impurities; and by the green color which their decoction, after having been cooled, gives with tincture of iodine (starch). When pure, the gum-resin is completely dissolved by the successive action of ether and water,* so that the amount of residue left by any specimen treated in the manner just spoken of indicates approximately the measure of the adulteration.

Properties. The officinal description is as follows. "In cylindrical pieces, sometimes hollow in the centre, one to two inches (25 to 50 mm.) in diameter, longitudinally striate on the surface; fracture flattish-conchoidal, smooth, of a waxy lustre; orange red, or in powder, bright yellow; inodorous; taste very acrid; the powder sternutatory. Gamboge is partly soluble in alcohol and in ether; when triturated with water, it yields a yellow emulsion, and forms, with solution of potassa, an orange red solution, from which, on the addition of hydrochloric acid, yellow resin is precipitated. Boiled with water, Gamboge yields a liquid which, after cooling,

* *Ceylon gamboge*, derived from the *Hebradendron Cambogioides* of Graham (*Cambogia gutta*, Linn., *Garcinia Morella*, De Cand., *G. pictoria*, Roxb.), is procured by incisions, or by cutting away a portion of the bark, and scraping off the juice which exudes. The specimens sent to Dr. Christison were in flattish or round masses, eight or nine inches in diameter, apparently composed of aggregated irregular tears, with cavities which are lined with a grayish and brownish powdery incrustation. It resembled coarse gamboge, and was identical in composition. In Ceylon it is used as a pigment and purgative. (*Christison.*)

does not become green with test-solution of iodine (abs. of starch)." *U. S.* From the brilliancy of its color, gamboge is highly esteemed as a pigment. It has no smell and little taste; but, after remaining a short time in the mouth, produces an acrid sensation in the fauces. Its sp. gr. is 1·221, and its chemical formula is given as $C_{20}H_{24}O_4$. Exposed to heat, it burns with a white flame, emitting much smoke, and leaving a light spongy charcoal. It is a gum-resin, without volatile oil. Christison has shown that the proportion of gum and resin varies in different specimens even of the purest drug. In one experiment, out of 100·8 parts he obtained 74·2 of resin, 21·8 of gum, and 4·8 of water. The gum is quite soluble in water, and of the variety denominated arabin. Flückiger, however, says that the gum is not identical with gum arabic, as its solution does not redden litmus, and is not precipitated by neutral acetate of lead, nor by ferric chloride, nor by silicate or biborate of sodium. By fusing purified gamboge resin with potash, Hlasiwetz and Barth (*Ann. Ch. und Pharm.*, 138, p. 61) obtained acetic and other acids of the same series, together with *phloroglucin*, $C_6H_3(OH)_3$, *pyrotartaric acid*, $C_5H_8O_4$, and *isuvitinic acid*, $C_6H_3,CH_3(COOH)_2$. Gamboge is readily and entirely diffusible in water, forming a yellow opaque emulsion, from which the resin is very slowly deposited. It yields its resinous ingredient to alcohol, forming a golden-yellow tincture, which is rendered opaque and bright yellow by the addition of water. Its solution in ammoniated alcohol is not disturbed by water. Ether dissolves about four-fifths of it, taking up only the resin. It is wholly taken up by alkaline solutions, from which it is partially precipitated by the acids. The strong acids dissolve it; the solution when diluted deposits a yellow sediment. The color, acrimony, and medicinal power of gamboge are thought to reside in the resin.

Prof. Hirschsohn gives a method for detecting gamboge in mixtures in *Phar. Zeit. f. Russl.*, 24, p. 609. (*A. J. P.*, 1885, p. 606.)

Medical Properties and Uses. Gamboge is a powerful, drastic, hydragogue cathartic, so very apt to produce nausea and vomiting and much griping when given in the full dose that it is almost never employed except in combination with other cathartics. In large quantities it is capable of causing fatal effects, and death has resulted from a drachm. The full dose is from two to six grains (0·13–0·4 Gm.), which in cases of tænia has been raised to ten or fifteen grains. It may be given in pill or emulsion, or dissolved in an alkaline solution. In the dose of five grains the resin is said to produce copious watery stools, with little or no uneasiness. If this be the case, it is probable that, as it exists in the gum-resin, its purgative property is somewhat modified by the other ingredients.

Off. Prep. Pilulæ Catharticæ Compositæ.

Off. Prep. Br. Pilula Cambogiæ Composita.

CAMPHORA. *U. S., Br.* *Camphor.*

$C_{10}H_{16}O$; 152. (CĂM'PHO-RĄ.) $C_{20}H_{16}O_2$; 152.

"A stearopten derived from Cinnamomum Camphora, F. Nees et Ebermaier (*Nat. Ord.* Lauraceæ), and purified by sublimation." *U. S.* "A stearoptene obtained from the wood of Cinnamomum Camphora, *Nees and Eberm.* (Camphora officinarum, *Nees*). Imported in the crude state, and purified by sublimation." *Br.*

Camphre, *Fr.;* Kampher, Kampfer, *G.;* Canfora, *It.;* Alcanfor, *Sp.*

The name of camphor has been applied to various concrete, white, odorous, volatile products, found in different aromatic plants, and resulting probably from chemical change in their volatile oil. But commercial camphor is derived exclusively from two plants, the *Camphora officinarum* of Nees or *Laurus Camphora* of Linnæus, and the *Dryobalanops Camphora;* the former of which yields our officinal camphor, the latter a product much valued in the East, but unknown in the commerce of this country and of Europe. A considerable quantity of camphor, said to be identical with the officinal, was a few years since obtained upon the Tenasserim Coast, in Farther India, by subliming the tops of an annual plant, abundant in that region, and thought to be a species of Blumia. This product, however, does not occur in general commerce. (*A. J. P.*, xvi. 56.) The Rev. Mr. Mason, an American missionary in Burmah, states that the Chinese settlers informed him that the same plant abounds in China, and that camphor is procured from it there. (*Proc. Acad. Nat. Sci. Phila.*, 1851, p. 201.) The following observations apply to the officinal camphor.

Gen. Ch. For characters of genus Cinnamon, see *Cinnamomum*. The genus Camphora as separated by Nees departs from the characters there given, in the segments of the perianth being completely deciduous, and falling off completely, leaving the berry resting upon the somewhat enlarged cup-shaped or disk-shaped, entire, or slightly serrate base or tube.

Camphora officinarum. Nees, *Laurin.* 88; Carson, *Illust. of Med. Bot.* ii. 29, pl. xxiv.—*Laurus Camphora.* Willd. *Sp. Plant.* ii. 478.—*Cinnamomum Camphora. B. & T.* 222. The camphor-tree is an evergreen of considerable size, having the aspect of the linden, with a trunk straight below, but divided above into many branches, which are covered with a smooth, greenish bark. Its leaves, which stand alternately upon long footstalks, are ovate-lanceolate, entire, smooth and shining, ribbed, of a bright yellowish green color on their upper surface, paler on the under, and two or three inches in length. The flowers are small, white, pedicelled, and collected in clusters, which are supported by long axillary peduncles. The fruit is a red berry, resembling that of the cinnamon. The tree is a native of China, Japan, and other parts of eastern Asia. It has been introduced into the botanical gardens of Europe, and is occasionally met with in our own conservatories.*

The leaves have when bruised the odor of camphor, which is diffused through all parts of the plant, and is obtained from the root, trunk, and branches by sublimation. The process is not precisely the same in all places. The following is said to be the one pursued in Japan.† The parts mentioned, particularly the roots and smaller branches, are cut into chips, which are placed with a little water in large iron vessels, surmounted by earthen capitals, furnished with a lining of rice-straw. A moderate heat is then applied, and the camphor, volatilized by the steam, rises into the capital, where it is condensed upon the straw. In China the comminuted plant is said to be first boiled with water until the camphor adheres to the stick used in stirring, when the strained liquor is allowed to cool; and the camphor which concretes, being alternated with layers of earth, is submitted to sublimation. In the island of Formosa, where the camphor-tree abounds, the chips are heated in a rough still. This is usually composed of a furnace surmounted with a trough or similar rude vessel, which is protected by clay. In this reservoir the chips are placed, with water upon them, and a perforated board luted upon the top; on this are set earthen pots. A fire having been lighted, steam rises through the chips and carries the camphor with it to deposit it in the pots. The crude camphor is taken to the towns in baskets and then put into large vats, with holes in the bottom, through which an oil escapes called *camphor-oil*, much used by the Chinese for medical purposes. It is said that of recent years hydraulic pressure is largely substituted for drainage, and that the camphor, thus drained, is packed in bags and exported. (*P. J. Tr.*, Dec. 1863, p. 280.)

Commercial History. Camphor, in the *crude* state, is brought to this country chiefly from Canton. It comes also from Batavia, Singapore, Calcutta, and frequently from London. All of it is probably derived originally from China and Japan. Two commercial varieties are found in the market. The cheapest and most abundant is the *Chinese camphor*, most of which is produced in the island of Formosa, and thence taken to Canton. It comes in chests lined with lead, each containing about 130 pounds. It is in small grains or granular masses, of a dirty-white color, and frequently mixed with impurities. It has occurred in commerce adulterated with chloride of ammonium. The other variety is variously called *Japan*, *Dutch*, or *tub*

* The camphor-tree sometimes attains a great age and an enormous size. A tree seen by Kämpfer, in Japan, in 1691, with a trunk 36 feet in circumference, was in the year 1826 described by Siebold as having a circumference of 50 feet. (*Japan as it was and is*, by R. Hildreth. Boston, 1855, p 337.) Dr. Geo. B. Wood saw a large tree growing in the open air at Naples, and had no doubt that it might be readily and perhaps profitably cultivated in the southern parts of our own country, and especially in California.

† For detailed description, see *P. J. Tr.*, xv. 167; also, *Proc. A. P. A.*, 1884, p. 133.

camphor, the first name being derived from the place of its origin, the second from the people through whom it was introduced into commerce, and the third from the recipient in which it is often contained. It has usually come from Batavia, to which port it was taken from Japan. Like the former variety, it is in grains or granular masses; but the grains are larger and of a pinkish color, and there are fewer impurities, so that it yields a larger product when refined.

Crude camphor, as brought from the East, is never found in the shop of the apothecary. It must be refined before it can be used for medicinal purposes. The process for refining camphor was first practised in Europe by the Venetians, who probably derived it from the Chinese. It was afterwards transferred to the Dutch, who long enjoyed a monopoly of this business; and it is only within a few years that the process has been generally known. It is now practised largely in this country, and the camphor refined in our domestic establishments is equal to any formerly imported. Crude camphor is mixed with about one-fiftieth of quicklime, and exposed, in an iron vessel placed in a sand-bath, to a gradually increasing heat, by which it is melted, and ultimately converted into vapor, which condenses in a suitable recipient.* Refined in this manner, it is usually in the form of large circular cakes, one or two inches thick, slightly convex on one side and concave on the other, and perforated in the centre.

Properties. "In white, translucent masses of a tough consistence and crystalline structure, readily pulverizable in the presence of a little alcohol, ether, or chloroform. It has the sp. gr. 0·990–0·995, melts at 175° C. (347° F.), boils at 205° C. (401° F.), sublimes without residue, and burns with a luminous, smoky flame. It has a penetrating odor, and a pungent taste, dissolves readily in alcohol, ether, chloroform, disulphide of carbon, benzin, fixed and volatile oils, and is sparingly soluble in water." *U. S.* Camphor has a peculiar, strong, penetrating, fragrant odor; and a bitter, pungent taste, with a slight sense of coolness. It is beautifully white and pellucid, somewhat unctuous to the touch, brittle, and yet possessed of a tenacity which renders its reduction to a fine powder very difficult, unless its cohesion be overcome by the addition of a minute proportion of alcohol, ether, chloroform, glycerin, essential or fatty oil, or other volatile liquid for which it has an affinity. It may be obtained in powder by pulverizing with an equal weight of sugar, by precipitating the tincture with water, or by grating and afterwards sifting it,† or better yet, by sublimation. The fracture of camphor is shining, and its texture crystalline. Its sp. gr. varies from 0·9857 to 0·996. When thrown in small fragments upon water, it assumes singular circulatory movements, which cease upon the addi-

* We are informed that the process is conducted in the following manner in some of the laboratories of Philadelphia. The vessels in which the camphor is put are of cast-iron, circular, from 12 to 15 inches or more in diameter, and 4 inches deep, with perpendicular sides, and a ledge at top, on which the cover rests. This consists of sheet-iron, with a hole through the centre about an inch in diameter, over which a small hollow cone of sheet-iron is placed loosely. The crude camphor mixed with the lime, the object of which is said to be to combine with the moisture present, which interferes with the due solidification of the camphor vapor, is placed in the iron vessels described, of which from 20 to 50 are arranged in a long sand-bath. Heat is then applied until the camphor melts, after which it is kept as nearly uniform as possible, so that the vaporation may take place regularly, without violent ebullition. The vapor condenses on the lower surface of the lid; and care is taken, by the occasional removal of the iron cone, and clearing of the opening by means of a knife, to allow the escape of any accidental excess of the vapor. They who desire to see minute details as to the mode of refining camphor practised in France, are referred to an article by M. Emile Perret, pharmacian at Moret, in the *Journ de. Pharm. et de Chimie* (Fév. 1868, p. 124).

† But the powder thus formed is apt to aggregate on keeping. To obviate this it is recommended to rub it up with a minute proportion of carbonate of magnesium, from 10 to 20 grains to the ounce; or, as suggested by the late Mr. Henry F. Fish, of New York, by pouring an alcoholic solution of camphor into water in which carbonate of magnesium is suspended; the proportion employed being 16 ounces of camphor to a drachm of the carbonate, suspended in a gallon of water. The powder is allowed to settle on a filter. (*A. J. P.*, Nov. 1870, p. 506.) Another method of accomplishing the same object, proposed by Mr. John C. Lowd, is to sublime camphor from a retort into a large chamber, and collect the powder. (*Ibid.*, March, 1872, p. 112.)

William F. Simes, of Philadelphia, sublimes camphor on a considerable scale as a preliminary process in making compressed camphor. His apparatus consists of a retort, which is connected with a large cooling chamber, in which are board partitions with openings alternately above and below, for the purpose of compelling the camphor vapor to pass over a circuitous route and come in contact with the cool air, which condenses it in very small particles. These collect upon the bottom and sides, and it forms, after sifting, a very uniform powder. For further details and improvements in this apparatus, see *N. R.*, 1882, p. 167.

tion of a drop of oil; and this property has been applied to the detection of grease in liquids, a very small proportion of which is sufficient to prevent the movements. Its volatility is so great that, even at ordinary temperatures, it is wholly dissipated if left exposed to the air. When it is confined in bottles, the vapor condenses on the inner surface, and, in large bottles partially filled, sometimes forms, after long standing, large and beautiful crystals. It melts at 175° C. (347° F.), boils at 204° C. (399·2° F.), and, in close vessels, sublimes unchanged. When allowed to concrete slowly from the state of vapor, it assumes the form of hexagonal plates. It is not altered by air and light. It readily takes fire, burning with a brilliant flame, with much smoke, and without residue. Water triturated with camphor dissolves, according to Berzelius, not more than 1000th part; which, however, is sufficient to impart a decided odor and taste to the solvent. By the intervention of sugar or magnesia, a much larger proportion is dissolved. (See *Aqua Camphoræ.*) Carbonic acid increases the solvent power of water, as also does the spirit of nitrous ether. Ordinary alcohol will take up 75 per cent. of its weight of camphor, which is precipitated upon the addition of water. Berzelius states that 100 parts of alcohol, of the sp. gr. 0·806, dissolve 120 parts at 10° C. (50° F.). It is soluble without change in ether, the volatile and fixed oils, strong acetic acid, and diluted mineral acids, and is extremely soluble in chloroform. Nitric acid on prolonged boiling with camphor oxidizes it into *camphoric acid*, $C_{10}H_{16}O_4$, and *camphoronic acid*, $C_9H_{12}O_5$. Schwanert's *camphresinic acid*, $C_{10}H_{14}O_{12}$, is, according to Kachler, a mixture of these two. Sulphuric acid in the proportion of ten parts to one gives, when heated with camphor, an oil isomeric with camphor, boiling at 200° C. (392° F.), and yielding a solid camphor when distilled repeatedly over solid caustic potash. Sulphuric acid in the proportion of four to one gives with camphor, according to Chautard, a volatile product which he calls *camphrene*, and to which Schwanert gives the formula $C_9H_{14}O$. Kachler (*Ann. Ch. und Pharm.*, 164, p. 90) considers, however, that camphrene is only *phorone* (a condensation product of acetone) with slight impurities. Alcoholic potash solution heated with camphor gives a derivative called *campholic acid*, $C_{10}H_{18}O_2$, a white solid, fusing at 95° C. (203° F.), and boiling at 250° C. (482° F.). Resins unite with it, forming a soft tenacious mass, in which the odor of the camphor is sometimes almost extinguished, and frequently diminished; and a similar softening effect results when it is triturated with the concrete oils.* Exposed to a strong heat, in close vessels, camphor is resolved into carbonic acid gas and hydrocarbons, among which cymol is especially to be recognized.

Camphor, $C_{10}H_{16}O$, and borneol, $C_{10}H_{18}O$,† are classified together as belonging to

* As this property of camphor may have a bearing, injuriously or otherwise, on pharmaceutical processes, it is desirable that the operator, as well as prescriber, should be aware of the degree of effect produced by different resinous substances which may be mixed with it. M. Planche has found that mixtures, formed by triturating powdered camphor with powdered *dragon's blood*, *guaiac*, *asafetida*, and *galbanum*, assume, and preserve indefinitely the pilular consistence; with *benzoin*, *tolu*, *ammoniac*, and *mastic*, though at first of a pilular consistence, afterwards become soft by exposure to the air; with *sagapenum* and *animé*, assume a permanently semi-liquid form; with *olibanum*, *opopanax*, *gamboge*, *euphorbium*, *bdellium*, *myrrh*, and *amber*, remain pulverulent though somewhat grumous; and with *tacamahac*, *resin of jalap*, *sandarac*, and *resinoid matter of cinchona*, preserve the form of powder indefinitely. The same experimenter observed that camphor loses its odor entirely when mixed with *asafetida*, *galbanum*, *sagapenum*, *animé*, and *tolu*; retains a feeble odor with *dragon's blood*, *olibanum*, *mastic*, *benzoin*, *opopanax*, *tacamahac*, *guaiac*, and *ammoniac*; while with the other resinous substances above mentioned, it either has its odor increased, or retains it without material change. (*Journ. de Pharm.*, xxiv. 226.)

In mixing camphor with other substances in the form of powder, it is best to first pulverize the camphor with the aid of a little alcohol, then to pulverize the other substances together, and lastly to mix the two powders gently; much rubbing with the pestle having the effect of consolidating the granules of the camphor. (*Procter.*)

† *Sumatra Camphor. Borneo Camphor. Dryobalanops Camphor. Baros Camphor. Borneol.* It has long been known that a variety of camphor is produced in the islands of Sumatra and Borneo, by a forest tree, which remained until a recent period undetermined. It was at length, however, described by Colebrook, and is now recognized in systematic works as *Dryobalanops Camphora*, or *D. aromatica*. It is a very large tree, often exceeding one hundred feet in height, with a trunk six or seven feet in diameter, and ranking among the tallest and largest trees in India.* It is found in Su-

* For a particular description of this tree, see a paper by Dr. W. H. De Vriese, of Leyden, in the *A. J. P.* (xxiv. 329), taken from Hooker's Journal of Botany. In this paper it is stated on the authority of Dr. Junghuhn, who witnessed the process of collection, that the camphor is deposited in very small quantities, in minute fis-

the group called in general *camphors*, and which occur with the *terpenes* or essential oils, $C_{10}H_{16}$, and are to be considered as oxidation products of these latter.

Borneol is an alcohol, yielding compound ethers when heated to about 200° C. (392° F.) with organic acids. It is a secondary alcohol, and therefore contains the group CH.OH linked to a more complex group. Secondary alcohols by oxidation yield *ketones*, by the change of the CH.OH group to CO. Common camphor bears this relation to borneol, and is therefore considered as a ketone, although not capable of being formed directly from borneol. The action of metallic sodium, however, upon common camphor, $C_{10}H_{16}O$, gives us borneol, $C_{10}H_{18}O$.

Genuine camphor is said to be sometimes adulterated with the artificial, which may be detected by the action of ammonia upon its alcoholic solution, causing a flocculent precipitate, which does not redissolve, and the quantity of which is proportionate to that of the artificial product in any mixture of the two. (*A. J. P.*, xxxiv. 189.) As a means of distinguishing from the artificial camphor resulting from the reaction between the oil of turpentine and hydrochloric acid, Mr. J. W. Bailey recommends that a drop of alcohol, holding a little of the camphor to be tested in solution, be allowed to evaporate on the slide of a microscope. The crystals then formed produced with polarized light beautiful colors, if of natural camphor, but not if of the artificial. (*Neues Repertorium*, xvi. 763, 1867.)

matra and Borneo, and is abundant on the north-west coast of the former island. The camphor exists in concrete masses, which occupy longitudinal cavities or fissures in the heart of the tree, from a foot to a foot and a half long, at certain distances apart. The younger trees are generally less productive than the old. The only method of ascertaining whether a tree contains camphor is by incision. A party proceed through the forest, wounding the trees, till they find one which will answer their purpose; and hundreds may be examined before this object is attained. When discovered, the tree is felled and cut into logs, which are then split, and the camphor removed by means of sharp-pointed instruments. It is stated that the masses are sometimes as thick as a man's arm; and that the product of a middling-sized tree is nearly eleven pounds; of a large one double that quantity. The trees which have been wounded and left standing often produce camphor seven or eight years afterwards. Mrs. Ida Pfeiffer states, in her *Second Journey round the World* (Am. ed., p. 183), that the camphor is also found in a concrete state under the bark, and is swept down with long brooms. The Dryobalanops yields also a fragrant straw-colored liquid, called in the East Indies *oil of camphor*, and highly valued as an external application in rheumatism and other painful affections. It is said to be found in trees too young to produce camphor, and is supposed to constitute the first stage in the development of this substance; as it occupies the cavities in the trunk which are afterwards filled with the camphor. It has been stated to hold a large portion of this principle in solution; and to yield an inferior variety by artificial concretion; but this was not true of a specimen in the possession of Dr. Christison. A specimen examined by Professor Procter deposited a small quantity of the camphor at a temperature near the zero of Fahrenheit. By the action of nitric acid, it may be combined with oxygen, and converted into camphor of the same character as that deposited by refrigeration. The whole tree is pervaded more or less by the camphor or the oil. The wood retains a fragrant smell, and, being on this account less liable to the attacks of insects, is highly esteemed for carpenter's work. The camphor-wood chests, occasionally brought to this country from the East Indies, are probably made out of the wood of the Dryobalanops.

Borneo camphor is also produced in Johore, a province of the Malay peninsula, where it is sold in four qualities. The first is composed of transparent crystals, generally a quarter of an inch and upwards in length; the second of brown crystals, inferior in size; the third of powdery coherent and slightly colored grayish crystals, which resemble Japanese camphor; the fourth quality is brownish, pulverulent, and looks like sea-shore sand. (See *P. J. Tr.*, xvii. 796.)

It has been supposed that this variety of camphor is occasionally brought into the markets of Europe and America; but this is a mistake; as the whole produce of the islands is engrossed by the Chinese, by whom it is so highly valued that it commands at Canton, according to Mr. Crawford, seventy-eight times, according to Mr. Reeves, one hundred times the price of ordinary camphor. A specimen which was sent to the late Prof. Joseph Carson from Canton as a curiosity, is in tabular plates of the size of a finger nail or smaller, of a foliaceous crystalline texture, white, somewhat translucent, of an odor analogous to that of common camphor, and yet decidedly distinct, and less agreeable. It has also a camphorous taste. It is more compact and brittle than ordinary camphor; and, though the pieces will often float for a time when thrown on water, yet they sink when thoroughly moistened, and deprived of adhering air. According to Dr. Christison, its sp. gr. is 1·009. It is easily pulverized without the addition of alcohol. It is, moreover, much less disposed to rise in vapor, and to condense on the inside of the bottle containing it; indeed, its value in China is largely dependent upon its being less volatile than the ordinary camphor, and hence preferable for embalming purposes.* Like ordinary camphor, it is fusible, very slightly soluble in water, and freely soluble in alcohol and in ether. Its formula is $C_{10}H_{18}O$.

---

sures between the fibres, from which it is scraped off by small splinters of wood, or by the nail; and the thickest and oldest trees seldom yield more than two ounces. This account as to the productiveness of the tree differs greatly from that of Colebrook, as stated in the note above.

* The statement that Borneo camphor *never* crystallizes on the side of the bottle or jar in which it is kept appears to be incorrect. (*P. J. Tr.*, xv. 796, 894.)

Medical Properties and Uses. Camphor does not seem to have been known to the ancient Greeks and Romans. Europe probably derived it from the Arabians, by whom it was employed as a refrigerant. Much difference of opinion has prevailed as to its mode of action; some maintaining its immediate sedative influence, others considering it as a direct and decided stimulant. Its operation appears to be primarily and chiefly directed to the cerebral and nervous systems; and the circulation, though usually affected to a greater or less extent, is probably involved, for the most part, through the brain. It acts, also, to a certain extent, as a direct irritant of the mucous membranes with which it is brought into contact, and may thus in some measure secondarily excite the pulse. The effects of the medicine vary with the quantity administered. In moderate doses it produces, in health, mental exhilaration, increased heat of skin, and occasional diaphoresis. The pulse is usually increased in fulness, but little, if at all, in force or frequency. According to the experiments of certain Italian physicians, it has a tendency to the urinary and genital organs, producing a burning sensation along the urethra, and exciting voluptuous dreams (*N. Am. Med. and Surg. Journ.*, ix. 442); and these experiments have been confirmed by the observations of Dr. Reynolds in a case of poisoning by camphor (*Brit. Am. Journ. of Med.*, June, 1846). Cullen, however, states that he has employed it fifty times, even in large doses, without having ever observed any effect upon the urinary passages. By many it is believed to calm irritation of the urinary and genital apparatus, and to possess antaphrodisiac properties. In its primary operation it allays nervous disorder, quiets restlessness, and produces a general placidity of feeling, and is thus highly useful in certain forms of disease attended with derangement of the nervous functions. In larger doses, it displays a more decided action on the brain, producing more or less giddiness and mental confusion, with a disposition to sleep; and in morbid states of the system, relieving pain, and allaying spasmodic action. In immoderate doses it occasions nausea, vomiting, anxiety, faintness, vertigo, delirium, insensibility, coma, and convulsions, which may end in death. The pulse, under these circumstances, is at first reduced in frequency and force (Alexander, *Experimental Essays*, p. 227); but, as the action advances, it sometimes happens that symptoms of strong sanguineous determination to the head become evident in the flushed countenance, inflamed and fiery eyes, and highly excited pulse. (*Quarin.*) In three cases of poisoning by camphor, reported by Schaaf, of Strasburg, the symptoms produced were violent and incessant convulsions, paleness and coolness of the surface, vomiting and frequent micturition, and finally stupor or coma. The patients were children, and the youngest, a girl of about eighteen months, died from the effects of the poison, of which she took about ten grains. (*Monthly Journ. of Med. Sci.*, Oct. 1850, p. 377.) There can be no doubt that camphor is absorbed; as its odor is observed in the breath and perspiration, and according to Dr. Reynolds, in the urine also, though the contrary has been asserted.

By its moderately stimulating powers, its diaphoretic tendency, and its influence over the nervous system, camphor is adapted to the treatment of diseases of a typhoid character, which combine, with the enfeebled condition of the system, a frequent irritated pulse, a dry skin, and much nervous derangement, indicated by restlessness, watchfulness, tremors, subsultus, and low muttering delirium. It is not, however, at present much used in serious disease, but is very extensively employed in various functional nervous disorders, such as hysteria, dysmenorrhœa, general nervousness, and even in nymphomania. It is much used in diarrhœa, in flatulence, spasmodic colic, etc., as a local stimulant to the alimentary canal. In some of these cases, advantage may be derived from combining it with opium. Camphor has also been employed internally to allay the strangury produced by cantharides.

It is much used locally as an anodyne, dissolved in alcohol, oil, or acetic acid, and frequently combined with laudanum. In rheumatic and gouty affections, and various internal spasmodic and inflammatory complaints, it often yields relief in this way. The ardor urinæ of gonorrhœa may be alleviated by injecting an oleaginous solution of camphor into the urethra; and the tenesmus from ascarides and dysentery, by administering the same solution in the form of enema. Twenty or thirty grains of camphor, added to a poultice, and applied to the perineum, allay the chordee which is a painful attendant upon gonorrhœa. Its vapor has been inhaled into the lungs with benefit in asthma and spasmodic cough; and a lump of it held to the nose is said to relieve coryza. It has been employed for the same purpose, and for nervous headache, in the form of powder snuffed up the nostrils. It enters into the composition of certain tooth-powders.

Camphor may be given in substance, in the form of bolus or pill, or diffused in water by trituration with various substances. The form of pill is objectionable; as in this state the camphor is with difficulty dissolved in the gastric liquor, and, floating on the top, is apt to excite nausea, or pain and uneasiness at the upper orifice of the stomach. Orfila states that, when given in the solid form, it is capable of producing ulceration in the gastric mucous membrane. The emulsion is almost always preferred. This is made by rubbing up the camphor with loaf sugar, gum arabic, and water; and the suspension will be rendered more complete and permanent by the addition of a little myrrh. Milk is sometimes used as a vehicle, but is objectionable, from its liability to become speedily sour. The aqueous solution is often employed where only a slight impression is desired. For this purpose, the *Aqua Camphoræ* of the U. S. Pharmacopœia is preferable to the solution made by simply pouring boiling water upon a lump of camphor, which is sometimes prescribed under the name of *camphor tea*. When chloroform is not inadmissible, an elegant preparation may be made by dissolving camphor in that liquid, in the proportion of two drachms of the former to a fluidrachm of the latter, and then mixing the solution with water by the intervention of the yolk of an egg.

The medium dose of camphor is from five to ten grains (0·33–0·65 Gm.); but, to meet various indications, it may be diminished to a single grain (0·065 Gm.) or increased to a scruple (1·3 Gm.). The injurious effects of an overdose are said to be best counteracted, after clearing out the stomach, by the use of opium.

Off. Prep. Aqua Camphoræ; Linimentum Camphoræ; Spiritus Camphoræ; Linimentum Belladonnæ; Linimentum Saponis; Linimentum Saponis Compositum; Mistura Chloroformi; Pulvis Morphinæ Compositus; Tinctura Opii Camphorata.

Off. Prep. Br. Aqua Camphoræ; Linimentum Aconiti; Linimentum Belladonnæ; Linimentum Camphoræ; Linimentum Camphoræ Compositum; Linimentum Chloroformi; Linimentum Hydrargyri; Linimentum Opii; Linimentum Saponis; Linimentum Sinapis Compositum; Linimentum Terebinthinæ; Linimentum Terebinthinæ Aceticum; Spiritus Camphoræ; Tinctura Camphoræ Composita; Unguentum Hydrargyri Compositum.

CAMPHORA MONOBROMATA. *U.S.* *Monobromated Camphor.*

$C_{10}H_{15}BrO$; 230·8. (CĂM'PHO-RĄ MŎN-O-BRŌ-MĀ'TĄ.) $C_{20}H_{15}BrO_2$; 230·8.

Bromated Camphor, Brominated Camphor, Brom-camphor; Camphre monobromé, *Fr.*; Monobrom Camphor, *G.*

This substance was discovered in 1861 by Th. Swarts, who prepared it by heating bibromide of camphor in a sealed tube to 100° C. It may also be made by heating for three hours in a sealed tube, with the water-bath, bromine and camphor in the proper chemical proportions. The crystalline mass is washed with water, recrystallized from alcohol after treatment with animal charcoal, washed with an alcoholic solution of potassa, then with much water, and finally recrystallized from a mixture of alcohol and ether. It is very easy to prepare the monobromide on a small scale in this way. There is, however, at all times a very great pressure upon the inside of the tube, and the attempt to practise the method upon a large scale is very apt to result in shattering the tubes. This has led to numerous experiments as to the best method of preparing it. Prof. Maisch (*A. J. P.*, 1872, p. 339) introduces 4 oz. bromine gradually into a retort, in which 13 oz. camphor have been previously placed. In 15 or 20 minutes a brisk reaction will commence. When this subsides, 8 or 9 oz. more bromine are to be poured in, in four portions, waiting after each addition until the reaction ceases. The liquid in the retort is now to be heated to about 132° C. (270° F.), then cooled, and sufficient petroleum benzin added to dissolve the crystalline mass. The crystals which are formed on cooling may be purified by recrystallization from benzin or hot alcohol. Various modifications of this process have been proposed. Prof. J. U. Lloyd (*A. J. P.*, April, 1875) directs the addition of water to the camphor and bromine in the retort, and boils the mixture for two hours, or until all of the water is evaporated. Then the contents are poured into a dish and treated with warm alcohol, and allowed to crystallize, the mother-liquor drained off and recrystallized from hot alcohol. C. C. Keller (*Schweiz. Wochensch. f. Pharm.*, 1880, p. 50) uses chloroform (instead of water, as proposed by Prof. Lloyd) with the camphor and bromine, and washes the crystals with absolute alcohol, crystallizing them finally from an ethereal solution. 300 parts of camphor yield 340 parts monobromated camphor.*

Properties. "Colorless, prismatic needles or scales, permanent in the air and unaffected by light, having a mild, camphoraceous odor and taste, and a neutral reaction. Almost insoluble in water; freely soluble in alcohol, ether, chloroform, hot benzin, and fixed oils; slightly soluble in glycerin. When heated, Monobromated Camphor slowly volatilizes; at 65° C. (149° F.) it melts, and may be sublimed at a slightly higher temperature. At 274° C. (525° F.) it boils and is completely volatilized with partial decomposition. If boiled with test-solution of nitrate of silver, it is decomposed and yields bromide of silver, amounting to 81·2 per cent. of the weight of Monobromated Camphor taken. It is soluble, without decomposition, in cold, concentrated sulphuric acid, and will again separate unaltered, if the solution be poured into water." *U. S.*

Medical Properties. It was first proposed as a medicine by Professor Deneffe, and has been used by various practitioners as a nervous sedative in delirium tremens, hysteria, convulsive irritation of teething, sleeplessness, etc. According to the experiments of Dr. Bourneville (*Le Progrès Médical*, 1874) and of Dr. Lawson (*The Practitioner*, Aug. 1874), it produces in mammals muscular weakness, passing into paralysis, very decided progressive reduction of temperature, decrease in the respiration rate, sleep passing into stupor, and finally death. Dr. Bourneville states that the vessels of the ear and eyelids in the rabbit are contracted. Its therapeutic action resembles, but is not identical with, that of other bromides; in the experience of Dr. H. C. Wood, it has seemed to be of especial value in spermatorrhœa. It is not safe to give it too freely, as in some cases its ingestion has been followed by epileptiform convulsions. The dose of it is 5 grains (·33 Gm.),† given in pill or emulsion, and repeated every hour for 2 or 3 doses if necessary. The emulsion may be made by dissolving it in six times its weight of expressed oil of almonds, and then forming an emulsion with gum and water in the usual manner.

CANELLÆ CORTEX. *Br.* *Canella Bark.*

(CĄ-NĔL'LÆ CŎR'TĔX.)

Canella, *U. S.*, 1870; Canelle blanche, *Fr.*; Weisser Zimmt, Canell, Weisser Canel, *G.*; Canella bianca, *It.*; Canela blanca, *Sp.*

"The bark of Canella alba, *Murray*, deprived of its corky layer and dried." *Br.*

Gen. Ch. *Calyx* three-lobed. *Petals* five. *Anthers* sixteen, adhering to an urceolate nectary. *Berry* one-celled with two or four seeds. *Willd.* (*Nat. Ord.* Canellaceæ.)

Canella alba. Willd. *Sp. Plant.* ii. 851; Carson, *Illust. of Med. Bot.* i. 24, pl. 16; *B. and T.* 26. This is the only species of the genus. It is an erect tree, rising sometimes to the height of fifty feet, branching only at the top, and covered with a whitish bark, by which it is easily distinguished from other trees in the woods where it grows. The leaves are alternate, petiolate, oblong, obtuse, entire, of a dark green color, thick and shining like those of the laurel, and of a similar odor. The

* *Chlorinated Camphor* ($C_{10}H_{15}Cl.O$), the counterpart of monobromated camphor, has been studied physiologically by F. Perrenot under the name of *Chlorure de Camphre* (*Thèse*, Lyon, 1886). He finds that it is not poisonous, but has distinct antiseptic properties, and recommends it as a substitute for iodoform and other antiseptics when ulcerated surfaces need a stimulant dressing.

† *Elixir of Monobromated Camphor* is proposed by Munday (*P. J. Tr.*, March 3, 1877). Monobromated camphor 3 parts, alcohol (90 per cent.) 120 parts, orange-flower water 80 parts, glycerin 100 parts. Mix the alcohol and glycerin; dissolve the monobromated camphor by the use of a gentle heat, and add the orange-flower water. It contains 1 per cent. of monobromated camphor.

flowers are small, of a violet color, and grow in clusters upon divided footstalks, at the extremities of the branches. The fruit is an oblong berry, containing one, two, or three black, shining seeds.

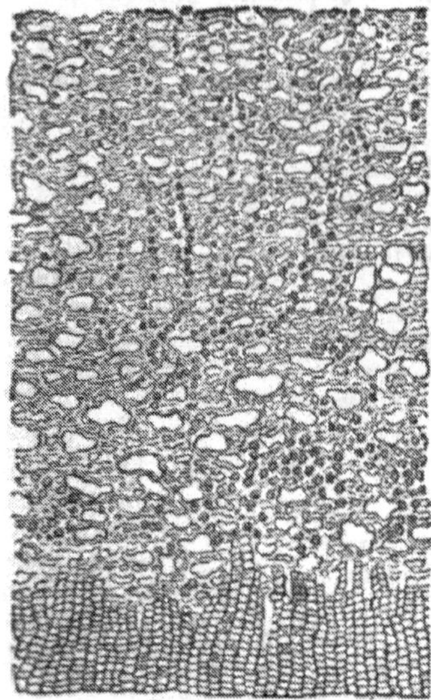

Transverse section.

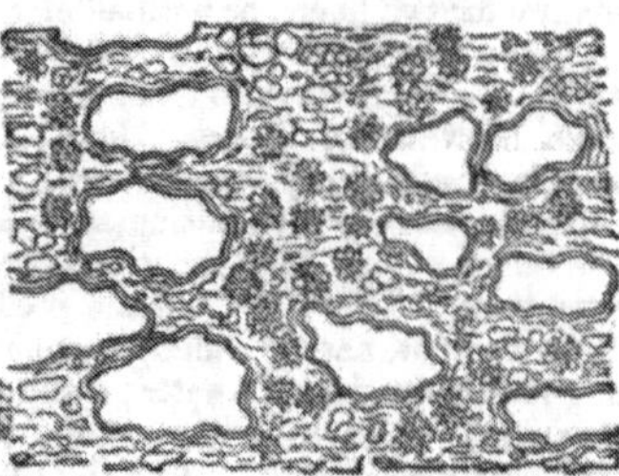

Showing rhapides of calcium oxalate in the liber.

Canella alba is a native of Florida, the Bahama Islands, and also of Jamaica and other West India islands. The bark of the branches, which is the part employed in medicine, is loosened and deprived of its epidermis by beating. After removal from the tree it is dried in the shade. It comes to us in pieces partially or completely quilled, occasionally somewhat twisted, of various sizes, from a few inches to two feet in length, from half a line to two or even three lines in thickness, and, in the quill, from half an inch to an inch and a half in diameter. It enters commerce solely from the Bahamas, where it is known as cinnamon bark, or as white wood bark.

Properties. Canella is of a pale orange yellow color externally, yellowish white on the inner surface, with an aromatic odor somewhat resembling that of cloves, and a warm, bitterish, very pungent taste. It is brittle, breaking with a short fracture, and yielding, when pulverized, a yellowish white powder. Boiling water extracts nearly one-fourth of its weight; but the infusion, though bitter, has comparatively little of the warmth and pungency of the bark. It yields all its virtues to alcohol, forming a bright yellow tincture, which is rendered milky by the addition of water. By distillation with water it affords a large proportion of a yellow or reddish, fragrant, and very acrid volatile oil. It contains, moreover, according to the analysis of MM. Petroz and Robinet, mannite, a peculiar very bitter extractive, resin, gum, starch, albumen, and various saline substances. Meyers and Reiche obtained twelve drachms of the volatile oil from ten pounds of the bark. They found it to consist of four different oils, the first being identical with the eugenol or eugenic acid of oil of cloves; the second is closely allied to the chief constituent of cajeput oil; the other oils require further examination. The bark yielded to Flückiger 0·74 per cent. of oil. Meyers and Reiche also obtained 8 per cent. of mannite and 6 per cent. of ash, chiefly calcium carbonate. (*Pharmacograph.*, 2d ed., p. 75.) Canella has been sometimes confounded with Winter's bark, from which, however, it differs both in sensible properties and composition. (See *Wintera.*) Mr. John P. Frey found by proximate analysis the following constituents: volatile oil, 1·28 per cent.; resin, 8·2 per cent.; mannit, 8 per cent.; ash, 8·9 per cent.; also starch, bitter principle, albumen, and cellulose. (*A. J. P.*, 1884, p. 1.)

Medical Properties and Uses. Canella is possessed of the ordinary properties of the aromatics, acting as a local stimulant and gentle tonic, and producing upon the stomach a warming cordial effect, which renders it useful as an addition to tonic or purgative medicines, in debilitated states of the digestive organs. It is scarcely ever prescribed except in combination. In the West Indies it is employed by the negroes as a condiment, and has some reputation as an antiscorbutic.

Off. Prep. Br. Vinum Rhei.

CANNABIS AMERICANA. *American Cannabis.*

(CĂN′NA̦-BĬS A̦-MĔR-Ĭ-CĀ′NA̦.)

"Cannabis sativa, Linné (*Nat. Ord.* Urticaceæ, Cannabineæ), grown in the Southern United States, and collected while flowering." *U. S.*

American Hemp, *U. S.* 1870; Chanvre américain, *Fr.;* Amerikanischer Hanf, *G.*

CANNABIS INDICA. *U. S., Br.* *Indian Cannabis.*

(CĂN′NA̦-BĬS ĬN′DĬ-CA̦.)

"The flowering tops of the female plant of Cannabis sativa, Linné (*Nat. Ord.* Urticaceæ, Cannabineæ), grown in the East Indies." *U. S.* "The dried flowering or fruiting tops of the female plants of Cannabis sativa; grown in India, and from which the resin has not been removed. It is known in India as Gunjah or Ganga." *Br.*

Hemp, Indian Hemp; Herba Cannabis Indicæ, *P. G.;* Chanvre Indien, *Fr.;* Indischer Hanf, *G.*

Gen. Ch. MALE. *Calyx* five-parted. *Stamens* five. FEMALE. *Calyx* one-leaved, rolled up. *Styles* two. *Lindley.*

Cannabis sativa. Linn. *Sp. Plant.* 1457; Griffith, *Med. Bot.* p. 572; *B. and T.* 231. Hemp is an annual plant, from four to eight feet or more in height, with an erect, branching, angular stem. The leaves are alternate or opposite, on long, lax footstalks, roughish, and digitate, with linear-lanceolate, serrated segments. The stipules are subulate. The flowers are axillary; the male in long, branched, drooping racemes; the female in erect, simple spikes. The stamens are five, with long pendulous anthers; the pistils two, with long, filiform, glandular stigmas. The fruit is ovate and one-seeded. The whole plant is covered with a fine pubescence, scarcely visible to the naked eye, and is somewhat viscid to the touch. The hemp plant of India, from which the drug is derived, has been considered by some as a distinct species, and named *Cannabis Indica;* but the most observant botanists, upon comparing it with our cultivated plant, have been unable to discover any specific difference. It is now, therefore, regarded merely as a variety, and is distinguished by the epithet *Indica.* Dr. Pereira states that, in the female plant, the flowers are somewhat more crowded than in the common hemp; but that the male plants in the two varieties are in all respects the same.

The American and true Indian hemp are respectively described as follows in the present edition U. S. P.

"Stem about six feet (2 m.) high, rough; leaves opposite below, alternate above, petiolate, digitate; the leaflets linear-lanceolate, serrate; diœcious, the staminate flowers in pedunculate clusters forming compound racemes; the pistillate flowers axillary, sessile and bracteate; odor heavy; taste bitter, slightly acrid." *U. S.*

"Branching, compressed, brittle, about two inches (5 cm.) long, with a few digitate leaves, having linear-lanceolate leaflets, and numerous, sheathing, pointed bracts, each containing two small, pistillate flowers, sometimes with the nearly ripe fruit, the whole more or less agglutinated with a resinous exudation. It has a brownish color, a peculiar, narcotic odor, and a slightly acrid taste." *U. S.*

C. sativa is a native of the Caucasus, Persia, and the hilly regions in the north of India. It is cultivated in many parts of Europe and Asia, and largely in our Western States. It is from the Indian variety exclusively that the medicine was formerly obtained; the heat of the climate in Hindostan apparently favoring the development of its active principle.* Dr. H. C. Wood having obtained a parcel

* On a visit to the botanical garden of Edinburgh, in the autumn of 1860, Dr. George B. Wood saw a full-grown specimen of *Cannabis sativa*, and was surprised to find that it was only about four feet high, had little or no odor, and was scarcely adhesive when handled. If this is the general character of the hemp plant in the north of Europe, it is not surprising that it should be destitute of the medicinal properties of the Indian plant. In Philadelphia, the plant attains a height usually of six or eight feet, has a decided narcotic odor, and exudes so much of its peculiar resin as to be very adhesive to the fingers. On this occasion Dr. Christison informed Dr. Geo. B. Wood, from information he had received from India, that the plant there cultivated in the hot plains does not yield hashish satisfactorily; but that this product is chiefly if not exclusively obtained from it

of the male plant from Kentucky, made an alcoholic extract of the leaves and tops, and, upon trying it on the system, found it effective in less than a grain, and, having inadvertently taken too large a dose, experienced effects which left no doubt of the powers of the medicine, and of the identity of its influence with that of the Indian plant. How far the female tops might have the same effect is left uncertain; but, if we are to judge from analogy with the Indian plant, they would be preferable to the male. (*Proc. Am. Philos. Soc.*, vol. xi. p. 226.) The results obtained by Dr. Wood were so decisive that, at the 1870 revision of our Pharmacopœia, the American plant and an extract were introduced into the materia medica catalogue; but none of the extract has been made for commercial purposes, and in the present Pharmacopœia, Extractum Cannabis Americanæ has been dropped.

The seeds, though not now officinal, have been used in medicine. They are about the eighth of an inch long, roundish-ovate, somewhat compressed, of a shining ash-gray color, and of a disagreeable, oily, sweetish taste. They yield by expression about 20 per cent. of a fixed oil, which has the drying property, and is used in the arts. They contain also uncrystallizable sugar and albumen, and when rubbed with water form an emulsion, which may be used advantageously in inflammations of the mucous membranes, though without narcotic properties. They are much used as food for birds, which are fond of them. They are generally believed to be in no degree poisonous; but M. Michaud relates the case of a child, in which serious symptoms of narcotic poisoning occurred after taking a certain quantity of them. It is probable that some of the fruit eaten by the child was unripe; as, in this state, it would be more likely to partake of the peculiar qualities of the plant itself. (*Annuaire de Thérap.*, 1860, p. 159.)

In Hindostan, Persia, and other parts of the East, hemp has long been habitually employed as an intoxicating agent. The parts used are the tops of the plant, and a resinous product obtained from it. The plant is cut after flowering, and formed into bundles from two to four feet long by three inches in diameter, which are sold in the bazaars under the name of *gunjah*. The *hashish* of the Arabs is essentially the same. The name *bang* is given to a mixture of the larger leaves and capsules without the stems. There is on the surface of the plant a resinous exudation to which it owes its clammy feel. Men clothed in leather run through the hemp fields, brushing forcibly against the plants, and thus separating the resin, which is subsequently scraped from their dress, and formed into balls. These are called *churrus*. In these different states of preparation, the hemp is smoked like tobacco, with which it is said to be frequently mixed. An infusion or decoction of the plant is also sometimes used as an exhilarating drink.

The imported *medicinal resin or extract of hemp*, directed by the U. S. Pharmacopœia of 1860, is made by evaporating a tincture of the dried tops. Dr. O'Shaughnessy directs it to be prepared by boiling the tops of the gunjah in alcohol until all the resin is dissolved, and evaporating to dryness by means of a water-bath. Mr. Robertson, of the Calcutta Medical College, prepares it by passing the vapor of boiling alcohol from the boiler of a still into the dried plant contained in a convenient receptacle, and evaporating the condensed liquor by a heat not exceeding 65·6° C. (150° F.). The Messrs. Smith, of Edinburgh, obtained a purer resin by the following process. Bruised gunjah is digested, first in successive portions of warm water, till the expressed liquid comes away colorless; and afterwards, for two days with a moderate heat, in a solution of carbonate of sodium, containing one part of the salt for two of the dried herb. It is then expressed, washed, dried, and exhausted by percolation with alcohol. The tincture, after being agitated with milk of lime containing one part of the earth for twelve of the gunjah used, is filtered; the lime is precipitated by sulphuric acid; the filtered liquor is agitated with animal charcoal, and again filtered; most of the alcohol is distilled off, and to the residue twice its weight

in the hilly regions. He said, moreover, that the story of the natives running through the hemp fields and collecting the resin on their clothing, from which it is afterwards scraped, is, if not quite untrue, at least apocryphal. He had been informed that the real mode of gathering it is to rub the hemp-tops between the hands, and, when the palms and fingers are sufficiently loaded with the resin, to scrape it off. It is possible, however, that different methods may be followed in different localities.

of water is added; the liquor is then allowed to evaporate gradually; and, finally, the resin is washed with fresh water until it ceases to impart a sour or bitter taste to the liquid, and is then dried in thin layers. Thus obtained, it retains the odor and taste of the gunjah, of which 100 pounds yield 6 or 7 of the extract. Much of the commercial extract is very impure, and is but partially soluble in alcohol.

Under the name of *Extractum Cannabis Purificatum*, the U. S. Pharmacopœia of 1860 directed a preparation made by evaporating a tincture of the crude extract, which, from its greater uniformity of strength, was preferable for prescription. The British Pharmacopœia directs the Extract of Indian Hemp to be prepared by macerating an avoirdupois pound of the dried tops of the hemp, in coarse powder, in four Imperial pints of rectified spirit, for seven days, then expressing, and evaporating to the proper consistence. From this a tincture is ordered to be prepared.

Properties. Fresh hemp has a peculiar narcotic odor, which is said to be capable of producing vertigo, headache, and a species of intoxication. It is much less in the dried tops, which have a feeble bitterish taste. According to Dr. Royle, *churrus* is when pure of a blackish-gray, blackish-green, or dirty olive color, of a fragrant and narcotic odor, and a slightly warm, bitterish, and acrid taste. Schlesinger found in the leaves a bitter substance, chlorophyll, green resinous extractive, coloring matter, gummy extract, extractive, albumen, lignin, and salts. The plant also contains volatile oil in very small proportion, which probably has narcotic properties. The resin obtained by T. & H. Smith, of Edinburgh, in 1846, has been thought to be the active principle, and has received the name of *cannabin*. It is neutral, soluble in alcohol and ether, and separable from the alcoholic solution by water as a white precipitate. Martino (*N. Rep. Pharm.*, 4, p. 529) obtained a resin fusing at 68° C. (154·4° F.), easily soluble in alcohol, ether, and volatile oils, difficultly soluble in aqueous alkalies and acids. By oxidation with nitric acid a product is formed, *oxycannabin*, $C_{20}H_{20}H_2O_7$, which, after purifying, is white and crystalline. Preobraschensky (*Pharm. Zeit. f. Russl.*, 1876, p. 705) believes that cannabis Indica contains the alkaloid nicotine; this has, however, not been confirmed, and is hardly probable, because the physiological actions of the two drugs differ very greatly. The taste of *cannabin* is warm, bitterish, acrid, somewhat balsamic, and its odor fragrant, especially when heated. From the effects on the system of the exhalations from fresh hemp, it was a very probable supposition that the plant owed its medical properties, in part at least, to a volatile principle. By repeated distillation of the same portion of water from relatively large quantities of hemp renewed at each distillation, M. J. Personne obtained a volatile oil, of a stupefying odor, and an action on the system such as to dispose him to think that it was the active principle of the plant. As the water distilled was strongly alkaline, he supposed that this volatile principle might be a new alkaloid; but the alkaline reaction was found to depend on ammonia; and the liquid obtained proved to be a volatile oil, lighter than water, of a deep amber color, a strong smell of hemp, and composed of two distinct oils, one colorless, with the formula $C_{18}H_{20}$, the other a hydride of the first, $C_{18}H_{22}$, which was solid, and separates from alcohol in plate-like crystals. For the former M. Personne proposes the name of *cannabene*. When this is inhaled, or taken into the stomach, a singular excitement is felt throughout the system, followed by a depression, sometimes amounting to syncope, with hallucinations which are generally disagreeable, but an action on the whole slighter and more fugitive than that of the resin. Siebold and Bradbury (*Year-Book of Pharmacy*, 1881, p. 453), by the process for nicotine, obtained *cannabinine* in the form of a varnish-like dry mass, which they assert is an alkaloid. Dr. Matthew Hay believes that there are several alkaloids in cannabis Indica, and he has obtained one, which he describes in *P. J. Tr.*, 1883, p. 998. *Tannate of cannabine* is now an article of commerce and made by Merck; it is asserted by Dr. Dornmüller to have soporific effects, but Dr. H. C. Wood has found it to be inert physiologically. Bombelon prepares pure *cannabine* by decomposing the tannate with oxide of zinc and extracting the cannabine as a greenish-brown, non-adhesive powder, which he asserts is more reliable than the tannate. (*Amer. Drug.*, 1884, p. 132.) The experiments of Warden and Weddell (*P. J. Tr.*, xv. 574) strongly indicate, however, that the active principle of hemp has not yet been isolated.

Medical Properties. Extract of hemp is a powerful narcotic, causing exhilaration, intoxication, delirious hallucinations, and, in its subsequent action, drowsiness and stupor, with little effect upon the circulation. It is asserted also to act as a decided aphrodisiac, to increase the appetite, and occasionally to induce the cataleptic state. In overdoses it may produce poisonous effects. In morbid states of the system, it has been found to cause sleep, to allay spasm, to compose nervous disquietude, and to relieve pain. In these respects it resembles opium; but it differs from that narcotic in not diminishing the appetite, checking the secretions, or constipating the bowels. It is much less certain in its effects; but may sometimes be preferably employed, when opium is contraindicated by its nauseating or constipating effects, or its disposition to produce headache, and to check the bronchial secretion. The complaints in which it has been specially recommended are neuralgia, gout, rheumatism, tetanus, hydrophobia, epidemic cholera, convulsions, chorea, hysteria, mental depression, delirium tremens, insanity, and uterine hemorrhage. Dr. Alexander Christison, of Edinburgh, affirms that it has the property of hastening and increasing the contractions of the uterus in delivery, and has employed it with advantage for this purpose. It acts very quickly, and without anæsthetic effect. It appears, however, to exert this influence only in a certain proportion of cases. (*Ed. Month. Journ. of Med. Sci.*, xiii. 117, and xv. 124.) The strength of the extract varies much as found in commerce, and therefore no definite dose can be fixed. When it is of good quality, half a grain or a grain (0·03–0·065 Gm.) will affect the system. The Messrs. Smith found two-thirds of a grain (0·04 Gm.) of their extract to produce powerful narcotic effects. In some instances it will be necessary to give as much as ten or twelve grains (0·65–0·80 Gm.) of the imported extract; and half an ounce (15·5 Gm.) of it has been taken without sensible effect. The proper plan is to begin with one-quarter or half a grain (0·016–0·03 Gm.), repeated at intervals of two, three, or four hours, and gradually increased until its influence is felt, and the strength of the parcel employed is thus ascertained. Afterwards the dose will be regulated by the ascertained strength; but, should a new parcel be employed, the same caution must be observed as to the commencing dose. A tincture is prepared by dissolving an ounce of the extract in a pint (Imp. meas.) of alcohol. A dose of this, equivalent to a grain of the extract, is about twenty minims (1·25 C.c.), or forty drops. Dr. O'Shaughnessy gave ten drops (0·6 C.c.) every half hour in cholera, and a fluidrachm (3·75 C.c.) every half hour in tetanus. As the resin is precipitated by water, the tincture should be administered in mucilage or sweetened water. Alarming effects have been produced by overdoses, and care should be taken to use only a tincture which has been tested carefully, by commencing with a small dose and gradually increasing it until its power is known.

Off. Prep. Extractum Cannabis Indicæ; Tinctura Cannabis Indicæ; Extractum Cannabis Indicæ Fluidum.

Off. Prep. Br. Extractum Cannabis Indicæ; Tinctura Cannabis Indicæ.

CANTHARIS, *U. S., Br.* *Cantharides.* [*Spanish Flies.*]

(CĂN'THA-RĬS.)

"Cantharis vesicatoria. De Geer. (*Class*, Insecta; *Order*, Coleoptera.) Cantharides should be kept in well-closed vessels, containing a little camphor." *U. S.* "The beetle, Cantharis vesicatoria, *De Geer*, dried." *Br.*

Cantharides, *P.G.;* Muscæ Hispanicæ; Cantharides, Cantharide, *Fr.;* Spanische Fliege, Kantharide, Canthariden, *G.;* Cantarelle, *It.;* Cantharidas, *Sp.*

The term *Cantharis* was employed by the ancient Greek writers to designate many coleopterous insects or beetles. Linnæus gave the title to a genus not including the officinal blistering insect, and placed this in the genus *Meloë*, which, however, has been since divided into several genera. Geoffrey made the Spanish fly (beetle)* the prototype of a new one called *Cantharis*, substituting *Cicindela* as the title of the Linnæan genus. Fabricius altered the arrangement of Geoffrey, and substituted *Lytta* for *Cantharis* as the generic name. The former was adopted by the London

* A *beetle* is to be distinguished from a *fly* by its having the first pair of wings converted into elytra, or wing-cases—*i.e.*, thickened and hardened for protection.

College, and at one time was in extensive use; but the latter, having been restored by Latreille, is now recognized in the British and American Pharmacopœias, and is universally employed. By this naturalist the vesicating insects were grouped in a small tribe, corresponding very nearly with the Linnæan genus Meloë, and distinguished by the title *Cantharidæ*. This tribe he divided into eleven genera, among which is Cantharis. Two others of these genera, *Meloë* properly so called, and *Mylabris*, have been employed as vesicatories. *Mylabris cichorii* is thought to be one of the insects described by Pliny and Dioscorides under the name of cantharides, and is to this day employed in Italy, Greece, the Levant, and Egypt; and another species, *M. pustulata*, is used for the same purpose in China. Mr. W. R. Warner has found 500 parts of *M. cichorii* to yield 2·13 parts of cantharidin, which somewhat exceeds the yield of Spanish flies (*A. J. P.*, xxviii. 195); and R. Wolff has obtained by ethereal extraction more than 4 parts of cantharidin in 500 of the *Lytta aspersa* of Buenos Ayres. The *M. cichorii* has been recently imported to some extent under the name of *Chinese blistering fly*. It is black, with the powder blackish gray and free from shining particles. *Meloë proscarabæus* and *M. majalis* have been occasionally substituted for cantharides in Europe, and *M. trianthemæ* is used in the upper provinces of Hindostan. Several species of Cantharis, closely analogous in medical properties, are found in various parts of the world; but *C. vesicatoria* is the only one recognized as officinal in the United States, Great Britain, and France. A second species, *C. vittata*, was introduced into our national Pharmacopœia, but has been discarded. Of this, and some other indigenous species, notice will be taken at the end of this article. At present we shall confine our observations to *C. vesicatoria.**

CANTHARIS. *Class* Insecta. *Order* Coleoptera. *Linn.*—*Family* Trachelides. *Tribe* Cantharidæ. *Latreille.*

Gen. Ch. *Tarsi* entire; *nails* bifid; *head* not produced into a rostrum; *elytra* flexible, covering the whole abdomen, linear, semicylindric; *wings* perfect; *maxillæ* with two membranous *laciniæ*, the external one acute within, subuncinate; *antennæ* longer than the head and thorax, rectilinear; first joint largest, the second transverse, very short; *maxillary palpi* larger at tip. (*Say.*)

Cantharis vesicatoria. Latreille, *Gen. Crust. et Insect.*, ii. p. 220. This beetle is from six to ten lines in length, by two or three in breadth, and of a beautiful, shining, golden green color. The head is large and heart-shaped, bearing two thread-like, black, jointed feelers; the thorax short and quadrilateral; the wing-sheaths long and flexible, covering brownish membranous wings. When alive, the Spanish flies have a strong, penetrating, fetid odor, compared to that of mice, by which swarms of them may be detected at a considerable distance. They attach themselves preferably to certain trees and shrubs, such as the white poplar, privet, ash, elder, and lilac, upon the leaves of which they feed. They abound most in Spain, Italy, and the south of France, but are found also in all the temperate parts of Europe, and in the west of Asia. According to the researches of Lichtenstein, the eggs are laid by the female in the latter part of June in small cylindrical holes made in the ground. A week later the larvæ hatch out. They are a millimetre long, with two long caudal threads, and of a brown color. After many efforts, M. Lichtenstein succeeded in getting them to feed on the honey contained in the stomach of bees. In a few days they changed into milk-white larvæ, and about a month after this buried themselves in the ground, to assume the chrysalis stage and to hatch out the following spring as perfected beetles. In the wild state the larvæ are said to mount up flowers and attach themselves to bees or other hymenopterous insects; carried by the bee to the hive, the larvæ feed upon the young bees and the honey and bee bread stored up for use. The beetles usually make their appearance in swarms upon the trees in May and June, when they are collected. The time preferred for the purpose is in the morning at sunrise, when they are torpid from the cold of the night, and easily let go their hold. Persons with their faces protected by masks, and their hands with gloves, shake the trees, or beat them with poles; and the insects are

* Those who wish to investigate the subject of vesicating insects generally are referred to the *P. J. Tr.* (Aug. 2, 1871), also *Proc. A. P. A.* (1876, p. 507).

received as they fall upon linen cloths spread underneath. They are then plunged into vinegar diluted with water, or exposed in sieves to the vapor of boiling vinegar, and, having been thus deprived of life, are dried either in the sun, or in apartments heated by stoves. This mode of killing the flies by the steam of vinegar is as ancient as the times of Dioscorides and Pliny. In some places they are gathered by smoking the trees with burning brimstone. It has been proposed by M. Lutrand to destroy them by the vapor of chloroform. When perfectly dry, they are introduced into casks or boxes, lined with paper and carefully closed, so as to exclude as much as possible the atmospheric moisture. According to M. Neutwich, the young fly has no vesicating power (*P. J. Tr.*, Nov. and Dec., 1870, p. 355); but this is denied by H. Beauregard. (*Ibid.*, xv. 873.)

Cantharides come chiefly from Spain, Italy, Sicily, and other parts of the Mediterranean. Considerable quantities are also brought from St. Petersburg, derived originally, in all probability, from the southern provinces of Russia, where the insect is very abundant. The Russian flies are most esteemed. They may be distinguished by their greater size, and their color approaching to that of copper.

In the United States are several species of Cantharis, which have been employed as substitutes for *C. vesicatoria*, and found equally efficient; but none of them are now recognized by our national Pharmacopœia; even *C. vittata*, which was at one time officinal, having been discarded. This we regret, as it seems to us that the native products of our country should always be encouraged when shown to be useful. We shall briefly notice all that have been submitted to experiment, and found to possess vesicating powers.

1. *Cantharis vittata.* Latreille, *Gen. Crust. et Insect.;* Durand, *Journ. of the Phil. Col. of Pharm.*, ii. 274, fig. 4. The *potato fly* * is rather smaller than *C. vesicatoria*, which it resembles in shape. Its length is about six lines. The head is light red, with dark spots upon the top; the feelers are black; the elytra or wing-cases are black, with a yellow longitudinal stripe in the centre, and with a yellow margin; the thorax is also black, with three yellow lines; and the abdomen and legs, which have the same color, are covered with a cinereous down. It inhabits chiefly the potato vine, and appears about the end of July or beginning of August, in some seasons very abundantly. It is found on the plant in the morning and evening, but during the heat of the day descends into the soil. The insects are collected by shaking them from the plant into hot water; and are afterwards carefully dried in the sun. They are natives of the Middle and Southern States. This species of Cantharis was first described by Fabricius in the year 1781, and was introduced to the notice of the profession by Dr. Isaac Chapman, of Bucks County, Pennsylvania, who found it equal if not superior to the Spanish fly as a vesicatory. The testimony of Dr. Chapman has been corroborated by that of many other practitioners. It may be applied to the same purposes, treated in the same manner, and given in the same dose as the foreign insect. Mr. W. R. Warner obtained 1·99 parts of cantharidin from 500 parts of this beetle, but by improved methods Mr. Fahnestock procured 1½ per cent. of the active principle. (*A. J. P.*, xxviii. 195; li. 298.) According to the researches of Prof. Jos. Leidy, the vesicating principle resides in the blood, the eggs, and a peculiar fatty matter of certain accessory glands of the generative apparatus. (*Am. Jour. of Med. Sci.*, Jan. 1860, p. 60); whilst H. Beauregard (*P. J. Tr.*, xv. 873) found that the blood, the seminal vesicules of the male, the eggs, and all parts of the generative organs of the female are active.

2. *Cantharis cinerea.* Latreille, *Gen. Crust. et Insect.;* Durand, *Journ. of the Phil. Col. of Pharm.*, ii. 274, fig. 5. The *ash-color cantharis* closely resembles the preceding species in figure and size; but differs from it in color. The elytra and body are black, without the yellow stripes that characterize *C. vittata*, and are entirely covered with a short and dense ash-colored down, which conceals the proper color of the insect. The feelers are black, and the first and second joints are very large in the male. This species also inhabits the potato plant, and is occasionally found on other plants, as the English bean and wild indigo. It is a native of

* According to the researches of L. Dembinski, the Colorado potato-beetle (*Doryphora decemlineata*) contains no cantharidin. (*A. J. P.*, 1877, p. 550.)

the Northern and Middle States. Illiger in 1801 discovered its vesicating properties; but Dr. Gorham was first to call public attention particularly to the subject, and to the fact of its equality in all respects with the potato fly, in a communication addressed, in the year 1808, to the Medical Society of Massachusetts.

3. *Cantharis marginata.* Latreille, *Gen. Crust. et Insect.;* Durand, *Journ. of the Phil. Col. of Pharm.*, ii. 274, fig. 6. This is somewhat larger than *C. vittata*, and of a different shape. The elytra are black, with the suture and margin ash-colored. The head, thorax, and abdomen are black, but nearly covered with an ash-colored down; and, on the upper part of the abdomen, under the wings, are two longitudinal lines of a bright clay color. The insect is usually found, in the latter part of summer, upon different species of Clematis, and frequents especially the lower branches which trail along the ground. Professor Woodhouse, of Philadelphia, first ascertained its vesicating properties; but it had previously been described by Fabricius as a native of the Cape of Good Hope. Dr. Harris, of Massachusetts, found it as efficient as any other species.

4. *Cantharis atrata.* Latreille, *Gen. Crust. et Insect.;* Durand, *Journ. of the Phil. Col. of Pharm.*, ii. 274, fig. 7. The *black cantharis* is smaller than the indigenous species already described; but resembles *C. marginata* in figure. Its length is only four or five lines. It is distinguished by its size, and its uniform black color. It frequents more especially the different species of Aster and Solidago, though it is found also on *Prunella vulgaris, Ambrosia trifida*, and some other plants. Mr. Durand met with considerable numbers of this insect near Philadelphia, in the month of September; and they continued to appear till the middle of October. They are common in the Northern and Middle States, but are not confined exclusively to this country, being found also in Barbary. Drs. Oswood and Harris, of New England, satisfactorily ascertained their vesicating powers. They are probably identical with the insect noticed as vesicatory by Prof. Woodhouse, under the name of *Meloë niger*.

5. *Cantharis Vulnerata.* Harrison Allen, *Medical Zoology*, 1st ed., p. 150. Dr. Geo. H. Horn states that this is so abundant upon the Pacific coast that he has often seen bushels of it covering the ground. It has a black body, an orange-colored head, sometimes with a broad black stripe down the middle, and black wing-cases. Dr. Horn found it medicinally very active, as was also the less plentiful *C. Melæna.*

Several other species have been discovered in the United States, but not yet practically employed. Among these are *C. æneas*, a native of Pennsylvania, discovered by Mr. Say; *C. politus* and *C. aszelianus*, inhabiting the Southern States; *C. Nuttalli*, a large and beautiful insect of Missouri, first noticed by Mr. Nuttall, and said to surpass the Spanish fly in magnitude and splendor; and *C. albida*, another large species, found by Mr. Say near the Rocky Mountains. Of these, *C. Nuttalli (Lytta Nuttalli*, Say, *Am. Entomol.*, i. 9) bids fair, at some future period, to be an object of importance in the western section of this country. The head is of a deep greenish color, with a red spot in front; the thorax is of a golden green; the elytra red or golden purple and somewhat rugose on their outer surface, green and polished beneath; the feet black; the thighs blue or purplish. The exploring party under Colonel Long ascertained the vesicating powers of this insect. It was found in the plains of the Missouri, feeding on a scanty grass. In one spot it was so numerous as to be swept away by bushels, in order that a place might be cleared for encamping. There are also a number of beetles found in the United States which are plentiful enough to be capable of affording a commercial article, and which are so closely allied to the genus Cantharis as to render it probable that they possess blistering properties. For an account of the more important, see *Proc. A. P. A.*, 1876, p. 506. Mr. J. O. Braithwaite found the *Mylabris bifasciata* of the Cape of Good Hope extremely rich in cantharidin, whilst its co-dweller, *M. lineata*, contained but little. (*P. J. Tr.*, xviii. 246.) *Huechys sanguinea*, or "*Chinese cantharides*" of the London market, is not active. (J. Moss, *P. J. Tr.*, xvii. 845.)

Properties. "About one inch (25 mm.) long, and a quarter of an inch (6 mm.) broad; with filiform antennæ, black in the upper part, and ample, membranous, transparent, brownish wings; elsewhere of a shining, coppery-green color; the powder is grayish brown and contains green, shining particles; odor strong and disagreeable." *U. S.* Dried Spanish flies preserve the form and color, and, to a certain extent, the disagreeable odor of the living insect. They have an acrid, burning, and urinous taste. Their powder is of a grayish brown color, interspersed with shining green particles, which are the fragments of the feet, head, and wing-cases. If kept perfectly dry, in well-stopped glass bottles, they retain their activity for a great length of time. A portion which had been preserved by Van Swieten for thirty years, in a glass vessel, was found still to possess vesicating properties. But, exposed to a damp air, they quickly undergo putrefaction; and this change takes place more speedily in the powder. Hence the insects should either be kept whole, and powdered as they are wanted for use, or, if kept in powder, should be well dried immediately after pulverization, and preserved in air-tight vessels. They should never be purchased in powder, as, independently of the consideration just mentioned, they may in this state be more easily adulterated. But, however carefully managed, cantharides are apt to be attacked by mites, which feed on the interior soft parts of the body, reducing them to powder, while the hard exterior parts are not affected. An idea was at one time prevalent that the vesicating property of the insect was not injured by the worm, which was supposed to devour only the inactive portion. But this has been proved to be a mistake. M. Farines, an apothecary of Perpignan, has satisfactorily shown that, though the hard parts left by these mites possess some vesicating power, and the powder produced by them still more, yet the sound flies are much stronger than either. Camphor, which has been recommended as a preservative, does not prevent the destructive agency of the worm.* It is stated by M. Farines that, when the flies are destroyed by the vapor of pyroligneous acid, instead of common vinegar, they acquire an odor which contributes to their preservation. Cantharides will bear a very considerable heat without losing the brilliant color of their elytra; nor is this color extracted by water, alcohol, ether, or the oils; so that the powder might be deprived of all its active principle, and yet retain the exterior characters unaltered. The wing-cases resist putrefaction for a long time, and the shining particles have been detected in the human stomach months after interment. Cantharides exhausted by ether are sometimes offered for sale. They are worthless, and are to be distinguished by their lack of substance and their yielding a nearly colorless ethereal tincture.

So early as 1778, Thouvenel attempted to analyze cantharides, and the attempt was repeated by Dr. Beaupoil in 1803; but no very interesting or valuable result was obtained till 1810, when Robiquet discovered in them a crystalline substance, which proved to be the vesicating principle of the insect, and received the name of *cantharidin.* The constituents, according to Robiquet, are—1, a green oil, insoluble in water, soluble in alcohol, and inert as a vesicatory; 2, a black matter, soluble in water, insoluble in alcohol, and inert; 3, a yellow viscid matter, soluble in water and alcohol, and without vesicating powers; 4, cantharidin; 5, a fatty matter, insoluble in alcohol; 6, phosphates of calcium and magnesium, acetic acid, and in the fresh insect, a small quantity of uric acid. Orfila afterwards discovered a volatile principle, upon which the fetid odor of the fly depends. It is separable by distillation with water. Prof. Dragendorff has found a volatile principle which acts on the system in the same manner as cantharidin. When powdered flies are moistened with water and distilled, the part which passes over, at or below 100° C. (212° F.), contains this principle. (*Chem. News*, May 31, 1867.) That the green coloring matter is chlorophyll seems to be shown by the experiments of Pocklington, who

* It appears from the experiments of M. Nivet that, though camphor does not preserve the entire fly from the attacks of the larvæ of the *Anthrenus*, it actually destroys the mites of the Cantharis so often found in the powder, and may, therefore, be introduced with advantage, in small lumps, into bottles containing powdered cantharides. (*Journ. de Pharm.*, xix. 604.) Carbonate of ammonium has also been recommended as a preservative. Pereira has found that a few drops of strong acetic acid, added to the flies, are very effectual. Among the best means of preserving them, whether whole or in powder, is the application of the process of Apert, which consists in exposing them, for half an hour, confined in glass bottles, to the heat of boiling water, which destroys the eggs of the insect, without impairing the virtues of the flies. (*Ibid.*, xxii. 246.) Of course the access of water to the flies should be carefully avoided. Lutrand recommends chloroform as the best preservative that he has tried. (*Journ. de Pharm.*, xviii. 214.) We have little doubt that exposure, in a confined vessel, to the vapor of carbolic acid, would be a perfect protection against all forms of insect life.

(*P. J. Tr.*, [3] iii. p. 681) found that when cantharides was treated with alcohol, ether, and bisulphide of carbon, the solutions yielded absorption spectra agreeing with that of chlorophyll.

Cantharidin is a white substance, in the form of crystalline scales, of a shining micaceous appearance, inodorous, tasteless, almost insoluble in water and in cold alcohol, but soluble in ether, chloroform, benzol, the oils, and in hot alcohol and acetic acid, which deposit it upon cooling.* It fuses at 210° C. (410° F.), and is volatilizable by heat without decomposition, and its vapor condenses in acicular crystals. As determined by the experiments of Mr. Wm. A. Guy, the subliming heat of isolated cantharidin is 100° C. (212° F.), or the temperature of boiling water. (*P. J. Tr.*, Feb. 1868, p. 373.) According to MM. Masing and Dragendorff, cantharidin, with the composition $C_{10}H_{12}O_4$, is capable of combining with water, and thus becomes cantharidic acid, $2(C_5H_6O_2.H_2O)$, or $C_{10}H_{14}O_5$, and in this state forms definite compounds with bases, such as $2(C_5H_6O_2.KHO) + H_2O$, and $2(C_5H_6O_2.NaHO) + H_2O$, which are crystallizable. These may be obtained by heating cantharidin with an alkaline solution. (*Journ. de Pharm. et de Chim.*, Janv. 1868, p. 79.) Cantharidin itself has been found to combine like an acid with the salifiable and earthy bases, forming soluble compounds with potassium, sodium, and lithium hydrates, salts of very sparing solubility, with baryta, strontia, and lime, and, with magnesia a salt, which, though feebly soluble in water (100 parts of water dissolving only 0·24 of the salt) (see *P. J. Tr.*, March 13, 1880), is much more largely dissolved in cold than in hot water, and in cold than hot alcohol. (For further details concerning the relations of cantharidin with bases, and the preparation of its salts, see *P. J. Tr.*, Oct. 1873, p. 282.) The most satisfactory test of cantharidin is its vesicating property. Notwithstanding the insolubility of this principle in water and cold alcohol, the decoction and tincture of cantharides have the medicinal properties of the insect; and Lewis ascertained that both the aqueous and alcoholic extracts acted as effectually in exciting vesication as the flies themselves, while the residue was in each case inert. Cantharidin consequently exists in the insect, so combined with the yellow matter as to be rendered soluble in water and cold alcohol. If, as stated by E. Dietrich (1883), formic acid is present in the Spanish fly, it is probable that the solution of the cantharidin is due to its presence. H. G. Greenish calls attention to the fact that much loss of cantharidin takes place in making the various pharmaceutical preparations through insufficient exhaustion by the use of the ordinary solvents. He obtained 0·822 per cent. of cantharidin from exhausted residues. Homolka records in *Ber. d. Chem. Ges.*, xix. 1082, the results of an investigation on the chemical decompositions of cantharidin.

Adulterations. These are not common. Occasionally other insects are added, purposely, or through carelessness. These may be readily distinguished by their different shape or color. Flies exhausted of their cantharidin by ether are said to have been substituted for the genuine. An account has been published of considerable quantities of variously colored glass beads having been found in a parcel of the drug; but this would be too coarse a fraud to be extensively practised. Pereira states that powdered flies are sometimes adulterated with euphorbium. According to the researches of Mr. Fahnestock (*A. J. P.*, 1879, p. 298), age destroys the activity of the drug without of necessity impairing its physical appearance.

* The solubilities of cantharidin were examined with great care by Professor Procter, with the following results. It is insoluble in water. Cold alcohol dissolves it slightly, hot alcohol freely. It is more soluble in ether, which also dissolves it more freely hot than cold. Chloroform, cold or hot, is its best solvent; and acetone ranks next to it in this respect. Olive oil, at 250° F., dissolves one-twentieth of its weight, and oil of turpentine, boiling hot, one-seventieth; and both deposit the greater portion on cooling. The olive oil solution after deposition vesicates, the terebinthinate does not. Strong acetic, sulphuric, and nitric acid dissolve it, with the aid of heat, and deposit it unchanged on cooling. It is also dissolved by solutions of potassa and soda, and to a small extent by a strong solution of ammonia. (*A. J. P.*, xxiv. 296.) Formic acid is said to be the best solvent.

Somewhat different results in relation to the solubility of cantharidin have been obtained by M. E. Rowan. Careful examination with distilled water showed that, when agitated for eight days at ordinary temperatures with pure cantharidin, it was capable of dissolving 0·0266 per cent. of that principle; boiling water dissolves 0·297 per cent.; boiling alcohol (99 Tralles) 2·168 per cent. (*Journ. de Pharm.*, Mai, 1873, p. 409.)

The percentage of cantharidin found in cantharides furnishes the best test of their virtues. Professor Procter succeeded, by means of chloroform, in isolating cantharidin with great facility. He treated the flies with chloroform by percolation, displacing the last portion by means of alcohol, and allowing the resulting solution to evaporate spontaneously. Cantharidin is thus obtained in crystals mixed with the green oil, the greater portion of which may be removed by bibulous paper. The residuary crystals are dissolved in a mixture of ether and alcohol, which, by the spontaneous evaporation of the ether, yield the cantharidin nearly pure. M. Mortreux, having ascertained that cantharidin is insoluble in bisulphide of carbon, proposed to use this fluid for removing the fatty matter associated with the cantharidin crystals obtained by the use of chloroform. He employed the same liquid in estimating the proportion of cantharidin, which he found to be about 20 centigrammes for 40 grammes of the flies, or half of one per cent. (*Journ. de Pharm. et de Chem.*, 3e sér., xlvi. 33, 1864.) Wittstein obtains it by digesting coarsely powdered flies repeatedly with water, straining through linen and expressing, allowing the liquid to settle for a day, separating the supernatant oil, adding a little wood charcoal, evaporating to dryness, treating the residue with ether so long as the solution affords a laminated substance on evaporation, evaporating the ethereal solution, treating the residue with cold alcohol of 80 per cent. for one day with frequent shaking, and finally drying the scales. (See *A. J. P.*, xxviii. 231.) Mr. Williams has obtained it by means of benzol. (*Ibid.*, xxvi. 340.)

Medical Properties and Uses. Internally administered, cantharides is a powerful irritant, with a peculiar direction to the urinary and genital organs. In moderate doses, this medicine sometimes acts as a diuretic, and generally excites some irritation in the urinary passages, which, if its use be persevered in, or the dose increased, often amounts to violent strangury, attended with excruciating pain, and the discharge of bloody urine. In still larger quantities, it produces, in addition to these effects, obstinate and painful priapism, vomiting, bloody stools, severe pains in the whole abdominal region, excessive salivation with a fetid cadaverous breath, hurried respiration, a hard and frequent pulse, burning thirst, exceeding difficulty of deglutition, sometimes a dread of liquids, frightful convulsions, tetanus, delirium, and death. Orfila has known twenty-four grains of the powder to prove fatal. Dissection reveals inflammation and ulceration of the mucous coat of the whole intestinal canal. According to M. Poumet, if the intestines be inflated, dried, cut into pieces, and examined in the sun between two pieces of glass, they will exhibit small shining yellow or green points, strongly contrasting with the matter around them. (*Journ. de Pharm.*, 3e sér., iii. 167.)* The poisonous effects are to be counteracted by emetics, cathartics, and opiates by the stomach and rectum. Dr. Mulock, of Dublin, recommends the officinal solution of potassa as an antidote, having found thirty drops given every hour an effectual remedy in strangury from blisters. (*Dub. Quart. Journ. of Med. Sci.*, N. S., vi. 222.) From the experiments of Schroff it seems that oils somewhat accelerate the poisonous action, probably by dissolving the cantharidin. (See *A. J. P.*, xxviii. 365.) By experiments upon dogs, M. Thouery, a French apothecary, has satisfied himself that animal charcoal possesses a real antidotal power. (*Journ. de Pharm.*, 1858, p. 65.) Notwithstanding their exceeding violence, cantharides have been long and beneficially used in medicine. Either these or other vesicating insects appear to have been given by Hippocrates in dropsy and amenorrhœa, in the latter of which complaints, when properly prescribed, they are a highly valuable remedy. They are also useful in obstinate gleet, leucorrhœa, and seminal weakness, and afford one of the most certain means of relief in incontinence of urine arising from debility or partial paralysis of the sphincter of the bladder. A case of diabetes is recorded in the *N. Am. Archives* (vol. ii. p. 175), in which recovery took place under the tincture of cantharides. They are used also in certain cutaneous eruptions, especially those of a scaly character, and in chronic

* Cantharidin may be detected in the body after death from poisoning. M. Dragendorff, contrary to the opinion that cantharidin is so rapidly decomposed in a case of poisoning as to render search for it futile, states that he has succeeded in finding it in the dead body of a cat three months after it had been taken, and is convinced that it might be discovered in the human corpse six months after burial. (*Journ. de Pharm.*, 1873, p. 443.)

eczema. Dr. Erven has employed them in scurvy (*Ann. de Thérap.*, 1845); and they have been found useful, internally administered, in obstinate ulcers. Their unpleasant effects upon the urinary passages are best obviated by the free use of diluent drinks, and, when not consequent upon great abuse of the medicine, may almost always be relieved by an anodyne injection, composed of laudanum with a small quantity of mucilaginous fluid. The dose of Spanish flies is one or two grains (0·065–0·13 Gm.) of the powder, which may be given twice a day, in the form of pill. The tincture, however, is more frequently employed.

Externally applied, cantharides excites inflammation in the skin, which terminates in a copious secretion of serum under the cuticle. It may be employed either as a rubefacient, or to produce a blister. In the former capacity it is seldom used, but as an epispastic it is preferred to all other substances.

Blisters were formerly employed to some extent as stimulants in certain low conditions of the system, and have even been used for the cure of remittent and intermittent fevers, the older writers asserting that they are capable of setting aside a paroxysm when so applied as to be in full operation at the period of its recurrence. At present they are used almost exclusively for revulsion. When they are allowed only to stay on long enough to irritate the skin, but not completely to blister, they are known as *flying blisters.* Used in this way, they are sometimes of service in neuralgias, applied directly over the seat of pain. Their chief value, is, however, found in cases of severe internal irritation. It is of great importance that the practitioner clearly comprehend the distinct uses of the rubefacient and the blister. The rubefacient is to be employed as a revulsive when the internal irritation is severe but is not connected with pronounced organic change. The immediate impression of a rubefacient, acting as it does upon a much larger surface than does the blister, is greater than that of the blister, but the permanent revulsive action is much less. The blister is, therefore, to be used when the internal disease is connected with inflammatory structural change. Thus, in a case of gastrodynia, a rubefacient is of much more service than a blister, whilst the blister is decidedly more effective in peritonitis. In a general wide-spread congestion of the lung the rubefacient is to be preferred to the blister, but in pneumonia the blister to the rubefacient. As, however, congestion of neighboring parts usually accompanies a localized inflammation, a rubefacient is sometimes to be employed as a temporary substitute for or adjuvant to a blister. The amount of serous discharge produced by blisters appears to be sometimes of service in almost directly evacuating local serous exudations. Thus, not rarely, repeated blistering affords the best treatment of a serous pleurisy. Possibly, however, even in these cases, the blister acts purely as a counter-irritant, as it certainly does in chronic rheumatic and other diseases of the joints. In all chronic joint inflammations the best results may often be obtained by a reblistering, extending, if necessary, over weeks and months. In some cases of skin disease blisters are capable of substituting their own action for the original morbid disease, and they are still occasionally used for this purpose in tinea capitis, obstinate herpes, and other affections. The length of time that a blister should be applied varies with the individual and with the position of the disease. In some constitutions they produce a poisonous impression, attended with frequent pulse, dryness of the mouth, subsultus tendinum, and even convulsion. Such symptoms are probably the results of an intense peripheral nervous irritation acting upon very susceptible centres. Such is not, however, the case with the strangury which may follow absorption of the cantharidin, and which is always the result of the direct action of the cantharidin upon the genito-urinary tract. In order to avoid such genito-urinary irritation, and also as much as possible the pain at the seat of application, the blister should be left on only until it distinctly reddens the skin, when a flaxseed poultice may be applied, and in the course of two or three hours the blister is formed. The time necessary for such reddening of the skin is usually from four to six hours, if the cantharidin be active. For further remarks upon the use of the blister, see *Ceratum Cantharidis.*

Off. Prep. Ceratum Cantharidis; Ceratum Extracti Cantharidis; Charta Cantharidis; Collodium cum Cantharide; Linimentum Cantharidis; Tinctura Cantharidis.

Off. Prep. Br. Acetum Cantharidis; Charta Epispastica; Emplastrum Calefaciens; Emplastrum Cantharidis; Liquor Epispasticus; Tinctura Cantharidis; Unguentum Cantharidis.

CAPSICUM. *U.S.* *Capsicum.*

(CĂP'SĮ-CŬM.)

"The fruit of Capsicum fastigiatum. Blume. (*Nat. Ord.* Solanaceæ.)" *U.S.* "The dried ripe fruit of Capsicum fastigiatum, *Blume.*" *Br.*

Capsici Fructus, *Br.;* Cayenne Pepper, African Pepper; Fructus capsici, *P.G.;* Piper Hispanicum; Pod Pepper, *E.;* Capsique, Piment des Jardins, Piment rouge, Poivre de Cayenne, Poivre de Guinée, Poivre d'Inde, *Fr.;* Spanischer Pfeffer, *G.;* Pepperone, *It.;* Pimiento, *Sp.*

Gen. Ch. Corolla wheel-shaped. *Berry* without juice. *Willd.*

Numerous species of Capsicum, inhabiting the East Indies and tropical America, are enumerated by botanists, the fruit of which, differing simply in the degree of pungency, may be indiscriminately used. *C. baccatum,* or bird pepper, and *C. frutescens,* are said to yield most of the Cayenne pepper brought from the West Indies and South America; and Ainslie informs us that the latter is chiefly employed in the East Indies. Both Pharmacopœias now recognize, as the source of capsicum, *C. fastigiatum,* a species growing in the East Indies, and on the coast of Guinea. The one most extensively cultivated in Europe and this country is *C. annuum.* The first three are shrubby plants, the last is annual and herbaceous.

Capsicum annuum. Willd. *Sp. Plant.* i. 1052; *B. & T.* 189. The stem of the annual capsicum is thick, roundish, smooth, and branching; rises two or three feet in height; and supports ovate, pointed, smooth, entire leaves, which are placed without regular order on long footstalks. The flowers are solitary, white, and stand on long peduncles at the axils of the leaves. The calyx is persistent, tubular, and five-cleft; the corolla, monopetalous and wheel-shaped, with the limb divided into five spreading, pointed, and plaited segments; the filaments, short, tapering, and furnished with oblong anthers; the germen, ovate, supporting a slender style which is longer than the filaments, and terminates in a blunt stigma. The fruit is a pendulous, pod-like berry, of various shape and size, light, smooth, and shining, of a bright scarlet, orange, or sometimes yellow color, with two or three cells, containing a dry, loose pulp, and numerous flat, kidney-shaped, whitish seeds.

Capsicum fastigiatum. Blume. *B. & T.* 188. This species resembles closely *C. annuum,* but is distinguished by the lobes of the corolla being more acute, and especially by the fruit and seeds. The latter are smaller than those of *C. annuum,* and the erect, narrowly ovoid, oblong pod is nearly cylindrical, one-half to three-quarters of an inch long, and of a bright orange scarlet color when ripe.

These plants are natives of the warmer regions of Asia and America, and are cultivated in almost all parts of the world both for culinary and medicinal purposes. *C. annuum* is chiefly grown in this country; its flowers appear in July and August, and the fruit ripens in October. The several varieties of it differ in the shape of the fruit. The most abundant is probably that with a large irregularly ovate berry, depressed at the extremity, which is much used in the green state for pickling. The medicinal variety is that with long, conical, generally pointed, recurved fruit, usually not thicker than the finger. Sometimes we meet with small, spherical, slightly compressed berries, not greatly exceeding a large cherry in size. When perfectly ripe and dry, the fruit is ground into powder, and brought into market under the name of *red* or *Cayenne* pepper. Our markets are also partly supplied from the West Indies. A variety of capsicum, consisting of very small, conical, pointed, exceedingly pungent berries, less than an inch, is imported from Liberia. It is probably the *Capsicum fastigiatum.* In England the fruit of *C. annuum* is frequently called *chillies.* The officinal description of the fruit of *C. fastigiatum* is as follows: "Conical, from half to three-quarters of an inch (12 to 18 mm.) long, supported by a flattish, cup-shaped, five-toothed calyx, with a red, shining, membranous and translucent pericarp enclosing two cells, and containing flat, reniform, yellowish seeds attached to a thick, central placenta. It has a peculiar odor, and an intensely hot taste." *U.S.*

Powdered capsicum is usually of a more or less bright red color, which fades upon exposure to light, and ultimately disappears. The color of the Liberia or African pepper, in powder, is a light brownish yellow. The odor is peculiar and somewhat aromatic, stronger in the recent than in the dried fruit. The taste is bitterish, acrid, and burning, producing a fiery sensation in the mouth, which continues for a long time. The pungency appears to depend on a peculiar principle, which was obtained, though not in a perfectly isolated state, by Braconnot, and named *capsicin*. It is obtained as a thick yellowish red liquid, but slightly soluble in water. When gently heated it becomes very fluid, and at a higher temperature is dissipated in fumes, which are extremely irritating to the respiration. It is evidently a mixed substance, consisting of resinous and fatty matters.

In 1876, Thresh isolated, however, a well-defined highly active principle, *capsaicin*, from the extract, which he obtained by exhausting Cayenne pepper with petroleum. From the red liquor dilute caustic alkali removes capsaicin, which is to be precipitated in minute crystals by passing carbonic acid through the alkaline solution. The crystals may be purified by recrystallizing them from either alcohol, ether, benzin, glacial acetic acid, or hot bisulphide of carbon; in petroleum capsaicin is but sparingly soluble, yet dissolves abundantly on addition of fatty oil. The latter being present in the pericarp is the reason capsaicin can be extracted by the above process. The crystals of capsaicin are colorless, and answer to the formula $C_9H_{14}O_2$; they melt at 59° C. (138·2° F.), and begin to volatilise at 115° C. (239° F.), but decomposition can only be avoided with great care. The vapors of capsaicin are of the most dreadful acridity, and even the ordinary manipulation of that substance requires much precaution. Felletar (*Journ. de Pharm.*, Avril, 1870, p. 347) first obtained from capsicum fruits a volatile alkaloid, which resembles conine in odor, but is distinguished by the different shape of its hydrochlorate crystals. Red oxide of lead is sometimes added to the powdered capsicum sold in Europe. It may be detected by digesting in diluted nitric acid, and precipitating the lead by sulphate of sodium. Capsicum is said to be sometimes adulterated with colored sawdust; to be recognized by the microscope. The cut represents the characteristic cells of capsicum. It is occasionally attacked by insects.

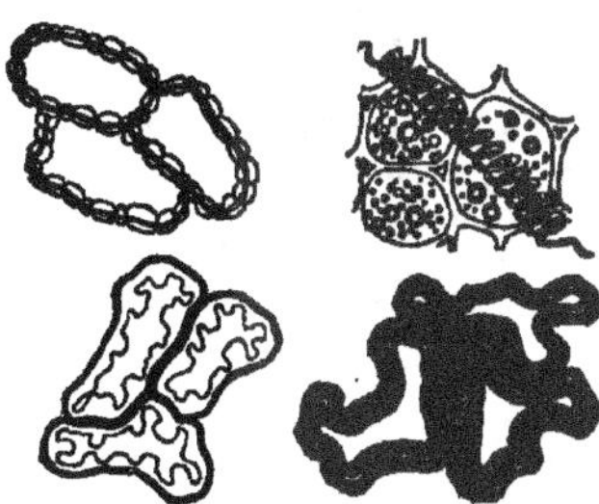

Medical Properties and Uses. Cayenne pepper is a powerful stimulant, producing when swallowed a sense of heat in the stomach, and a general glow over the body, without any narcotic effect. Its influence upon the circulation, though considerable, is not in proportion to its local action. It is much employed as a condiment, and proves highly useful in correcting the flatulent tendency of certain vegetables, and aiding their digestion. Hence the advantage derived from it by the natives of tropical climates, who live chiefly on vegetable food. In the East Indies it has been used from time immemorial. From a passage in the works of Pliny, it appears to have been known to the Romans. As a medicine it is useful in cases of enfeebled and languid stomach, and is occasionally prescribed in dyspepsia and atonic gout, particularly when attended with much flatulence, or occurring in persons of intemperate habits. It has also been given as a stimulant in palsy and certain lethargic affections. To the sulphate of quinine it forms an excellent addition in some cases of intermittents, in which there is a great want of gastric susceptibility. Upon the same principle of rousing the susceptibility of the stomach, it may prove useful in low forms of fever, as an adjuvant to tonic or stimulant medicines. Its most important application, however, is to the treatment of malignant sore throat and scarlet fever, in which it is used both internally and as a gargle. The following formula was employed in malignant scarlatina, with great advantage, in the West Indies, where this application of the remedy originated. Two tablespoonfuls (31·1 Gm.) of the powdered pepper, with a teaspoonful (3·9 Gm.) of common salt, are infused for an hour in a pint of boiling liquid, composed of equal parts of water and vinegar. This is strained when cool through a fine linen cloth, and given in the dose of a tablespoonful (15 C.c.) every half hour. The same preparation is also used as a gargle. It is, however, only to the worst cases that the remedy is applied so energetically. In milder cases of scarlatina, with inflamed or ulcerated throat, much relief and positive advantage often follow the employment of the pepper in a more diluted state. Capsicum has been advantageously used in sea-sickness, in the dose of a teaspoonful (3·9 Gm.), given in some convenient vehicle on the first occurrence of nausea. It is thought also to have been beneficial in hemorrhoidal affections. It has long been used as a stomachic stimulant in the enfeebled digestion of drunkards, and has been recommended in delirium tremens, in which, when taken early, it is said sometimes to produce sleep, and thus to cut short the disease. (Dr. Lyons, *Med. Press and Circ.*, April 18, 1866.)

Applied externally, Cayenne pepper is a powerful rubefacient, very useful in local rheumatism, and in low forms of disease, where a stimulant impression upon the surface is demanded. It has the advantage of acting speedily without endangering vesication. It may be applied in the form of cataplasm, or more conveniently and efficiently as a lotion, mixed with heated spirit. The powder or tincture, brought into contact with a relaxed uvula, often acts very beneficially. The tincture has also been used advantageously in chilblain. The ethereal extract (*Oleoresina Capsici, U. S.*) is powerfully rubefacient.

The dose of the powder is from five to ten grains (0·33–0·65 Gm.), which is most conveniently given in the form of pill. Of an infusion prepared by adding two drachms to half a pint of boiling water, the dose is half a fluidounce (15 C.c.). A gargle may be prepared by infusing half a drachm of the powder in a pint of boiling water, or by adding half a fluidounce of the tincture to eight fluidounces of rose-water.

Off. Prep. Extractum Capsici Fluidum; Oleoresina Capsici; Tinctura Capsici.
Off. Prep. Br. Tinctura Capsici.

CARBO. *Carbon.*

C; 12. (CĂR'BŌ.) C; 6.

Pure Charcoal; Carbone, *Fr., It.;* Kohlenstoff, *G.;* Carbon, *Sp.*

Carbon is an element of great importance, and very extensively diffused in nature. It exists in large quantity in the mineral kingdom, and is the most abundant constituent of animal and vegetable matter. In the crystallized state it constitutes the diamond; and, more or less pure, it forms the substances called graphite, or black lead, plumbago, anthracite and bituminous coal, coke, animal charcoal, and vegetable charcoal. Combined with oxygen it forms *carbon dioxide*, or *carbonic acid gas*, which is a constituent of the atmosphere, and present in many natural waters, especially those which have an effervescing quality. United with oxygen and a base it forms the carbonates, among others *carbonate of calcium*, which is one of the most abundant minerals. There are three allotropic conditions of carbon, represented respectively by the diamond, graphite, and charcoal.

The *diamond* is found principally in India, Brazil, and Cape Colony, South Africa. Several diamonds have been found in the gold regions of Georgia and North Carolina. This gem is perfectly transparent, and the hardest and most brilliant substance in nature. Its sp. gr. is about 3·5. It is fixed and unalterable in the fire, provided air be excluded; but is combustible in air or oxygen, the product being the same as when charcoal is burned, namely, carbon dioxide.

Next to diamond, graphite or plumbago is the purest natural form of carbon. Graphite is the substance of which black-lead crucibles and pencils are made. It is found in greatest purity in the mine of Borrowdale, in England; but it also occurs very pure in this country, and in extensive deposits at Ticonderoga, N. Y., Stourbridge, Mass., and in Canada. In physical characters it is utterly different from the diamond; it crystallizes in hexagonal plates, is very soft and unctuous, of 2 to 2·5 sp. gr., and generally contains a little ash. It was formerly supposed to be a carbide of iron; but, in very pure specimens, it is nearly free from iron, which must, therefore, be deemed an accidental impurity. *Anthracite*, the purest variety of natural coal, occurs in different parts of the world, but particularly in the State of Pennsylvania. It contains from 90 to 95 per cent. of carbon, and several per cent. of ash. *Bituminous coal* is another variety, containing, besides the fixed or free carbon, some 10 to 15 per cent. of volatile hydrocarbons or gas-making material. When this is driven off by the process of charring, as in the manufacture of coal gas, a kind of mineral charcoal, called *coke*, is obtained, very useful in the arts as a fuel. When peat is charred, it is converted into *peat charcoal*, which forms a cheap disinfectant and deodorizer, applicable to the purification of hospitals, dissecting rooms, factories, privies, etc.

Carbon may be obtained in a state approaching to purity by several processes. One method is to expose lampblack to a full red heat in a close vessel. It may also be obtained, in a very pure state, by passing the vapor of volatile oils through an ignited porcelain tube; whereby the hydrogen and oxygen of the oil will be dissipated, and the charcoal left in the tube. The purest black is now made from natural gas in western Pennsylvania and in Ohio. This lampblack is miscible with water, does not color ether, and is free from oily matter.

Properties. Carbon, in its uncrystallized state, is an insoluble, infusible solid, generally of a black color, and without taste or smell. It burns when sufficiently heated, uniting with the oxygen of the air, and generating carbonic acid gas. Its sp. gr. in the solid state, apart from its pores when in mass, is 3·5; but with the air of the pores included, it is only 0·44. It is a very unalterable and indestructible substance, and has great power in resisting and correcting putrefaction in other bodies. When properly prepared, it possesses the property of absorbing the coloring and odorous principles of most liquids. (See *Carbo Animalis.*) Its other physical properties differ according to its source, and peculiar state of aggregation. As a chemical element it enjoys a very extensive range of combination. It forms two compounds with oxygen, *carbon dioxide* (carbonic acid gas) and *carbon monoxide* (carbonous oxide). With hydrogen it forms a number of compounds, called *hydrocarbons*, of which the most interesting, excluding hypothetical radicals, are light carburetted hydrogen or marsh-gas, olefiant gas, the light and concrete oils of wine, the hydrocarbons constituting petroleum, and the various essential oils. With nitrogen it constitutes cyanogen, the compound radical of hydrocyanic or prussic acid; and united in minute proportion with iron it forms steel.

To notice all the forms of the carbonaceous principle would be out of place in this work. We shall, therefore, restrict ourselves to the consideration of those which are officinal, namely, *animal charcoal* and *wood charcoal.*

CARBO ANIMALIS. *U.S., Br.* *Animal Charcoal.*

(CĂR'BŌ ĂN-Ĭ-MĀ'LĬS.)

"Animal [*sic*] charcoal prepared from bone." *U.S.* "The residue of bones, which have been exposed to a red heat without access of the air." *Br.*

Bone Black, Ivory Black, *Br.;* Charbon animal, Noir d'Os, *Fr.;* Thierische Kohle, Knochen Kohle, Beinschwarz, Thierkohle, *G.;* Carbone animale, *It.;* Carbon animal, *Sp.*

The animal charcoal employed in pharmacy and the arts is usually obtained from bones, by subjecting them to a red heat in close vessels. The residue of the ignition is a black matter, which, when reduced to powder, forms *bone-black*, sometimes incorrectly called *ivory-black.* Ivory by carbonization will furnish a black, which, on account of its fineness and intensely black color, is more esteemed than the ordinary bone-black; but it is much more expensive.

In manufacturing bone-black, the bones, first boiled in water to separate the fat, are subjected to destructive distillation in iron cylinders, connected with vessels which receive the ammoniacal liquor, called *bone-spirit*, together with a dark tarry liquid (*bone-oil*), this being a secondary product of the operation. When the bone-spirit ceases to come over, the residue is charred bone, or bone-black. Bone consists of animal matter with phosphate and carbonate of calcium. In consequence of the decomposition of the animal matter involved in this destructive distillation, the nitrogen and hydrogen, united as ammonia, and a part of the charcoal, in the form of carbonic acid gas, distil over; while the remainder of the charcoal is left in the cylinder, intermingled with the calcareous salts. M. Deiss, of Paris, proposes bisulphide of carbon as a solvent for the fat of bones; as it furnishes a larger and better product of fat, and renders the bones fitter for producing a good bone-black. (*Chem. Gaz.*, April 1, 1856.) This form of animal charcoal necessarily contains phosphate and carbonate of calcium.

Properties. Animal charcoal is in the form of "dull black, granular fragments, or a dull black powder, odorless and nearly tasteless, and insoluble in water or alcohol. When ignited, it leaves a white ash, amounting to at least 86 per cent. of the original weight, which should be completely soluble in hydrochloric acid, with the aid of heat." *U. S.* It is, however, more dense and less combustible than vegetable charcoal; from which, moreover, it may be distinguished by burning a small portion of it on a red-hot iron, when it will leave a residuum imperfectly acted on by sulphuric acid; whereas the ashes from vegetable charcoal readily dissolve in this acid, forming a bitterish solution.

Animal charcoal by no means necessarily possesses the decolorizing property; as this depends upon its peculiar state of aggregation. If a piece of pure animal matter is carbonised, it usually enters into fusion, and from the gaseous matter which is extricated, becomes porous and cellular. The charcoal formed has generally a metallic lustre, and a color resembling that of black lead. It has, however, little or no decolorizing power, even though finely pulverized.

The decolorizing power of vegetable charcoal was first noticed by Lowitz, of St. Petersburg; and that of animal charcoal by Figuier, of Montpellier, in 1811. In 1822 the subject was ably investigated by Bussy, Payen, and Desfosses. The power is generally communicated to charcoal by igniting it in close vessels, but not always. The kind of charcoal, for example, obtained from substances which undergo fusion during carbonization scarcely possesses the property, even though it may be afterwards finely pulverized. The property in question is possessed to a certain extent by wood charcoal;* but is developed in it in a much greater degree by burning it with some chemical substance, which may have the effect of reducing it to an extreme degree of fineness. The most powerful of all the charcoals for discharging colors are those obtained from certain animal matters, such as dried blood, hair, etc., by first carbonising them in connection with carbonate of potassium, and then washing the product with water. Charcoal, thus prepared, seems to be reduced to a state of extremely minute division, and is, therefore, very porous. The next most powerful decolorizing charcoal is *bone-black*, in which the separation of the carbonaceous particles is effected by the phosphate of calcium present in the bone. Vegetable substances also may be made to yield a good charcoal for destroying color, provided, before carbonization, they be well comminuted, and mixed with pumice stone, chalk, flint, or other similar substance in a pulverized state.

The following table, abridged from one drawn up by Bussy, denotes the relative decolorizing power of different charcoals.

KINDS OF CHARCOAL.	Decolorising power on Syrup.	Decolorising power on Indigo.
Bone-black	1	1
Bone charcoal treated with an acid	1·6	1·8
Lampblack, not ignited	3·3	4
Charcoal, from acetate of potassium	4·4	5·6
Blood ignited with phosphate of calcium	10	12
Lampblack ignited with carbonate of potassium	10·6	12·2
Blood ignited with chalk	11	18
White of egg ignited with carbonate of potassium	15·5	34
Glue ignited with carbonate of potassium	15·5	36
Bone charcoal, formed from bone deprived of phosphate of calcium by an acid, and subsequently ignited with carbonate of potassium	20	45
Blood ignited with carbonate of potassium	20	50

* Dr. Stenhouse divides decolorizing charcoals into three classes. First, pure charcoals, which, being in a state of minute division, decolorise by their porosity alone. Second, those which, like aluminised charcoal and artificial bone-black, decolorise solely by the bases they contain, acting as mordants. Third, those which, like bone-black, decolorise, partly by the mineral matter, and partly by the minutely divided charcoal they contain. (*P. J. Tr.*, Jan. 1857, p. 366.)

In order to determine the commercial value of animal charcoal, M. Corenwinder has proposed to ascertain its power of absorbing lime from a solution of saccharate of lime of determinate strength. The value is in proportion to the absorbing power of the charcoal. A given weight of the charcoal to be tested is left in contact, for an hour, with a given volume of the solution of the saccharate, taken in excess. The liquid is then filtered, and a small measure of it saturated with dilute sulphuric acid of known strength. The less the acid necessary for this purpose, the greater the amount of lime absorbed, and the better the animal charcoal. (*Chem. Gaz.*, 1854, p. 16; *Scientific American*, April 22, 1876; *Arch. d. Pharm.*, 1887, p. 133; *Proc. A. P. A.*, 1887, p. 205.)

Spent animal charcoal, which has been used by the sugar refiners, may have its decolorizing power restored by calcination, which destroys the organic matters that have become fixed in it; and it is stated that it may be submitted to this process twenty times before becoming unfit for use. According to Pelouze, the same object may be accomplished by subjecting it to a weak solution of carbonate of potassium or of sodium. In removing the coloring matter, the alkaline solution becomes yellow. After its action the animal charcoal must be carefully washed, first with boiling water, and afterwards with acidulated water. But a process devised by MM. Leplay and Cuisinier is probably more effectual. The charcoal, without being removed from the cylinders, is thoroughly washed, treated by steam to remove viscous substances, and then percolated successively, 1, by a weak alkaline solution, which removes salts and some coloring matters; 2, by weak hydrochloric acid, which, in removing a certain amount of salts of lime, liberates coloring matter; 3, again with a weak alkaline solution to carry off the remaining coloring matter; and 4, lastly by a solution of biphosphate of calcium, by which the decolorizing power of the charcoal is restored. (Dr. F. C. Calvert, *A. J. P.*, 1865, p. 263.)

Animal charcoal is capable of taking the bitter principles from infusions and tinctures, and iodine from liquids which contain it in solution. Its power, however, of acting on solutions and chemical compounds is much more decided in its purified state, as shown by both Warington and Weppen. (See *Carbo Animalis Purificatus*; see, also, *Ephemeris*, 1885, p. 721.)

Bone-black consists of about 90 per cent. of phosphate and carbonate of calcium, and 10 per cent. of charcoal.

Pharm. Uses. Animal charcoal is used in pharmacy for decolorizing vegetable principles, such as gallic acid, quinine, morphine, veratrine, etc., and in the arts, principally for clarifying syrups in sugar refining, for depriving spirits distilled from grain of the peculiar volatile oil, called *fusel oil*, which imparts to them an unpleasant smell and taste, as first distilled, and for the filtration of petroleum residuums in the manufacture of petrolatum and petroleum jellies. (See *Petrolatum.*) The manner in which it is used as a decolorizer is to mix it with the substance to be decolorized, and to allow the mixture to stand for some time. The charcoal unites with the coloring matter, and the solution by filtration is obtained white and transparent. Its use, however, in decolorizing the organic alkalies and other vegetable principles, no doubt causes a loss by absorption; since it has been shown by the experiments of M. Lebourdais, mentioned under the head of purified animal charcoal, that several of these principles may be obtained by the sole action of charcoal. For most pharmaceutical operations, and for use as an antidote, animal charcoal must be purified by hydrochloric acid from phosphate and carbonate of calcium. (See *Carbo Animalis Purificatus.*) According to Guthe, a German chemist, bone charcoal, without purification, is to be preferred as a decolorizer, in all cases in which the calcareous salts exert no injurious effect.

Off. Prep. Carbo Animalis Purificatus.

CARBO ANIMALIS PURIFICATUS. *U.S., Br.* *Purified Animal Charcoal.*

(CÄR'BŌ ĂN-I-MĀ'LĬS PŪ-RI-FI-CĀ'TŬS.)

Charbon animal purifié, *Fr.;* Gereinigte Knochen Kohle, *G.*

"Animal Charcoal, in No. 60 powder, *two parts;* Hydrochloric Acid, *three parts;*

Water, *a sufficient quantity.* Pour the Hydrochloric Acid, previously mixed with *fifteen* (15) *parts* of Water, upon the Animal Charcoal, and digest the mixture on a water-bath, for twenty-four hours, occasionally stirring. Pour off the supernatant liquid, and digest the undissolved portion with *fifteen* (15) *parts* of Water for two hours. Transfer the mixture to a strainer, and, when the liquid portion has run off, wash the residue with Water until the washings cease to be affected by test-solution of nitrate of silver. Dry the product, heat it to dull redness in a closely covered crucible, and, when cool, keep it in well-stopped bottles." *U. S.*

"Take of Bone Black, in powder, *sixteen ounces* [avoirdupois]; Hydrochloric Acid *ten fluidounces;* Distilled Water *a sufficiency.* Mix the Hydrochloric Acid with a pint of the Water, and add the Bone Black, stirring occasionally. Digest at a moderate temperature for two days, agitating from time to time; collect the undissolved charcoal on a calico filter, and wash with Distilled Water till what passes through gives scarcely any precipitate with nitrate of silver. Dry the charcoal, and then heat it to redness in a covered crucible." *Br.*

Animal charcoal, as it is made by charring bones, necessarily contains bone-phosphate and carbonate of calcium, the presence of which does no harm in some decolorizing operations; but, in delicate chemical processes, these salts may be dissolved or decomposed, and thus become a source of impurity. It is on this account that animal charcoal requires to be purified from its calcareous salts; and this is accomplished by diluted hydrochloric acid, which dissolves the phosphate and decomposes the carbonate. According to Dr. Stenhouse, aluminized vegetable charcoal may be substituted for purified animal charcoal, and is equally efficacious as a decolorizer. (See page 367.)

Properties. Purified animal charcoal is "a dull black powder, odorless and tasteless, and insoluble in water, alcohol, or other solvents. When ignited at a high temperature with a little red oxide of mercury and with free access of air, it leaves at most only a trace of residue. If 1 part be digested with 2 parts of hydrochloric acid and 6 parts of water, the filtrate, after being supersaturated with water of ammonia, should remain unaffected by test-solution of magnesium (abs. of phosphate)." *U. S.*

It has been shown by Mr. Robert Warington that bitter vegetable substances, including the organic alkalies, are removed from solution by passing through purified animal charcoal, especially when the action is assisted by heat. M. Weppen finds that a similar effect is produced by it in removing resins from tinctures, tannic acid and bitter principles from astringent and bitter infusions, and certain metallic salts from their solutions. Purified animal charcoal, thus employed, has been resorted to by M. Lebourdais as an agent for obtaining the active principles of plants. A decoction or infusion of the plant is either boiled with or filtered through the charcoal, which takes up, more or less completely, the bitter and coloring principles. The charcoal, after having been washed and dried, is treated with boiling alcohol, which dissolves the principles taken up. Finally, the alcohol is distilled off, and the principles are obtained in a separate state. In this way digitalin, ilicin, scillitin, columbin, colocynthin, arnicine, strychnine, quinine, and other principles have been obtained by M. Lebourdais. (*Chem. Gaz.*, Nov. 15, 1848.) In relation to the method of M. Lebourdais, see a paper by Mr. J. S. Cobb. (*A. J. P.*, 1851.) Dr. A. B. Garrod has proposed purified animal charcoal as an antidote to vegetable and animal poisons, with which it appears to combine. According to his experiments, common bone-black has not one-fifth of the powder possessed by the purified substance; and vegetable charcoal and lampblack are nearly or quite useless. The amount of the antidote proposed by Dr. Garrod is half an ounce for each grain of a vegetable organic alkali. Dr. Alfred Taylor deems the results of Dr. Garrod inconclusive. Prof. B. H. Rand, of this city, made some interesting observations in relation to the antidotal powers of purified animal charcoal, and proved that poisonous doses of the strongest vegetable poisons may be swallowed with impunity, if mixed with that substance. (*Med. Exam.*, Sept. 1848.) It has also been recommended as an antidote for phosphorus (*N. Y. Med. Record*, 1874, p. 68), but its value is very doubtful.

In using animal charcoal for decolorizing active vegetable principles, great caution should be observed, as much loss is often incurred by the absorption of those principles by the charcoal.

CARBO LIGNI. *U. S., Br.* *Charcoal.*

(CĂR'BŌ LĬG'NĪ.)

"Charcoal prepared from soft wood." *U. S.* "Wood charred by exposure to a red heat without access of air." *Br.*

Wood Charcoal, Vegetable Charcoal; Carbo Pulveratus, *P. G.;* Carbo Præparatus, Carbo e Ligno; Charbon végétal, Charbon de Bois, *Fr.;* Holzkohle, Präparirte Kohle, *G.;* Carbone di Legno, *It.;* Carbon de Lena, *Sp.*

Preparation on the Large Scale. Billets of wood are piled in a conical form, and covered with earth and sod to prevent the free access of air; several holes being left at the bottom, and one at the top of the pile, in order to produce a draught to commence the combustion. The wood is then kindled from the bottom. In a little while the hole at the top is closed, and, after the ignition is found to have pervaded the whole pile, those at the bottom are stopped also. The combustion taking place with a smothered flame, the volatile portions of the wood, consisting of hydrogen and oxygen, are dissipated; while the carbon, in the form of charcoal, is left.

In this process for the carbonization of wood, all the volatile products are dissipated; and a portion of the charcoal itself is lost by combustion. Wood, thus carbonized, yields not more than 17 or 18 per cent. of charcoal. A better method is to char the wood in iron cylinders, when it yields from 22 to 23 parts in 100 of excellent charcoal; and, at the same time, the means are afforded for collecting the volatile products, consisting of pyroligneous acid, empyreumatic oil, and tar. This process for obtaining charcoal has been described under another head. (See *Acidum Aceticum.*) A method of preparing charcoal by subjecting wood to over-heated steam has been invented by M. Violette. When the temperature of the steam is 300° C. (572° F.), the wood is converted into a peculiar charcoal, called *red charcoal*, which is intermediate in its qualities between wood and ordinary charcoal. When the temperature is lower, the carbonization is incomplete; when higher, the product is black charcoal. The steam process yields a uniform charcoal for a given temperature, which may be easily regulated, and a product about double that obtained in closed cylinders. Charcoal, prepared in closed cylinders, yields ten times as much ash as that ordinarily made. Charcoal contains *carbon*, in proportion to the temperature at which it is formed; varying from 65 per cent. when made at 250° C. (482° F.), to 80 per cent. at 400° C. (752° F.). The gaseous matter present is always inversely as the temperature of carbonization. Thus, for charcoal made at 300° C. (572° F.), it is one-third of its weight; at 350° C. (662° F.), one-fourth. (*Journ. de Pharm.*, 1851, p. 35.)

Mr. E. C. C. Stanford has called attention to a variety of vegetable charcoal, obtained by charring a species of sea-weed, *Laminaria digitata*, gathered on the shores of the Hebrides, which, although, on account of the large proportion of carbonate of calcium contained in it (20 per cent.), unfit for use in refining sugar, possesses more of the deodorizing and decolorizing power than animal charcoal itself, which, with the exception referred to, it closely resembles in chemical composition. (*P. J. Tr.*, 1867, p. 186.)

Preparation for Medicinal Use. M. Belloc recommends charcoal for this purpose to be obtained from poplar shoots, cut at the time the sap rises, and deprived of their bark. The carbonization should be performed in cast-iron vessels at a red-white heat. The product is a light and brilliant charcoal, which must be purified by being macerated for three or four days in water, frequently renewed. It is then dried, powdered, and placed in bottles, which should be well stopped. The charcoal most esteemed in Philadelphia, for medicinal purposes, is that prepared by the Messrs. Dupont, near Wilmington, Delaware, for the manufacture of gunpowder. It is made from young willow shoots of two or three years' growth.

Properties. Charcoal is a black, shining, brittle, porous substance, tasteless and inodorous and insoluble in water. It is a good conductor of electricity, but a bad one of heat. It possesses the remarkable property of absorbing many times its own bulk of certain gases. When exposed to the air after ignition, it increases rapidly in weight, absorbing from 12 to 14 per cent. of moisture. As ordinarily prepared, it contains the incombustible part of the wood amounting to 1 or 2 per cent., which is left as ashes when the charcoal is burned. These may be removed by digesting the charcoal in diluted hydrochloric acid, and afterwards washing it thoroughly with boiling water.

Medical Properties, etc. Powdered charcoal is disinfectant and absorbent. It is employed with advantage in diarrhœa as an absorbent, and in dyspepsia with fetid breath and eructations. It was given in dysentery by the late Dr. Robert Jackson, who found it to have the effect of soothing the patient, and improving the character and consistence of the stools. It is also useful, in the form of injection, in putrid discharges from the uterus. M. Belloc recommends it strongly in gastralgia, and especially pyrosis, in which, if it fails to remove the disease, it abates the pain, nausea, and vomiting; and his observations have been confirmed by a committee of the French Academy of Medicine. As a remedy in obstinate constipation, Dr. Daniel, of Savannah, speaks of it in high terms. He also found it useful in nausea and constipation of pregnancy. On the other hand, some practitioners have found charcoal to confine the bowels. Dr. Wilson, of New Zealand, speaks highly of it in the diarrhœa of measles, and in epidemic cholera. Dr. Newman recommends it as a dressing to wounds and ulcers. Mr. Wormald, of St. Bartholomew's Hospital, has made a useful application of the disinfecting power of dry charcoal, in what he calls the *charcoal quilt*. This consists of two sheets of cotton wadding, quilted together in small segments, with a tolerably thick layer of powdered charcoal between them. The quilts, thus prepared, may be of any size, so as to fit a gangrenous sore or stump. Its use as an ingredient of poultices is noticed under *Cataplasma Carbonis*. Several of its varieties are used as tooth-powder. Those generally preferred are the charcoals of the cocoa-nut shell and of bread. It is said that charcoal proves useful in preserving the teeth by absorbing the acid sometimes morbidly present in the mucus of the mouth. The dose of charcoal varies from one to four teaspoonfuls (3·9–15·5 Gm.) or more. Dr. Daniel gave it in his case of constipation in doses of a tablespoonful (15·5 Gm.), repeated every half hour. *Charcoal biscuits* have been prepared, containing 15 or 20 per cent. of charcoal in fine powder, whilst *charcoal lozenges*, either with charcoal alone or associated with bismuth, have been employed with asserted good results in certain forms of gastric disturbances.

For internal use charcoal is preferred by some in the *granular form*. Mr. W. Lascelles Scott employs the following method of preparing it. He prefers the wood of the box, willow, or linden, which, after being charred, should be allowed to cool out of contact with air, then boiled for some time in diluted hydrochloric acid, and afterwards, having been thoroughly washed with pure water, in a little weak ammonia. The fragments are again ignited, and then quickly powdered, and passed through a sieve of 80 or 100 apertures to the inch. Nine pounds of this powder are mixed with one pound of pure sugar passed through a 30 sieve, and 4 ounces of gum arabic in impalpable powder. The whole is then moistened with a few ounces of warm distilled water, to which have been added an ounce and a quarter of tincture of benzoin, and a little mucilage. The mass is now granulated on flat steam pans, in the usual manner, at a temperature of 101·6°–107·2° C. (215° or 225° F.). When perfectly dry it is sifted, and secured in well-stopped bottles. (*Chem. News*, 1867, p. 204.)

Charcoal has been employed with good effect, as a deodorizer, in dissecting-rooms, placed in open pans through the room. It has the advantage over the chlorides that it has no smell. When it loses its effect, it may be recalcined. Water for long voyages is kept sweet by having a little powdered charcoal added to each cask.

Dr. Stenhouse has devised a process for combining alumina with common vegetable charcoal, forming what he calls *aluminized charcoal*, which is an economical substitute for purified animal charcoal, and equally efficacious as a decolorizer. It is prepared by digesting finely powdered charcoal with sufficient of the solution of sulphate of aluminium to give an impregnation of 7·5 per cent. of alumina. The whole is evaporated to dryness, and ignited in a covered Hessian crucible, until the water and acid have been dissipated. Aluminized charcoal is perfectly black, though thoroughly impregnated with anhydrous alumina, and only requires to be carefully pulverized to be ready for use. (*P. J. Tr.*, 1857, p. 364.) On similar principles, Dr. Stenhouse prepares his *artificial bone-black*, by impregnating powdered wood charcoal with 7·5 per cent. of phosphate of calcium, by digesting it in a solution of this salt in hydrochloric acid, evaporating to dryness, and igniting in covered vessels. This charcoal decolorizes well, but can be used only for neutral solutions.

Charcoal may act either as an oxidizer or deoxidizer; and these contrary powers seem to depend upon its having for oxygen a medium affinity, which enables it to take that element from some bodies, and to yield it to others, or at least by its porosity to facilitate atmospheric oxidation. Thus, it is known to reduce several oxides; while, on the other hand, it aids powerfully in the oxidation of animal matter. The bodies of two dogs having been laid in an open box on a bed of charcoal, a few inches deep, and covered by the same material, were kept by Mr. John Turnbull, of Glasgow, for six months in his laboratory, without emitting any perceptible effluvium; and, when they were examined at the end of this time, scarcely anything remained but the bones. Dr. Stenhouse, who relates this experiment, has confirmed it by observations of his own, and believes that the animal matter thus treated, undergoes putrefaction; though the products, by their rapid oxidation and absorption, are prevented from contaminating the air. He, therefore, considers charcoal not to be antiseptic, but the very opposite. (*Chem. Gaz.*, 1854, p. 132.)

The study of the absorbent and oxidizing properties of charcoal led Dr. Stenhouse to apply it to the purpose of preventing the access of noxious effluvia to the lungs in respiration. This object he proposed to effect by covering the nose and mouth with what he called the *charcoal respirator*. The instrument consists of a layer of coarsely powdered charcoal, a quarter of an inch thick, between two sheets of silvered wire gauze, covered with thin woollen cloth, by means of which the temperature of the inspired air is greatly increased. The frame is made of thin sheet-copper; but the edges of lead padded and lined with velvet so as to fit the lower part of the face. Dr. Stenhouse considered his respirator to act as an air filter, and to be peculiarly adapted to protect the wearer against infectious diseases. (*P. J. T.*, 1855, p. 328.) This instrument must not be confounded with Jeffrey's wire ventilator, which is intended solely to warm the air before entering the lungs.

Off. Prep. Cataplasma Carbonis, *Br.*

CARBONEI BISULPHIDUM. *U.S.* *Bisulphide of Carbon.* [*Disulphide of Carbon.*]

CS_2; 76. (CĂR-BŌ′NĒ-Ī BĪ-SŬL′PHĮ-DŬM.) CS_2; 38.

"Bisulphide of Carbon should be kept in well-stopped bottles, in a cool place, remote from lights or fire." *U. S.*

Carboneum Sulfuratum, Alcohol Sulfuris, *P.G.*; Carbonii Bisulphidum; Carbon Sulphide, Sulfure de Carbone, *Fr.*; Schwefelkohlenstoff, *G.*

This compound, corresponding to carbon dioxide (carbonic acid gas), CO_2, is prepared by the direct combination of carbon and sulphur at a moderate red heat. To effect this, charcoal is heated to redness in a vertical cylinder, while sulphur is admitted through a lateral tubulure near the bottom. As the sulphur melts and vaporizes, it combines with the carbon, and the carbon disulphide formed distils over through a series of condensing tubes, which, while they serve to collect the crude carbon disulphide, allow of the escape of the hydrogen sulphide formed at the same time. The crude product is then rectified, first over a solution of chlorinated lime to break up any hydrogen sulphide gas remaining, and then repeatedly either over mercury, mercuric chloride, anhydrous cupric sulphate, or over a pure fatty oil, which withdraws from it all free sulphur and bad-smelling sulphur compounds. Obach experimented with permanganate of potassium as a purifying agent, as was suggested by Allary. He finds it well adapted for use on a small scale in combination with mercury, sulphur, mercuric sulphate. (*N. R.*, 1883, p. 21.)

The manufacture of carbon disulphide has within late years assumed large proportions. In the works of Deiss at Pantin, near Marseilles, France, 500 kilogrammes are turned out daily, and their annual production in 1880 exceeded 1,200,000 kilogrammes.

It is used in the arts for the extraction of oils from different oil-seeds, for the extraction of sulphur from some varieties of sulphur ores, for the cleansing of wool and recovering the fat, in the manufacture of india-rubber goods as a solvent for the caoutchouc, for the extraction of perfumes, and latterly on an enormous scale in France as a remedy against the *phylloxera*, or grape pest, using it either directly or to produce the alkaline xanthogenates (sulphocarbonates).

Properties. "A clear, colorless, highly refractive liquid, very diffusive, having a strong, characteristic odor, a sharp, aromatic taste, and a neutral reaction. It is insoluble in water; soluble in alcohol, ether, chloroform, and fixed or volatile oils. Sp. gr. 1·272. It vaporizes abundantly at ordinary temperatures, is highly inflammable, boils at 46° C. (114·8° F.), and, when ignited, burns with a blue flame, producing carbonic and sulphurous acids. It should not affect the color of blue litmus paper moistened with water (abs. of sulphurous acid). A portion evaporated spontaneously in a glass vessel should leave no residue (sulphur). Test-solution of acetate of lead agitated with it should not be blackened (abs. of hydrosulphuric acid)." *U. S.*

Medical Properties. Bisulphide of carbon is a powerful poison, but is not used as an internal remedy. According to M. Delpech, the workmen exposed to the fumes of the bisulphide are affected with headache, vertigo, and over-excitement of the nervous system, as evinced by voluble talking, incoherent singing, or immoderate laughter, or sometimes by weeping; and a continuance of the exposure is apt to cause at length a state of cachexia, characterized by general weakness, loss of sexual appetite, dulness of sight and hearing, and impairment of memory. M. S. Cloëz has made with it experiments on some of the smaller animals, as rats and rabbits, which were confined under a bell-glass with some cotton saturated with the bisulphide. In a few moments the animal exhibited signs of its action in great excitement, followed by retarded movements, with some convulsive shocks, then fell on its side and died in five minutes from the beginning. Congestion of the lungs and of the cavities of the heart, without any cerebral lesion, while the right auricle continued to contract two hours after apparent death, were the phenomena observed on dissection. (*Lancet*, Sept. 1866, p. 267.) The swallowing by a man, with suicidal intent, of a half an ounce of bisulphide of carbon was followed in half an hour by absolute unconsciousness, very rapid, feeble pulse, slow and stertorous respiration, cold and clammy surface of body, and insensitive conjunctiva, with mobile pupils. Two hours later, death occurred. The blood was found fluid, and there were no marked lesions of irritation in the gastro-intestinal mucous membrane. (*Lancet*, July 17, 1886.) India-rubber workers, by whom the sulphide is largely used, are said to suffer frequently from paralytic symptoms. (*Lancet*, Jan. 1886.)

Externally, the bisulphide has been used as a counter-irritant and local anæsthetic. In enlarged lymphatic glands, Dr. Turnbull has used it with asserted good success. He applies it by means of a bottle with a proper sized mouth, containing a fluid-drachm of the bisulphide, imbibed by a piece of sponge. The skin over the gland is first well moistened with water. He employed the vapor also with benefit in deafness, when dependent on want of nervous energy, and a deficiency of wax. For this purpose, the bottle containing the bisulphide is made with a neck to fit the meatus, and, being applied to the ear, is held there until considerable warmth is produced. The remedy has been used often with very good results, in a similar manner, in facial and other neuralgias and various local pains. It causes a good deal of smarting, but its disagreeable odor is the chief objection to it. M. Chiandi Bey finds that a solution of bisulphide of carbon (three parts per thousand) is a most energetic antiseptic, killing microbes and arresting all fermentation; he proposes its use in zymotic diseases internally, and its free employment as a cheap, active disinfectant. (*Compt.-Rendus*, xcix.)

CARDAMOMUM. *U. S., Br.* *Cardamom.*

(CĂR-DA-MŌ-MŬM.)

"The fruit of Elettaria Cardamomum. Maton. (*Nat. Ord.* Zingiberaceæ.)" *U. S.*
"The dried ripe seeds of the Malabar Cardamom, Elettaria Cardamomum, *Maton.*

The seeds are best kept in their pericarps, in which condition they are imported; but when required for use they should be separated and the pericarps rejected." *Br.*

Cardamomi Semina, *Br.;* Fructus (Semen) Cardamomi Minoris, *P.G.;* Cardamomum Minus, Cardomomum Malabarism; Malabar Cardamoms; Cardamomes, Petit Cardamome, *Fr.;* Cardamomen, Kleine Cardamomen, *G.;* Cardamomo minore, *It.;* Cardamomo menor, *Sp.;* Ebil, *Arab.;* Kakelah seghar, *Pers.;* Capalaga, *Malay;* Gujaratii elachi, *Hindoost.*

The subject of Cardamom has been involved in some confusion and uncertainty, both in its commercial and botanical relations. The name has been applied to the aromatic capsules of various Indian plants belonging to the family of Scitamineæ. Three varieties have long been designated by the several titles of the *lesser*, *middle*, and *larger*—*cardamomum minus*, *medium*, and *majus;* but these terms have been used differently by different writers, so that their precise signification remains doubtful. To the late Dr. Pereira we are mainly indebted for the clearing up of this confusion. It is well known that the *lesser cardamom* of most writers is the variety recognized by the Pharmacopœias, and generally kept in the shops. The other varieties, though circulating to a greater or less extent in European and Indian commerce, are little known in this country.* The following remarks have reference exclusively to the genuine Malabar, or officinal cardamom.

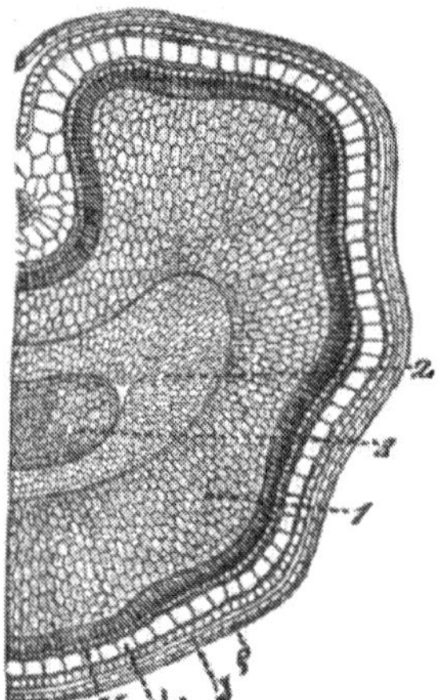

Cardamom seed. 1, perisperm; 2, endosperm; 3, embryo; *s*, inner seed-coat; *j*, oil-cells; *s*, seed-coat; *t*, outer seed-coat. (After Berg.)

Linnæus confounded, under the name of *Amomum Cardamomum*, two different vegetables,—the genuine plant of Malabar, and another growing in Java. These were separated by Willde-

* The following is a sketch of the non-officinal cardamoms, compiled chiefly from the publications of Pereira and of Flückiger and Hanbury.

1. *Ceylon Cardamom.* This has been denominated variously *cardamomum medium, cardamomum majus*, and *cardamomum longum*, and is sometimes termed in English commerce *wild cardamom.* It is the *large cardamom* of Guibourt. In the East it is sometimes called *grains of Paradise;* but it is not the product known with us by that name. (See p. 371, 7.) It is derived from a plant cultivated in Candy, in the island of Ceylon, and also growing wild in the forests of the interior, which was designated by Sir James Edward Smith *Elletaria major*, but is now generally acknowledged to be only a variety of the officinal plant. This plant was described by Pereira in *P. J. Tr.* (ii. 388). The fruit is a lanceolate-oblong, acutely triangular capsule, somewhat curved, about an inch and a half long and four lines broad, with flat and ribbed sides, tough and coriaceous, brownish or yellow ash-colored, having frequently at one end the long, cylindrical, three-lobed calyx, and at the other the fruit-stalk. It is three-celled, and contains angular, rugged, yellowish red seeds, of a peculiar fragrant odor and spicy taste. Its effects are analogous to those of the officinal cardamom.

2. *Round Cardamom.* This is probably the Αμωμον of Dioscorides, and the *Amomi uva* of Pliny, and is believed to be the fruit of *Amomum Cardamomum* (Willd.), growing in Sumatra, Java, and other East India islands. The capsules are usually smaller than a cherry, roundish or somewhat ovate, with three convex sides, more or less striated longitudinally, yellowish or brownish white, and sometimes reddish, with brown, angular, cuneiform, shrivelled seeds, which have a spicy camphorous flavor. They are sometimes, though rarely, met with connected in their native clusters, constituting the *amomum racemosum*, or *amome en grappes* of the French. They are similar in medicinal properties to the officinal, but are seldom used except in the southern parts of Europe.

3. *Java Cardamom.* The plant producing this variety is supposed to be the *Amomum maximum* of Roxburgh, growing in Java and other Malay islands in the East. The capsules are oval, or oval-oblong, often somewhat ovate, from eight to fifteen lines long, and from four to eight broad, usually flattened on one side and convex on the other, sometimes curved, three-valved, and occasionally imperfectly three-lobed, of a dirty grayish brown color, and coarse fibrous appearance. When soaked in water, they exhibit as their distinguishing character from nine to thirteen ragged membranous wings along their whole length, which distinguish them from all other varieties. The seeds have a feebly aromatic taste and smell. This variety of cardamom affords but a very small proportion of volatile oil, is altogether of inferior quality, and, when imported into London, is usually sent to the continent.

4. *Madagascar Cardamom.* This is the *Cardamomum majus* of Geiger and some others, and is thought to be the fruit of *Amomum angustifolium* of Sonnerat, growing in marshy grounds in Madagascar. The capsule is ovate, pointed, flattened on one side, striated, with a broad circular scar at the bottom, surrounded by an elevated, notched, corrugated margin. The seeds have an aromatic flavor analogous to that of officinal cardamom.

5. *Bengal Cardamom.* The fruit of *Amomum subulatum*, Roxb., sometimes known by the name

now, who conferred on the former Sonnerat's title of *Amomum repens*, while he retained the original name for the latter, though not the true cardamom plant. In the tenth volume of the Linnean Transactions, 1811, Mr. White, a British Army Surgeon in India, published a very minute description of the Malabar plant, which he had enjoyed frequent opportunities of examining in its native state. From this description, Dr. Maton inferred that the plant, according to Roscoe's arrangement of the Scitamineæ, could not be considered an *Amomum;* and, as he was unable to attach it to any other known genus, he proposed to construct a new one with the name of *Elettaria*, derived from *elettari* or *elatari*, the Malabar name of this vegetable. Sir James Smith afterwards suggested the propriety of naming the new genus *Matonia*, in honor of Dr. Maton; and the latter title, having been adopted by Roscoe, obtained a place in former editions of the London and U. S. Pharmacopœias. The celebrated Dr. Roxburgh described the Malabar cardamom plant as an *Alpinia*, with the specific name *Cardamomum*. As doubts were entertained of the necessity for the new genus proposed by Maton, Roxburgh was followed in the London and U. S. Pharmacopœias, and the fruit was referred to *Alpinia Cardamomum*. This decision, however, has been revised in the later editions of the U. S. and British Pharmacopœias. Finally Roscoe has arranged it with the abandoned genus *Renealmia* of Linnæus, which he has restored.

Gen. Ch. Corolla with the tube filiform and the inner limb one-lipped. *Anther* naked. *Capsule* often berried, three-celled, three-valved. *Seeds* numerous, arillate. *Blume.*

Elettaria Cardamomum. Maton; *B. & T.*, 267.—*Alpinia Cardamomum.* Roxburgh.—*Amomum Repens.* Sonnerat; Willd. *Sp. Plant.* i. 9.—*Renealmia Cardamomum.* Roscoe, *Monandrous Plants.* Figured in *Linn. Trans.* x. 248, and Carson's *Illust. of Med. Bot.* ii. 55. The cardamom plant has a tuberous horizontal root or rhizome, furnished with numerous fibres, and sending up from eight to twenty erect, simple, smooth, green and shining, perennial stems, which rise from six to twelve feet in height, and bear alternate sheathing leaves. These are from nine inches to two feet long, from one to five inches broad, elliptical-lanceolate, pointed,

of Winged Bengal Cardamom. *Morung elachi*, or *Buro elachi*, is about an inch in length, obscurely three-sided, ovoid or somewhat obconic, with nine narrow, jagged ridges or wings (best seen after soaking in water) upon its distal end, which terminates in a truncate bristly nipple. The pericarp is coarsely striated, of a deep brown, splitting into three valves, disclosing a three-lobed mass of seeds, 60 to 80 in number, agglutinated by their viscid saccharine anthers.

6. *Nepal Cardamom* is produced by an Amomum of undetermined species, and resembles the Bengal cardamom, except in having a long tubular calyx on its summit, and in being usually attached to a stalk.

7. *Grains of Paradise. Grana Paradisi.* Under this name and that of *Guinea grains*, and *Malegueta*, or *Mallaguetta pepper*, are found in commerce small seeds of a round or ovate form, often angular, and somewhat cuneiform, minutely rough, brown externally, white within, of a feebly aromatic odor when rubbed between the fingers, and of a strongly hot and peppery taste. Two kinds of them are known in the English market, one larger, plumper, and more warty, with a short conical projecting tuft of pale fibres on the umbilicus; the other smaller and smoother, and without the fibrous tuft. The latter are the most common. It is probable that one of the varieties is produced by *Amomum Grana Paradisi* of Sir J. E. Smith, and the other by Roscoe's *Amomum Melegueta.* (Pereira's *Mat. Med.*, 3d ed., p. 1134.) Dr. W. F. Daniell, who has published (*P. J. Tr.*, xiv. 312 and 356) an elaborate paper on the Amoma of Western Africa, states that the true Mallaguetta pepper is obtained exclusively from varieties of the same species, to which belong the *Amomum Grana Paradisi* of Afzelius, and the *A. Melegueta* of Roscoe; while the *A. Grana Paradisi* of Sir J. E. Smith is a different plant, and yields a different product. These grains are imported from Guinea, and other parts of the western coast of Africa. Similar grains are taken to England from Demerara, where they are obtained from a plant cultivated by the negroes, supposed to have been brought from Africa, and believed by Dr. Pereira to be the *Amomum Melegueta* of Roscoe. (*Ibid.*, vi. 412.) At the international exhibition of 1862, at London, Dr. Geo. B. Wood noticed a specimen of similar grains, under the name of grains of Paradise, sent from the island of Trinidad. Their effects on the system are analogous to those of pepper; but they are seldom used except in veterinary practice, and to give artificial strength to spirits, wine, beer, and vinegar. In the same journal (ii. 443), Dr. Pereira points out seven distinct scitamineous fruits, to which the name of grains of Paradise has been applied by different authors. J. C. Thresh made a proximate analysis of the seeds, and found volatile oil, resin, tannin, starch, albuminoids, and an active principle in the form of a straw-colored, viscid, odorless fluid, pungent, but not so hot as capsaicin. (*P. J. Tr.*, 1884, p. 297.) Fredk. Schwartz found in the seeds a reddish-brown acrid resin, and an oil having a burning aromatic taste, upon which the virtues probably depend. (*A. J. P.*, 1886, p. 118.)

Other products of different Scitamineæ, which have received the name of cardamom, are described; but the above are all that are known in commerce, or likely to be brought into our drug markets.

entire, smooth, and dark green on the upper surface, glossy and pale sea-green beneath, with strong midribs, and short footstalks. The flower-stalk proceeds from the base of the stem, and lies upon the ground, with the flowers arranged in a panicle. The calyx is monophyllous, tubular, and toothed at the margin; the corolla monophyllous and funnel-shaped, with the inferior border unilabiate, three-lobed, and spurred at the base. The fruit is a three-celled capsule, containing many seeds.

This valuable plant is a native of the mountains of Malabar, where it springs up spontaneously in the forests after the removal of the undergrowth, and is very extensively cultivated by the natives. The curious reader may find a detailed account of the method of culture in the *A. J. P.*, 1877, p. 605. The plant begins to yield fruit at the end of the fourth year, and continues to bear for several years afterwards. The capsules when ripe are picked from the fruit stems, dried over a gentle fire, and separated by rubbing with the hands from the footstalks and adhering calyx.

Thus prepared, they are ovate-oblong, from three to ten lines long, from two to four thick, three-sided with rounded angles, obtusely pointed at both ends, longitudinally wrinkled, and of a yellowish white color. The seeds which they contain are small, angular, irregular, rough as if embossed upon their surface, of a brown color, easily reduced to powder, and thus separable from the capsular covering, which, though slightly aromatic, is much less so than the seeds, and should be rejected when the medicine is administered. The seeds constitute about 74 parts per cent. by weight. According to Pereira, three varieties are distinguished in commerce:—1, the *shorts*, from three to six lines long, from two to three broad, browner and more coarsely ribbed, and more highly esteemed than the others; 2, the *long-longs*, from seven lines to an inch in length by two or three lines in breadth, elongated, and somewhat acuminate; and 3, the *short-longs*, which are somewhat shorter and less pointed than the second variety. The odor of cardamom is fragrant, the taste warm, slightly pungent, and highly aromatic. "Ovoid or oblong, from two-fifths to four-fifths of an inch (1 to 2 cm.) long, obtusely triangular, rounded at the base, beaked, longitudinally striate; of a pale buff color, three-celled, with a thin, leathery, nearly tasteless pericarp and a central placenta. The seeds are reddish brown, angular, transversely rugose, depressed at the hilum, surrounded by a thin, membranous arillus, and have an agreeable odor and a pungent aromatic taste." *U. S.* Cardamom yields its virtues to water and alcohol, but more readily to the latter. The seeds contain 4·6 per cent. of volatile oil, 10·4 of fixed oil, 2·5 of a salt of potassa mixed with a coloring principle, 3·0 of starch, 1·8 of azotised mucilage, 0·4 of yellow coloring matter, and 77·3 of ligneous fibre. (Trommsdorff.) The volatile oil is colorless, of an agreeable and very penetrating odor, and of a strong aromatic, burning, camphorous, and bitterish taste. It is dextrogyrate, and consists essentially of a terpene, $C_{10}H_{16}$. From old specimens of oil Dumas and Peligot claim to have obtained crystals of *terpine*, $C_{10}H_{16} + 3H_2O$, while Flückiger has obtained a crystalline deposit from Ceylon oil which he considers identical with common camphor. The sp. gr. of the oil is between 0·92 and 0·94. It cannot be kept long without undergoing change, and finally, even though excluded from the air, loses its peculiar odor and taste. If ether be made to percolate through the powdered seeds, and the liquor obtained be deprived of the ether, a light greenish brown fluid remains, consisting almost exclusively of the volatile and fixed oils. It has the odor of cardamom, and keeps better than the oil obtained by distillation. (*A. J. P.*, xxi. 116.) The seeds should be powdered only when wanted for use; as they retain their aromatic properties best while in the capsules.

Cardamoms are not often adulterated; but an instance has been mentioned by Mr. G. W. Kennedy, as having occurred under his own observation, in which orange seeds and unroasted grains of coffee were mixed with the cardamoms to the extent of nearly 4 per cent. (*A. J. P.*, 1872, p. 389.)

Medical Properties and Uses. Cardamom is a warm and grateful aromatic, less heating and stimulating than some others belonging to the class, and very useful as an adjuvant or corrective of cordial, tonic, and purgative medicines. Throughout the East Indies it is largely consumed as a condiment. It was known to the ancients, and derived its name from the Greek language. In this country it is employed chiefly as an ingredient in compound preparations.

Off. Prep. Tinctura Cardamomi; Tinctura Cardamomi Composita; Pulvis Aromaticus; Extractum Colocynthidis Compositum; Tinctura Gentianæ Composita; Tinctura Rhei; Tinctura Rhei Dulcis; Vinum Aloes.

Off. Prep. Br. Extractum Colocynthidis Compositum; Pulvis Cinnamomi Compositus; Pulvis Cretæ Aromaticus; Tinctura Cardamomi Composita; Tinctura Gentianæ Composita; Tinctura Rhei; Vinum Aloes.

CARUM. *U.S., Br.* *Caraway.*

(CĂ'RŬM.)

"The fruit of Carum Carvi. Linné. (*Nat. Ord.* Umbelliferæ, Orthospermæ.)" *U.S.* "The dried fruit of Carum Carui." *Br.*

Carui Fructus, *Br.;* **Caraway Fruit; Fructus Carvi**, *P.G.;* **Cumin des Prés, Carvi**, *Fr.*, *It.*, **Gemeiner Kümmel, Kümmel**, *G.;* **Alcaravea**, *Sp.*

Gen. Ch. Fruit ovate-oblong, striated. *Involucre* one-leafed. *Petals* keeled, inflexed-emarginate. *Willd.*

Carum Carui. Willd. *Sp. Plant.* i. 1470; *B. & T.* 121. This plant is biennial and umbelliferous, with a spindle-shaped, fleshy, whitish root, and an erect stem, about two feet in height, branching above, and furnished with doubly pinnate, deeply incised leaves, the segments of which are linear and pointed. The flowers are small and white, and in erect terminal umbels, which are accompanied with an involucre, consisting sometimes of three or four leaflets, sometimes of one only, and are destitute of partial involucre.

The caraway plant is a native of Europe, growing wild in meadows and pastures, and cultivated in many places. It has been introduced into this country. The flowers appear in May and June, and the seeds, which are not perfected till the second year, ripen in August. The root, when improved by culture, resembles the parsnep, and is used as food in the north of Europe. The seeds are the part used in medicine. They are collected by cutting down the plant, and threshing it on a cloth. Our markets are supplied partly from Europe, partly from our own gardens. The American seeds are usually rather smaller than the German. Under the name of *Ajowan*, the fruit of the *Carum Ajowan*, Bentham & Hooker (*Ammi Copticum*, Linn.) are largely used in India. They are $\frac{1}{10}$ to $\frac{1}{16}$ of an inch long, and resemble the fruits of common parsley, but are distinguished by their odor, and their surface being very rough from numerous, very minute tubercles. They contain about 4 per cent. of a volatile oil, which has the odor of the oil of thyme, and contains thymol: it may be used as an aromatic carminative. (See *Brit. Med. Journ.*, June 6, 1885.)

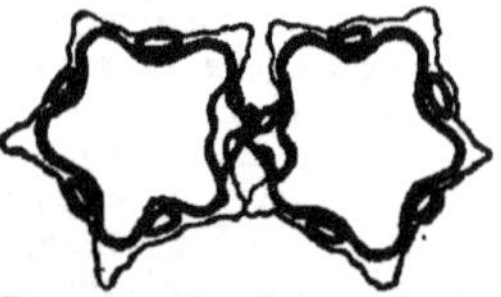

Transverse section of caraway, showing oil-tubes.

Caraway seeds (half-fruits) are about two lines in length, slightly curved, with five longitudinal ridges, which are of a light yellowish color, while the intervening spaces are dark brown. "Oblong, laterally compressed, about one-sixth of an inch (4 mm.) long, usually separated into the two mericarps, and these curved, narrower at both ends, brown, with five yellowish, filiform ribs, and with six oil-tubes." *U.S.* They have an agreeable aromatic smell, and a sweetish, warm, spicy taste. These properties depend on an essential oil, which they afford largely by distillation. (See *Oleum Cari.*) The residue is insipid. They yield their virtues readily to alcohol, and more slowly to water.

Medical Properties and Uses. Caraway is a pleasant stomachic and carminative, occasionally used in flatulent colic, and as an adjuvant or corrective of other medicines. The dose in substance is from a scruple to a drachm (1·3–3·9 Gm.). An infusion may be prepared by adding two drachms of the seeds to a pint of boiling water. The volatile oil, however, is most employed. (See *Oleum Cari.*) The seeds are baked in cakes, to which they communicate an agreeable flavor, while they stimulate the digestive organs.

Off. Prep. Tinctura Cardamomi Composita.

Off. Prep. Br. Aqua Carui; Confectio Opii; Confectio Piperis; Oleum Carui; Pulvis Opii Compositus; Tinctura Cardamomi Composita; Tinctura Sennæ.

CARYOPHYLLUS. *U.S., Br.* *Cloves.*

(CĂR-Y̆-O-PHY̆L'LUS.)

"The unexpanded flowers of Eugenia caryophyllata. Thunberg. (*Nat. Ord.* Myrtaceæ.)" *U. S.* "The dried flower-bud of Eugenia caryophyllata." *Br.*

Caryophyllum, *Br.;* Caryophilli, *P. G.;* Caryophylli Aromatici; Girofle, Clous aromatiques, Clous de Girofles, *Fr.;* Gewurznelken, Nägelein, *G.;* Garofani, *It.;* Clavos de Especia, *Sp.;* Cravo da India, *Portug.;* Kruidnagel, *Dutch;* Kerunfel, *Arab.*

Gen. Ch. Tube of the *calyx* cylindrical; limb, four-parted *Petals* four, adhering by their ends in a sort of calyptra. *Stamens* distinct, arranged in four parcels in a quadrangular fleshy hollow, near the teeth of the calyx. *Ovary* two-celled, with about twenty ovules in each cell. *Berry* one or two celled, one or two seeded. *Seeds* cylindrical or half-ovate. *Cotyledons* thick, fleshy, convex externally, sinuous in various ways internally. *Lindley. De Cand.*

Eugenia caryophyllata. Willd. *Sp. Plant.* ii. 965; *B. & T.* 112.—*Caryophyllus aromaticus.* Linn. *Sp. Plant.*, 735; De Cand. *Prodrom.* iii. 262; Carson, *Illust. of Med. Bot.* i. 43, pl. 37. This small tree is one of the most elegant of those inhabiting the islands of India. It has a pyramidal form, is always green, and is adorned throughout the year with a succession of beautiful rosy flowers. The stem is of hard wood, and covered with a smooth, grayish bark. The leaves are about four inches in length by two in breadth, obovate-oblong, acuminate at both ends, entire, sinuated, with many parallel veins on each side of the midrib, supported on long footstalks, and opposite. They have a firm consistence, and a shining green color, and when bruised are highly fragrant. The flowers are disposed in terminal corymbose panicles, and exhale a strong, penetrating, and grateful odor.

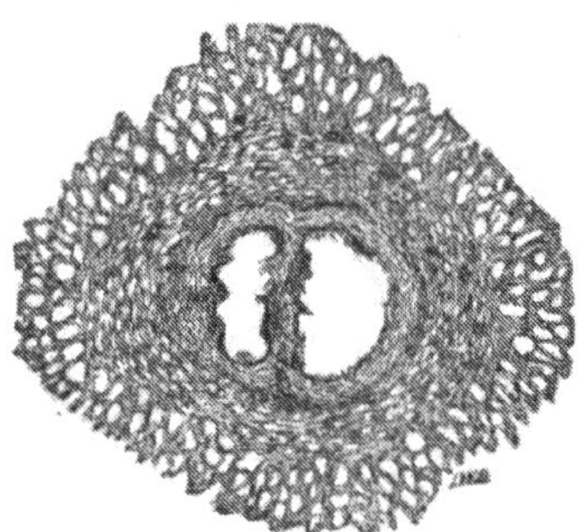

Transverse section of calyx-tube of clove.

The natural geographical range of the clove is extremely limited, being confined to the Molucca Islands. According to Flückiger, the cloves were known in western Europe as early as the sixth century, long before the discovery of the Moluccas by the Portuguese. After the conquest of the Molucca Islands by the Dutch, the monopolizing policy of that commercial people led them to extirpate the trees in nearly all the islands except Amboyna and Ternate, which were under their immediate inspection. Notwithstanding, however, their jealous vigilance, a French governor of the Isles of France and Bourbon, named Poivre, succeeded, in the year 1770, in obtaining plants from the Moluccas, and introducing them into the colonies under his control. Five years afterwards, the clove-tree was introduced into Cayenne and the West Indies, in 1803 into Sumatra, and in 1818 into Zanzibar. It is now cultivated largely in these and other places; and commerce has ceased to depend on the Moluccas for supplies of this spice.*

The unexpanded flower-buds are the part of the plant employed under the ordinary name of cloves.† They are first gathered when the tree is about six years old. The fruit has similar aromatic properties, but much weaker. The buds are at first white, then become green, and then bright red, when they must be at once collected, which is done sometimes by hand-picking, sometimes by beating the trees with bamboos, and catching the falling buds. In the Moluccas they are said to be sometimes immersed in boiling water, and afterwards exposed to smoke and arti-

* Cloves from Cayenne, and from various West India islands, as Martinique, Guadaloupe, and Trinidad, have been for several years circulating in commerce. Dr. Geo. B. Wood saw a specimen from Para, in Brazil, at the international exhibition at London (1862). They were lighter colored than those from the East Indies.

† The peduncles of the flowers have been sometimes employed. They possess the odor and taste of the cloves, though in a less degree, and furnish a considerable quantity of essential oil. The French call them *griffes de girofles.*

ficial heat, before being spread out in the sun. In Zanzibar, Cayenne, and the West Indies, they are dried simply by solar heat.

Cloves appear to have been unknown to the ancients. They were introduced into Europe by the Arabians, and were distributed by the Venetians. After the discovery of the southern passage to India, the trade in this spice passed into the hands of the Portuguese; but was subsequently wrested from them by the Dutch, by whom it was long monopolized. Within a few years, however, the extended culture of the plant has thrown open the commerce in cloves to all nations. The United States derive much of their supply from the West Indies and Guiana; but the great source of cloves have been recently the islands of Zanzibar and Pemba, on the east coast of Africa. In 1872 the clove orchards in Zanzibar were nearly destroyed by a hurricane, but it is said that they have been replanted. The Molucca cloves are said to be thicker, darker, heavier, more oily, and more highly aromatic than those cultivated elsewhere. They are known by the name of *Amboyna cloves.* The *Bencoolen cloves*, from Sumatra, are deemed equal if not superior by the English druggists.

Properties. Cloves in shape resemble a nail, with a round head with four spreading points beneath it. "About half an inch (12 mm.) long, dark brown, consisting of a subcylindrical, solid and glandular calyx-tube, terminated by four teeth, and surmounted by a globular head, formed by four petals, which cover numerous, curved stamens and one style." *U. S.* Their color is externally deep brown, internally reddish; their odor strong and fragrant; their taste hot, pungent, aromatic, and very permanent. The best cloves are large, heavy, brittle, and exude a small quantity of oil on being pressed or scraped with the nail. When light, soft, wrinkled, pale, and of feeble taste and smell, they are inferior. Those from which the essential oil has been distilled are sometimes fraudulently mixed with the genuine. In powdered cloves this fraud appears to be extensively practised, and its detection is almost impossible.

Trommsdorff obtained from 1000 parts of cloves 180 of volatile oil, 170 of a peculiar tannin, 130 of gum, 60 of resin, 280 of vegetable fibre, and 180 of water. M. Lodibert afterwards discovered a fixed oil, aromatic and of a green color, and a white resinous substance which crystallizes in fasciculi, composed of very fine diverging silky needles, without taste or smell, soluble in ether and boiling alcohol, and exhibiting neither alkaline nor acid reaction. This substance, called by M. Bonastre *caryophyllin*, was found in the cloves of the Moluccas, of Bourbon, and of Barbadoes, but not in those of Cayenne, from which, however, it has since been procured. To obtain it, the ethereal extract of cloves is treated with water, and the white substance thrown down is separated by filtration, and treated repeatedly with ammonia to deprive it of impurities. The most recent determination of its formula by Mylius (*D. Chem. Ges.*, 1873, p. 1053) makes it $C_{20}H_{32}O_2$. Dr. Theod. Martius obtains it cheaply by exposing cloves, previously deprived as far as possible of oil by distillation with water, to distillation at a higher temperature, redistilling the brown liquid obtained until the distillate nearly ceases to have the taste or smell of cloves, and then purifying the residue by washing with water, and treating it with boiling alcohol and animal charcoal repeatedly, until the caryophyllin, which is deposited by the alcohol on cooling, is perfectly white. (See *A. J. P.*, xxxii. 65.) M. Dumas has discovered another crystalline principle, which forms in the water distilled from cloves, and is gradually deposited. Like caryophyllin, it is soluble in alcohol and ether, but differs from that substance in becoming red when touched with nitric acid. M. Bonastre proposed for it the name of *eugenin.* (*Journ. de Pharm.*, xx. 565.) It has the formula $C_{10}H_{12}O_2$, and is isomeric with eugenol or eugenic acid, a constituent of oil of cloves. Water extracts the odor of cloves with comparatively little of their taste. All their sensible properties are imparted to alcohol; and the tincture when evaporated leaves an excessively fiery extract, which becomes insipid if deprived of the oil by distillation with water, while the oil which comes over is mild. Hence it has been inferred that the pungency of this aromatic depends on a union of the essential oil with the resin. *Caryophyllic acid*, $C_{20}H_{32}O_6$, is obtained by gradually adding caryophyllin to fuming nitric acid, kept cool by immersing the vessel in water until crystals begin to separate; these are purified by dissolving them in ammonia, precipitating with hydrochloric acid, and redissolving in alcohol and crystallizing. For an account of the oil and its constituents, see *Oleum Caryophylli.* The infusion and oil of cloves are reddened by nitric acid, and rendered blue by tincture of chloride of iron; facts of some interest, as morphine gives the same reactions.

Medical Properties and Uses. Cloves are among the most stimulant of the aromatics, but, like others of this class, act less upon the system at large than on the part to which they are immediately applied. They are sometimes administered in substance or infusion to relieve nausea and vomiting, correct flatulence, and excite languid digestion; but their chief use is to assist or modify the action of other medicines. They enter into several officinal preparations. Their dose in substance is from five to ten grains (0·33–0·65 Gm.).

The French Codex directs a *tincture of cloves* to be prepared by digesting for six days, and afterwards filtering, a mixture of four ounces of powdered cloves and sixteen of alcohol of 31° Cartier. Three ounces to the pint of alcohol is a sufficiently near approximation.

Off. Prep. Tinctura Lavandulæ Composita; Tinctura Rhei Aromatica; Vinum Opii.

Off. Prep. Br. Infusum Aurantii Compositum; Infusum Caryophylli; Mistura Ferri Aromatica; Oleum Caryophylli; Vinum Opii.

CASCARILLA. *U. S., Br.* *Cascarilla.*

(CĂS-CA-RĬL′LA.)

"The bark of Croton Eluteria. Bennett. (*Nat. Ord.* Euphorbiaceæ.)" *U. S.*
"The dried bark of Croton Eluteria." *Br.*

Cascarillæ Cortex, *Br.;* Cascarilla Bark; Cortex Cascarillæ, *P.G.;* Cortex Eluteriæ, Cortex Thuris; Chacrille, Ecorce éleuthérienne, Cascarille, *Fr.;* Cascarillrinde, Cascarilla, Kaskarillrinde, *G.;* Cascariglia, *It.;* Chacarila, *Sp.*

Gen. Ch. MALE. *Calyx* cylindrical, five-toothed. *Corolla* five-petalled. *Stamens* ten to fifteen. FEMALE. *Calyx* many-leaved. *Corolla* none. *Styles* three, bifid. *Capsule* three-celled. *Seed* one. *Willd.*

There has been much confusion in relation to the different species of Croton growing in the West Indies, and as to which of them the Cascarilla of the shops is to be ascribed. At present, however, it is generally admitted that this bark, which is brought exclusively from the Bahama Islands, is the product of *Croton Eluteria;* and, though it is probable that the proper *C. Cascarilla* may at one time have yielded a portion of its bark to commerce, at present little or none is derived from that species. The London College committed the error, which it afterwards corrected, of recognizing *C. Cascarilla* of Don as the source of it. This botanist mistook the *Copalchi bark* of Mexico, which is produced by *Croton Pseudo-China* of Schiede, and somewhat resembles cascarilla, for the genuine bark, and hence proposed to transfer the specific name of Cascarilla to the Mexican plant.*

Croton Eluteria. Bennett, *Journ. of the Linn. Soc.* iv. 29; Daniell, *P. J. Tr.* 2d ser., iv. 145, figured at p. 150; *B & T.* 238.—*Clutia Eluteria.* Woodv. *Med. Bot.* 3d ed., iv. 633, t. 223. As described by Dr. W. F. Daniell, who resided in the Bahama Islands, this, though commonly a shrub of from three to five feet high, sometimes appears in the form of a small tree with a stem from four to eight inches

* *Copalchi bark* has been mistaken not only for cascarilla, but also for a variety of cinchona. Portions of it, having been taken to Europe, attracted the attention both of pharmacologists and physicians. Two kinds were noticed; one, in small slender quills, of an ash color, bearing some resemblance to a variety of pale cinchona, but having the flavor of cascarilla, and burning with a similar odor; the other in larger quills, with a thick cork-like epidermis, very bitter, and yielding an aromatic odor when burnt. The former is the product of *Croton Pseudo-China;* the latter is of unknown origin, but conjecturally referred to *C. suberosum.* Mr. J. E. Howard states that the quilled copalchi bark contains a bitter alkaloid, soluble in ether, and precipitable as a white hydrate from its acid solution. (*P. J. Tr.*, xiv. 319.) Copalchi bark is an aromatic tonic, employed in Mexico in intermittents, and capable of useful application in all cases requiring a mild aromatic bitter. Dr. Stark has employed it advantageously in feeble states of digestion with irritable bowels, and found it, in one or two cases, to exhibit antiperiodic properties. It may be given in infusion, made with half an ounce of the bark to a pint of water, in the dose of one or two fluidounces three times a day. (*Ed. Med. and Surg. Jour.*, April, 1849, p. 410; see, also, *P. J. Tr.*, 1886, p. 917.)

in diameter.* The stem is straight, and marked at intervals with white or grayish stains. The leaves are petiolate, from two to three inches in length by an inch or more in breadth, often somewhat cordate at the base, obtusely acuminate, pale or grayish green above, and densely covered beneath with shining silvery scales, appearing white at a distance. They are smaller and narrower in the plants of arborescent growth. The flowers, which have a delicious odor, are monœcious, small, white, petiolate, and closely set in simple terminal or axillary spikes. The shrub is a native of the Bahamas, scarce at present in the island of New Providence, but still abundant in Andros, Long, and Eleutheria islands, from the latter of which it derived its botanical title. Daniell calls the plant *sweet-wood.* The name of *seaside balsam* belongs to another species, *C. Balsamiferum* of Linnæus, which grows in the Bahamas and other West India islands, and owes its name to the exudation of a balsamic juice from its young branches when wounded.

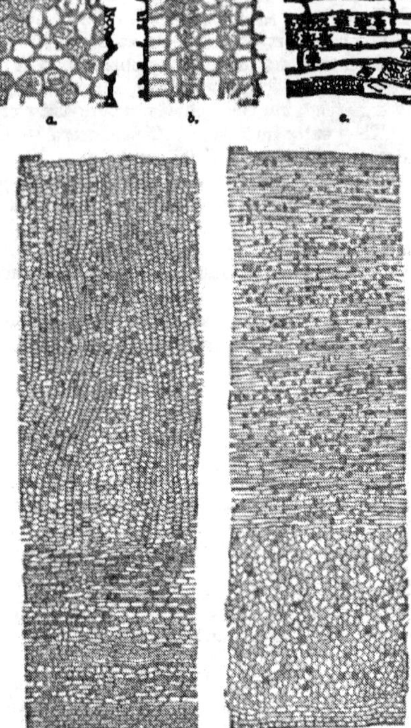

Figs. *a*, *c*, highly magnified sections, showing raphides and starch granules and a bast-cell; *b*, longitudinal section highly magnified, showing raphides and starch granules; *d*, transverse section moderately magnified; *e*, longitudinal section.

Croton Cascarilla. Bennett, *Journ. of the Linn. Soc.* iv. 30.—*Clutia Cascarilla.* Linn. *Sp. Plant.* ed. 1, p. 1042.—*Ricinoides elæagnifolia.* Catesby, *Hist. Carolin.* ii. t. 46. As described by Daniell, this is a shrub of from four to six feet, much branched, with a pale grayish green stem, without the white stains of the former species. The leaves are petiolate, long, narrow, lanceolate, tapering towards each end, pointed, with flat, or somewhat undular margins, above smooth and green, beneath pale and very hairy. The flowers are monœcious, in simple terminal spikes, with small white petals tinged with yellow. They are very fragrant. The plant is a native of the Bahamas, and is said also to grow in Hayti. In the Bahamas it is much scarcer than formerly, and is said by Dr. Daniell to yield at present none of the cascarilla of commerce, of which much was formerly derived from it. This species seems to have been confounded by some with *Croton lineare* of Jacquin, which grows in the Bahamas and most of the West India islands, where it is known by the name of *wild rosemary*, owing probably in part to its fragrant smell, but still more to its narrow linear leaves with reflected margins.

* The plant referred to in very early editions of this work, as having been seen by Dr. Wright in Jamaica, and called by him *C. Eluteria*, is, according to Mr. Bennett, a distinct species, *C. Sloanei*, which was confounded by Linnæus with the genuine cascarilla plant, under the name of *Clutia Eluteria*. The genuine plant was first described by him in his *Hortus Cliffortianus* (pp. 486–7), from a specimen in Clifford's herbarium in the British Museum, and afterwards apparently confused with a Jamaica specimen sent to him by Patrick Brown, from the latter of which the description of his *Clutia Eluteria* was drawn up, which is quite inapplicable to the original plant. It is the *C. Sloanei* also that was described by Schwartz in his *Flora Indiæ Occidentalis* (p. 1188), under the name of *Croton Eluteria*, and probably the same that was figured by Dr. Carson in his *Illust. of Med. Bot.* ii. 34, pl. 78. (See *P. J. Tr.*, 1859, pp. 132–3.)

Cascarilla is brought to this market from the West Indies, and chiefly, as we have been informed, from the Bahamas. It comes in bags or casks. We have observed it in the shops in two forms, so distinct as to merit the titles of varieties. In one, the bark is in rolled pieces of every size, from three or four inches in length and half an inch in diameter to the smallest fragments, covered externally with a dull whitish or grayish white epidermis, which in many portions is partially, sometimes wholly removed, leaving a dark brown surface, while the inner surface has a chocolate color, and the fracture is a reddish brown. The small pieces are sometimes curled, but have a distinct abrupt edge as if broken from the branches. The second variety consists entirely of very small pieces, not more than an inch or two in length, very thin, without the white epidermis, not regularly quilled, but curved more or less in the direction of their length, often having a small portion of woody fibre attached to their inner surface, and appearing precisely as if shaved by a knife from the stem or branches. Whether these two varieties are derived from distinct species, or differ only from the mode of collection, it is difficult to determine. The officinal description of cascarilla is as follows. "In quills or curved pieces, about one-twelfth of an inch (2 mm.) thick, having a grayish, somewhat fissured, easily detached, corky layer, the remaining tissue being dull brown, and the inner surface smooth. It breaks with a short fracture, having a resinous and radially striate appearance; when burned, it emits a strong, aromatic odor; its taste is warm and very bitter." *U. S.*

Properties. Cascarilla has an aromatic odor, rendered much more distinct by friction, and a warm, spicy, bitter taste. It is brittle, breaking with a short fracture. When burnt it emits a pleasant odor, closely resembling that of musk, but weaker and more agreeable. This property serves to distinguish it from other barks. It was analyzed by Trommsdorff, and more recently by M. Duval, of Liseux, in France. The constituents found by the latter were albumen, a peculiar kind of tannin, a bitter crystallizable principle called *cascarillin*, a red coloring matter, fatty matter of a nauseous odor, wax, gum, volatile oil, resin, starch, pectic acid, chloride of potassium, a salt of lime, and lignin. The oil, according to Trommsdorff, constitutes 1·6 per cent., is of a greenish yellow color, a penetrating odor analogous to that of the bark, and of the sp. gr. 0·938. It is probably a mixture of two oils, one of which is oxygenated. Gladstone (*Jahresbr. der Pharm.*, 1872, p. 450) gives to the hydrocarbon of cascarilla oil the composition of oil of turpentine. To obtain cascarillin, M. Duval treated the powdered bark with water, added acetate of lead to the solution, separated the lead by sulphuretted hydrogen, filtered, evaporated with the addition of animal charcoal, filtered again, evaporated at a low temperature to a syrupy consistence, and, having allowed the semi-liquid substance thus obtained to harden by cooling, purified it by twice successively treating it, first with a little cool alcohol, to separate the coloring and fatty matters, and afterwards with boiling alcohol and animal charcoal. The last alcoholic solution was allowed to evaporate spontaneously. Thus obtained, cascarillin is white, crystalline, inodorous, bitter, very slightly soluble in water, soluble in alcohol and ether. (*Journ. de Pharm.*, 3e sér., viii. 96.) It melts at 205° C. (401° F.), is not volatile nor a glucoside. Its composition answers to the formula $C_{12}H_{18}O_4$. Dr. P. E. Alessandri regards *cascarilline* as an alkaloid, and obtains it economically by mixing powdered cascarilla with sufficient 3 per cent. aqueous solution of oxalic acid to cover it, shaking the mixture, and heating it to 140° F., then allowing it to cool, expressing the mixture and saturating the filtered liquor with ammonia, then evaporating at a low temperature to two-thirds of its bulk, allowing it to cool, and separating any deposit. The clear liquid is then shaken with ether, which takes up the cascarilline, and which may be obtained through evaporation of the ethereal liquid. (*L'Orosi*, v. 1; *P. J. Tr.*, 1882, p. 993.) R. A. Cripps was unable to obtain the alkaloid by Alessandri's method, and suggests that the bitterness of the so-called cascarilline might be due to adherent resin. (*P. J. Tr.*, 1886, p. 1103.) Either alcohol or water will partially extract the active matters of cascarilla; but diluted alcohol is the proper menstruum.

Medical Properties and Uses. This bark is aromatic and tonic. It was known in Germany so early as the year 1690, and was much used as a substitute for Peruvian bark by those who were prejudiced against that febrifuge in the treatment of remittent and intermittent fevers. It has, however, lost much of its reputation, and is now employed only where a pleasant and gently stimulant tonic is desirable; as in dyspepsia, chronic diarrhœa and dysentery, flatulent colic, and other cases of debility of the stomach or bowels. It is said to promote the flow of milk in the lower animals, and has been proposed with a view to the same effect in the human subject. It is sometimes advantageously combined with the more powerful bitters. It may be given in powder or infusion. The dose of the former is from a scruple to half a drachm (1·3–1·95 Gm.), which may be repeated several times a day. Prof. Procter published a formula for a fluid extract, which contains the virtues of a troyounce of the bark in a fluidounce. (*A. J. P.*, 1863, p. 113.) In consequence of its pleasant odor when burnt, some smokers mix it in small quantity with their tobacco; but it is said, when thus employed, to occasion vertigo and intoxication.

Off. Prep. Br. Infusum Cascarillæ; Tinctura Cascarillæ.

CASSIA FISTULA. *U. S., Br.* *Cassia Fistula.* [*Purging Cassia.*]

(CĂS'SI-Ą FĬS'TŪ-LĄ.)

"The fruit of Cassia Fistula. Linné. (*Nat. Ord.* Leguminosæ, Cæsalpinieæ.)" *U. S.* "The pulp obtained from the recently imported pods of Cassia Fistula." *Br.*

Cassiæ Pulpa, *Br.;* Cassia Pulp; Fructus Cassiæ Fistulæ; Casse officinale, Casse en Batons, Pulpe de Casse, Casse mondée, Casse, *Fr.;* Rohrenkassie, Purgiercassie, Fistelkassie, *G.;* Cassia, *It.;* Cana Fistula, *Sp.*

Gen. Ch. *Calyx* five-leaved. *Petals* five. *Anthers*, three upper sterile, three lower beaked. *Lomentum. Willd.*

The tree which yields the purging cassia is ranked by some botanists as a distinct genus, separated from the Cassia, and denominated *Cathartocarpus.* (See *Lindley's Flor. Med.*, 262.)

Cassia Fistula. Willd. *Sp. Plant.* ii. 518; Carson, *Illust. of Med. Bot.* i. 24, pl. 26.; *B. & T.* 87.—*Cathartocarpus Fistula.* Persoon, *Synops.* i. 459. This is a large tree, rising to the height of forty or fifty feet, with a trunk of hard, heavy wood, dividing towards the top into numerous spreading branches, and covered with a smooth ash-colored bark. The leaves are commonly composed of five or six pairs of opposite leaflets, which are ovate, pointed, undulated, smooth, of a pale green color, from three to five inches long, and supported upon short petioles. The flowers are large, of a golden yellow color, and arranged in long, pendent, axillary racemes. The fruit consists of long, cylindrical, woody, dark brown, pendulous pods, which, when agitated by the wind, strike against each other, and produce a sound that may be heard at a considerable distance.

This species of Cassia is a native of Upper Egypt and India, whence it is generally supposed to have been transplanted to other parts of the world. It is at present very extensively diffused through the tropical regions of the old and new continents, being found in Insular and Continental India, Cochin-China, Egypt, Nubia, the West Indies, and the warmer parts of the continent of America. The fruit is the officinal portion of the plant. It is imported from the East and West Indies, chiefly the latter, and from South America.

Properties. Cassia pods are a foot or more in length, straight, or but slightly curved, cylindrical, less than an inch in diameter, with a woody shell, externally of a dark brown color, and marked with three longitudinal shining bands, extending from one end to the other, two of which are in close proximity, appearing to constitute a single band, and the third is on the opposite side of the pod. These bands mark the place of junction of the valves of the legume, and are represented as sometimes excavated in the form of furrows. There are also circular depressions at unequal distances. The officinal description is as follows. "Cylindrical, eighteen to twenty-four inches (45 to 60 cm.) long, nearly one inch (25 mm.) in diameter, blackish brown, somewhat veined, the sutures smooth, forming two longitudinal bands; indehiscent, internally divided transversely into numerous cells, each containing a glossy seed imbedded in a blackish brown, sweet pulp." *U. S.* The pods brought from the East Indies are smaller, smoother, have a blacker pulp, and are more esteemed than those from the West Indies.

We have seen a quantity of pods in this market sold as cassia pods, which were an inch and a half in diameter, flattened on the sides, exceedingly rough on the outer surface, and marked by three longitudinal very elevated ridges, corresponding to the bands or furrows of the common cassia. The pulp was rather nauseous, but in other respects seemed to have the properties of the officinal purging cassia. They correspond exactly with a specimen of the fruit of *Cassia Brasiliana* brought from the West Indies, and were probably derived from that plant.

The heaviest pods, and those which do not make a rattling noise when shaken, are to be preferred; as they contain a larger portion of the pulp, which is the part employed. This should be black and shining, and have a sweet taste. It is apt to become sour if long exposed to the air, or mouldy if kept in a damp place. The pulp is extracted from the pods by first bruising them, then boiling them in water, and afterwards evaporating the decoction; or, when the pods are fresh, by opening them at the sutures, and removing the pulp by a spatula.

Cassia pulp has a slight rather sickly odor, and a sweet mucilaginous taste. From the analysis of M. Henry it appears to contain sugar, gum, a substance analogous to tannin, a coloring matter soluble in ether, traces of a principle resembling gluten, and a small quantity of water.

Medical Properties and Uses. Cassia pulp is laxative, and may be advantageously given in small doses in cases of habitual costiveness. In quantities sufficient to purge, it occasions nausea, flatulence, and griping. In this country it is rarely prescribed, except as an ingredient in the confection of senna, which is a pleasant and useful laxative preparation. The dose of the pulp as a laxative is one or two drachms (3·9–7·8 Gm.), as a purge one or two ounces (31·1–62·2 Gm.).

Off. Prep. Confectio Sennæ.

CASTANEA. *U.S.* *Castanea.* [*Chestnut.*]

(CĂS-TĀ'NĘ-Ą.)

"The leaves of Castanea vesca, Linné (*Nat. Ord.* Cupuliferæ), collected in September or October, while still green." *U.S.*

Folia Castaneæ; Feuilles de Châtaignier, Feuilles de Marronier, Châtaigne, *Fr.;* Kastanie, Kastanienblätter, *G.;* Castagna, *It.;* Castaña, *Sp.*

Gen. Ch. MALE. *Ament* naked. *Calyx* none. *Corolla* five-petalled. *Stamens* ten to twenty. FEMALE. *Calyx* five or six-leaved, muricate. *Corolla* none. *Germs* three. Stigma pencil-formed. *Nuts* three, included in an echinated calyx. *Willd.*

This is a very small genus, separated from the original Fagus of Linn., including only two or three recognized species; the *Castanea vesca* of Europe and North America, and *C. pumila* of the United States, which will be found described in Part II. of the present work. The European and American chestnut-trees are known under the same botanical title; as no points of difference can be found between them, which botanists in general are willing to recognize as authorizing distinct specific designations. The late Dr. Geo. B. Wood, however, believed, for reasons given below, that they are distinct trees, differing in origin, and as much entitled to distinct names as the European and American white oaks, or indeed any other analogous species of the two continents. Thus, the general aspect of the two trees is such that the accustomed eye will at a glance recognize the difference, though it might be difficult to say in what exactly the difference consists. The much greater size and somewhat peculiar shape of the fruit of the European, or, as it is commonly called, in this country, the Spanish Chestnut, is another very striking distinction, and, if permanent, should, we think, be admitted as a sufficient specific character. Besides, the European tree does not lose its distinctive character, under complete change of circumstances. Transplanted into North America, and propagated by the seed, it has retained, through a succession of generations, the original superiority in the size of its fruit, which, had the tree been of the same species as the American, would have almost certainly more or less deteriorated.

Castanea vesca. Willd.; Michaux, *N. American Sylva*, iii. 9. *Castanea Americana.* Persoon. (See *Mérat and De Lens.*) The American chestnut is, under favorable circumstances, one of our largest and most magnificent native trees. Michaux states that he had measured several trees, the trunks of which, at six feet from the ground, were fifteen or sixteen feet in circumference, and their stature equal to that of the loftiest trees of the forest. So great a size, however, is rare. Its leaves, which are the officinal portion, serve also at once to distinguish the tree. They are from four to ten inches long by about two in breadth, oblong-elliptical, sharp at the end, strongly and somewhat unequally serrated, with prominent parallel nerves beneath, of a brilliant color, and firm consistence. The only leaves that are liable to be confounded with them are those of the chestnut-oak, which have a very similar form and structure, but are at once distinguishable by the rounded crenate projections on the edge, instead of the sharp serratures of the chestnut. The male flowers are whitish, and disposed on axillary peduncles, four or five inches long; the fertile aments similarly disposed, but less conspicuous. The fruit is a spherical burr, an inch or two in diameter, and very prickly, containing two or three brown nuts, the appearance of which is too well known to require description here. When perfectly ripe, it opens and lets fall the seeds. The bark is very peculiar and characteristic in its appearance, with a longitudinal arrangement of its fibres. The wood is firm and elastic, though not compact, with a remarkable power of resisting decomposition from the weather, and therefore very valuable for posts and rails in fencing. It is not well fitted for fuel, in consequence of a great disposition to snap in the fire, and to throw off burning particles to a considerable distance.

The American chestnut is spread largely through the eastern portions of the United States, from New Hampshire to the mountainous districts of Virginia, North and South Carolina, Georgia, and Tennessee, where it abounds; as also in the Middle States of New Jersey and Pennsylvania, though rare in the maritime parts of Virginia and the other Southern States. The leaves should be collected after perfect maturity, and before beginning to decay in autumn.

The European species is distributed in the south of Europe very much as the American is with us, preferring hilly regions, and abounding in Spain, the south and west of France, Switzerland, and Italy. It sometimes attains an enormous magnitude, and Michaux describes one, growing at Sancerre in France, which at six feet from the ground is thirty feet in circumference, and six hundred years ago was known as the *Great Chestnut*. Though supposed to be more than one thousand years old, its trunk is perfectly sound, and its branches are annually loaded with fruit. Much larger than this is the celebrated chestnut of Mount Etna, of which the trunk is said to be one hundred and sixty feet in circumference, though hollow in the centre, so that the tree lives by its bark. (*Mérat and De Lens.*) In Europe the young chestnut is much used for making hoops, for which it is preferred to all other wood on account of resisting the effects of air and moisture. For this purpose it is much cultivated in Europe, and cut when large enough. But the tree is still more valuable on account of its large nuts, which are much used as food, being a favorite on the table of the rich, and often the main dependence of the poor peasant, who considers himself well-off when possessed of a few healthy chestnut-trees. Whole provinces are said to be supported by this fruit. Though cultivated in small numbers in this country, they have not been so extensively introduced as they ought to be, chiefly, in all probability, from their difficulty of propagation. The inner bark of the chestnut has been vaunted in Europe as a remedy in dysentery. (*Mérat and De Lens.*)

Properties. The leaves, which have already been described, are so flexible and tenacious that it is difficult to powder them. In preparing them for the action of a solvent, they must be comminuted by cutting and bruising them in a mortar. They are not, therefore, well fitted for percolation. (*Maisch.*) They have little smell, and a slightly astringent, and scarcely bitterish taste, so that they are not offensive to children. They yield their virtues freely to water, and, probably, less so to alcohol. John B. Turner found in chestnut leaves chlorophyll, tannin, gallic acid, gum, and albumen. (*A. J. P.*, 1879, p. 542.) In addition to these constituents, L. J. Steltzer found carbonates, chlorides, and phosphates of potassium, calcium, magnesium, and iron, and a trace of resin and fat. (*A. J. P.*, 1880, p. 294.)

Medical Uses. The only remedial use of the leaves, so far as we have learned, has been in the treatment of hooping-cough. Their effects on the system do not appear to have been carefully studied; but their sensible properties do not indicate the possession of any extraordinary physiological power. A communication from Mr. G. C. Close, of Brooklyn, N. Y., calling attention to their efficacy in hooping-cough, made to the American Pharmaceutical Association, at the meeting of 1862, was the first intimation that has come to our notice of their claims to consideration as a medicine. Enough of favorable reports have been since published to indicate that the leaves have some control over the disease, but their use has not become general in the profession.

The leaves may be administered in infusion or fluid extract. Dr. Unzicker prepared an infusion with three or four drachms of the leaves and a pint of boiling water, and gave of it, well sweetened, as much as the child would drink.

Off. Prep. Extractum Castaneæ Fluidum.

CATAPLASMATA. *Cataplasms.*

(CĂT-A-PLĂS′MA-TA.)

Poultices, *E.;* Cataplasmes, *Fr.;* Umschläge, Breiumschläge, *G.*

Cataplasms or *poultices** are moist substances intended for external application, of such a consistence as to accommodate themselves accurately to the surface to which they are applied, without being so liquid as to spread over the neighboring parts, or so tenacious as to adhere firmly to the skin. As they are in this country seldom made by the apothecary, they were not deemed by the compilers of the U. S. Pharmacopœia proper objects for officinal direction. The ounce used in the following processes is the avoirdupois.

CATAPLASMA CARBONIS. *Br.* *Charcoal Poultice.*

(CĂT-A-PLĂS′MA CÄR-BŌ′NĬS.)

Cataplasme au Charbon, *Fr.;* Kohlenumschlag, *G.*

"Take of Wood Charcoal, in powder, *half an ounce;* Crumb of Bread *two ounces;* Linseed Meal *one ounce and a half;* Boiling Water *ten fluidounces.* Macerate the Bread in the Water for ten minutes near the fire, then mix, and add the Linseed Meal gradually, stirring the ingredients, that a soft poultice may be formed. Mix with this half the charcoal, and sprinkle the remainder on the surface of the poultice." *Br.*

Charcoal, recently prepared, has the property of absorbing those principles upon which the offensive odor of putrefying animal substances depends. In the form of poultice, it is an excellent application to foul and gangrenous ulcers, correcting their fetor, and improving the condition of the sore. It should be frequently renewed.

CATAPLASMA CONII. *Br.* *Hemlock Poultice.*

(CĂT-A-PLĂS′MA CO-NĪ′Ī.)

Cataplasme avec la Ciguë, *Fr.;* Schierling-Umschlag, *G.*

"Take of Juice of Hemlock *one fluidounce;* Linseed Meal *four ounces;* Boiling Water, *ten fluidounces.* Evaporate the hemlock juice to half its volume, add this to the linseed meal and water previously mixed, and stir them together." *Br.*

This cataplasm may be advantageously employed as an anodyne application to cancerous, scrofulous, syphilitic, and other painful ulcers; but its liability to produce narcotic effects, in consequence of the absorption of the active principle of the hemlock, should not be overlooked. (See *A. J. P.*, 1873, p. 177.)

CATAPLASMA FERMENTI. *Br.* *Yeast Poultice.*

(CĂT-A-PLĂS′MA FER-MĔN′TĪ.)

Cataplasme avec le Levûre de Bière, *Fr.;* Hefenumschlag, *G.*

"Take of Beer Yeast *six fluidounces;* Wheaten Flour *fourteen ounces;* Water,

* *Spongio Piline* is a thick cloth into which sponge in very small pieces has been felted, and a layer of rubber applied upon the surface. It is used as a substitute for a poultice by simply soaking a piece of the desired size in warm or hot water, and, after wiping the rubber side dry, applying at once, using a bandage to keep it in place if necessary. Moisture is retained a long time, evaporation being prevented by the rubber coating. If desired, Fluid Extract of Belladonna, Conium, or any similar preparation, may be added in proper quantity to the warm water.

heated to 100° F., *six fluidounces.* Mix the Yeast with the Water, and stir in the Flour. Place the mass near the fire till it rises." *Br.*

By exposing a mixture of yeast and flour to a gentle heat, fermentation takes place, and carbonic acid gas is extricated, which causes the mixture to swell, and is the source of its peculiar virtues. The yeast cataplasm is gently stimulant, and is sometimes applied with benefit to foul and gangrenous ulcers, the fetor of which it corrects, while it hastens the separation of the slough.

CATAPLASMA LINI. *Br.* *Linseed Poultice.*

(CĂT-Ą-PLĂŞ′MĄ LĪ′NĪ.)

Cataplasma Emolliens, s. Communis; Flaxseed Poultice; Cataplasme de Farine de Lin, Cataplasme simple (commun), *Fr.;* Leinsamen-Umschlag, *G.*

"Take of Linseed Meal *four ounces;* Boiling Water *ten fluidounces.* Mix the Linseed Meal gradually with the Water, with constant stirring." *Br.*

The flaxseed meal which remains after the expression of the oil is sometimes employed; this is called *cake meal;* but that which has not been submitted to pressure is decidedly preferable, and answers an excellent purpose when mixed with boiling water, without other addition. Fresh lard or olive oil, spread upon the surface of the poultice, serves to prevent its adhesion to the skin, and to preserve its softness.

The use of this and other emollient cataplasms is to relieve inflammation, or to promote suppuration. They act mainly by the sedative influence of their moisture and by excluding the air. An extensively employed poultice is prepared by heating together milk and the crumb of bread. The milk should be quite sweet, and fresh lard should be incorporated with the poultice. Mush made with the meal of Indian corn also forms an excellent emollient cataplasm.*

CATAPLASMA SINAPIS. *Br.* *Mustard Poultice.*

(CĂT-Ą-PLĂŞ′MĄ SĮ-NĀ′PĬS.)

Sinapismus, *P. G.;* Cataplasma Rubefaciens; Sinapisme, Cataplasme de Moutarde, Cataplasme rubéfiant, *Fr.;* Senfteig, *G.*

"Take of Mustard, in powder, 2½ ounces [av.], or a sufficiency; Linseed Meal 2½ ounces [av.]; Boiling Water, Water, of each a sufficiency. Mix the mustard with two or three ounces of lukewarm water; mix the linseed meal with six to eight ounces of boiling water; add the former to the latter, and stir them together." *Br.*

The simplest and most effectual mode of preparing a mustard poultice, plaster, or *sinapism,* as it is variously termed, is to mix the powdered mustard of the shops, diluted with flour or flaxseed according to the exigencies of the case, with a sufficient quantity of warm water to give it a due consistence. Vinegar never increases its efficiency, and, in the case of the black mustard seed, has been ascertained by MM. Trousseau and Blanc to diminish its rubefacient power. The same may be said of alcohol. A boiling temperature is also injurious, by interfering with the development of the volatile oil or acrid principle. (See *Sinapis.*)

The mustard poultice is a very powerful rubefacient, producing at once a sense of warmth, which increases until it becomes an almost insufferable burning, and leaving after removal an intensely red burning surface, followed, if the application has been sufficiently prolonged, by desquamation or vesication. In some cases of low vitality even obstinate ulcers and gangrene have resulted from the protracted action of mustard. A poultice composed of pure black mustard should rarely be left on more than from fifteen to twenty minutes, one of white mustard from twenty to thirty minutes, whilst one of half strength may be applied from thirty to forty-five minutes. On some susceptible skins a mustard plaster is tolerated for only a very few minutes. In cases of insensibility or of excessive internal irritation, care is necessary not to allow the application to continue too long, as violent inflammation followed by obstinate ulceration may result. It is remarkable that in the conditions just spoken of a mustard plaster may at the time of its application seem to have no effect whatever,

* A substitute for linseed meal poultices has been prepared by saturating a piece of thick felt paper with a decoction of linseed and drying. When intended to be used, the prepared paper is dipped in hot water. It swells considerably, and is applied to the desired part, covered with waxed paper, rubber tissue, or oiled silk, fastened with bandages, and allowed to remain 12 hours. (Volkhausen, *Pharm. Ztg.,* 1879, p. 95.)

leaving the surface white and painless, and yet, when reaction occurs, furious inflammation, ending, it may be, in sloughing, may result. A severe inflammation produced by mustard is more painful and more obstinate than one caused by cantharides. In children particular care is necessary in the application of mustard. The poultice should be thickly spread on linen, muslin, or thick paper, and may be covered with gauze or unsized paper in order to prevent its adhesion to the skin. If hairs are present they should be removed by the razor. Sinapisms may be employed whenever a speedy rubefacient impression is desired. (See *Charta Sinapis.*)

CATAPLASMA SODÆ CHLORINATÆ. *Br.* *Chlorine Poultice.*

(CĂT-A-PLĂS'MA SŌ'DÆ CHLŌ-RI-NĀ'TÆ.)

"Take of Solution of Chlorinated Soda *two fluidounces;* Linseed Meal *four ounces;* Boiling Water *eight fluidounces.* Mix the Linseed Meal gradually with the Water, and add the Solution of Chlorinated Soda, with constant stirring." *Br.*

This is an excellent application to sloughing and other fetid ulcers, to correct the smell, and afford a moderate stimulation.

CATECHU. *U. S., Br.* *Catechu.*

(CĂT'E-CHŪ—kăt'e-kū.)

"An extract prepared from the wood of Acacia Catechu. Willdenow. (*Nat. Ord.* Leguminosæ, Mimoseæ)" *U. S.* "An extract of the leaves and young shoots of Uncaria Gambir (Nauclea Gambir)." *Br.*

Catechu Pallidum, Pale Catechu, Cutch, Terra Japonica, Catechu Nigrum; Cachou, *Fr.;* Catechu, Katechu, Pegu Catechu, *G.;* Catecu, Cateiu, Catto, *It.;* Catecu, *Sp.;* Cutt, *Hindostanee.*

The British Pharmacopœia has entirely rejected the proper catechu, which in the former edition was recognized under the inappropriate name of Catechu Nigrum, retaining by the name of Catechu a product which, though analogous to catechu, is entirely distinct, being derived from a different plant, and known commonly by a different name, that, namely, of gambir. We treat in the text of the proper catechu, and, in a note, of gambir among the catechus not recognized by the U. S. Pharmacopœia.

Acacia Catechu. Willd. *Sp. Plant.* iv. 1079; Carson, *Illust. of Med. Bot.* i. 32, pl. 24; *B. & T.* 95. According to Mr. Kerr, whose description has been followed by most subsequent writers, *Acacia Catechu* is a small tree, seldom more than twelve feet in height, with a trunk one foot in diameter, dividing towards the top into many close branches, and covered with a thick, rough, brown bark. The leaves, which stand alternately upon the younger branches, are composed of from fifteen to thirty pairs of pinnæ nearly two inches long, each of which is furnished with about forty pairs of linear leaflets, beset with short hairs. At the base of each pair of pinnæ is a small gland upon the common footstalk. Two short recurved spines are attached to the stem at the base of each leaf. The flowers are in close spikes, which arise from the axils of the leaves, and are about four or five inches long. The fruit is a lanceolate, compressed, smooth, brown pod, with an undulated thin margin, and contains six or eight roundish flattened seeds, which when chewed emit a nauseous odor.

This species of Acacia is a native of the East Indies, growing abundantly in various provinces of Hindostan, and in the Burmese Empire. Pereira says that it is now common in Jamaica. Like most others of the same genus, it abounds in astringent matter, which may be extracted by decoction. Catechu is an extract from the wood of the tree.

This drug had been long known before its source was discovered. It was at first called *terra Japonica*, under the erroneous impression that it was an earthy substance derived from Japan. When ascertained by analysis to be of vegetable origin, it was generally considered by writers on the Materia Medica to be an extract of the *betel nut*, which is the fruit of a species of palm, denominated *Areca Catechu.* Its true origin was made known by Mr. Kerr, assistant surgeon of the civil hospital in Bengal, who had an opportunity of examining the tree from which it was obtained, and observing the process of extraction. According to Mr. Kerr, the manufacturer, having cut off the exterior white part of the wood, reduces the interior brown or reddish-colored portion into chips, which he then boils in water in unglazed earthen vessels, till all the soluble matter is dissolved. The decoction thus obtained is evaporated first by artificial heat, and afterwards in the sun, till it has assumed a thick consistence, when it is spread out to dry upon a mat or cloth, being, while yet soft, divided by means of a string into square or quadrangular pieces. The account subsequently given by Dr. Royle, of the preparation of the extract in Northern India, is essentially the same. The process, as he observed it, was completed by the pouring of the extract into quadrangular earthen moulds. Our countryman, the Rev. Howard Malcom, states, in his "Travels in South-Eastern Asia," that catechu is largely prepared from the wood of *Acacia Catechu* near Prome, in Burmah. Two kinds, he observes, are prepared from the same tree; one *black*, which is preferred in China, and the other *red*, which is most esteemed in Bengal. It is said that the unripe fruit and leaves are also sometimes submitted to decoction.

The name *catechu* in the native language signifies the *juice of a tree*, and appears to have been applied to astringent extracts obtained from various plants. According to the U. S. Pharmacopœia, however, the term is properly restricted to the extract of *Acacia Catechu;* as it was not intended to recognize all the astringent products which are floating in Asiatic commerce; and those from other sources than the Acacia, though they may occasionally find their way into our shops, do so as an exception to the general rule. A minute account of the diversified forms and exterior characters which officinal catechu presents as produced in different localities, would rather tend to perplex the reader than to serve any good practical purpose. These characters are, moreover, frequently changing, as the drug is procured from new sources, or as slight variations may occur in the mode of its preparation. Commerce is chiefly supplied with catechu from Bahar, Northern India, and Nepaul through Calcutta, from Canara through Bombay, and from the Burmese dominions. We derive it directly from Calcutta, or by orders from London, and it is sold in our markets without reference to its origin. It is frequently called *cutch* by the English traders, a name derived, no doubt, from the Hindoostanee word *cutt.**

* In order not to embarrass the text unnecessarily, we have thrown together, in the form of a note, the following observations upon the varieties of catechu; those being first considered which are probably derived from *Acacia Catechu*, and, therefore, recognized as officinal in the U. S. Pharmacopœia.

1. *Officinal Catechu. U.S.*

The following, so far as we have been able to distinguish them, are the varieties of officinal catechu to be found in the markets of Philadelphia.

1. *Plano-convex Catechu. Cake Catechu.* This is in the form of circular cakes, flat on one side, convex on the other, and usually somewhat rounded at the edge, as if the soft extract had been placed in saucers, or vessels of a similar shape, to harden. As found in the retail shops, it is generally in fragments, most of which, however, exhibit some evidences of the original form. The cakes are of various sizes, from two or three to six inches or more in diameter, and weighing from a few ounces to nearly two pounds. Their exterior is usually smooth and dark brown; but we have seen a specimen in which the flat surface exhibited impressions as if produced by coarse matting. The color internally is always brown, sometimes of a light yellowish brown or chocolate color, but more frequently dark reddish brown, and sometimes almost black. The cakes are almost always more or less cellular in their interior; but in this respect great diversity exists. Sometimes they are very porous, so as almost to present a spongy appearance, sometimes compact and nearly uniform; and this difference may be observed even in the same piece. The fracture is sometimes rough and dull, but in the more compact parts is usually smooth and somewhat shining; and occasionally a piece split in one direction will exhibit a spongy fracture, while in another it will be shining and resinous, indicating the consolidation of the extract in layers. This variety of catechu is often of good quality. It is common at present in our market, but we have been unable to trace its origin accurately. There can be little doubt, from its internal character, that it comes from the East Indies, and is the product of *A. Catechu:* but no accounts that we have seen of the preparation of the drug, in particular geographical sites, indicate this particular shape; and it is not impossible that portions of it may be formed out of other varieties of catechu by a new solution and evaporation.

2. *Pegu Catechu.* This is the product derived from the Burmese dominions, and named from that section of the country whence it is exported. It enters commerce, probably in general through Calcutta, in large masses, sometimes of one cwt., consisting of layers of flat cakes, each wrapped in leaves, said to be those of the *Nauclea Brunonis.* In this form, however, we do not see it in the shops; but almost always in angular, irregular fragments, in which portions of two layers sometimes cohere with leaves between them, indicating their origin. It is characterized by its compactness, shining fracture, and blackish brown or dark port-wine color, so that when finely broken it

Properties. Catechu, as it comes to us, is in masses of different shapes, some in balls more or less flattened, some in circular cakes, some saucer-shaped, others

bears considerable resemblance to kino. This is an excellent variety of catechu, and is not unfrequent in the shops.

3. *Catechu in Quadrangular Cakes.* This is scarcely ever found in the shops in its complete form, and the fragments are often such that it would be impossible to infer from them the original shape of the cake. This is usually between two and three inches in length and breadth, and somewhat less in thickness, of a rusty brown color externally, and dark brown or brownish gray within, with a somewhat rough and dull fracture, but, when broken across the layers in which it is sometimes disposed, exhibiting a smoother and more shining surface. Guibourt speaks of the layers as being blackish externally and grayish within, and bearing some resemblance to the bark of a tree, a resemblance, however, which has not struck us in the specimens which have fallen under our notice. There is little doubt that this variety comes from the provinces of Bahar and Northern India, where the preparation of the drug was witnessed by Mr. Kerr and Dr. Royle, who both speak of it as being brought, when drying, into the quadrangular form. It has been called *Bengal Catechu*, because exported from that province.

Pale catechu, so far as the term is not applied to *gambir*, may be considered as belonging to this variety. A specimen with this name, which was sent from India to the great London exhibition, and which Dr. G. B. Wood had an opportunity of examining, was in oblong rectangular pieces, or fragments of such pieces, about three and a half inches long by an inch and a half in breadth, of a dirty yellowish color within, and an earthy fracture, quite free from gloss, and bearing a much stronger resemblance to gambir than to ordinary catechu.

4. *Catechu in Balls.* We have seen this in two forms—one consisting of globular balls about as large as an orange, very hard and heavy, of a ferruginous aspect externally, very rough when broken, and so full of sand as to be gritty under the teeth; the other in cakes, originally, in all probability, globular, and of about the same dimensions, but flattened and otherwise pressed out of shape before being perfectly dried, sometimes adhering two together, as happens with the lumps of Smyrna opium, and closely resembling in external and internal color, and in the character of their fracture, the quadrangular variety last described. The former kind is rare, and the specimens we have seen had been twenty years in the shop, and had very much the appearance of a factitious product. The latter is in all probability the kind known formerly as the *Bombay catechu;* as Dr. Hamilton, and, more recently, Major Mackintosh, in describing the mode of preparing catechu on the Malabar coast, of which Bombay is the entrepot, say that, while the extract is soft, it is shaped into balls about the size of an orange.

2. *Catechus not recognized in the U. S. Pharmacopœia.*

1. **Catechu,** *Br. Gambir. Terra Japonica. Pale Catechu.* An astringent extract is abundantly prepared in certain parts of the East Indies, under the name of *gambir* or *gambeer*, and imported into Europe and America under that of terra Japonica. The plant from which it is obtained, called by Mr. Hunter, who first minutely described it, *Nauclea Gambir*, but by Roxburgh, De Candolle, and others, *Uncaria Gambir*, is a climbing shrub of the natural order Rubiaceæ of Jussieu, Cinchonaceæ of Lindley. (*B. & T.* 139.) It is a native of Malacca, Sumatra, Cochin-China, and other parts of Eastern Asia, and is largely cultivated in the islands of Bintang, Singapore, and Prince of Wales. The gambir is prepared by boiling the leaves and young shoots in water, and evaporating the decoction either by artificial or solar heat. When of a proper consistence, it is spread out into flat cakes in moulds or otherwise, and then cut into small cubes, which are dried in the sun. Sometimes these cohere into a mass when packed before being quite dry.

Gambir is in cubes, with sides about an inch square, is light and porous, so that it floats when thrown in water, is deep yellowish, or reddish brown externally, but pale yellowish within, presents a dull earthy surface when broken, is inodorous, and has a strongly astringent, bitter, and subsequently sweetish taste. It softens and swells up when heated, and leaves a minute proportion of ashes when burnt. It is partially soluble in cold water, and almost wholly so in boiling water, which deposits a portion upon cooling. Duhamel, Ecky, and Procter dissolved 87·5 per cent. of it in cold water by means of percolation. (*A. J. P.*, xvi. 166.) Nees von Esenbeck found it to consist of from 36 to 40 per cent. of catechu-tannic acid, a peculiar principle called *catechuin*, *catechin*, or catechuic acid, gum or gummy extractive, a deposit like the cinchonic red, and 2·5 per cent. of lignin. *Catechuic acid*, when perfectly pure, is snow-white, of a silky appearance, crystallizable in fine needles, unalterable if dry in the air, fusible by heat, very slightly soluble in cold water with which it softens and swells up, soluble in boiling water which deposits it on cooling, and soluble also in alcohol and ether. It very slightly reddens litmus paper, and, though coloring the solution of chloride of iron green, and producing with it a grayish green precipitate, differs from tannic acid in not affecting a solution of gelatin. It bears considerable analogy to gallic acid in its relations to the metallic salts, but does not, according to Neubauer, bear the same relation to the tannic acid of catechu that gallic acid does to that of galls. On the contrary, instead of resulting from the oxidation of tannic acid, it is by heat converted into a substance analogous to tannin. (*A. J. P.*, xxviii. 329 and 331; from *Liebig's Annalen*, xcvi. 337.) The very great discordance of different authors as to its formula seems to be explained by some recent experiments of Etti (*Liebig's Ann.*, 186, p. 327), who shows that *catechin*, $C_{19}H_{18}O_8$, readily gives at 100° C. (212° F.), or even when kept for some time over sulphuric acid, an anhydride, $C_{38}H_{34}O_{15}$, and at 160° C. (320° F.) a second anhydride, $C_{38}H_{32}O_{14}$, which, mixed in varying proportions, explain the varying results. Gautier (*Journ. de Pharm. et de Chim.*, 1878, p. 368) assigns to catechin the formula $C_{21}H_{18}O_8$.

Several varieties of gambir are described. Sometimes it is in oblong instead of cubical pieces, without differing in other respects from the ordinary kind; sometimes in small circular cakes, or short cylindrical pieces, heavier than water, of a pale reddish yellow color, moderately astringent, gritty under the teeth, and quite impure; sometimes in very small cubes, distinguishable by the

cubical or oblong, or quite irregular, and of every grade in size, from small angular pieces, which are evidently fragments of the original cakes, to lumps which weigh one or two pounds. The color is externally of a rusty brown more or less dark, internally varying from a pale reddish or yellowish brown to a dark liver color. In some specimens it is almost black, in others somewhat like the color of port wine, and in others again, though rarely, dull red like annotta. The extract has been distinguished into the *pale* and *dark* varieties; but there does not appear to be sufficient ground for retaining this distinction, at least in relation to the proper catechu obtained from the wood of *A. Catechu.* Catechu is inodorous, with an astringent and bitter taste, followed by a sense of sweetness. It is brittle, and breaks with a fracture which is rough in some specimens, in others uniform, resinous, and shining. That which is preferred in our market is of a dark color, easily broken into small angular fragments, with a smooth glossy surface, bearing some resemblance to kino. Catechu is often mixed with sand, sticks, and other impurities. From 200 parts of Bombay catechu, Sir H. Davy obtained 109 parts of tannic acid, 68 of extractive, 13 of mucilage, and 10 of insoluble residue. The same quantity of Bengal catechu yielded 97 of tannic acid, 73 of extractive, 16 of mucilage, and 14 of insoluble residue. Other experimenters have obtained results somewhat different. The proportion of tannic acid, which may be considered the efficient principle, varies from about 30 to 55 per cent. in the different varieties of the drug. The portion designated by Davy as extractive is said to contain, if it does not chiefly consist of, a principle discovered by Buchner, and now called *catechin*, *catechuin*, or *catechuic acid*, to which Etti gives the formula $C_{19}H_{18}O_8$. To prepare pure catechin, Etti (*loc. cit.*) proceeds as follows.

black color they afford with tincture of iodine, indicating the admixture of sago, or other amylaceous matter; and, finally, in circular cakes of the size of a small lozenge flat on one side, and somewhat convex on the other, of a pale pinkish yellowish white color, and a chalky feel. This is most highly esteemed by the natives in India. (*Pereira.*) None of these varieties occur to any extent in our commerce. At the Edinburgh Forestry Exhibition in 1885, the Maharajah of Johore exhibited specimens labelled "gambier produced in Johore." The first quality, which was "*makan*" (for eating), was in regular cubes, externally cassia brown color, internally pale cinnamon brown, and yielded 32 per cent. of tannic acid; the second quality was in badly-formed cubes, externally brown and black, internally cinnamon, and yielded 30 per cent. of tannic acid; the third quality was in dull brown, well-shaped cubes, internally pale brown, and yielded 19 per cent. of tannic acid. The oblong or *parallelopiped gambier* was of a uniform dull brown, very hard and strong, and yielded only 2 per cent. of tannic acid. Mr. MacEwan believes that the low percentage of tannin was due to the decoction not having been subjected to prolonged boiling, which favors the decomposition of catechin, with the formation of catechu-tannic acid.

Gambir was probably the substance first brought from the East under the name of *terra Japonica.* It is largely consumed in the East by the betel-chewers. Great quantities are imported into Europe, where it is used for tanning, calico-printing, dyeing, etc. In this country it is also largely consumed by the calico-printer. It is a strong astringent, and applicable to the same purposes as the officinal catechu.

2. *Areca Catechu.* This is obtained from the *areca nut*, or *betel nut*, which is the seed of *Areca Catechu*, a palm cultivated in all parts of India. (See Part II.) It is prepared by boiling the nuts in water, and evaporating the decoction. There are two varieties; one of a black color, very astringent, mixed with paddy husks and other impurities, and obtained by evaporating the first decoction; the other, yellowish brown, of an earthy fracture, and pure, resulting from the evaporation of a decoction of the nuts which had been submitted to the previous boiling. The first is called *kassu*, the other *coury*. (Heyne, *Tracts, etc., on India.*) They are prepared in Mysore, and Ainslie states that both varieties are sold in the bazaars of Lower India, and used for the same purpose as the officinal catechu by the native and European practitioners. They are also much used for chewing by the natives. But they are seldom exported, and it is uncertain whether they find their way into European or American commerce. Pereira thought he had identified the *kassu* with a variety of catechu derived from Ceylon, where he had been informed that an extract of the areca nut is prepared. It was in circular flat cakes, from two to three inches in diameter, scarcely an inch thick, covered on one side with paddy husks, and internally blackish brown and shining, like Pegu catechu.

Guibourt and Pereira describe other varieties, which we have not met with, and which are probably rare. One of these is the *Siam catechu*, in conical masses shaped like a betel nut, and weighing about a pound and a half. Its fracture is shining and liver-colored, like that of hepatic aloes; in other respects it resembles Pegu catechu. Another is the *black mucilaginous catechu* of Guibourt, in parallelopipeds, an inch and a half in length by an inch in breadth. Internally it is black and shining, and its taste is mucilaginous and feebly astringent. A third is the *dull reddish catechu* of Guibourt, in somewhat flattened balls, weighing three or four ounces, of a dull reddish, wavy, and often marbled fracture. Many years since an extract like this was brought to Philadelphia upon speculation by a merchant from Calcutta, but it is not now in the market. Lastly, there is a *pale* or *whitish* catechu, in small roundish or oval lumps, with an irregular surface, dark or blackish brown externally, very pale and dull internally, and of a bitter, astringent and sweetish taste, with a smoky flavor. It is unknown in commerce.

Catechu is dissolved in eight times its weight of boiling water, and the liquid, after being strained through a cloth, is left for some days until the insoluble catechin has subsided. The crude catechin is collected in a linen cloth and submitted to the action of a screw-press, then dissolved in a sufficient amount of dilute alcohol, and the filtered solution is shaken up with ether as long as any catechin is thereby dissolved; and after the ether has been removed by distillation the residue is taken up with distilled water, and the solution is left for a few days, when the catechin crystallizes out in an almost colorless state. After pressure in a cloth it is again dissolved in boiling water, when a yellowish white body remains behind, which appears to be *quercetin.* The deep red liquid remaining behind after the catechin has been dissolved out with ether contains *catechu red*, $C_{36}H_{34}O_{15}$. The *tannic acid* is of the variety which precipitates iron of a greenish black color, and differs from most of the other varieties in not yielding grape-sugar when digested with dilute sulphuric acid. It is not, therefore, a glucoside. It precipitates gelatin, but not tartar emetic (*Kane*), and is not, like the tannic acid of galls, converted into gallic acid by exposure to the air. It may be distinguished by the name of *catechu-tannic acid.* Catechu is almost wholly soluble in a large quantity of water, to which it imparts a brown color. The extractive or catechuic acid is much less soluble than the astringent principle, which may be almost entirely separated from it by the frequent application of small quantities of cold water. Boiling water dissolves it much more readily than cold, and deposits it of a reddish brown color upon cooling. Both principles are readily dissolved by alcohol or proof spirit, and also by ether. For the important reactions of catechu, see *Acidum Tannicum.*

The importations of *cutch* or catechu and terra japonica or gambir for purposes of tanning and calico printing are quite large, amounting in 1887 to 25,598,212 pounds.

M. de Meyer affirms that the best method of detecting adulteration of catechu is to treat the suspected drug with ether. Catechu of good quality, after repeated treatment with ether, loses 53 per cent. of its weight, and the dried residue weighs only 47 per cent. of the catechu employed. If this be exceeded, the drug must be proportionately impure. (*Journ. de Pharm.*, Juin, 1870, p. 479.) A. Jossart (*Journ. Pharm. d'Anvers*, 1881, p. 41) examined a catechu which was adulterated with 60 to 65 per cent. of ferrous carbonate.

Medical Properties and Uses. Catechu is a powerful astringent. The dark-colored is somewhat more powerful than the light, and is therefore usually preferred; but the light, being rather sweeter, is chosen by the Malays, Hindoos, and other East Indians, who consume vast quantities of this extract by chewing it, mixed with aromatics and a small proportion of lime, and wrapped in the leaf of the *Piper Betel.* Catechu may be advantageously used in most cases where astringents are indicated. The complaints to which it is best adapted are diarrhœa dependent on debility or relaxation of the intestinal mucous membrane, and passive hemorrhages, particularly that from the uterus. A small piece held in the mouth and allowed slowly to dissolve, is an excellent remedy in relaxation of the uvula, and the irritation of the fauces and troublesome cough which depend upon it. Applied to spongy gums, in the state of powder, it sometimes proves useful; and it has been recommended as a dentifrice in combination with powdered charcoal, Peruvian bark, myrrh, etc. Sprinkled upon the surface of indolent ulcers, it is occasionally beneficial, and is much used in India for the same purpose, in the form of an ointment. An infusion of catechu may be used as an injection in obstinate gonorrhœa, gleet, and leucorrhœa, and we have found it highly beneficial, when thrown up the nostrils, in arresting epistaxis. The dose is from ten grains to half a drachm (0·65–1·95 Gm.), which should be frequently repeated, and is best given with sugar, gum arabic, and water.*

* ***Fluid Extract of Catechu.*** Prof. Procter suggested the following formula for a *fluid extract of catechu* based on the solvent power of glycerin over this extract. Eight *troyounces* of pure catechu, in moderately coarse powder, are mixed in a mortar with *four fluidounces* of glycerin so as to form a paste, to which enough diluted alcohol is added to make a pint. The liquid is poured into a bottle, shaken occasionally for twenty-four hours, and then strained through muslin. Each fluidrachm of the fluid extract represents thirty grains of catechu. (*Proc. A. P. A.*, 1863, p. 241.)

Off. Prep. Tinctura Catechu Composita.

Off. Prep. Br. Infusum Catechu; Pulvis Catechu Compositus; Tinctura Catechu; Trochisci Catechu.

CAULOPHYLLUM. *U. S.* *Caulophyllum.* [*Blue Cohosh.*]

(CÂU-LO-PHŸL'LUM.)

"The rhizome and rootlets of Caulophyllum thalictroides. Michaux. (*Nat. Ord.* Berberidaceæ.)" *U. S.*

Pappoose Root, Squaw Root, Blueberry Root.

Gen. Ch. Sepals 6, with three small bractlets at the base, ovate-oblong. *Petals* 6, thick and gland-like, somewhat kidney-shaped or hooded bodies, with short claws much smaller than the sepals, one at the base of each of them. *Stamens* 6: *anthers* oblong. *Pistil* gibbous, style short. *Stigma* minute and unilateral. *Ovary* bursting soon after flowering by the pressure of the two erect, enlarging seeds and withering away. The spherical *seeds* naked on their thick seed-stalks, looking like drupes; the fleshy integument turning blue; albumen of the texture of horn. (*Gray's Manual.*)

Caulophyllum thalictroides. Michaux. *Leontice thalictroides.* Linn. This is an indigenous, perennial, herbaceous plant, with matted, knotty rhizomes, from which rises a single smooth stem, about two feet high, naked till near the summit, where it sends out a large triternately compound leaf, and ending in a small raceme or panicle of greenish yellow flowers, at the base of which is often a smaller biternate leaf. The whole plant when young, as well as the seeds, which are about as large as peas, is glaucous. It is the only known species of the genus. It is found in most parts of the United States, growing in moist rich woods.

Properties. The root stock is the only part used. It has a sweetish, pungent taste, and yields its virtues to water and alcohol. It is officinally described as follows. "Rhizome about four inches (10 cm.) long, and about one-fourth to two-fifths of an inch (6 to 10 mm.) thick, bent; on the upper side with broad, concave stem-scars and short, knotty branches; externally gray brown, internally whitish, tough and woody. Rootlets numerous, matted, about four inches (10 cm.) long, and one twenty-fifth of an inch (1 mm.) thick, rather tough; nearly inodorous; taste sweetish, slightly bitter, and somewhat acrid." *U. S.*

Caulophyllum was examined by Mayer, who found it to contain *saponin.* (*A. J. P.*, 1863, p. 99.) A. E. Ebert subsequently made an investigation of its constituents, and found albumen, gum, starch, phosphoric acid, extractive, two resins, coloring matter, and a body analogous to saponin. The *caulophyllin* of the eclectics is made in the usual way, by pouring a concentrated alcoholic tincture into water and collecting, washing, and drying the resinous precipitate. Prof. J. U. Lloyd purified the substance which Ebert described as analogous to saponin, and for distinction terms it *leontin.* (See *Drugs and Medicines of North America*, vol. ii. p. 152.)

Medical Properties. Caulophyllum has been scarcely used at all by the general medical profession, although the so-called eclectic or homœopathic practitioners claim for it peculiar valuable properties. It is said to be sedative, antispasmodic, and oxytocic, and to have the power when uterine inertia occurs during labor to cause the contractions to become very severe, without altering their general character as does ergot. It is also alleged to be capable of arresting threatened abortion, to be very efficacious in hysteria, in amenorrhœa, in dysmenorrhœa, menorrhagia, uterine subinvolution, etc.; also to be capable of originating uterine contractions and producing abortion. For a detailed description of the various more or less contradictory powers ascribed to it, the reader is referred to *Lloyd's Drugs and Medicines of North America*, vol. ii. p. 155. It is given in decoction, infusion, or tincture, the first two being made in the proportion of an ounce to a pint of water, the last of four ounces to a pint of spirit. The dose of the decoction or infusion is one or two fluidounces, of the tincture one or two fluidrachms. Leontin has also been used in doses of one drachm of the one per cent. solution.

CERA ALBA. *U. S., Br.* *White Wax.*

(CĒ'RĄ ĂL'BĄ.)

"Yellow wax bleached." *U. S.* "Yellow wax bleached by exposure to moisture air, and light." *Br.*

Cire blanche, *Fr.*; Weisses Wachs, *G.*; Cera bianca, *It.*; Cera blanca, *Sp.*

CERA FLAVA. *U. S., Br.* *Yellow Wax.*

(CĒ'RĄ FLĀ'VĄ.)

"A peculiar, concrete substance, prepared by Apis mellifica. Linné. (*Class*, Insecta; *Order*, Hymenoptera.)" *U. S.* "Prepared from the honeycomb of the Hive Bee, Apis mellifica." *Br.*

Cera Citrina; Beeswax; Cire jaune, *Fr.*; Gelbes Wachs, *G.*; Cera gialla, *It.*; Cera amarilla, *Sp.*

Wax is a product of the common bee, *Apis mellifica* of naturalists, which constructs with it the cells of the comb in which the honey and larvæ are deposited. It was at one time doubted whether the insect elaborated the wax by its own organs, or merely gathered it from vegetables. The question was set at rest by Huber, who fed a swarm of bees exclusively on honey and water, and found that they formed a comb consisting of wax. This, therefore, is a proper secretion of the insect. It is produced in the form of scales under the rings of the belly. But wax also exists in plants, bearing in this, as in other respects, a close analogy to the fixed oils. It is, however, the product of the bee only that is recognized by the Pharmacopœias.* This is directed in two forms: 1, that of *yellow wax* procured immediately from the comb; and, 2, that of *white wax* prepared by bleaching the former. We shall consider these separately, and afterwards give an account of *vegetable wax.*

1. CERA FLAVA, or *Yellow Wax.* This is obtained by slicing the comb taken from the hive, draining and afterwards expressing the honey, and melting the residue in boiling water, which is kept hot for some time in order to allow the impurities to separate, and either subside or be dissolved by the water. When the liquid cools the wax concretes, and, having been removed and again melted in boiling water, is strained and poured into pans or other suitable vessels. The labor-saving device is sometimes adopted of stretching a strainer of cheese-cloth upon a hoop, and wedging the latter down into the hot mixture below the level of the water; as this cools, the melted wax slowly rises through the cloth, and thus a perfectly clean cake of wax is formed on top on cooling. It is usually brought to market in round flat cakes of considerable thickness. The druggists of Philadelphia are supplied chiefly from the Western States and North Carolina, especially the latter, and from Cuba and California.

* *China wax*, called *pe-la* by the Chinese, resembles spermaceti in whiteness and crystalline appearance, but is distinguished by greater hardness and friability, and a somewhat fibrous fracture. It melts at about 83° C. (181° F.), is very slightly soluble in alcohol or ether, is insoluble in cold oil of turpentine and rectified petroleum, but is dissolved with the aid of heat, and very soluble in benzol. These solubilities distinguish it from spermaceti. (*P. J. Tr.*, xiv. 9.) It was formerly supposed to be of vegetable origin, but has been ascertained to be the product of an insect belonging to the genus Coccus, which fixes itself to the branches of a certain tree, and investing them closely, becomes imbedded in a waxy material, which is scraped off with the insects, and constitutes the crude wax. It is purified by melting and straining. (Hanbury, *P. J. Tr.*, xii. 476.) The tree from which the wax is obtained has been ascertained to be the *Fraxinus Chinensis* of Roxburgh. (*Ibid.*, Sept. 1, 1859, p. 176.)

Mr. T. T. Cooper, in his "Travels of a Pioneer" in China, gives some interesting statements as to the production of this wax, which are the result of his own personal observations. It is chiefly the province of S'zchuan which is the seat of this industry; the cultivation of the China wax being a source of great wealth to this province, second only in importance to the silk culture. The "wax trees" are all cut down at the height of 8 feet, leaving no branches, the trunks being about as thick as a man's thigh, and sending forth shoots in the spring. The insects are cultivated in a different province, that of Yunnan, whence vast quantities of the eggs are sent annually to S'zchuan, where they are received in little balls of the size of a pea. These are suspended, enclosed in young leaves, to the shoots of the tree in March. In about two months the larvæ appear, and feeding on the leaves soon attain the size of small butterflies, which spread themselves in immense numbers over the branches, which are whitened by them, so as to seem covered with feathery snow. The grub, as it advances to the chrysalis form, buries itself in a white secretion by which all the branches are coated an inch in thickness. These are then cut off near the stem and divided into small pieces, which are tied in bundles, and put into large caldrons, where they are boiled in water till all the wax melts and rises to the surface. It is then skimmed off and run into moulds where it hardens. In the form thus produced, it is spread over the Empire, where it is used for candles and as medicine. (*P. J. Tr.*, 1872, p. 569; also vol. xv., 1885, p. 755.)

Properties. Yellow wax is "a yellowish or brownish yellow solid, having an agreeable, honey-like odor, and a faint, balsamic taste. It is brittle when cold, but becomes plastic by the heat of the hand. It melts at 63°–64° C. (145·4°–147·2° F.), and congeals with a smooth and level surface. Sp. gr. 0·955 to 0·967.* It is insoluble in water, but soluble in 35 parts of ether and in 11 parts of chloroform; also soluble in oil of turpentine, and in fixed or volatile oils. Cold alcohol dissolves it only partially, but it is almost completely soluble in boiling alcohol. If 1 Gm. of Wax be boiled, for half an hour, with 40 Gm. of solution of soda (sp. gr. 1·180), the volume being preserved by the occasional addition of water, the Wax should separate, on cooling, without rendering the liquid opaque, and no precipitate should be produced in the filtered liquid by hydrochloric acid (abs. of fats or fatty acids, Japan wax, resin); nor should the same reagent produce a precipitate in water which has been boiled with a portion of the Wax (abs. of soap). If 5 Gm. of Wax be heated in a flask, for fifteen minutes, with 25 Gm. of sulphuric acid to 160° C. (320° F.), and the mixture diluted with water, no solid, wax-like body should separate (abs. of paraffin)." *U. S.*

Various adulterations have been practised, most of which may be readily detected. Meal, earth, and other insoluble substances are at the same time discovered and separated by melting and straining the wax. When the fracture is smooth and shining instead of being granular, the presence of resin may be suspected. This is dissolved by cold alcohol, while the wax is left untouched. Yellow wax is frequently adulterated with a mixture of paraffin and rosin; such wax is usually translucent on the edges. Dr. A. W. Miller has observed that when a large quantity of paraffin is present the upper surface of the cake is concave, whilst pure yellow wax presents either a plane or slightly convex surface. For other adulterating substances used, and the modes of detecting them, see the remarks which follow on white wax.

Yellow wax is used chiefly as an ingredient of plasters and cerates.

2. Cera Alba, *Bleached Yellow Wax*, or *White Wax.* The color of yellow wax is discharged by exposing it, with an extended surface, to the combined influence of air, light, and moisture. The process of bleaching is carried on to a considerable extent in this country. The wax, previously melted, is made to fall in streams upon a revolving cylinder, kept constantly wet, upon which it concretes, forming thin riband-like layers. These, having been removed, are spread upon linen cloths stretched on frames, and exposed to the air and light, care being taken to water and occasionally turn them. In a few days they are partially bleached; but, to deprive the wax completely of color, it is necessary to repeat the whole process once, if not oftener. When sufficiently white, it is melted and cast into small circular cakes. The color may also be discharged by chlorine; but the wax is said to be somewhat altered.† White wax sometimes contains one or more free fatty acids,

* Dieterich has modified Hagar's method of taking the specific gravity of wax, as follows. A piece of wax is heated on the edge of a colorless flame, so that drops of melted wax may fall into alcohol placed in a saucer. Having thus obtained about a dozen wax-pearls, they are allowed to dry thoroughly by allowing them to remain on blotting-paper for 24 hours. Eight portions of diluted alcohol are prepared, of the following specific gravities respectively: 0·960; 0·961; 0·962; 0·963; 0·964; 0·965; 0·966; 0·967; and the pearl is dropped into these liquids in turn. The specific gravity of the wax is of course the same as the specific gravity of that liquid in which the pearl remains floating indifferently in any part of the vessel. (See *Remington's Practice of Pharmacy*, page 68. *Lovi's beads.*) Dieterich examined hundreds of specimens annually, and found the wax to vary in sp. gr. from 0·963 to 0·966. He also determined the specific gravities of the following substances used to adulterate wax: white wax, 0·973; cera japonica, Japan wax, 0·975; ceresin, half white, 0·920; ozokerite, crude, 0·952; rosin, common, 1·108; cacao butter, 0·980–0·981; pure rosin, 1·045; beef suet, 0·952–0·953; yellow wax, 0·963-0·964; ceresin, white, 0·918; ceresin, yellow, 0·922; spermaceti, 0·960; French rosin, 1·104-1·105; paraffin, med. hard, 0·913–0·914; stearin, A No. 1, 0·971–0·972; mutton suet, 0·961. (*Arch. d. Pharm.*, 1882, p. 55.)

† The following process for purifying wax by steam has been patented by M. Cassgrand, in France, and is said to have been employed advantageously. Wax melted by steam is passed along with the steam through a coiled tube or worm, is received into a double bottom heated by steam, where it is washed with water, and is then raised by a pump into another pan, also heated by steam, where it is again washed with water; and the whole operation is repeated three or four times; the wax being allowed to rest for about four or five minutes in the upper pan after each operation, and, after the last one, an hour or two for the subsidence of impurities. The wax is then granulated by means of cold water, allowed to dry for two or three days, and then exposed to light and air. The whole process is completed in a few days. (See *A. J. P.*, xxvi. 525.)

consequent probably upon the employment of alkalies in bleaching it, which render it an unfit ingredient in the unctuous preparations of certain salts. Of these acids it may be deprived by means of alcohol.

Perfectly pure wax is white, shining, diaphanous in thin layers, inodorous, insipid, harder and less unctuous to the touch than the yellow, soft and ductile at 35° C. (95° F.), and fusible at 65° C. (149° F.), retaining its fluidity at a lower temperature. According to Saussure, its sp. gr. in the solid state is 0·966. The U. S. Pharmacopœia describes it as "a yellowish white solid, generally in form of circular cakes, about four inches (10 cm.) in diameter, somewhat translucent in thin layers, having a slightly rancid odor and an insipid taste. It melts at about 65° C. (149° F.). Sp. gr. 0·965–0·975. In other respects it has the characteristics and answers to the tests mentioned under Yellow Wax (see *Cera Flava*)." *U. S.* By a great heat it is partly volatilized, partly decomposed; and, when flame is applied to its vapor, it takes fire and burns with a clear bright light. It is insoluble in water, and in cold alcohol or ether, but is slightly soluble in boiling alcohol and ether, which deposit it in a great measure upon cooling. The volatile and fixed oils dissolve it with facility, resin readily unites with it by fusion, and soaps are formed by the action of soda and potassa in solution. It is not affected by the acids at ordinary temperatures, but is converted into a black mass when boiled with concentrated sulphuric acid. Bleached wax contains, according to Lewy's analysis, 80·2 per cent. of carbon, 13·4 of hydrogen, and 6·4 of oxygen. It is a mixture of three different substances, which may be separated from one another by alcohol, viz.: 1, *myricin*, insoluble in boiling alcohol, and consisting chiefly of myricyl palmitate, $C_{16}H_{31}(C_{30}H_{61}O_2)$,—that is, a compound of *palmitic acid*, $C_{16}H_{31}O.OH$, and *myricyl alcohol*, $C_{30}H_{61}OH$; 2, *cerotic acid*, $C_{27}H_{54}O_2$ (formerly called *cerin* when obtained only in an impure state), which is dissolved by boiling alcohol, but crystallizes out on cooling; 3, *cerolein*, which remains dissolved in the cold alcoholic liquid. This latter is probably a mixture of fatty acids, as indicated by its acid reaction. It has not been investigated fully, however. (See results of Schwalb's analysis, *Jour. Chem. Soc.*, 1887, p. 124.)

Wax has been variously adulterated. *White lead* sinks to the bottom of the vessel when the wax is melted. *Starch*, *meal*, and other *insoluble substances* remain behind when the wax is dissolved in oil of turpentine or benzin; and the starch is known by producing a blue color with iodine added to water in which the wax has been boiled. *Water*, which is said to be sometimes fraudulently incorporated with it, by agitation when partially melted, is driven off by heat. *Fatty substances* render lime-water turbid, when agitated with it and allowed to stand. For the detection of stearin and stearic acid, M. Lebel dissolves the suspected wax in two parts of oil, beats the cerate thus formed with its weight of pure water, and then adds a few drops of solution of subacetate of lead. If stearin is present, there is an immediate decomposition, and the mixture acquires an extraordinary solidity from the formation of stearate of lead. (*Journ. de Pharm.*, 3e sér., xv. 302.) Vogel proposes chloroform as a means of detecting the adulteration with fatty matters. That liquid dissolves only 25 per cent. of wax, but stearin and stearic acid completely. If, therefore, wax, treated with 6 or 8 parts of chloroform, loses more than one-quarter of its weight, it may be considered as impure. (*Ibid.*, xvii. 374.) Overbeck detects stearic acid by the abundant effervescence produced from the escape of carbonic acid, when a small portion of the suspected wax is boiled in a solution composed of one part of carbonate of sodium and fifty of distilled water. (*P. J. Tr.*, xi. 128.) Fehling detects *stearic acid* and *resin* by boiling one part of the wax in twenty of alcohol, filtering the solution when cold, and then adding water. If either of these substances be present, there will be a flocculent precipitate, whereas if the wax be pure there will scarcely be an observable turbidness. The natural fats, as *tallow*, *suet*, *lard*, etc., are not amenable to this test; but it may be applied by first saponifying them, and thus converting them into the fatty acids, as the stearic. But, as wax itself is somewhat liable to be affected, it is necessary to avoid too strong an alkaline solution, and too long boiling in the process. To obviate such a result, 30 grains of the wax are to be boiled with two or three fluidounces of water containing 6 grains of pure hydrate of soda, and the mass saturated with a very dilute acid, and heated. The wax is then to be separated, dried between folds of blotting-paper, and treated as above for stearic acid. (*Neues Repert. für Pharm.*, viii. 78.) For the detection of rosin cold alcohol is sufficient. It dissolves the rosin, and yields it on evaporation, attended with a very small portion of pure wax, which yields 2·4 per cent. to cold alcohol. (Ed. Davies, *A. J. P.*, 1870, p. 537.) F. Jean states that a few drops of sulphuric acid added to the melted wax, adulterated with rosin, cause a red color, or, if only 1 per cent. be present, a greenish tint. (*A. J. P.*, 1881, p. 307.) To detect *paraffin*, which is another adulteration said to be frequent, Prof. Landolt, of Bonn, heats the wax with fuming sulphuric acid (*Nordhausen*), which destroys the wax, converting it into a black jelly-like mass, while the paraffin is left as a transparent layer on the surface. (See *A. J. P.*, xxxiv. 35.) M. Lies Bodart detects the same impurity by a somewhat complex process, based on the etherification of the wax; the paraffin being left sufficiently pure to enable its proportion to be estimated. For the particulars of the process, the reader is referred to the *Journ. de Pharm. et de Chim.* (4e sér., iii. 287, 1866). A simpler method is that of M. Dullo, who treats the adulterated wax with ether. If this dissolves more than 50 per cent., the presence of paraffin is indicated. M. Payen resorts to the point of fusion as a means of detecting paraffin. This substance melts at a lower temperature than wax, and lowers the melting point of wax with which it is mixed. (*Ibid.*, 4e sér., ii. 233.) White wax should not melt below 65·5° C. (150° F.); yellow not below 60° C. (140° F.). (*Br.*) *Japan wax* is said also to be largely employed for adulterating beeswax; so that sometimes but little of the product of the bee is to be found in the mixture. To detect Japan wax, M. Dullo boils together for a minute 10 Gm. (150 grains) of wax, 120 Gm. of water, and 1 of soda. If there be Japan wax present, a soap will immediately form, which will slowly solidify on cooling. Beeswax does not saponify under these circumstances. (*Ibid.*, 4e sér., i. 448.) Ceresin, a principle obtained from ozokerit (see Part II.), is also employed as an adulterant, and is manufactured largely for that purpose in Vienna. It is only native paraffin, and of course answers to the tests for that substance. There are other less precise methods of detecting adulterations. Thus, spermaceti and lard render wax softer and less cohesive, of a smoother and less granular fracture, and of a different odor when heated. The melting point and specific gravity are lowered by tallow, suet, and lard. Legrip's cereometer is based upon the altered specific gravity of wax when adulterated. Any one may apply this principle by making such a mixture of alcohol and water that pure wax will neither sink nor rise in it, but remain wherever placed. (See page 391.) Adulterated wax would either swim or sink in this liquid. Pereira says that pure wax is yellowish white; and that the white wax in circular cakes always contains spermaceti, added to improve its color.

Medical Properties and Uses. Wax has little effect upon the system. Under the impression that it sheathes the inflamed mucous membrane of the bowels, it was formerly prescribed in diarrhœa and dysentery; and it is mentioned by Dioscorides as a remedy in the latter complaint; but at the present time, we suppose, no one would think of employing wax for such purposes. Its sole use in modern medicine is in the formation of ointments, cerates, plasters, and suppositories, surgical dressings, etc., in which it acts mechanically, either giving stiffness or serving to protect from water. It is an ingredient in almost all the officinal cerates, which owe to it their general title.

3. VEGETABLE WAX. Many vegetable products contain wax. It exists in the pollen of numerous plants, and forms the bloom or glaucous powder which covers certain fruits, and the coating of varnish with which leaves are sometimes supplied. In some plants it is so abundant as to be profitably extracted for use. Such is the *Ceroxylon Andicola*, a lofty palm growing in the South American Andes. Upon the trunk of this tree, in the rings left by the fall of the leaves, is a coating of wax-like matter, about one-sixth of an inch thick, which is removed by the natives, and employed in the manufacture of tapers. It contains, according to Vauquelin, two-thirds of a resinous substance, and one-third of pure wax. Two kinds of wax are collected

in Brazil, one called *carnauba*,* from the leaves of the *Copernicus cerifera*, a palm, which forms large forests in the province of Ceara, the other *ocuba*, from the fruit of a shrub of the province of Para. (*Journ. de Pharm.*, 3e sér., v. 154.)† A form of vegetable wax sometimes seen in this country is that derived from *Myrica cerifera*, and commonly called *myrtle wax*. The *wax myrtle* is an aromatic shrub, from one to twelve feet high, growing in the United States, from New England to Louisiana, and flourishing especially on the sea-coast. The fruit, which grows in clusters closely attached to the stems and branches, is small, globular, and covered with a whitish coat of wax, which may be separated for use. Other parts of the plant are said to possess medical virtues. The bark of the root is acrid and astringent, and in large doses emetic, and has been popularly employed in jaundice. The process for collecting the wax is simple. The berries are boiled in water, and the wax, melting and floating on the surface, is either skimmed off and strained, or allowed to concrete as the liquor cools, and then removed. To render it pure, it is again melted and strained, and cast into large cakes. It is collected in New Jersey, North Carolina, and New England, and particularly in Rhode Island.

Myrtle wax is of a pale grayish green color, somewhat diaphanous, more brittle and unctuous to the touch than beeswax, of a feeble odor, and a slightly bitterish taste. It is about as heavy as water, and melts, according to Dr. G. E. Moore, at from 46·6° C.–48·8° C. (116° F.–120° F.). It is insoluble in water, scarcely soluble in cold alcohol, soluble, excepting about 13 per cent., in twenty parts of boiling alcohol, which deposits the greater portion on cooling, soluble also in boiling ether, and slightly so in oil of turpentine. It is readily saponifiable with the alkalies. By Dr. John it was found to consist, like beeswax, of cerin and myricin, containing 87 per cent. of the former and 13 of the latter; but a more accurate analysis by Dr. Moore gives as its constituents one part of palmitin and four of palmitic acid, with a

* *Carnauba Wax* is collected by cutting out the leaf buds, drying and beating them, and melting the powder thus detached in water. According to Nevil Story Maskelyne, it consists chiefly of melissyl-alcohol, $C_{30}H_{62}O$, which saponifies, another alcohol, $C_{25}H_{48}O$, and small quantities of resin and a substance melting at 150° C. (221° F.). Berard believes it to be composed of free cerotic acid and melissyl ether. It is hard, brittle, and buff-colored, yellow, or greenish, resembling the resins more than wax, and melts at 89° C. (192° F.), which is much higher than the fusing point of other kinds of vegetable wax. "It takes a fine polish when rubbed with any soft material," does not receive impressions from the finger at the natural temperature of the hand, and is adapted for polishing furniture, either alone or mixed with wax. 2,000,000 pounds of it are said to be annually produced in Brazil, where it is largely used, mixed with tallow, in making candles, etc.

Under the name of *Ocotilla wax*, Miss H. C. De S. Abbott has described (*A. J. P.*, Feb. 1885) a wax which she has obtained from the bark of the *Fouquieria splendens*, and believes to be a new variety. A wax which is said to be used, under the name of *Arbol de la Cera*, in Mexico not only for domestic purposes, but also as a remedy in diarrhœa and jaundice, is that obtained by boiling the fruit of the *Myrica jalapensis* in water. It is greenish or yellow, more brittle and unctuous than bees' wax, has a feeble odor, a slightly bitter taste, and a density nearly equal to that of water, and melts at 43°; but on exposure the fusing point rises to 47·5°. It is wholly soluble in boiling ether, insoluble in water, sparingly soluble in cold alcohol, and dissolves in twenty parts of boiling alcohol, depositing the greater part on cooling; alkalies saponify it readily. (*A. J. P.*, xv. 339, 1885.)

† *Japan Wax.* A substance under this name has been imported into Europe in considerable quantities, either directly from Japan, or through the Chinese ports. It is obtained from the berries of the *Rhus Succedaneum* of Linnæus, and in small amount from the *R. Sylvestris* and *R. Vernicifera*, or lacquer plant. The partially dried berries are crushed, winnowed, steamed, placed in hemp cloth bags, steamed again, and pressed in a wooden wedge press. They yield about 15 per cent. of a coarse greenish tallowy mass. It has come in two forms, the one, as originally distinguished by Mr. Hanbury, of circular cakes, about four inches in diameter, and an inch thick, flat on one side and somewhat convex on the other; the second, as brought directly from Japan, of large rectangular blocks, which are packed in chests. It bears a considerable resemblance to purified beeswax, but is not quite so white, having a slightly yellowish tint, is softer, more friable, and has a somewhat rancid smell and taste. Its melting point is below that of wax, varying from 49° C. (120° F.), as stated by Prof. Procter, to 52° C. (125° F.), and even 55° C. (131° F.), as observed in different specimens by Mr. Hanbury. Meyer noticed a sample melting at 42° C. (107° F.). It is much more soluble in alcohol than is beeswax, is saponifiable with the alkalies, and is said to contain palmitic acid. It has been employed in the preparation of candles, which yield as brilliant light as those made of common wax. It has been found useful in the preparation of cerates, etc.

From Roucher's experiments it appears that there are two melting points of this wax, one corresponding closely with Prof. Procter's results, while the same wax rapidly heated to a point above that of fusion and then allowed to cool, if plunged into water at 42° C., melts into a transparent liquid; consequently melting at a point 12° C. below its freezing point in its ordinary state, which was 54° C.; the two temperatures being about equivalent in Fahrenheit's scale to 107° and 129°. (*P. J. Tr.*, Aug. 1872, p. 122.)

little laurin or lauric acid. (*Am. Journ. of Sci. and Arts*, 1852, p. 319.) The green color and bitterness depend upon distinct principles, which may be separated by boiling with ether. On cooling, the wax is deposited colorless, while the ether remains green. The color is ascribed by Dr. Moore to chlorophyll.

Medical Properties and Uses. This variety of wax has been popularly employed in the United States as a remedy for dysentery; and we are told by Dr. Fahnestock that he found great advantage from its use in numerous cases during an epidemic prevalence of that complaint. He gave the powdered wax in doses of a teaspoonful (3·75 C.c.) frequently repeated, mixed with mucilage or syrup. (*Am. Journ. of Med. Sci.*, ii. 313.) It is occasionally substituted by apothecaries for beeswax in the formation of plasters, and is used in the preparation of tapers and candles. It is somewhat fragrant when burning, but emits a less brilliant light than common lamp oil.

Off. Prep. of White Wax. Ceratum; Ceratum Cetacei; Charta Cantharidis; Unguentum Aquæ Rosæ.

Off. Prep. Br. Charta Epispastica; Unguentum Cetacei; Unguentum Simplex.

Off. Prep. of Yellow Wax. Ceratum Cantharidis; Ceratum Extracti Cantharidis; Ceratum Resinæ; Emplastrum Asafœtidæ; Emplastrum Picis Burgundicæ; Emplastrum Picis Canadensis; Emplastrum Resinæ; Unguentum; Unguentum Mezerei.

Off Prep. Br. Cera Alba; Emplastrum Calefaciens; Emplastrum Cantharidis; Emplastrum Galbani; Emplastrum Picis; Emplastrum Saponis Fuscum; Pilula Phosphori; Unguentum Cantharidis; Unguentum Hydrargyri Compositum; Unguentum Picis Liquidæ; Unguentum Resinæ; Unguentum Sabinæ; Unguentum Terebinthinæ.

CERATA. *Cerates.*

(CE-RĀ'TA.)

Cérats, Cérèotés, *Fr.;* Cerate, Wachssalben, *G.*

These are unctuous substances consisting of oil or lard, mixed with wax, spermaceti, or resin, to which various medicaments are frequently added. Their consistence, which is intermediate between that of ointments and of plasters, is such that they may be spread at ordinary temperatures upon linen or leather, by means of a spatula, and do not melt or run when applied to the skin. In preparing them, care should usually be taken to select the oil or lard perfectly free from rancidity. In reference to the wax, too, there would seem to be a choice, as experience has shown that cerates made with yellow wax keep longer unchanged than those made with white or bleached wax, probably because there is in yellow wax some principle which corrects the tendency of fatty matters to become rancid. (F. Bringhurst, *A. J. P.*, 1869, p. 59.) The liquefaction should be effected by a very gentle heat, which may be applied by means of a water-bath; and during the refrigeration the mixture should be well stirred, and the portions which solidify on the sides of the vessel should be made to mix again with the liquid portion, until the whole assumes the proper consistence, or, as some prefer, the melted cerate is allowed to cool quickly without stirring. When a large quantity is prepared, the mortar or other vessel into which the mixture may be poured for cooling, should be previously heated by means of boiling water. It has been proposed to substitute paraffin for wax in the preparation of the cerates, but the great tendency to produce granulations in the finished cerate has largely prevented its use. It is, we think, unfortunate that this class of preparations has been abandoned in the British Pharmacopœia; the several cerates having been rejected, or transferred to the class of Ointments. Independently of the connection between the name and one of the characteristic constituents of the cerates, there is a ground of difference between them and the ointments in their consistence; that of the cerates being such as to render them especially suitable for spreading on linen, while that of ointments is peculiarly adapted to innunction.*

* Dr. W. H. Mielcke (*Pharm. Centralb.*, 1881, Nos. 20, 21) proposes a new class of preparations, to which he has given the name "*Steatins,*" "*Steatinum.*" These are about the consistence of cerates, of varied composition, and contain usually a considerable portion of tallow. The *Steatinum Iodoformi* offers a fair specimen of the class. "Take of mutton tallow 18 parts, expressed oil of nutmeg 2 parts, iodoform, in fine powder, 1 part. Melt the tallow and add the other ingredients." For other formulas, see *A. J. P.*, 1881, p. 404.

CERATUM. *U. S.* *Cerate.*

(CE-RĀ'TŬM.)

Ceratum Adipis, *U. S.* 1860; Ceratum Simplex, *U. S.* 1850; Cérat simple, *Fr.;* Einfaches Cerat, Wachssalbe, *G.*

"White Wax, *thirty parts* [or three ounces av.]; Lard, *seventy parts* [or seven ounces av.], To make *one hundred parts* [or ten ounces av.]. Melt them together, and stir the mixture constantly until cool." *U. S.*

Cerate, or, as it is usually called, *simple cerate*, has been changed very slightly in the last revision; the proportion of wax has been slightly decreased; formerly it was 33·3 per cent., it is now 30 per cent. This change will be regarded by many as an improvement. In the preparation of this cerate, peculiar care should be taken that the oleaginous ingredient be entirely free from rancidity, and that the heat employed be not sufficient to produce the slightest decomposition; for the value of the preparation depends on its perfect blandness. To avoid change, it should be put up in small jars, and covered closely with tin foil so as to exclude the air. It is used for dressing blisters, wounds, etc., in all cases in which the object is to prevent the contact of air and preserve the moisture of the part, and at the same time to avoid all irritation. It is sometimes improperly employed as the vehicle of substances to be applied by inunction. For this purpose lard should be used in winter, and simple ointment in summer; the cerate having too firm a consistence. George W. Sloan recommends simple cerate as a pill excipient for certain oxidizable substances and special uses. (*Proc. A. P. A.*, 1884.)

The simple ointment, Unguentum Simplex, of the British Pharmacopœia is very nearly equivalent to this preparation, but contains some olive oil. It will be described among the ointments.

CERATUM CAMPHORÆ. *U. S.* *Camphor Cerate.*

(CE-RĀ'TŬM CĂM'PHO-RÆ.)

"Camphor Liniment, *three parts* [or fifteen minims]; Olive Oil, *twelve parts* [or one fluidrachm]; Cerate, *eighty-five parts* [or four hundred grains], To make *one hundred parts* [or about one ounce]. Mix the Camphor Liniment and the Olive Oil, and incorporate with the Cerate." *U. S.*

This is a new officinal preparation; it was introduced primarily for use in making cerate of subacetate of lead by the extemporaneous process. It will no doubt be found useful for its own sake as a slightly stimulating dressing. If a stronger cerate is needed, sixty grains of camphor may be melted by as low heat as possible with one ounce of cerate and stirred until cold.

CERATUM CANTHARIDIS. *U. S.* *Cantharides Cerate.* *Blistering Cerate.*

(CE-RĀ'TŬM CAN-THĂR'I-DĬS.)

Emplastrum Cantharidis, *Br.;* Cantharides Plaster; Emplastrum Cantharidum (Vesicatorium) Ordinarium, *P.G.;* Emplastrum Epispasticum, s. Vesicatorium, s. Vesicans; Emplâtre de Cantharides, Emplâtre vésicatoire, *Fr.;* Spanischfliegen Pflaster, Blasenpflaster, *G.*

"Cantharides, in No. 60 powder, *thirty-five parts* [or seven ounces av.]; Yellow Wax, *twenty parts* [or four ounces av.]; Resin, *twenty parts* [or four ounces av.]; Lard, *twenty-five parts* [or five ounces av.], To make *one hundred parts* [or twenty ounces av.]. To the Wax, Resin, and Lard, previously melted together and strained through muslin, add the Cantharides, and, by means of a water-bath, keep the mixture in a liquid state, for half an hour, stirring occasionally. Then remove it from the water-bath, and stir constantly until cool." *U. S.*

The British Pharmacopœia directs of Cantharides, in powder, *twelve ounces* [avoirdupois]; Yellow Wax, and Prepared Suet, each, *seven ounces and a half;* Prepared Lard *six ounces;* and Resin *three ounces;* melts the Wax, Suet, and Lard together, by a water-bath, and adds the Resin previously melted; then introduces the Cantharides, mixes the whole thoroughly, and continues to stir the mixture while cooling.

This is the common well-known *blistering plaster*. As it can be readily spread without the aid of heat, it is properly a cerate, and is, therefore, correctly named in the U. S. Pharmacopœia. The process now officinal differs but slightly from that of the U. S. P. 1870. The quantity of lard is about 4 per cent. less, thus making the cerate a trifle stronger. It is essentially the same as prepared by the two processes; though the U. S. formula has a decided advantage over the British, in keeping the mixture of the flies and the other ingredients for some time at an elevated temperature, while in the latter they are allowed to cool after being mixed with the fatty matters. Care was formerly considered requisite, in making the cerate, not to injure the flies by heat. It was, therefore, recommended that they should not be added to the other ingredients until immediately before these begin to stiffen, after having been removed from the fire; and, though this direction has been omitted, no provision is made for the continued application of heat. From the experiments of Mr. Donovan (*Dublin Med. Press*, Aug. 1840), and those of Professor Procter (*A. J. P.*, xiii. 302, and xxiv. 296), it may be inferred that the vesicating principle of Spanish flies is not injured or dissipated by a heat under 148·8° C. (300° F.), and that an elevated temperature, instead of being hurtful, is positively advantageous in the preparation of the cerate. The cantharidin is thus more thoroughly dissolved by the oleaginous matter, and consequently brought more efficiently into contact with the skin, than when retained in the interior of the tissue of the fly. Another advantage, stated by Donovan, is that the moisture, usually existing to a certain extent in all the ingredients of the cerate, is thus dissipated, and the preparation is less apt to become mouldy, or otherwise to undergo decomposition. Instead, therefore, of waiting until the melted wax, resin, and lard begin to stiffen, it is better to add the powder before the vessel is removed from the fire. Mr. Donovan recommends that, as soon as the other ingredients are melted, the powdered flies should be added, and the mixture stirred until the heat is shown by a thermometer to have risen to 121·1° C. (250° F.), when the vessel is to be removed from the fire, and the mixture stirred constantly until cool. At the heat mentioned, ebullition takes place in consequence of the escape of the moisture contained in the materials. In the cerate thus prepared, the active matter has been dissolved by the lard, and the powder may be separated, if deemed advisable, by straining the mixture before it solidifies. Care should be taken that the temperature be not so high as to decompose the ingredients; and it would be better to keep it within 100° C. (212° F.), by means of a water-bath, as in the U. S. process, than to incur any risk from its excess. Violent irritation and even vesication of the face of the operator are stated to have resulted from exposure to the vapors of the liquid, at a temperature of 121·1° C. (250° F.). (*P. J. Tr.*, ii. 391.) From an experiment, however, of Professor Procter, it appears that, though cantharidin begins to volatilize slightly at 121·1° C. (250° F.), and rapidly rises in vapor and sublimes at from 205·5° C. to 211·1° C. (402° F. to 412° F.), yet it is not decomposed unless by increasing the heat considerably above the last-mentioned point. (*A. J. P.*, xxiv. 296 and 298.) It is desirable that the flies should be very finely pulverized. Coarsely-powdered cantharides should not be used, because of the imperfect and unequal distribution of the vesicating agent. Powdered euphorbium is said to be sometimes fraudulently added.

The cerate will always raise a blister in ordinary conditions of the system, if the flies are good, and not injured in the preparation. It should be spread on soft leather, though linen or even paper will answer the purpose when that is not to be had. An elegant mode of preparing it for use is to spread a piece of leather, of a proper size, first with adhesive plaster, and afterwards with the cerate, leaving a margin of the former uncovered, in order that it may adhere to the skin. Heat is not requisite, and should not be employed in spreading the cerate. Some sprinkle powdered flies upon the surface of the plaster, press them lightly with a roller, and then shake off the portion which has not adhered; but, if the flies originally employed were good, this addition is superfluous. The habit of applying over the surface with a brush an ethereal tincture of cantharides, which leaves a thin coating of extract, renders the preparation more certain.

Upon the application of the plaster, the skin should be moistened with warm vinegar or other liquid. In adults, when the full action of the flies is desired, and the object is to produce a permanent effect, the application should be continued for eight hours, and on the scalp for twelve hours. In very delicate persons, however, or those subject to strangury, or upon parts of a loose texture, or when the object is merely to produce a blister to be healed as quickly as possible, the plaster should remain no longer than is necessary for the production of full redness of the skin, which generally occurs in five or six hours, or even in a shorter time. It should then be removed, and followed by a flaxseed poultice, or some other emollient dressing, under which the cuticle rises, and a full blister is usually produced. By this management the patient will generally escape strangury, and the blister will very quickly heal after the discharge of the serum.* In young children, cantharides sometimes produce alarming and even fatal ulceration, if too long applied, and from two to four hours are usually sufficient for any desirable purpose. When the head, or other very hairy part, is to be blistered, an interval of ten or twelve hours should, if possible, be allowed between the shaving of the part and the application of the plaster; so that the abrasions may heal, and some impediment be offered to the absorption of the flies. After the blister has been formed, it should be opened at the most depending parts, and, the cuticle being allowed to remain, should be dressed with simple cerate; but, if it be desirable to maintain the discharge for a short time, resin cerate should be used, and the cuticle removed if it can be done without inconvenience. When it is wished that the blistered surface should heal as soon as possible, and with the least inconvenience to the patient, Dr. Maclagan recommends a dressing of cotton wadding; an emollient poultice being first applied for two hours after the removal of the blistering cerate, the cuticle then cut, and the surface afterwards covered with the cotton, with its raw surface next the skin. Should the dressing become soaked, so much of the cotton may be removed as can be done without disturbing the cuticle, and a new batch applied. The cotton is to be allowed to remain until the old cuticle spontaneously separates. The simple application of Goulard's cerate seems to us, however, preferable to the method of Dr. Maclagan. The effects of an issue may be obtained by employing savine ointment, or the ointment of Spanish flies, as a dressing. If much inflammation take place in the blistered surface, it may be relieved by emollient poultices, weak lead-water, or Goulard's cerate. When there is an obstinate indisposition to heal, we have found nothing so effectual as zinc ointment with two to four grains of carbolic acid to the ounce.

Various preparations of cantharides have been proposed and employed as substitutes for the cerate. They consist for the most part of cantharidin, more or less pure, either dissolved in olive oil and applied to the skin by means of a piece of paper saturated with it, or incorporated with wax and spread in a very thin layer upon fine waxed cloth, silk, or paper, constituting the *blistering cloth*, *blistering paper*, *vesicating taffetas*, etc., of the shops. The advantages of these preparations are that they occupy less space, are more portable, and, being very pliable, are more easily adapted to irregularities of the surface. Absolutely pure cantharidin is expensive and not requisite;† as extracts of cantharides, made with ether, alcohol, or boiling water, will answer every purpose. Henry and Guibourt give the following formula. Digest powdered cantharides in ether, distil off the ether, evaporate the residue by means of a salt-water bath, until ebullition ceases, melt the mass which remains with twice its

* The late Dr. M. B. Smith, of Philadelphia, informed us that he had frequently employed uva ursi, as a preventive of strangury from blisters, and had never found it to fail. He gave a small wineglassful of the officinal decoction (see *Decoctum Uvæ Ursi*) every hour, commencing two hours after the application of the blister. Camphor is sometimes incorporated with the blistering cerate to prevent strangury, though with doubtful effect. A plan proposed by M. Vée is to spread over the surface of the plaster, when ready for delivery, by means of the finger, a saturated solution of camphor in ether. The ether evaporates, leaving a thin coating of camphor uniformly diffused. (*Journ. de Pharm.*, 3e sér., viii. 68.) Guyot Dannecy believes camphor to be useless in this connection, and recommends dusting the blister with bicarbonate of sodium and powdered cantharides in equal parts. The late Dr. Joseph Hartshorne, of Philadelphia, was in the habit, in cases where he apprehended strangury, of directing four grains of opium and twenty of camphor to be mixed with the cerate of a blister of large size, and experienced the happiest effects from the addition.

† Dragendorff (*A. J. P.* 1872, p. 273) recommends *cantharidate of sodium*. M. E. Delpech (*A. J. P.*, xlii. 240) proposes the use of *cantharidate of potassium* in substance or solution. He prepares it by dissolving two parts of cantharides in 150 parts of alcohol, and adding 1-6 parts of caustic potash dissolved in a very little water. The whole becomes a crystalline mass from which the alcohol may be separated by pressure. See also R. Rother, *Chicago Pharmacist*, Nov. 1872.

weight of wax, and spread the mixture upon waxed cloth. The *waxed cloth* may be prepared by spreading upon linen or muslin a mixture composed of 8 parts of white wax, 4 of olive oil, and 1 of turpentine, melted together. An extract of cantharides of a buttery consistence, said to act very efficiently when applied by means of paper greased with it, is prepared by digesting 4 parts of flies with one part of strong acetic acid, and 16 of alcohol, straining, filtering, and evaporating at a moderate heat. A preparation which received the favorable report of a committee of the Society of Pharmacy, at Paris, is the following, proposed by M. Dubuison. Four parts of a hydro-alcoholic extract of the flies, made by maceration, are mixed with an aqueous solution of one part of pure gelatin, so as to obtain a solution of suitable consistence, which is then applied upon a piece of extended waxed cloth, care being taken that the brush should always have the same direction. When the first layer has dried, a second and a third are to be applied in the same manner. The gelatin renders the cloth more adhesive and less deliquescent. The hydro-alcoholic extract is preferred to the alcoholic, because it contains less of the green oil, which does not readily mix with the other ingredients. The committee, however, preferred the aqueous extract, as cheaper and more active. This taffeta has been tried, and found to raise blisters in four hours. (*Journ. de Pharm.*, 3e sér., viii. 67.) For very speedy vesication, an infusion of the flies in strong acetic acid is sometimes employed. None of these preparations are likely to supersede the cerate, but the demand for them has been met by introducing into the Pharmacopœia the Charta Cantharidis and the Collodium cum Cantharide.

Off. Prep. Emplastrum Picis cum Cantharide, *U. S.*

CERATUM CETACEI. *U. S.* *Spermaceti Cerate.*

(CE-RĀ'TŬM CE-TĀ'CE-Ī.)

Emplastrum Spermatis Ceti, Ceratum Labiale Album; Cérat de Blanc de Baleine, Onguent blanc, *Fr.;* Wallrath-Cerat, *G.*

"Spermaceti, *ten parts* [or one ounce av.]; White Wax, *thirty-five parts* [or three and a half ounces av.]; Olive Oil, *fifty-five parts* [or five and a half ounces av.], To make *one hundred parts* [or ten ounces av.]. Melt together the Spermaceti and Wax; then add the Olive Oil, previously heated, and stir the mixture constantly until cool." *U. S.*

The direction to heat the oil before adding it to the other ingredients is important. If added cold, it is apt to produce an irregular congelation of the wax and spermaceti, and thus to render the preparation lumpy. The cerate is employed as a dressing for blisters, excoriated surfaces, and wounds, and as the basis of more active preparations. When the ingredients are pure and sweet, it is perfectly free from irritating properties. The present formula contains a little less spermaceti than that of U. S. P. 1870. From experiments made by Mr. J. B. Barnes, it appears that this cerate keeps much better when made of unbleached materials, than when prepared with olive oil and wax previously bleached. (*P. J. Tr.*, 1861, p. 352.)

CERATUM EXTRACTI CANTHARIDIS. *U. S.* *Cerate of Extract of Cantharides.*

(CE-RĀ'TŬM EX-TRĂC'TĪ CAN-THĂR'I-DĬS.)

Cérat d'Extrait de Cantharides, *Fr.;* Cantharidenextract-Cerat, *G.*

"Cantharides, in No. 60 powder, *thirty parts* [or six ounces av.]; Resin, *fifteen parts* [or three ounces av.]; Yellow Wax, *thirty-five parts* [or seven ounces av.]; Lard, *thirty-five parts* [or seven ounces av.]; Alcohol, *a sufficient quantity*. Moisten the Cantharides with *eighteen parts* [or four fluidounces] of Alcohol, and pack firmly in a cylindrical percolator; then gradually pour on Alcohol, until *one hundred and eighty parts* [or two and a half pints] of percolate are obtained, or until the Cantharides are exhausted. Distil off the Alcohol by means of a water-bath, transfer the residue to a tared capsule and evaporate it, on a water-bath, until it weighs *fifteen parts* [or three ounces av.]. Add to this the Resin, Wax, and Lard, previously melted together, and keep the whole at a temperature of 100° C. (212° F.) for fifteen minutes. Lastly, strain the mixture through muslin, and stir it constantly until cool." *U. S.*

This preparation of the Pharmacopœia of 1860, adopted from a formula of Mr. Wm. R. Warner, published in the *A. J. P.*, 1860, p. 11, was intended as a substitute for the old Ceratum Cantharidis, from which it differs mainly in containing an alcoholic extract of the flies instead of the flies themselves. If the percolation be well conducted, so as to exhaust the cantharides, of which the active matter is soluble in alcohol, this cerate ought theoretically to be more effective than the old blistering cerate; as the active principles are separated from the inert matter of the flies which envelops them in the natural state, and must in some measure interfere with their action; and it is said that its superior efficacy has been practically ascertained. It is to be used in the same manner as the cerate of cantharides.

CERATUM PLUMBI SUBACETATIS. *U.S.* *Cerate of Subacetate of Lead.* [*Goulard's Cerate.*]

(CĘ-RĀ'TŬM PLŬM'BĪ SŬB-ĂÇ-Ę-TĀ'TĬS.)

Unguentum Glycerini Plumbi Subacetatis, *Br.;* Unguentum Plumbi Subacetatis Compositum; Compound Ointment of Subacetate of Lead; Unguentum Plumbi, *P.G.;* Ceratum cum Subacetate Plumbico; Cérat de Saturne, Saturné de Goulard, *Fr.;* Bleisalbe, Bleicerat, *G.*

"Solution of Subacetate of Lead, *twenty parts* [or one ounce av.]; Camphor Cerate, *eighty parts* [or four ounces av.], To make *one hundred parts* [or five ounces av.]. Mix them thoroughly. This Cerate should be freshly prepared, when wanted for use." *U.S.*

The British Pharmacopœia of 1867 takes *six fluidounces* of the Solution of Subacetate of Lead, *eight ounces* [avoirdupois] of White Wax, *a pint* [Imperial measure] of Oil of Almonds, and *sixty grains* of Camphor. The wax and four-fifths of the oil are melted by means of a water-bath, and the solution of subacetate of lead added gradually, stirring as the mixture cools; the camphor dissolved in the remaining fifth of the oil is then added, and the whole mixed thoroughly.

The process now officinal differs from that of U. S. P. 1870, experience having shown the futility of all expedients to prevent rancidity. The camphor cerate keeps well with care, but it can be readily made extemporaneously, and thus dispensed in a fresh, non-irritating condition. This plan was proposed by Prof. Remington, and adopted by the Pharmacopœia committee of the Philadelphia College of Pharmacy.

This cerate received the name by which it is commonly known from M. Goulard, by whom it was employed and recommended. It immediately begins to assume a yellowish color, and after a short time becomes so rancid as to be scarcely fit for use. Hence it should be prepared in small quantities at once. The addition of a few drops of acetic acid prevents the yellow color from remaining permanent. The late Mr. Jacob Bell found it more satisfactory when made with yellow wax. (*P. J. Tr.*, 1859, p. 459.) Eggenfels, a German pharmaceutist, recommends the following method of proceeding to prevent its change of color. The wax and oil are melted in a water-bath; the solution of subacetate of lead, previously heated, is added in small portions successively, and the mixture well stirred, and digested for some time; a partial saponification takes place, and an emulsion afterwards; and the cerate retains its white color. (See *A. J. P.*, 1861, p. 408.) It is used chiefly in excoriations, burns, scalds, and chilblains, and in cutaneous eruptions. Wherever there is an acute active inflammation of the skin it is a most efficient remedy.

CERATUM RESINÆ. *U.S.* *Resin Cerate.* [*Basilicon Ointment.*]

(CĘ-RĀ'TŬM RĘ-ȘĪ'NÆ.)

Unguentum Resinæ, *Br.;* Ointment of Resin, Unguentum Basilicum; Cérat de Résine anglais, *Fr.;* Harzcerat, *G.*

"Resin, *thirty-five parts* [or seven ounces av.]; Yellow Wax, *fifteen parts* [or three ounces av.]; Lard, *fifty parts* [or ten ounces av.], To make *one hundred parts* [or twenty ounces av.]. Melt them together at a moderate heat, strain the mixture through muslin, and allow it to cool without stirring." *U. S.*

"Take of Resin, in coarse powder, *eight ounces;* Yellow Wax *four ounces;* Simple Ointment *sixteen ounces.* Melt with a gentle heat, strain the mixture while hot through flannel, and stir constantly while it cools." *Br.*

This preparation does not differ greatly from that formerly officinal; it contains now about 1 per cent. less wax, and 6 per cent. less lard. An improvement has been made in the manipulation, however, in directing the ointment not to be stirred, a better consistence being secured by this change. The straining is directed in consequence of the impurities which resin often contains. Resin cerate, commonly called *basilicon ointment*, is much used as a gently stimulant application to blistered surfaces, indolent ulcers, burns, scalds, and chilblains. We have found no application more effectual in disposing the ulcers which follow burns, to heal.*

Off. Prep. Ceratum Sabinæ; Linimentum Terebinthinæ.

Off. Prep. Br. Linimentum Terebinthinæ.

CERATUM SABINÆ. *U. S.* *Savine Cerate.*

(CĒ-RĀ′TŬM SA-BĪ′NÆ.)

Unguentum Sabinæ, *Br.;* Ointment of Savine, Unguentum Sabinæ, *P.G.;* Cérat de Sabine, *Fr.;* Sadebaum Salbe, *G.*

"Fluid Extract of Savine, *twenty-five parts* [or five ounces av.]; Resin Cerate, *ninety parts* [or eighteen ounces av.]. Melt the Resin Cerate by means of a water-bath, add the Fluid Extract of Savine, and continue the heat until the alcohol has evaporated; then remove the heat, and stir constantly until cool." *U. S.*

"Take of Fresh Savine Tops, bruised, *eight ounces;* White Wax *three ounces;* Prepared Lard *sixteen ounces.* Melt the Lard and Wax together on a water-bath, add the Savine, and digest for twenty minutes. Then remove the mixture, and express through calico." *Br.* The U.S. preparation is identical with that formerly officinal.

As the savine used in this country is generally brought from Europe in the dried state, we are compelled to resort to a mode of preparing the cerate different from that usually employed in Europe. In the Pharmacopœia of 1850, the dried savine was simply mixed, in powder, with resin cerate previously softened; and the proportion used was one part of the powder to six parts of the cerate. Nor did we find the preparation thus made to be "intolerably acrid and almost caustic," as Dr. Duncan described it. On the contrary, it answered very well the purpose for which it was used, that of maintaining the discharge from blistered surfaces. The process, however, of the present edition of the Pharmacopœia is certainly more elegant than the former, and probably, if the fluid extract has been carefully made, yields a more effective product. A cerate, prepared in the same manner as the former cerate, from the leaves of the red cedar (*Juniperus Virginiana*), is sometimes substituted for that of savine, but is less efficient. Prepared according to the process of the British Pharmacopœia, savine cerate has a fine deep green color, and the odor of the leaves. It should be kept in closely-covered vessels.

Savine cerate is preferable to the ointment of Spanish flies as a dressing for perpetual blisters, from the circumstance that it has no tendency to produce strangury. The white coating which forms, during its use, upon the blistered surface should be occasionally removed, as it prevents the contact of the cerate. It is sometimes applied to seton cords, to increase the discharge.

CEREVISIÆ FERMENTUM. *Br.* *Beer Yeast.*

(CĔR-Ē-VĬS′Ĭ-Æ FĔR-MĔN′TŬM.)

"The ferment obtained in brewing beer, and produced by Saccharomyces (Torula, *Turpin*) cerevisiæ, *Meyen.*" *Br.*

Fermentum, *U. S.* 1870; Levûre de Bière, Levûre, *Fr.;* Bierhefen, Oberhefe, *G.;* Fermento di Cervogia, *It.;* Espuma de Cerveza, *Sp.*

* *Ceratum Resinæ Compositum, U. S.* 1870. *Compound Resin Cerate.* Deshler's Salve; Cérat de résine composé, *Fr.* "Take of Resin, Suet, Yellow Wax, each, *twelve troyounces;* Turpentine *six troyounces;* Flaxseed Oil *seven troyounces.* Melt them together, strain the mixture through muslin, and stir it constantly until cool." *U. S.* 1870. This is somewhat more stimulating than the Ceratum Resinæ, but is applicable to similar purposes, particularly to the treatment of indolent ulcers. Under the name of *Deshler's salve,* it is popularly employed in some parts of the United States. It should be kept well protected from the air, in consequence of its liability when exposed to acquire a tough consistence. It was officinal in 1870, but was dropped at the last revision.

This is the substance which rises, in the form of froth, to the surface of beer, and subsides, during the process of fermentation. A similar substance is produced during the fermentation of other saccharine liquids.

It is flocculent, frothy, somewhat viscid, semifluid, of a dirty yellowish color, a sour vinous odor, and a bitter taste. At the temperature of 60° or 70° F., in a close vessel or damp atmosphere, it soon undergoes putrefaction. Exposed to a moderate heat it loses its liquid portion, becomes dry, hard, and brittle, and may in this state be preserved for a long time, though with the loss of much of its peculiar power. *Yeast cakes* are made by putting yeast into sacks, washing it with water, then submitting it to pressure, and ultimately drying it.

Yeast is insoluble in alcohol or water. Its ultimate composition, according to Schlossberger (*Ann. Chem. und Pharm.*, 51, p. 199), is carbon 49·9 per cent, hydrogen 6·6 per cent., nitrogen 12·1 per cent., and oxygen 31·4 per cent. Its proximate constituents are albuminoids, cellulose, fats, and resinous substances. Its bitterness is attributable to a principle derived from the hops. The property for which it is chiefly valued is that of exciting the vinous fermentation in saccharine liquids, and in various farinaceous substances. This property it owes to its nitrogenous ingredient; for, if separated from this, it loses its powers as a ferment, and reacquires them upon its subsequent addition. It is also rendered ineffective by strong alcohol, by several of the acids, as sulphuric and concentrated acetic acids, by various other substances, and by a heat of 212°. At a high temperature the yeast is decomposed, affording products similar to those which result from the decomposition of animal matters. From experiments by Mr. Horace T. Brown, it would appear that the degree of atmospheric pressure has much influence upon the progress of the alcoholic fermentation, which is considerably retarded by a diminution of that pressure. (*P. J. Tr.*, Jan. 1874, p. 615.)

Besides alcohol and carbonic acid, which are the characteristic products of the vinous fermentation, various other substances are generated in smaller or larger proportions. Pasteur has shown that while 94 to 95 per cent. of the sugar decomposes into ethyl alcohol and carbon dioxide, the other 5 or 6 per cent. decomposes by secondary reactions, yielding *glycerin*, 2·5 to 3·6 per cent., and *succinic acid*, 0·4 to 0·7 per cent. The higher homologues of ethyl alcohol are also produced in small amount, forming the fusel oil or the raw spirit.

The opacity of yeast is due to the presence of a microscopic fungus, first discovered in it by Leuwenhoek in 1680. As originally announced by Thénard in 1803, this yeast plant is the cause of the alcoholic fermentation. It consists of numerous cells, irregular, roundish, or cylindrical in shape, separate, joined into rows, or budding one from the other. During fermentation the yeast plant multiplies very rapidly: and when the fermentation is very active the plant rises to the surface, constituting the so-called *top yeast* of the brewer; when the process is restrained by cold the yeast settles and constitutes *bottom yeast*. Top and bottom yeast have a tendency to produce the form of fermentation by which they were developed. It is most probable that the yeast plant is the mycelium, or early vegetative stage, of more than one species of mucor or mould; and some authorities recognize various species of the yeast fungus. The name of *Torula*, or *Torula cerevisiæ*, was first given to the yeast plant, which was subsequently called *Mycoderma vini;* Dr. M. Reess, in his elaborate work (*Botan. Untersuch. Alkoholsgährungspilze*, Leipsic, 1870), makes a distinct genus of it, *Saccharomyces*, including many species.

There have been three theories in regard to fermentation: 1st, that it is a chemical process; 2d, that it is of galvanic origin; 3d, that it is the result of the vital actions of the yeast plant. The chemical theory founded by Trommsdorff and Meissner has been very ably advocated by Liebig, but, chiefly owing to the labors of Pasteur, the vital theory is now almost universally accepted.

Medical Properties. Yeast has been highly commended as a stimulant remedy in *typhoid*, *hectic*, and other similar fevers, but is at present very rarely used. In some of these cases it has been given with great asserted advantage in doses of a pint (472 C.c.) a day. It still continues to be employed to a considerable extent as a remedy against successive eruptions of boils, in doses of an ounce (30 C.c.) three times a day. Locally applied it is probably stimulant, although it may be the products of fermentation rather than the yeast which give the peculiar value to the "yeast poultice."

Off. Prep. Br. Cataplasma Fermenti.

CERII OXALAS. *U. S., Br.* *Oxalate of Cerium.*

$Ce_2(C_2O_4)_3 . 9H_2O$; 708. (CĒ′RI-Ī ŎX′Ą-LĂS.) $Ce_2O_3, 3C_2O_3 . 9HO$; 354.

"A salt which may be obtained as a precipitate by adding solution of oxalate of ammonia to a soluble salt of cerium." *Br.*

Cerium Oxalicum, Oxalas Ciricus; Oxalate de Cérium, *Fr.;* Oxalsaures Ceroxydal, Cerium Oxalat, *G.*

Cerium is a metal, which was discovered in 1803 by Berzelius and Hisinger, and about the same time by Klaproth, who, however, described it as an earth. By the two former chemists it was recognized as a metal, and named cerium in honor of the goddess Ceres. It was obtained from a Swedish mineral, formerly from its great weight called *heavy stone of Bastnas* (Bastnas Schwerstein), but now named *cerite*, after the metal extracted from it. Besides cerite, it has been found in several other minerals, as *gadolinite*, *orthite*, etc., in the north of Europe, a number of different minerals from Greenland, and *allanite* near Bethlehem, in Pennsylvania. It is not easy to obtain it pure in the metallic state, as its oxides and salts are difficult of reduction. Berzelius describes it as in the form of pulverulent masses, of a deep chocolate-brown, which exhibit, however, under the burnisher a metallic appearance, and a dark gray color. Hildebrand and Norton have since prepared it in large quantity by the electrolysis of its chloride. It is a bad conductor of electricity. Heated in the air it takes fire before the point of ignition, and burns vividly, passing to the state of peroxide. At ordinary temperatures it is oxidized in a moist atmosphere, giving out a strong and disagreeable smell of hydrogen. In water, especially when moderately heated, it rapidly oxidizes with the evolution of hydrogen, and the water does not become alkaline. There are two oxides of cerium hitherto considered as the protoxide and sesquioxide. (According to more recent investigators, cerium forms a sesquioxide and a dioxide only, so that cerous oxalate, which is the officinal salt, is an oxalate of the sesquioxide, a fact recognized in the Pharmacopœia of 1880.) Sulphur and phosphorus combine with it. Of its compounds two only have been introduced into medicine, the nitrate and oxalate, of which the latter was recognized for the first time officinally in the last edition of the British Pharmacopœia, and in the U. S. Pharmacopœia of 1870.

Oxalate of cerium may be obtained from cerite, and Prof. F. F. Mayer, of New York, gives a process for the purpose, of which the following is an outline.

The mineral consists of silicates of cerium, lanthanum, and didymium, with numerous other substances in smaller proportion, the oxide of cerium constituting about 39 per cent. of the whole. The powdered mineral is made into a paste with sulphuric acid, and then heated over a lamp until the mass ceases to swell up, and no longer absorbs sulphuric acid very cautiously added. Upon the cooling of the mass, it is powdered, and exposed in a crucible to the heat of an anthracite fire until it assumes a pale brownish red color. It is now lixiviated first with hot water and then with nitric acid, and the solution treated with sulphuretted hydrogen in order to get rid of various metals by precipitation. To the clear liquid some hydrochloric acid is first added, and then a solution of oxalic acid, the former of which holds in solution the oxalate of calcium produced, the latter throws down oxalates of cerium and other metals. The precipitate, having been washed with warm water, is formed into a paste with a quantity of carbonate of magnesium equal to half that of the mineral employed; and the paste is dried on porous fire brick, finely powdered, and calcined till it becomes of a cinnamon color. It now contains all of the cerium in the form of ceroso-ceric oxide. To separate this the mass is treated with an excess of nitric acid, the solution evaporated to get rid of the excess of acid, then diluted with warm water, and lastly poured into a vessel containing boiling water acidulated with a little more than half of one per cent. of sulphuric acid. A yellow precipitate of basic sulphate of cerium is formed, while a little of the neutral sulphate, and all the lanthanum and didymium, remain dissolved. The precipitate is now dissolved in stronger sulphuric acid, the solution digested with a few crystals of hyposulphite of sodium, in order to reduce the ceroso-ceric oxide of cerium to cerous oxide, and the liquid, having been filtered, is treated with solution of oxalic acid, which causes a precipitate of oxalate of cerium. This is washed with warm water, and dried. (*A. J. P.*, 1860, p. 4.)

Oxalate of cerium is "a white, slightly granular powder, permanent in the air, odorless and tasteless, insoluble in water or alcohol, but soluble in hydrochloric acid. On heating the salt to a dull red heat, a yellow or yellowish-red residue of oxide of cerium is left (a brown color would indicate the presence of oxide of didymium). On boiling the salt with solution of potassa, filtering, supersaturating a portion of the cold filtrate with acetic acid, and adding test-solution of chloride of calcium, a white precipitate is obtained, soluble in hydrochloric acid. The other portion of the filtrate should not yield a precipitate on the addition of an excess of test-solution of chloride of ammonium (aluminium), or of test-solution of sulphide of ammonium (zinc). On dissolving the salt in hydrochloric acid, no effervescence should occur (abs. of carbonate), and the solution should not be precipitated or rendered turbid by hydrosulphuric acid (abs. of metallic impurities)." *U. S.* As usually seen in commerce it has a pinkish tinge, due to the presence of a trace of a compound of didymium. The British Pharmacopœia states that "if the salt be boiled with solution of potash and filtered, the filtrate is not affected by solution of chloride of ammonium, but, when supersaturated with acetic acid, it gives with chloride of calcium a white precipitate, soluble in hydrochloric acid." When heated to dull redness it yields a reddish brown powder, which is wholly soluble without effervescence in boiling hydrochloric acid, and the resulting solution gives with solution of sulphate of potassium a white crystalline precipitate. *Br.*

Medical Properties. The oxalate of cerium is supposed to act in a manner very similar to the subnitrate of bismuth. It was originally brought forward by Sir James Y. Simpson as a remedy in the vomiting of pregnancy, and has been extensively used in this affection, and also in gastric disturbances of various diseases, such as phthisis, uterine disorder, hysteria, dyspepsia, pyrosis, etc. To a less extent it has been used in intestinal inflammatory diseases. Prof. Simpson also considered it to be a good nervine tonic, and used it with great asserted advantage in chorea. The dose is a grain (0·065 Gm.), doubled if necessary, and repeated three times a day, or more frequently if a return of the vomiting should seem to require it. It may be given in pill or suspended in water.

Nitrate of cerium has also been employed, though not officinal. The late Dr. Simpson believed it to act as a nervine tonic, and has seen it useful in chronic intestinal eruption, irritable dyspepsia with gastrodynia and pyrosis, and chronic vomiting generally, as well as in that of pregnancy. The dose is the same as that of the oxalate, though it would be prudent to begin with a smaller quantity, as, being a soluble salt, it might be more disposed to irritate in overdoses.

CETACEUM. *U. S., Br.* *Spermaceti.*

(CE-TĀ'CE-ŬM.)

"A peculiar, concrete, fatty substance, obtained from Physeter macrocephalus. Linné. (*Class*, Mammalia; *Order*, Cetacea.)" *U. S.* "A concrete fatty substance, obtained, mixed with oil, from the head of the Sperm Whale, Physeter macrocephalus. It is separated from the oil by filtration and pressure, and afterwards purified." *Br.*

Ambre blanc, Blanc de Baleine, Spermaceti, Cétine, *Fr.;* Wallrath, Spermacetis, *G.;* Spermaceti, *It.;* Esperma de Ballena, *Sp.*

The spermaceti whale is from sixty to eighty feet long, with an enormous head, not less in its largest part than thirty feet in circumference, and constituting one-third of the whole length of the body. The upper part of the head is occupied by large cavities, separated by cartilaginous partitions, and containing an oily liquid, which, after the death of the animal, concretes into a white spongy mass consisting of spermaceti mixed with oil. This mass is removed, and the oil allowed to separate by draining. The crude spermaceti, obtained from a whale of the ordinary size, is more than sufficient to fill twelve large barrels. It still contains much oil and other impurities, from which it is freed by expression, washing with hot water, melting, straining, and repeated washing with a weak boiling lye of potash. Common whale oil and the oil of other cetaceous animals contain small quantities of spermaceti, which they slowly deposit on standing.*

Spermaceti is in white, pearly, semitransparent masses; of a neutral reaction; of a crystalline foliaceous texture; friable, soft, and somewhat unctuous to the touch; slightly odorous; insipid; of the sp. gr. 0·943; fusible at 44·5° C. (112° F.) (*Bostock*), not under 38° C. (100° F.) (*Br.*); volatilisable at a high temperature without change, *in vacuo*, but partially decomposed if the air is admitted; inflammable; insoluble in water; soluble in small proportion in boiling alcohol, ether, and oil of turpentine, but deposited as the liquids cool; and in the fixed oils; not affected by the mineral acids, except sulphuric, which decomposes and dissolves it; rendered yellowish and rancid by long exposure to hot air, but capable of being again purified by washing with a warm lye of potash. "Sp. gr. about 0·945. It melts near 50° C. (122° F.), and congeals near 45° C. (113° F.). It is soluble in ether, chloroform,† disulphide of carbon, and in boiling alcohol; but slightly soluble in cold benzin." *U. S.* As found in the shops it is not chemically pure, containing a fixed oil, and often a peculiar coloring principle. From these it is separated by boiling in alcohol, which on cooling deposits it in crystalline scales. Thus purified, it does not melt under 49° C. (120° F.), is soluble in 40 parts of boiling alcohol of the sp. gr. 0·821 (*Thenard*), and is harder, more shining, and less unctuous than ordinary spermaceti.

Spermaceti is a mixture of various fats. When recrystallized from alcohol as just described, the purified *cetin* is obtained, while the alcohol on evaporation deposits an oil (mechanically admixed sperm oil), the *cetin-elaine* of Berzelius, which saponified yields *cetin-elaic acid*, an acid resembling but distinct from oleic acid. The cetin which crystallizes out of the alcohol is essentially *cetyl palmitate*, $C_{16}H_{33}(C_{16}H_{31}O_2)$,—that is, a compound of *cetyl alcohol* (*ethal of Chevreul*), $C_{16}H_{33}OH$. and *palmitic acid*, $C_{16}H_{32}O_2$. According to Heintz, however, there are small amounts of other fats with the cetin; fats containing the acids, *stearic*, $C_{18}H_{36}O_2$, *myristic*, $C_{14}H_{28}O_2$, and *lauro-stearic*, $C_{12}H_{24}O_2$, and the alcohol radicles corresponding to these acids.

Medical Properties and Uses. Spermaceti has been given as a demulcent in irritations of the mucous membranes; but it possesses no peculiar virtues, and its internal use has generally been abandoned. It may be reduced to powder by the addition of a little alcohol or almond oil, or administered in emulsion, conveniently made by mixing the spermaceti, first with half its weight of olive oil, then with powdered gum arabic, and lastly with water gradually added. It is an ingredient of many ointments and cerates.

Off. Prep. Ceratum Cetacei; Charta Cantharidis; Unguentum Aquæ Rosæ.

Off. Prep. Br. Charta Epispastica; Unguentum Cetacei.

CETRARIA. *U. S., Br.* *Cetraria.* [*Iceland Moss.*]

(CE-TRĀ'RI-A).

"Cetraria Islandica. Acharius. (*Nat. Ord.* Lichenes.)" *U. S.* "The dried lichen, Cetraria Islandica." *Br.*

Lichen Islandicus, *P.G.;* Mousse d'Islande, Lichen d'Islande, *Fr.;* Isländisches Moos, Isländische Flechte, Lungenmoos, *G.;* Lichene islandico, *It.;* Liquen islandico, *Sp.;* Iceland Lichen.

Gen. Ch. Plant cartilagino-membranous, ascending or spreading, lobed, smooth,

* According to W. Gilmour, *sperm oil* should contain not less than 4 per cent. of cetin, and if much less be obtained by the following process, adulteration has been practised. Shake one part by weight of sulphuric acid (sp. gr. 1·84) with four parts of the oil; allow to stand 20 minutes, shaking twice; add 3 ounces of distilled water; shake this thoroughly, and allow to stand 16 to 20 hours; dilute with 3 or 4 times its volume of distilled water; agitate thoroughly. On standing the cetin floats upon the top, and can readily be skimmed off, washed, dried, and weighed. (*P. J. Tr.*, vii. 328.)

† In consequence of its solubility in chloroform, stains made by dropping it on cloth may be quickly removed by that liquid.

and naked on both sides. *Apothecia* shield-like, obliquely adnate with the margin, the disk colored, plano-concave; border inflexed, derived from the frond. *Loudon's Encyc.*

Cetraria Islandica. Acharius, *Lichenog. Univ.* 512; *B. & T.* 302.—*Lichen Islandicus.* Woodv. *Med. Bot.* p. 803, t. 271. Iceland moss is foliaceous, erect, from two to four inches high, with a dry, coriaceous, smooth, shining, laciniated frond or leaf, the lobes of which are irregularly subdivided, channelled and fringed at their edges with rigid hairs. Those divisions upon which the fruit is borne are dilated. The color is olive-brown or greenish gray above, reddish at the base, and lighter on the under than the upper surface. The fructification is in flat, shield-like, reddish brown receptacles, with elevated entire edges, placed upon the surface of the frond near its border. The plant is found in the northern latitudes of the old and new continents, and on the elevated mountains farther south. It received its name from the abundance with which it prevails in Iceland. It is also abundant on the mountains and in the sandy plains of New England. "It should be freed from pine leaves, mosses and other lichens, which are frequently found mixed with it." *U. S.*

The dried moss is of diversified color, grayish white, brown, and red, in different parts, with less of the green tint than in the recent state. It is officinally characterised as follows. "From two to four inches (5 to 10 cm.) long, foliaceous, with fringed and channelled lobes, brownish above, whitish beneath, brittle and inodorous; when softened in water, cartilaginous, and having a slight odor; its taste is mucilaginous and bitter." It is inodorous, and has a mucilaginous, bitter taste. Macerated in water, it absorbs rather more than its own weight of the fluid, and, if the water be warm, renders it bitter. Boiling water extracts all its soluble principles. The decoction thickens upon cooling, and acquires a gelatinous consistence, resembling that of starch in appearance, but without its viscidity. After some time the dissolved matter separates, and when dried forms semi-transparent masses, insoluble in cold water, alcohol, or ether, but soluble in boiling water, and in solution forming a blue compound with iodine. *Lichenin*, or *Lichen Starch*, $C_{12}H_{20}O_{10}$, resembles starch in its general characters, but differs from it in some respects. Berzelius found in 100 parts of Iceland moss 1·6 of chlorophyll, 3·0 of a peculiar bitter principle, 3·6 of uncrystallizable sugar, 3·7 of gum, 7·0 of the apotheme of extractive, 44·6 of the peculiar starch-like principle, 1·9 of the bilichenates of potassium and calcium mixed with phosphate of calcium, and 36·2 of amylaceous fibrin—the excess being 1·6 parts.

The starch-like substance named lichenin has been found to consist of two distinct proximate principles, one, for which the name of lichenin may be retained, while for the other no particular designation has been chosen, but which we may call *lichenoid*. According to Th. Berg (*Thèse de Dorpat*, 1872), cetraria yields 35·15 per cent. of the mixed principles, of which 20 per cent. is of lichenin, and 11·5 of the so-called lichenoid. To separate them, a decoction of the moss, concentrated to a small bulk, and still hot, is treated by alcohol at 85°. The lichenoid is deposited in flocculi, which gradually unite in a viscid mass. This, being washed by alcohol, until it ceases to be bitter, and then dried, yields a light friable matter partly soluble in cold water, with which it forms a yellow, limpid solution. To deprive it of mineral and coloring substances, it is dissolved in a little water, and precipitated afresh by alcohol. Lichenin is insoluble in cold water, but swells up and easily dissolves in hot water. It is insoluble in alcohol and in ether. It is only tinged by iodine. Lichenoid is, on the contrary, colored blue by that reagent. It is in part dissolved in cold water; and the undissolved part is equally colored blue by iodine. It is, like lichenin, insoluble in alcohol and ether. Both substances have strong analogies with starch, yet are distinct. For a further account of these principles, see *Journ. de Pharm.*, 1873, p. 154.

The name of *cetrarin* has been conferred on the bitter principle. The following process for obtaining it is that of Dr. Herberger. The moss, coarsely powdered, is boiled for half an hour in four times its weight of alcohol of 0·883. The liquid when cool is expressed and filtered, and treated with diluted hydrochloric acid, in the proportion of three drachms to every pound of moss employed. Water is then added in the quantity of about four times the bulk of the liquid, and the mixture left for a night in a closed matrass. The deposit which forms is collected on a filter, allowed to drain as much as possible, and submitted to the press. To purify it, the mass, while still moist, is broken into small pieces, washed with alcohol or ether, and treated with two hundred times its weight of boiling alcohol, which dissolves the cetrarin, leaving the other organic principles by which it has hitherto been accompanied. The greater part is deposited as the liquor cools, and the remainder may be obtained by evaporation. By this process one pound of moss yielded to Dr. Herberger 133 grains of cetrarin. This principle is white, not crystalline, light, unalterable in the air, inodorous, and exceedingly bitter, especially in alcoholic solution. Its best solvent is absolute alcohol, of which 100 parts dissolve 1·7 of cetrarin at the boiling temperature. Ether also dissolves it, and it is slightly soluble in water. Its solutions are quite neutral to test-paper. It is precipitated by the acids, and rendered much more soluble by the alkalies. Concentrated hydrochloric acid changes its color to a bright blue. It precipitates the salts of iron, copper, lead, and silver. In the dose of two grains, every two hours, it has been used successfully in intermittent fever. (*Journ. de Pharm.*, xxiii. 505.) Drs. Schnedermann and Knop have ascertained that the cetrarin above referred to consists of three distinct substances; 1, *cetraric acid*, $C_{18}H_{16}O_8$, which is the true bitter principle, crystallizable, and intensely bitter; 2, a substance resembling the fatty acids, called *lichen-stearic acid*, $C_{14}H_{24}O_3$, the crystals of which melt at 120° C. (248° F.); and, 3, a green coloring substance, which they name *thallochlor*. These principles are obtained perfectly pure with great difficulty. (*Ann. der Pharm.*, lv. 144.)

The gum and starch contained in the moss render it sufficiently nutritive to serve as food for the Lapps and Icelanders, who employ it powdered and made into bread, or boiled with milk, after having partially freed it from the bitter principle by repeated maceration in water. As suggested by Berzelius, the bitterness may be entirely extracted by macerating the powdered moss, for 24 hours, in twenty-four times its weight of a solution formed with 1 part of an alkaline carbonate and 375 parts of water, then decanting the liquid, and repeating the process with an equal quantity of the solution. The powder, being now dried, is perfectly sweet, and has been used to some extent in pharmacy as a substitute for acacia. It lacks one important quality of the latter, however,—*i.e.*, adhesiveness, and it must be entirely devoid of bitterness, if it is to be used for this purpose.

Medical Properties and Uses. Iceland moss is demulcent, nutritious, and tonic, and well calculated for affections of the mucous membrane of the lungs and bowels, with debility of the digestive organs, or of the system generally. Hence it has been found useful in chronic catarrhs, and other chronic pulmonary affections attended with copious puruloid expectoration, in dyspepsia, in chronic dysentery and diarrhœa, and in the debility succeeding acute disease, or dependent on copious purulent discharge from external ulcers. At one time it possessed much reputation as a remedy in pulmonary consumption. It had long been employed in this disease, and in hæmoptysis, by the Danish physicians, before it became generally known. In the latter half of the last century it came into extensive use, and numerous cures supposed to have been effected by it are on record. We now know that it acts only as a mild, nutritious, demulcent tonic, and can exercise no specific influence over the tuberculous affection, though it may be of some value in relieving irritated conditions of the bronchial mucous membrane.

It is usually employed in the form of decoction. (See *Decoctum Cetrariæ.*) By some writers it is recommended to deprive it of the bitter principle by maceration in water or a weak alkaline solution, before preparing the decoction; but we thus reduce it to the state of a simple demulcent, or mild article of diet, in which respect it is not superior to the ordinary farinaceous or gummy substances used in medicine. The powder is sometimes given in the dose of thirty grains or a drachm (1·95–3·9 Gm.); and a preparation at one time obtained some repute, in which the ground moss was incorporated with chocolate, and used at the morning and evening meal as an ordinary beverage.

Off. Prep. Decoctum Cetrariæ.

CHARTÆ. *Papers.*

(CHĂR'TÆ.)

Papiers sparadrapiques, *Fr.;* Medicamentirte Papiere, *G.*

This class of preparations, long officinal in the French Codex, was some time since adopted into the British Pharmacopœia, but was not introduced into that of the United States until the revision of 1870.

CHARTA CANTHARIDIS. *U.S. Cantharides Paper.*

(CHĂR'TA CAN-THĂR'I-DĬS.)

Charta Epispastica, *Br.;* Blistering Paper, Charta Vesicatoria; Papier épispastique, Papier à Vésicatoire aux Cantharides, *Fr.;* Spanischfliegen-Papier, *G.*

"White Wax, *eight parts* [or four ounces av.]; Spermaceti, *three parts* [or one and a half ounces av.]; Olive Oil, *four parts* [or two fluidounces]; Canada Turpentine, *one part* [or half an ounce av.]; Cantharides, in No. 40 powder, *one part* [or half an ounce av.]; Water, *ten parts* [or five fluidounces]. Mix all the substances in a tinned vessel, and boil gently for two hours, constantly stirring. Strain through a woollen strainer without expressing, and, by means of a water-bath, keep the mixture in a liquid state in a shallow, flat-bottomed vessel with an extended surface. Coat strips of sized paper with the melted plaster, on one side only, by passing them successively over the surface of the liquid; when dry, cut the strips into rectangular pieces." *U. S.*

"Take of White Wax *four ounces;* Spermaceti *one and a half ounces;* Olive Oil *two fluidounces;* Resin *three-quarters of an ounce;* Canada Balsam *one-quarter of an ounce;* Cantharides, in powder, *one ounce;* Distilled Water *six fluidounces.* Digest all the ingredients, excepting the Canada Balsam, in a water-bath for two hours, stirring them constantly; then strain, and separate the plaster from the watery liquid. Mix the Canada Balsam with the plaster melted in a shallow vessel, and pass strips of paper over the surface of the hot liquid, so that one surface of the paper shall receive a thin coating of the plaster. It may be convenient to employ paper ruled so as to indicate divisions each of which is one square inch." *Br.* The weights employed in this process are avoirdupois, and the measures Imperial.

This was intended as a convenient substitute for the common blistering plaster, and, if equally effectual, would be frequently preferred, from being already spread, as well as for its greater cleanliness and facility of application. The proportion of flies, however, is considerably less. From this cause it must be very greatly inferior in blistering power, and consequently less certain; this is a point which has been determined by experience; although it is said that, when properly applied, so as to insure close adhesion to the skin, it is not less efficient than the British plaster, or the *Cerate of Cantharides* of the U. S. Pharmacopœia. (*Med. Times and Gaz.*, 1867, p. 284.) It has been so seldom used, however, since its introduction, that it would seem hardly proper to venture an opinion upon its value.

CHARTA POTASSII NITRATIS. *U.S. Nitrate of Potassium Paper.*

(CHĂR'TA PO-TĂS'SI-Ī NĪ-TRĀ'TĬS.)

Papier nitré, *Fr.*

"Nitrate of Potassium, *twenty parts* [one ounce av.]; Distilled Water, *eighty parts* [four fluidounces]. Dissolve the Nitrate of Potassium in the Distilled Water. Immerse strips of white, unsized paper in the solution and dry them. Keep the paper in securely closed vessels." *U. S.*

This is a new officinal preparation, and is identical with the *Charta Nitrata* of the German Pharmacopœia; it is sometimes called *asthma paper.* Care should be taken to dissolve thoroughly all of the nitrate of potassium, so that it shall not be deposited upon the paper in large particles, and thus interfere with the slow and steady combustion of the paper.

Medical Properties. This paper is an excellent remedy, which in many cases of asthma affords much relief. It is used by burning in front of the patient, who inhales its fumes. Its efficacy is much increased by saturating it with fluid extract of belladonna and drying. Paper thus prepared must be used with some caution.

CHARTA SINAPIS. *U. S.* *Mustard Paper.*

(CHÄR'TĄ SĮ-NĀ'PĬS.)

Papier sinapisé, *Fr.;* Senfpapier, *G.*

"Black Mustard, in No. 60 powder; Benzin, Solution of Gutta-percha, each, *a sufficient quantity.* Pack the Mustard tightly in a conical percolator, and gradually pour Benzin upon it until the percolate ceases to produce a permanent, greasy stain upon blotting paper. Remove the powder from the percolator, and dry it by exposure to the air. Then mix it with so much of Solution of Gutta-percha as may be necessary to give it a semi-liquid consistence, apply the mixture, by means of a suitable brush, to one side of a piece of rather stiff, well sized paper, so as to cover it completely, and allow the surface to dry. Each square inch (or 6·5 square centimeters) of paper should contain about *six* (6) *grains* or *forty* (40) *centigrammes* of Mustard. Before being applied to the skin, the Mustard Paper should be dipped in warm water for about fifteen seconds." *U. S.*

"Take of Mustard, in powder, *one ounce;* Solution of Gutta-percha *two fluidounces*, or *a sufficiency.* Mix the Mustard with the Gutta-percha Solution so as to form a semi-fluid mixture, and having poured this into a shallow, flat-bottomed vessel, such as a dinner plate, pass strips of cartridge-paper over its surface, so that one side of the paper shall receive a thin coating of the mixture. Then lay the paper on a table with the coated side upwards, and let it remain exposed to the air until the coating has hardened. Before being applied to the skin, let the Mustard Paper be immersed for a few seconds in tepid water." *Br.*

The British preparation is at fault in not providing for the extraction of the fixed oil of mustard by previously percolating with benzin or carbon disulphide, otherwise the paper will be greasy, giving to the plaster an untidy appearance, and causing it to adhere to the skin. Solution of gutta-percha is unsuited for use in this preparation on account of want of adhesiveness, and tendency of the mixture, when dry, to crack and peel off. We have used instead a solution of 1 part of pure rubber in 30 of equal parts of bisulphide of carbon and benzin. On the large scale, by means of a plaster-spreading apparatus a uniform coat of this solution may be applied to paper. As the latter passes out from under the apparatus, a sieve containing the powdered mustard is shaken over it; this is fixed by the adhesive coat and firmly retained after the evaporation of the volatile liquids in a warm place. The application of the powdered mustard must be properly regulated according to the speed with which the machine delivers the coated paper. The paper is cut into pieces of convenient size, and needs only to be wetted to be ready for use.

Owing to the fact that the large manufacturers can put mustard paper upon the market at such low rates that it pays the apothecary better to buy, than to prepare it, Charta Sinapis, so far as we can learn, is rarely made in the retail stores. Experience has shown that the ready-made mustard papers err rather from too much than from too little activity. Moreover, their action cannot be regulated with the same nicety as can that of the mustard poultice. Unless in the case of travellers and of others who must wait upon themselves, the domestic application is preferable. The mustard leaves can rarely be borne for more than ten or fifteen minutes.

CHELIDONIUM. *U. S.* *Chelidonium.* [*Celandine.*]

(ÇHĔL-Į-DŌ'NĮ-ŬM.)

"Chelidonium majus. Linné. (*Nat. Ord.* Papaveraceæ.)" *U. S.*

Herba Chelidonii, *P.G.;* Tetterwort; Chélidoine, Herbe à l'Hirondelle, *Fr.;* Schöllkraut, *G.*

Celandine is a perennial herbaceous plant, growing wild in this country, about old houses and in rocky places; supposed to have been introduced from Europe, where it is indigenous. It is one or two feet high, bears pinnate leaves and small peduncled umbels of yellow flowers, and, when wounded, emits a yellow, opaque juice. The whole plant is used. It has a faint unpleasant odor, and a bitter, acrid, durable taste, which is stronger in the roots than in the leaves. The odor is nearly lost by drying, but the taste remains. The yellow juice is bitter and exceedingly acrid, and when applied to the skin produces inflammation and even vesication. It is officinally described as follows: "Root several-headed, branching, red-brown. Stem about twenty inches (50 cm.) long, light green, hairy; leaves about six inches (15 cm.) long, petiolate, the upper ones smaller and sessile, light green, on the lower side glaucous, lyrate-pinnatifid, the pinnæ ovate-oblong, obtuse, coarsely crenate or incised, and the terminal one often three-lobed; flowers in small, long-peduncled umbels with two sepals and four yellow petals; capsule linear, two-valved, and many-seeded."

The plant, analyzed by MM. Chevallier and Lassaigne, afforded a bitter resinous substance of a deep yellow color; a kind of gum resin of an orange-yellow color, and bitter, nauseous taste; mucilage; albumen; and various saline substances, besides free malic acid and silica. Dr. Probst, of Heidelberg, afterwards found in it a peculiar acid denominated *chelidonic acid;* two alkaline principles, one of which forms neutral salts with the acids, and is called *chelerythrine* (*chelerythria*) in consequence of the intense redness of its salts, the other unites with but does not neutralize the acids, and is named *chelidonine* (*chelidonia*); and lastly a neutral crystallizable, bitter principle, which from its yellow color he calls *chelidoxanthin.* Chelerythrine appears to be an acrid narcotic poison. (*Annal. der Pharm.*, xxix. 113.) It has been shown by Dr. James Schiels, of St. Louis, to be identical with *sanguinarine,* and may be prepared in the same manner. (See *Sanguinaria.*) Zwenger isolated another acid, which he names *chelidoninic acid,* although both Walz and Kraut consider it to be only succinic acid. (*A. J. P.*, 1861, p. 7.) Schmidt considers chelidoninic acid to be identical with ethylene-succinic acid. (*Arch. d. Pharm.*, 1886, p. 531.)

Medical Properties and Uses. Celandine is an acrid purgative, possessed also of diuretic, and perhaps diaphoretic and expectorant, properties. In overdoses it produces unpleasant effects, and is by some considered poisonous. By the ancients it was much esteemed as a remedy in jaundice; and it has been found useful in the same complaint by some modern physicians. It was the chief ingredient of the old *decoctum ad ictericos* of the Edinburgh Pharmacopœia. It has been given also in other complaints, especially those of a scrofulous character, affecting the mesenteric and lymphatic glands, the skin, and the eyes. The yellow juice is often applied to corns and warts, which it destroys by stimulating them beyond their vital powers, and is said to be very useful in eczema, urticaria, and other itching eruptions. The fresh herb is also applied locally about the pelvis, with asserted benefit, in amenorrhœa, and is much used in the south of Europe as a vulnerary. The dose of the dried root or herb is from thirty grains to a drachm (1·9–3·9 Gm.), that of the fresh root one or two drachms (3·9–7·8 Gm.), and the same quantity may be given in infusion. The watery extract and expressed juice have also been employed. The dose of the former is from five to ten grains, of the latter from ten to twenty drops, to be gradually increased.

CHENOPODIUM. *U. S.* *Chenopodium.* [*American Wormseed.*]

(CHĔ-NO-PŌ'DI-ŬM.)

"The fruit of Chenopodium ambrosioides. Linné. *Var.* anthelminticum. Gray. (*Nat. Ord.* Chenopodiaceæ.)" *U. S.*

Fructus Chenopodii Anthelmintici; Semences de Chénopode anthelmintique, *Fr.;* Amerikanischer Wurmsamen, *G.*

Gen. Ch. *Calyx* five-leaved, four-cornered. *Corolla* none. *Seed* one, lenticular, superior. *Willd.*

Chenopodium anthelminticum. Willd. *Sp. Plant.* i. 1304; Barton, *Med. Bot.* ii. 183; *B. & T.* 216. This is an indigenous perennial plant, with an herbaceous, erect, branching, furrowed stem, which rises from two to five feet in height. The leaves are alternate or scattered, sessile, oblong-lanceolate, attenuated at both ends, sinuated and toothed on the margin, conspicuously veined, of a yellowish green color, and dotted on their under surface.* The flowers are very numerous, small, of the same color with the leaves, and arranged in long, leafless, terminal panicles, composed of slender, dense, glomerate, alternating spikes.

This species of Chenopodium, known commonly by the names of *wormseed* and *Jerusalem oak,* grows in almost all parts of the United States, but most vigorously

* Dr. H. Paschkis has made an elaborate study of the microscopic structure of this leaf. (*P. J. Tr.*, 1881, p. 44.)

and abundantly in the southern section. It is usually found in the vicinity of rubbish, along fences, in the streets of villages, and in open grounds about the larger towns. It flowers from July to September, and ripens its seeds successively through the autumn. The whole herb has a strong, peculiar, offensive, yet somewhat aromatic odor, which it retains when dry. All parts of the plant are occasionally employed; but the fruit only is strictly officinal. This should be collected in October.*

Wormseed, as found in the shops, is in small grains, not larger than the head of a pin, irregularly spherical, very light, of a dull, greenish yellow, or brownish color, a bitterish, somewhat aromatic, pungent taste, and possessed in a high degree of the peculiar smell of the plant. These grains, when deprived, by rubbing them in the hand, of a capsular covering which invests the proper seed, exhibit the shining, blackish surface of the obtusely-edged seed. They abound in a volatile oil, upon which their sensible properties and medical virtues depend, and which is obtained by distillation. (See *Oleum Chenopodii.*) The same oil impregnates to a greater or less extent the whole plant.

Medical Properties and Uses. Wormseed is one of our most efficient indigenous anthelmintics, and is thought to be particularly adapted to the expulsion of the round worms in children. A dose of it is usually given before breakfast in the morning, and at bedtime in the evening, for three or four days successively, and then followed by calomel or some other brisk cathartic. If the worms are not expelled, the same plan is repeated. The medicine is most conveniently administered in powder, mixed with syrup, in the form of an electuary. The dose for a child two or three years old is from one to two scruples (1·3–2·6 Gm.). The volatile oil is more frequently given than the fruit in substance; though its offensive odor and taste sometimes render it of difficult administration. The dose for a child is from five to ten drops (0·3–0·6 C.c.) mixed with sugar, or in the form of emulsion. A tablespoonful (15 C.c.) of the expressed juice of the leaves, or a wineglassful (60 C.c.) of the decoction prepared by boiling an ounce of the fresh plant in a pint of milk, with the addition of orange-peel or other aromatic, is sometimes substituted in domestic practice for the ordinary dose of the fruit and oil.

The fruit of *Chenopodium ambrosioides*, which is very prevalent in the Middle States, is said to be used indiscriminately with that of *C. anthelminticum*, and to be employed in Brazil, under the name of *Herba Santa Maria*, as an anthelmintic and in pectoral complaints. (*P. J. Tr.*, ix. 713.) It may be distinguished by its odor, which is weaker and less offensive, and to some persons agreeable. The plant itself is often confounded with the true wormseed, from which it differs in having its flowers in leafy racemes. This Chenopodium has been employed in Europe as a remedy in nervous affections, particularly chorea. A cupful of an infusion (ʒii to 10f℥) is said to have been given with excellent results, morning and evening.

C. Botrys, or *Jerusalem oak*, is another indigenous species, possessing anthelmintic virtues. It is said to have been used in France with advantage in catarrh and humoral asthma.

CHIMAPHILA. *U. S.* *Chimaphila.* [*Pipsissewa.*]

(CHI-MĂPH'I-LA.)

"The leaves of Chimaphila umbellata. Nuttall. (*Nat. Ord.* Ericaceæ.)" *U. S.*

Prince's Pine, Wintergreen; Herbe de Pyrole ombellée, *Fr.*; Doldenblüthiges Harnkraut, Wintergrün, *G.*

Gen. Ch. *Calyx* five-toothed. *Petals* five. *Style* very short, immersed in the germ. *Stigma* annular, orbicular, with a five-lobed disk. *Filaments* stipitate; stipe discoid, ciliate. *Capsules* five-celled, opening from the summits, margins unconnected. *Nuttall.*

* *C. anthelminticum* is cultivated to a considerable extent in Maryland, twenty or thirty miles north of Baltimore. The seeds are sown in small beds of rich mould early in spring, and during the month of June the young plants are pulled up, and set out in ridges three feet apart, with intervals of from six to ten inches. The plants do not require to be renewed oftener than once in four or five years. The crop of the second year is more productive than that of the first. The plant is fit for distillation during the first half of September. The distillation is carried on in the same neighborhood. The whole herbaceous part of the plant is used. It is said to yield from 1·5 to 2 per cent. of the oil, and the produce of an acre will yield 20 pounds. (See *A. J. P.*, xxii. 304.)

This genus was separated from *Pyrola* by Pursh. It embraces two species, *C. umbellata* and *C. maculata*, which are both indigenous, and known by the common title of *winter-green*. The generic title is formed of two Greek words, χειμα winter, and φιλος a friend. *C. umbellata* only is officinal.

Chimaphila umbellata. Barton, *Med. Bot.* i. 17; Carson, *Illust. of Med. Bot.* i. 62, pl. 53.—*Pyrola umbellata*. Willd. *Sp. Plant.* ii. 622; Bigelow, *Am. Med. Bot.* ii. 15.—*Chimaphila corymbosa*. Pursh. *B. & T.* 165. The pipsissewa is a small evergreen plant, with a perennial, creeping, yellowish root (rhizome), which gives rise to several simple, erect or semiprocumbent stems, from four to eight inches in height, and ligneous at their base. The leaves are wedge-shaped, somewhat lanceolate, serrate, coriaceous, smooth, of a shining, sap-green color on the upper surface, paler beneath, and supported upon short footstalks, in irregular whorls, of which there are usually two on the same stem. The flowers are disposed in a small terminal corymb, and stand upon nodding peduncles. The calyx is small and divided at its border into five teeth or segments. The corolla is composed of five roundish, concave, spreading petals, which are of a white color tinged with red, and exhale an agreeable odor. The stamens are ten, with filaments shorter than the petals, and with large, nodding, bifurcated, purple anthers. The germ is globular and depressed, supporting a thick and apparently sessile stigma, the style being short and immersed in the germ. The seeds are numerous, linear, chaffy, and enclosed in a roundish, depressed, five-celled, five-valved capsule, having the persistent calyx at the base.

This humble but beautiful evergreen is a native of the northern latitudes of America, Europe, and Asia. It is found in all parts of the United States. It grows under the shade of woods, and prefers a loose sandy soil, enriched by decaying leaves. The flowers appear in June and July. All parts of the plant are endowed with active properties. The leaves and stems are kept in the shops.

C. maculata, or *spotted winter-green*, probably possesses similar virtues. The character of the leaves of the two plants will serve to distinguish them. Those of *C. maculata* are lanceolate, rounded at the base, where they are broader than near the summit, and of a deep olive green, veined with greenish white; those of the officinal species are broadest near the summit, gradually narrowing to the base, and of a uniform shining green.

Properties. Pipsissewa, when fresh and bruised, exhales a peculiar odor. The leaves have been already described. Their taste is pleasantly bitter, astringent, and sweetish; that of the stems and root unites with these qualities a considerable degree of pungency. Boiling water extracts the active properties of the plant, which are also imparted to alcohol. The leaves have been examined by Mr. Samuel Fairbank, who found in them gum, starch, sugar, extractive, pectic acid, tannic acid, resin, fatty matter, chlorophyll, yellow coloring matter, lignin, a peculiar whitish substance which he calls *chimaphilin*, and various inorganic substances, as potassa, lime, magnesia, chloride of sodium, and sulphuric, phosphoric, and silicic acids. The chimaphilin was obtained by agitating a tincture with chloroform, allowing the mixture to stand, removing the lighter liquid, and allowing the chloroformic solution to evaporate. A yellow crystalline substance was left, which, purified by solution in alcohol, filtration, and spontaneous evaporation, constituted the substance in question. It was also obtained by simply distilling the stems with water. It is in beautiful, golden yellow, acicular crystals, inodorous, tasteless, fusible, volatilizable unchanged, insoluble or nearly so in water, soluble in alcohol, ether, chloroform, and the fixed and volatile oils, and possessed of neither acid nor alkaline properties. (*Journ. and Trans. of the Md. Col. of Pharm.*, March, 1860.) The active principle of the leaves seems to have been isolated by E. S. Beshore (*A. J. P.*, 1887, p. 125) by treatment of the powdered leaves with petroleum spirit. He obtained white crystals, melting at 236° C., sparingly soluble in cold or boiling 90 per cent. alcohol, sparingly soluble in ether, benzin, chloroform, and cold glacial acetic acid; more soluble in hot glacial acetic acid. An ultimate analysis gave the formula $C_{10}H_{18}O$. He also obtained the golden yellow crystalline principle of Fairbank both from the leaves and the stems. He considers it distinct from the one described above.

Medical Properties and Uses. This plant is diuretic, tonic, and astringent. It was employed by the aborigines in various complaints, especially scrofula, rheumatism, and nephritic affections. From their hands it passed into those of the European settlers, and was long a popular remedy in certain parts of the country, before it was adopted by the profession. The first regular treatise in relation to it that has come to our knowledge, was the thesis of Dr. Mitchell, published in the year 1803; but it was little thought of till the appearance of the paper of Dr. Sommerville, in *Lond. Med.-Chir. Trans.*, vol. v. It has been particularly recommended in dropsy attended with disordered digestion and general debility, and is usually very acceptable to the stomach, but it cannot be relied on, and is at present very little used in this complaint. Other disorders, in which it is said to have proved useful, are calculous and nephritic affections, and in general all those complaints of the urinary passages for which uva ursi is prescribed. It is much esteemed by some practitioners as a remedy in scrofula, both before and after the occurrence of ulceration; and it has certainly proved highly advantageous in obstinate ill-conditioned ulcers and cutaneous eruptions, supposed to be connected with the strumous diathesis. In these cases it is used both internally, and locally as a wash. It is best administered in the form of the officinal fluid extract, which may readily be made into a syrup. The dose is two fluidrachms (7·5 C.c.) three or four times a day. The decoction was formerly preferred.

Off. Prep. Extractum Chimaphilæ Fluidum.

CHINOIDINUM. *U.S.* *Chinoidin.* [*Quinoidin.*]

(CHĬN-ŎĬ'DĬ-NŬM.)

"A mixture of alkaloids, mostly amorphous, obtained as a by-product in the manufacture of the crystallizable alkaloids from Cinchona." *U. S.*

Chinoidine, Quinoidine, Precipitated Extract of Bark, Amorphous Quinine; Quinine brute ou amorphe, *Fr.*

This preparation is a *revived* officinal. It was adopted in the edition of the Pharmacopœia for 1830 under the name of impure sulphate of quinia, but was abandoned in the edition of 1840 on account of the difficulty of ascertaining its purity, and we think it unfortunate that the Committee of Revision have decided to introduce it in the present Pharmacopœia, for it is now very variable in quality and the tests introduced are not quantitative. The wisdom of deviating from the rule to adopt the *ina* termination for the Latin title of the alkaloids, and *ine* for the English name, in this case is also not apparent, for although it is a mixture, the officinal description clearly defines it as a mixture of *alkaloids*, and hence it should have the alkaloidal termination, and not that of the neutral principles. The term chinoidine was first applied to all of the amorphous alkaloids found in and existing naturally in cinchona bark, but it is now used to define a complex body consisting not only of the natural amorphous alkaloids, but those which are artificial and accidental in the derivative products resulting from the application of heat. Upon the evaporation of the mother-liquor left after the crystallization of sulphate of quinine in the preparation of that salt, a dark-colored substance is obtained, having the appearance of an extract. Sertürner supposed that he had discovered a new alkaline principle in this product; but his conclusions were invalidated by the experiments of MM. Henry and Delondre, which went to prove that the alkaline matter contained in it consisted of quinine and cinchonine, obscured by admixture with a yellowish substance that interfered with their crystallization. Nevertheless, under the name of *quinoidine* or *chinoidine*, given to the supposed new alkaloid by Sertürner, there has been long employed in Europe a substance precipitated from the mother-liquor of sulphate of quinine by means of an alkaline carbonate, having a yellowish white or brownish color, and, when moderately heated, agglutinating into a mass of resinous appearance. This substance was found by Dr. F. L. Winckler to contain an uncrystallizable alkaline principle, having the same molecular weight as quinine, and differing from that alkaloid only in the want of the property of crystallization, and in forming uncrystallizable salts with the acids. (*Pharm. Centralb.*, May, 1847, p. 310.) Liebig afterwards proved it to be identical in composition with ordinary quinine, to which he considered it as bearing the same relation that uncrystallizable sugar bears to the crystallizable. Pasteur has found that ordinary quinoidine, or amorphous quinine, consists of two alkaloids, derivatives from quinine and cinchonine, with which they are respectively isomeric, though differing in being uncrystallizable, and named, in view of their origin, *quinicine* and *cinchonicine*. The pure amorphous quinine of Liebig is the former of these alkaloids. The *amorphous quinine*, as Liebig calls it, is entirely soluble in diluted sulphuric acid and in alcohol; and, if its solution in a diluted acid yields upon the addition of ammonia exactly as much precipitate as there was of the original substance dissolved, it may be considered pure. (*A. J. P.*, xviii. 181.) We have been informed that, in an extensive chemical manufacturing establishment in Philadelphia, the loss by quinoidine in the preparation of sulphate of quinine has much diminished since the introduction of steam heat, showing the agency of heat in converting the crystallizable into the uncrystallizable salt; by the use of vacuum apparatus this loss might be still further diminished.

Properties. The U. S. Pharmacopœia describes chinoidine as "a brownish black, or almost black solid, breaking, when cold, with a resinous, shining fracture, becoming plastic when warmed, odorless, having a bitter taste and an alkaline reaction. Almost insoluble in water, freely soluble in alcohol, chloroform, and diluted acids; partially soluble in ether and in benzol. The solutions have a very bitter taste. If Chinoidin be triturated with boiling water, the liquid, after filtration, should be clear and colorless, and should remain so on the addition of an alkali (abs. of alkaloidal salts). On ignition, Chinoidin should not leave more than 0·7 per cent. of ash." *U. S.*

A simple method of purification consists in dissolving the chinoidine in diluted hydrochloric acid, adding water and precipitating with an alkali, washing and drying.*

Tinctura Chinoidini is made, by the German Pharmacopœia, by simply dissolving 2 parts of chinoidine in one of hydrochloric acid and 17 of alcohol, sp. gr. ·894.

Hydrochlorate of Chinoidine is made by heating 1 part of purified chinoidine with 4 parts of distilled water, adding sufficient diluted hydrochloric acid to complete the solution, filtering, evaporating, and powdering the residue. Zimmer furnishes the German market with the purified hydrochlorate, under the name of *Chininum amorphum muriaticum purum*. It has been largely used medicinally. For formulas for various salts of chinoidine, see *N. R.*, 1882, p. 11, or *Proc. A. P. A.*, 1882, p. 417.

Medical Properties. Chinoidine is undoubtedly possessed of decided antiperiodic properties, but in these it is inferior to the cinchona alkaloids. It is, moreover, much more apt to disagree with the stomach, and is uncertain in its dose, so that, notwithstanding its great cheapness, it is but rarely used. From thirty grains to a drachm (1·9–3·9 Gm.) may be given in the interparoxysmal periods of an intermittent, and its action closely watched.

* *Purified Chinoidine.* The following process has been adopted by the Dutch Society for the Advancement of Pharmacy. Digest one part of chinoidine with two parts of benzol on a water-bath. Pour off the clear solution and wash the residue with one part of benzol. Agitate the united clear liquids with a small excess of diluted hydrochloric acid, allow the mixture to subside, remove the acid liquid, and add solution of soda until fairly alkaline. A portion of the filtered solution is now tested by adding a few drops of concentrated solution of sodium hyposulphite; if a precipitate occurs which does not disappear on further dilution with water, the solution has not been sufficiently purified; then the whole solution must be purified by adding hyposulphite until a permanent precipitate is no longer produced. The liquid is then heated on a water-bath mixed with solution of soda in excess, the precipitate washed with water, and dried. (*N. R.*, 1882, p. 11.)

The objection to the above process is, that it is sometimes difficult to entirely get rid of the odor of benzol. Dr. J. E. De Vrij proposes the following improvement. One hundred parts of chinoidine are boiled during ten minutes with a diluted solution of soda, with constant stirring. When cold, the alkaline liquid is poured off, and the remaining chinoidine washed with a little water. Three hundred parts of water are now added to the washed chinoidine, the whole heated to boiling, and then mixed very slowly with the *least necessary quantity of nitric acid* to obtain a homogeneous dark-colored solution; great care must be observed not to add one drop too much of nitric acid. The still alkaline liquid is set aside for 12 hours to separate. The upper layer is poured off as clear as possible, and the lower layer washed with water until a brownish black insoluble mass remains, which is worthless. The united liquids are filtered, water added, and if turbidity results, still more water until the addition ceases to produce cloudiness. The liquid is then filtered, and an excess of soda added, which precipitates the chinoidine. This is washed with water, and the mass heated carefully until free from water. (*Amer. Drug.*, 1884, p. 134.)

CHIRATA. *U. S., Br.* Chirata.

(CHI-RĀ'TA.)

"Ophelia Chirata. Grisebach. (*Nat. Ord.* Gentianaceæ.)" "The dried plant Ophelia Chirata, *Griesb.; Wallich, Plant. asiat. Gentiana Chirata*, collected when the fruit begins to form." *Br.*

Chirette, *Fr.;* Chiretta, *G.*

Gen. Ch. Corolla withering, rotate, in æstivation twisted to the right; with glandular hollows protected by a fringed scale upon the segments. *Anthers* not changing. *Stigmas* sessile. *Capsules* conical; one-celled, with spongy placentæ upon the sutures. *Seeds* indefinite, minute. *Lindley.*

Agathotes Chirayta. Don, *Lond. Philos. Mag.* 1836, p. 76.—*Gentiana Chirayta.* Fleming, *Asiat. Research.* xi. 167.—*Ophelia Chirata.* Grisebach. *B. & T.* 183.

The *chirayta* or *chiretta* is an annual plant, about three feet high, with a branching root, and an erect, smooth, round stem, branching into an elegant leafy panicle, and furnished with opposite, embracing, lanceolate, very acute, entire, smooth, three or five-nerved leaves. The flowers are numerous, peduncled, yellow, with a four-cleft calyx having linear acute divisions, the limb of the corolla spreading and four-parted, four stamens, a single style, and a two-lobed stigma. The capsules are shorter than the permanent calyx and corolla. The plant is a native of Nepaul, and other parts of Northern India. The whole of it is gathered when the flowers begin to decay.*

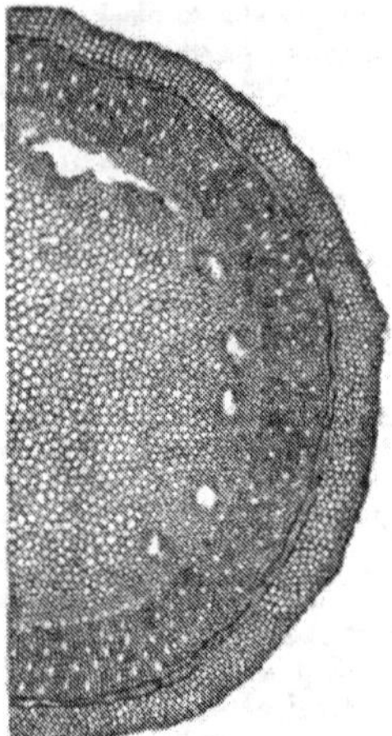

Chiretta, transverse section.

The dried plant is imported into Europe in bundles, consisting mainly of the stems, with portions of the root attached. The stems contain a yellowish pith. The drug is officinally described as a "root nearly simple, about three inches (75 mm.) long; stem branched, nearly forty inches (1 m.) long, slightly quadrangular above; leaves opposite, sessile, ovate, entire, five-nerved; flowers numerous, small, with a four-lobed calyx and corolla; the whole plant smooth, pale brown, inodorous and intensely bitter." *U. S.* It imparts its virtues to water and alcohol; and they are retained in the extract. According to Lassaigne and Boissel, the stems contain resin, a yellow bitter substance, brown coloring matter, gum, and various salts. Flückiger and Höhn, who have subsequently examined the stems and roots, have extracted from them sugar, wax, chlorophyll, soft resin, tannin, an acid which they name *ophelic*, possessing the formula $C_{13}H_{20}O_{10}$, and a peculiar bitter substance, denominated *chiratin*, $C_{26}H_{48}O_{15}$. The acid is syrupy, deliquescent, yellowish brown, at first slightly sour, afterwards intensely bitter. It is soluble in water with some turbidness, probably owing to resin mixed with it, and completely soluble in alcohol, or a mixture of this with ether. It decomposes certain salts, and forms amorphous compounds with acids. Chiratin is a yellow, hygroscopic powder, but feebly crystallizable, very bitter, sparingly soluble in cold water, more so in hot water, and readily dissolved by alcohol and ether. It is neutral to test-paper, and yields a copious precipitate with tannic acid. By the action of acids, chiratin is separated into ophelic acid, and a yellowish brown, amorphous substance, bitter, scarcely soluble in water, readily soluble in spirit, and not reducing copper

* In the Indian bazaars the name chiretta is applied to various dried gentianaceous plants; the most important of these is the *Ophelia angustifolia*. It yields the *Paharee* or *Hill chiretta*, which is distinguished by its inferior bitterness, and its rectangular, winged stems, whose section presents a thick woody ring and a centre nearly or entirely hollow, with only traces of pith. A false chirata, which has also found its way into the London markets, and resembles the officinal variety in having a well-developed pith, but which is completely lacking in bitterness, is affirmed to be the product of *Ophelia alata*. (*P. J. Tr.*, xvii. 903.)

solutions, as the ophelic acid does. Höhn gives it the formula $C_{13}H_{24}O_{3}$, and names it *chiratogenin*. (*P. J. Tr.*, Aug. 1870, p. 106.)

Medical Properties and Uses. Chiretta has long been used in India. It has been introduced into Europe, and appears to be highly esteemed, but has not been employed to any considerable extent in this country. Its properties are those of the pure bitters, and probably do not differ from those of the other members of the family of Gentianaceæ. (See *Gentiana.*) Like these, in overdoses it nauseates and oppresses the stomach. Some have supposed that, in addition to its tonic properties, it exerts a peculiar influence over the liver, promoting the secretion of bile and correcting it when deranged, and restoring healthy evacuations in cases of habitual costiveness. It has been used in dyspepsia, and in the debility of convalescence, and generally in cases in which corroborant measures are indicated. In India it has been successfully employed in intermittents and remittents, combined with the seeds of *Guilandina Bonducella.* It may be given in powder, infusion, tincture, or extract. The dose in substance is twenty grains (1·3 Gm.). A fluid extract may be made in the same manner as that of gentian.

Off. Prep. Extractum Chiratæ Fluidum; Tinctura Chiratæ.

Off. Prep. Br. Infusum Chiratæ; Tinctura Chiratæ.

CHLORAL. *U.S., Br.* *Chloral.* [*Hydrate of Chloral.*]

C_2HCl_3O, H_2O; 165·2. (CHLŌ'RĂL.) $C_4HCl_3O_2, 2HO$; 165·2.

"Chloral should be preserved in glass-stoppered bottles, in a cool and dark place." *U. S.* "Chloral, produced by the action of dry chlorine gas on anhydrous alcohol, purified by treatment, first with sulphuric acid and afterwards with a small quantity of lime, and finally converted into hydrous chloral by the addition of water." *Br.*

Chloral Hydras, *Br.* Hydrous Chloral; Chloralum Hydratum Crystallisatum, *P.G.;* Hydrate de Chloral, *Fr.;* Chloral Hydrat, *G.*

In adopting the name chloral to designate the hydrate of chloral, the U. S. Pharmacopœia has unfortunately perpetuated an inaccuracy which neither the English, the Germans, nor the French follow in their usage, the term *hydrate* being always employed as it should be. The fact that water is absolutely necessary to allow of the crystallization of the preparation, and to give it medicinal character, should be recognized in the name. As custom has sanctioned the usage here in the present article, whenever the term chloral is used, the hydrate is intended; and whenever the uncombined substance is referred to, it is designated *anhydrous chloral.*

Perhaps no medicine has come so rapidly into extensive use as that now under consideration. Though discovered by Liebig so long since as 1832, and afterwards investigated by Dumas, who determined its chemical formula, it was not until 1869 that its remedial properties were first made known by their discoverer, Dr. Otto Liebreich, of Berlin; in 1878 the consumption of chloral was estimated at one ton daily in England and America alone.

Anhydrous Chloral. In preparing anhydrous chloral, the simple method originally employed by Liebig, of acting directly on alcohol by chlorine, is generally preferred, even, we believe, by the larger manufacturers; though a more complex proceeding has been suggested by Stædeler, of distilling together proximate vegetable principles, as fecula, sugar, etc., with black oxide of manganese and hydrochloric acid, whereby the chlorine acts *in statu nascendi.* The following details of the manufacture of chloral hydrate as carried out on a commercial scale have been supplied by E. Schering, of Berlin, who has been for some years the largest manufacturer of it. Absolute alcohol in lots of 50 pounds is placed in large glass flasks and saturated with chlorine, which is passed in a continuous stream for 6 to 8 weeks. The chlorine is led into cold alcohol at first, and when no more is absorbed, the alcohol is heated at first gently and then to 60° C. (140° F.). When saturated, the mixture formed is agitated with sulphuric acid at a temperature of 60° C. (140° F.) for several hours, during which time most of the hydrochloric acid escapes. The separated chloral is then rectified over calcium carbonate. The pure chloral so obtained is then mixed in glass flasks with the necessary amount of water, and the resulting hydrate either cast into cakes or purified by crystallization. As solvents for this purpose certain of the side products of the chloral manufacture after being purified and rectified, are used, for instance, ethylen and ethyliden chlorides. Or in their absence chloroform is used; petroleum benzin, and bisulphide of carbon have also been recommended. (See also *A. J. P.*, 1873, p. 413.)* According to Gerhardt, the formula of anhydrous chloral is C_2Cl_3HO; in other words, aldehyd C_2H_4O, in which 3 atoms of hydrogen have been replaced by 3 atoms of chlorine. The alcohol C_2H_6O may be supposed to give up 2 atoms of its hydrogen to form aldehyd, which exchanges 3 of its atoms of hydrogen for 3 atoms of the chlorine, the hydrogen forming hydrochloric acid with 3 other atoms of the chlorine. The name of chloral was derived from the *chlor*ine and *al*cohol from which it is formed. The anhydrous chloral thus formed is a colorless liquid, of penetrating disagreeable odor, of little taste, of the sp. gr. 1·502, and boiling at 94° C. (201·2° F.). It is soluble in ether or chloroform without change.

Meta-chloral. By continued contact of anhydrous chloral and concentrated sulphuric acid, a change is effected in the chloral, by which it becomes a solid insoluble in water, which is designated as *insoluble chloral*, or *meta-chloral.* It is tasteless, of a white color resembling porcelain, and insoluble in alcohol and ether. Its formula is $C_6H_3Cl_9O_3$, being formed by the union of three molecules of chloral. It is stated that when perfectly pure, chloral does not become polymerised; the change is also said to be prevented by the addition of a little chloroform. When heated to 180° C., metachloral distils with reversion to liquid chloral. (Allen, *Com. Org. Analysis*, 2d ed., i. p. 171.)

Alcoholate of Chloral. A compound obtained by M. Roussin, which he announced as pure hydrate of chloral, was found by M. Personne to contain no water, but to be in fact a compound of alcohol and chloral, and is now known by the name of *alcoholate of chloral*, C_2HCl_3O,C_2H_6O. It results directly from the action of absolute alcohol on anhydrous chloral, and is now known to be formed as a stage in the manufacture of chloral from alcohol. As it is very likely to be confounded with chloral hydrate, the following points of difference should be noted. It forms white crystals melting at 46° C. (114·8° F.), and boils at 113·5° C. (236° F.), while chloral hydrate crystals melt at 48°–49° C. (118.4°–120·2° F.), and boil at 97·5° C. (207° F.); chloral alcoholate melts without complete solution when warmed with two volumes of water, and, on cooling, congeals below the surface of the water, while chloral hydrate is soluble in one and one-half times its weight of water; chloral alcoholate, gently heated with nitric acid of 1·2 sp. gr., is violently attacked, while chloral hydrate is scarcely acted on; chloral-alcoholate, heated on platinum foil, inflames readily, while chloral hydrate scarcely burns. (Allen, *Commerc. Org. Analysis*, 2d ed., i. p. 172.)

The three forms of chloral, the *anhydrous*, the polymeric *meta-chloral*, and the *alcoholate*, described above, have been more or less introduced into the European markets, and have required some notice to prevent them from being confounded with the hydrate, which is alone officinal. The following observations will be confined to this compound; and the reader will note that whether the simple term chloral, or the exact designation, hydrate of chloral, is used, the same substance is intended.

Properties of Hydrate of Chloral, or Chloral, *U. S.* This results from simply mixing anhydrous chloral with water. Acicular crystals soon form, which consist of a molecule each of the chloral and water, constituting hydrate of chloral, or officinal chloral. As employed in the United States, this comes, we believe, exclusively from Europe, and chiefly from Germany, with the exception of that produced by Dr. E. R. Squibb, of Brooklyn. It occurs in commerce mainly in two forms, in distinct crystals, which is the officinal form, or in crystalline plates, about three lines in thickness, broken into small, irregular, angular pieces, so as to be readily introduced into broad-mouthed bottles. These pieces, while retaining their tabular form, are somewhat translucent, but usually covered with a white powder, which somewhat conceals that property. This is the more common form and the cheaper; but the crystals are to be preferred, as their purity may be relied on. Chloral is

* Page states that a larger yield of chloral will be obtained if the alcohol used in its preparation be treated first with 5 per cent. of ferric chloride or thallium chloride. (*Amer. Drug.*, 1885, p. 44.)

white, of a peculiar pungent odor, and an acrid pungent taste, especially affecting the velum pendulum. The odor has been compared to that of an over-ripe melon. Exposed to the air it very slowly volatilizes, and, like camphor, when enclosed in a bottle, covers the interior surface with numerous minute crystallizations. The boiling point of the pure crystals, obtained from their solution in bisulphide of carbon, is 97·5° C. (207° F.). If the boiling point be under 95° C., it indicates an under-hydrated preparation; if above 98° C., an over-hydrated one. (E. R. Squibb.) The pure hydrate does not take fire when heated in a spoon, but evaporates without residue. With the aid of heat, its solution may be effected readily in chloroform; and the solution, on cooling, deposits it in beautiful crystals, which are generally needle-shaped; but, when deposited from bisulphide of carbon, they are prisms. The watery solution is prone to decomposition, which is ultimately attended with the development of algæ. Chloral should not, therefore, be kept long in this state. (Dr. E. Labbée, *Arch. Gén.*, Sept. 1870, p. 31.) In its relation to acids and alkalies it is neutral, or, according to E. Schering, slightly acid when perfectly pure. When equal parts of chloral in crystals and of camphor in small fragments are shaken together in a bottle, and allowed to stand, they liquefy, forming a clear solution. When chloral and sulphuric acid are mixed, the temperature is greatly reduced. A solution of chloral hydrate dissolves morphine, quinine, and most of the vegetable alkaloids. (R. F. Fairthorne, *A. J. P.*, Oct. 1871, p. 447.) When ammonium sulphide is added to an aqueous solution of chloral hydrate, the mixture rapidly turns yellow, and, after passing through several shades of color, finally becomes dark brown. From this liquid diluted sulphuric acid throws down a bulky brown precipitate. This, purified from precipitated sulphur and dried, is a light brown powder of the composition $C_{12}H_{24}S_{13}N_4O_6$. Hydrogen sulphide gas forms a sulphydrate by its action on chloral. These reactions are important, as the detection of metallic poisons in toxicological cases by hydrogen sulphide has been complicated by the presence of chloral hydrate. A still more important chemical reaction of chloral is that which takes place when the hydrate, or either of its other forms, is placed under the influence of an alkali. Chloroform is developed, and along with it a formate of the alkali employed. Thus, in a strong solution of potassa, put a pinch of powdered chloral, and almost instantly the odor of chloroform becomes sensible, and some oil-like globules of chloroform are visible at the bottom of the vessel. The reaction is as follows:

$$\underset{\text{Chloral hydrate}}{C_2HCl_3O,H_2O} + \underset{\text{potassium hydrate}}{KOH} = \underset{\text{chloroform}}{CHCl_3} + \underset{\text{potassium formate}}{CHO.OK} + \underset{\text{water}}{H_2O.}$$

This relation of chloral to chloroform would serve as a ready test of the former, and may be used also to determine its quality; for pure hydrate of chloral ought by calculation to yield 76·35 per cent. of chloroform, and the best known yields, according to the table of Mason, 71·5 (72·20 Selden) per cent. If, therefore, the product of chloroform should fall much below the latter percentage, the parcel acted on is probably impure. For other methods of assaying chloral hydrate, see Allen, *Com. Org. Analysis*, i. pp. 174 and 175. When blood is agitated with chloral, it produces the same change, and the smell of chloroform becomes sensible after a time; and Richardson was able to collect a certain quantity by distillation. (*Labbée.*) Important pathological inferences have been drawn from this result. The following tests of purity are given in the U. S. Pharmacopœia. "Separate, rhomboidal, colorless, and transparent crystals, slowly evaporating when exposed to the air, having an aromatic, penetrating, and slightly acrid odor, a bitterish, caustic taste, and a neutral reaction. Freely soluble in water, alcohol, or ether; also soluble in four parts of chloroform, in glycerin, benzol, benzin, disulphide of carbon, fixed or volatile oils. It liquefies when mixed with carbolic acid or with camphor. Its aqueous solution soon acquires an acid reaction, but its alcoholic solution remains neutral. At about 58° C. (136° F.), it melts to a clear liquid of sp. gr. 1·575, which solidifies to a crystalline mass at a temperature between 35° and 50° C. (95° and 122° F.). At about 78° C. (172° F.) it begins to yield vapors of water and of anhydrous chloral, and it boils at 95° C. (203° F.). When dissolved in water and treated, while hot, with solution of potassa or of soda, or with water of ammonia, a vaporous, milky mixture of chloroform is obtained, with a formate in solution. If the addition of the water of ammonia be made in a test-tube, after adding a few drops of test-solution of nitrate of silver, a silver mirror will be obtained upon the glass. An aqueous solution, treated with test-solution of sulphide of ammonium, gives a reddish-brown precipitate. Chloral should be dry, and should not readily attract moisture in ordinarily dry air;* when dissolved in diluted alcohol it should not redden blue litmus paper (abs. of acids), nor be precipitated upon addition of a few drops of nitric acid, and of test-solution of nitrate of silver (abs. of hydrochloric acid). Warmed in contact with an equal volume of sulphuric acid, it liquefies, but should not blacken; and, when vaporized by heat, no residue should remain. It should not dissolve in less than 4 times its weight of chloroform at 15° C. (59° F.), (difference from alcoholate). A portion, in a test-tube, containing a fragment of broken glass, held in water nearly boiling should boil at about 97° C. (206·6° F.) (difference from alcoholate, which boils at 115° C. (239° F.), and evidence of due hydration). If 1 Gm. be dissolved in 2 C.c. of distilled water, the solution warmed, and about 8 C.c. (or a slight excess) of solution of potassa added, the mixture filtered clear through wet filter paper, and the filtrate treated with test-solution of iodine until it is yellowish, no yellow, crystalline precipitate (iodoform) should appear, even after standing half an hour (abs. of alcoholate of chloral)." *U. S.*

Medical Properties and Uses. When chloral is ingested in full therapeutic dose (from 15 to 30 grains), it produces in from ten minutes to half an hour a quiet, placid sleep, which usually continues about three hours, when it ceases, generally without any unpleasant symptom during its progress, or after its termination. In some instances the ordinary doses fail to cause sleep, and in others the sleep is attended with dreams and hallucinations, and followed by unpleasant symptoms, like those which often succeed other hypnotics, especially opium; such as nausea, headache, unpleasant nervous disorder, etc. These diversities may be ascribed in part to peculiarity of constitution; but more frequently, in all probability, they are owing to morbid conditions existing at the time, which oppose themselves to the proper action of the choral. In an individual in health chloral will probably almost always induce a calm sleep, differing little from the natural. Moreover, these unpleasant symptoms are now much more rarely produced than formerly, and there can be but little doubt that they have often been due to impurities in the drug. The pulse is in this degree of action not affected, or is rendered a little slower; the pupil is contracted, but becomes normal so soon as the subject is awakened; the respiration is deep, full, and regular. When larger amounts are given, the sleep is much deeper, and may pass into profound coma; the respirations fall in number; the pulse is weakened and rendered slower, but may become rapid and irregular if the dose has been toxic; the temperature is reduced; the muscular system is relaxed, and both sensibility and reflex action are diminished. If a fatal dose has been given, all these symptoms are intensified: with coma, intense muscular relaxation, weak, thready pulse, and a pupil contracted at first, but afterwards dilated, the victim gradually sinks into death, paralyzed and anæsthetic. The immediate cause of death is generally a paralytic arrest of respiration; but in many cases there appears to be a simultaneous arrest of the cardiac action, and it is very possible that fatal syncope may at times occur. At post-mortem examination, congestion of the meninges and substance of the brain and cord, and of the lungs, is commonly found. The blood is thought by Richardson (*Med. Times and Gaz.*, Sept. 4, 1870) to coagulate less firmly than normal.

After the brain the motor tract of the spinal cord, including the respiratory centre, is most sensitive to the action of chloral. The loss of voluntary muscular power and the lessening of reflex activity which the drug produces, are the result of this spinal influence. Upon the sensory tract of the cord chloral acts with much less vigor, while the nerves and muscles practically escape its influence. Of course any

* M. Guerin adds his testimony to the necessity for only dispensing chloral hydrate which has been recrystallized and which is in the form of distinct crystals. He examined many samples, and found acidity in the cake variety, due, as he believes, to the formation of hydrochloric and formic acids, produced by the action of water retained in the cake during the manufacture, and this remaining in contact with the confused mass of crystals excites decomposition. (*Archiv d. Pharm.* 1886, p. 253.)

agent which produces sleep in some measure relieves pain, but the anæsthetic influence of chloral is far from pronounced, and often patients on waking will complain bitterly of pain suffered during sleep.

The physiological action of chloral may be summed up as follows. Upon the cerebrum it acts as a most powerful and certain hypnotic; in full doses it acts as an intense depressant upon the centres at the base of the brain, and upon the spinal cord, causing slowing and weakness of the heart's action, probably vaso-motor paralysis, slowing of the respiration, and muscular weakness, lessening of reflex activity, with a certain amount of anæsthesia; in fatal doses it causes death generally by arresting respiration through paralysis of the nerve-centres, and finally stopping the heart in diastole. Its action in very small doses is uncertain, but there is considerable evidence to indicate that it irritates or stimulates the spinal and the cardiac, and even the vaso-motor, centres. On the vagi and on the motor nerve trunks it has no marked influence. Clinical experience indicates that chloral acts as a depressant to the heart-muscle; although some authorities believe the influence of the drug upon the heart is not direct, but exerted through the nerve-centres. Chloral has little effect on the secretions, though it is said somewhat to increase the secretion of urine. In man, it is stated by Bouchut that, in accordance with his observations, this secretion is not only increased, but has been found also augumented in density; at the same time reducing the cupro-potassic liquor, and rendered brown by potassa or subnitrate of bismuth; as if a temporary glycosuria were produced. Formic acid has never been found in the urine as a result of the taking of chloral. (*Arch. Gén.*, Sept. 1870, p. 346.)

Action as Chloral. The conversion of chloral by alkalies in solution into chloroform and formic acid first suggested its use in medicine to Liebreich (*Wiener Medizinische Wochenschrift*, August, 1869); and the theory that its action is really due to chloroform generated by the alkalinity of the blood has been received with favor by Personne and other writers, but there are very many facts which militate against the truth of this supposition. Thus chloroform cannot be detected either in the blood, breath, or excretions of chloralized animals, although chloroform at once manifests itself when it is administered, and in the so-called "salt frogs" of Cohnheim, after substitution of warm salt water for the blood of the animal, chloral acts as upon the normal batrachian.

Chloral, especially when used continuously, is said to produce in some individuals serious disturbances. Such are vaso-motor paralysis, transient skin neurosis, acute purpura, and great prostration of the heart's action, sometimes amounting to paralysis of that organ; and sometimes ending fatally, even though the doses of the chloral used were within the limits ordinarily deemed safe. For a full discussion of these phenomena, see H. C. Wood's *Therapeutics*. Dr. Hawkes, though a strong advocate for the use of chloral, has found it repeatedly prejudicial in the general paralysis of mania and in elderly persons with feeble circulation and impaired nutrition. There can be no doubt that great caution should be practised in administering the drug when the heart is very weak, or the general powers much enfeebled. Dr. Jolly relates two cases in which 5 grammes (about 76 grains), given every night, caused death, in one case after the fifth dose, and, in the second, after the thirteenth, without abnormal symptoms until after the last dose, when the action of the heart and respiration suddenly ceased, and the patient died. (*New York Med. Journ.*, Nov. 1872.) These cases would appear to justify the statement that there is a possible cumulative action of the drug. Although 480 grains have been recovered from, Dr. Fuller has recorded a case in which a single dose of thirty grains proved fatal in a young lady, and two others in which the same quantity caused alarming symptoms in similar circumstances; so that the highest dose to begin with in ordinary diseases, especially in delicate women, should not exceed twenty grains. In poisoning by chloral, if the case be seen early, the stomach should be thoroughly evacuated by an emetic or the stomach-pump, and the system afterwards supported by cardiac and respiratory stimulants, as milk punch, carbonate of ammonium, etc. Atropine, digitalis, and strychnine should be administered freely, and the same general measures taken to sustain the respiration as are usually practised in opium poisoning. Atropine is undoubtedly of value when there is failure of respiration, and care should always be taken to maintain the bodily temperature. Artificial respiration should be practised when necessary. Care also should be exercised to maintain the bodily temperature by external heat. Dr. Liebreich recommends strychnine as an antidote; having found that poisonous doses of the two substances, introduced into the same animal, neutralize each other's operation, and no serious effect ensues.

From what has been said it will be readily perceived that the two great indications for this remedy are to procure sleep and to relax spasm. In pure nervous insomnia, and in the same affection attendant on other diseases, as in acute fevers, active congestion of the brain, cerebral inflammation, mania, delirium tremens, etc., it is superior to opium; fifteen to twenty or twenty-five grains (1–1·3 or 1·565 Gm.) are generally sufficient for a commencing dose, to be repeated in half the quantity in an hour, if the first dose fail. The sleep is usually calm and undisturbed for three or four hours, and may be renewed, if required, by the repetition of the dose. When the sleeplessness is due to pain, opium is much more effective than chloral. The combination of chloral and morphia is often very useful in procuring sleep for the suffering. As an anæsthetic, chloral should never be employed; the intravenous use of it as practised to some extent in France is most dangerous and absolutely unjustifiable. In spasmodic affections chloral is one of the most powerful remedies known. In tetanus and in strychnine poisoning it is singularly useful, but must be given in very large doses. In hysteria, severe chorea, and other functional or spinal convulsions, it is no less efficient. In epilepsy and other forms of cerebral convulsions chloral is of less service, although it is frequently employed with benefit in puerperal convulsions. In local spasms it is often of service, and has been used with success in strangulated hernia, spasm of the glottis, spasmodic croup, asthma, hiccough, and even in incontinence of urine. Chloral is possessed of very decided antiseptic properties; a solution of the strength of 30 grains to the ounce will preserve animal tissues for a long time. Locally applied, chloral is stimulating and antiseptic, and may occasionally be used with very good results in the treatment of foul sores, irritable ulcers, etc., which need stimulation. The solution may vary from five to thirty-one grains to the ounce, according to the exigencies of the case. Dr. A. M. Fauntleroy states that if powdered chloral be sprinkled on adhesive plaster and the whole heated sufficiently to adhere to the skin, and applied whilst warm, there is produced an increasing burning, and in about ten minutes a blister is formed.

Pharmaceutical Preparations. Chloral is best administered in solution with syrup of orange flowers, or in simple solution. The French sometimes employ *chloral cream*, made of chloral hydrate 5 parts, water 15 parts, white sugar finely powdered 100 parts, flavored with mint, orange, or vanilla. One grain of chloral is contained in 24 grains of the cream, and a teaspoonful is equivalent to about 3 grains of chloral. This preparation keeps well, and the dose may be dissolved in a little water. *Chloral liniment* may be made by dissolving 6 parts of chloral in 30 parts oil of sweet almonds. *Chloral ointment*, 6 parts chloral, 3 parts white wax, 27 parts lard; the lard and wax are melted at a gentle heat, the chloral added in powder and dissolved. (See *Chloral Camphoratum*, Part II.) *Chloral plaster*, to produce counter-irritant effects, is prepared by spreading powdered chloral on Burgundy pitch plaster.

CHLOROFORMUM PURIFICATUM. *U.S.* *Purified Chloroform.*

$CHCl_3$; 119·2. (CHLŌ-RO-FŌR'MŬM PŪ-RI-FI-CĀ'TŬM.) C_2HCl_3; 119·2.

Chloroformum, *Br.;* Chloroformium, *P.G.;* Formylum Trichloratum; Chloroforme pur, *Fr.;* Reines Chloroform, *G.*

"Commercial Chloroform, *two hundred parts* [or seventy fluidounces]; Sulphuric Acid, *forty parts* [or eleven and a half fluidounces]; Carbonate of Sodium, *ten parts* [or five ounces av.]; Lime, in coarse powder, *one part* [or half an ounce av.]; Alcohol, *two parts* [or two and a quarter fluidounces]; Water, *twenty parts* [or ten fluidounces]. Add the Acid to the Chloroform and shake them together, occasionally, during twenty-four hours. Separate the lighter liquid and add to it the Carbonate of Sodium previously dissolved in the water. Agitate the mixture thoroughly for half an hour and set it aside; then separate the Chloroform from the supernatant layer, mix it with the Alcohol, transfer it to a dry retort, add the Lime, and, taking care that the temperature in the retort does not rise above 67·2° C. (153° F.), distil, by means of a water-bath, into a well-cooled receiver, until the residue in the retort is reduced to *two parts* [or six fluidrachms]. Keep the product in glass-stoppered bottles, in a cool and dark place." *U. S.*

"Take of Chlorinated Lime *ten pounds* [avoirdupois]; Rectified Spirit *thirty fluidounces* [Imperial measure]; Slaked Lime *a sufficiency;* Water *three gallons* [Imp. meas.]; Sulphuric Acid *a sufficiency;* Chloride of Calcium, in small fragments, *two ounces* [av.]; Quick Lime *half an ounce;* Distilled Water *nine fluidounces* [Imp. meas.]; Ethylic Alcohol *a sufficiency*. Place the Water and the Spirit in a capacious still, and raise the mixture to the temperature of 100° F. (37°·8 C.). Add the Chlorinated Lime and five pounds [av.] of the Slaked Lime, mixing thoroughly. Connect the still with a condensing worm encompassed by cold water, and terminating in a narrow-necked receiver; and apply heat so as to cause distillation, taking care to withdraw the fire the moment that the process is well established. When the distilled product measures fifty ounces, the receiver is to be withdrawn. Pour its contents into a gallon [Imp. meas.] bottle half filled with Water, mix well by shaking, and set at rest for a few minutes, when the mixture will separate into two strata of different densities. Let the lower stratum, which constitutes crude chloroform, be washed by agitating it in a bottle with three [fluid]ounces of the Distilled Water. Allow the Chloroform to subside, withdraw the water, and repeat the washing with the rest of the Distilled Water, in successive quantities of three [fluid]-ounces at a time. Agitate the washed Chloroform for five minutes in a bottle with an equal volume of pure Sulphuric Acid, allow the mixture to settle, and transfer the upper stratum of liquid to a bottle containing a little alkaline water. After agitation transfer the chloroform to a dry bottle containing the Chloride of Calcium mixed with half an ounce of Quick Lime. Mix well by agitation. After the lapse of an hour decant the chloroform into a flask, connect the flask with a Liebig's condenser, and distil over the Pure Chloroform by means of a water-bath. Add one per cent. by weight of Ethylic Alcohol. Preserve the product in a cool place, in a bottle furnished with an accurately ground stopper.

"The lighter liquid which floats on the Crude Chloroform after its agitation with water, and the washings with distilled water, should be preserved, and employed in a subsequent operation." *Br.*

In the U. S. Pharmacopœia of 1850 a process was given for preparing chloroform; but as this is never made on a small scale by the apothecary, but purchased of the manufacturer, it was very properly transferred, at the next revision, to the Materia Medica Catalogue. But, as the chloroform of commerce is often impure, and, though fitted for external use, and for various pharmaceutical purposes, is, in this impure state, unfit for use as a respiratory anæsthetic agent, it was deemed advisable to introduce a formula by which its purification, if required, might be readily effected. This process is the first of those above given. The process of the British Pharmacopœia is for the preparation of the chloroform *ab initio*, with directions which secure its purity if complied with. In this process, the reaction by which the chloroform is produced takes place between the chlorinated lime and the alcohol; the slaked lime, which is added in accordance with the directions in the late Dublin Pharmacopœia, being intended probably to lessen the production of the chlorinated pyrogenous oil, the amount of which is greater, according to Soubeiran and Mialhe, in proportion to the relative excess of the chlorine to the lime employed. The use of this earth is stated by some chemists to give rise to Dutch liquid, or ethene chloride, $C_2H_4Cl_2$, and to increase the product at the expense of its purity.* As first distilled, the chloroform is very impure, and is directed to be washed first with ordinary water, and afterwards with distilled water, which separate alcohol, chlorine, and probably

* According to Gehe & Co. (June, 1881), the yield of pure chloroform is nearly 8 per cent. of the amount of chloride of lime used; this being the average product during several months' manufacture of chloroform.

other contaminating substances. In consequence of the density of the chloroform and its insolubility in water, it readily subsides, forming a distinct layer which may be easily separated. The crude product, after having been freed from alcohol by the washing with water, is purified from the chlorinated pyrogenous oil, which comes over with the chloroform, by agitation with an equal volume of sulphuric acid, which ought to be *pure* and *colorless*, and at least of the density 1·840. The oil is charred and destroyed by the acid, which becomes yellow or reddish brown, and is partially changed into sulphurous acid. To remove the latter acid, as well as any water present, the chloroform, which floats on the surface of the acid, is removed and agitated well with chloride of calcium and quick lime, then again submitted to distillation, and one per cent. of absolute alcohol added to preserve the chloroform from decomposition. According to Gregory and Kemp, of Edinburgh, by whom the use of sulphuric acid for this purpose was proposed, chloroform is effectually purified from the pyrogenous oil by agitation with this acid if strong and pure. So long as a ring, darker than the rest of the acid, appears, after rest, at the line of contact between the acid and the chloroform, the agitation must be repeated; and the oil is known to be fully separated when the acid remains colorless. Black oxide of manganese has been employed to separate the sulphurous acid; but, in this case, the chloroform is apt to become, after the lapse of a few weeks, of a delicate pink color, which sometimes disappears and then returns. This coloration depends upon the presence of manganese, and forms an objection to the use of the black oxide as a purifier.

In the U. S. process the method of purification is somewhat different. Instead of equal measures of the impure chloroform and sulphuric acid and an agitation for only 5 minutes, the commercial chloroform is shaken occasionally for 24 hours with but one-fifth of its weight of the acid. To remove any water and acid that may be present, instead of chloride of calcium and lime, a little stronger alcohol is mixed with the chloroform in a dry retort, and then lime in coarse powder is added, and the mixture is distilled to dryness.

It sometimes happens that the chloroform purified with sulphuric acid, though apparently pure at first, will not keep, but, after some time, becomes so loaded with chlorine and hydrochloric acid as to be altogether unfit for respiration. Dr. Christison ascertained that, if the sulphuric acid employed contain hyponitric acid, the chloroform changes in less than 24 hours. The idea has been entertained that it would be necessary to abandon sulphuric acid as a purifying agent; but experience has shown that, with certain precautions, it may be safely used; and its efficiency in getting rid of the empyreumatic impurity is so great that it is still much employed for the purpose. The British Council endeavors to escape the difficulty by using a large quantity of the acid, and allowing but very brief contact; while in the U. S. process the same end is arrived at by employing a comparatively small quantity of the acid, with a much longer period for its operation. In any case, however, the acid should be strong and pure, and especially free from any of the nitrogen acids; and care should afterwards be taken to remove every particle of the sulphuric or sulphurous acid, as is done in the officinal processes, by lime and carbonate of sodium. Dr. Squibb attributes the fact, that chloroform purified by concentrated sulphuric acid does not keep well, to the very purity attained. He believes that perfectly pure chloroform is prone to decomposition, and is rendered more stable by the addition of a small proportion of alcohol, so as to reduce its density to the officinal standard, 1·49. This he effects by adding alcohol in the proportion of ten drops to each fluidounce of good chloroform of maximum density. This recommendation is carried into effect in the U. S. process, and explains the addition of alcohol before distillation. Dr. Gregory also attributes the tendency to decomposition to its purity, and to the action of sunlight; having found that those portions which he had purified with the greatest care were soonest decomposed under the influence of light.

As chloroform of great purity is *usually* to be purchased in the market, it is not necessary for the pharmacist to apply the officinal process of purification to every parcel that he may meet; but it is in the highest degree incumbent on him to sell none for inhalation which is not so pure as to stand the tests given in the Pharmacopœia, and if he can obtain none so pure, then to purify it himself. All pure specimens, moreover, should be kept distinct, and labelled with the officinal title of Purified Chloroform, for the sake of distinction.

The intermediate formation of chloral as a result of the reaction between alcohol and chlorinated lime suggested the preparation of chloroform from chloral, which has of late years been produced in immense quantities. The advantages which were anticipated by decomposing pure chloral hydrate with alkalies have not altogether been realized, for the product is much more expensive, and the claim of greater stability has not been sustained, as it requires just as much alcohol to preserve it as that made in the usual way.

Chloroform is now made on a large scale both in this country and in Germany by the distillation of acetone with chlorinated lime: indeed, this process has latterly almost entirely replaced the manufacture from alcohol. Liebig, as long ago as 1832, described the reaction, but it was thought to be not adapted for commercial use. In 1882 the manufacture was begun on a commercial scale at Mannheim, Germany, and since June, 1885, in this country. In July, 1885, a patent was taken out by G. Michaelis, of Albany, for the manufacture of chloroform from the liquid products resulting from the decomposition of crude acetates at high temperatures. These liquid products are acetone and other higher ketones. The purified chloroform from acetone has a small quantity of alcohol added to prevent decomposition and bring it to Pharmacopœia requirements. Pure methyl alcohol, on the other hand, does not yield chloroform. The erroneous statements on this point generally current are probably due to the fact that commercial wood spirit contains a large percentage of acetone.

Damoiseau (*Comptes-Rendus*, vol. xcii. p. 42, 1881; *N. R.*, 1881, p. 71) describes a new method of making chloroform, by passing chlorine, mixed with the proper proportion of methyl chloride, through a long tube containing animal charcoal, heated from 250° C. to 350° C. (482° F. to 662° F.).

Pettenkofer inferred, from numerous experiments on the manufacture of chloroform, that very different quantities are obtained, on different occasions, from the same amount of materials, and the same process. The yield is less, the longer the mixture is allowed to stand before distillation, and is greater when the heat of the mixture is between 57·2° C. (135° F.) and 75° C. (167° F.) than at either a lower or higher temperature. When the latter degree is exceeded, the chloroform contains more chlorine. (*Buchner's Neues Repert.*, x. 103.)

Discovery and History. Chloroform was discovered by Mr. Samuel Guthrie, of Sackett's Harbor, N. Y., in 1831, and about the same time by Soubeiran in France, and Liebig in Germany. Guthrie obtained it by distilling a gallon from a mixture of three pounds of chlorinated lime and two gallons of alcohol of the sp. gr. 0·844, and rectifying the product by redistillation, first from a great excess of chlorinated lime, and afterwards from carbonate of potassium. (*Silliman's Journal*, vol. xxi., Jan. 1832, p. 64.) In a subsequent letter to Professor Silliman, dated Feb. 15, 1832, Mr. Guthrie states that the substance which he had obtained, "distilled off sulphuric acid, has the specific gravity of 1·486, or a little greater, and may then be regarded as free from alcohol; and if a little sulphuric acid which sometimes contaminates it be removed by washing it with a strong solution of carbonate of potassium, it may then be regarded as *absolutely pure*." (*Ibid.*, vol. xxii., July, 1832, p. 105.) It is thus evident that Mr. Guthrie obtained, in a pure state, the substance now called chloroform; but he erroneously supposed his product to be the well-known oily liquid of the Dutch chemists, which it greatly resembles, and for the preparation of which he believed he had fallen on a cheap and easy process. Under this impression, he called the substance, in his communications, *chloric ether*, one of the names by which *Dutch liquid*, or *Ethene dichloride*, is designated. He was induced to make the preparation from noticing, in Professor Silliman's Elements of Chemistry, a reference to the Dutch liquid as a grateful diffusible stimulant, when properly diluted with alcohol and water.

Properties. Chloroform is "a heavy, clear, colorless, diffusive liquid, of a characteristic, pleasant, ethereal odor, a burning, sweet taste, and a neutral reaction. Soluble in about 200 parts of water, and, in all proportions, in alcohol or ether; also in benzol, benzin, fixed or volatile oils. Sp. gr. 1·485–1·490 at 15° C. (59°

F.). It boils at 60° to 61° C. (140° to 142° F.), corresponding to the presence of three-fourths (¾) to one (1) per cent. of alcohol." *U. S.* According to Remys (*Archiv der Pharm.*, 3, v. 31), pure chloroform has the sp. gravity of 1·500 at 15° C. (59° F.). Besnou gives the densities of various mixtures of alcohol and the purest commercial chloroform at 4·5° C. (40° F.) as follows:

Specific Gravity.	Chloroform, per cent.	Alcohol, per cent.	Specific Gravity.	Chloroform, per cent.	Alcohol, per cent.
1·4945	100·0	0·0	1·4772	97·5	2·5
1·4908	99·5	0·5	1·4602	95·0	5·0
1·4874	99·0	1·0	1·4262	90·0	10·0
1·4845	98·5	1·5	1·4090	87·5	12·5

When pure, it has no action on potassium, except to cover the surface of the metal with small bubbles of gas. Chloroform is a powerful antiseptic. It does not, like creasote, coagulate albumen. It is scarcely acted on by sulphuric acid in the cold, but dissolves readily in alcohol and ether. The alcoholic solution, when moderately diluted with water, forms an aromatic, saccharine liquid of a very grateful taste. A strong alcoholic solution is decomposed by abundance of water, the chloroform separating and subsiding, and the alcohol uniting with the water. It is liable to decomposition by sunlight, or even diffused daylight; and hence the propriety of keeping it in bottles, covered with dark paper, in a rather dark place. Chloroform has extensive solvent powers, being capable of dissolving caoutchouc, gutta-percha, mastic, elemi, tolu, benzoin, and copal. Amber, sandarac, lac, and wax are only partially soluble. It also dissolves iodine, bromine, the organic alkalies, the fixed and volatile oils, most resins, and fats. It dissolves sulphur and phosphorus sparingly. It possesses the power of dissolving a large quantity of camphor, and furnishes the means of administering that medicine in an elegant form. As a general solvent, it has the advantage over ether of not being inflammable; the inflammability of the latter being the cause of frequent accidents. For an extensive list of substances, soluble, insoluble, and partly soluble in chloroform, see a paper by M. Lepage, of Gisors, France, copied into *A. J. P.*, 1852, p. 147.* It has been found by J. B. Barnes that chloroform has the power of preventing the alcoholic, lactic, and other fermentations, probably by killing the organisms that provoke these processes. Twenty minims preserved sixteen ounces of malt, to which two drachms of yeast had been added, as long as the experiment lasted. The same quantity kept fresh eight fluidounces of milk in a warm place for five days. Mucilage and infusions were preserved for weeks with one minim or even less to the ounce. Similar results were reached by Mr. F. J. Barrett and others. (*P. J. Tr.*, 1874, pp. 441, 442, 455.) The active properties of chloroform forbid its use as a preservative of medicinal infusions, but from milk it could always be removed by boiling. A. Muns (*P. J. Tr.*, 1875, p. 967) proposes the employment of chloroform as a test between chemical and living ferments, since he has found it to have no effect upon the former, though absolutely destructive to the latter.

Composition. Chloroform is composed of one atom of carbon, one of hydrogen, and three of chlorine. Its simplest derivation in theory is from marsh-gas (*methane*), CH_4, whence it is often called *trichloro-methane.* While it can be thus produced, by the action of chlorine upon marsh-gas, in practice, it is formed either

* The following table of the solubility of the several alkaloids and their salts in chloroform, prepared with great care by A. Schlimpert, may be of some practical use. At 17·7° C. (64° F.) 100 parts of chloroform dissolve

Morphine	1·66	Sulphate of cinchonine	3·00	Caffeine	11·00
Acetate of morphine	1·66	Chinoidine	25·30	Digitaline	1·25
Quinine	15·00	Veratrine	11·60	Brucine	14·00
Sulphate of quinine	0·00	Atropine	33·00	Aconitine	22·00
Hydrochlorate of quinine	11·10	Strychnine	14·10	Santonin, pure	23·00
Cinchonine	2·50	Nitrate of strychnine	6·60	Santonin, impure	33·30

(*A. J. P.*, 1860, p. 160; from *Archiv de Pharm.*, Nov. 1859, p. 151.)

from alcohol by the action of bleaching-powder, from chloral by an alkaline hydrate, or latterly from acetone and bleaching powder.

The reactions are sometimes complex, but if the temperature be carefully kept at from 70° C. (158° F.) to 73° C. (163·4° F.), they are essentially as follows:

$$C_2H_6O + CaOCl_2 = CaCl_2 + C_2H_4O + H_2O;$$

that is, one molecule of bleaching-powder, reacting with one of alcohol, yields one of calcium chloride, one of aldehyd, and one of water. The aldehyd formed is then further decomposed according to the reaction:

$$2(C_2H_4O) + 6(CaOCl_2) = 3CaCl_2 + 3Ca(OH)_2 + 2(C_2HCl_3O);$$

that is, two molecules of aldehyd, reacting with six of bleaching-powder, yield three of calcium chloride, three of calcium hydrate, and two of chloral. The chloral is, however, decomposed by the free base calcium hydrate according to the reaction:

$$2(C_2HCl_3O) + Ca(OH)_2 = Ca(CHO_2)_2 + 2(CHCl_3);$$

that is, two molecules of chloral, reacting with one of calcium hydrate, yield one of calcium formate and two of chloroform. The reaction for the manufacture from acetone is simpler:

$$2C_3H_6O + 3Ca(OCl)_2 = 2CHCl_3 + 2Ca(OH)_2 + Ca(C_2H_3O_2)_2.$$

Impurities and Tests. Chloroform is liable to contain alcohol and ether, both of which lower its specific gravity. If it have a less density than 1·38, it will float instead of sinking in a mixture of equal weights of concentrated sulphuric acid and water, after it has cooled. M. Mialhe has proposed the following test for the presence of alcohol. Drop into distilled water a small quantity of the chloroform. If pure, it will remain transparent at the bottom of the glass; but, if it contain even a small proportion of alcohol, the globules will acquire a milky appearance. Soubeiran's method was to agitate almond oil and chloroform together in a tube. If the chloroform be pure, it remains clear; if it contain as much as 5 or 6 per cent. of alcohol, it becomes milky. (*Journ. de Pharm.*, Août, 1860, p. 95.) Prof. Procter detected alcohol by adding the suspected chloroform to an oxidizing mixture of bichromate of potassium and sulphuric acid. If alcohol be present, the deep orange color of the chromic mixture will gradually become green; if absent, no change of color will take place. (*A. J. P.*, 1856, p. 213.) Hoffmann's violet has been recently suggested as a test. If a small portion is added to chloroform containing alcohol, the solution is colored a deep purple. Boettger recommends adding to the chloroform a solution of molybdic acid in pure, strong sulphuric acid, when even a trace of alcohol will cause an intense blue color. (1879.) A. C. Oudemans, Jr., affirms that the percentage of alcohol may be correctly estimated by the power of the suspected liquid to dissolve cinchonine (*A. J. P.*, 1873, p. 223), and gives the table inserted in the note below.* The most injurious impurities are the chlorinated pyrogenous oils, already alluded to. These are different as obtained from methylic or normal chloroform. The oil, obtained by Soubeiran and Mialhe from methylic chloroform, is an oleaginous, yellow liquid, lighter than water, and of a peculiar nauseous empyreumatic odor, perceptible in the methylic chloroform itself. In commercial chloroform it is sometimes present to the amount of 6 per cent. It is easily set on fire, and burns with a smoky flame, chlorine being among the products of its combustion. The oil procured from normal chloroform, which contains it in the amount of about one-fifth

* Percentage of Alcohol.	Percentage of Cinchonine by weight, at 17° C.	Difference between it and pure Chloroform.	Percentage of Alcohol.	Percentage of Cinchonine by weight, at 17° C.	Difference between it and pure Chloroform.
0	0·28	0	6	3·39	40
1	0·90	62	7	3·79	36
2	1·46	56	8	4·15	33
3	1·99	53	9	4·48	28
4	2·49	47	10	4·76	...
5	2·96	43	11	......	...

The cinchonine is best prepared by precipitating a weak alcoholic solution of a pure salt of the alkaloid by ammonia.

of 1 per cent. only, is essentially different from the methylic chloroform oil. It is heavier than water, and has an acrid, penetrating odor, unlike that of the other oil. When the vapor of these oils is inspired or even smelt, it causes, according to Dr. Gregory, distressing sickness and headache. These pyrogenous oils are detected and removed by *pure* and *strong* sulphuric acid. Chloroform, when pure, upon being mixed with an equal volume of this acid, does not color it; but, when contaminated with these oils, gives the acid a color, varying from yellow to reddish brown, according to the amount of impurity. Alcohol also is detected and removed by sulphuric acid. In applying this test, several fluidounces of chloroform should be used; as a slight change of color cannot be easily seen in a test-tube, and care must be taken to see that mechanical impurities like cork-dust, dirt, etc., have been filtered out of the specimen, or the acid will be discolored from this cause. A still more delicate test of the oily impurities, according to Dr. Gregory, is the smell which they leave. If chloroform, thus contaminated, be poured upon the hand, it quickly evaporates, leaving the oily impurities, recognizable by their offensive odor, now no longer covered by that of the chloroform. The pure substance, rubbed on the skin, quickly evaporates, and leaves scarcely any smell. Chloroform sometimes contains Dutch liquid, which may be discovered by adding an alcoholic solution of potassa; when the mixture, if this impurity be present, will heat and give off a permanent gas, which is *acetyl chloride*, C_2H_3OCl. (*Geuther.*)* Fuming nitric acid, heated with chloroform to 90° C. (194° F.) for 120 hours, forms a new substance, *chloropicrine*. (*Journ. de Pharm.*, 4e sér., xv.)

Certain conclusions of Prof. John M. Maisch upon the subject of chloroform, drawn from a series of practical and experimental observations, are worthy of notice. Chloroform may be made of the sp. gr. 1·5, or perhaps somewhat heavier, and this is its density when pure; but it will not keep so well as when of the officinal strength from 1·490 to 1·494. When pure, or even of the sp. gr. of about 1·49, it is quickly decomposed in direct sunlight, and more slowly in diffused daylight; and the presence of water, however small in quantity, favors the decomposition. The products of its decomposition are hydrochloric acid and phosgene gas. If, however, it be perfectly excluded from the light, it will keep indefinitely; Wiggers having preserved some, unaltered, for fifteen years. According to Schacht, moreover, pure chloroform will resist even sunlight, if in a perfect vacuum. To prevent the decomposition of chloroform the most effectual means is the addition of alcohol. If reduced by this to the sp. gr. 1·480 or 1·484, it will keep well in diffused daylight, and, for a time at least, even in the sun's rays, if perfectly free from moisture. At the sp. gr. 1·475 or lower, it remains unaffected whether in diffused light or in the sun, and whether the bottles be damp or dry. The measures, therefore, to secure chloroform from decomposition are two, either of which will answer; first, to keep it perfectly secluded from light, from the moment of rectification; or, secondly, to reduce the sp. gr. to 1·475 by alcohol, as suggested by Dr. Squibb. Sulphuric acid will not decompose chloroform in the dark; in the light it evolves hydrochloric acid. One of the best criteria of its purity is a constant boiling point. When of the sp. gr. 1·496, it boils at 67° C. (152·6° F.). A slight acid reaction in chloroform is not easily detected, as litmus is quite insoluble in that fluid. It is best observed by allowing a few drops of chloroform to evaporate spontaneously with one drop of an aqueous solution of litmus duly neutralized. The color will be changed to reddish. After becoming acid, chloroform may be readily regenerated, by agitating it with solution of carbonate of sodium, and distilling from a little unslaked lime. From what has been said above, chloroform to be kept for use should have the sp. gr. 1·475, and if denser than this, should be brought to it by the addition of alcohol. It is best kept in cork-stoppered bottles. As the cork is not acted on by chloroform, if it become yellow and softened, it will indicate the presence of an acid, and thus act as a test. (*A. J. P.*, 1868, p. 289.)

Boettger states that chloroform altered by the sun's rays, containing hydrochloric acid and having a chlorinous odor, may be restored and made fit for inhalation by

* In relation to chloroform, see the paper of Soubeiran and Mialhe, *Journ. de Pharm.*, July, 1849, copied into *A. J. P.*, xxi. 313; also the paper of Dr. Gregory, *Chem. Gaz.*, May 15, 1850.

agitation with a few fragments of caustic soda, and that the fluid may be kept exposed to light, if protected in the same way. (*Ibid.*, Sept. 1866, p. 473; from *Journ. de Pharm.*, Avril, 1864.) M. Jaillard (*Journ. de Pharm.*, 4, sér. xxii., p. 305) states that he has frequently found both hydrochloric and formic acids in chloroform exposed for sale. He employs nitrate of silver as a test, using an excess of the reagent; he filters out the precipitated chloride, and boils, when, if formic acid be present, black metallic silver is deposited.

Officinal Tests. The U. S. Pharmacopœia directs that "if 5 C.c. of Purified Chloroform be thoroughly agitated with 10 C.c. of distilled water, the latter, when separated, should not affect blue litmus paper (abs. of acids), nor test-solution of nitrate of silver (chloride), nor test-solution of iodide of potassium (free chlorine). If a portion be digested, warm, with solution of potassa, the latter should not become dark colored (abs. of aldehyde). On shaking 10 C.c. of the Chloroform with 5 C.c. of sulphuric acid, in a glass-stoppered bottle, and allowing them to remain in contact for twenty-four hours, no color should be imparted to either liquid. If a few C.c. be permitted to evaporate from blotting-paper, no foreign odor should be perceptible after the odor of Chloroform ceases to be recognized." *U. S.* These tests imply the presence of but a minute proportion of alcohol, and the total absence of chlorine and those volatile and empyreumatic substances which constitute the most injurious impurities of chloroform. A heat that would be felt through the bottle, on the admixture of sulphuric acid with chloroform, would evince the presence of too much alcohol or water. The want of discoloration from the contact of the two liquids shows the absence of empyreumatic oily matter; but a very slight discoloration might proceed from the alcohol present, and would not, therefore, be a material objection. A color bordering on that of madeira wine would imply an objectionable amount of impurities. The volatile impurities are less volatile than chloroform, and would consequently be the last to escape on the evaporation of the liquid. Impure chloroform, therefore, leaves a foreign odor behind it when allowed to evaporate from the hand, and especially when from a porcelain plate, in the amount and manner indicated; and if a specimen stand this test well, it may be considered as free from noxious volatile impurity. The slight foreign aroma without pungency, which is given out under these circumstances, is of no injurious significance. It is stated that chloroform made from chloral may be distinguished from other chloroform by its remaining colorless when the sulphuric acid test is employed, and by its leaving no aromatic residue when evaporated, evidences of its absolute purity. It has been claimed that this chloral chloroform does not undergo decomposition, but this has been proved not to be correct. (*A. J. P.*, xlii. 409.)

Medical Properties and Uses. Chloroform, when applied locally, is very irritant and produces decided pain, which may be followed by some numbness and local anæsthesia. If the chloroform be prevented from evaporating, its prolonged contact with the skin is apt to produce blistering. Taken internally, it is absorbed and acts upon the general system. The rapidity of its absorption, and, to some extent, its general effects, depend upon the method in which it is administered. It is commonly exhibited by the mouth or by inhalation. Taken into the stomach in doses of 15 to 25 drops (0·24–0·38 C.c.), it induces only gastric symptoms, chiefly due to its irritant properties; but when there is excessive flatulence, colic, or gastralgia, it not only causes an increased peristalsis and expulsion of any flatus present, but evinces a distinct local narcotic influence by quieting pain and spasm. Taken in doses of 1 to 2 fluidrachms (3·75–7·5 C.c.), it produces a narcotism similar to that seen when it is administered by inhalation, the narcotism, however, developing and passing off much more slowly than in the latter case. Chloroform, as prepared by Mr. Guthrie, was used internally as early as 1832 by Professor Ives and Dr. Nathan B. Ives, of New Haven, in asthma, spasmodic cough, scarlet fever, and atonic quinsy, with favorable results. (*Silliman's Journ.*, xxi. 406, 407.) It was employed by Dr. Formby, of Liverpool, in hysteria, in 1838; by Mr. Tuson, of London, in cancer and neuralgic affections, in 1843; and by M. Guillot, of Paris, in asthma, in 1844. The first case in which it was employed in inhalation is related by Professor Ives, of New Haven, under date of the 2d of Jan. 1832. The case was one of pulmonic disease, attended with general debility and difficult respiration, and was effectually relieved. (*Silliman's Journ.*, vol. xxi., Jan. 1832, p. 406.) In March, 1847, the action of the pure substance by inhalation was tried on the lower animals, by M. Flourens, and its effects on the spinal marrow described. In November of the same year, Dr. Simpson, of Edinburgh, after experimenting with a number of anæsthetic agents in order to discover a substitute for ether, tried chloroform at the suggestion of Mr. Waldie, and, having found its effects favorable, brought it forward as a new remedy for pain, by inhalation in surgery and midwifery. The advantages which he conceived it to possess over ether were the smallness of the dose, its more prompt action, more agreeable effects, less tenacious odor, greater cheapness, and greater facility of exhibition.

The usual effects produced by a full dose of chloroform, administered by inhalation, are the rapid production of coma, relaxation of the muscles, slow and often stertorous breathing, upturning of the eyes, and total insensibility to agents which ordinarily produce acute pain. The effect on the heart's action is somewhat variable, but the pulse is usually quickened, with a more or less marked loss of volume and firmness. Sometimes frothing of the mouth takes place, and, more rarely, convulsive twitches of the face and limbs. The insensibility is generally produced in one or two minutes, and usually continues for five or ten minutes; but the effect may be kept up for many hours, provided the inhalation be cautiously renewed from time to time. As a general rule, no recollection is retained of anything that occurred during the state of insensibility. In some cases sensibility is distinctly affected before consciousness, but the loss is rarely complete enough to be of any practical value; so that it is almost always necessary to produce unconsciousness before the surgeon can commence his operation.

The dose of chloroform for inhalation is a fluidrachm (3·75 C.c.), equivalent to 250 drops, or more, to be repeated in two minutes, if the desired effect should fail to be produced. The most convenient inhaler is a handkerchief, loosely twisted into the form of a bird's nest, which, after having been imbued with the chloroform, is held to the mouth and nose. The use of this simple inhaler insures a due admixture of atmospheric air with the vapor of the chloroform. The patient should always be in the horizontal posture. The moment insensibility is produced, which should be brought on *gradually*, the inhalation should be suspended; and, if consciousness return too soon, it should be cautiously renewed. In all cases an experienced assistant should attend to the administration of the chloroform and to nothing else, watching the state of the respiration and pulse. The moment there is the least snoring or failure of the pulse, the vapor should be withdrawn. As shown by Claude Bernard, the hypodermic use of morphine greatly prolongs the anæsthesia caused by chloroform. Chloroform should not be administered to persons subject to epilepsy, affected with organic disease of the heart, or predisposed to syncope. Even with the greatest care, there is always danger in the anæsthetic use of this agent. It is estimated (*Med. Times and Gaz.*, 1870; *Pacific Med. Journ.*, June, 1869) that death occurs once in 3000 inhalations on an average. In very many fatal cases the operation has been a very trifling one, and death has occurred in the most robust, and in those who had previously taken the anæsthetic without bad effects. The advantages which chloroform has over ether are in its greater rapidity of action, and in the fact that it is less prone to produce, as an after-effect, much nausea and vomiting. The greater safety of ether, however, more than counterbalances these advantages, so that a large proportion of surgeons believe the use of chloroform unjustifiable, except under especial circumstances. The reason that ether is so much safer than chloroform lies not chiefly in the greater power of the latter agent, but in the fact that it is directly paralyzant to the heart, whilst ether is primarily stimulant to that viscus. Experiments show that in the lower animals the arterial pressure steadily falls during the administration of the chloroform, whilst under ether it rises, and clinical experience abundantly demonstrates that the effects of these agents upon the circulation in man and in the lower animals are identical. As chloroform accidents usually occur very suddenly, the patient should always be closely watched. In most instances a peculiar pallor of the face is the first evidence of danger. The remedies for the accident are placing the patient at an angle of 45°, with the head downward, or even completely inverting the person, cold air fanned upon the face, cold water poured upon the head, sinapisms to the feet, frictions and heat to the body and extremities, and ammonia to the nostrils. If respiration ceases, the tongue should be seized with the artery-forceps, and pulled forward from off the glottis, and artificial respiration vigorously performed. When the patient can swallow, strong alcoholic drinks may be given with advantage. Dr. Halfourd has proposed the injection of liq. ammonia into the veins, and it has been successfully practised in one or two cases; and if circumstances favor it, intravenous injections of the tincture of digitalis may be employed. Faradaic irritation of the body should also be practised, and in some cases faradization of the phrenic nerve has seemed to be of service. Sometimes chloroform produces unpleasant remote effects; such as abolition of smell, perversion of taste, and loss of tonicity in the bladder and rectum.

In midwifery chloroform is believed to be safer than in surgery, and its use is very extensive. It certainly tends to increase the danger of post-partum hemorrhage, but this tendency can be overcome by the administration of ergot after the head has come well down upon the perineum. It is frequently stated that no case of death has occurred from its administration during labor; but this appears to be a mistake. On account of its power of producing muscular relaxation, chloroform is frequently employed in general and local spasms. In setting fractured bones, in reducing dislocations or strangulated hernias, etc., the surgeon frequently employs it, and it is often used by the physician in hiccough, chorea, hooping-cough, hysteria, the paroxysm of asthma, angina pectoris, biliary and nephritic colic, tetanus, poisoning from strychnine, hydrophobia, and the paroxysm of tic douloureux. In these cases it is superior to ether, when a very prompt action is desirable.

As chloroform is powerfully sedative, and ether powerfully stimulant, it was very naturally supposed that, by combining them, the depressing effects of the former might be counteracted by the latter; but experience has not confirmed the suggestion of theory in this case; as fatal effects have several times followed the joint administration of the two anæsthetics. This result may be in part explained by the more rapid volatilization of the chloroform, which may cause it to reach the surface of absorption with comparatively little admixture of the ethereal vapor, as suggested by Mr. Robert Ellis. (*Med. Times and Gaz.*, March 9, 1867.)

Locally, chloroform is employed as a very prompt, active counter-irritant and narcotic in neuralgia, colic, etc., and deep injections of it in the neighborhood of painful nerve trunks have been practised by Dr. Roberts Bartholow with asserted good effects.

M. Fournié has found that the vapor from a mixture of equal measures of glacial acetic acid and chloroform is even more effectual, as a local anæsthetic, than that of pure chloroform; producing complete insensibility of the skin in five minutes, if applied from a bottle heated simply by the hand. (*P. J. Tr.*, 1862, p. 385.)

Chloroform may be gelatinized by agitating it with an equal weight of white of egg in the cold. In three hours it takes the gelatinous form. A stronger preparation may be made by shaking together, in a bottle, four parts of chloroform and one of white of egg, and placing the mixture in water at 60° C. (140° F.). In four minutes the gelatinization is completed. *Gelatinized chloroform* may be applied to the skin, spread on linen, or by friction.

Chloroform, in vapor, may be used as a topical application to the rectum. M. Ehrenreich employed it with success in tenesmus. A drachm may be vaporized by the heat of warm water from a bottle, fitted with a flexible tube, inserted into the bowel. It may be applied to the skin in the form of a vapor douche, according to the method of Dr. Hardy, of Dublin. (See *Ranking's Abstract*, No. 19, p. 287.) Prof. Langenbeck, of Berlin, prefers chloroform to tincture of iodine, as an injection for the radical cure of hydrocele.

When an overdose of chloroform is taken by the mouth, it is essential to empty the stomach by the pump or siphon tube, and then treat the case much as in serious narcosis from inhalation. In a case of suicide by swallowing chloroform, in which death took place in about thirty-four hours, the lining membrane of the larynx and trachea was found inflamed, the bronchi were loaded with a dirty-gray purulent fluid, the lungs were inflamed as in the first stage of pneumonia, and the brain and its membranes congested; but these morbid appearances are not constant.

In relation to the preparations, consisting of chloroform and alcohol, which have been used under the name of "chloric ether," the reader is referred to *Spiritus Chloroformi.**

Off. Prep. and Pharm. Uses. Mistura Chloroformi; Spiritus Chloroformi; Pilula Phosphori.

Off. Prep. Br. Aqua Chloroformi; Linimentum Chloroformi; Spiritus Chloroformi; Tinctura Chloroformi Composita; Tinctura Chloroformi et Morphinæ.

CHLOROFORMUM VENALE. *U. S.* *Commercial Chloroform.*

(CHLŌ-RO-FŌR'MŬM VE-NĀ'LĒ.)

"A liquid containing at least 98 per cent. of Chloroform." *U. S.*

Chloroforme vénal, *Fr.;* Käufliches Chloroform, *G.*

The employment of commercial chloroform should be restricted to preparations for external application, or as a solvent. "Commercial Chloroform has nearly the same sensible properties as Purified Chloroform (see *Chloroformum Purificatum*). Its sp. gr. should not be lower than 1·470. If 1 C.c. be agitated with 20 C.c. of distilled water, the latter, when separated, should not render test-solution of nitrate of silver more than slightly turbid (limit of foreign chlorine compounds). When shaken with an equal volume of sulphuric acid, the subsiding, acid layer should not become quite black within twenty-four hours. A portion evaporated should leave no fixed residue." *U. S.*

Off. Prep. and Pharm. Uses. Chloroformum Purificatum; Linimentum Chloroformi; Collodium cum Cantharide; Liquor Gutta-Perchæ.

CHONDRUS. *U. S.* *Irish Moss.*

(CHŎN'DRUS.)

"Chondrus crispus, Lyngbye, and Chondrus mammilosus, Greville. (*Nat. Ord.* Algæ.)" *U. S.*

Carrageen, *P. G.;* Caragahen, Fucus Crispus; Carragaheen, Mousse marine pertée, *Fr.;* Irländisches Moos, Perlmoos, Knorpeltang, *G.*

Gen. Ch. Frond cartilaginous, dilating upwards into a flat, nerveless, dichotomously divided expansion, of a purplish or livid-red color. *Fructification*, subspherical capsules in the substance of the frond, rarely supported on little stalks, and containing a mass of minute free seeds. *Greville.*

Chondrus crispus. Greville, *Alg. Brit.* 129, t. 15; *B. & T.* 305.—*Sphærococcus crispus.* Agardh.—*Fucus crispus.* Linn. The *Irish moss*, or *carrageen* as it is frequently called, consists of a flat, slender, cartilaginous frond, from two to twelve inches in length, dilated as it ascends until it becomes two or three lines in width, then repeatedly and dichotomously divided, with linear, wedge-shaped segments, and more or less curled up so as to diminish the apparent length. The capsules are somewhat hemispherical, and are imbedded in the disk of the frond. The plant grows upon rocks and stones on the coast of Europe, and is especially abundant on the southern and western coasts of Ireland, where it is collected. It is also a native of the United States, and is said to be gathered largely on the southern sea-coast of Massachusetts, where it is partly torn from the rocks, and partly collected upon the beach, on which it is thrown up during storms. It is prepared for market by spreading it out high on the beach, to dry and bleach in the sun. (Aug. P. Melzar, *Proc.*

* *Chlorodyne.* An empirical remedy under this name was first used in London, but is now in some of its imitations very largely employed in various parts of the world. Many formulas are extant. The following has been extensively used in Philadelphia. Hydrochlorate of morphine 8 grains, water f℥ss, hydrochloric acid f℥ss, chloroform f℥iss, tincture of cannabis Indica f℥i, hydrocyanic acid, U. S. P., ♏xii, alcohol f℥ss, oil of peppermint ♏ij, oleoresin of capsicum ♏i. The hydrochlorate of morphine and water are heated in a flask with the hydrochloric acid until a clear solution is produced, then the other ingredients are mixed together, and when the first solution is cold the mixture added to it. This is a dangerous remedy, and should be used with great care in three to ten drop doses for an adult. (See *Mistura Chloroformi et Opii, Part II., National Formulary.*)

A. P. Ass., 1860.) An elaborate account of the plant, its distribution on the sea-coast of Massachusetts, and of the mode of gathering and curing it, is given by Mr. G. Hubert Bates, of Scituate, Mass. (*U. S. Agricultural Report*, 1866; also *A. J. P.*, 1868, p. 417.) There is evidence to prove that some of the moss in the market has been bleached by the use of permanganate of potassium and hyposulphite of sodium by the same process as that used for bleaching sponge. (See *Spongia Decolorata, Part II., National Formulary.*) Herr Schack was led to suspect this through discovering the presence of sulphurous acid in a German specimen. (*Pharm. Zeitung*, 1886, p. 87.)

When collected, it is washed and dried. In the fresh state it is of a purplish color, but, as found in the shops, is yellowish or yellowish white, with occasionally purplish portions. It is officinally described as "yellowish or white, horny, translucent; many-forked; when softened in water, cartilaginous; segments flat, wedge-shaped, or linear; at the apex emarginate or two-lobed; it has a slight sea-weed odor, and a mucilaginous, somewhat saline taste. One part of it boiled for ten minutes with 30 parts of water, yields a solution which gelatinizes on cooling." *U. S.* It swells in cold water, but does not dissolve. Boiling water dissolves a large proportion of it, and the solution, if sufficiently concentrated, gelatinizes on cooling. According to Feuchtwanger, it contains starch and pectin, with compounds of sulphur, chlorine, and bromine, and some oxalate of calcium. Herberger found 79·1 per cent. of pectin, and 9·5 of mucus, with fatty matter, free acids, chlorides, etc., but neither iodine nor bromine. M. Dupasquier discovered in it both of these elements, which had generally escaped attention in consequence of their reaction, as soon as liberated, upon the sulphide of sodium resulting from the decomposition of the sulphate of sodium of the moss when charred. (*Journ. de Pharm.*, 3e sér., iii. 113.) The pectin Pereira thought peculiar, and proposed to call *carrageenin.* It is distinguished from gum by affording, when dissolved in water, no precipitate with alcohol; from starch, by not becoming blue with tincture of iodine; from pectin, by yielding no precipitate with acetate of lead, and no mucic acid by the action of nitric acid. M. Ch. Blondeau gives the name of *goëmine* to a substance obtained by boiling carrageen (*goémon, Fr.*) for several hours in distilled water, and precipitating the mucilaginous liquid by alcohol. The precipitate, being redissolved in water, yields on evaporation thin, transparent, elastic plates, resembling ichthyocolla, which soften and swell up on contact with cold water. This substance, which is probably complex, is without smell or taste, neutral to test-paper, and dissolves completely in alkaline liquids. Blondeau's analysis gave 21·80 per cent. of carbon, 4·87 of hydrogen, 21·36 of nitrogen, 2·51 of sulphur, and 49·46 of oxygen. Flückiger, who analyzed this mucilage with care, found in it *no* sulphur, and only 0·88 per cent. of nitrogen. The drug itself yielded not more than 1·012 per cent. of nitrogen. (*Pharmacographia*, 2d ed., p. 748.)* Carrageenin is said to have been used as a substitute for acacia under the name of *imitation gum arabic;* the latter occurs in three forms, white, light yellow, and yellow. They all have similar properties, swelling up like tragacanth when mixed with cold water; but not forming a clear solution unless the mixture is boiled; in this latter respect differing from tragacanth or albumen; iodine did not give a blue color, and alcohol did not precipitate the solution, even when 50 per cent. of it was added. It has mild adhesive properties. (E. C. Federer, *Pharm. Era*, 1887, p. 146.)

The mucilage of Irish moss has come into considerable use at this time (1888) as an emulsifying agent. (See *Mucilago Chondri in Part II., from the National Formulary;* Emlen Painter, *Proc. A. P. A.*, 1887, p. 578; A. J. Staudt, *A. J. P.*, 1888, p. 170.)

Carrageen is nutritive and demulcent, and, being easy of digestion and not unpleasant to the taste, forms a useful article of diet in cases in which the farinaceous preparations, such as tapioca, sago, barley, etc., are usually employed. It has been

* Most species of sea-weed contain a mucous substance analogous to, if not identical with, that of carrageen, but are not available for use on account of their disagreeable taste. In France the *Gigartina aciculosus* is said to be extensively sold as carrageen. (Dragendorff, *Jahresb.*, 1874, p. 42.)

particularly recommended in chronic pectoral affections, scrofulous complaints, dysentery, diarrhœa, and disorders of the kidneys and bladder. It may be used in the form of decoction, made by boiling a pint and a half of water with half an ounce of the moss down to a pint. Sugar and lemon-juice may usually be added to improve the flavor. Milk may be substituted for water, when a more nutritious preparation is required. It is recommended to macerate the moss for about ten minutes in cold water before submitting it to decoction. Any unpleasant flavor that it may have acquired from the contact of foreign substances is thus removed.

CHRYSAROBINUM. *U. S., Br.* *Chrysarobin.*

(CHRȲS-A-RO-BĪ'NŬM.)

"A mixture of proximate principles, commonly misnamed Chrysophanic Acid, extracted from Goa-powder,* a substance found deposited in the wood of the trunk of Andira Araroba. Aguiar. (*Nat. Ord.* Leguminosæ, Papilionaceæ.)" *U. S.* "The medullary matter of the stem and branches of Andira araroba, *Aguiar.;* dried, powdered, and purified; containing more or less chrysophanic acid according to age and condition, and yielding much chrysophanic acid by oxidation." *Br.*

Goa Powder, Araroba, Poh di Bahia; Poudre de Goa, *Fr.;* Goa-Pulver, *G.*

Chrysarobin, or Araroba, has long been used as a medicine in Brazil, and exported in considerable quantities to Portugal, whence it found its way through the Portuguese colonies into Eastern commerce. In the East Indies it is usually known as Goa Powder. Indeed, the identity of the two powders was first proved in 1875 by Dr. J. F. Dasilva Lima. (*P. J. Tr.*, v. 724, 801, 806.)

Chrysarobin has been supposed to be yielded by certain lichens, but was shown by Dr. R. A. Monteiro to be obtained from a leguminous tree abundant in the forests of the Brazilian province of Bahia, which was referred by Mr. E. M. Holmes to the genus Cæsalpinia, but which was determined by studies made in its native forests by Dr. J. M. de Aguiar to be an undescribed species of Andira.

Andira Araroba, Aguiar, is a large tree, attaining a height of 100 feet, with a smooth trunk, and a spheroidal, not very bushy head. The wood is yellowish, with numerous longitudinal canals, besides abundant irregular interspaces or lacunæ, in which the chrysarobin is found. (See *P. J. Tr.*, ix. 755; x. 42, 814.) The oldest trees yield the largest amount of the powder; the parts containing it are finely chipped or scraped off. The workmen who procure it often suffer severely from irritation of the eyes and face.

Properties. "A pale orange yellow, crystalline powder, permanent in the air, odorless and tasteless, almost insoluble in water, only slightly soluble in alcohol, readily soluble in ether and in boiling benzol. When heated to about 162° C. (323·6 F.), it melts, and may be partially sublimed. On ignition it is wholly dissipated. In solutions of alkalies it is soluble with a yellowish red or reddish yellow color, which is changed to red by passing air through the liquid. Sulphuric acid dissolves it with a deep blood-red color; on pouring the solution into water, the substance separates again unchanged." *U. S.* As first obtained, chrysarobin is stated to be of a pale primrose yellow, but it rapidly darkens with age, so that in commerce it varies from a dull ochre color to a dark chocolate or maroon-brown. It is sometimes a rather fine powder, but is usually more or less agglomerated, and not rarely contains fragments of woody tissue. Its taste is bitter. It is insoluble in water and most menstrua, but yields as much as 80 per cent. of its weight to solutions of caustic alkalies and to benzol. The British Pharmacopœia requires that it shall be "almost entirely soluble in 150 parts of hot rectified spirit." Attfield analyzed Goa powder, and found, along with 2 per cent. of resin, 5·5 per cent. of woody fibre, and 7 per cent. of bitter extractive, 80 to 84 per cent. of what he considered to be chrysophanic acid; but Liebermann and Siedler showed that this was not chrysophanic acid at all, but a substance easily convertible into the acid, which substance

* Dr. C. Rice (*American Druggist*, 1886) states that chrysarobin, as at present sold, is not as strong as that which was in the market some five or six years ago, and suggests that the powder contains some substance still more active than chrysarobin, supporting his supposition by the statement of Gehe, that the mother liquid left after the crystallization of chrysarobin has in it a very active substance.

they called *chrysarobin*, and gave to it the formula $C_{30}H_{26}O_7$. (*A. J. P.*, 1879, p. 80.) When chrysarobin is distilled with zinc dust it yields methyl-anthracene, $C_{15}H_{12}$.

Medical Uses. When taken internally in sufficient amount, chrysarobin acts as a decided gastro-intestinal irritant, producing large, very watery, brownish stools, and repeated vomiting without much nausea. Dr. J. A. Thompson (*N. R.*, 1877, p. 167) states that it acts efficiently in doses of 20 to 25 grains (1·3–1·565 Gm.) for the adult, 10 grains (0·65 Gm.) for children 12 years of age, 6 grains (0·4 Gm.) for babies. He believes it to have practical value as affording a very prompt and efficient means of clearing out the whole primæ viæ, and of causing very large discharges of bile. It is, however, not probable that it will be used to any extent as an internal remedy.

Chrysarobin has been long used in South America and India as a remedy in skin diseases, but the attention of the general profession was first called to it in 1874 by Sir Joseph Fayrer. It is frequently applied in psoriasis and very chronic eczema, by being rubbed up with water into a dough, which is spread over the diseased spot after it is as far as possible freed from scales by washing. As soon as the dough is dry, it should be covered with a layer of collodion or solution of gutta-percha, and the whole allowed to remain for several days, when it is removed by washing and renewed. In using chrysarobin, care must be observed not to allow it to come in contact with the clothes, as it leaves an indelible stain. It is at present employed largely in the preparation of chrysophanic acid.*

Off. Prep. Unguentum Chrysarobini.

CIMICIFUGA. *U. S., Br. Cimicifuga.* [*Black Snakeroot.*]

(CĬM-Ĭ-CĬF'Ū-GĄ.)

"The rhizome and rootlets of Cimicifuga racemosa. Elliott. (*Nat. Ord.* Ranunculaceæ." *U. S.* "The dried rhizome and rootlets of Cimicifuga racemosa, *Elliott* (Actæa racemosa, *Linn.*)." *Br.*

Actææ Radix; Black Cohosh; Racine d'Actée à Grappes, *Fr.;* Schwarze Schlangenwurzel, *G.*

Gen. Ch. Calyx four or five-leaved. *Petals* four to eight, deformed, thickish, sometimes wanting. *Capsules* one to five, oblong, many-seeded. *Seeds* squamose. *Nuttall.*

Cimicifuga racemosa. Torrey, *Flor.* 219; Carson, *Illust. of Med. Bot.* i. 9, pl. 3. —*C. serpentaria.* Pursh, *Flor. Am. Sept.* p. 372.—*Actæa racemosa.* Willd. *Sp. Plant.* ii. 1139.—*Macrotys racemosa.* Eaton's *Manual*, p. 288; *B. & T.* 8. This is a tall stately plant, having a perennial root, and a simple herbaceous stem, which rises from four to eight feet in height. The leaves are large, and ternately decomposed, having oblong-ovate leaflets, incised and toothed at their edges. The flowers are small, white, and disposed in a long, terminal, wand-like raceme, with occasionally one or two shorter racemes near its base. The calyx is white, four-leaved, and deciduous; the petals are minute, and shorter than the stamens; the pistil consists of an oval germ and sessile stigma. The fruit is an ovate capsule containing numerous flat seeds.

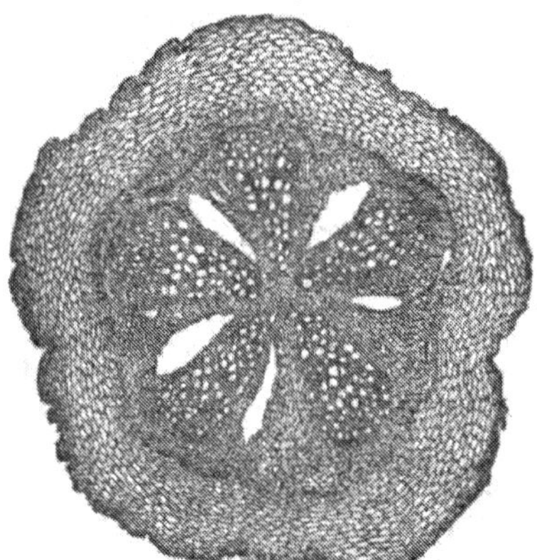

Transverse section of Cimicifuga; rootlet showing five ligneous rays.

The *black snakeroot*, or *cohosh* as this plant is sometimes called, is a native of the United States, growing in shady or rocky woods from Canada to Florida, and flowering in June and July. The root is the part employed.

* Liebermann described (*Ber. d. Chem. Ges.*, 1888, p. 447) several compounds obtained from alizarin and purpurin by reduction, which, from their similarity of composition to chrysarobin, he proposes to call *anthrarobins*. The commercial anthrarobin, prepared from commercial alizarin, has been tried by Dr. G. Behrend and Professor Köbner with favorable results in psoriasis, pityriasis, papulous syphilis, herpes tonsurans, and eczema marginatum.

Properties. The dried root consists of a thick, irregularly bent or contorted body or caudex, from one-third of an inch to an inch in thickness, often several inches in length, furnished with many slender radicles, and rendered exceedingly rough and jagged in appearance by the remains of the stems of successive years, which to the length of an inch or more are frequently attached to the root. It is officinally described as follows. "The rhizome is horizontal, hard, two inches (5 cm.) or more long, about one inch (25 mm.) thick, with numerous stout, upright or curved branches, terminated by a cup-shaped scar, and with numerous, wiry, brittle, obtusely quadrangular rootlets, about one-twelfth of an inch (2 mm.) thick; the whole brownish-black, nearly inodorous, and having a bitter, acrid taste. Rhizome and branches have a smooth fracture, with a large pith, surrounded by numerous, sub-linear, whitish wood-rays, and a thin, firm bark. The rootlets break with a short fracture, have a thick bark, and contain a ligneous cord branching into about four rays." *U. S.* The odor, though not strong, is peculiar and rather disagreeable, and is gradually lost by keeping. The root yields its virtues to boiling water. It was found by Mr. Tilghman, of Philadelphia, to contain gum, starch, sugar, resin, wax, fatty matter, tannic and gallic acids, a black coloring matter, a green coloring matter, lignin, and salts of potassa, lime, magnesia, and iron. (*A. J. P.*, vi. 20.) It no doubt also contains, when fresh, a volatile principle, with which its virtues may be in some degree associated; as we are confident that it is more efficacious in the recent state, than when long kept. In fact, Mr. George H. Davis, in a more recent analysis, has separated by distillation a small proportion of volatile oil, having decidedly the peculiar odor of the root. Mr. Davis also found, in addition to the principles above mentioned, albumen and extractive among the organic, and silica among the inorganic constituents. The sugar, moreover, noticed by him was of the uncrystallizable variety, and the resin of two kinds, one soluble in alcohol but not in ether, the other soluble in both these menstrua. (*A. J. P.*, xxxiii. 396.)

A crystallizable principle has been obtained from the root by Mr. T. Elwood Conard. After failing to obtain any volatile principle from the fresh root by distillation, he prepared a strong tincture of the root, treated this with the solution of subacetate of lead, which precipitated resin, tannin, and coloring matters, then filtered, and precipitated the lead by sulphuretted hydrogen in excess, and allowed the tincture to evaporate spontaneously; and, finally, having treated the residuary powder with benzin, afterwards washed it with water, dissolved it to saturation in strong alcohol, and treated the solution with alumina. The mixture was allowed to evaporate to a dry mass, which was nearly exhausted with alcohol. The solution, being allowed to evaporate, left behind a crystalline mass, somewhat resembling alum. This substance has little taste on account of its extreme insolubility in the saliva; but in alcoholic solutions has very strongly the acrid taste characteristic of the fresh root. The crystals are very soluble in cold, and more so in hot alcohol, soluble also in chloroform, and slightly in ether. They are fusible and inflammable. They are neutral, possessing neither acid nor alkaline properties. Their effects on the system were not examined. (*A. J. P.*, 1871, p. 151.) L. F. Beach (*A. J. P.*, 1876, p. 385) obtained from commercial resin of cimicifuga (the so-called cimicifugin or macrotin) a crystalline principle by Conard's process. M. S. Falck (*A. J. P.*, 1884, p. 459) found in the juice of the fresh plant a crystalline principle resembling the principle announced by Conard. On the other hand, neither F. H. Trimble (*A. J. P.*, 1878, p. 468) nor Profs. Warder or Coblentz were able to obtain a crystalline principle, while C. S. Gallaher obtained crystals of cane sugar from the fluid extract. (*A. J. P.*, 1887, p. 545.) In view of these

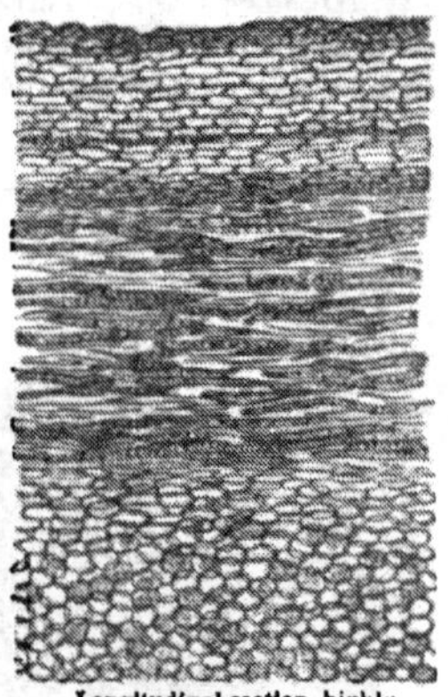
Longitudinal section, highly magnified.

* For a detailed description of the microscopic character of the root, see *A. J. P.*, 1884, p. 460.

facts, it would appear that the active principle is a resinous amorphous body. (See *Drugs and Medicines of North America*, vol. i. p. 264.)

Medical Properties and Uses. In 1831 cimicifuga was introduced to the notice of the profession by Dr. Young, and, although used to a considerable extent since that time, very little is known of its real influence upon the system. In overdoses it is said to cause general relaxation, vertigo, tremors, decided reduction of the pulse; occasionally it vomits, but its emetic action is never violent, and is probably simply the result of a mild gastric irritation. It certainly in large doses produces giddiness, with intense headache and prostration. It has been found by Dr. R. Hutchinson to cause in frogs complete anæsthesia by a direct action upon the sensory side of the spinal cord. The same observer noted that toxic doses produce in mammals slowing of the pulse with fall of the arterial pressure, results which appear to be in part due to a direct depressant action upon the heart-muscle or its ganglia, in part to a paralysis of the vaso-motor centre. It has been used in the past in rheumatism, dropsy, hysteria, phthisis, and various other affections, but at present is employed almost exclusively in the treatment of the St. Vitus's dance of childhood, in which it is an efficient remedy.

It may be given in substance, decoction, tincture, or extract. The dose of the powder is from a scruple to a drachm (1·3–3·9 Gm.). The *decoction* has been much used, but is thought by some not to contain all the virtues of the root. An ounce of the bruised root may be boiled for a short time in a pint of water, and one or two fluidounces (30–60 C.c.) given for a dose. From half a pint to a pint of the decoction may be taken without inconvenience during the day. The *tincture* is officinally made in the proportion of twenty parts in one hundred of alcohol, and given in the dose of one or two fluidrachms (3·75–7·5 C.c.). The fluid extract when properly made from good root is, however, the best preparation. The dose of it is from a half to one fluidrachm (1·9–3·75 C.c.) three or four times a day in water. The practitioners calling themselves eclectics use, under the name of *cimicifugin*, or *macrotin*, an impure resin obtained by precipitating a saturated tincture of the root with water. It is given in the dose of a grain or two (0·065–0·13 Gm.). The names, however, are inappropriate, as they should be reserved for the pure active principle or principles when discovered. (See *N. J. Med. Reporter*, viii. 247.)

Off. Prep. Extractum Cimicifugæ Fluidum; Tinctura Cimicifugæ.

CINCHONA. *U. S., Br.* *Cinchona.*

(CĬN-CHŌ'NA.)

"The bark of any species of Cinchona (*Nat. Ord.* Rubiaceæ, Cinchoneæ), containing at least 3 per cent. of its peculiar alkaloids." *U. S.* "The dried bark of Cinchona Calisaya, *Weddell;* Cinchona officinalis, *Linn.;* Cinchona succirubra, *Pavon;* Cinchona lancifolia, *Mutis;* and other species of Cinchona from which the peculiar alkaloids of the bark may be obtained." *Br.*

Cinchonæ Cortex, *Br.;* Peruvian Bark; Cinchona Bark; Quinquina, *Fr.;* China, Peruvianische Rinde, *G.;* China, *It.;* Quina, *Sp.*

Varieties.

CINCHONA FLAVA. *Yellow Cinchona.* [*Calisaya Bark.*] *U. S.* "The bark of the trunk of Cinchona Calisaya, Weddell. (*Nat. Ord.* Rubiaceæ, Cinchoneæ), containing at least 2 per cent. of quinine." *U. S.*

Cinchonæ Flavæ Cortex, *Br.;* *Yellow Cinchona Bark.*

CINCHONA RUBRA. *Red Cinchona.* [*Red Bark.*] *U. S.* "The bark of the trunk of Cinchona succirubra, Pavon. (*Nat. Ord.* Rubiaceæ, Cinchoneæ), containing at least 2 per cent. of quinine." *U. S.* "The dried bark of the stem and branches of cultivated plants of Cinchona succirubra, *Pavon.*" *Br.*

Cinchonæ Rubræ Cortex, *Br.;* *Red Cinchona Bark.*

Botanical History.

Though the Peruvian bark was introduced into Europe so early as 1640, it was not till the year 1737 that the plant producing it was known to naturalists. In that year La Condamine, on a journey to Lima, through the province of Loxa, had an opportunity of examining the tree, of which, upon his return, he published a description in the Memoirs of the French Academy. Soon afterwards Linnæus gave it the name of *Cinchona officinalis*, in honor of the Countess of Cinchon, who is said to have first taken the bark to Europe; but, in his description of the plant, he united the species discovered by La Condamine with *C. pubescens*, a specimen of which had been sent to him from Santa Fé de Bogota. For a long time it was not known that more than one species existed; and *C. officinalis* continued, till a comparatively recent period, to be recognized by the Pharmacopœias as the only source of the Peruvian bark of commerce. But a vast number of plants belonging to the Linnæan genus Cinchona were in the course of time discovered; and the list became at length so unwieldy and heterogeneous, that botanists were compelled to distribute the species into several groups, each constituting a distinct genus, and all associated in the natural family of Cinchonaceæ. Among these genera, the *Cinchona* is that which embraces the true Peruvian bark trees, characterised by the production of the alkaloids, quinine, cinchonine, etc., as well as by certain botanical peculiarities, among which the most distinctive is probably the dehiscence of the capsule from the base towards the apex, or from below upward. The new genera *Exostemma* and *Buena* embrace species which have been, perhaps, most frequently referred to as Cinchonas; but they are sufficiently characterized, the former by the projection of the stamens beyond the corolla, a peculiarity which has given name to the genus, the latter by the different shape of the corolla, the separation of the calyx from the fruit at maturity, and the opening of the capsule from above downward. More recently Weddell has separated several generally admitted species from Cinchona, and instituted a new genus, which he proposes to name *Cascarilla*. This includes the former *Cinchona magnifolia* of Ruiz and Pavon (*C. oblongifolia* of Mutis), the *C. stenocarpa* of Lambert, the *C. acutifolia* of Ruiz and Pavon, the *C. oblongifolia* of Lambert, the *C. macrocarpa* of Vahl, and the *C. cava* of Pavon, which differ from the true Cinchona in having the dehiscence of the capsules from the apex towards the base, or from above downward, and the barks of which contain neither of the alkaloids above referred to. (Weddell, *Hist. Nat. des Quinquinas*, p. 77.) With this brief preliminary notice, we shall proceed to consider the true Cinchonas. It may be proper, however, first to say, that the botanists who have personally observed these plants, besides La Condamine, of whom we have before spoken, are chiefly Joseph de Jussieu, who in the year 1739 explored the country about Loxa, and gathered specimens still existing in the cabinets of Europe; Mutis, who in 1772 discovered Cinchona trees in New Granada, and afterwards, aided by his pupil, Zea, made further investigations and discoveries in the same region; Ruiz and Pavon, who in 1777 began a course of botanical inquiries in the central portions of Lower Peru, and discovered several new species; Humboldt and Bonpland, who visited several of the Peruvian bark districts, and published the results of their observations after 1792; Pöppig, who travelled in Peru so late as 1832, and published an account of his journey about the year 1835; Weddell, whose researches in Bolivia are so well known, and have been so productive of valuable information in relation to the Calisaya bark and allied species; whilst Karsten, Caldas, Martius, Ledger, and other intrepid explorers have in later times largely added to our information.

Gen. Ch. Calyx with a turbinate tube, and a persistent five-toothed limb. *Corolla* with a round tube, a five-parted limb, and oblong lobes valvate in æstivation. *Stamens* with short filaments inserted into the middle of the tube, and linear anthers entirely closed. *Stigma* bifid, subclavate. *Capsule* ovate or oblong, somewhat furrowed on each side, bilocular, crowned with the calyx, septicidal-dehiscent, with the mericarps loosened from the base towards the apex, the introflexed part disjoined. *Placentæ* elongated. *Seeds* numerous, erect, imbricated upward, compressed, winged, with a membranous margin, and a fleshy albumen.—The plants composing this genus are trees or shrubs. The leaves are opposite, upon short petioles with flat margins, and are attended with ovate or oblong, foliaceous, free, deciduous stipules. The flowers are terminal, in corymbose panicles, and of a white or purplish rose color. *De Candolle.*

The genuine Cinchona trees are natives exclusively of South America.* In that continent, however, they are widely diffused, extending from the 19th degree of south latitude, considerably south of La Paz, in Bolivia, to the mountains of Santa Marta, or, according to Weddell, to the vicinity of Caracas, on the northern coast, in about

* *Transplanting of the Cinchona trees, and Cultivation in new Sites.* For a long time after the discovery of the virtues of Peruvian bark, no attempt appears to have been made to transplant to other countries the trees which produced it. In 1737, La Condamine collected a large number of young plants, with a view of conveying them to Europe; but, after having descended the Amazon in safety for more than a thousand leagues, they were washed overboard, near the mouth of that river, from the boat containing them, and were all lost. After this failure, though the idea of transplanting the Cinchonas was occasionally suggested, nothing was done until 1846–7, when Dr. Weddell, now celebrated for his successful exploration of the region of the Calisaya bark, sent some seeds to France, which were planted with success in the Jardin des Plantes, and thus supplied some of the conservatories of Europe with specimens of the plant. But the first successful effort, with a view to great practical results, was made in 1853, by the Dutch government, by whom Mr. Hasskarl, formerly superintendent of the Botanical Garden in Java, was sent to South America on this important mission. A number of young Cinchona plants were sent by him directly across the Pacific to Batavia, which they reached before the close of 1854. From these, and from seeds obtained from other sources, which were planted in the mountains of Java, in sites selected for their supposed conformity in climate with the native locality of the Cinchona, have sprung numerous plantations.

Stimulated by the suggestions of Dr. Royle, and by the partial success of the Dutch, the English government engaged, in 1859, the services of Mr. Clements B. Markham, who proceeded to Bolivia, in South America, and, after almost incredible hardships, arising partly from the nature of the country and partly from the jealousy of the native authorities, succeeded in collecting and transmitting to England upwards of 400 Calisaya plants. Most of these, however, were so much injured, on their way from England to India, by the excessive heat of the Red Sea, that very few, on their arrival in Hindostan, had sufficient life remaining to grow when planted. Happily, the deficiency was supplied by seeds of *C. Calisaya* sent from Java, where they were produced, to Calcutta, at the request of the English Governor-General. (De Vrij, *P. J. Tr.*, 1863, p. 440.) Whilst Mr. Markham was in Bolivia, other agents were collecting other species in Peru and Ecuador, whence seeds of the pale and red bark Cinchonas reached India, and, being planted in the selected sites, proved to be very productive.

The sites selected for the Cinchona plantations were in the Neilgherry Hills, in Southern India, in the Presidency of Madras, at the junction of the East and West Ghauts, near the Sanitary Station of Ootacamund, at heights varying from 5000 to 7450 feet above the sea. These positions unite the peculiar characters of the native region of the Cinchonas in the Andes, not only as regards elevation and latitude, but also as to atmospheric moisture, an excess of which, for the greater portion of the year, seems essential to the perfection of these trees. But, though a certain excess of atmospheric moisture is necessary, yet the trees do not grow well in a wet soil, as Mr. Cross, who personally inspected the region in the Andes where the best barks are obtained, found the Cinchona plants only on the dry slopes, and never on wet ground. He remarked, moreover, that constant dampness of the atmosphere is unfavorable, as a certain amount of dry weather is necessary for the ripening of the capsules. In regard to the temperature, which is about the same throughout the year, he observed that during the hottest days the thermometer rose to 59° or 60° F., falling to 46° or 48° F. at night; but at the upper limit it ranged, during the day, from 46° to 48°, and at night fell to 35° or 36° F. (*A. J. P.*, 1867, p. 161.)

Besides the Neilgherry Hills, other sites were selected for experimental plantations; and, since the first introduction of the Cinchona trees, their culture has been extended to various points from Hakgalla, in the island of Ceylon, to the Himalaya Mountains; as in the Wynaad, the Coorg, the hills of Travancore, and especially at Peermede in the Presidency of Madras; in Sikkim and Darjeeling in the Presidency of Bengal; at Lingmulla in the Presidency of Bombay; and in the valley of Kangra in the Punjab; from the southern to the northern extremity of British India. The culture has especially flourished in Ceylon; but the attempt has collapsed in St. Helena.

Besides the general fact of the success of the culture, other results, as unexpected as they are important, have been obtained within the last few years. It was ascertained at an early period, that the productiveness of these plants in alkaloids had not been diminished by transplanting; it is now known that this productiveness has in fact been very considerably increased. Another highly important result is the discovery by Mr. MacIvor, that the yield in alkaloids is greatly augmented by a certain treatment of the trees. It had been noticed that the cinchona alkaloids, especially in any other form than that of sulphate, were apt, on exposure to the direct light of the sun, to become reddened by the generation of coloring matter, at the expense of the alkaloid. It was a very natural inference that a similar change might take place in the living plant, as a consequence of which the proportion of alkaloids they were capable of producing, might be greatly diminished. To obviate this presumed effect, Mr. MacIvor was induced to make the experiment of covering the stems of the growing trees with a layer of moss, so as completely to protect the bark against the influence of sunlight. The result was favorable beyond all expectation; and the yield of the bark thus protected in alkaloids is said to be doubled, tripled, or increased even in larger proportion. A tree can thus be made continuously productive; for if a slip is removed longitudinally from the trunk, from top to bottom, by covering the decorticated portion with moss, the bark is renewed, at least as rich as previously in the alkaloids, while from time to time other strips may be taken, till the whole of the old bark is removed, and the new ready for removal by a repetition of the same process; and the tree is thus preserved indefinitely, probably for the whole normal length of its life. The practical difficulty with the process is that it requires skilled workmen, not always attainable, and hence the "coppicing system" still largely prevails in India.

the 10th degree of north latitude. They follow, in this distance, the circuitous course of the great mountain ranges, and for the most part occupy the eastern slope of the second range of the Cordilleras. Those which yield the bark of commerce grow at various elevations upon the Andes, seldom less than 4000 feet above the sea, and require a temperature considerably lower than that which usually prevails in tropical countries.

There has been much difficulty in properly arranging the species of Cinchona. One source of the difficulty is the varying shape of the leaves of the same species, according to the degree of elevation upon the mountainous declivities, to the severity or mildness of the climate, the greater or less humidity of the soil, and to various circumstances in the growth of individual plants. Even the same tree often produces foliage of a diversified character; and a person, not aware of this fact, might be led to imagine that he had discovered different species from an examination of the leaves from one and the same branch. The fructification partakes, to a certain extent, of the same varying character. Lambert, in his "*Illustration of the genus Cinchona*," published in 1821, after admitting with Humboldt the identity of several varieties which had received specific names from other botanists, described nineteen species. De Candolle enumerated only sixteen. Lindley admits twenty-one known species, and five doubtful. Weddell describes twenty-one species, including eight new ones of his own, and two doubtful, and excluding several before admitted by other writers,

Under it the trees are cut down, not too close to the ground, when young shoots put up abundantly. It has been experimentally found best to allow only two of these shoots to remain, and that the bark contains the maximum of alkaloid in the eighth year of growth. A third method of gathering cinchona bark largely practised in India and Java, is by shaving or scraping with a sharp tool the external bark of the growing tree so as to leave the lighter untouched. This has been found especially applicable to young trees, in which the second growth of bark is rapidly formed, and contains 20 to 50 per cent. more alkaloid than that which has been taken off. It seems to be a general opinion among the planters that shaving checks the growth of the tree after it is five years old, so that from three to five years is the age at which it is best practised. (*P. J. Tr.*, xv. 65.)

In Bolivia cinchona trees are cultivated to a considerable extent. In 1884 it was estimated that there were nearly seven millions of trees planted on the sides of the valleys or ridges of the Andes, between three and four thousand feet above the sea. The root bark is thinner and much less easily separated than that of the stem, but is carefully preserved, as it has been found to yield a better percentage of alkaloid than does the stem bark.

At present (1887) the Java plantations are very flourishing, and excellent results have been obtained by grafting the shoots of Ledgeriana upon young plants belonging to a species of little value. As much as thirteen per cent. of quinine is said to be obtained from this bark. The trees are by some planters uprooted when ten or twelve years old, and the root bark removed along with that of the trunk and branches. Scraping is also practised with great success.

A very important result of the culture in India has been the appearance of hybrids. One which has received the name of *C. angustifolia* has been found to contain in its bark 11 per cent. of alkaloids, whilst a second form, believed to be a cross between *C. officinalis* and *C. Calisaya*, has been called *C. pubescens* and yielded a bark containing 12·2 per cent. of alkaloids. The culture of bark in India may be considered as fully established, although Markham affirms that the greed for immediate results has been disastrous and that the plantations are not in as good condition as formerly. The total yield of bark by Ceylon and India for the season of 1879 and 1880 was 1,172,060 pounds. The quality of the bark seems to be superior to that of South America, whilst the financial success has been such that 70 per cent. a year is said to be sometimes returned, and Mr. Markham affirms that the plantations have entirely paid for themselves, principal and interest. (For further information in regard to the culture of Cinchonas in India, see *Peruvian Bark*, by C. R. Markham. London, John Murray, 1880; also *P. J. Tr.*, xi. 244; also vols. xv., xvi., and xvii.)

Owing to the worthlessness of many of the species of Cinchona first introduced into Java, the Dutch have reaped success more slowly than the English; but by destroying the progeny of the first imports and introducing from India other more valuable species the Java plantations have at last been made to flourish, and in 1879 and 1880 yielded 70,088 pounds of good bark. Attempts have also been made to introduce the new culture into the West India island of Jamaica. Various special difficulties have environed the attempts at Cinchona culture in Jamaica; thus, in 1874, 60,000 trees were destroyed by a hurricane. Nevertheless, progress has been made, and about 21,000 pounds of the bark found its way from Jamaica to the London market in the season of 1879–80.

The French have been less successful than the Dutch and English. The first plants taken by Weddell from Peru to Paris all perished. Subsequently trials have been made in the Isle of Bourbon, and at Guadeloupe, but with what final results we do not know. In Algiers, where situations believed to be suitable were selected for plantations among the mountains, no satisfactory results have yet been attained. The Brazilians have had somewhat better success near Rio Janeiro, and it is said that plants have been introduced into the Azores, which are growing well. (Soubeiran, *Journ. de Pharm.*, Feb. 1868, p. 189.)

which he joins to his new genus Cascarilla. (For further information, see foot-note p. 430.)

Until recently, it was impossible to decide from which species of Cinchona the several varieties of bark were respectively derived. The former references of the yellow bark to *C. cordifolia*, of the pale to *C. lancifolia*, and of the red to *C. oblongifolia*, have been very properly abandoned in all the Pharmacopœias. It is now universally admitted that the officinal barks, known in the market by these titles, are not the product of the species mentioned. It is stated by Humboldt that the property of curing agues belongs to the barks of all the Cinchonas with hairy and woolly blossoms, and to these alone. All those with smooth corollas belong to the genus Cascarilla of Weddell. Within a few years much light has been thrown upon the botanical history of the different varieties of bark, and at present most if not all of the valuable varieties can be traced to their sources. The following species are acknowledged by the Pharmacopœia of the United States.

1. *Cinchona Calisaya.* Weddell, *Hist. Nat. des Quinquinas*, p. 30, t. 3. This is a lofty tree, with a trunk often two feet or more in diameter, and a summit usually rising above the other trees of the forest. The leaves are petiolate, oblong or lanceolate-obovate, from three to six inches long and one or two in breadth, obtuse, acute or slightly attenuated at the base, softish, above smooth, of a velvety aspect, and obscurely green, beneath smooth and of a pale emerald hue, with scrobiculi at the axils of the veins, but scarcely visible on the upper surface. The stipules are about as long as the petioles, oblong, very obtuse, and very smooth. The flowers are in ovate or subcorymbose panicles. The calyx is pubescent, with a cup-shaped limb, and short triangular teeth; the corolla is rose-colored, with a cylindrical tube about four lines long, and a laciniate limb fringed at the edges; the stamina are concealed in the tube, with anthers more than twice as long as the filaments. The fruit is an ovate capsule scarcely as long as the flower, enclosing elliptical lanceolate seeds, the margin of which is irregularly toothed, with a fimbriated appearance. The tree grows in the forests, upon the declivities of the Andes, at the height of 6000 or 7000 feet above the ocean, in Bolivia and the southernmost part of Peru.

A variety of this species, described by Weddell under the name of *Josephiana*, is a mere shrub, not more than twelve feet high, with a slender stem, erect branches, and a strongly adherent bark. This variety is found in some places covering extensive surfaces destitute of forest trees. Weddell supposes that these tracts had once been covered with forests, which, having been destroyed by fires, have been succeeded by this stunted growth springing from the roots, and prevented from receiving its full development by the want of protection from other trees.

Mr. Markham states that the natives recognise three varieties of the Calisaya: 1. *Calisaya amarilla* or *fina* (*a. vera* of Weddell); 2. *C. morada* (*C. Boliviana*, Wedd.); and 3. *C. verde* or *alta*, a very large tree, growing lower in the valley than the other varieties, and distinguished by having the veins of the leaves never purple, but always green. (*A. J. P.*, 1866, p. 422.) By the discovery of this species, the long unsettled point of the botanical source of Calisaya bark has been determined. The immense consumption of that bark, and the wasteful methods pursued by the bark-gatherers, have caused the rapid destruction of the tree; and many years ago it had disappeared from the neighborhood of inhabited places, except in the form of a shrub. Weddell was compelled to make long journeys on foot through the forests, by paths scarcely opened, before he could get a sight of the tree in its full vigor.

2. *Cinchona Condaminea.* Humb. and Bonpl. *Plant. Equin.* i. p. 33, t. 10; Lindley, *Flor. Med.* 414; Carson, *Illust. of Med. Bot.* i. 53, pl. 45.—*Cinchona officinalis.* Linn.; Hooker, *Bot. Mag.* t. 5364. This tree, when full grown, has a stem about eighteen feet high and a foot in thickness, with opposite branches, of which the lower are horizontal, and the higher rise at their extremities. The bark of the trunk yields when wounded a bitter astringent juice. The leaves are of variable shape, but generally ovate-lanceolate, about four inches in length by less than two in breadth, smooth and scrobiculate at the axils of the veins beneath. The flowers are in axillary, downy, corymbose panicles. The tree grows on the declivities of the mountains, at an elevation of from about a mile to a mile and a half, and in a mean

temperature of 67° F. It was seen by Humboldt and Bonpland in the neighborhood of Loxa, and is said also to grow near Guancabamba and Ayavaca in Peru. It is now admitted to be the source of the *crown bark of Loxa*. Weddell considers as varieties of this species, though with some hesitation, as he has never seen them alive, the following: 1, *Candolli* (*C. macrocalyx* of Pavon and De Candolle); 2, *lucumæfolia* (*C. lucumæfolia* of Pavon and Lindley); 3, *lancifolia* (*C. lancifolia* of Mutis), hereafter referred to as a distinct species; and, 4, *Pitayensis*, growing in New Granada.* The last mentioned variety has subsequently been raised by Weddell to the rank of a distinct species.

3. *C. micrantha.* Ruiz and Pavon, *Fl. Peruv.* ii. 52, t. 194; Lindley, *Flor. Med.* 412; Carson, *Illust. of Med. Bot.* i. 52, pl. 44. This is a large tree, forty feet high, with oblong leaves, from four to twelve inches in length and from two to six in breadth, scarcely acute, smooth, shining on the upper surface, and scrobiculate at the axils of the veins beneath. The flowers are in terminal, loose leafless panicles, and are smaller than those of any other species except *C. lancifolia.* (*Lindley.*) The tree grows, according to Ruiz and Pavon, in the mountains near Chicoplaya, Monson, and Puebla de San Antonio, according to Pöppig, at Cuchero, and, according to Weddell, in the Peruvian province of Carabaya, and in Bolivia. Ruiz states that its bark is always mixed with that sent into the market from the provinces of Panatahuas, Huamilies, and Huanuco. The Edinburgh and Dublin Colleges ascribed to it the *cinchona cinerea*, the *gray* or *silver bark* of the British commerce; and the U. S. Pharmacopœia recognizes it as one of the sources of pale bark, as it undoubtedly is.

Cinchona succirubra, Pavon, which was officinally recognized in the U. S. Pharmacopœia of 1870, and, as the source of the genuine red bark, is scarcely less important than either of the preceding, has, within a few years, acquired additional value from the great success with which it has been propagated in the Highlands of Hindostan.

4. *C. succirubra.* Pavon, *MS.*; Howard, *Pharm. Journ. and Trans.*, Oct. 1856, p. 209, with a figure.—*C. ovata*, var. *erythroderma.* Weddell, *Hist. Nat. des Quinquinas*, p. 60. This species has been satisfactorily ascertained to produce the proper officinal red bark, the origin of which remained so long unknown, or at least undetermined. The name of *C. succirubra* originated with Pavon, having been applied by him, in an unpublished manuscript, to an undescribed species yielding the bark called *cinchona colorada de Huaranda*, which has been shown to be identical with officinal red bark; while a specimen of the plant itself, in the collection of Ruiz and Pavon at Kew, upon examination by Mr. J. E. Howard, of London, proved to correspond exactly with a specimen of the red bark tree which that gentleman had received from South America. The same plant was described by Weddell, in his *Natural History of the Cinchonas*, as a variety of *C. ovata*, under the designation of *Cinchona ovata*, var. *erythroderma*, and was conjectured by him to be the source of red bark, though he did not at the time feel justified in giving a decided opinion.

* Botanists seem disposed to return to the old Linnæan designation of this species, *Cinchona officinalis*, of which three varieties are recognized, under the names of *Bonplandiana*, *Uritusinga*, and *Crespilla*, all yielding the crown barks. Of these the *Bonplandiana* seems to have been most successfully transplanted, as upwards of 750,000 are now growing in the plantations of British India. (*Bronghton.*) The varieties of this species seem to flourish best at a greater elevation than the *C. succirubra*, growing at heights from 5500 or 6000 feet even to 8350 feet above the level of the sea. The effect of the moss in increasing the productiveness of this species in alkaloids has been highly satisfactory. (*Markham.*) Instead, however, of cinchonine being the prominent alkaloid of this species, as in the pale barks of Loxa, the quinine has been found most abundant in the Indian bark, and, though the former alkaloid is generally present, yet it is usually in small proportion. Indeed, Mr. Broughton states that the trees of the variety Bonplandiana yield a bark nearly equal to the fine Calisaya bark of Bolivia, and superior in some respects for manufacturing purposes to the richer red barks, as it yields its alkaloids more readily in a free state, in consequence of the smaller amount of resin and coloring matter contained in it. The following results were obtained by Mr. Broughton in the chemical examination of the bark of this species. The dried bark of the trunk yielded altogether in alkaloids (hydrated) 3·6 per cent., of which 2·8 per cent. was quinine (or of alkaloid soluble in ether), and only 0·8 per cent. was of cinchonine and cinchonidine jointly; and 2·8 per cent. of crystallized sulphate of quinine was obtained. Another specimen was even more productive, yielding 3·0 per cent. of quinine. The bark of the same species, which had been renewed in six months under the mossing process, gave a total of alkaloids (hydrated) 6 8 per cent., of which 4·8 was of quinine, and 2·0 of cinchonine and cinchonidine jointly; and 4·1 per cent. of crystallised sulphate of quinine was obtained. (*P. J. Tr.*, 1867, p. 241.)

This point, however, having been subsequently determined, and the plant elevated to the dignity of a new species, Mr. Howard proposed at first to name it *Cinchona erythroderma*, not only from courtesy to Dr. Weddell, but also from the appropriateness of the name itself, implying the redness of the bark; but Pavon's name of *succirubra* was afterwards preferred on the ground of priority, being itself also (red-juiced) expressive of a quality of the tree. This species is, when full-grown, of great magnitude; but almost all the older trees have been destroyed, and few now remain with a stem so much as a foot in diameter. The branches have a silvery epidermis, corresponding with that of the red bark in quills as often seen in the market. The leaves are ovate, varying greatly in size, often as much as nine inches by six, narrowing towards the base, somewhat membranaceous, pubescent beneath, and green on both sides. The tree inhabits a region in the present republic of Ecuador, on the western slope of Chimborazo, the seaport of which is the town of Guayaquil.*

Commercial History.

For more than a century after Peruvian bark came into use, it was procured almost exclusively from the neighborhood of Loxa. In a memoir published in 1738, La Condamine speaks of the bark of Rhiobambo, Cuença, Ayavaca, and Jaen de Bracomoros. Of these places, the first two, together with Loxa, lie within the ancient kingdom of Quito, at the southern extremity; the others are in the same vicinity, within the borders of Peru. The drug was shipped chiefly at Payta, whence it was carried to Spain, and thence spread over Europe. Beyond the limits above mentioned, the Cinchona was not supposed to exist, till, in the year 1753, a gentleman of Loxa discovered it, while on a journey to Santa Fé de Bogota, in numerous situations along his route, wherever, in fact, the elevation of the country was equal to that of Loxa, or about 6500 feet above the level of the sea. This discovery extended through Quito into New Granada, as far as two degrees and a half north of the equator. But no practical advantage was derived from it; and the information lay buried in the archives of the viceroyalty, till subsequent events brought it to light. To Mutis belongs the credit of making known the existence of the Cinchona in New Granada. He first discovered it in the neighborhood of Bogota, in 1772. A botanical expedition was afterwards organized by the Spanish government, with the view of exploring this part of their dominions, and the direction was given to Mutis. Its researches eventuated in the discovery of several species of Cinchona in New Granada; and a commerce in the bark soon commenced, which was carried on through the ports of Carthagena and Santa Martha.

To these sources another was added about the same time (1776), by the discovery of the Cinchona in the centre of Peru, in the mountainous region about the city of Huanuco, which lies on the eastern declivity of the Andes, northeast of Lima, at least six degrees south of the province of Loxa. To explore this new locality, another botanical expedition was set on foot, at the head of which were Ruiz and Pavon, the distinguished authors of the Flora Peruviana. These botanists spent several years in that region, during which time they discovered numerous

* Botanists are far from being in concord in regard to the naming of the species of the genus Cinchona. As previously mentioned, the experiments made in India have shown that the trees have a remarkable tendency to hybridize, and Kuntze, as the result of studies made in the India plantations, has concluded that there are but four true species, namely, *C. Weddelliana*, Kuntze, nearly answering to *C. Calisaya*, Weddell; *C. Paviana*, Kuntze, including *C. micrantha*, Ruiz and Pavon, with various allied forms; *C. Howardiana*, Kuntze, including *C. succirubra*, Pavon, and other species of various authors; and *C. Pahudiana*, Howard. (*Cinchona, Arten, Hybriden, und Cultur der Chininbäume*, Leipzig, 1878.) The conspectus on p. 431 of the principal species of Cinchona is taken from the *Pharmacographia*. It seems to represent more nearly, as well as more concisely, the present state of our knowledge than does much of the matter in previous editions of the United States Dispensatory, and is consequently substituted for the latter.

Markham in his recent work gives the following synopsis of the valuable species.

I. C. officinalis, var. α. Condaminea, β. Bonplandia, γ. Crispa, } yielding crown bark.

II. C. succirubra, Pavon, yielding red bark.

III. C. pitayensis, C. lancifolia, C. cordifolia, } yielding colombian bark.

IV. C. nitida, C. micrantha, C. Peruviana, } yielding gray bark.

V. C. Calisaya, yielding yellow bark.

Conspectus of the Principal Species of Cinchona.

Species (excluding sub-species and varieties) according to Weddell.	Where Figured.	Native Country.	Where Cultivated.	Product.
I. Stirps Cinchonæ officinalis.				
1. Cinchona officinalis, Hook.	Bot. Mag. 5364.	Ecuador (Loxa).	India, Ceylon, Java.	Loxa or Crown Bark, Pale Bark.
2. " macrocalyx, Pav.	Howard, N. Q.	Peru.		Ashy Crown Bark. The sub-species *C. Palton* affords an important sort called *Palton Bark* much used in the manufacture of quinine.
3. " lucumæfolia, Pav.	Do.	Ecuador, Peru.		
4. " lanceolata, R. et P. (?)	Do.	Peru.		Carthagena Bark, confounded with Palton Bark, but is not so good.
5. " lancifolia, Mutis.	Karsten tab. 11, 12.	New Granada.	India.	Columbian Bark. Imported in large quantities for manufacture of quinine. The soft Columbian Bark is produced by Howard's var. *oblonga*.
6. " amygdalifolia, Wedd.	Wedd. tab. 6.	Peru, Bolivia.		A poor bark, but not now imported.
II. Stirps Cinchonæ rugosæ.				
7. Cinchona pitayensis, Wedd.	Karst. tab. 22. (*C. Trianæ.*)	New Granada (Popayan)	India.	Pitayo Bark. Very valuable; used by makers of quinine; it is the chief source of quinidine.
8. " rugosa, Pav.	Howard, N. Q.	Peru.		Bark unknown, probably valueless.
9. " Mutisii, Lamb.	Do.	Ecuador.		Bark not in commerce, contains only aricine.
10. " hirsuta, R. et P.	Wedd. tab. 21.	Peru.		
11. " carabayensis, Wedd.	Wedd. tab. 19.	Peru, Bolivia.		Bark not collected.
12. " Pahudiana, How.	Howard, N. Q.	Peru.	India, Java.	A poor bark, yet of handsome appearance; propagation of tree discontinued.
13. " asperifolia, Wedd.	Wedd. tab. 20.	Bolivia.		Bark not collected.
14. " umbellulifera, Pav.	Howard, N. Q.	Peru.		Bark not known as a distinct sort.
15. " glandulifera, R. et P.	Do.	Peru.		Do.
16. " Humboldtiana, Lamb.	Do.	Peru.		False Loxa Bark, Jaen Bark. A very bad bark.
III. Stirps Cinchonæ micranthæ.				
17. Cinchona australis, Wedd.	Wedd. tab. 8.	South Bolivia.		An inferior bark, mixed with Calisaya.
18. " scrobiculata, H. et B.	Do.	Peru.		Bark formerly known as *Red Cusco Bark* or *Santa Ana Bark*.
19. " peruviana, How.	Howard, N. Q.	Peru.	India.	Gray Bark, Huanuco or Lima Bark. Chiefly consumed on the Continent.
20. " nitida, R. et P.	Do.	Peru.	India.	
21. " micrantha, R. et P.	Do.	Peru.	India.	
IV. Stirps Cinchonæ Calisayæ.				
22. Cinchona Calisaya, Wedd.	Wedd. tab. 9.	Peru, Bolivia.	India, Ceylon, Java, Jamaica, Mexico.	Calisaya Bark, Bolivian Bark, Yellow Bark. The tree exists under many varieties, bark also very variable.
23. " elliptica, Wedd.		Peru (Carabaya).		Carabaya Bark. Bark scarcely now imported. *C. euneura*, Miq. (flower and fruit unknown), may perhaps be this species.
V. Stirps Cinchonæ ovatæ.				
24. Cinchona purpurea, R. et P.	Howard, N. Q.	Peru (Huamalies)		Huamalies Bark. Not now imported.
25. " rufinervis, Wedd.	Do.	Peru, Bolivia.		Bark, a kind of light Calisaya.
26. " succirubra, Pav.	Do.	Ecuador.	India, Ceylon, Java, Jamaica.	Red Bark. Largely cultivated in British India.
27. " ovata, R. et P.	Do.	Peru, Bolivia.	India (?), Java (?).	Inferior Brown and Gray Barks.
28. " cordifolia, Mutis.	Karsten tab. 8.	New Granada, Peru.		Columbian Bark (in part). Tree exists under many varieties; bark of some used in manufacture of quinine.
29. " tucujensis, Karst.	Karsten tab. 9.	Venezuela.		Maracaibo Bark.
30. " pubescens, Vahl.	Wedd. tab. 16.	Ecuador, Peru, Bolivia.		Arica Bark (Cusco Bark from var. *Pelletieriana*). Some of the varieties contain aricine. *C. caloptera*, Miq., is probably a var. of this species.
31. " purpurascens, Wedd.	Wedd. tab. 18.	Bolivia.		Bark unknown in commerce.

species. Lima became the entrepot for the barks collected around Huanuco; and hence probably originated the name of Lima bark, so often conferred, in common language, not only upon the varieties received through that city, but also upon the medicine generally.

Soon after the last-mentioned discovery, two additional localities of the Cinchona were found; one at the northern extremity of the continent near Santa Martha,* the other very far to the south, in the provinces of La Paz and Cochabamba, then within the viceroyalty of Buenos Ayres, now in the republic of Bolivia. These latter places became the source of an abundant supply of excellent bark, which received the name of Calisaya. It was sent partly to the ports on the Pacific, partly to Buenos Ayres.

The consequence of these discoveries was a vast increase in the supply of bark, which was now shipped from the ports of Guayaquil, Payta, Lima, Arica, Buenos Ayres, Carthagena, and Santa Martha. At the same time the average quality was probably deteriorated; for, though many of the new varieties were possessed of excellent properties, yet equal care in superintending the collection and assorting of the bark could scarcely be exercised in a field so much more extended. The varieties now poured into the market soon became so numerous as to burden the memory if not to defy the discrimination of the druggist; and the best pharmacologists found themselves at a loss to discover any permanent peculiarities which might serve as the basis of a proper and useful classification. This perplexity has continued more or less to the present time; though the discovery of the alkaloidal principles has presented a ground of distinction before unknown. The restrictions upon the commerce of South America, by directing the trade into irregular channels, had also a tendency to deteriorate the character of the drug. Little attention was paid to a proper assortment of the several varieties; and not only were the best barks mixed with those of inferior species and less careful preparation, but the products of other trees, bearing no resemblance to the Cinchona, were sometimes added, having been artificially prepared so as to deceive a careless observer. The markets of this country were peculiarly ill-furnished. The supplies, being derived chiefly, by means of a contraband trade, from Carthagena and other ports on the Spanish Main, or indirectly through the Havana, were necessarily of an inferior character; and most of the good bark which reached us was imported by our druggists from London, whither it was sent from Cadiz. A great change, however, in this respect, took place after the ports on the Pacific were opened to our commerce. The best kinds of bark were thus rendered directly accessible to us; and the trash which formerly glutted our markets is now in great measure excluded. Our ships trading to the Pacific run along the American coast from Valparaiso to Guayaquil, stopping at the intermediate ports of Coquimbo, Copiapo, Arica, Callao, Truxillo, etc., from all which they probably receive supplies. Much good bark has of late also been imported from Carthagena, and other ports of the Caribbean Sea, being brought down the Magdalena River from the mountainous regions of New Granada; and, since the completion of the railroad across the Isthmus, large quantities reach this country by way of Panama, to which place they are brought chiefly from the Pacific ports of Buenaventura and Guayaquil. An additional source of supply has recently been opened through the Amazon; a considerable quantity of bark having been taken to the London market from the port of Para, in Brazil, brought down that river, probably, from the Peruvian province of Huanuco. According to Mr. Howard, the bark thus obtained is of inferior quality, yielding but a small proportion of alkaloids. (*P. J. Tr.*, Dec. 1863, p. 248.)†

The persons who collect the bark are called in South America *Cascarilleros.*

* In relation to this locality of the Cinchonas, we are informed that Dr. Ernst, President of a Scientific Society of Caracas, in an excursion from that place, discovered on the slopes of several mountains, groups of the *Cinchona cordifolia*, var. *rotundifolia*, Weddell, *C. rotundifolia* of Pavon, at the height of 4500 feet above the sea. The bark of this tree is said to be the variety known in commerce as the *Ashy Crown bark*, one of the Loxa barks. The bark was found to contain 0·5 per cent. of quinine, and 0·67 of cinchonine. (*A. J. P.*, 1870, p. 449.)

† An interesting history of the commerce in the Cinchona barks, by Dr. H. A. Weddell, will be found in the *A. J. P.* (xxvi. 539, Nov. 1854), originally from his *Voyages dans le Nord de la Bolivie*, Paris, 1853.

Considerable experience and judgment are requisite to render an individual well qualified for this business. He must not only be able to distinguish the trees which produce good bark from those less esteemed, but must also know the proper season and age at which a branch should be decorticated, and the marks by which the efficiency or inefficiency of any particular product is indicated. The bark gatherers begin their work with the setting in of the dry season in May. Sometimes they first cut down the tree, and afterwards strip off the bark from the branches; in other instances they decorticate the tree while standing. The former plan is said to be the most economical; as, when the tree is cut down, the stump pushes up shoots which in the course of time become fit for decortication, while, if deprived of its bark, the whole plant perishes. The operator separates the bark by making a longitudinal incision with a sharp knife through its whole thickness, and then forcing it off from the branch with the back of the instrument. Other means are resorted to, when the trunk or larger limbs are decorticated. According to Pöppig, the bark is not separated until three or four days after the tree is felled. It must then be speedily dried, as otherwise it becomes deteriorated. For this purpose it is taken out of the woods into some open place, where it is exposed to the sun. In drying it rolls up, or becomes quilled; and the degree to which this effect takes place is proportionate directly to the thinness of the bark, and inversely to the age of the branch from which it was derived. In packing the bark for exportation, it often happens that several different kinds are introduced in the same case. The packages are, in commercial language, called *seroons*. As found in this market they are usually covered with a case of thick and stiff ox-hide, lined within by a very coarse cloth, apparently woven out of some kind of grass.

The Cinchona forests, being in very thinly inhabited districts, do not, for the most part, belong to individuals, but are open to the enterprise of all who choose to engage in the collection of the bark. The consequence is, that the operations are carried on without reference to the future condition of this important interest; and the most wasteful modes of proceeding are often adopted.

The bitterness of the Cinchona is not confined to its bark. The leaves and flowers also have this property, which in the former is associated with acidity, in the latter with a delicious aroma, which renders the air fragrant in neighborhoods where the trees abound. The wood is nearly tasteless; but the bark of the root has the same virtues as that of the trunk.*

It was at one time supposed that the leaves might have sufficient of the active principles of the bark to justify their use in medicine; but, though they have proved useful as a tonic, experiment has not shown them to be possessed of decided antiperiodic powers, and, on chemical examination, they have yielded but a small proportion of the characteristic alkaloids.

Classification.

To form a correct and lucid system of classification is the most difficult part of the subject of bark. An arrangement founded on the botanical basis is liable to the objection, that the product of the same species may vary according to the age of the bark and the situation of the tree; and, besides, is at present scarcely practicable;

* Dr. De Vrij, on examining a specimen of *C. Pahudiana*, grown in Java, obtained from the bark of the stem 1·274 per cent. of alkaloids (cinchonidine and cinchonicine, without any quinine), and afterwards from the bark of the root, 2·818 per cent. of alkaloids, of which 1·849 was quinine. Another specimen, only two years old, yielded to him from the bark of the stem 0·09 per cent. of alkaloid, without a trace of quinine; while from the root, treated so as to separate all the woody fibres, he obtained 1·941 per cent. of alkaloids, of which more than three-fourths was quinine. Four other species yielded, for the most part, analogous results. *C. Calisaya* of Java gave 3·676 per cent. of alkaloids from bark of the stem, and 4·430 from that of the root; the same species from Hindostan 1·89 to 3·10; *C. lancifolia* of Java 4·18 to 2·94; *C. succirubra*, No. 1, from Ootacamund (East India) 2·10 to 2·00; *C. succirubra* from the same place 2·65 to 7·514; and *C. micrantha* from Ootacamund 2·791 to 4·166. The result of all his experiments justified, he thought, an appeal to his government to devote a small portion of ground to the cultivation of the *C. Pahudiana*, with the view of obtaining quinine from the roots when two years old; as he believed that the alkaloids might then be profitably obtained; but his application was not favorably received: and the correctness of his inference remains still undetermined. (*Journ. de Pharm.*, Janv. 1869, pp. 17-23.)

as, though our knowledge of the source of the several varieties has very much extended, it is still defective on some points.

The Spanish merchants adopted a classification, dependent partly on the place of growth or shipment, and partly on the inherent properties or supposed relative value of the bark. So long as the sources of the drug were very confined, and the varieties few, this plan answered the purposes of trade; but at present it is quite inadequate; and, though some of the names originally conferred upon this principle are still retained, they are often uncertain or misapplied.

Perhaps, on the whole, the best arrangement for pharmaceutical and medicinal purposes is that founded upon difference of color. It is true that dependence cannot be placed upon this property alone; as barks of a similar color have been found to possess very different virtues; and, between the various colors considered characteristic, there is an insensible gradation, so that it is not always possible to decide where one ends and the other begins. Still, it has been found that most of the valuable barks may be arranged, according to their color, in three divisions, which, though mingling at their extremes, are very distinctly characterized, in certain specimens, by peculiarity not only in color, but also in other sensible properties, and even in chemical constitution. The three divisions alluded to are the *pale*, the *yellow*, and the *red*. This arrangement has been adopted in the Br. Pharmacopœia; and the U. S. recognizes the yellow and red, and under Cinchona any colored bark containing at least 3 per cent. of alkaloids. Until recently, as almost all the highly-esteemed barks were brought from the Pacific coast of South America, and those from the northern coast were deemed inferior, it was only the former that were recognized under the three divisions referred to. Of late, however, some of the best barks, and most productive in alkaloids, have been brought from India and Java; so that the restriction of the officinal barks to the Pacific coast was abandoned at the late revision of the U. S. Pharmacopœia; and the much better rule was adopted of recognizing all the Cinchona barks as officinal which might contain three per cent. of their proper alkaloids. Nevertheless, the former officinal varieties have been retained. In describing, therefore, the different kinds of barks, we shall treat first, under the officinal titles of *pale*, *yellow*, and *red*, of those originally brought only from the ports of the Pacific; while those coming to us from the northern ports of New Granada and Venezuela will be subsequently considered under the heading of *Carthagena barks*, by which name they have been generally known in commerce. The commercial name will be given whenever a knowledge of it can be useful. It is proper to state that the different barks are often mingled in the same package, and that, in deciding upon the character of a seroon, the druggist is guided rather by the predominance than the exclusive existence of certain distinctive properties.

1. Pale or Gray Bark.

The epithet *pale*, applied to the barks of this division, is derived from the color of the powder. The French call them *quinquinas gris*, or gray barks, from the color of the epidermis. They come into the market in cylindrical pieces, of variable length from a few inches to a foot and a half, sometimes singly, sometimes doubly quilled, from two lines to an inch in diameter, and from half a line to two or three lines in thickness. The kinds which were formerly deemed the finest are about the size of a goose-quill; but experience has shown that the young barks are not the most efficient. Their exterior surface is usually more or less rough, marked with transverse and sometimes with longitudinal fissures, and of a grayish color, owing to adhering lichens. The shade is different in different samples. Sometimes it is a light gray, approaching to white, sometimes dull and brown, sometimes a grayish fawn, and frequently diversified by the intermixture of the proper color of the epidermis with that of the patches of lichens. The interior surface, in the finer kinds, is smooth; in the coarser, occasionally rough and somewhat ligneous. Its color is a brownish orange, sometimes inclining to red, sometimes to yellow, and, in some inferior specimens, of a dusky hue. The fracture is usually smooth, with some short filaments on the internal part only. In the coarser barks it is more fibrous. The color of the powder is a pale fawn, which is of a darker hue in the inferior kinds. The taste is moderately bitter and somewhat astringent, without being disagreeable or nauseous. Authors speak also of an acidulous and aromatic flavor. The better kinds have a feeble odor, which is distinct and agreeably aromatic in powder and decoction. The pale barks are chemically characterized by containing *a much larger proportion of cinchonine and quinidine or cinchonidine than of quinine;* and their infusion does not yield a precipitate with solution of sulphate of sodium. Their appearance generally indicates that they were derived from the smaller branches. They are collected in the provinces about Loxa, or in the country which surrounds the city of Huanuco, northeast of Lima, and are probably derived chiefly from *Cinchona Condaminea*, *C. nitida*, and *C. micrantha*.

There are several commercial varieties of pale bark, obtained from different sources, and differing more or less in properties. The most highly esteemed of these is the *Loxa bark*, the finest specimens of which are sometimes called *crown bark of Loxa*, from the impression that they have the same origin and character with the bark formerly selected with great care for the use of the King of Spain and the royal family. The pale bark collected about Huanuco is named either *Lima bark*, because taken to that city for commercial distribution, or *Huanuco bark*, from its place of collection. The former name has been more common in this country, where, indeed, this commercial variety has not unfrequently been confounded with the Loxa bark. Other pale barks are the *Jaen* and *Huamilies barks*, which are scarcely known as distinct varieties in the United States.*

In this country, the pale bark has fallen into disuse. As it yields little quinine, it is not employed in the manufacture of the sulphate of that alkaloid, which has almost superseded the bark as a remedy in intermittents; and the red or yellow bark is preferred by physicians when it is necessary to resort to the medicine in substance. There is no doubt, however, that *cinchonine*, *quinidine*, and *cinchonidine* possess febrifuge properties little inferior, so that the pale bark may come into more extensive use for the preparation of the other alkaloids.

2. Yellow Bark.

The officinal term yellow bark is applicable only to the valuable variety of the drug called commercially *Calisaya*, a name which has been said, though erroneously, to be derived from a province in Bolivia, near the city of La Paz, where the bark is collected.† By the druggists *Calisaya bark* is arranged in two sub-varieties, the quilled and the flat, which sometimes come mixed together in the same seroon, sometimes separate. It is called by the French *quinquina jaune royal* (royal yellow bark), from its resemblance to a variety formerly collected for the Spanish king.

The *quilled Calisaya* (*Calisaya arrolada* of the Spanish Americans) is in pieces from three inches to two feet long, from a quarter of an inch to two or three inches in diameter, and of equally variable thickness. The epidermis is of a brownish color, diversified or concealed by silvery white, whitish, or yellowish lichens, is marked by longitudinal wrinkles and transverse fissures, and is often partially separated, and generally easily separable from the proper bark. In the larger kinds, it is thick, rough, deeply indented by the transverse fissures, which often surround the quills, and is composed of several layers, separated from each other by a reddish brown membrane. The epidermis yields a dark red powder, and is tasteless and inert. It is desirable, therefore, to get rid of it before the bark is powdered, as the medicine is thus procured of greater strength. The bark itself, without the epidermis, is from one to two lines in thickness, compact, of a short-fibrous texture, and when broken presents shining points, apparently the termination of small fibres running

* For an elaborate description of numerous varieties of Pale Bark, see fourteenth edition of the United States Dispensatory. This is omitted here as unnecessary, because barks are no longer purchased by their physical appearance, but by their yield of alkaloids on analysis.

† No such province exists in Bolivia. According to M. Laubert, the name is a corruption of *collisalla*, said to be derived from *colla*, a remedy, and *salla*, a rocky country. (*Journ. de Pharm.*, xxii. 614.) Weddell refers the origin of the name to the words *colli* and *saya*, which in the Quichua language signify *red* and *sort*, and have probably been applied from the redness which the outer denuded surface of the bark assumes in drying, or from the red color which the leaves sometimes exhibit.

longitudinally, which, examined by the microscope, are found, when freed from a salmon-colored powder that surrounds them, to be yellow and transparent. When the bark is powdered, they readily separate, in the form of spicula, which, like those of cowhage, insinuate themselves into the skin, and produce a disagreeable itching and irritation. The color of the bark is brownish yellow with a tinge of orange, the taste less astringent than that of the pale bark, but much more bitter; and the bitterness is somewhat peculiar. The external part of the proper bark is more bitter and astringent, and consequently stronger in medicinal power, than the internal. The odor is faint, but when the bark is boiled, resembles that of the pale varieties. The small quills closely resemble some of the pale barks, but may be distinguished by their very bitter taste. The U. S. Pharmacopœia thus describes quilled Calisaya. "The quills are either single or double, varying in length, and from one-half to two inches (1 to 5 cm.) in diameter; the bark is from one-sixteenth to one-eighth of an inch (1·5 to 3 mm.) in thickness; it is covered with a grayish cork marked by longitudinal and transverse fissures, about one inch (25 mm.) apart and forming irregular meshes with raised edges. The inner surface is cinnamon-brown and finely striate from the bast-fibres." *U. S.*

The *flat Calisaya* (*Calisaya plancha* of the Spaniards), which is derived from the large branches and trunk, is in pieces of various lengths, either quite flat, or but slightly curved, and generally destitute of the epidermis, which has been obviously removed through its own want of adhesiveness to the proper bark, and not by a knife, as is the case with some inferior barks in other respects resembling the Calisaya. "The flat pieces vary in length and width; are from one-sixth to two-fifths of an inch (4 to 10 mm.) in thickness, almost entirely deprived of the brown, corky layer, compact, of a tawny-yellow color; outer surface marked with shallow, conchoidal depressions and intervening, rather sharp ridges; inner surface closely and finely striate; the transverse fracture showing numerous, very short and rigid, glistening fibres, which are radially arranged, and rarely in small groups. The powder has a light cinnamon-brown color, and a slightly aromatic but persistently bitter taste." *U. S.* The inner surface is like that of the quilled pieces; the outer is irregular, marked with confluent longitudinal furrows and ridges, and somewhat darker colored than the inner, being of a brownish fawn, frequently diversified with darker stains. The bark is of uniform fracture throughout, generally thicker than the quilled, more fibrous in its texture, less compact, less bitter, and possessed of less medicinal power. Though weaker than the proper bark of the quills, it is usually, in equal weight, more valuable than that variety, because free from the useless epidermis. This variety of yellow bark is now (1889) practically out of the American market.

The officinal yellow bark is characterized by its strongly bitter taste, with little astringency; by its fine brownish yellow, somewhat orange color, which is still brighter in the powder; and by *containing a large proportion of quinine with very little cinchonine.* The salts of quinine and lime are so abundant, that a strong infusion of it instantly affords a precipitate when crystals of sulphate of sodium are added. (Guibourt, *Hist. des Drogues*, 4éme ed., iii. 131.)* "The true yellow Cinchona Bark should not be confounded with other Cinchona barks of a similar color, but having the bast-fibres in bundles or radial rows, and breaking with a splintery or coarsely fibrous fracture." *U. S.*

Until the recent most valuable researches of Weddell, nothing was known with certainty as to the particular species which yields Calisaya bark. At present there is no variety of which, in this respect, we have more accurate knowledge. The genuine bark is derived from the newly described species, named *C. Calisaya;* but the bark of *C. Boliviana*, another of the species discovered by Weddell, is sometimes

* For descriptions of varieties of yellow bark, see 14th edition U. S. Dispensatory. A *false bark* has been sometimes mixed with the genuine Calisaya, which it resembles so closely as not to be easily distinguished by the eye. According to Weddell, it is the bark of *Gomphosia chlorantha*, a lofty tree, growing in the same forests where the *Calisaya* is found. It is distinguished by a peculiar odor, and by exhibiting in its transverse section, under the microscope, "a peculiar fasciculate disposition of the cortical fibres, and some vessels gorged with a ruby-colored juice." It does not contain a particle of alkaloid, but yields a volatile oil on which its odor depends. (Howard, *P. J. Tr.*, xiv. 318.)

mixed with it in the same seroons. It is produced exclusively in Bolivia, formerly upper Peru, and in the southern portion of the adjoining Peruvian province of Carabaya. Before these countries were separated from Spain, it was shipped as well from Buenos Ayres as from the ports on the Pacific; but at present it comes only from the latter. As first announced in this work, from information derived from merchants long personally engaged in commercial transactions on the Pacific coast of South America, the bark is brought from the interior to the port of Arica, whence it is sent to various other ports on the coast. The interior commerce in the drug has its centre chiefly in the town of La Paz. The trade in this bark has been much diminished, in consequence partly of its greater scarcity, partly of restrictions by the Bolivian government.

It is generally supposed to have been first introduced into commerce towards the end of the last century, and it was probably not known by its present name till that period; but La Condamine states that the Jesuits of La Paz, at a period anterior to the discovery of the febrifuge of Loxa, sent to Rome a very bitter bark by the name of *quinaquina*, which, though supposed by that traveller to have been derived from the Peruvian balsam tree, was very probably, as conjectured by Guibourt, the true cinchona. Besides, Pomet, in his *History of Drugs*, published in 1694, speaks of a bark more bitter than that of Loxa, obtained from the province of Potosi, which borders upon that of La Paz; and Chomal also states that the cinchona tree inhabited the mountains of Potosi, and produced a bark more esteemed than that which grew in the province of Quito. (Guibourt, *Journ. de Pharm.*, xvi. 235.) It is possible that, though known at this early period, it may have gone out of use; and its re-introduction into notice, towards the end of the last century, may have been mistaken for an original discovery.

3. Red Bark.

The name of this variety is very appropriately applied; as the color is usually distinct both in the bark and the powder. In South America it is called *cascarilla roxa* and *colorada*. Some writers have divided it into several sub-varieties; but, in relation to the true red bark, there does not seem to be ground for such division in any essential difference of properties. Like the *Calisaya*, it comes in quills and flat pieces, which are probably derived from different parts of the same tree. It is imported in chests.

Some of the pieces are entirely rolled, some partially so, as if they had been taken from half the circumference of the branch; others are nearly or quite flat. They vary greatly in size, the quill being sometimes less than half an inch in diameter, sometimes as much as two inches; while the flat pieces are occasionally very large and thick, as if derived from the trunk of a tree. They are covered with a reddish brown or gray, sometimes whitish epidermis, which is rugged, wrinkled longitudinally, and in the thicker pieces marked with furrows, which in some places penetrate to the surface of the proper bark. In many specimens, numerous small roundish or oblong eminences, called warts, may be observed upon the outer surface. Beneath the epidermis is a layer, dark red, brittle and compact, which possesses some bitterness and astringency, but much less than the interior parts. These are woody and fibrous, of a more or less lively brownish red color, which is usually very distinct, but in some specimens passes into orange and even yellowish brown; so that it is not always possible to distinguish the variety by this property alone. The taste is bitter and astringent, and the odor similar to that of other good barks. Red bark is chemically distinguished by *containing considerable quantities of both quinine and cinchonine*. It yields a turbid salmon-colored decoction with water. Mr. Howard, in examining slender sections of a fine specimen of red bark under the microscope, noticed numerous stellate groups of crystals diffused irregularly throughout its substance, which he believed to consist of quinovate of quinine, formed during the drying of the bark. He also noticed other crystalline forms which he ascribed to the quinovates severally of cinchonine, quinidine, and cinchonidine. (*P. J. Tr.*, May, 1865, p. 584.)* The U. S. Pharmacopœia thus describes red bark. "In quills and in

* For description of varieties of Red Bark, see fourteenth edition of U. S. Dispensatory.

flat or inflexed pieces, varying in length and width, and from one-eighth to one-half of an inch (3 to 12 mm.) in thickness; compact; of a deep brown-red color; outer surface covered with numerous, suberous warts and ridges, or longitudinally and somewhat transversely fissured; inner surface rather coarsely striate; transverse fracture short-fibrous; the bast-fibres in interrupted, radial lines; the powder deep brown-red, slightly odorous, astringent and bitter. Red Cinchona should not be confounded with other Cinchona barks, having an orange-red color, and breaking with a coarse, splintery fracture. Thin, quilled Red Cinchona of a light red-brown color should be rejected." *U. S.*

NON-OFFICINAL OR CARTHAGENA BARKS.

Under this head may be classed all the Cinchona barks brought from the northern Atlantic ports of South America. In commerce, they are variously called *Pitaya, Bogota, Carthagena, Maracaybo*, and *Santa Martha barks*, according to the place in the vicinity of which they are collected, or the particular port at which they may be shipped. Formerly these barks were for the most part of inferior quality, and were therefore not recognized in the Pharmacopœias; but the deficient supply and consequent high price of Calisaya have directed enterprise into other quarters; and large quantities of very good bark were thrown into commerce from New Granada, derived chiefly from the neighborhood of Bogota and Popayan, and brought down the river Magdalena. Since the completion of the railroad across the Isthmus of Panama, considerable quantities have been brought to us by that route, being shipped from the port of Buenaventura, on the Pacific coast. There can be little doubt that the commerce in these barks will continue and increase; as some of them are inferior in their yield of alkaloids only to the Calisaya, if even to that variety, and the region from which they are procured is almost virgin soil. It has appeared to us, from an examination of such of them as have come under our notice, that they may all, at least with one exception, be referred without violence to some one or another of the varieties of Carthagena bark already recognized; but these better kinds formerly seldom reached the market; because, partaking of the general reputation of the inferior barks from the same region, it was feared that they might not pay the cost of importation. Most of the Carthagena barks are characterized by a soft, whitish or yellowish white epidermis, which may be easily scraped by the nail, and which, though often more or less completely removed, almost always leaves behind traces sufficient to indicate its character. Those of them which may, in other respects, bear some resemblance to Calisaya, are in general readily distinguishable by this character of the epidermis when it remains, and, when it is wanting, by the peculiar appearance of the outer surface, showing that the exterior coating has been scraped off, or shaved off with a knife. They all contain the alkaloids in greater or less proportion, though they differ much in this respect. In reference to the relative proportion of the different alkaloids, they have nothing in common, except perhaps that they yield proportionately more cinchonine, cinchonidine, and quinidine than the Calisaya, resembling, in this respect, the pale and red barks. Inferior barks, with the soft, white epidermis, are found on the western coast of South America, where they are known as *white barks*;* but they seldom reach us. In the state of

* *Paytine* or *Paytina*. Having been requested by a merchant to examine for quinine a *white bark* from the Pacific port of *Payta*, Dr. O. Hesse, in the year 1870, discovered that the bark contained alkaloids, but not one of those proved to exist in the proper Cinchona barks. The alkaloid specially noticed by him, may be prepared from the alcoholic extract, by treating this with soda, and agitating with ether, which dissolves the alkaloid with some coloring matter. The ethereal liquid, agitated with dilute sulphuric acid, furnishes a solution of the sulphate. This is decolorized by a little animal charcoal, almost neutralised with heat by ammonia, then, after cooling, is treated with iodide of potassium, until this ceases to produce a precipitate. The salt thus formed is entirely deposited in 24 hours. Separated from the mother-water, it is treated with dilute solution of soda, and shaken with ether. This, holding the alkaloid in solution, is separated from the heavier liquid; and, having been washed with water, yields, on spontaneous evaporation, the alkaloid in fine colorless crystals. Dr. Hesse gives the new alkaloid the name of *paytine*, after the port whence the bark was obtained. Paytine is in well-defined prismatic crystals. It has a bitter taste. It melts at 156° C., and distils partially at a higher temperature, leaving a carbonaceous residue. It is very soluble in alcohol, ether, benzin, and chloroform, but little soluble in water and alkaline solution. According to the analysis of Hesse it is represented by the formula $C_{21}H_{24}N_2O$ for the pure anhydrous alkaloid, with the addition of one mol. of water in the crystals. It seems to be without poisonous properties, as dogs have taken it freely without evil results. It has not been tried on man; but is a good sub-

powder, the inferior Carthagena barks were formerly, and are still, to a certain extent, kept in the shops, and sold for tooth-powder, etc., under the name of *common bark.* They have not unfrequently been substituted, either fraudulently or by mistake, for the better kinds.

The Carthagena barks were formerly classified, according to their color, into the *yellow, orange, red,* and *brown ;* but this mode of distinction must now be abandoned; for these varieties of color may be found in the barks identical in other respects, and derived from the same species of Cinchona. The well characterized Carthagena barks may all be referred to one of the three following varieties.

1. *Hard Carthagena Bark. Hard Yellow Carthagena Bark. Yellow Bark of Santa Fé. Common Yellow Carthagena Bark.—China flava dura.* Von Bergen. *Quinquina de Carthagène jaune pâle.* Guibourt. This is in pieces of various size and form, sometimes wholly or partially quilled, and sometimes flat; and the flat pieces present the appearance of having been warped in drying, being frequently curved longitudinally backward, and sometimes also in the transverse direction or spirally. The quills are from three to eight lines in diameter, from half a line to a line and a half thick, and from five to nine and rarely fifteen inches long. The flat pieces are thicker, from half an inch to two inches broad, and from four to eight and sometimes twelve inches in length. As found in this market, the bark is sometimes in small, irregularly square or oblong, flattish, and variously warped pieces, from one to four inches long, and from one to three lines in thickness, mixed with small quills or fragments of quills; the former appearing as if chipped from the trunk or larger branches, the latter evidently derived from the small branches. In this shape it was treated of in some former editions of this work, as a distinct variety, under the name of *Santa Martha Bark,* which it at one time held in the market; but a closer examination has convinced us that it is the same bark as the one above described, though collected in a different manner. The quills are generally more covered with the whitish epidermis than the flat pieces, in which it is often nearly or quite removed. The inner surface of the latter, though sometimes smooth, is often rough and splintery, as if forcibly separated from the wood. The color of the proper bark is a pale, dull, brownish yellow, darker in parcels which have been long kept; and the surface often appears as if rubbed over with powdered bark. The texture is rather firm and compact, and the fracture abrupt, without being smooth or presenting long splinters. The taste is bitter and nauseous. This variety of bark is now universally ascribed to *C. cordifolia.*

2. *Fibrous Carthagena Bark. Fibrous Yellow Carthagena Bark. Spongy Carthagena Bark. Bogota Bark. Coquetta Bark.—Quinia naranjanda.* Mutis.—*Quinquina orangé.* Humboldt.—*China flava fibrosa.* Von Bergen.—*Quinquina Carthagène spongieux.* Guibourt. This is in quills or half-quills, or is slightly rolled; and there are comparatively few pieces which are quite flat, even among the largest barks. The quills are from half an inch to an inch and a half in diameter, and of extremely variable length, with a yellowish brown epidermis, often covered with crustaceous lichens so as to render the surface of the bark whitish and smooth, and exhibiting not unfrequently longitudinal and transverse fissures. The larger barks, which are much the most frequent in commerce, are usually from six to twelve inches long, from one to two inches broad, and from two to five lines in thickness; but they often vary much from these dimensions, being sometimes in the smallest fragments, and sometimes forming semi-cylinders four or five inches in diameter, a foot and a half long, and nine lines thick. They are usually without epidermis, which has been scraped off, or pared off with a knife, leaving the surface smooth and uniform in the former case, and somewhat angular in the latter. Sometimes, however, the

ject for therapeutical experiment, especially in miasmatic fevers. According to Dr. Hesse, the bark which yields it, though bearing a superficial resemblance to the Calisaya, cannot, from its interior structure, have been the product of a Cinchona. The bark is in pieces about one foot long, two inches broad, and two or three lines thick; and consists mainly of greenish yellow cells, between which is lodged, in large quantities, a white pulverulent matter. It has so little firmness that its fibres are crushed under the pressure of the finger-nail. It has been found to contain another alkaloid besides paytine; but this has not been examined. For further particulars about the alkaloid see the *Journ. de Pharm.*, Nov.-Dec. 1870, p. 389.

epidermis either partially or wholly remains, when it generally exhibits the soft whitish surface characteristic of most of the Carthagena barks. The bark is very fibrous, presenting generally, when broken, long, sometimes stringy splinters, though the outer edge of the fracture is occasionally short from the cellular, or remains of the suberous coat. Its texture is loose, soft, and spongy under the teeth, and the bark itself is usually light. The color both of the trimmed outer surface, and the inner, and of the bark itself, varies from an ochreous or light brownish yellow, to orange, and red; but, for the most part, it presents more or less of the orange tint, which induced Mutis to give it the title of *orange bark*. The red color is found especially in the largest barks. The larger pieces are sometimes marked on the outside with a deep spiral impression, produced probably by a climbing plant winding around the stem of the tree. The color of the powder is yellowish, with not unfrequently an orange tint. The taste is more or less bitter, but varies in this respect extremely; some barks being almost insipid, while others have a very decided taste. There can be little doubt that these barks are all derived from the *Cinchona lancifolia* of Mutis. It is asserted that the red variety of the bark is obtained from trees which grow side by side with those which yield the yellow or orange.

The productiveness of the fibrous bark in alkaloids varies greatly in the different specimens. Thus, while some have yielded scarcely any product, others have been found to afford more than three per cent. They probably contain all the cinchona alkaloids; but some have been found more abundant in one, and others in another. Thus, the red is said to be especially rich in quinidine (cinchonidine); a Pitaya bark, which we believe to belong to the fibrous Carthagena, has yielded a very large product of quinine; while, in not a few specimens which have been examined, the cinchonine predominates. (*A. J. P.*, xxv. 308.) It is probable that the richness in these principles depends in some degree on the natural position of the plants; those growing in low situations being less productive than those higher on the mountains.*

A specimen labelled *yellow bark of Loxa*, brought from South America several years since by Dr. Dillard, of the U. S. Navy, and said to be used in Loxa for making extract of bark, presents characteristics closely analogous to those of fibrous Carthagena bark, sufficiently so to justify the supposition that it was derived from the same species of Cinchona; and we have seen a specimen sent hither from Guayaquil, which has the same character, and is so rich in alkaloids as to be worked with advantage.†

3. *Hard Pitaya Bark.—Pitaya Condaminea Bark.* Pereira.—*Quinquina brun de Carthagène. Quinquina Pitaya, ou de la Colombia, ou d'Antioquia.* Guibourt. This bark, though seen by Guibourt so long since as 1830, did not come into general notice until some years afterwards. Much of it has been imported into Philadelphia, coming sometimes through Carthagena, and sometimes over the Isthmus of Panama, whither it is brought from Buenaventura. The following description is drawn from an examination of the bark contained in several seroons that have come under our notice. It is in small irregular pieces, from less than an inch to about four inches long, which are obviously the fragments of larger pieces

* Karsten states that the bark of *C. lancifolia*, which on the average yields 2·5 per cent. of sulphate of quinine and from 1·0 to 1·5 per cent. of sulphate of cinchonine, often yields neither, and sometimes 4·5 per cent. of the two. The bark of the young branches yields much less than that of the trunk. (*A. J. P.*, xxx. 534.)

† *Fibrous Carthagena Bark.* The following is an abbreviation of Von Bergen's description of this variety. In shape and dimensions it does not materially differ from the preceding; but the flatter pieces are almost always a little rolled, or curved laterally. The epidermis is in general either in part or wholly rubbed off. When it is present, the outer surface is nearly smooth, only marked here and there with faint irregular transverse fissures and longitudinal furrows. Its color varies from a dirty whitish gray to yellowish, but is sometimes more or less dark. When the outer surface is rubbed off, as is almost always the case in the flat pieces, the color is nearly pure ochre yellow. Where the whole thickness of the outer coat is wanting, as happens here and there in spots, the surface is dark cinnamon, or dark ochre yellow, and commonly dull or powdery. The inner surface is usually even, but sometimes irregular and splintery, and always harsh to the fingers, leaving small splinters sticking in the skin when drawn over it. It is of a nearly pure ochre yellow color, and is very powdery. The fracture distinguishes this variety from the preceding, and from all others. The longitudinal fracture is strikingly fibrous, and in the flat pieces the fragments still hang together by connecting fibres.

both quilled and flat. Dr. Pereira states that he had pieces more than a foot in length. In thickness it varies from less than a line to four or five lines. Most of

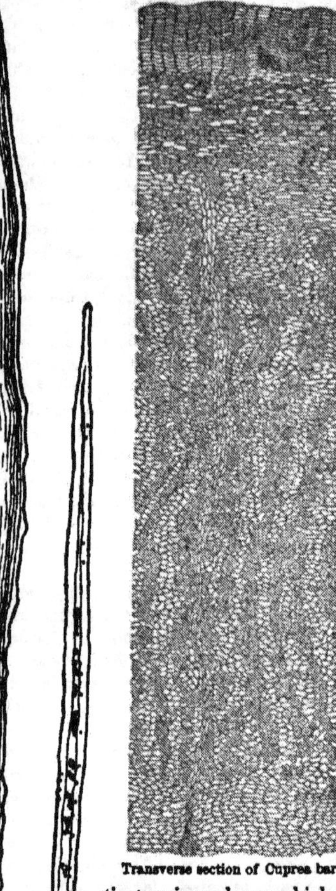

Highly magnified section of Cuprea bark, showing bast-cells.

Transverse section of Cuprea bark.

Bast-cells from Carthagena and Cuprea barks.

the fragments are covered with the whitish, soft epidermis, characteristic of the Carthagena barks; but some of them have a dark brown epidermis, rugose with innumerable cracks in all directions; and others are partially or wholly destitute of the outer covering, presenting generally, in the denuded part, a dark uniform or somewhat wrinkled surface. The inner surface is finely and compactly fibrous, and of a dull yellowish brown color with a reddish tinge; and the whole of the liber or true bark has the same color and texture. But outside of the liber there is in many pieces a very distinct resinous layer, which is sometimes of considerable thickness, and, when cut across by a knife, exhibits a dark reddish brown, shining surface. The resinous layer is the most striking peculiarity of the bark, though not present in all of the pieces, which sometimes consist of the liber alone. The fracture is towards the interior shortly fibrous, towards the exterior often smooth, in consequence of the layer just referred to. The whole bark is rather hard, compact, and heavy; differing in this respect very decidedly from the last mentioned variety. It has more resemblance to the hard Carthagena, from which, however, it differs by its deeper and redder color, its much more developed resinous coat, and its occasional grater-like epidermis. The taste is very bitter, and the yield in alkaloids considerable. Mr. Weightman informed us that he had obtained from it an average product of 1·6 per cent. of sulphate of quinine, and 0·34 of sulphate of cinchonine, independently of the amorphous or uncrystallizable alkaloidal matter. It must, therefore, be ranked among the efficient barks, though not so productive as the fine variety of fibrous bark denominated soft Pitaya. It contains also a large proportion of resin.

This bark comes from the mountain of Pitaya near Popayan, and the particular seroons examined by ourselves were said to have been brought down the Magdalena River from the town of Honda. It is referred by Dr. Pereira and Mr. Howard to the *Cinchona Condaminea*, var. *Pitayensis* of Weddell, of which that author has made a distinct species, under the name of *Cinchona Pitayensis.* (*Ann. des Sci. Nat.*, May, 1849.)*

CUPREA BARK.—As early as 1820, a Brazilian surgeon, by the name of Remijio, pointed out to his countrymen that the bark of certain small trees or shrubs growing in Brazil were as effective as the Peruvian bark in malarial fevers, and ever since in Brazil these plants have been known by the names of *Quinia de Sera*, or *Quinia de Remijio.* St. Hiliare (*Plantes Us. Bras.*) placed these shrubs in the genus Cinchona, as *C. Remijiana*, *ferruginea*, and *Vellozii;* but De Candolle (*Prodromus*, iv. 357) erected for them a new genus, Remijia, which has since been universally recognized by botanists. It is distinguished from Cinchona by the fruit capsules opening semi-loculicidally, by its peltate seeds, and by its inflorescence in elongated axillary racemes with opposite fascicles of flowers. In 1857 a new bark appeared in the London market, but only within the last few years has this so-called *Cuprea bark* appeared in large quantities. After its value became known the search for it in South America became very active; indeed, in Colombia a "fever" is said to have broken out, which has caused agriculture to be neglected and deranged the business of the country, whilst in London the supply has been so great as to break the whole cinchona market. Mr. S. G. Rosengarten informs us that the bark reaches this country from London, and also directly from Colombia. There are two distinct regions which yield it: one is the lower part of the basin of the Magdalena River, in the province of Santander, the trees growing in the mountain chain of La Paz, and the port of export being Bucaramanga; the other the basin of the Orinoco, among the mountains which constitute the eastern branch of the Cordillera of the Andes.

Bentham states that the genus Remijia comprises 13 species; according to the researches of José Triana, but two of these, *R. Purdieana*, Wedd. (*Ann. Sci. Nat.*, 3e sér., xi. p. 272), and *R. pedunculata*, Triana (*Cinchona pedunculata*, Karsten), yield the Cuprea bark of commerce. (*P. J. Tr.*, April, 1882.) An exceedingly important fact connected with these trees is that they grow in a dry climate, and in position a little above the level ot the sea, and hence without doubt could be cultivated in many intertropical countries where the Cinchonas will not grow. They would in all probability flourish within the limits of the United States.

The specimens of Cuprea bark which have been furnished us as typical by the Messrs. Rosengarten are composed of pieces varying from half an inch to 3 or 4 inches in length, from a quarter to a twelfth of an inch in thickness, strong and hard, varying from a yellowish to a red cinnamon color, and having a somewhat cupreous tint, distinctly curled, *very smooth* upon their inner surface, on their outer surface smoothish, or in the larger specimens rough, with the epidermis usually adherent; marked, except in the very large pieces, with fine wrinkles, and sometimes with transverse or spiral grooves, which are sometimes quite shallow, but often are deeply and sharply cut. The texture is dense and hard, the fracture is short, not fibrous, and free from spicules. The microscopic characters differ from that of the true Cinchonas in the bast-cells being small and with their cavity widely open, not obliterated by secondary layers. The figure represents a bast-cell obtained from a Carthagena bark, and one from Cuprea bark equally magnified. The shaved transverse section of Cuprea bark is further characterized by a peculiar horny appearance different from that of the true Cinchonas. The bark is also remarkable for its density, which Arnaud gives as from 1·128 to 1·18, and consequently sinks in water.

Cuprea bark varies in the percentage of quinine it contains. The Messrs. Rosengarten state that the yield in their laboratories has been from 1 to 2 per cent., and that usually the bark is remarkably free from inferior alkaloids. The complete absence of cinchonidine is said to be characteristic of them. Messrs. D. Howard and

* More minute descriptions of the Carthagena barks may be found in the foot-notes to the fourteenth edition of the U. S. Dispensatory.

I. Hodgkin, Dr. B. H. Paul, and Mr. Cownley and Mr. T. G. Whiffen almost simultaneously announced the discovery of a new alkaloid, *homoquinine* or *ultra-quinine*, which there is some reason for believing is a double salt of quinine and quinidine. (*Chem. News*, xlv. 6.) The characteristic chemical product is the alkaloid *cinchonamine*, whose right to a separate existence seems to be well established. (See page 460.)

False Barks.

Before dismissing the subject of the varieties of Cinchona, it is proper to observe that numerous barks have at various times been introduced into the market, and sold as closely resembling or identical with the febrifuge of Peru, which experience has proved to differ from it materially, both in chemical composition and in medical virtues. These barks are generally procured from trees formerly ranked among the Cinchonas, but now arranged in other genera. They are distinguished from the true Peruvian bark by the absence of its peculiar alkaloids. Hence they are readily distinguished by means of *Grahe's test*. This depends upon the fact that the cinchona alkaloids and barks containing them yield, when heated, beautiful purplish vapors, condensing into a similarly colored tar. (See p. 464, note.) Hesse's method of testing is probably the best: it consists in extracting the bark by slightly acidulated water, solidifying the liquid with the powdered bark, and heating in a large test-tube. If the bark be a true Cinchona, the vapors will be unmistakable. The microscopic character of the false barks also distinguish them from the genuine. Among them are—1, a bark known to the French pharmaceutists by the name of *quinquina nova*, or *new bark*, the product of *Cascarilla oblongifolia*,* which, though at one time thought to be possessed of some virtues, has been proved to be worthless; 2, the *Caribæan bark*, from *Exostemma Caribæa*; 3, the *St. Lucia bark*, or *quinquina piton* of the French, derived from *Exostemma floribunda*; and, 4, a bark of uncertain botanical origin, called in France *quinquina bicolore*, and in Italy *china bicolorata*, and sometimes erroneously named *Pitaya bark*. Of these the last only is known in this country. A considerable quantity of it was some time since imported into New Orleans, whence a portion reached this city. The specimen in our possession is in quills, for the most part singly, but in some instances doubly rolled, from eight or ten inches to more than two feet in length, and from a quarter of an inch to an inch or more in diameter. The outer surface is of a dull grayish olive color, with numerous large oval or irregular spots, much lighter colored, sometimes even whitish and slightly depressed beneath the general surface, as if a layer of the epidermis had fallen off within their limits. It is to this appearance that the bark owes the name of *bicolorata*. The color of the internal surface is deep brown or almost blackish; that of the fresh fracture, brownish red. The bark is hard, compact, and thin, seldom as much as a line thick, and breaks with a short rough fracture. It is inodorous, and has a very bitter taste, not unlike that of some of the inferior kinds of Cinchona.†

The inner bark of an Indian species of *Hymenodictyon*, formerly considered as a Cinchona, and named *C. excelsa*, has been supposed to possess properties analogous to those of genuine cinchona. It has been chemically examined by Mr. Broughton, who succeeded in obtaining from it a pure crystalline principle, ascertained to be identical with *æsculin*, the characteristic principle of *Æsculus Hippocastanum*, or common horse-chestnut. He could find no trace of any of the cinchona alkaloids. (*P. J. Tr.*, March, 1868, p. 418.)

Bark Structure. The general structure of Cinchona barks does not differ from that of other barks, though in some of their microscopical details they are peculiar. The true epidermis is found only upon the growing twigs, and is never present in the commercial cinchona; the so-called epidermis of the various Cinchona barks of

* For minute description of this bark, see fourteenth edition U. S. Dispensatory.

† An elaborate study of this bark by Mr. Hodgkin (*P. J. Tr.*, xv. 217) leads him to the conclusion that it is yielded by a Remijia, for which he proposes the name of *bicolorata*. Its bast-cells are stated by Hesse to be arranged in groups of eight or ten, some of the cells being oval and lignified with a small cavity, whilst others are polygonal and almost completely lignified. (*A. J. P.*, 1887, 77.) Hesse affirms that it contains none of the cinchona alkaloids, but a peculiar alkaloid; which may be the *pitaynine* isolated from it by Perette in 1834–5.

commerce being really the outer corky layer, the *exophlœum*, or *outer bark* of botanists. Within it is the *mesophlœum*, or *middle bark;* and innermost of all, the *endophlœum*, *inner bark*, or *liber*. The tuberous outer bark is composed of flat, thick-walled cells, and in some Cinchonas, instead of forming a distinct outer coating, sends processes into the mesophlœum, or it may occur in scattered islets through the middle bark. Under these circumstances, the middle bark may finally altogether be supplanted; if now the exophlœum be shed or rubbed off, a bark is finally left composed entirely of liber, as is the case, for example, with the large, flat pieces of true Calisaya. The middle bark, when present, is formed out of irregular parenchymatous cells, among which may, in some species, be seen the so-called latex vessels, composed of soft, elongated, unbranched cells, more or less completely fused together into channels. In old bark these latex vessels are often entirely obliterated. The parenchymatous cells sometimes contain minute starch granules, and occasionally single cells may be found, having crystals of oxalate of lime, or a softish, reddish, resinoid mass, in their interiors. These constitute the so-called *crystal* and *resin cells* of authors.

The endophlœum is divided by distinct medullary rays into wedge-like masses of parenchymatous tissue, containing the liber, or bast-cells, which, on section, are seen to be thick-walled, with a faint yellowish tint. The liber-cells are the most distinctive feature of Cinchona barks. (See p. 453.) "They are elongated and bluntly pointed at their ends, but never branched, mostly spindle-shaped, straight, or slightly curved, and not exceeding in length 3 mm. They are consequently of a simpler structure than the analogous cells of most other officinal barks. They are about ⅙ to ⅛ mm. thick, their transverse section exhibiting a quadrangular rather than a circular outline. Their walls are strongly thickened by numerous secondary deposits, the cavity being reduced to a narrow cleft, a structure which explains the brittleness of the fibres. The liber fibres are either irregularly scattered in the liber rays, or they form radial lines transversely intersected by narrow strips of parenchyma, or they are densely packed in short bundles. It is a peculiarity of Cinchona barks that these bundles consist always of a few fibres (3 to 5 or 7), whereas in many other barks (as cinnamon) analogous bundles are made up of a large number of fibres."* (*Pharmacographia*, p. 356.)

It has been asserted that crystals of salts of the alkaloids can be seen with the microscope in Cinchona bark, but this is an error. These crystals are only to be found in sections which have been boiled in a dilute solution of caustic alkali, and then washed with water, and are probably alkaloids that have been set free by the decomposition of the quinovates by the potassium or sodium.

Various attempts have been made to identify the different species of Cinchona by the structure of their barks, and we append in a foot-note† the analyses of Prof.

* Any one desirous of studying these bast-cells can easily separate them by boiling fragments of the bark in dilute nitric acid until thoroughly pulpified and then teasing out with needles.

† PROF. MAISCH'S ANALYSIS.

1.—*Bast fibres single, sometimes in groups of 2, or rarely more; medium-sized.*

C. Calisaya. Laticiferous ducts in young bark; no resin-cells; old bark with prominent secondary cork; medullary rays narrow.

C. glandulifera. Laticiferous ducts in 1 or 2 rows; resin-cells few; bast rays narrow; medullary rays large-celled.

2. *Bast fibres single, or oftener in groups; not in distinct radial lines.*

C. micrantha. No laticiferous ducts; resin-cells few or none; bast fibres medium; medullary rays narrow.

C. purpurea. Laticiferous ducts in 1 or 2 rows; resin-cells numerous; bast fibres thin, with some incomplete fibres; medullary rays broadly wedge-shaped at end.

C. pubescens. Laticiferous ducts in 1 row; resin-cells numerous; bast fibres large, variable, with incomplete fibres; medullary rays broad.

3. *Bast fibres in interrupted single or double radial lines.*

C. succirubra. Laticiferous ducts in 1 row, in old bark often filled with cells; bast and medullary rays narrow; bast fibres medium.

C. officinalis. Laticiferous ducts thin, soon obliterated; resin-cells none; bast fibres medium; medullary rays narrow.

C. Pitayensis. Laticiferous ducts none; resin-cells few or none; bast fibres thin; medullary rays mostly narrow, wedge-shaped at end.

C. cordifolia. Laticiferous ducts none; resin-cells few; bast fibres small, with some incomplete fibres; medullary rays large-celled.

Maisch and Mr. J. C. Reeve. The constancy of the characters is, however, very doubtful, and in some studies of commercial barks, owing to the contradictory characters presented, we have found it impossible to apply the asserted facts, so as to determine by the microscope from what species the bark had been procured.

Chemical History.

In the analysis of Cinchona bark, the attention of chemists was at first directed exclusively to the action of water and alcohol upon it, and to the determination of the relative proportions of its gummy or extractive and resinous matter. The presence of tannin and of various alkaline or earthy salts in minute quantities was afterwards demonstrated. Fourcroy made an elaborate analysis, which proved the existence of other principles in the bark besides those previously ascertained. Dr. Westring was the first who attempted the discovery of an active principle in the bark, on which its febrifuge virtues might depend; but he was not successful. Seguin afterwards pursued the same track, and endeavored, by observing the effects of various reagents, to discover the relative value of different varieties of the drug; but his conclusions have not been supported by subsequent experiment. M. Deschamps, an apothecary of Lyons, obtained from bark a crystallizable salt of lime, the acid of which Vauquelin afterwards separated, and called *kinic acid.* The latter chemist also pushed to a much further extent the researches of Seguin as to the influence of reagents, and arrived at the conclusion that those barks were most efficient which gave precipitates with tannin or the infusion of galls. Reuss, of Moscow, succeeded in isolating a peculiar coloring matter from red bark, which he designated by the name of *cinchonic red*, and obtained a bitter substance which probably consisted in part of the peculiar alkaline principles subsequently discovered. The first step, however, towards the discovery of cinchonine and quinine appears to have been taken by the late Dr. Duncan, of Edinburgh, so early as 1803. He believed the precipitate, afforded by the infusion of cinchona with that of galls, to be a peculiar vegetable principle, and accordingly denominated it *cinchonine.* Dr. Gomez, a Portuguese physician, convinced that the active principle of bark resided in this cinchonine, but

C. lancifolia. Laticiferous ducts none; resin-cells many; bast fibres medium, with some incomplete fibres; medullary rays large-celled.

C. nitida. Laticiferous ducts none; resin-cells few or none; bast fibres mostly thin, but many thick or medium; medullary rays narrow.

C. Peruviana. Laticiferous ducts (in 1 row) and resin-cells small; bast fibres small, many incompletely filled.

4. *Bast fibres in nearly uninterrupted radial lines.*

C. scrobiculata. Laticiferous ducts in 1 or 2 rows; resin-cells and bast fibres numerous; medullary rays large-celled.

Mr. Reeve's Analysis.

1. *Resin-cells absent.*

Laticiferous ducts present (in young bark); thickest fibres observed average ·095 mm. in diameter; fibres mostly separate. *C. Calisaya.*

Laticiferous ducts present (sometimes obscured in old bark); thickest fibres average ·085 mm. in diameter: fibres in lines, and occasionally groups of 2 to 8. *C. succirubra.*

Laticiferous ducts present (soon obliterated). *C. officinalis.*

2. *Resin-cells few or none* (i.e., *they vary*).

Laticiferous ducts absent; thickest fibres ·10 mm. in diameter; fibres in groups of 2 or 3, in elder barks of more; medullary rays thin and indistinct. *C. micrantha.*

Laticiferous ducts absent; thickest observed fibres average ·075 mm.; thin fibres, mostly in single lines; section in places or sometimes entirely light gray. *C. Pitayensis.*

3. *Resin-cells present.*

Laticiferous ducts absent; thickest fibres average ·084 mm.; numerous resin-cells; fibres in line or groups of 2 to 4, with some staff-cells; medullary rays large-celled. *C. lancifolia.*

Laticiferous ducts absent: thickest fibres average ·078 mm.; resin-cells few; medullary rays large-celled; fibres small (sometimes few), in mostly single lines of 2 to 4, with some staff-cells; in some regions the fibres are dark red-brown, becoming bright rose-red with KOH. *C. cordifolia.*

Laticiferous ducts present; thickest observed fibres average ·106 mm.; numerous resin-cells; medullary rays broadly wedge-shaped; fibres in groups of 3 to 5, with some staff-cells. *C. purpurea.*

Laticiferous ducts present: numerous resin-cells; medullary rays broad; fibres large, in groups of 2 to 3, with staff-cells. *C. pubescens.*

Laticiferous ducts present; numerous resin-cells; fibres very numerous, in uninterrupted, usually single lines. *C. scrobiculata.*

Same as last, but few resin-cells. *C. glandulifera.*

Resin-cells, laticiferous ducts, and fibres small, many fibres incompletely filled in lines of 2 to 6. *C. Peruviana.*

mixed with impurities, instituted experiments upon some pale bark, which resulted in the separation of a white crystalline substance, considered by him to be the pure *cinchonine* of Dr. Duncan. It was obtained by the action of potassa upon an aqueous infusion of the alcoholic extract of the bark, and was undoubtedly the principle now universally known by the name of *cinchonine* or *cinchonia*. But Dr. Gomes was ignorant of its precise nature, considering it to be analogous to resin. M. Laubert afterwards obtained the same principle by a different process, and described it under the name of *white matter*, or *pure white resin*. To Pelletier and Caventou was reserved the honor of crowning all these experiments, and applying the results which they obtained to important practical purposes. In 1820, they demonstrated the alkaline character of the principle discovered by Gomes and Laubert, and gave it definitively the name of *cinchonine*. They discovered in the yellow or Calisaya bark another alkaline principle, which they denominated *quinine*. Both these bases they proved to exist in the barks, combined with *kinic* or *quinic acid*, in the state of *kinate of cinchonine and of quinine*. It was, moreover, established by their labors that the febrifuge property of bark depends upon the presence of these two principles. In 1833, MM. O. Henry and Delondre discovered a new alkaloid, but afterwards, finding its composition in its anhydrous state the same as that of quinine, concluded that it was a hydrate of that base. About 1844, Winckler announced anew the existence of the same principle which he considered distinct, and named *chinidine;* and, under the similar title of *quinidine*, it has now taken its place among the cinchona alkaloids. In 1853, M. Pasteur found that what had been considered as quinidine consisted in fact of two alkaloids, for one of which he retained the name of quinidine, and called the other *cinchonidine;* and, on pushing his investigations further, he ascertained that no less than six alkaloids may be obtained from different varieties of Peruvian bark; namely, *quinine* and *quinidine* isomeric with each other, *cinchonine* and *cinchonidine* also isomeric, and two others, derivatives from the preceding through the agency of heat, viz., *quinicine* from quinine, and *cinchonicine* from cinchonine, each being isomeric with the alkaloid from which it is derived.* The termination *a* or *ia* has heretofore been adopted by American and English chemists to distinguish the organic alkaloids from other organic proximate principles, the names of which terminate in *in* or *ine*, the terms quinine and cinchonine becoming *quinia* and *cinchonia*. On the same principle, *quinidine*, *quinicine*, *cinchonidine*, and *cinchonicine* were called respectively *quinidia*, *quinicia*, *cinchonidia*, and *cinchonicia*. The Committee of Revision of the Pharmacopœia, 1880, have, however, accepted the custom of continental writers, and the *a* and *ia* termination has been dropped and *ine* substituted.

At the present time, 1888, the following alkaloids are recognized, as either existing naturally, or produced artificially, from the Cinchona, Cuprea, or allied barks.

Natural Alkaloids. 1. QUININE, $C_{20}H_{24}N_2O_2$. 2. QUINIDINE (*Conchinine of Hesse*), $C_{20}H_{24}N_2O_2$. 3. CINCHONINE, $C_{19}H_{22}N_2O$. 4. CINCHONIDINE, $C_{19}H_{22}N_2O$. (These four alkaloids are the most important, and the only ones used medicinally.) 5. *Quinamine*, $C_{19}H_{24}N_2O_2$. 6. *Quinidamine* or *Conquinamine* (*Conchinamine of Hesse*), $C_{19}H_{24}N_2O_2$. 7. *Homoquinine* or *Ultra-quinine*, $C_{19}H_{22}N_2O_2$. 8. *Hydroquinine*, $C_{20}H_{26}N_2O_2$. 9. *Hydroquinidine*, $C_{20}H_{26}N_2O_2$. 10. *Hydrocinchonidine*, $C_{19}H_{24}N_2O$. 11. *Cinchonamine*, $C_{19}H_{24}N_2O$. 12. *Paytine*, $C_{21}H_{24}N_2OH_2O$. 13. *Homocinchonine*, $C_{19}H_{22}N_2O$. 14. *Homocinchonidine*, $C_{19}H_{22}N_2O$. 15. *Cinchotine*, $C_{19}H_{24}N_2O$. 16. *Cusconine*, $C_{23}H_{26}N_2O_4 2H_2O$. 17. *Concusconine*, $C_{23}H_{26}N_2O_4$. 18. *Cusconidine*. 19. *Aricine* (*Cinchovatine of Manzini*), $C_{23}H_{26}N_2O_4$. 20. *Paricine*, $C_{16}H_{18}N_2O$. 21. *Paytamine*. 22. *Dihomocinchonine*. 23. *Dicinchonine*, $C_{38}H_{44}N_4O_2$. 24. *Diquinidine* (*Diconchinine of Hesse*), $C_{40}H_{46}N_4O_3$. 25. *Javanine*. 26. *Cincholine*. 27. *Chairamine*, $C_{22}H_{26}N_2O_4$. 28. *Conchairamine*, $C_{22}H_{26}N_2O_4$. 29. *Conchairamidine*, $C_{22}H_{26}N_2O_4$.

The Artificial Alkaloids at present known are: 1. *Quinicine*, $C_{20}H_{24}N_2O_2$. 2. *Diquinicine*, $C_{40}H_{46}N_4O_3$. 3. *Cinchonicine*, $C_{19}H_{22}N_2O$. 4. *Dicinchonicine*, $C_{38}H_{42}N_4O$. 5. *Quinamicine*, $C_{19}H_{24}N_2O_2$. 6. *Quinamidine*, $C_{19}H_{24}N_2O_2$. 7.

* It is unfortunate that in Germany some confusion yet exists in the names adopted for the cinchona alkaloids. Cinchonidine is frequently called *chinidine*, and Hesse insists on calling quinidine *conchinine*.

Protoquinamicine, $C_{17}H_{20}N_2O_2$. 8. *Apoquinamine*, $C_{19}H_{22}N_2O$. 9. *Homocinchonicine*, $C_{19}H_{22}N_2O$. 10. *Hydrocinchonine*, $C_{20}H_{26}N_2O$. 11. *Chairamidine*, $C_{22}H_{26}N_2O_4$.

Chinoidine or *Quinoidine* is a term now applied to the resinous substance, consisting not only of the *amorphous* natural alkaloids, but to those which are produced artificially, through the action of heat and acids upon the crystalline alkaloids. It is now officinal. The other constituents of Cinchona bark are *Kinic* or *Quinic*, *Kinovic* or *Quinovic*, *Cinchotannic* or *Quinotannic* acids, *Kinovin* or *Quinovin*, *Cinchonic red*, volatile butyraceous oil in small quantity, red and yellow coloring matter. These constituents will now be considered in detail.

Quinine, *Quinidine*, *Cinchonine*, *Cinchonidine*, or their sulphates, having been made officinal, will be treated of under separate heads (see Index). *Quinicine* and *Cinchonicine*, being derivatives of quinine and cinchonine, will be considered under their respective sources.

QUINAMINE, *Quinamia*, $C_{19}H_{24}N_2O_2$. Dr. O. Hesse discovered this cinchona alkaloid in the bark of *C. succirubra* from Darjeeling in 1872. He has since found it in all of the East Indian succirubra barks, as well as in the barks of *C. nitida*, *C. Calisaya*, var. *Schuhkrafft*, *C. erythrantha*, *C. erythroderma*, *C. rosulenta*, and *C. Calisaya* (Para bark). De Vrij (*L'Union Pharm.*, 1877, p. 204; *N. R.*, 1877, p. 300) has published a process for its preparation. It crystallizes in very long, asbestos-like, white prisms, without water of crystallization. It is insoluble in water, and solution of potassa or ammonia; is readily dissolved by hot alcohol, which deposits it in crystals, and less readily by diluted alcohol. Ether dissolves it rather easily at ordinary temperature, more readily when boiling hot, and gives it up crystallized on cooling and evaporation. In alcoholic solution it has an alkaline reaction. It neutralizes sulphuric and hydrochloric acids, forming with the latter an amorphous salt, but with the former one that crystallizes with difficulty in hexagonal scales and short prisms. Its solution is dextrogyrate. Its reaction with chloride of gold is very characteristic; the solution of the chloride producing with it a yellowish white precipitate, which soon becomes purple, and separates gold; the supernatant liquid assuming a purplish red, and afterwards a brown color. (For other characters, see *A. J. P.*, 1872, p. 302.)

QUINIDAMINE, *Quinidamia* (*Conchinamine of Hesse*), $C_{19}H_{24}N_2O_2$, is found in *C. rosulenta* and *C. succirubra*, and probably exists in other species of red bark. It crystallizes in long, brilliant prisms, which melt at 123° C. (253·4° F.). A crystalline hydriodide has been produced. Like quinamine, its gold salt soon decomposes.

HOMOQUININE, $C_{19}H_{22}N_2O_2$, was discovered in 1881 simultaneously, by D. Howard and J. Hodgkin, B. H. Paul, A. J. Cownley and T. G. Whiffen (*P. J. Tr.*, 1881, p. 497; 1882, p. 905). It was named by Howard, and Hesse states that J. A. Tod observed the alkaloid in 1880. It is obtained from the Cuprea bark, and was first noticed by Paul and Cownley on account of the readiness with which it crystallized from its ethereal solution. It exists in the bark sometimes to the extent of 0·3 per cent. *Ultraquinine* is the name suggested for *Homoquinine* by Whiffen, on account of its extreme lævogyrate properties. It is freely soluble in alcohol and chloroform, sparingly in ether, from which it crystallizes in proportion as it can take up water. (*Hesse.*) It is also soluble in diluted sulphuric acid, producing fluorescence, and gives, with chlorine water and ammonia, a green coloration (thalleioquin). The sulphate coincides exactly in properties with sulphate of quinine except in its behavior with ether. Its tartrate closely resembles tartrate of cinchonidine. Homoquinine and its salts behave towards polarized light like quinine. Dr. O. Hesse is convinced of the identity of the alkaloid *cupreine* discovered by Paul and Cownley, and he believes that homoquinine is merely a compound of quinine with cupreine. (*P. J. Tr.*, 1886, p. 641.)

HYDROQUININE, $C_{20}H_{26}N_2O_2$, according to Hesse, dissolves freely in alcohol and ether, and gives the thalleioquin reaction with chlorine water and ammonia like quinine. (*P. J. Tr.*, 1882, p. 904.)

HYDROQUINIDINE (hydroconchinine), $C_{20}H_{26}N_2O_2 + 2\frac{1}{2}H_2O$, is crystalline, dissolving freely in hot alcohol and in chloroform, but less freely in ether. It gives the thalleioquin reaction like quinine. (*P. J. Tr.*, 1882, p. 904.)

HYDROCINCHONIDINE, $C_{19}H_{24}N_2O$, bears the same relation to cinchonidine that hydroquinine does to quinine. It is found associated with homocinchonidine in commercial cinchonidine. (*A. J. P.*, 1883, p. 20.)

CINCHONAMINE, $C_{19}H_{24}N_2O$. This alkaloid was discovered in 1881 by M. Arnaud in Cuprea bark. It exists in the proportion of 0·2 per cent., and is usually associated with cinchonine. His process is to treat the bark with milk of lime, dry the mixture, exhaust with boiling alcohol, distil off the alcohol, and take up the residue with diluted hydrochloric acid; hydrochlorate of cinchonamine crystallizes out, hydrochlorate of cinchonine remaining in solution. Cinchonamine is insoluble in cold water, soluble in 30 parts of alcohol, more soluble in hot alcohol, and in 100 parts of ether. It is dextrogyrate. For formulas for salts of cinchonamine, see *A. J. P.*, 1884, p. 156. Physiologically, cinchonamine, according to the experiments of Sée and Bochefontaine, has six times the toxic power of quinine, and has decided sialagogue properties. (*P. J. Tr.*, 1885, p. 791.)

PAYTINE, $C_{21}H_{24}N_2O,H_2O$, was discovered by Hesse in the white Payta bark. PAYTAMINE is an amorphous alkaloid accompanying *Paytine.*

HOMOCINCHONINE, $C_{19}H_{22}N_2O$, *the Cinchonodine of Koch*, is obtained from the bark of *C. rosulenta*; it is lævogyrate, and crystallizes from its alcoholic solution in large prisms. It has been mistaken for *aricine.*

DIHOMOCINCHONINE, $C_{38}H_{44}N_4O_2$, is an amorphous alkaloid obtained from *C. rosulenta.* It is dextrogyrate.

HOMOCINCHONIDINE, $C_{19}H_{22}N_2O$, is also obtained from *C. rosulenta.* It crystallizes in large prisms, and forms a neutral sulphate containing six molecules of water, which may be had in commerce. Its existence is denied by Skraup.

CUSCONINE, $C_{23}H_{26}N_2O_4.2H_2O$, was discovered by Leverköhn. It is a constituent of the cusco bark, *C. pubescens* var. *Pelletieriana*, and Hesse has recently found it in Cuprea bark. It is nearly insoluble in water, soluble in 35 parts of ether, more easily in alcohol, very soluble in chloroform. It may be distinguished from other cinchona alkaloids by forming with sulphuric acid a neutral sulphate, which is amorphous, gelatinous, and yellow, and insoluble in an excess of the acid.

CONCUSCONINE, $C_{23}H_{26}N_2O_4$, discovered by Hesse. It is tasteless.

CUSCONIDINE is an amorphous alkaloid found in cusco bark, accompanying cusconine.

ARICINE, $C_{23}H_{26}N_2O_4$. *Cinchovatine.* This alkaloid, found in cusco bark, and quite recently in Cuprea bark, was formerly believed by Hesse to be identical with cinchonidine. Pelletier and Cariol obtained *aricine* as far back as 1829 (see note, p. 308, 14th ed. U. S. D.). Its separate existence is now not doubted. It crystallizes in prisms, and its salts are of sparing solubility.

PARICINE, $C_{16}H_{18}N_2O$, is found with quinamine in the bark of *C. succirubra* of Darjeeling, and, according to Hesse, it may be separated from all the cinchona alkaloids with which it may be associated in solution by treating with carbonate of sodium, which precipitates paricine first.

DICINCHONINE, $C_{38}H_{44}N_4O_2$, exists in the bark of *C. rosulenta* and *C. succirubra*, and may also be obtained by fractional precipitation from the mixed amorphous alkaloids before melting, but not from commercial chinoidine.

DIQUINIDINE, *Diconchinine of Hesse*, $C_{40}H_{46}N_4O_3$, is found principally in chinoidine which has been obtained from barks containing quinine and quinidine. It is dextrogyrate, produces a fluorescent solution with diluted sulphuric acid, and gives the thalleioquin reaction.

JAVANINE, obtained by Hesse from *C. Calisaya* var. *Javanica.*

CINCHOLINE, a pale yellow, liquid alkaloid, having an odor recalling that of quinoline or chinoline, discovered by Hesse in 1882. (See *P. J. Tr.*, May 6, 1882.)

CHAIRAMINE, $C_{22}H_{26}N_2O_4$, discovered by Hesse in *Remijia Purdieana*, occurs in white needles, which are readily soluble in ether and chloroform. (*Ann. d. Chem.*, 225, p. 211.)

CONCHAIRAMINE, $C_{22}H_{26}N_2O_4 + H_2O + C_2H_6O$, also discovered by Hesse, crystallises with both water and *alcohol of crystallization*. It is soluble in hot alcohol, ether, and chloroform. The alcoholate dissolves in sulphuric acid containing molybdic acid, giving a brown coloration, which soon becomes intensely green. (*Ann. d. Chem.*, 225, p. 211.)

CONCHAIRAMIDINE, $C_{22}H_{26}N_2O_4 + H_2O$, crystallizes in white needles, and is very soluble in ether, chloroform, alcohol, benzene, and acetone. (*Ann. d. Chem.*, 225, p. 211.)

Of the artificial bases, QUINAMICINE and QUINAMIDINE are isomeric; they are both amorphous, and are produced by heating quinamine in contact with diluted sulphuric acid. If the action of sulphuric acid be continued at 120° C. (248° F.) to 130° C. (266° F.), an amorphous brownish substance is formed which may be precipitated by carbonate of sodium, and is insoluble in ether. Hesse has named this PROTO-QUINAMICINE.

DIQUINICINE, $C_{40}H_{46}N_4O_3$, also termed *diconchinine* and *apodiquinidine*, is one of the chief amorphous alkaloids in commercial chinoidine; its formula indicates its relation to quinine or quinidine. By deducting one molecule of water from a double molecule of either there results diquinicine; thus, $2C_{20}H_{24}N_2O_2 - H_2O = C_{40}H_{46}N_4O_3$.

DICINCHONICINE, $C_{38}H_{42}N_4O$?, *dichonchonine* or *apodicinchonine*, is derived from cinchonine and cinchonidine, and found in commercial chinoidine. It probably exists in bark in an amorphous condition.

APOQUINAMINE is isomeric with homocinchonine, and is prepared by boiling quinamine or quinamidine with hydrochloric acid for a short time. It is white, amorphous, soluble in ether, alcohol, and diluted hydrochloric acid. HOMOCINCHONICINE is prepared from homocinchonidine just as cinchonicine and quinicine are from cinchonine and quinine,—*i.e.*, by heating their sulphates.

HYDROCINCHONINE, $C_{19}H_{24}N_2O$, discovered by Caventou, is obtained by treating cinchonine with potassium permanganate. It is soluble in 1300 parts of water, more soluble in alcohol and ether. The statement that it may be found in commercial cinchonine has not been confirmed.

The other constituents of Cinchona bark are of less importance.

Kinic Acid (*Cinchonic* or *Quinic Acid*), $C_7H_{12}O_6$. This acid was isolated as early as 1785 by Hofmann, an apothecary of Leer, who obtained it from the calcium salt from cinchona. It exists in a number of important plants,—ivy, oak, elm, ash, coffee, etc. It may be desirable to procure the alkaloids in the state of saline combination in which they exist in the bark; since it is possible that they may exert an influence over the system in this state, somewhat different from that produced by their combinations with the sulphuric or other mineral acid. As it is impossible to procure the kinates immediately from the bark in a pure state, it becomes necessary first to obtain the kinic acid separately, which may thus become of some practical importance. We shall, therefore, briefly describe the mode of procuring it, and its characteristic properties. It is most usually prepared from the kinate of calcium, the residue obtained in the manufacture of sulphate of quinine (see *Quininæ Sulphas*) by decomposing an aqueous solution of kinate of calcium with oxalic acid, filtering out the precipitated oxalate of calcium, and evaporating the filtrate to the crystallizing point; or by evaporating the infusion of bark to a solid consistence, and treating the extract with alcohol, we have in the residue a viscid matter consisting chiefly of mucilage with kinate of calcium, which is insoluble in alcohol. If an aqueous solution of this substance be formed, and allowed to evaporate at a gentle heat, crystals of the kinate will be deposited, which may be purified by a second crystallization. The salt thus obtained, being dissolved in water, is decomposed by means of oxalic acid, which precipitates the lime, and leaves the *kinic acid* in solution. This may be procured in the crystalline state by spontaneous evaporation, though as usually prepared it is in the form of a thick syrupy liquid. The crystals are transparent and colorless, sour to the taste, and readily soluble in alcohol and in water. By heating kinic acid or a kinate with manganese dioxide and sulphuric acid, we get yellow crystals of *kinone*, better known as *quinone*, $C_6H_4O_2$; a reaction which may be used for ascertaining the presence of kinic acid. The kinates of cinchonine and quinine may be obtained either by the direct combination of their constituents, or by the mutual decomposition of the sulphates of those alkaloids and kinate of calcium. *Kinate of cinchonine* has a bitter and astringent taste, is very soluble in water, is soluble also in alcohol, and is crystallized with difficulty. *Kinate of quinine* is also very soluble in water, but less so in rectified alcohol. Its taste is very bitter, resembling that of yellow bark. It crystallizes in beautiful stellate groups, which are opaque or semi-transparent. The salt is with difficulty obtained free from color, and only by employing the ingredients in a state of extreme purity. (*Ann. de Chim. et de Phys.*, Juillet, 1829.) Lautemann found, in experiments upon himself, that kinic acid, when taken into the system, undergoes a conversion into hippuric acid, and in this state escapes with the urine. (*Ann. der Chem. und Pharm.*, cxxv. 9.) M. Rabuteau has investigated the physiological properties of kinic acid, and has found it closely to resemble the ordinary vegetable acids, being harmless in its effects on the system, and forming with water a refreshing drink like lemonade. Like other vegetable acids, also, it is decomposed in the system, forming, when taken in the state of an alkaline salt, a carbonate of the alkali in the blood, and rendering that fluid alkaline. (*Am. Journ. of Med. Sci.*, Oct. 1872, p. 524.) Kinic acid is said by Zwenger to have been found in the leaves of *Vaccinium Myrtillus*. (*A. J. P.*, March, 1861, p. 128.)

Quinovin or *Kinovin*. *Kinovic Bitter*, $C_{30}H_{48}O_8$. Originally discovered in the false bark called quinquina nova or new bark, this substance has since been found in the Calisaya bark, and probably exists, in greater or less proportion, in all the Cinchona barks. It was detected by De Vrij not only in the bark, but also in the wood and leaves of *C. Calisaya* and *C. lucumæfolia*. (*Journ. de Pharm.*, Avril, 1860, pp. 225 and 258.) It is white, uncrystallizable, almost insoluble in water, but readily dissolved by alcohol and ether. It is very bitter, and, as it is asserted to have no febrifuge virtues, may on this account mislead the judgment in relation to the activity of the bark in which it may be found. Some barks are said to owe their bitterness mainly to this ingredient. Winckler gives, as a certain test of its presence in any bark, the sulphate of copper, which is indifferent to infusion of bark containing none of this principle, but detects the smallest proportion of it by producing a dirty green color, soon followed by the deposition of a fine similarly colored powder. This is a salt of copper, and has a very bitter and metallic taste. (See *A. J. P.*, xxv. 343.)

Kinovin in alcoholic solution was shown in 1859 by Hlasiwetz to be resolved by means of hydrochloric acid gas into kinovic acid, $C_{24}H_{38}O_4$, and an uncrystallizable sugar *mannitan*, $C_6H_{12}O_5$, by assimilation of H_2O. The formation of kinovic acid takes place more easily if kinovin is placed in contact with sodium amalgam and spirit of wine, when after 12 hours mannitan and kinovate of sodium are formed. (*Pharmacographia*, 2d ed., p. 364.)

Kinovic or *Quinovic Acid*, resulting as before stated from the decomposition of kinovin, and possessing the formula $C_{24}H_{38}O_4$, is white, in rhomboidal crystals, insoluble in water, but slightly soluble in ether, somewhat more so in boiling alcohol, but very soluble in ammonia and the fixed alkalies. All its solutions are decidedly bitter. Its acid properties are feeble, yet it is capable of decomposing the alkaline carbonates. (*Journ. de Pharm.*, Nov. 1859, p. 386.) De Vrij proposes the following method of isolating kinovin. Macerate powdered cinchona with a very weak solution of caustic potassa or soda, precipitate the filtered liquid with an acid, redissolve the precipitate in milk of lime to separate the cinchonic red, filter and precipitate the solution boiling hot with hydrochloric acid, separate the precipitate, wash it, express as much as possible, and lastly dry it on porous stones, and powder it. Thus prepared, the kinovic bitter forms soluble compounds with magnesia and lime, and has been employed, in this mode of combination, as a tonic in the hospital of Batavia, with encouraging success. (*Ibid.*, Avril, 1860, p. 258.) Dr. Kerner (*Deutsche Klin.*, xx. p. 81) speaks very favorably of kinovic acid, as an excellent and at the same time perfectly safe tonic, which produces no narcotic symptoms, and given to adults, in the quantity of half or three-quarters of an ounce, causes not the slightest ill effect. He prefers it in the form of kinovate of calcium, of which 40 grains (2·6 Gm.) is the average dose. (*Am. Journ. of Med. Sci.*, Oct. 1869, p. 543.)

A bitter principle was extracted from Calisaya bark by Winckler. He named it *kinovic bitter;* but, having been supposed to possess acid properties, it was after wards denominated *quinovic* or *kinovic acid*. The compounds are, however, distinct, although associated.

By the experiments of Henry, Jr., and Plisson, it may be considered as established that the alkaloids of the different varieties of bark are combined at the same time with kinic acid, and with one or more of the coloring matters, which, in relation to these substances, appear to act the part of acids. This idea was originally suggested by Robiquet. (*Journ. de Pharm.*, xii. 282, 369.) The compounds of quinine, cinchonine, etc., with the coloring matter, are scarcely soluble in water, while their kinates are very soluble.

The odor of bark appears to depend on a *volatile oil*, which Fabroni and Trommsdorff obtained by distillation with water. The oil floated on the surface of the water, was of a thick consistence, and had a bitterish, acrid taste, with the odor of bark.

The *fatty matter*, which was first obtained pure by M. Laubert, is of a greenish color as obtained from the pale bark, orange yellow from the yellow. It is insoluble in water, soluble in boiling alcohol, which deposits a part of it on cooling, very soluble in ether even cold, and saponifiable with the alkalies.

The *cinchonic red* of Reuss, the *insoluble red coloring matter* of Pelletier and Caventou, $C_{28}H_{22}O_{14}$, is reddish brown, insipid, inodorous, largely soluble in alcohol, especially when hot, and almost insoluble in ether or water, though the latter dissolves a little at the boiling temperature. The acids promote its solubility in water. It precipitates tartar emetic, but not gelatin; but if treated with a cold solution of potassa or soda, or by ammonia, lime, or baryta, with heat, and then precipitated by an acid, it acquires the property of forming an insoluble compound with gelatin. It yields protocatechuic acid when fused with caustic potash. It is most abundant in the red bark (over 10 per cent.), and least so in the pale.

The *yellow coloring matter* has little taste, is soluble in water, alcohol, and ether, precipitates neither gelatin nor tartar emetic, and is itself precipitated by subacetate of lead.

CINCHOTANNIC ACID. *Tannic acid*, *tannin*, or *soluble red coloring matter* of Pelletier and Caventou, has been considered as possessing all the properties which characterize the proximate vegetable principles associated together under the name cinchotannic acid. It has a brownish red color and an austere taste, is soluble in water and alcohol, combines with metallic oxides, and produces precipitates with the salts of iron, which vary in color according to the variety of bark, being deep green with the pale bark, blackish brown with the yellow, and reddish brown with the red. It also forms white precipitates with tartar emetic and gelatin, and readily combines with atmospheric oxygen, becoming insoluble. It must, however, differ materially from the tannic acid of galls, which could not exist in aqueous solutions containing cinchonine and quinine without forming insoluble compounds with them. Rembold has shown that when cinchotannic acid is boiled with diluted sulphuric acid cinchonic red is produced, sugar being formed at the same time.

CINCHOCEROTIN, $C_{27}H_{46}O_2$. This substance was discovered by Dr. Kerner in flat Calisaya bark from South America. He obtained it in white, very light, crystalline scales. It is not soluble in boiling water, nor in hydrochloric, dilute sulphuric, or glacial acetic acid, but dissolves readily in ether, chloroform, and alcohol. (*A. J. P.*, 1883, p. 357.)

Incompatibles. Of the relations of bark to the several solvents employed in pharmacy we shall speak hereafter, under the heads of its infusion, decoction, and tincture; where we shall also have an opportunity of mentioning some of the more prominent substances which afford precipitates with its liquid preparations. It is sufficient at present to state that all the substances which precipitate the infusion of bark do not by any means necessarily affect its virtues; as it contains several inert ingredients which form insoluble compounds with bodies that do not disturb its active principles. As *tannic acid* forms with the alkaloids compounds insoluble in water, it is desirable that substances containing this acid in a free state should not be prescribed in connection with the infusion or decoction of bark; for, though these insoluble tannates might be found efficacious if administered, yet, being precipitated from the liquid, they would be apt to be thrown away as dregs, or at any rate would communicate, if agitated, an unpleasant turbidness. The same may be said of the *tincture* and *compound solution of iodine*, which form insoluble compounds with all the cinchona alkaloids, and of the *alkalies*, *alkaline carbonates*, and *alkaline earths*, which precipitate these alkaloids from their aqueous solution.

Estimation of Value. It is evident, from what has been said, that an infusion of bark, on account of the tannin-like principle which it contains, may precipitate gelatin, tartar emetic, and the salts of iron, without having a particle of cinchonine, quinine, or other alkaloid in its composition; and that consequently any inference as to its value, drawn from these chemical properties, would be fallacious; but, as the active principles are thrown down by the tannic acid of galls, no bark can be considered good which does not afford a precipitate with the infusion of this substance.*

It is impossible to determine, with accuracy, the relative proportion of the active ingredients in the different varieties of cinchona; as the quantity is by no means uniform in different specimens of the same variety. The results of the most recent experiments have been already stated under the head of the several varieties of bark described. But it is highly important, in relation to any particular sample of bark, to be able to ascertain its medicinal efficiency, which is measured by the quantity of the peculiar cinchona alkaloids it may contain. The U. S. Pharmacopœia for the first time in its history gives a process for assaying Cinchona bark; this is deemed necessary because of the impossibility of judging of the quality of the bark by its physical appearances. The manufacturing chemist never trusts to anything short of a careful chemical assay, and Cinchona bark should never be dispensed or used without having its quality tested or certified to by a competent authority. The following process of assay was contributed to the Committee of Revision by Prof. A. B. Prescott, of Ann Arbor, Mich., who acknowledges valuable assistance from Dr. W. M. Mew, Chemical Service U.S.A., Medical Museum, Washington, D. C. It is based upon De Vrij's method, and will give sufficiently accurate results for the uses of the pharmacist. Each manufacturer and quinologist usually has a process of his own, which he carefully keeps secret, and a method which will accurately differentiate the quantities of the alkaloids is usually difficult and unreliable in the hands of the inexperienced.

"Assay of Cinchona Bark. I. *For Total Alkaloids.* Cinchona, in No. 80 powder, and fully dried at 100° C. (212° F.), *twenty grammes*; Lime, *five grammes*; Diluted Sulphuric Acid, Solution of Soda, Alcohol, Distilled Water, each, *a sufficient quantity.* Make the Lime into a milk with 50 C.c. of Distilled Water, thoroughly mix therewith the Cinchona, and dry the mixture completely at a temperature not above 80° C. (176° F.). Digest the dried mixture with 200 C.c. of Alcohol, in a flask, near the temperature of boiling, for an hour. When cool, pour the mixture upon a filter of about six inches (15 cm.) diameter. Rinse the flask and wash the filter with 200 C.c. of Alcohol, used in several portions, letting the filter drain after use of each portion. To the filtered liquid add enough Diluted Sulphuric Acid to render the liquid acid to test-paper. Let any resulting precipitate (sulphate of calcium) subside; then decant the liquid, in portions, upon a very small filter, and wash the residue and filter with small portions of Alcohol. Distil or evaporate the filtrate to expel all the Alcohol, cool, pass through a small filter, and wash the latter with Distilled Water slightly acidulated with Diluted Sulphuric Acid, until the washings are no longer made turbid by Solution of Soda. To the filtered liquid, concentrated to the volume of about 50 C.c., when nearly cool, add enough Solution

* *Grahe's test.* A test of the Cinchona barks, containing one or more of their characteristic alkaloids, has been proposed by Grahe. It is founded on the fact, that, when these barks are exposed to destructive distillation, a product is obtained of a bright carmine color, which is yielded by no other bark under the same circumstances, and not by cinchona unless it contain one or more of its peculiar alkaloids. Nor do the pure alkaloids afford it; but, if mixed with a little acetic, kinic, tannic, citric, or tartaric acid, they exhibit the reaction, showing that in the bark it takes place between the alkaloids and organic acids contained in it. Grahe applies the test by heating a piece of the bark weighing from five to ten grains in an ordinary test-tube, and gradually increasing the heat to redness. Whitish smoke, and watery vapor condensing on the surface of the tube, are first given off, which are soon followed by the appearance of redness in the fumes, and by the deposition, an inch above the heated part, of a red pulverulent film, which is gradually changed into a thick, oily liquid, running down the glass in drops or streaks of a fine carmine color. (*Chemisches Centralblatt*, Feb. 17, 1858, p. 97.) For further information see p. 443.

of Soda to render it strongly alkaline. Collect the precipitate on a wetted filter, let it drain, and wash it with small portions of Distilled Water (using as little as possible), until the washings give but a slight turbidity with test-solution of chloride of barium. Drain the filter by laying it upon blotting or filter papers until it is nearly dry. Detach the precipitate carefully from the filter and transfer it to a weighed capsule, wash the filter with Distilled Water acidulated with Diluted Sulphuric Acid, make the filtrate alkaline by Solution of Soda, and, if a precipitate result, wash it on a very small filter, let it drain well and transfer it to the capsule. Dry the contents of the latter at 100° C. (212° F.) to a constant weight, cool it in a desiccator and weigh. The number of grammes multiplied by *five* (5), equals the percentage of total alkaloids in the Cinchona.

"II. *For Quinine.* To the total alkaloids from 20 grammes of Cinchona, previously weighed, add Distilled Water acidulated with Diluted Sulphuric Acid, until the mixture remains for ten or fifteen minutes after digestion, just distinctly acid to test-paper. Transfer to a weighed beaker, rinsing with Distilled Water, and adding of this enough to make the whole weigh *seventy* (70) *times* the weight of the alkaloids. Add now, in drops, Solution of Soda previously well diluted with Distilled Water, until the mixture is exactly neutral to test-paper. Digest at 60° C. (140° F.) for five minutes, then cool to 15° C. (59° F.) and maintain at this temperature for half an hour. If crystals do not appear in the glass vessel, the total alkaloids do not contain quinine in quantity over *eight* (8) *per cent.* of their weight (corresponding *to nine* (9) *per cent.* of sulphate of quinine crystallized). If crystals appear in the mixture, pass the latter through a filter not larger than necessary, prepared by drying two filter papers of two to three and a half inches (5 to 9 cm.) diameter, trimming them to an equal weight, folding them separately, and placing one within the other so as to make a plain filter four-fold on each side. When the liquid has drained away, wash the filter and contents with Distilled Water of a temperature of 15° C. (59° F.), added in small portions, until the entire filtered liquid weighs *ninety* (90) *times* the weight of the alkaloids taken. Dry the filter, without separating its folds, at 60° C. (140 F.), to a constant weight, cool, and weigh the inner filter and contents, taking the outer filter for a counter-weight. To the weight of effloresced sulphate of quinine so obtained, add 11·5 per cent. of its amount (for water of crystallization), and add 0·12 per cent. of the weight of the entire filtered liquid (for solubility of the crystals at 15° C.) 59° F. The sum in grammes, multiplied by *five* (5), equals the percentage of crystallized sulphate of quinine equivalent to the quinine in the Cinchona." *U. S.*

The Br. Pharmacopœia gives the following method for testing Red Cinchona bark.

"*Test.* When used for purposes other than that of obtaining the alkaloids or their salts, it should yield between five and six per cent. of total alkaloids, of which not less than half shall consist of quinine and cinchonidine, as estimated by the following methods.

"1. *For Quinine and Cinchonidine.* Mix 200 grains of red cinchona bark in No. 60 powder with sixty grains of hydrate of calcium; slightly moisten the powders with half an ounce of water; mix the whole intimately in a small porcelain dish or mortar; allow the mixture to stand for an hour or two, when it will present the characters of a moist, dark brown powder, in which there should be no lumps or visible white particles. Transfer this powder to a six-ounce flask, add three fluidounces of benzolated amylic alcohol,* boil them together for about half an hour, decant and drain off the liquid on to a filter, leaving the powder in the flask; add more of the benzolated amylic alcohol to the powder, and boil and decant as before; repeat this operation a third time; then turn the contents of the flask on to the filter, and wash by percolation with more of the benzolated amylic alcohol until the bark is exhausted. If, during the boiling, a funnel be placed in the mouth of the flask, and another flask filled with cold water be placed in the funnel, this will form a convenient condenser, which will prevent the loss of more than a small quantity of the boiling liquid. Introduce the collected filtrate while still warm into a stoppered glass separator; add

* "Made by mixing together three volumes of benzol and one of amylic alcohol, and decanting the supernatant fluid from any deposited water." *Br.*

to it twenty minims of diluted hydrochloric acid, mixed with two fluidrachms of water; shake them well together, and when the acid liquid has separated this may be drawn off, and the process repeated with distilled water slightly acidulated with hydrochloric acid, until the whole of the alkaloids have been removed. The acid liquid thus obtained will contain the alkaloids as hydrochlorates, with excess of hydrochloric acid. It is to be carefully and exactly neutralized with ammonia while warm, and then concentrated to the bulk of three fluidrachms. If now about fifteen grains of tartarated soda, dissolved in twice its weight of water, be added to the neutral hydrochlorates, and the mixture stirred with a glass rod, insoluble tartrates of quinine and cinchonidine will separate completely in about an hour; and these collected on a filter, washed, and dried, will contain eight-tenths of their weight of the alkaloids, quinine and cinchonidine, which, divided by 2, represents the percentage of those alkaloids. The other alkaloids will be left in the mother-liquor.

"2. *For Total Alkaloids.* To the mother-liquor from the preceding process add solution of ammonia in slight excess. Collect, wash, and dry the precipitate, which will contain the other alkaloids. The weight of this precipitate divided by 2, and added to the percentage weight of the quinine and cinchonidine, gives the percentage of total alkaloids." *Br.*

The German Pharmacopœia gives the following method. "The powdered bark is assayed as follows: Shake 20 Gm. of it strongly and repeatedly with a mixture of 10 Gm. of water of ammonia, 20 Gm. of alcohol, and 170 Gm. of ether, and, after a day, decant 120 Gm. of the clear liquid. To this liquid add 3 C.c. of volumetric hydrochloric acid, remove the ether by distillation or evaporation, and again add, if necessary, enough hydrochloric acid to render the solution acid. Then filter, and mix the cold filtrate with 3·5 C.c. of volumetric solution of potassa. When the alkaloids have subsided, drop more of the solution of potassa into the clear supernatant liquid, until nothing more is thrown down. Finally, collect the whole of the precipitate on a filter, and wash it repeatedly with small portions of water, until drops of the wash water allowed to come in contact with the surface of a cold, aqueous, neutral, saturated solution of sulphate of quinine no longer produce a turbidity. When the alkaloids have drained, press them gently between bibulous paper, and, having dried them sufficiently in the air to permit their being removed to a watch-glass, dry them completely, first over sulphuric acid, and, finally, by means of a water-bath. The weight of alkaloids procured by this method should not be less than 0·42 Gm. When a small portion of the same is boiled with 300 parts of water, the filtrate, after cooling, should yield flakes of quinine. When to 5 parts of this solution, after being cooled and decanted, 1 part of chlorine water is added, and water of ammonia immediately dropped in, the liquid should acquire a beautiful green color."* *Ph. Germ.*

* *Dr. E. R. Squibb's Method of Assaying Cinchona Bark.* Take of the powdered cinchona 5 grammes = 77·16 grains; lime, well burnt, 1·25 grammes = 19·29 grains; amylic alcohol, stronger ether, purified chloroform, normal solution of oxalic acid, normal solution of sodium and water, of each a sufficient quantity, or, double all the quantities throughout, as well as size of vessels, etc., if the barks be poor, or if it be desired to divide the errors of manipulation. Add to the lime contained in a 10 Cm. = 4-inch capsule, 30 C.c. = 1 fluidounce of hot water, and when the lime is slaked, stir the mixture, add the cinchona, stir very thoroughly, and digest in a warm place for a few hours, or overnight. Then dry the mixture at a low temperature on a water-bath, rub it to powder in the capsule, and transfer it to a flask of 100 C.c. = 3·3 fluidounces capacity, and add to it 25 C.c. = ⅚ fluidounce of amylic alcohol. Cork the flask, and digest in a water-bath at a boiling temperature, and with frequent vigorous shaking for four hours. Then cool, and add 60 C.c. = 2 fluidounces of stronger ether, sp. gr. 0·728, and again shake vigorously and frequently during an hour or more. Filter off the liquid through a double filter of 10 Cm. = 4 inches diameter, into a flask of 150 C.c. = 5 fluidounces capacity, and transfer the residue to the filter. Rinse out the flask on to the filter with a mixture of 10 volumes of amylic alcohol and 40 of stronger ether, and then percolate the residue on the filter with 15 C.c. = half a fluidounce of the same mixture, added drop by drop from a pipette to the edges of the filter and surface of the residue. Return the residue to the flask from whence it came, add 30 C.c. = 1 fluidounce of the amylic alcohol and ether mixture, shake vigorously for five minutes or more, and return the whole to the filter. Again percolate the residue with 15 C.c. of the menstruum, applied drop by drop from a pipette as before. Then put the filter and residue aside, that it may be afterward tested in regard to the degree of exhaustion. Boil off the ether from the filtrate in the flask by means of a water-bath, taking great care to avoid igniting the ether vapor, and also to avoid explosive boiling by having a long wire in the flask. When boiled down as far as practicable in the flask, transfer the remainder to a tared capsule of 10 Cm. = 4 inches diameter, and continue the evaporation on a water-bath until the contents are

It is usually sufficient to ascertain the quantity of total alkaloids in bark, for this is really a test of the efficacy of the bark for pharmaceutical purposes; for all the organic alkaline principles contained in it are efficient as medicines, and in all probability in a nearly equal degree. But, for manufacturing purposes, it is necessary to push the investigation further, and ascertain the proportion of the several alkaloids in the mixture.

From the most recent and carefully conducted assays, it appears that the best officinal yellow Calisaya bark, the finest red bark, and the finest fibrous Carthagena bark (*soft Pitaya*) are about equal in their amount of alkaloids, each containing from 3 to 4 per cent., and the Indian and Java barks frequently exceed these yields; De Vrij obtained from bark of *C. officinalis* grown at Ootacamund total alkaloids as high as 11·96 per cent. (9·1 per cent. of which was quinine). The highest yield yet recorded was obtained by De Vrij from Ootacamund bark, 13·5 per cent., the greater part of which was quinine.* Between these and the barks of lowest

reduced to about 6 grammes = 92 grains. Transfer this to a flask of 100 C.c. = 3·3 fluidounces capacity, rinsing the capsule into the flask with not more than 4 C.c. = 64 minims of amylic alcohol. Then add 6 C.c. = 96 minims of water, and 4 C.c. = 64 minims of normal solution of oxalic acid, and shake vigorously and frequently during half an hour. Pour the mixture while intimately mixed on to a well-wetted double filter of 12 Cm. = 4½ inches diameter, and filter off the watery solution from the amylic alcohol into a tared capsule of 10 Cm. = 4 inches diameter. Wash the filter and contents with 5 C.c. = 80 minims of water, applied drop by drop from a pipette to the edges of the filter and surface of the amylic alcohol. Then pour the amylic alcohol back into the flask over the edge of the filter and funnel, rinsing the last portion in with a few drops of water. Add 10 C.c. = 160 minims of water, and 1 C.c. = 16 minims of normal solution of oxalic acid; again shake vigorously for a minute or two, and return the whole to the wetted filter, and filter off the watery portion into the capsule with the first portion. Return the amylic alcohol again to the flask, and repeat the washing with the same quantities of water and normal oxalic solution. When this has drained through, wash the filter and contents with 5 C.c. = 80 minims of water, applied drop by drop from a pipette. Evaporate the total filtrate in the capsule on a water-bath, at a low temperature, until it is reduced to about 15 grammes = 241 grains, and transfer this to a flask of 100 C.c. = 3·3 fluidounces capacity, rinsing the capsule into the flask with 5 C.c. = 80 minims of water. Add 20 C.c. = 66 fluidounces of purified chloroform, and then 6·1 C.c. = 98 minims of normal solution of sodium, and shake vigorously for five minutes or more. While still intimately mixed by the shaking, pour the mixture upon a filter of 12 Cm. = 4½ inches diameter, well wetted with water. When the watery solution has passed through, leaving the chloroform on the filter, wash the filter and chloroform with 5 C.c. = 80 minims of water, applied drop by drop. Then transfer the chloroform solution, by making a pin-hole in the point of the filter, to another filter of 10 Cm. = 4 inches diameter, well wetted with chloroform, and placed over a tared flask of 100 C.c. = 3·3 fluidounces capacity. Wash the watery filter through into the chloroform-wet filter with 5 C.c. = 80 minims of purified chloroform, and when this has passed through into the flask, wash the chloroform-wet filter also with 5 C.c. = 80 minims of chloroform applied drop by drop to the edges of the filter. When the whole chloroform solution of alkaloids is collected in the flask, boil off the chloroform to dryness in a water-bath, when the alkaloids will be left in watery groups of radiating crystals adhering over the bottom and sides of the flask. Place the flask on its side in a drying stove, and dry at 100° C. = 212° F. to a constant weight. The weight of the contents multiplied by 20 gives the percentage of the total alkaloids of the cinchona in an anhydrous condition, to within ·1 or ·2 of 1 per cent. if the process has been well managed.

* *Quinetum.* Under this name a compound is produced in India and other Eastern countries, which consists of the mixed alkaloids of Red Bark, the object being to produce a cheap febrifuge which will answer all practical purposes and save the cost of refining. The following formula has been adopted by the Dutch Society for the Advancement of Pharmacy: "Red Cinchona bark (the bark of the trunk of *Cinchona succirubra*, grown in Java or India, and containing at least 6 per cent. of alkaloids), in fine powder, 1000 parts; normal hydrochloric acid (volumetric standard), 1000 parts; oxalic acid, 12 parts; solution of soda, q. s.; water, q. s.

"Macerate the cinchona with the hydrochloric acid and 3000 parts of water for at least 12 hours, occasionally stirring. Pour the mixture into a percolator, the lower orifice of which is closed by a linen plug, and, as soon as the liquid runs off clear, displace with water until the liquid running from the percolator is no longer precipitated (though it may be colored) by solution of soda.

"To the strained liquid (which may amount to perhaps 8000 parts) add the oxalic acid dissolved in a little water, and then add *carefully*, under continued stirring, just enough solution of soda until the precipitate which forms at first separates in coherent flakes. Separate this precipitate (which consists of oxalate of calcium and cinchona-red) by pouring off as much of the still acid clear liquid as is possible, and filter the remainder. To the united liquids add now an excess of solution of soda, let it settle, and collect the precipitate upon a moistened double filter. Wash it with a weak soda solution until the washings have only a light-red color; then wash with the least possible quantity of water, until the washings begin to have a bitter taste. Let the precipitate drain, dry it in the air, and powder it.

"Quinetum is completely soluble in strong, warm alcohol. When 3·1 grammes of quinetum are dissolved in 10 C.c. of normal hydrochloric acid, this solution must be clear, and, on the addition of 2 grammes of Rochelle salt, must yield a precipitate which, when dried, should amount to *at least* 65 per cent. of the weight of the quinetum dissolved." (*N. R.*, 1862, p. 10)

value there is every grade of productiveness, down to a mere trace of alkaloidal matter.*

The quantities of cinchona and other barks used in the manufacture of quinine, imported into the United States during the years 1884, '85, '86, and '87, according to the U. S. Bureau of Statistics, were—in 1884, 2,580,052 lbs.; in 1885, 3,513,391 lbs.; in 1886, 4,454,368 lbs.; and in 1887, 4,788,044 lbs. The maximum importation in any year for ten years past was in 1879, when 6,388,641 lbs. were imported.

Medical Properties and Uses. This valuable remedy was unknown to the civilized world till about the middle of the seventeenth century, though the natives of Peru are generally supposed to have been long previously acquainted with its febrifuge powers. Humboldt, however, is of a different opinion. In his Memoir on the Cinchona forests, he states that it is unknown as a remedy to the Indians inhabiting the country where it grows; and, as these people adhere pertinaciously to the habits of their ancestors, he concludes that it never was employed by them. They have generally the most violent prejudices against it, considering it poisonous, and in the treatment of fever prefer the milder indigenous remedies. Ruiz and Pavon, however, ascribe the discovery to the Indians; and Tschudi states, in his Travels in Peru (*Am. ed.*, ii. 280), that the inhabitants of the Peruvian forests drink an infusion of the green bark as a remedy in intermittent fever.† On the other hand, the statements of Humboldt have recently been confirmed by the travellers Markham and Spence, the former remarking that the native Indian doctors do not use the bark, and the latter that the Cascarilleros of Ecuador believe that their red bark is used solely for dyeing. It is uncertain whether, as Jussieu stated in 1739, the Jesuit fathers received their knowledge from the Indians, or, as Humboldt believes, discovered the virtues of the drug for themselves, having been led to make trial of it by its extreme bitterness. The Countess of Cinchon, wife of the Viceroy of Peru, having in her own person experienced the beneficial effects of the bark, is said, on her return to Spain in the year 1640, to have first introduced the remedy into Europe. Hence the name of *pulvis Comitissæ*, by which it was first known. After its introduction, it was distributed and sold by the Jesuits, who are said to have obtained for it the price of its weight in silver. From this circumstance it was called *Jesuit's powder*, a title which it long retained. In 1653, Dr. Chifflet, physician to the Archduke Leopold, directed the attention of all Europe to the bark by his work entitled *Pulvis Febrifugus Orbis Americani.* This gave rise to a very active controversy; the high price of the drug aiding very greatly those who opposed its introduction. According to Sturm, twenty doses in 1658 cost sixty florins. It seems first to have been advertised in England for sale in 1658 by a James Thomson, and by 1660 it was much employed. It still, however, encountered much prejudice and ignorance, and was not made officinal in the London Pharmacopœia until 1677. Sir Robert Talbot (or Talbor) used it as a secret remedy with so much address and success that in 1679 he cured Charles II. of a tertian, and subsequently sold his secret to Louis XIV. of France, who published it in 1681.

When taken into the stomach, bark usually excites in a short time a sense of warmth in the epigastrium, which often diffuses itself over the abdomen and even the breast, and is sometimes attended with considerable gastric and intestinal irritation. Nausea and vomiting are sometimes produced, especially if the stomach was previously in an inflamed or irritated state. Purging, moreover, is not an unfrequent attendant upon its action. After some time has elapsed, the circulation often

* To obviate the disadvantages arising from the variable strength of bark, M. Guillermond recommends to fix on an appropriate strength, as indicated by the percentage of quinine, below the highest yet much above the lowest, and either to select bark of this strength, or to bring that employed to the medium strength, by adding a stronger or weaker bark, as the case may require, in due proportion. He recommends as this standard the yield of 3·2 per cent. of sulphate of quinine. This is to be treated by alcohol till entirely exhausted, and the tincture evaporated so as to yield an extract which shall exactly represent the virtues of the bark, and shall always have the same strength. From this extract all the preparations of bark are to be made, which will thus always be uniform in strength. (*Journ. de Pharm.*, Août, 1863, p. 124.)

† Tschudi also observes that he has found the fresh bark more efficacious than the dried; as, in less than half the usual dose, it not only effects cures in a short time, but insures the patient against the return of the disease.

experiences its influence, as exhibited in the somewhat increased frequency of pulse; and, if the dose be repeated, the whole system becomes more or less affected, and all the functions undergo a moderate degree of excitement. Its action upon the nervous system is often evinced by a sense of tension, or fulness, or slight pain in the head, singing in the ears, and partial deafness, which are always experienced by many individuals when brought completely under its influence. The effects above mentioned entitle bark to a place among the tonics, and it is usually ranked at the very head of this class of medicines. It has, however, certain, at present inscrutable, powers, which enable it to combat the action of malaria. It is, therefore, *antiperiodic*, but why it is so is at present entirely unknown. At present it is never itself employed in intermittents, and for the details of its action upon the system the reader is referred to the article upon the sulphate of quinine. As a tonic, bark is advantageously employed in chronic diseases connected with debility; as, for example, in scrofula, dropsy, passive hemorrhages, certain forms of dyspepsia, obstinate cutaneous affections, amenorrhœa, chorea, hysteria; in fact, whenever a corroborant influence is desired, and no contraindicating symptoms exist. But in all these cases it greatly behooves the physician to examine well the condition of the system, and, before resorting to the tonic, to ascertain the real existence of an enfeebled condition of the functions, and the absence of such local irritations or inflammations, especially of the stomach or bowels, as might be aggravated by its use. In doubtful cases, we have been in the habit of considering the occurrence of profuse sweating during sleep as an indication for its use, and, under these circumstances, have prescribed it very advantageously, in the form of sulphate of quinine, in acute rheumatism, and in the advanced stages of protracted fevers. Cinchona bark was formerly used in doses of 10 grains to a drachm (0·65 Gm. to 3·9 Gm.), but at present is never exhibited in its crude state.

Off. Prep. of Yellow Bark. Extractum Cinchonæ; Extractum Cinchonæ Fluidum; Infusum Cinchonæ; Tinctura Cinchonæ.

Off. Prep. of Red Bark. Tinctura Cinchonæ Composita.

Off. Prep. of Red Bark. Br. Decoctum Cinchonæ; Extractum Cinchonæ Liquidum; Infusum Cinchonæ Acidum; Mistura Ferri Aromatica; Tinctura Cinchonæ; Tinctura Cinchonæ Composita.

CINCHONIDINÆ SULPHAS. *U.S., Br.* *Sulphate of Cinchonidine.*

(CĬN-ÇHO-NI-DĪ'NÆ SŬL'PHĂS.)

$(C_{20}H_{24}N_2O)_2 H_2SO_4 . 3H_2O$; 768.* $(C_{20}H_{12}NO)_2, HO, SO_3 3HO$; 384.

"The neutral sulphate of an alkaloid prepared from certain species of Cinchona, chiefly Red Cinchona." *U. S.* "The sulphate of an alkaloid obtained from the bark of various species of Cinchona." *Br.*

Sulphate of Cinchonidia; Schwefelsaures Cinchonidin, *G.*; Sulfate de Cinchonidine, *Fr.*

This is a new officinal, which has largely come into use lately. It is prepared from the mother-liquors obtained in the manufacture of sulphate of quinine, and is separated from the sulphates of the other alkaloids by fractional crystallization. The British-India and Javanese cultivated red barks usually contain large quantities of cinchonidine. Of the South American barks, probably the Colombian varieties yield the largest proportion of cinchonidine. Owing to some confusion in naming cinchonidine and quinidine, this alkaloid is sometimes incorrectly called in Germany *chinidine*. Skraup's researches on the composition of cinchonine and cinchonidine (1879) established the correctness of the formula $C_{19}H_{22}N_2O$, instead of the long accepted formula of Pasteur (1853), $C_{20}H_{24}N_2O$. Skraup's formula has been confirmed by Hesse, and is now generally accepted among chemists. The French Codex of 1884 uses it, but the British Pharmacopœia of 1885 retains the old formula.

Properties. Sulphate of cinchonidine occurs in "white, silky, lustrous needles, or thin quadratic prisms, odorless, having a very bitter taste, and a neutral or faintly alkaline reaction. Soluble in 100 parts of water and in 71 parts of alcohol at 15° C. (59° F.), in 4 parts of boiling water, in 12 parts of boiling alcohol, freely in

* The formula now accepted is that of Skraup, $(C_{19}H_{22}N_2O)_2H_2SO_4.6H_2O$; 794.

acidulated water and in 1000 parts of chloroform (the undissolved portions becoming gelatinous); very sparingly soluble in ether or benzol. At 100° C. (212° F.) the salt loses its water of crystallization. From a dilute aqueous solution the salt crystallizes with 13·13 per cent. (6 to 7 mol.) of water of crystallization; from a concentrated aqueous solution with 7·03 per cent. (3 to 4 mol.). On ignition, the salt is dissipated without leaving a residue. The aqueous solution of the salt yields, on addition of water of ammonia, a white precipitate (Cinchonidine) which requires a large excess of ammonia to dissolve it, and which is soluble in about 75 times its weight of ether. With test-solution of iodide of mercury and potassium, the aqueous solution yields a curdy precipitate, and with test-solution of chloride of barium a white precipitate insoluble in hydrochloric acid. The moderately dilute aqueous solution of the salt, acidulated with sulphuric acid, should not show more than a slight blue fluorescence (abs. of more than traces of sulphate of quinine or of quinidine). The salt should not be colored by the addition of sulphuric acid (abs. of foreign organic matters). If 1 Gm. be dried at 100° C. (212° F.) until it ceases to lose weight, the residue, cooled in a desiccator, should weigh not less than 0·92 Gm. If 0·5 Gm. of the salt be digested with 20 C.c. of cold distilled water, 0·5 Gm. of tartrate of potassium and sodium added, the mixture macerated, with frequent agitation, for one hour at 15° C. (59° F.), then filtered, and a drop of water of ammonia added to the filtrate, not more than a slight turbidity should appear (abs. of more than 0·5 per cent. of sulphate of cinchonine, or of more than 1·5 per cent. of sulphate of quinidine)." *U. S.*

Cinchonidine. The alkaloid itself is not officinal; as usually seen it is in white, light, pulverulent masses. It is crystallizable, soluble in 1680 parts of cold and in a somewhat smaller quantity of hot water, in about 20 parts of alcohol and 70 parts of ether. It melts at 206·5° C. (404° F.), and becomes a solid mass of crystals at 190° C. (374° F.). The *acid sulphate* (sometimes called *bisulphate*) is much more soluble in water than the officinal sulphate. The *salicylate of cinchonidine* is neutral and crystalline, insoluble in cold water, sparingly in hot water, easily soluble in alcohol and diluted alcohol. It may be prepared by the direct combination of salicylic acid with the alkaloid. (Rosengarten, *A. J. P.*, 1879, p. 616.) The *hydrobromate* has been employed by Prof. Gubler hypodermically. (*N. R.*, 1879, p. 366.)*

Medical Properties. So far as our knowledge goes, this alkaloid influences the system similarly to quinine; the only difference being seemingly that it is less powerful. It may be given in a dose one-third greater than those of quinine, but should not be relied on in very severe cases.

CINCHONINA. *U. S.* *Cinchonine.* [*Cinchonia.*]

$C_{20}H_{24}N_2O$; 308.† (CĬN-CHŌ-NĪ'NĂ.) $C_{20}H_{12}NO$; 154.

"An alkaloid prepared from different species of Cinchona." *U. S.*

This alkaloid is introduced for the first time into the U. S. Pharmacopœia. The sulphate has had an extensive use, is again officinal, and is the source from whence this alkaloid is usually prepared. Cinchonine is most conveniently precipitated from an aqueous solution of sulphate of cinchonine by water of ammonia. Several processes have been employed for the preparation of cinchonine. One of the simplest is the following. Powdered pale bark is submitted to the action of sulphuric or hydrochloric acid very much diluted, and the solution obtained is precipitated by an excess of lime. The precipitate is collected on a filter, washed with water, and treated with boiling alcohol. The alcoholic solution is filtered while hot, and de-

* *Benzoate of Cinchonidine* may be made by Byasson's process. Sixty parts of benzoic acid are dissolved in two hundred parts of alcohol, and poured into a porcelain vessel containing three thousand parts of boiling distilled water; two hundred parts of cinchonidine sulphate are dissolved in two thousand parts of water, using sufficient diluted sulphuric acid to effect the solution; this is precipitated with ammonia, and washed with a small quantity of cold water; the moist precipitate of cinchonidine is added to the hot solution of benzoic acid, and filtered while hot. The solution must be made faintly alkaline by the cautious addition of ammonia. On cooling, the cinchonidine benzoate separates in the form of small, thin, prismatic needles, resembling cinchonidine sulphate. The yield is about two hundred parts. (*Phar. Rec.*, 1884, p. 45.)

† Skraup's formula is now generally accepted, $C_{19}H_{22}N_2O$; 294.

posits the cinchonine when it cools. A further quantity is obtained by evaporation. If not perfectly white, it may be made so, by converting it into a sulphate with dilute sulphuric acid, then treating the solution with animal charcoal, filtering, precipitating by an alkali, and redissolving by alcohol in the manner already mentioned. It may also be obtained from the mother-waters of sulphate of quinine by diluting them with water, precipitating with ammonia, collecting the precipitate on a filter, washing and drying it, and then dissolving it in boiling alcohol, which deposits the cinchonine in a crystalline form upon cooling. It may be still further purified by a second solution and crystallization. Its formula is now generally accepted as $C_{19}H_{22}N_2O$, the molecular weight of which is 294, as proposed by Skraup, instead of the older formula, $C_{20}H_{24}N_2O$, of Pasteur.

Properties. This alkaloid occurs in "white, somewhat lustrous prisms or needles, permanent in the air, odorless, at first nearly tasteless, but developing a bitter after-taste, and having an alkaline reaction. Almost insoluble in cold or hot water, soluble in 110 parts of alcohol at 15° C. (59° F.), in 28 parts of boiling alcohol, 371 parts of ether, 350 parts of chloroform, and readily soluble in diluted acids, forming salts of a very bitter taste. At about 250° C. (482° F.) it melts and turns brown with partial sublimation. On ignition, the alkaloid is dissipated without leaving a residue. A solution of the alkaloid in diluted sulphuric acid, should not exhibit more than a faint blue fluorescence (abs. of more than traces of quinine or quinidine). On precipitating the alkaloid from this solution by water of ammonia, it is very sparingly dissolved by the latter (difference from and abs. of quinine), and requires at least 300 parts of ether for solution (difference from quinine, quinidine, and cinchonidine). The salt should not be colored, or but very slightly colored, by the addition of sulphuric acid (abs. of foreign organic matter)." *U. S.* Waddington found it to sublime readily, without change, in perfectly characteristic crystals. (*P. J. Tr.*, March, 1868, p. 414.)* Its alkaline character is very decided, as it neutralizes the strongest acids. Of the salts of cinchonine, the sulphate, nitrate, hydrochlorate, phosphate, and acetate are soluble in water. The neutral tartrate, oxalate, and gallate are insoluble in cold water, but soluble in hot water, alcohol, or an excess of acid. Winkler has shown that cinchonine is rendered uncrystallizable or amorphous by sulphuric acid in excess, aided by heat; a fact of importance in the preparation of the sulphate of this alkaloid. (*Chem. Gaz.*, March 15, 1848.) Cinchonine is but little more soluble in carbonic acid water than in pure water, and does not, like quinine, yield crystals of the carbonate on exposure of its carbonic acid solution. (*Comptes-Rendus*, Nov. 7, 1853, p. 727.) It differs from quinine by its rotating the plane of polarization to the right, by the want of fluorescence in its solutions, and by its failing to give the *thalleioquin* test.

Exposed to the air, cinchonine does not suffer decomposition, but very slowly absorbs carbonic acid gas, and acquires the property of effervescing slightly with acids. It is precipitated sulphur yellow by the terchloride of gold. Chlorine water dissolves it or any of its salts without change; but if ammonia be now added, a white precipitate is produced. It is thus distinguishable from quinine. (See *Quinine.*) Dr. J. W. Bill, U.S.A., proposes ferrocyanide of potassium as a very delicate test of cinchonine. If added to the solution of a salt of this alkaloid, it produces a yellowish white curdy precipitate, which is dissolved upon the application of a gentle heat, but is again deposited, when the liquid cools, as an abundant crop of golden yellow crystals. No other alkaloid exhibits the same reaction. A cloudy precipitate is produced by the same reagent with a salt of quinine; but this does not happen when the ferrocyanide is in excess; and, if the precipitate be dissolved by heat, no subsidence takes place on cooling. Hence, in the application of this test to cinchonine, a slight excess of the ferrocyanide should be added. (*Am. Journ. of Science and Arts*, July, 1858, p. 108.)

By the action of permanganate of potassium cinchonine is decomposed, with the

* It is asserted that the hydrochlorates of quinine, cinchonine, and quinidine, heated on a slip of platinum, short of combustion, emit a purple vapor like iodine. Neither the alkaloids nor their sulphates have this property; but the addition of one-tenth of hydrochlorate will cause the evolution of the colored vapor. (*Journ. de Pharm. et de Chim.*, 4e sér., iii. 397.)

effect of producing, at first, an entirely distinct neutral principle, *cinchotenine*, $C_{18}H_{20}N_2O_3+3H_2O$, and an alkaloid, which the authors named *hydrocinchonine*, $C_{19}H_{24}N_2O$, as it differs from cinchonine (cinchonia) only in having two additional atoms of hydrogen. The cinchotenine, when further oxidized by the same reagent, yields quinoline and pyridine derivatives (see Part II.), as *cinchonic* (quinoline-carbonic) *acid*, $C_9H_6N(COOH)$, and *cinchomeronic* (pyridine-dicarbonic) *acid*, $C_5H_3N(COOH)_2$.

Medical Properties. The physiological action of cinchonine is similar to but less powerful than that of quinine. Thus, Conzen (quoted by Husemann) has found that its action on infusoria and on fermentation is similar to but weaker than that of its sister alkaloid, and that on the movements of the white blood-corpuscles its influence seems transient. Upon dogs, according to Bernatzik's experiments, the lethal dose of cinchonine is to that of quinine as 5 is to 4. As an antiperiodic or tonic, cinchonine exerts an influence similar to that of quinine, but is probably about one-third weaker than that alkaloid, and must be used in correspondingly larger dose.

CINCHONINÆ SULPHAS. *U.S.*, *Br.* *Sulphate of Cinchonine.*

(CĬN-CHŌ-NĪ'NÆ SŬL'PHĂS.)

$(C_{20}H_{24}N_2O)_2H_2SO_4.2H_2O$; 750.* $(C_{20}H_{12}NO)_2.HO,SO_3.2HO$; 375.

"The sulphate of an alkaloid obtained from the bark of various species of Cinchona and Remijia." *Br.*

Cinchoniæ Sulphas, *Pharm.* 1870; Cinchoninum Sulfuricum, *P.G.*; Sulfate de Cinchonine, *Fr.*; Schwefelsaures Cinchonin, *G.*

The process officinal in U. S. P. 1870 is as follows. "Take of the mother-water, remaining after the crystallisation of Sulphate of Quinine, in the process for preparing that salt, *a convenient quantity*; Solution of Soda, Alcohol, Diluted Sulphuric Acid, Animal Charcoal, in fine powder, each, *a sufficient quantity*. To the mother-water add gradually, with constant stirring, Solution of Soda, until the liquid becomes alkaline. Collect on a filter the precipitate formed, wash it with water, and dry it. Then wash it with successive small portions of alcohol, to remove other alkaloids which may be present. Mix the residue with eight times its weight of water, and, having heated the mixture, add gradually Diluted Sulphuric Acid until it is saturated and becomes clear. Then boil the liquid with Animal Charcoal, filter it while hot, and set it aside to crystallize. Lastly, drain the crystals, and dry them on bibulous paper. By evaporating the mother-liquid, more crystals may be obtained." *U. S.*

In consequence of its greater solubility, Sulphate of Cinchonine remains behind in the mother-waters, when sulphate of quinine crystallizes, in the process for preparing the latter salt. To separate it from other substances contained in the mother-waters, it is decomposed by solution of soda, which is preferable to potassa, as it forms a very soluble salt, with sulphuric acid, whereas the sulphate of potassium, being of difficult solubility, might fall with the precipitated cinchonine. The precipitate may be safely washed with small portions of alcohol, as the alkaloid is almost insoluble in that liquid when cold. It is next reconverted into the sulphate; and the solution, having been boiled with *unpurified* animal charcoal to decolorize it, and at the same time neutralize any possible excess of sulphuric acid which might interfere with the crystallization of the salt, is filtered while hot, and then allowed to stand. It is peculiarly important that there should be no excess of sulphuric acid while the solution is exposed to heat, as, under this influence, the alkaloid is much disposed to become uncrystallizable. Hence the advantage of using unpurified animal charcoal or bone-black, as the carbonate of calcium contained in it neutralizes any excess of the acid. The sulphate of cinchonine, held in solution by the liquid while hot, is deposited by it upon cooling in crystals.

It may be prepared also by first obtaining cinchonine from one of the pale barks; treating this with water acidulated with sulphuric acid, added gradually till the alkaloid is dissolved; then boiling with purified animal charcoal, filtering the solution while hot, and setting it aside to crystallize.

* Skraup's formula $(C_{19}H_{22}N_2O)_2H_2SO_4.2H_2O$; 732, is now accepted instead of the officinal one.

There are two sulphates of cinchonine, the neutral and the acid-sulphate. The officinal salt is the neutral sulphate. It is in "hard, white, shining prisms of the clino-rhombic system, permanent in the air, odorless, having a very bitter taste and a neutral or faintly alkaline reaction. Soluble in about 70 parts of water and in 6 parts of alcohol at 15° C. (59° F.), in 14 parts of boiling water, 1·5 parts of boiling alcohol, 60 parts of chloroform, and easily so in diluted acids; insoluble in ether or benzol. At 100° C. (212° F.) the salt loses its water of crystallization, and at about 240° C. (464° F.) it melts with partial sublimation. On ignition, the salt is dissipated without leaving a residue. The aqueous solution of the salt yields a curdy precipitate with test-solution of iodide of mercury and potassium. With water of ammonia it yields a white precipitate (Cinchonine) which is very sparingly soluble in an excess of ammonia (difference from quinine), and not soluble in less than 300 parts of ether (difference from quinine, quinidine, and cinchonidine).* With test-solution of chloride of barium it yields a white precipitate insoluble in hydrochloric acid. A moderately dilute solution of the salt, acidulated with sulphuric acid, should not show more than a faint blue fluorescence (abs. of more than traces of sulphate of quinine or of quinidine). If 1 Gm. be dried at 100° C. (212° F.), until it ceases to lose weight, the residue, cooled in a desiccator, should weigh not less than 0·952 Gm. If the salt, dried at a gentle heat, be macerated, for half an hour, with frequent agitation, with 70 times its weight of chloroform at 15° C. (59° F.), it should wholly, or almost wholly, dissolve (any more than traces of sulphate of quinine or sulphate of cinchonidine remaining undissolved). It should not be colored by contact with sulphuric acid (abs. of foreign organic matters)." *U. S.* The *acid sulphate*, or *bisulphate*, $C_{19}H_{22}N_2OH_2SO_4,3H_2O$, is prepared by adding sulphuric acid to the neutral sulphate. According to Baup, 100 parts are soluble in 45 parts of water and in 100 parts of absolute alcohol; it is insoluble in ether. It crystallizes in rhombic octahedrons.

Medical Properties and Uses. It is now determined that sulphate of cinchonine has the same remedial properties as sulphate of quinine, but must be given in somewhat larger dose. As a tonic it may be given in the dose of a grain or two (0·065–0·13 Gm.) three or four times a day; as an antiperiodic, 15 grains to 40 grains (1·0–2·6 Gm.) may be given between the paroxysms. It may be taken in pill or solution made by the addition of dilute sulphuric acid, in the proportion of a minim or two drops for each grain of the salt. To lessen the bitterness in taste, it may be given suspended in syrup, without the use of any acid, or with a few grains of powdered liquorice added to the mixture.

CINNAMOMUM. *U. S.* *Cinnamon.*

(CĬN-NẠ-MŌ′MŬM.)

"The inner bark of the shoots of Cinnamomum Zeylanicum, Breyne (Ceylon Cinnamon); or the bark of the shoots of one or more undetermined species of Cinnamomum grown in China (Chinese Cinnamon). (*Nat. Ord.* Lauraceæ.)" *U. S.* "The dried inner bark of shoots from the truncated stocks or stools of the cultivated cinnamon tree, Cinnamomum zeylanicum, *Breyn.* Imported from Ceylon, and distinguished in commerce as Ceylon Cinnamon." *Br.*

Cinnamomi Cortex, *Br.;* Cinnamon Bark; Cortex Cinnamomi Zeylonici; Cinnamomum Acutum, s. Verum; Cannelle de Ceylon, Cannelle, *Fr.;* Brauner Canel, Zeylonzimmt, Zimmt, *G.;* Canella, *It.;* Canela, *Sp.;* Kurundu *Cingalese;* Karua puttay, *Tamil.*

Cassia.—Cortex Cinnamomi, *P.G.;* Cinnamomum Chinense, Cassia Cinnamomea; Cassia Lignea; Cassia Bark; Casse, Cannelle de Chine, *Fr.;* Cassienzimmt, Zimmtkassie, Chinesischer (Gemeiner) Zimmt, *G.;* Canellina, *It.;* Casia, *Sp.*

The U. S. Pharmacopœia embraces, under the title of Cinnamon, not only the bark of that name obtained from the island of Ceylon, which is the only variety recognized in the British Pharmacopœia, but also the commercial cassia, which is im-

* A test, distinguishing between the sulphates of quinine and of cinchonine, has been announced by M. Palm, of Russia, in the polysulphide of potassium prepared by boiling solution of potassa with an excess of sulphur. When a solution of this sulphide is added to a boiling solution of sulphate of quinine, the latter, however small the quantity present, is thrown down as a red terebinthinate mass, which hardens on cooling, and then assumes the appearance of a resin; while with sulphate of cinchonine a white powder is precipitated containing sulphur. (*Journ. de Pharm.*, Mai, 1864.)

ported from China; and, as the two products, though very different in price, and somewhat in flavor, possess identical medical properties and are used for the same

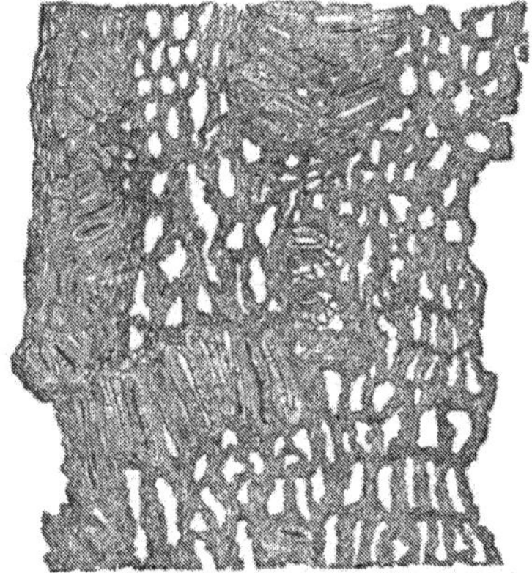

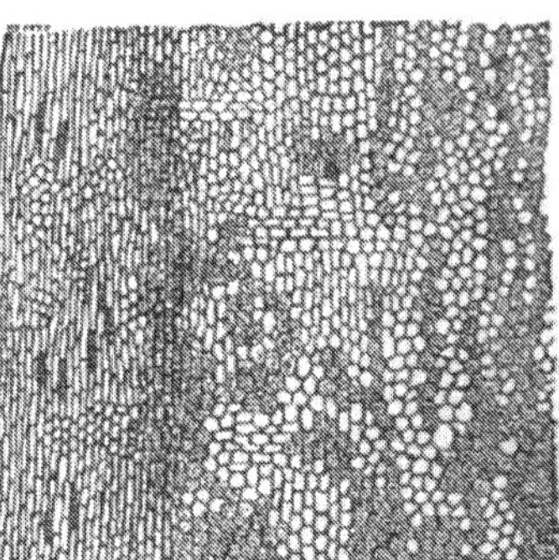

Fig. 1.—True Cinnamon, transverse section (very highly magnified). Cassia Bark, longitudinal section.

purposes, there seems to be no necessity for giving them distinct officinal designations. Indeed, the barks of all the species of the genus Cinnamomum, possessing analogous properties, are as much entitled to the common name of cinnamon, as the barks of the Cinchonas are to the name of cinchona, and the juice of different species of Aloe to that of aloes. Both *cinnamomum* and *cassia* were terms employed by the ancients, but whether exactly as now understood it is impossible to determine. The term *cassia*, or *cassia lignea*, has been generally used in modern times to designate the coarser barks analogous to cinnamon. It was probably first applied to the barks from Malabar, and afterwards extended to those of China and other parts of Eastern Asia. It has been customary to ascribe *cassia lignea* to the *Laurus Cassia* of Linnæus; but the specific character given by that botanist was so indefinite, and based on such imperfect information, that the species has been almost unanimously abandoned by botanists. The barks sold as cinnamon and cassia in different parts of the world are derived from various species of Cinnamomum. We shall describe only the two species recognized in the U. S. Pharmacopœia.

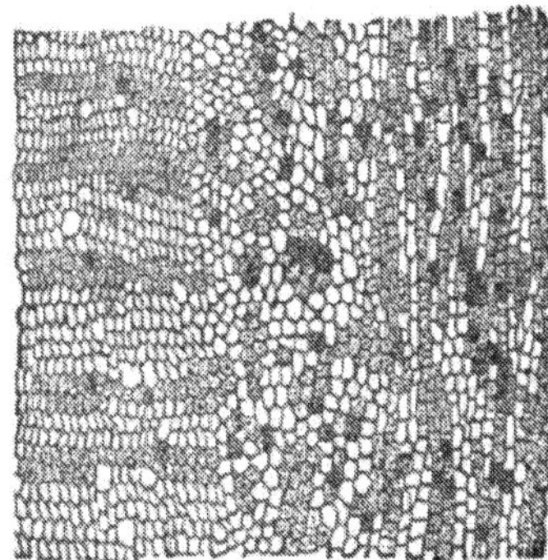

Cassia Bark, transverse section.

Gen. Ch. Flowers hermaphrodite or polygamous. *Perianth* six-cleft, the upper half of each segment deciduous. *Stamens* nine, with four-celled anthers, six (opposite the perianth-segments) opening inwards without glands, three (opposite three of the above) opening outwards and bearing a gland on each side at the base. *Staminodia* three (opposite the three other outer stamens), with capitate or cordate abortive anthers. *Berry* resting on the enlarged six-lobed base of the perianth." (Bentham, *Flora Hongkongensis.*) As thus defined, the genus Cinnamomum does not include the genus Camphora; for the modification of character necessary to do this, see *Camphora.*

1. *Cinnamomum Zeylanicum.* Nees, *Laurineæ,* 52; Lindley, *Flor. Med.* 329; Hayne, *Darstel. und Beschreib., etc.* xii. 263.—*Laurus Cinnamomum.* Linn. This is a tree about 20 or 30 feet high, with a trunk from 12 to 18 inches in diameter, and covered with a thick, scabrous bark. The branches are numerous, strong, horizontal,

and declining; and the young shoots are beautifully speckled with dark green and light orange colors. The leaves are opposite for the most part, coriaceous, entire, ovate, or ovate-oblong, obtusely pointed, and three-nerved, with the lateral nerves vanishing as they approach the point. There are also two less obvious nerves, one on each side arising from the base, proceeding towards the border of the leaf, and then quickly vanishing. The footstalks are short and slightly channelled, and, together with the extreme twigs, are smooth and without the least appearance of down. In one variety, the leaves are very broad and somewhat cordate. When mature, they are of a shining green upon their upper surface, and lighter colored beneath. The flowers are small, white, and arranged in axillary and terminal panicles. The fruit is an oval berry, which adheres like the acorn to the receptacle, is larger than the black currant, and when ripe has a bluish brown surface, diversified with numerous white spots.

The tree emits no smell perceptible at any distance. The bark of the root has the odor of cinnamon with the pungency of camphor, and yields this principle upon distillation. The leaves have a spicy odor when rubbed, and a hot taste. A volatile oil distilled from them has been introduced into commerce.* The petiole has the flavor of cinnamon. It is a singular fact that the odor of the flowers is to people in general disagreeable, being compared by some to the scent exhaled from newly-sawn bones. The fruit has a terebinthinate odor when opened, and a taste in some degree like that of Juniper berries. A fatty substance, called *cinnamon-suet*, is obtained from it when ripe, by bruising and then boiling it in water, and removing the oleaginous matter which rises to the surface, and concretes upon cooling. It is the prepared bark that constitutes the genuine cinnamon.

This species is a native of Ceylon, where it has long been cultivated. It is said also to be a native of the Malabar Coast, and has at various periods been introduced into Java, the Isle of France, Bourbon, the Cape Verds, Brazil, Cayenne, several of the West India islands, and Egypt, and in some of these places is at this time highly productive, especially in Cayenne, where the plant was flourishing so early as 1755. It is exceedingly influenced, as regards the aromatic character of its bark, by the circumstances of soil, climate, and mode of culture. Thus, we are told by Marshall that in Ceylon, beyond the limits of Negombo and Matura, in the western and southern parts of the island, the bark is never of good quality, being greatly deficient in the aromatic flavor of the cinnamon; and that even within these limits it is of unequal value, from the various influence of exposure, soil, shade, and other circumstances.

2. *C. aromaticum.* Nees, *Laurineæ*, 52; Lindley, *Flor. Med.* 330.—*C. Cassia.* Blume, Ed. Ph.; Hayne, *Darstel. und Beschreib., etc.* xii. 23.—*Laurus Cassia.* Aiton, *Hort. Kew.* ii. 427.—Not *Laurus Cassia* of Linn. This is of about the same magnitude as the former species, and, like it, has nearly opposite, shortly petiolate, coriaceous, entire leaves, of a shining green upon the upper surface, lighter colored beneath, and furnished with three nerves, of which the two latter vanish towards the point. The leaves, however, differ in being oblong-lanceolate and pointed, and in exhibiting, under the microscope, a very fine down upon the under surface. The footstalks and extreme twigs are also downy. The flowers are in narrow, silky panicles. The plant grows in China, Sumatra, and other parts of Eastern Asia, and is said to be cultivated in Java. It is believed to be the species which furnishes, wholly or in part, the Chinese cinnamon or cassia brought from Canton, and is supposed to be the source of the *cassia buds*.

Besides the two species above described, others have been thought to contribute to the cinnamon and cassia of commerce. In 1839 (*Madras Journ. Lit. & Sci.*, No. 22), Dr. Wight stated that in his belief cinnamon was derived from 12 to 18 specially distinct trees. *C. inners*, Reinw., is distinguished from *C. Zeylanicum* by

* The *cinnamon leaf oil*, as imported into Great Britain, is of two kinds, one containing a considerable quantity of a fatty fixed oil, perhaps cinnamon-suet from the fruit, the other a pure volatile oil. The oil is said to be obtained by distilling the leaves after maceration in sea-water. It resembles the oil of cloves and pimento in sensible properties, having a brownish color, a penetrating, fragrant odor, and a very pungent taste. According to Stenhouse, it is of the sp. gr. 1·053, has an acid reaction, and consists of eugenic acid, a neutral substance with the formula $C_{10}H_{16}$, and a minute proportion of benzoic acid. (*P. J. Tr.*, xiv. 319.)

the nervation of its leaves, which are also paler and thinner than those of the officinal plant, of which, however, it is probably only a variety. It yields the so-called *wild cinnamon* of Japan. *C. Loureirii* of Nees, growing in the mountains of Cochin-China, near Laos, and in Japan, affords, according to Loureiro, a cinnamon of which the finest kind is superior to that of Ceylon. *C. nitidum*, growing in Ceylon, Java, and on the continent of India, is said to have been the chief source of the drug known formerly by the name of *Folia Malabathri*, and consisting of the leaves of different species of Cinnamomum mixed together. *C. Culilawan* of the Moluccas yields the aromatic bark called culilawan, noticed in Part II. of this work; and similar barks are obtained from another species of the same region, named *C. rubrum*, and from *C. Sintoc* of Java. *Massoy-bark*, from which an aromatic volatile oil is obtained called *oil of massoy*, is the product of *C. Kiamis*. (Gmelin, *Handbook*, xiv. 380.) In the mountains of Eastern Bengal, at a height of 1000 to 4000 feet, flourish *C. obtusifolium*, Nees, *C. pauciflorum*, Nees, and *C. Tamala*, W., and these afford quantities of a bark which is brought to Calcutta for shipment under the name of *cassia lignea*, or *cassia*.

Culture, Collection, Commerce, etc. Our remarks under this head will first be directed to the cinnamon of Ceylon, in relation to which we have more precise information than concerning that obtained from other sources. The bark was originally collected exclusively from the tree in a wild state; but the Dutch introduced the practice of cultivating it, which has been continued since the British came into possession of the island. The principal cinnamon gardens are in the vicinity of Columbo. The seeds are planted in a prepared soil at certain distances; and, as four or five are placed in a spot, the plants usually grow in clusters like the hazel-bush. In favorable situations they attain the height of five or six feet in six or seven years; and a healthy bush will then afford two or three shoots fit for peeling, and every second year afterwards from four to seven shoots in a good soil. The cinnamon harvest commences in May, and continues till late in October. The first object is to select shoots proper for decortication, and those are seldom cut which are less than half an inch or more than two or three inches in diameter. The bark is divided by longitudinal incisions, of which two are made in the smaller shoots, several in the larger, and is then removed in strips by means of a suitable instrument. The pieces are next collected in bundles, and allowed to remain in this state for a short time, so as to undergo a degree of fermentation, which facilitates the separation of the epidermis. This, with the green matter beneath it, is removed by placing the strip of bark upon a convex piece of wood, and scraping its external surface with a curved knife. The bark now dries and contracts, assuming the appearance of a quill. The peeler introduces the smaller tubes into the larger, and connects them also endwise, thus forming a congeries of quills which is about forty inches long. When sufficiently dry, these cylinders are collected into bundles weighing about thirty pounds, and bound together by pieces of split bamboo. The commerce in Ceylon cinnamon was formerly monopolized by the East India Company; but the cultivation is now unrestricted, and the bark may be freely exported upon the payment of a fixed duty. It is assorted in the island into three qualities, distinguished by the designations of *first*, *second*, and *third*. The inferior kinds, which are of insufficient value to pay the duty, are used for the preparation of oil of cinnamon.

Immense quantities of cinnamon are exported from China, the finest of which is little inferior to that of Ceylon, though the mass of it is much coarser. It passes in commerce under the name of *cassia*, and is said by Mr. Reeves to be brought to Canton from the province of Kwangse, where the tree producing it grows very abundantly. (*Trans. Medico-Bot. Soc.*, 1828, p. 26.) It has already been stated that this tree is supposed to be the *Cinnamomum aromaticum;* but we have no positive proof of the fact. Travellers inform us that cinnamon is also collected in Cochin-China; but that the best of it is monopolized by the sovereign of the country. It is supposed to be obtained from the *Cinnamomum Loureirii* of Nees, the *Laurus Cinnamomum* of Loureiro. According to Siebold, the bark of the large branches is of inferior quality and is rejected; that from the smallest branches resembles the Ceylon cinnamon in thickness, but has a very pungent taste and smell, and is little esteemed; while the intermediate branches yield an excellent bark, about a line in thickness, which is even more highly valued than the cinnamon of Ceylon, and yields a sweeter and less pungent oil. (*Annal. der Pharm.*, xx. 280.) Cinnamon of good quality is said to be collected in Java; and considerable quantities of inferior quality have been thrown into commerce, as *cassia lignea*, from the Malabar Coast. Manilla and the Isle of France are also mentioned as sources whence this drug is supplied. Little, however reaches the United States from these places. The island of Martinique, Cayenne, and several of the West India islands, yield to commerce considerable quantities of cinnamon of various qualities. That of Cayenne is of two kinds, one of which closely resembles, though it does not quite equal, the aromatic of Ceylon, the other resembles the Chinese. The former is supposed to be derived from plants propagated from a Ceylonese stock, the latter from those which have sprung from a tree introduced from Sumatra.

By far the greater proportion of cinnamon brought to this country is imported from China. It is entered as *cassia* at the custom-house, while the same article brought from other sources is almost uniformly entered as cinnamon. Much of it is afterwards exported.

From what source the ancients derived their cinnamon and cassia is not certainly known. Neither the plants nor their localities, as described by Dioscorides, Pliny, and Theophrastus, correspond precisely with our present knowledge; but in this respect much allowance must be made for the inaccurate geography of the ancients. It is not improbable that the Arabian navigators, at a very early period, conveyed this spice within the limits of Phœnician and Grecian, and subsequently of Roman commerce.

Properties. *Ceylon cinnamon* is in long cylindrical fasciculi, composed of numerous quills, the larger enclosing the smaller. In the original sticks, which are somewhat more than three feet in length, two or three fasciculi are neatly joined at the end, so as to appear as if the whole were one continuous piece. The finest is of a light brownish yellow color, almost as thin as paper, smooth, often somewhat shining, pliable to a considerable extent, with a splintery fracture when broken. It has a pleasant fragrant odor, and a warm, aromatic, pungent, sweetish, slightly astringent, and highly agreeable taste. When distilled it affords but a small quantity of essential oil, which, however, has an exceedingly grateful flavor. It is brought to this country from England; but it is costly. The inferior sorts are browner, thicker, less splintery, and of a less agreeable flavor, and are little if at all superior to the best Chinese. The finer variety of *Cayenne cinnamon* approaches in character that above described, but is paler and in thicker pieces, being usually collected from older branches. That which is gathered very young is scarcely distinguishable from the cinnamon of Ceylon. "*Ceylon Cinnamon* is in long, closely-rolled quills, composed of eight or more layers of bark of the thickness of paper; pale yellowish-brown; outer surface smooth, marked with wavy lines; inner surface scarcely striate; fracture splintery; odor fragrant; taste sweet and warmly aromatic." *U. S.**

Chinese cinnamon, or *Cassia*, is in tubes from one-eighth of an inch to an inch in diameter, usually single, sometimes double, but very rarely more than double. In some instances the bark is rolled very much upon itself, in others is not even completely quilled, forming segments more or less extensive of a hollow cylinder. It is of a redder or darker color than the finest Ceylon cinnamon, thicker, rougher, denser, and breaks with a shorter fracture. It has a stronger, more pungent and astringent, but less sweet and grateful taste, and, though of a similar odor, is less agreeably fragrant. It is the kind almost universally kept in our shops. Of a similar character is the cinnamon imported directly from various parts of the East Indies. But under the name of cassia have also been brought to us very inferior kinds of cinnamon, collected from the trunks or large branches of the trees, or injured by want of care in keeping, or perhaps derived from inferior species. It is said that cinnamon from which the oil has been distilled is sometimes fraudulently mixed with the genuine. These inferior kinds are detected, independently of their greater thickness and coarseness of fracture, by their deficiency in the peculiar sensible proper-

* For an account of the cultivation of *C. Zeylanicum*, see *P. J. Tr.*, xi. 261.

ties of the spice. "*Chinese Cinnamon* (Cassia Bark) is in quills about one twenty-fifth of an inch (1 mm.) or more in thickness; nearly deprived of the corky layer; brown, outer surface somewhat rough; fracture nearly smooth; odor and taste analogous to that [*sic*] of Ceylon Cinnamon, but less delicate." *U. S.*

The *Pharmacographia* gives the following tests for distinguishing powdered cassia from powdered cinnamon, and for recognizing the inferior varieties of cassia. Make a decoction of powdered cinnamon of known genuineness, and one of similar strength of the suspected powder; when cool and strained, test a fluidounce of each with one or two drops of tincture of iodine. A decoction of cinnamon is but little affected, but in that of cassia a deep blue-black tint is immediately produced. The cheap kinds of cassia known as *cassia vera* may be distinguished from the more valuable Chinese cassia as well as from cinnamon by their richness in mucilage; this can be extracted by cold water as a thick glairy liquid, giving dense ropy precipitates with corrosive sublimate or neutral acetate of lead, but not with alcohol.

Microscopic Structure. Ceylon cinnamon usually consists simply of liber, the outer coatings having been stripped off during its preparation for market. Three layers are distinguishable in the liber. "1. The external surface, which is composed of one to three rows of large thick-walled cells (Fig. 1), forming a coherent ring; it is only interrupted by bundles of liber fibres, which are obvious even to the unaided eye. 2. The middle layer is built up of about 10 rows of parenchymatous thin-walled cells, interrupted by much larger cells containing deposits of mucilage, while other cells not larger than those of the parenchyme itself are loaded with essential oil. 3. The innermost layer exhibits the same thin-walled but smaller cells, yet intersected by narrow somewhat darker medullary rays, and likewise interrupted by cells containing either mucilage or essential oil, instead of bundles of liber fibres. Fibres mostly isolated are scattered through the two inner layers, the parenchyme of which abounds in small starch granules accompanied by tannic matter. On a longitudinal section the length of the liber fibres becomes more evident, as well as oil-ducts and gum-ducts." (*Pharmacographia.*)

The coarser cassia bark, or cassia lignea, usually has some of the external or corky layer adherent to it, and always the parenchymatous mesophlœum or middle bark; but the liber constitutes the chief mass. Isolated liber fibres and thick-walled cells (stone-cells) are scattered even through the outer layers of a transverse section. In the middle zone they are numerous, but do not form a coherent sclerenchymatous ring as in Ceylon cinnamon. The innermost part of the liber shares the structural character of cinnamon, with difference due to age, as, for instance, the greater development of the medullary rays. Oil-cells and gum-ducts are likewise distributed in the parenchyme of the former. The finest cassia or Chinese cinnamon has the three layers described in Ceylon cinnamon, but is readily distinguished by the adherent outer parenchymatous and suberous layer.

Chemical Composition. According to the analysis of Vauquelin, cinnamon contains a peculiar volatile oil, tannin, mucilage, a coloring matter, an acid, and lignin. The tannin is of the variety which yields a greenish black precipitate with the salts of iron. Jas. A. Ferguson (1887), in the Laboratory of the Philadelphia College of Pharmacy, determined the ash of several samples of Ceylon cinnamon, finding an average of 4 per cent., while in powdered *cinnamon cassia* he found 2·8 and 2·5 per cent. (*A. J. P.*, 1887, pp. 278 and 279.) The oil obtained from the Cayenne cinnamon was found to be more biting than that from the Ceylonese, and at the same time to be somewhat peppery. Buchols found in 100 parts of *cassia lignea*, 0·8 of volatile oil, 4·0 of resin, 14·6 of gummy extractive (probably including tannin), 64·3 of lignin and bassorin, and 16·3 of water including loss. This aromatic yields its virtues wholly to alcohol, and less readily to water. At the temperature of boiling alcohol very little of the oil rises, and an extract prepared from the tincture retains, therefore, the aromatic properties. For an account of the volatile oil, see *Oleum Cinnamomi.*

Medical Properties and Uses. Cinnamon is among the most grateful and efficient of the aromatics. It is warm and cordial to the stomach, carminative, astringent, and, like most other substances of this class, more powerful as a local than as a general stimulant. It is seldom prescribed alone, though, when given in powder or infusion, it will sometimes allay nausea, check vomiting, and relieve flatulence. It is chiefly used as an adjuvant to other less pleasant medicines, and enters into a great number of officinal preparations. It is often employed in diarrhœa, in connection with chalk and astringents, and has recently been recommended as peculiarly efficacious in uterine hemorrhage. The dose of the powder is from ten grains to a scruple (0·65–1·3 Gm.).

CASSIA BUDS. This spice consists of the calyx of one or more species of Cinnamomum, surrounding the young germ, and, as stated by Dr. Martius, on the authority of the elder Nees, about one-quarter of the normal size. It is produced in China; and Mr. Reeves states that great quantities of it are brought to Canton from the province which affords cassia. The species which yields it is in all probability the same with that which yields the bark, though it has been ascribed by Nees to *Cinnamomum Loureirii*. In favor of the former opinion is the statement of Dr. Christison, that *C. aromaticum*, cultivated in the hot-houses of Europe, bears a flower-bud which closely resembles the cassia bud when at the same period of advancement. Cassia buds have some resemblance to cloves, and are compared to small nails with round heads. The enclosed germen is sometimes removed, and they are then cup-shaped at top. They have a brown color, with the flavor of cinnamon, and yield an essential oil upon distillation. They may be used for the same purposes as the bark.

Off. Prep. Tinctura Cinnamomi; Infusum Digitalis; Pulvis Aromaticus; Syrupus Rhei; Tinctura Cardamomi Composita; Tinctura Catechu Composita; Tinctura Lavandulæ Composita; Tinctura Rhei Aromatica; Vinum Opii.

Off. Prep. Br. Aqua Cinnamomi; Decoctum Hæmatoxyli; Infusum Catechu; Oleum Cinnamomi; Pulvis Catechu Compositus; Pulvis Cinnamomi Compositus; Pulvis Cretæ Aromaticus; Pulvis Kino Compositus; Tinctura Cardamomi Composita; Tinctura Catechu; Tinctura Cinnamomi; Tinctura Lavandulæ Composita; Vinum Opii.

COCAINÆ HYDROCHLORAS. *Br.* *Hydrochlorate of Cocaine.*

(CŌ-CA-Ī'NÆ HȲ-DRO-CHLŌ'RĂS.)

$C_{17}H_{21}NO_4, HCl.$

"The hydrochlorate of an alkaloid obtained from the leaves of Erythroxylon Coca, *Lamarck*." *Br.*

The British Pharmacopœia has introduced this valuable compound into the revision of 1885. "It may be obtained by agitating with ether an aqueous solution of an acidulated alcoholic extract, made alkaline with carbonate of sodium; separating and evaporating the ethereal liquid, purifying the product by repeating the treatment with acidulated water, carbonate of sodium, and ether; decolorizing; neutralizing with hydrochloric acid, and recrystallizing." *Br.* For other processes, see *Erythroxylon*. The following characters and tests are from the British Pharmacopœia.

Properties. "In almost colorless acicular crystals or crystalline powder, readily soluble in water, alcohol, and ether. Its solution in water has a bitter taste; gives a yellow precipitate with chloride of gold; and a white precipitate with carbonate of ammonium, soluble in excess of the reagent. Its solution produces on the tongue a tingling sensation followed by numbness. The aqueous solution dilates the pupil of the eye. It dissolves without color in cold concentrated acids, but chars with hot sulphuric acid. The solution yields little or no cloudiness with chloride of barium or oxalate of ammonium. Ignited in the air it burns without residue." *Br.*

The physiological and therapeutic properties of coca leaf depend, so far as we know at present, chiefly upon the alkaloid cocaine. They will be fully discussed under the head of *Erythroxylon*, to which article the reader is referred for information. The dose of the salts of cocaine may be set down at from ¼ to 1 grain.

Off. Prep. Br. Lamellæ Cocainæ.

COCCUS. *U. S., Br.* *Cochineal.*

(cŏc'cŭs.)

"The dried female of Coccus cacti. Linné. (*Class* Insecta; *Order* Hemiptera.)" *U. S.* "The dried female insect, Coccus Cacti, reared on Opuntia cochinillifera, *Mills*, and on other species of Opuntia." *Br.*

Coccionella, *P. G.;* Cochenille, *Fr., G.;* Scharlachwurm, *G.;* Cocciniglia, *It.;* Cochinilla, *Sp.*

The coccus is a genus of hemipterous insects, having the snout or rostrum in the breast, the antennæ filiform, and the posterior part of the abdomen furnished with bristles. The male has two erect wings, the female is wingless. The *C. Cacti* is characterized by its depressed, downy, transversely wrinkled body, its purplish abdomen, its short and black legs, and its subulate antennæ, which are about one-third of the length of the body. (*Rees's Cyclopædia.*) Another species, *C. Ilicis*, which inhabits a species of oak, is collected in the mountainous parts of the Morea, in Greece, and used as a dye-stuff in the East, under the name of *kermes*, *chermes*, or *alkermes*. The dried insects are nearly globular, smooth, about the size of a pea, and of a reddish brown color. They yield a carmine-colored powder, and with a salt of tin, a fine scarlet-red dye. They probably contain carminic acid, though we have met with no analysis of them. The Coccus Cacti is found wild in Mexico and Central America, inhabiting different species of Cactus and allied genera of plants, and is said to have been discovered also in some of the West India islands, and the southern parts of the United States. In Mexico, particularly in the provinces of Oaxaca and Guerrero, it is an important object of culture. The Indians form plantations of the *nopal* (*Opuntia cochinillifera*), upon which the insect feeds and propagates. During the rainy season, a number of the females are preserved under cover, upon the branches of the plant, and, after the cessation of the rains, are distributed upon the plants without. They perish quickly, after having deposited their eggs. These, hatched by the heat of the sun, give origin to innumerable minute insects, which spread themselves over the plant. The males, of which, according to Mr. Ellis, the proportion is not greater than one to one hundred or two hundred females, being provided with wings and very active, approach and fecundate the latter. After this period, the females, which before moved about, attach themselves to the leaves, and increase rapidly in size; so that, in the end, their legs, antennæ, and probosces are scarcely discoverable; and they appear more like excrescences on the plant than distinct animated beings. They are now gathered for use, by detaching them by means of a blunt knife, a quill, or a feather; a few being left to continue the race. They are destroyed either by dipping them enclosed in a bag into boiling water, or by the heat of a stove. In the former case they are subsequently dried in the sun. The males, which are much smaller than the full-grown females, are not collected. It is said that of the wild insect there are six generations every year, furnishing an equal number of crops; but the domestic is collected only three times annually, the propagation being suspended during the rainy season, in consequence of the inability of the insect to support the inclemency of the weather. The insect has been taken from Mexico to the Canary Islands; and very large quantities of cochineal have been delivered to commerce from the island of Teneriffe.* Its culture is said to have proved successful in Java and Algeria, but unprofitable in Spain.†

Cochineal is defined in the U. S. Pharmacopœia as follows: "About one-fifth of an inch (5 mm.) long; of a purplish-gray or purplish-black color; nearly hemispherical; somewhat oblong and angular in outline; flat or concave beneath; convex above; transversely wrinkled; easily pulverizable, yielding a dark-red powder. Odor faint; taste slightly bitterish. It contains a red coloring matter soluble in

* Various species of Opuntia are adapted to the support of the cochineal insect, especially those which are very juicy, with few thorns and a thick skin. It is the *O. Ficus Indica* which is chiefly cultivated in Teneriffe, the dry but hot climate of which is peculiarly adapted to the growth both of the plant and the insect. For an account of the mode of rearing the cochineal insect in the Canary Islands, see *P. J. Tr.*, Sept. 1871; in Central America, see *A. J. P.*, 1873, p. 39; *N. R.*, 1880, p. 175.

† In Asia Minor, in the vicinity of Oushak, are great quantities of an insect, closely resembling the Coccus Cacti, which feed on a species of Cistus; but it is unknown whether any portion has been introduced into general commerce. (*A. J. P.*, xxxv. 455.)

water, alcohol, or water of ammonia, slightly soluble in ether, insoluble in fixed and volatile oils. On macerating Cochineal in water, the insect swells up, but no insoluble powder should be separated." *U. S.*

As kept in the shops, the finer cochineal, *grana fina* of Spanish commerce, is in irregularly circular or oval, somewhat angular grains, about one-eighth of an inch in diameter, convex on one side, concave or flat on the other, and marked with several transverse wrinkles. Two varieties of this kind of cochineal are known to the druggist, distinguished by their external appearance. One is of a reddish gray color, formed by an intermixture of the dark color of the insect with the whiteness of a powder by which it is almost covered, and with patches of a rosy tinge irregularly interspersed. From its diversified appearance, it is called by the Spaniards *cochinilla jaspeada*. It is the variety commonly kept in our shops. The other, *cochinilla renegrida*, or *grana nigra*, is dark-colored, almost black, with only a minute quantity of the whitish powder between the wrinkles. The two are distinguished in our markets by the names of *silver grains* and *black grains*. Some suppose the difference to arise from the mode of preparation; the gray cochineal consisting of the insects destroyed by a dry heat; the black, of those destroyed by hot water, which removes the external whitish powder. According to Mr. Faber, who derived his information from a merchant residing in the neighborhood where the cochineal is collected, the silver grains consist of the impregnated female just before she has laid her eggs; the black, of the female after the eggs have been laid and hatched. (*A. J. P.*, xviii. 47.) There is little or no difference in their quality.* Another and much inferior variety is the *grana sylvestra*, or wild cochineal, consisting partly of very small separate insects, partly of roundish or oval masses, which exhibit, under the microscope, minute and apparently new-born insects, enclosed in a white or reddish cotton-like substance. It is scarcely known in our drug market.

Cochineal has a faint heavy odor, and a bitter slightly acidulous taste. Its powder is of a purplish carmine color, tinging the saliva intensely red. According to Pelletier and Caventou, it consists of a peculiar coloring principle, a peculiar animal matter constituting the skeleton of the insect, stearin, olein, an odorous fatty acid, and various salts. Tyrosin, a crystallizable animal principle, has been found by De la Rue. (*Gmelin*, xiii. 358.) It was also analyzed by John, who called the coloring principle *cochinilin*. It is, however, universally known now as *carminic acid*, and has the composition $C_{17}H_{18}O_{10}$. Hlasiwetz and Grabowski (*Ann. Chem. und. Ph.*, 141, p. 329) have shown that it is a glucoside, and is decomposed by boiling with diluted sulphuric acid into a non-fermentable sugar and *carmine red*, $C_{11}H_{12}O_7$. Carminic acid is of a brilliant purple-red color, unalterable in dry air, is decomposed at temperatures over 136° C. (276·8° F.), is very soluble in water, soluble in cold, and more so in boiling alcohol, insoluble in ether, and without nitrogen. It is obtained by macerating cochineal in ether, and treating the residue with successive portions of boiling alcohol, which on cooling deposits a part of the carminic acid, and yields the remainder by spontaneous evaporation. It may be freed from a small proportion of adhering fatty matter by dissolving it in alcohol of 40° Baumé, and then adding an equal quantity of ether. The pure carminic acid is deposited in the course of a few days. Prof. Liebermann found that the coating of the silver cochineal consisted of a peculiar wax, which he named *coccerin*, $C_{30}H_{60}(C_{31}H_{61}O_3)_2$; this is soluble in benzol, but nearly insoluble in ether. (*P. J. Tr.*, 1885, p. 186; from *Berichte.*) The watery infusion of cochineal is of a violet-crimson color, which is brightened by the acids and deepened by the alkalies. The coloring matter is readily precipitated. The salts of zinc, bismuth, and nickel produce a lilac precipitate, and those of iron a dark purple approaching to black. The salts of tin, especially the nitrate and chloride, precipitate the coloring matter of a brilliant scarlet, and form the basis of those splendid scarlet and crimson dyes, which have rendered cochineal so valuable in the arts. With alumina the coloring matter forms the pigment called

* *Cake cochineal* is the name given to a variety of the drug, produced in the Argentine Republic. A specimen, examined by Dr. Stark, was in flat cakes about a quarter of an inch thick, and, under the microscope, was seen to consist chiefly of the cochineal insect, mixed with small portions of the thorns and epidermis of the cactus, in consequence of careless gathering. It is inferior for dyeing purposes to the ordinary variety. (*P. J. Tr.*, xiv. 346.)

lake. The finest *lakes* are obtained by mixing the decoction of cochineal with freshly prepared gelatinous alumina. The pigment called *carmine* is the coloring matter of cochineal precipitated from the decoction by acids, the salts of tin, etc., or by animal gelatin, and when properly made is of the most intense and brilliant scarlet. J. J. Hess proved that if fatty matters found in cochineal were removed by treatment with alcohol, a much more brilliant carmine could be produced. He found in Guatemala cochineal 17 per cent. of a crystalline stearopten, in Java cochineal 7 per cent., and in Canary cochineal 18 per cent. (Dingler, *P. J. Tr.*, 235, 88; *N. R.*, 1880, p. 338.) The degree of coloring power in cochineal may be approximately measured by the decolorizing effect produced by solution of permanganate of potassium. For a method of applying this process, the reader is referred to a paper by J. M. Merrick, of Boston, in *A. J. P.*, 1871, p. 263; from *Amer. Chem.* (April, 1871).

Cochineal has been adulterated by causing certain heavy substances, such as powdered talc, carbonate of lead, and sulphate of barium, by shaking in a bag or otherwise, to adhere, by means of some glutinous material, to the surface of the insects, and thus increase their weight. Cochineal yields 1·5 per cent. of ashes. Five specimens of the drug have been examined, which left in their ashes respectively 8, 12, 16, 18, and 25 per cent. of the salt of baryta. (*A. J. P.*, 1870, p. 220.) The fraud may be detected by the absence, under the microscope, of a woolly appearance, which characterizes the white powder upon the surface of the unadulterated insect. Metallic lead, which is said frequently to exist in fine particles in the artificial coating, may be discovered by powdering the cochineal, and suspending it in water, when the metal will remain behind. Grains of a substance artificially prepared to imitate the dried insect have been mixed with the genuine in France. A close inspection will serve to detect the difference. (*Journ. de Pharm.*, 3e sér., ix. 110.) Vermilion and chrome-red (dichromate of lead) are said also to have been largely used in the adulteration of carmine, to the extent sometimes of 60 or even 70 per cent. (*P. J. Tr.*, 1860, p. 547.) There can be no difficulty in detecting them by the appropriate tests. Starch has been used, according to Prof. Maisch, for the same purpose in the United States, and in one specimen he found 57·14 per cent. (*A. J. P.*, xxxiii. 18.)

The importations of cochineal are diminishing, owing to the gradual replacement of this dye by the newer azo colors. The annual importations for 1884, '85, '86, and '87 were 681,996 lbs., 783,382 lbs., 665,779 lbs., and 492,304 lbs., respectively, against more than twice as much ten years ago.

Medical Properties, etc. Cochineal is supposed by some to possess anodyne properties, and has been highly recommended in hooping-cough and neuralgic affections, but is probably useless. In pharmacy it is employed to color tinctures and ointments. To infants with hooping-cough, cochineal in substance is given in the dose of about one-third of a grain (0·02 Gm.) three times a day. The dose of a tincture, prepared by macerating one part of the medicine in eight parts of diluted alcohol, is for an adult from twenty to thirty drops (1·25–1·9 C.c.), twice a day. In neuralgic paroxysms, Sauter gave half a tablespoonful (7·5 C.c.), with the asserted effect of curing the disease.

Off. Prep. Tinctura Cardamomi Composita.

Off. Prep. Br. Tinctura Cardamomi Composita; Tinctura Cinchonæ Composita; Tinctura Cocci.

CODEINA. *U. S., Br.* *Codeine.* [*Codeia.*]

$C_{18}H_{21}NO_3.H_2O$; 317. (CŌ-DE-Ī'NA.) $C_{36}H_{21}NO_6.2HO$; 317.

"An alkaloid prepared from Opium." *U. S.* "An alkaloid contained in opium." *Br.*

Codeinum, *P.G.;* Codeine, *Fr.;* Codeïn, *G.*

Codeine was discovered in 1832 by Robiquet in the hydrochlorate of morphine prepared according to the process of Gregory. It exists in opium combined like morphine with meconic acid, and is extracted along with that alkaloid in the preparation of the hydrochlorate. (See *Morphina.*) When the solution of the mixed hydrochlorates of morphine and codeine is treated with ammonia, the former alkaloid is precipitated, and the codeine, remaining in solution, may be obtained by evaporation and crystallization. It may be purified by treating the crystals with hot ether, which dissolves them, and yields the codeine in colorless crystals on spontaneous evaporation. Codeine is the methyl derivative of morphine, as shown in the formula $C_{17}H_{18}(CH_3)NO_3$. It may be formed artificially from morphine by treating this latter successively with methyl iodide and fixed alkali. (Grimaux, 1881, *Jour. Chem. Soc.*, 44, 358.) Codeine occurs in "white, or yellowish-white, more or less translucent, rhombic prisms, somewhat efflorescent in warm air, odorless, having a slightly bitter taste and an alkaline reaction. Soluble in 80 parts of water at 15° C. (59° F.) and in 17 parts of boiling water; very soluble in alcohol and in chloroform; also soluble in 6 parts of ether and in 10 parts of benzol, but almost insoluble in benzin. When heated to 120° C. (248° F.), Codeine loses its water of crystallization. At about 150° C. (302° F.) it melts, and, on ignition, it is completely dissipated. Codeine is dissolved by sulphuric acid containing 1 per cent. of molybdate of sodium, to a liquid having, at first, a dirty green color, which, after a while, becomes pure blue and gradually fades, within a few hours, to pale yellow. On dissolving Codeine in sulphuric acid, a colorless liquid results, which, on the addition of a trace of ferric chloride, and gentle warming, becomes deep blue. An aqueous solution of Codeine, added to test-solution of mercuric chloride, should produce no precipitate; and if Codeine be added to nitric acid of sp. gr. 1·200, it will dissolve to a yellow liquid which should not become red (difference from and abs. of morphine)." *U. S.* When added in excess to boiling water, the undissolved portion melts and sinks to the bottom, having the appearance of an oil. It may be separated from morphine by a solution of potassa or soda, which dissolves the morphine, and leaves the codeine. It has an alkaline reaction on test-paper, and combines with acids to form salts, some of which are crystallizable, particularly the nitrate. Its capacity of saturation is almost identical with that of morphine. According to Robiquet, 1 part of hydrochloric acid is saturated by 7·837 of codeine, and by 7·88 of morphine. It is distinguishable, however from the latter principle by the different form of its crystals, which are octohedral, by its solubility in boiling ether, greater solubility in water, and insolubility in alkaline solutions, and by not assuming a red color with nitric acid, or a blue one with ferric salts. Tincture of galls precipitates from its solutions a tannate of codeine. Crystallized from a watery solution, it contains about 6 per cent. of water, which is driven off at 100° C. (212° F.). The crystals obtained from a solution in ether contain no water.

Medical Properties. It is probable that pure codeine is a very feeble alkaloid, tolerated by the human system in very large doses. On the other hand, cases of severe poisoning have been published, and experimenters have claimed for it a very powerful influence upon the lower animals. As late as 1874, Dr. Myrtle reported the instance of a man who was almost killed by four grains of codeine, prepared by Messrs. Smith, of Edinburgh. (*Br. Med. Journ.*, 1874, i. 478.) The symptoms were first vascular excitement and exhilaration, then depression, with great anxiety, nausea and vomiting, cold pale, moist skin, slight contraction of the pupil, and delirious sleeplessness. On the other hand, Dr. S. Weir Mitchell took five grains of codeine without effect, save some nausea, slight giddiness, and cerebral heaviness, and a trifling acceleration of the pulse; whilst we have given codeine prepared by Powers & Weightman, of Philadelphia, in doses of eight grains a day without distinct effect. It is very evident that commercial codeine has been and probably still is of varying composition, and the results frequently obtained have been produced by coherent alkaloids. Mr. Wm. Weightman informs us that nearly the whole product of their laboratory goes to France, where it appears to be largely used as a calmative drug, free from many of the objections to opium, but in no way comparing with it in power. Within the last year or two it has been highly lauded in the treatment of diabetes mellitus, and cases of recovery under its use reported. In the grave form of this disorder we have seen it fail to exert any perceptible influence, but the evidence is sufficient to demand a fair trial of the remedy in any individual case. On account of its frequent contamination, care should be exercised as to the commencing dose, but no effect at all is to be expected from less than one grain (0·06 Gm.), and this dose may be rapidly increased until some symptoms are produced. It may be given in pill or in syrupy solution.

COLCHICI RADIX. *U. S.* *Colchicum Root.*

(CŎL'CHI-CĪ RĀ'DĬX—kŏl'kĭ-sī.)

"The Corm of Colchicum autumnale. Linné. (*Nat. Ord.* Melanthaceæ.)" *U. S.* "The fresh corm of Colchicum autumnale, collected about the end of June or beginning of July; and the same stripped of its coats, sliced transversely, and dried at a temperature not exceeding 150° F. (65°·5 C.)." *Br.*

Colchici Cormus, *Br.;* Colchicum Corm; Bulbus s. Tuber Colchici; Meadow-Saffron Root, Bulbe de Colchique, de Safran bâtard, *Fr.;* Zeitlosenknollen, *G.*

COLCHICI SEMEN. *U. S.* *Colchicum Seed.*

(CŎL'CHI-CĪ SĒ'MĔN—kŏl'kĭ-sī.)

"The seed of Colchicum autumnale. Linné. (*Nat. Ord.* Melanthaceæ.)" *U. S.* "The seeds of Colchicum autumnale, *Linn.*, collected when fully ripe, which is commonly about the end of July or beginning of August; and carefully dried." *Br.*

Colchici Semina, *Br.;* Colchicum Seeds; Semen Colchici, *P.G.;* Semences de Colchique, Colchique, *Fr.;* Zeitlose, Herbst-Zeitlose, Zeitlosensamen, *G.;* Colchico, *It.*, *Sp.*

Gen. Ch. A *spathe.* *Corolla* six-parted, with a tube proceeding directly from the root. *Capsules* three, connected, inflated. *Willd.*

Colchicum autumnale. Willd. *Sp. Plant.* ii. 272; Woodv. *Med. Bot.* p. 759, t. 258. This species of Colchicum, often called *meadow-saffron*, is a perennial bulbous plant, the leaves of which appear in spring, and the flowers in autumn. Its manner of growth is peculiar, and deserves notice as connected in some measure with its medicinal efficacy. In the latter part of summer, a new bulb, or *cormus* as the part is now called, begins to form at the lateral inferior portion of the old one, which receives the young offshoot in its bosom, and embraces it half round. The new plant sends out fibres from its base, and is furnished with a radical spathe, which is cylindrical, tubular, cloven at top on one side, and half under ground. In September, from two to six flowers, of a lilac or pale-purple color, emerge from the spathe, unaccompanied with leaves. The corolla consists of a tube five inches long, concealed for two-thirds of its length in the ground, and of a limb divided into six segments. The flowers perish by the end of October, and the rudiments of the fruit remain under ground till the following spring, when they rise upon a stem above the surface, in the form of a three-lobed, three-celled capsule. The leaves of the new plant appear at the same time; so that in fact they follow the flower instead of preceding it, as might be inferred from the order of the seasons in which they respectively show themselves. The leaves are radical, spear-shaped, erect, numerous, about five inches long, and one inch broad at the base. In the mean time, the new bulb has been increasing at the expense of the old one, which, having performed its appointed office, perishes; while the former, after attaining its full growth, sends forth shoots, and in its turn decays. The old bulb, in its second spring, and a little before it perishes, sometimes puts forth one or more small bulbs, which are the sources of new plants.

C. autumnale is a native of the temperate parts of Europe and of Northern Africa, growing in moist pastures and meadows. Attempts have been made to introduce its culture into this country, but with no great success; though small quantities of the bulb, of apparently good quality, have been brought into the market. The flowers possess virtues similar to the bulb and seeds.

COLCHICI RADIX. The medicinal virtue of the bulb depends much upon the season at which it is collected. Early in the spring, it is too young to have fully developed its peculiar properties; and, late in the fall, it has become exhausted by the nourishment afforded to the new plant. The proper period for its collection is from the early part of June, when it has usually attained perfection, to the middle of August, when the offset appears.* It may be owing, in part, to this inequality at different seasons, that entirely opposite reports have been given of its powers. Krapf ate whole bulbs without inconvenience; Haller found the bulbs entirely void of taste

* Dr. Christison, however, has found the roots collected in April to be more bitter than those gathered in July, and conjectures that the common opinion of their superior efficacy at the latter season may not be well founded. Prof. Schroff states, as the result of his observation, that the autumn root is much stronger than that dug in summer. (See *A. J. P.*, xxix. 324.)

and acrimony; and we are told that in Carniola the peasants use it as food with impunity in the autumn. On the other hand, there can be no doubt of its highly irritating and poisonous nature, when fully developed, under ordinary circumstances. Perhaps soil and climate may have some influence in modifying its character.

The bulb is often used in the fresh state in the countries where it grows; as it is apt to be injured in drying, unless the process is carefully conducted. The usual plan is to cut the bulb, as soon after it has been dug up as possible, into thin transverse slices, which are spread out separately upon paper or perforated trays, and dried with a moderate heat. The reason for drying it quickly, after removal from the ground, is that it otherwise begins to vegetate, and a change in its chemical nature takes place; and such is its retentiveness of life, that, if not cut in slices, it is liable to undergo a partial vegetation even during the drying process. Dr. Houlton recommends that the bulb be stripped of its dry coating, carefully deprived of the bud or young bulb, and then dried whole. It is owing to the high vitality of the bud that the bulb is so apt to vegetate. During desiccation there is great loss of weight, 70 per cent. being the average for a number of years in the laboratory of Messrs. Allen & Hanburys, in London.

Properties. The recent bulb or cormus of *C. autumnale* resembles that of the tulip in shape and size, and is covered with a brown membranous coat. Internally it is solid, white and fleshy, and, when cut transversely, yields, if mature, an acrid milky juice. There is often a small lateral projection from its base, which is the bud for the development of a new plant: this bud is frequently broken off in drying. When dried, and deprived of its external membranous covering, the corm is of an ash-brown color, convex on one side, and somewhat flattened on the other, where it is marked by a deep groove, extending from the base to the summit. As found in our shops it is always in the dried state, sometimes in segments made by vertical sections of the bulb, but generally in transverse circular slices, about the eighth or tenth of an inch in thickness, with a notch at one part of their circumference. "About one inch (25 mm.) long, ovoid, flattish and with a groove on one side; externally brownish and wrinkled; internally white and solid; often in transverse slices, reniform in shape, and breaking with a short, mealy fracture; inodorous; taste sweetish, bitter and acrid. Colchicum root which is very dark colored internally, or breaks with a horny fracture, should be rejected." *U. S.* The cut surface is white, and of an amylaceous aspect. Examined with the microscope, the corm is seen to be composed of large irregular cells, full of ovoid, angular, sometimes compound, starch grains, and interspersed with spiral vessels in vascular bundles. The odor of the recent bulb is said to be hircine. It is diminished but not lost by drying. The taste is bitter, hot, and acrid. The active principle is an alkaloid, *Colchicine*, the chemical history of which we give in full in a foot-note below.* Wine and vinegar extract

* The alkaloid of colchicum has been a subject of some controversy. According to Geiger and Hesse, to whom has been ascribed the credit of determining its precise nature, *colchicine* (*colchicia*) is crystallizable, and has a very bitter and sharp taste, but is destitute of the extreme acrimony of veratrine, and does not, like that principle, excite violent sneezing when applied to the nostrils. It differs also in being more soluble in water, and less poisonous. To a kitten eight weeks old, one-tenth of a grain was given dissolved in dilute alcohol. Violent purging and vomiting were produced, with apparently severe pain and convulsions, and the animal died at the end of twelve hours. The stomach and bowels were found violently inflamed, with effusion of blood through their whole extent. A kitten somewhat younger was destroyed in ten minutes by only the twentieth of a grain of veratrine; and, on examination after death, marks of inflammation were found only in the upper part of the œsophagus. The alkaloid was obtained from the seeds by a process similar to that employed in the preparation of hyoscyamine from hyoscyamus. (See *Hyoscyamus*.) A simpler process is to digest the seeds of meadow-saffron in boiling alcohol, precipitate with magnesia, treat the precipitated matter with boiling alcohol, and finally filter and evaporate.

The nature of the active principle of colchicum subsequently engaged the attention of L. Oberlin. Upon repeating the process of Geiger and Hesse, he was unable to obtain a crystallizable product, and came to the conclusion that the substance obtained by them was complex. By acidifying its watery solution by sulphuric or hydrochloric acid, and concentrating until the liquid became intensely yellow, he obtained, upon the addition of water, a yellowish white precipitate, which, when well washed and freed from coloring matter, dissolved readily in alcohol or ether, and crystallised with facility. The crystalline product thus obtained he proposed to call *colchiceine*. It is a neutral substance, contains no acid, crystallizes in pearly lamellæ, is almost insoluble in cold water, to which, however, it imparts a slight bitterness, is more soluble in boiling water, and readily dissolves in alcohol, ether, methylic alcohol, and chloroform. It is dissolved by concentrated sul-

all the virtues of the bulb. Dr. A. T. Thomson states that the milky juice of fresh colchicum produces a fine blue color, if rubbed with the tincture of guaiac, and that the same effect is obtained from an acetic solution of the dried bulb. He considers

phuric, hydrochloric, and nitric acids, becoming yellow, by acetic acid without change of color, and by ammonia and potassa. It is not altered or precipitated by acetate or subacetate of lead, nitrate of silver, mercuric chloride, or infusion of galls, but is rendered green by sesquichloride of iron. It was found to be very poisonous to rabbits, killing an animal in 12 hours in the dose of about one-seventh of a grain, and in a few minutes in five times that quantity. (*Comptes-Rendus*, Dec. 1856, p. 1199.)

Subsequently Mr. J. E. Carter, of Philadelphia, has made some experiments which appear to invalidate the conclusions of Oberlin as to the nature of colchicine, and to confirm the previous opinion of its alkaloid character. Mr. Carter used the bulb, instead of the seeds, which had previously in general been made the subject of experiment. He employed two processes for the extraction of the alkaloid, but found the following most productive. The dried and powdered bulb was exhausted by alcohol of 0·835 by means of percolation; the tincture thus obtained was evaporated to the consistence of syrup; water acidulated with acetic acid was added, and the liquor, after filtration, was nearly neutralized with ammonia, and then precipitated by solution of tannic acid; the precipitated tannate, after being well washed, was rubbed with five times its weight of freshly prepared hydrated oxide of lead, small quantities of alcohol being added from time to time during the trituration; the whole was then filtered, and the filtered liquid evaporated at a gentle heat. Twenty grains were thus obtained from three pounds of the dried root. Thus obtained, *colchicine* was yellowish in mass, nearly white in powder, inodorous, bitter without being acrid, not sternutatory, soluble in water hot or cold, still more so in dilute acids and alkaline solutions, very soluble in alcohol and chloroform, sparingly so in pure ether, and insoluble in benzol. Mr. Carter did not succeed in crystallising it. It was alkaline to test-paper, neutralised the acids, and with sulphuric acid formed a crystallizable salt. The most delicate test appeared to be that of sulphuric acid and nitre. A piece of nitre, added to its solution in sulphuric acid, produced a beautiful blue color, changing to green, dark brown or purple, and finally reddish yellow. (For a further account of Mr. Carter's experiments, see *A. J. P.*, 1858, p. 209.)

Since Mr. Carter's experiments, others have engaged in the same inquiry. Ludwig confirms the statements of Oberlin. Hubler, operating on the unbruised seeds by a process similar to that of Mr. Carter with the cormus, for the details of which we refer to *A. J. P.* (1866, p. 105), obtained an amorphous substance, soluble without residue in water and in alcohol, of an odor like that of hay, and very bitter. It had no effect on test-paper; its solution was precipitated yellow by chloride of gold, and white by corrosive sublimate; mineral acids and alkalies turned it yellow; at 140° C. (284° F.) it melted, with no other observable change except in color, which became brown; and its composition was represented by the formula $C_{17}H_{19}NO_5$. When treated with acids it yielded crystallizable bodies, but these, instead of salts, were a new product, isomeric with colchicine, but in character resembling if not identical with the colchiceine of Oberlin, which is therefore a result of change in the colchicine. Both these substances are poisonous.

Mr. Carter's statement has been fully confirmed by Prof. J. M. Maisch, who made a very careful examination of a portion of the colchicine obtained by Mr. Carter, and kept as a specimen, with the following results. It was an amorphous powder; of a light yellow color, a faint odor, and intense bitterness; sparingly soluble in ether, and readily in water and alcohol. The aqueous solution was slightly turbid, probably from the decomposition by time and exposure of a portion of the colchicine into resin and colchiceine. Heated on platinum foil, it melted, and at a higher temperature took fire, and burned without residue. It restored the blue color of reddened litmus, and even neutralized sulphuric acid in very minute proportion. It answered to the best tests of colchicine, namely, 1, the effect on its solution of both acids and alkalies, which cause it to assume a yellow color, and, 2, the violet and blue color produced by oxidising agents on the dry colchicine. When treated first with concentrated sulphuric acid, and then with nitric acid or a fragment of a nitrate, it went through a series of changes of color, ending in yellow. The same effect resulted from sulphuric acid with a trace of chromate or bichromate of potassium, sesquichloride of iron, or binoxide of lead; the first two causing a green color with the solution, through the intermixture of their yellowishness with the blue developed. The colchicine also answered to the following tests of the alkaloids, giving precipitates with iodohydrargyrate of potassium, phosphomolybdic acid, and tannic acid.

Hertel (1881) considers that ordinary colchicine contains several resinous impurities and colchiceines. His description of the several compounds is as follows: *Colchicine*, $C_{17}H_{23}NO_6$, is colorless or yellow, soluble in water, alcohol, and chloroform, of a saffron-like odor and bitter taste, precipitated by tannin, slowly decomposes with formation of ammonia; *Colchiceine*, $C_{17}H_{21}NO_5 + 2H_2O$, is in inodorous white crystals, soluble in alcohol, chloroform, and hot water, with slight acid reaction; on redissolving in water the colchicine extracted with chloroform, a brown resin remains. This *Colchicoresin*, $C_{51}H_{60}N_2O_{16}$, is amorphous, soluble in chloroform and alcohol, insoluble in ether. Acted upon with mineral acids, it decomposes into two resins, one soluble in 30 to 40 per cent. alcohol, and the other, *Betacolchicoresin*, $C_{34}H_{38}NO_{10}$, insoluble.

Houdés and Zeisel have obtained colchicine in a crystalline condition. (*Jour. Chem. Soc.*, 1884, p. 1055; *A. J. P.*, 1883, p. 268.) C. J. Bender, on the other hand, doubts the genuineness of Houdés's crystals, and states that the colchicine as obtained by Hertel, Dragendorff, and himself is amorphous. (*Amer. Drug.*, 1885, p. 162.)

The inference from these experiments is that the active principle of colchicum, known by the name of colchicine, is an alkaloid, but that its salts in solution, on being kept, or evaporated, especially if heat is used, are decomposed, and converted into resin and colchiceine, the latter of which crystallizes; and, as this is isomeric with colchicine, the probability is that the resin has the same composition. In preparing colchicum pharmaceutically, if it be desired to retain the colchicine

the appearance of this color, when the slices are rubbed with a little distilled vinegar and tincture of guaiac, as a proof that the drug is good and has been well dried. Dr. J. M. Maclagan has shown that this change of color is produced with the albumen, which is not affected if previously coagulated; so that the value of the test consists simply in proving that the drying has not been effected at a heat above 180°, or the temperature at which albumen coagulates. A very deep or large notch in the circumference of the slices is considered an unfavorable sign; as it indicates that the bulb has been somewhat exhausted in the nourishment of the offset. The decoction yields a deep blue precipitate with solution of iodine, white precipitates with acetate and subacetate of lead, mercurous nitrate, and nitrate of silver, and a slight precipitate with tincture of galls. The value of colchicum is best tested by its bitterness.

Medical Properties and Uses. When taken internally in therapeutic dose, colchicum usually produces no other symptoms than intestinal pains and looseness of the bowels. In some rare cases it is said to give rise to copious diuresis or diaphoresis instead of purging. When larger amounts are exhibited, the purging is more pronounced, and there may be also vomiting. With these symptoms there may be some depression, which seems to be due to the gastro-intestinal irritation rather than to the direct action of the poison. In an overdose, it may produce dangerous and even fatal effects. Excessive nausea and vomiting, abdominal pains, purging and tenesmus, great thirst, sinking of the pulse, coldness of the extremities, and general prostration, with occasional symptoms of nervous derangement, such as headache, delirium, and stupor, are among the results of its poisonous action. A peculiarity of its influence is that when its dose is increased beyond a certain point there is not a corresponding increase in the rapidity of the fatal issue. This is probably because it kills not by a direct influence upon the heart or nervous system, but by causing gastro-enteritis. On post-mortem examination the alimentary mucous membrane is found much inflamed.

Colchicum was well known to the ancients as a poison, and is said to have been employed by them as a remedy in gout and other diseases. Störck revived its use among the moderns. He gave it as a diuretic and expectorant in dropsy and humoral asthma; and on the continent of Europe it acquired considerable reputation in these complaints; but the uncertainty of its operation led to its general abandonment, and it had fallen into almost entire neglect, when Dr. Want, of London, again brought it into notice by attempting to prove its identity with the active ingredient of the *eau médicinale d'Husson*, so highly celebrated as a cure for gout. In James's Dispensatory, printed in 1747, it is said to be used in gout as an external application. The chief employment of the meadow-saffron is at present in the treatment of gout and rheumatism, in which experience has abundantly proved it to be a highly valuable remedy. We have, within our own observation, found it especially useful in these affections, when of a shifting or neuralgic character. It sometimes produces relief without obviously affecting the system; but it is more efficient when it evinces its influence upon the skin or alimentary canal. Professor Chelius states that it changes the chemical constitution of the urine in arthritic patients, producing an evident increase of the uric acid. Dr. Maclagan has found it greatly to increase the proportion both of urea and uric acid in the urine, and, where these previously existed in the blood, to separate them from it. (*Ed. Monthly Journ. of Med. Sci.*, N. S., v. 23.) But Graves and Gardner affirm that the urates diminish under its influence, and in a very careful and extended research Dr. A. B. Garrod found that its action upon the uric acid elimination is very irregular and uncertain. Dr. Elliotson successfully treated a case of prurigo with the wine of colchicum, given

unchanged, both acids and alkalies should be avoided, especially when heat is employed. Of the officinal preparations, the two fluid extracts contain the colchicine as in nature; the acetic extract has a portion at least of colchiceine in its composition. In the wines, when kept, the colchicine probably passes gradually into colchiceine. (*A. J. P.*, 1867, p. 97.) But it has not been proved that these latter preparations are in any degree less efficacious remedially; and in the absence of all experience to the contrary, the inference is that colchiceine may have all the powers of colchicine; for the acetic extract, and the wines after being long kept, have often been used in practice, without having been found less effectual than other preparations of colchicum.

in the dose of half a drachm (1·9 C.c.) three times a day, and continued for three weeks; and it has been found useful in urticaria and other cutaneous affections, probably of a gouty nature. At various times colchicum has been used in various diseases, but in modern practice is employed almost solely in gout. Even in rheumatism it is at present rarely administered. It is generally given in the state of vinous tincture (see *Vinum Colchici Radicis*); but there are various other officinal preparations, any one of which may be used efficiently. The dose of the dried bulb is from two to eight grains (0·13–0·52 Gm.), which may be repeated every four or six hours till its effects are obtained.

COLCHICI SEMEN.—The seeds of the meadow-saffron ripen in summer, and should be collected about the end of July or beginning of August. They never arrive at maturity in plants cultivated in a dry soil, or in confined gardens. (*Williams.*) They are nearly spherical, about the eighth of an inch in diameter, of a reddish brown color externally, white within, and of a bitter acrid taste. "Sub-globular, about one-twelfth of an inch (2 mm.) thick, very slightly pointed at the hilum; reddish-brown, pitted, internally whitish; very hard and tough; inodorous; bitter and somewhat acrid." *U. S.* They are chiefly composed of a gray horny albumen, constituted of very thick-walled cells, and surrounded by a closely adherent testa. The leafless embryo is very small, and is situated close to the surface opposite the strophiole. Dr. Williams, of Ipswich, England, first brought them into notice in 1820 as superior to the bulb. Prof. Schroff, however, has found that their activity is inferior to that of the dried bulb, dug in autumn (*A. J. P.*, xxix. 324); and recent studies indicate that they contain only a very small percentage of alkaloid. A wine, fluid extract, and tincture of the seeds are directed in the U. S. Pharmacopœia. Their dose is about the same as that of the bulb.

Off. Prep. of the Root. Extractum Colchici Aceticum; Extractum Colchici Radicis Fluidum; Vinum Colchici Radicis.

Off. Prep. of the Corm. Br. Extractum Colchici; Extractum Colchici Aceticum; Vinum Colchici.

Off. Prep. of the Seed. Extractum Colchici Seminis Fluidum; Tinctura Colchici Seminis; Vinum Colchici Seminis.

Off. Prep. of the Seeds. Br. Tinctura Colchici Seminum.

COLLODIUM. *U. S., Br.* *Collodion.*

(CQL-LŌ'DĮ-ŬM.)

Collodion, *Fr.*; Collodium, *G.*

"Pyroxylin, *four parts* [or half an ounce av.]; Stronger Ether, *seventy parts* [or 11 fluidounces 5 fluidrachms]; Alcohol, *twenty-six parts* [or 3 fluidounces 7 fluidrachms], To make *one hundred parts* [or about one pint]. To the Pyroxylin, contained in a tared bottle, add the Alcohol and let it stand for fifteen minutes; then add the Ether, and shake the mixture until the Pyroxylin is dissolved. Cork the bottle well, and set it aside until the liquid has become clear. Then decant it from any sediment which may have formed, and transfer it to bottles, which should be securely corked. Keep the Collodion in a cool place, remote from lights or fire." *U. S.*

"Take of Pyroxylin *one ounce* [avoirdupois]; Ether *thirty-six fluidounces* [Imperial measure]; Rectified Spirit *twelve fluidounces* [Imp. meas.]. Mix the Ether and the Spirit, and add the Pyroxylin. Set aside for a few days, and, should there be any sediment, decant the clear solution. Keep it in a well-corked bottle." *Br.*

Collodion is a solution of gun cotton. On account of the facility with which ether evaporates, it is the better menstruum for remedial purposes; but gun cotton will not dissolve in that liquid when quite pure, and the addition of a little alcohol is necessary. Formerly the U. S. Pharmacopœia directed that the gun cotton be prepared at the time of making the collodion, giving directions for the purpose, but at the revision of 1870 the process of the British Pharmacopœia was substantially adopted, a formula for the preparation of pyroxylin being given separately in the Pharmacopœia. The present formula differs very slightly from that of 1870, containing a little more pyroxylin and alcohol. (See *Pyroxylin.*) A change has been made, however, in directing the collodion to be decanted from the sediment. In the

Pharm. 1870 the sediment was directed to be re-incorporated with the clear collodion, and the result was the making of a tougher film. This sediment consists of undecomposed filaments of cotton, and these become partially felted, as the ethereal liquid evaporates, and the film is forming; this direction of the former Pharmacopœia was usually disregarded, although for many purposes the cloudy film is to be preferred.

Collodion is a transparent, colorless liquid, of a syrupy consistence, and ethereal smell. When applied to a dry surface, the ether quickly evaporates, and a transparent film is left, having remarkable adhesiveness and contractility. On account of the great volatility of ether, collodion must be kept in bottles well stopped. When insecurely kept, the liquid thickens and becomes less fit for the use of the surgeon. The thickened liquid sometimes contains acicular crystals, as was first observed by Mr. Higginson, of London, and afterwards by Prof. Leidy, of this city. The addition of a small quantity of ether will generally restore the collodion to its original condition.

Collodion was first applied to the purposes of surgery by Dr. J. Parker Maynard,* of Boston, when a student of medicine, in January, 1847. It is employed for holding together the edges of incised wounds, for covering ulcers or abraded or diseased surfaces, chilblains, chapped nipples, etc., with an impervious film not acted upon by water, and for encasing parts which require to be kept without relative motion. It is applied, brushed over the part, or by means of strips of muslin. In whatever way applied, the solvent quickly evaporates, and leaves the solid adhesive material. The rigid film thus formed contracts with a good deal of force. This property adapts collodion for certain purposes, such as drawing together the edges of wounds, exciting pressure on buboes, etc. When, however, the surgeon desires simply to protect a surface, a flexible, non-contracting film is preferable, and the officinal *Collodion flexile* should be used.

Collodion has been variously medicated, and thus made the vehicle of several important medicines for external application. *Iodized collodion* has been proposed by Dr. C. Fleming, for the purpose of obtaining the specific effects of iodine in a rapid manner, especially on tumors. It is made by dissolving from ten to twenty grains of iodine in a fluidounce of collodion. M. Aran has proposed a *ferruginous collodion*, made of equal parts of collodion and tincture of chloride of iron, as a remedy in erysipelas.† A *caustic collodion* may be prepared by dissolving 4 parts of corrosive sublimate in 30 of collodion. Dr. Macke, of Sorau, has used this preparation for destroying nævi materni. The eschar formed is one or two lines in thickness, and separates in from three to six days, leaving but a trifling cicatrix. (See *A. J. P.*, May, 1858, for formulas in which collodion is made the vehicle of iodine, belladonna, sulphur, etc.) All these medicated collodions are most conveniently applied by means of a camel's-hair brush. Collodion is also much used in photography.‡

Off. Prep. Collodium Flexile; Collodium Stypticum.

Off. Prep. Br. Collodium Flexile.

* Dr. Maynard recommended the following formula. Take of sulphuric acid of sp. gr. 1·850 *two parts*, and of nitric acid of sp. gr. 1·450 *one part*. Mix them, and, having permitted the heat to fall to about 100° F., add raw cotton to saturation. Let it macerate for one or two hours; then pour off the acids, wash the cotton till the washings cease to affect litmus paper, and dry thoroughly. The gummy matter thus formed is now to be dissolved in ether of the sp. gr. about ·750, or in a mixture of three parts of pure ether and one part of alcohol of 95 per cent. Two ounces of cotton will make about a pint of collodion. (*Bost. Med. and Surg. Journ.*, 1866, p. 39.)

† *Pavesi's Styptic Collodion.* Collodion, 100 parts; Carbolic acid, 10 parts; Pure tannin, 5 parts; Benzoic acid, 3 parts. Agitate till thoroughly mixed. On evaporation it leaves a brown pellicle, adhering strongly to tissues, and effecting instant coagulation of the blood and albumen.

Iodoform Collodion is made, according to Moleschott, by dissolving 1 part of iodoform, in fine powder, in 15 parts of flexible collodion. It is recommended for relieving pain caused by gout, and for orchitis, pericarditis, etc.

‡ *Silk Collodion.* M. Persoz, the younger, prepares a collodion by bringing silk to the condition of the material from which the worm spins its thread. This he does by dissolving it in a solution of chloride of zinc, and then separating the solvent by means of dialysis. The chloride passes through the parchment of a dialyser, leaving the silk substance in a soft fibreless state. The material thus obtained is said to be applicable to photographic purposes. Before it could be used as collodion, it would be necessary to dissolve it in a volatile liquid, which would evaporate spontaneously on application to the surface. (See *A. J. P.*, 1867, p. 182.)

COLLODIUM CUM CANTHARIDE. *U.S.* *Collodion with Cantharides.* [*Cantharidal Collodion.*]

(CQL-LŌ'DI-ŬM CŬM CAN-THĂR'I-DĔ.)

Collodium Vesicans, *Br.;* Blistering Collodion; Collodium Cantharidatum, *P.G.;* Collodium Cantharidale, s. Vesicans; Collodion vésicant (cantharidé), *Fr.;* Blasenziehendes Collodium, *G.*

"Cantharides, in No. 60 powder, *sixty parts;** Flexible Collodion, *eighty-five parts;* Commercial Chloroform, *a sufficient quantity.* Pack the powder firmly in a cylindrical percolator, and gradually pour Commercial Chloroform upon it, until *two hundred and fifty* (250) *parts* of tincture are obtained, or until the Cantharides are exhausted. Recover, by distillation on a water-bath, about *two hundred* (200) *parts* of the Chloroform, and evaporate the residue in a capsule, by means of a water-bath. until it weighs *fifteen* (15) *parts.* Dissolve this in the Flexible Collodion, and let it stand at rest for forty-eight hours. Finally, pour off the clear portion from any sediment which may have been deposited, and transfer it to bottles, which should be securely corked. Keep the Cantharidal Collodion in a cool place, remote from lights or fire." *U. S.*

"Take of Blistering liquid (see *Liquor Epispasticus*) *twenty fluidounces* [Imp. meas.]; Pyroxylin *one ounce* [av.]. Add the Pyroxylin to the liquid in a stoppered bottle, and shake them together until the former is dissolved." *Br.*

The officinal process differs considerably in the manipulation from that of the U. S. P. 1870, although the finished preparation is not essentially different. Chloroform is used to extract the cantharidin from the powdered cantharides, by percolation; the chloroform is afterwards recovered by distillation, and the oily residue containing the vesicant is dissolved in the collodion. The efficiency of chloroform as a solvent of cantharidin has been shown by Professor Procter. The original process of M. Ilisch was to exhaust, by percolation, a pound of cantharides, with a mixture consisting of a pound of ether and three ounces of acetic ether; and in two ounces of this liquid to dissolve 25 grains of gun cotton. Professor Procter states that it has been found more advantageous to exhaust the flies with ether, distil off the ether, and mix the oily residue with collodion already prepared of the proper consistence (*A. J. P.*, xxiv. 303); and this is probably a better formula than the officinal, if care is used in recovering the ether to avoid contact with flame. Mr. Charles S. Rand (*A. J. P.*, xxii. 18) states that Ilisch's preparation, made with double the proportion of ether, vesicates equally well, and proposes the addition of about 1 per cent. of Venice turpentine, which he has found to prevent the disagreeable and sometimes painful contraction of the collodion upon drying. The preparation may be kept indefinitely, in an opaque glass-stoppered bottle, without change; but, on exposure to the light, the greenish coloring matter of the flies bleaches, and the liquid becomes yellowish.†

Cantharidized Collodion may be made from cantharidin by dissolving four grains of cantharidin in one thousand grains of flexible collodion.

Cantharidal collodion is a very convenient epispastic remedy. It may be applied to the surface by means of a camel's-hair brush, and, after the evaporation of the ether, which takes place in less than a minute, may be reapplied if the surface should not be well covered. It produces a blister in about the same time as the ordinary cerate, and has the advantages that it is applied with greater facility, is better adapted to cover uneven surfaces, and retains its place more certainly. According to Mr. Rand, if the evaporation of the ether be restrained by a piece of oiled silk immediately after its application, it will act much more speedily.

COLLODIUM FLEXILE. *U. S., Br.* *Flexible Collodion.*

(CQL-LŌ'DI-ŬM FLĔX'I-LĔ.)

Collodium Elasticum, *P.G.;* Collodion élastique, *Fr.;* Elastisches Collodium, *G.*

"Collodion, *ninety-two parts;*‡ Canada Turpentine, *five parts;* Castor Oil, *three*

* As the liquid ingredients in this preparation are more conveniently weighed than measured, the equivalent measures have been omitted.

† *Croton Oil Collodion* is made by mixing equal weights of croton oil and flexible collodion. (*Report on Revision of U. S. Pharm., A. P. A.,* 1880.)

‡ As the liquid ingredients in this preparation are more conveniently weighed than measured, the equivalent measures have been omitted.

parts, To make *one hundred parts*. Mix them, and keep the mixture in a well-corked bottle, in a cool place, remote from lights or fire." *U. S.*

"Take of Collodion *twelve fluidounces* [Imperial measure]; Canada Balsam *half an ounce;* Castor Oil *quarter of an ounce*. Mix, and keep in a well-corked bottle." *Br.*

The contractility of the collodion film has long been felt as a drawback to its use simply for the purposes of protection. Mr. C. S. Rand, of Philadelphia, proposed to obviate this by dissolving one part of gun cotton and three of Venice turpentine in twenty parts of ether. To give more flexibility to the film, M. Sourisseau, of Kaiserberg, suggested the addition of one part of elemi to twelve of collodion. According to Mr. Startin, of London, opacity and elasticity may be imparted at the same time, by adding from half a drachm to a drachm of lard, or some similar fatty matter, previously dissolved in ether, to an ounce of collodion. The qualities of softness and elasticity may also be given by combining collodion with castor oil, in the proportion of thirty parts to two, agreeably to the plan of M. Guersant, who found it useful, thus modified, in erysipelas; and the proportion of castor oil may be increased if thought desirable. This is the method preferred by the French Codex. An elastic collodion, somewhat similar, in which, besides castor oil, Venice turpentine and white wax are ingredients, has been proposed by E. Lauras. (*P. J. Tr.*, xii. 303.) According to MM. Cap and Garot, the most successful way for obtaining an elastic collodion is to mix two parts of glycerin with one hundred of collodion. *Glycerized collodion* is exceedingly supple, does not crack and scale off from the skin, and accommodates itself to the motions of the part. In order to imitate the color of the skin, an ethereal tincture of turmeric or saffron may be added, so as to produce the desired tint. Dr. Meller has proposed a solution of shellac in highly rectified alcohol, so as to have a gelatinous consistence, as a substitute for collodion. Of all these plans, probably that followed in the officinal directions is the best. Dr. Tournie recommends, in superficial cervical adenitis with redness, painting the part with several layers of flexible collodion every two days. (*Med. Times and Gaz.*, 1874, p. 540.)

COLLODIUM STYPTICUM. *U. S.* *Styptic Collodion.*

(CQL-LŌ'DĮ-ŬM STȲP'TĮ-CŬM.)

Styptic Colloid, Xylostyptic Ether; Collodion styptique, *Fr.*

"Tannic Acid, *twenty parts* [or eighty grains av.]; Alcohol, *five parts* [or twenty-six minims]; Stronger Ether, *twenty parts* [or one hundred and ten minims]; Collodion, *fifty-five parts* [or four and a half fluidrachms], To make *one hundred parts* [or about one fluidounce]. Place the Tannic Acid in a tared bottle, add the Alcohol, Ether, and Collodion, and agitate until the Tannic Acid is dissolved. Keep the product in well corked bottles, in a cool place, remote from lights or fire." *U. S.*

This new officinal is a modification of the *styptic colloid* of Dr. B. W. Richardson, of London (*P. J. Tr.*, 1867, p. 29), a preparation which has had considerable use, particularly in hospitals. Experience has shown, however, that Dr. Richardson's formula contained too little tannin; the quantity has been increased in the U. S. process to twenty per cent.; but this is more than will dissolve. The manipulation in the officinal formula might be improved by directing the tannic acid to be rubbed into a smooth paste in a mortar with sufficient alcohol, before introducing into the bottle. This would enable the pharmacist to prepare it extemporaneously. When applied on wounded or abraded surfaces, it soon loses the ether and alcohol, and a firm coating is left, in which, besides the tannin and colloidal substance, are the coagulated blood and secretions from the surface, forming a covering for the part by which the air is excluded. The liquid is applied with a camel's-hair brush, or by means of cotton saturated with it, to the edges of wounds closed by stitches, to ulcerated surfaces and bleeding parts. If it be desired to make a special impression on the diseased surface, carbolic acid, creasote, iodine, morphine, etc., may be incorporated with the styptic fluid.*

* *Carbolised Styptic Colloid.* In this preparation advantage is taken of the antiseptic and styptic properties of carbolic acid, and a very effective hæmostatic results. It is made by adding ten per cent. of carbolic acid to officinal styptic collodion.

COLOCYNTHIS. *U. S.* *Colocynth.*

(CŎL-Q-CȲN'THIS.)

"The fruit of Citrullus Colocynthis, Schrader (*Nat. Ord.* Cucurbitaceæ), deprived of its rind." *U. S.* "The dried peeled fruit, freed from seeds, of Citrullus Colocynthis, *Schrod.*" *Br.*

Colocynthidis Pulpa, *Br.;* Colocynth Pulp; Fructus Colocynthidis, *P.G.;* Poma Colocynthidis; Pulpe de Coloquinte; Coloquinte, *Fr.;* Coloquintenapfel, Koloquintenmark, Koloquinten, *G.;* Coloquintida, *It., Sp.*

Gen. Ch. MALE. *Calyx* five-toothed. *Corolla* five-parted. *Filaments* three. FEMALE. *Calyx* five-toothed. *Corolla* five-parted. *Pistil* three-cleft. *Seeds* of the *gourd* with a sharp edge. *Willd.*

Cucumis Colocynthis. Willd. *Sp. Plant.* iv. 611; Woodv. *Med. Bot.* p. 189, t. 71.—*Citrullus Colocynthis*, Royle's Mat. Med. The *bitter cucumber* is an annual plant, bearing considerable resemblance to the common watermelon. The stems, which are herbaceous and beset with rough hairs, trail upon the ground, or rise upon neighboring bodies, to which they attach themselves by their numerous tendrils. The leaves, which stand alternately on long petioles, are triangular, many-cleft, variously sinuated, obtuse, hairy, of a fine green color on the upper surface, rough and pale on the under. The flowers are yellow, and appear singly at the axils of the leaves. The fruit is a globular pepo, of the size of a small orange, yellow and smooth when ripe; and contains, within a hard, coriaceous rind, a white, spongy, medullary matter, enclosing numerous ovate, compressed, white or brownish seeds.

The plant is a native of Turkey, and abounds in the islands of the Archipelago. It grows also in various parts of Africa and Asia. Burckhardt, in his travels across Nubia, found the country covered with it; Thunberg met with it at the Cape of Good Hope; and Ainslie says that it grows in many parts of Lower India, particularly in sandy places near the sea. It is said to be cultivated in Spain, to abound in Morocco and in the neighboring countries, and even to have been collected in Japan. The fruit is gathered in autumn, when it begins to become yellow, and, having been peeled, is dried quickly in a stove or by the sun. Thus prepared, it is imported from the Levant. Small quantities are said to be imported into England from Mogador in the form of brown, unpeeled globular gourds.*

The so-called Persian colocynth of the London markets is very small, and has apparently been compressed in a fresh state, so that the position of the seeds is perceptible through the dry pulp. The microscopic structure and the proportion of the pulp to the seed appear to be the same as in other colocynths. (*P. J. Tr.*, xvi. p. 107.)

Properties. As kept in the shops, colocynth is in the shape of whitish balls about the size of an orange, very light and spongy, and abounding in seeds which constitute three-fourths of their weight. The seeds are somewhat bitter, but possess little activity, and, according to Captain Lyon, are even used as food in the north of Africa.† When the medicine is prepared for use, they are separated and rejected, the pulpy or medullary matter only being employed. This has a very feeble odor, but a nauseous and intensely bitter taste. The U. S. Pharm. thus describes colocynth. "From two to four inches (5 to 10 cm.) in diameter; globular; white or yellowish-white; light; spongy; readily breaking into three wedge-shaped pieces, each containing, near the rounded surface, many flat, ovate, brown seeds; inodorous; taste intensely bitter. Hard and dark colored Colocynth should be rejected. The pulp, when used, should be deprived of the seeds." *U. S.* Water and alcohol extract the

* In Union Village, Lebanon, Ohio, the Shakers formerly prepared an extract from a hybrid between the colocynth and the watermelon. The two plants were placed close to each other, and the hybrid resulting yielded the second year a gourd resembling a watermelon, but very bitter, and affording an abundant extract. This is stated to be equal in purgative properties to that of colocynth, but at present it is not manufactured.

† Dr. Nachtigal confirms this statement of Captain Lyon; but with the qualification, that, before being eaten, the seeds are deprived of their coating by some mechanical means, and the kernels are heated to the boiling point, then washed with cold water, dried, and powdered. Professor Flückiger found a bitter principle in the testa, which accounts for its rejection as food, though rendering improper the rejection of the seed in preparing the extract. He found in the kernels about 45 per cent. of fixed oil and 18 per cent. of albumen. (*A. J. P.*, 1872, p. 538.)

virtues of colocynth. It is a matter of importance to be able to determine whether the drug miller who usually powders colocynth is careful to reject the seeds. If the seeds have been ground with the mass, the microscope will show the presence of numerous albuminous granules derived from the cotyledons. (W. T. Clark, *P. J. Tr.*, vii. 509.) These are best found by putting a small amount of the powder on the glass slide, adding a drop of water, and gently rubbing the cover glass over it: fragments of the double-walled embryo sac showing on the outer side, elongated, more or less hexagonal, thin-walled cells, and on the inner side irregular, tabular, thick-walled cells. Powdered colocynth containing a large number of starch granules has suffered adulteration. Vauquelin obtained the bitter principle of colocynth in a separate state, and called it *colocynthin.* According to Meissner, 100 parts of the dry pulp of colocynth contain 14·4 parts of colocynthin, 10·0 of extractive, 4·2 of fixed oil, 13·2 of a resinous substance insoluble in ether, 9·5 of gum, 3·0 of pectic acid (pectin), 17·6 of gummy extract derived from the lignin by means of potassa, 2·7 of phosphate of calcium, 3·0 of phosphate of magnesium, and 19·0 of lignin, besides water.* Colocynthin is obtained by boiling the pulp in water, evaporating the decoction, treating the extract thus procured with alcohol, evaporating the alcoholic solution, and submitting the residue, which consists of the bitter principle and acetate of potassium, to the action of a little cold water, which dissolves the latter, and leaves the greater part of the former untouched. Mr. Bastick obtained it by exhausting the pulp with cold water, heating the solution to ebullition, adding subacetate of lead so long as a precipitate was produced, filtering the liquor when cold, adding dilute sulphuric acid gradually until it no longer occasioned a precipitate, boiling to expel free acetic acid, filtering to separate sulphate of lead, evaporating cautiously nearly to dryness, extracting the colocynthin from the residuum by strong alcohol, which left the salts, and finally evaporating the alcoholic solution. The following process, employed by Dr. Walz, probably yields it in a purer state.

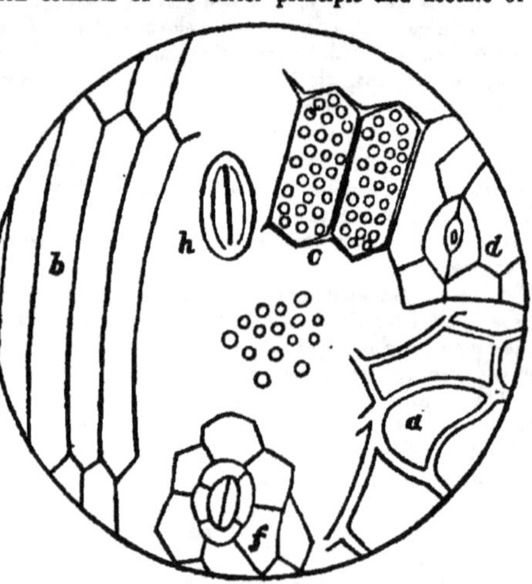

470 Diameters.

a, inner layer of embryo sac; *b*, outer layer of ditto; *c*, cells of palisaded layer with granules; *d*, stomata from cotyledon; *e*, granules from cotyledons; *f*, epidermis of rind; *h*, starch granule (side view).

Colocynth is exhausted by alcohol of 0·84, the tincture evaporated to dryness, the residue treated with water, and the solution precipitated first with acetate and afterwards with subacetate of lead. The yellow filtered liquor is then treated with sulphuretted hydrogen to separate the lead, and, after filtration, with solution of tannic acid, which throws down a compound of tannic acid and colocynthin. This is dissolved in alcohol, the tannin thrown down by subacetate of lead, the excess of lead separated, and the liquid digested with animal charcoal, filtered, and evaporated. The residue, washed with anhydrous ether, is pure colocynthin. This is yellowish, somewhat translucent, brittle and friable, fusible by a heat below 100° C. (212° F.), inflammable, more soluble in alcohol than in water, but capable of rendering the latter intensely bitter. M. Mouchon states that it is insoluble in ether. It is neither acid nor alkaline; but its aqueous

* Dr. Walz supposes that he has found another peculiar principle, *colocynthitin.* It was obtained by treating with ether the alcoholic extract previously exhausted by water, decolorizing the ethereal solution with animal charcoal, evaporating to dryness, and dissolving the residue in anhydrous alcohol, which deposited it in crystals on spontaneous evaporation. It is white and tasteless, and is probably a resin. (*N. Jahrbuch der Pharm.*, xvi. 10.)

solution gives with infusion of galls a copious white precipitate. Its formula, according to Dr. Walz, is $C_{56}H_{84}O_{23}$. Upon the same authority it is a glucoside, being resolved, by the action of sulphuric acid, into sugar and a peculiar resinous substance termed *colocynthein*. Henke doubts the probability of colocynthin being a glucoside, and states that it is uncrystallizable; he reviews the methods of previous investigators, and obtained by his own process but 0·66 per cent. of colocynthin. (*Archiv d. Pharm.*, 1883, p. 200; *A. J. P.*, 1883, p. 301.) According to Johannson, colocynthin, when heated with diluted sulphuric acid, yields colocynthein, elaterin, and bryonin. (*A. J. P.*, 1885, p. 451.)* An infusion of colocynth, made with boiling water, gelatinizes upon cooling. Neumann obtained from 768 parts of the pulp, treated first with alcohol and then with water, 168 parts of alcoholic and 216 of aqueous extract.

Medical Properties and Uses. The pulp of colocynth is a powerful drastic, hydragogue cathartic, producing, when given in large doses, violent griping, and sometimes bloody discharges, with dangerous inflammation of the bowels. Death has resulted from a teaspoonful and a half of the powder. (*Christison.*) Even in moderate doses it sometimes acts with much harshness, and is, therefore, seldom prescribed alone. By some writers it is said to be diuretic. It was frequently employed by the ancient Greeks and the Arabians, though its drastic nature was not unknown to them. Among the moderns it is occasionally used in obstinate dropsy, and in various affections depending on disordered action of the brain. In combination with other cathartics it loses much of its violence, but retains its purgative energy, and in this state is extensively employed. The compound extract of colocynth is a favorite preparation with many practitioners; and, combined with calomel, extract of jalap, and gamboge, it forms a highly efficient and safe cathartic, especially useful in congestion of the portal circle and torpidity of the liver. (See *Pilulæ Catharticæ Compositæ.*) The dose of colocynth is from five to ten grains (0·33–0·65 Gm.). It is best administered in minute division, effected by trituration with gum or farinaceous matter. The active principle has sometimes been employed, and, in the impure state in which it is prepared by the process of M. Emile Mouchon, may be given in the dose of a grain (·065 Gm.).†

Thunberg states that the fruit of *C. Colocynthis*, at the Cape of Good Hope, is rendered so mild by being properly pickled, that it is eaten both by the natives and the colonists; but, as it is thus employed before attaining perfect maturity, it is possible that the drastic principle may not have been developed.

Off. Prep. Extractum Colocynthidis.

Off. Prep. Br. Extractum Colocynthidis Compositum; Pilula Colocynthidis Composita; Pilula Colocynthidis et Hyoscyami.

CONFECTIONES. *Confections.*

(CON-FĔC-TI-Ō'NĒS—kon-fĕk-she-ō'nēz.)

Electuaries; Conserves, Electuaires, Saccharolés mous, *Fr.*; Conserven, Latwergen, *G.*

Under the general title of Confections, the Pharmacopœias include all those preparations having the form of a soft solid, in which one or more medicinal substances are incorporated with saccharine matter, with a view either to their preservation or more convenient administration. But two confections have been retained in the present revision of the U. S. Pharmacopœia. The old division into Conserves and Electuaries has been abandoned; but, as there is some ground for the distinction, we shall make a few general remarks upon each division, before proceeding to the consideration of the individual preparations.

* According to Ernst Johannson (*Inaug. Diss.*, Dorpat, 1884), colocynthin can readily be found in the alvine discharges, and in the body after poisoning by it, by the following tests: $\frac{1}{50}$ milligramme will give with concentrated sulphuric acid a reddish-yellow color, deepening into red; Froehde's reagent strikes with $\frac{1}{50}$ milligramme a cherry-red color; one part of ammonium vanadanate in 200 parts of concentrated sulphuric acid make with $\frac{1}{50}$ milligramme a blood-red spot surrounded by a bluish tint; alcohol with sulphuric acid strikes a yellow color, not altered by warming; selenosulphuric acid (H_2SeSO_3) does the same; basic acetate of lead and tannic acid precipitate by weak solutions.

† For further processes for preparing colocynthin, see U. S. D., fourteenth edition, or *A. J. P.*, xxviii. 166; 1863, 116.

CONSERVES consist of recent vegetable substances and refined sugar beaten into a uniform mass. By means of the sugar, the vegetable matter is enabled to resist for some time the decomposition to which it would otherwise be exposed in the undried state, and the properties of the recent plant are thus retained to a certain extent unaltered. But, as active medicines even thus treated undergo some change, and those which lose their virtues by desiccation cannot be long preserved, the few conserves now retained are intended rather as convenient vehicles of other substances than for separate exhibition. The sugar used in their preparation should be reduced to a fine powder by pounding and sifting, as otherwise it will not mix uniformly with the other ingredients.

ELECTUARIES are mixtures consisting of medicinal substances, especially dry powders, combined with syrup or honey, in order to render them less unpleasant to the taste, and more convenient for internal use. They are usually prepared extemporaneously; and it is only when their complex nature renders it convenient to keep them ready made in the shops, or some peculiarity in the mode of mixing the ingredients requires attention, that they become proper objects for officinal direction. Their consistence should not be so soft, on the one hand, as to allow the ingredients to separate, nor so firm, on the other, as to prevent them from being swallowed without mastication. Different substances require different proportions of syrup. Light vegetable powders usually require twice their weight, gum-resins two-thirds of their weight, resins somewhat less, mineral substances about half their weight, and deliquescent salts not more than one-tenth. Should the electuary be found, after having been kept for a short time, to swell up and emit gas, it should be beaten over again in a mortar, so that any portion of the sugar which may have crystallized may be again accurately incorporated with the other ingredients. Should it, on the contrary, become dry and hard from the mutual reaction of its constituents, more syrup should be added, so as to give it the requisite consistence. If the dryness result from the mere evaporation of the aqueous part, water should be added instead of syrup, and the same remark is applicable to the conserves. To prevent the hardening of electuaries, the French writers recommend the use of syrup prepared from brown sugar, which is less apt to crystallize than that made from the refined. Molasses would answer the same purpose; but its taste might be objectionable. Some employ honey, but this is not always acceptable to the stomach. Glycerin might sometimes be used with advantage.*

CONFECTIO OPII. *Br.* *Confection of Opium.*

(CON-FĔC'TI-Ō Ō'PI-Ī—kon-fĕk'she-ō.)

Electuarium Theriaca, *P. G.;* Confection (Electuaire) opiacé, Thériaque, *Fr.;* Opiumlatwerge, Theriak, *G.*

"Take of Compound Powder of Opium *one hundred grains;* Syrup *three hundred grains.* Mix." *Br.*

This preparation was dropped in the last revision of the U. S. Pharm. It was intended as a substitute for those exceedingly complex and unscientific preparations, formerly known by the names of *theriaca* and *mithridate*, which have been expelled from modern pharmacy. It was an officinal of the London and Edinburgh Col-

* *Confectio Aromatica. Aromatic Confection.* (Electuarium Aromaticum; Électuaire, Confection aromatique, *Fr.;* Aromatische Latwerge, Gewürzlatwerge, *G.*) "Take of Aromatic Powder *four troyounces;* Clarified Honey *four troyounces*, or *a sufficient quantity*. Rub the Aromatic Powder with Clarified Honey until a uniform mass of the proper consistence is obtained." *U. S.* 1870. The aromatic confection has been abandoned in the U. S. and Br. Pharmacopœias, probably because readily prepared extemporaneously. It affords, nevertheless, a convenient means of administering the spices contained in it, and an agreeable vehicle for other medicines. The 1870 U. S. formula differed favorably from that of 1850 in the omission of the saffron; and the place of the syrup of orange peel has been economically supplied by using a larger proportion of honey. The confection is given in debilitated states of the stomach. The dose is from ten to sixty grains (0·65–3·9 Gm.)."

Confectio Aurantii Corticis. Confection of Orange Peel. (Conserva Aurantii; Conserve d'Ecorce d'Orange, *Fr.;* Apfelsinenschalen-Conserve, *G.*) "Take of Sweet Orange Peel, recently separated from the fruit by grating, *twelve troyounces;* Sugar [refined] *thirty-six troyounces.* Beat the Orange Peel with the Sugar, gradually added, until they are thoroughly mixed." *U. S.* 1870. This confection, like the preceding, has been dropped in the U. S. and Br. Pharmacopœias. It is not used as frequently as it deserves to be. It is, when well made, a grateful aromatic vehicle or adjunct for tonic and purgative powders.

leges, and, after having been discarded in the first British Pharmacopœia, was adopted in the last edition. The preparation is a combination of opium with spices, which render it more stimulant, and more grateful to a debilitated stomach. It may be given in atonic gout, flatulent colic, diarrhœa unattended with inflammation, and other diseases requiring the use of a stimulant narcotic. Added to Peruvian bark or sulphate of quinine, it increases the efficacy of this remedy in obstinate cases of intermittent fever. One grain of opium is contained in about thirty-six grains of the U. S. confection of 1870,* and in about forty grains of the British.

The dose is from five to twenty grains (0·325 to 1·3 Gm.).

CONFECTIO PIPERIS. *Br.* *Confection of Pepper.*

(CON-FĔC'TI-Ō PĬ'PĔR-ĬS.)

Electuarium Piperis; Electuaire de Poivre, *Fr.*; Pfefferlatwerge, *G.*

"Take of Black Pepper, in fine powder, *two ounces;* Caraway Fruit, in fine powder, *three ounces;* Clarified Honey *fifteen ounces.* Rub them well together in a mortar." *Br.* This preparation was intended as a substitute for *Ward's paste,* which acquired some reputation in Great Britain as a remedy in piles and ulcers of the rectum. To do good, it must be continued, according to Mr. Brodie, for two, three, or four months. The dose is from one to two drachms (3·9 to 7·8 Gm.), repeated two or three times a day. Its stimulating properties render it inapplicable to cases attended with much inflammation.

CONFECTIO ROSÆ. *U. S.* *Confection of Rose.*

(CON-FĔC'TI-Ō RŌ'ŞÆ.)

Confectio Rosæ Gallicæ, *Br.;* Confection of Roses; Conserva Rosarum; Conserve de Rose rouge, *Fr.;* Rosen-Conserve, *G.*

"Red Rose, in No. 60 powder, *eight parts* [or one ounce av.]; Sugar, in fine powder, *sixty-four parts* [or eight ounces av.]; Clarified Honey, *twelve parts* [or one and a half ounces av.]; Rose Water, *sixteen parts* [or two fluidounces], To make *one hundred parts* [or twelve and a half ounces]. Rub the Red Rose with the Rose Water heated to 65° C. (149° F.), then gradually add the Sugar and Honey, and beat the whole together until thoroughly mixed." *U. S.*

"Take of Fresh Red-Rose Petals *one pound;* Refined Sugar *three pounds.* Beat the Petals to a pulp in a stone mortar; add the Sugar, and rub them well together." *Br.*

This preparation differs from that formerly officinal only in a slight increase, 4 per cent., in the quantity of sugar; this is rather an improvement.

In the British process the unblown petals only are used, and these should be deprived of their claws; in other words, the rose-buds should be cut off a short distance above their base, and the lower portion rejected. In the last three editions of the U. S. Pharmacopœia, dried roses have been substituted for the fresh, as the latter are not brought to our market. The process is very similar to that of the French Codex. We have been informed, however, that much of the confection of roses made in Philadelphia on the large scale is prepared from the fresh petals of the hundred-leaved rose and others, by beating them into a pulp with sugar, as in the British process. An excuse for this deviation from the officinal formula is, that the confection thus made has greater adhesiveness than the officinal, and is therefore better fitted for the formation of pills.

This confection is slightly astringent, but is almost exclusively used as a vehicle of other medicines, or to impart consistence to the pilular mass.

Off. Prep. Br. Pilula Aloes Barbadensis; Pilula Aloes et Asafœtidæ; Pilula Aloes et Ferri; Pilula Aloes Socotrinæ; Pilula Ferri Carbonatis; Pilula Hydrargyri; Pilula Plumbi cum Opio.

* "Take of Opium, in fine powder, *two hundred and seventy grains;* Aromatic Powder *six troyounces;* Clarified Honey *fourteen troyounces.* Rub the Opium with the Aromatic Powder, then add the Honey, and beat the whole together until thoroughly mixed." *U. S.* 1870.

CONFECTIO ROSÆ CANINÆ. *Br.* *Confection of Hips.*

(CON-FEC'TI-Ō RŌ'ṢÆ CA-NĪ'NÆ.)

Confectio Cynosbati, Conserva Cynorrhodi; Conserve de Cynorrhodon, *Fr.;* Hainbutten-Conserve, *G.*

"Take of Hips deprived of their seed-like fruits *one pound;* Refined Sugar *two pounds.* Beat the Hips to a pulp in a stone mortar, and rub the pulp through a sieve, then add the sugar, and rub them well together." *Br.*

This preparation is acidulous and refrigerant, and is used in Europe for forming more active medicines into pills and electuaries. On standing it is apt to develop saccharine crystals, and is therefore not so eligible as confection of rose.

CONFECTIO SCAMMONII. *Br.* *Confection of Scammony.*

(CON-FEC'TI-Ō SCAM-MŌ'NI-Ī.)

Electuaire ou Confection de Scammonée, *Fr.;* Scammonium-Latwerge, *G.*

"Take of Resin of Scammony, in powder, *six ounces;* Ginger, in fine powder, *three ounces;* Oil of Caraway *one-quarter of a fluidounce;* Oil of Cloves *one-eighth of a fluidounce;* Syrup *six fluidounces;* Clarified Honey *three ounces.* Rub the powders with the Syrup and the Honey into a uniform mass, then add the Oils and mix." *Br.* The ounce used in this process is the avoirdupois ounce.

The confection is actively cathartic in the dose of half a drachm or a drachm (1·9 or 3·9 Gm.), but is very little used.

CONFECTIO SENNÆ. *U. S., Br.* *Confection of Senna.*

(CON-FEC'TI-Ō SĔN'NÆ.)

Electuarium e Senna, *P. G.;* Electuarium de Senna Compositum, Electuarium Lenitivum; Electuaire de Séné composé, Électuaire lénitif, *Fr.;* Senna-Latwerge, *G.*

"Senna, in No. 60 powder, *ten parts;* Coriander, in No. 40 powder, *six parts;* Cassia Fistula, bruised, *sixteen parts;* Tamarind, *ten parts;* Prune, sliced, *seven parts;* Fig, bruised, *twelve parts;* Sugar, in fine powder, *fifty parts;* Water, *sixty parts,* To make *one hundred parts.* Place the Cassia Fistula, Tamarind, Prune, and Fig in a close vessel with *forty-five* (45) *parts* of the Water, and digest for three hours, by means of a water-bath. Separate the coarser portions with the hand, and rub the pulpy mass, first through a coarse hair sieve, and then through a fine one, or through a muslin cloth. Mix the residue with the remainder of the Water, and, having digested the mixture for a short time, treat it as before, and add the product to the pulpy liquid first obtained. Then, by means of a water-bath, dissolve the Sugar in the pulpy liquid, and evaporate the whole until it weighs *eighty-four* (84) *parts.* Lastly, add the Senna and Coriander, and incorporate them thoroughly with the other ingredients while yet warm." *U. S.*

"Take of Senna, in fine powder, *seven ounces;* Coriander Fruit, in fine powder, *three ounces;* Figs *twelve ounces;* Tamarind *nine ounces;* Cassia Pulp *nine ounces;* Prunes *six ounces;* Extract of Liquorice *one ounce;* Refined Sugar *thirty ounces;* Distilled Water *a sufficiency to make seventy-five ounces.* Boil the Figs and Prunes gently with twenty-four [fluid]ounces of Distilled Water in a covered vessel for four hours; then, having added more Distilled Water to make up the quantity to its original volume, mix the Tamarind and Cassia Pulp, digest for two hours, and rub the softened pulp of the fruits through a hair sieve, rejecting the seeds and other hard parts. To the pulped product add the Sugar and Extract of Liquorice and dissolve them with the aid of a little heat; while the mixture is still warm, add to it gradually the mixed Senna and Coriander powders, and mix the whole thoroughly, making the weight of the resulting Confection seventy-five ounces either by evaporation or by the addition of more Distilled Water." *Br.* The ounce employed in the British process is the avoirdupois ounce.

The Confection of Senna, when correctly made, is an elegant preparation, and keeps well if properly secured. The present U. S. process differs from that of 1860 in preparing the pulps, as suggested in former editions of this Dispensatory, instead of taking them already prepared. There may be difficulty, however, in the evaporation to 84 parts, particularly if the pulpy drugs are of good quality. The present preparation contains nearly 20 per cent. more sugar than that officinal in 1870, and nearly 2 per cent. more senna. It is not uncommon to omit the cassia pulp in the preparation of the confection, as the pods are not always to be found in the market. But, as this is next to senna the most active ingredient, the omission is to be regretted. Cassia fistula is now readily procured in commerce, and there can be no excuse for its omission. It has also been proposed to substitute the fluid extract of senna for the crude drug (*A. J. P.*, xliii. 123); but, as the fluid extract is of such uncertain quality, the leaves themselves are certainly preferable.

This is one of our best and most pleasant laxatives, being admirably adapted to cases of habitual costiveness, especially in pregnant women and persons affected with piles. It is also very useful in constipation during convalescence from acute disease. The dose is two drachms (7·8 Gm.), to be taken at bedtime.

CONFECTIO SULPHURIS. *Br.* *Confection of Sulphur.*

(CON-FĔC′TI-Ō SŬL′PHŪ-RĬS.)

Electuarium Sulphuris; Électuaire de Soufre, *Fr.*; Schwefel-Latwerge, *G.*

"Take of Sublimed Sulphur *four ounces* [avoirdupois]; Acid Tartrate of Potassium, in powder, *one ounce* [av.]; Syrup of Orange Peel *four fluidounces;* Tragacanth, in powder, *eighteen grains.* Rub them well together." *Br.*

This is merely a mode of administering the two laxatives, sulphur and bitartrate of potassium; and the relative proportion of the latter is so small that it can have little effect. The addition of tragacanth is due to a suggestion of Mr. Peter Boa, who found that without it a syrupy layer of liquid formed on top of the confection. (*P. J. Tr.*, 1882, p. 682.) The dose is from one to two drachms (3·9 to 7·8 Gm.) or more.

CONFECTIO TEREBINTHINÆ. *Br.* *Confection of Turpentine.*

(CON-FĔC′TI-Ō TĔR-Ē-BĬN′THI-NÆ.)

Electuarium Terebinthinatum; Électuaire térébinthiné, *Fr.*; Terpentinol-Latwerge, *G.*

"Take of Oil of Turpentine *one fluidounce;* Liquorice Root, in powder, *one ounce* [avoirdupois]; Clarified Honey *two ounces* [av.]. Rub the Oil of Turpentine with the Liquorice, add the Honey, and mix to a uniform consistence." *Br.*

Confections might be multiplied indefinitely upon the principle which appears to have been adopted here, that, namely, of giving a convenient formula for the administration of medicines. The effects of this confection are those only of the oil of turpentine. The dose may be from a half a drachm to a drachm (1·9 to 3·9 Gm.).

CONII FOLIA. *Br.* *Conium Leaves.*

(CO-NĪ′Ī FŌ′LI-Ă.)

"The fresh leaves and young branches of Conium maculatum; gathered from wild British plants when the fruit begins to form." *Br.*

Hemlock Leaves; Herba Conii, *P.G.*; Herba Cicutæ Majoris; Feuilles de grande Ciguë (de Ciguë officinale), *Fr.*; Schierlingskraut, Schierlings-Blätter, *G.*

CONIUM. *U.S.* *Conium.* [*Hemlock.*]

(CO-NĪ′ŬM.)

"The full-grown fruit of Conium maculatum. Linné. (*Nat. Ord.* Umbelliferæ, Campylospermæ), gathered while yet green." *U.S.* "The fruit of Conium maculatum, *Linn.*, gathered when fully developed, but while still green, and carefully dried." *Br.*

Conii Fructus, *Br.*; Hemlock Fruit; Fruits de grande Ciguë, Ciguë ordinaire, Grand Ciguë, *Fr.*; Gefleckter Schierling, Schierlingsfrüchte, *G.*; Cicuta, *It.*, *Sp.*

Gen. Ch. Partial involucre halved, usually three-leaved. *Fruit* nearly globular, five-streaked, notched on both sides. *Willd.*

Conium maculatum. Willd. *Sp. Plant.* i. 1395; Bigelow, *Am. Med. Bot.* i. 113; Woodv. *Med. Bot.* p. 104, t. 42. This is an umbelliferous plant, having a biennial spindle-shaped whitish root, and an herbaceous branching stem, from three to six feet high, round, hollow, smooth, shining, slightly striated, and marked with brownish purple spots. The lower leaves are tripinnate, more than a foot in length, shining, and attached to the joints of the stem by sheathing petioles; the upper are smaller, bipinnate, and inserted at the division of the branches; both have channelled footstalks, and incised leaflets, which are deep green on their upper surface and paler beneath. The flowers are very small, white, and disposed in compound terminal umbels. The general involucre consists of from three to seven lanceolate, reflected leaflets, whitish at their edges; the partial involucre, of three or four, oval, pointed, spreading, and on one side only. There are five petals, cordate, with their points inflected, and nearly equal. The stamens are spreading, and about as long as the corolla; the styles diverging. The fruit, commonly called seeds, is roundish-ovate, a line and a half or rather less in length by a line in breadth, striated, and composed of two plano-convex, easily separable parts, which have on their outer surface five crenated ribs separated by slightly wrinkled furrows. On cross-section the absence of oil-ducts becomes apparent, and a deep furrow upon the commissural face of the albumen gives a reniform appearance. As kept in the shops, the mericarps are usually separated. They are thus described in the U. S. Pharmacopœia. "About one-eighth of an inch (3 mm.) long; broadly ovate; laterally compressed; gray-green; often divided into the two mericarps, each with five crenate ribs, without oil-tubes, and containing a seed which is grooved on the face; odor and taste slight. When triturated with solution of potassa, Conium gives off a strong, disagreeable odor." *U. S.*

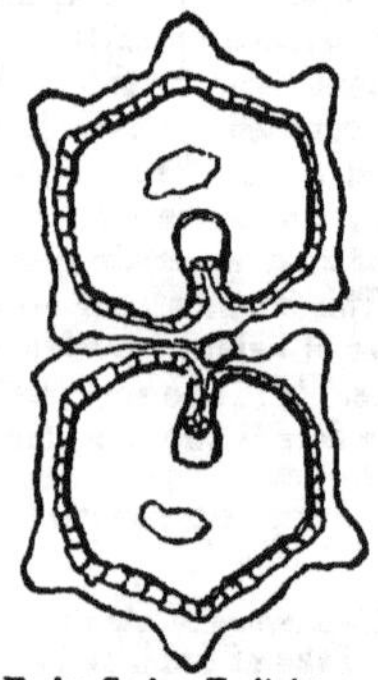

Unripe Conium Fruit, transverse section.

Conium is a native of Europe, and has become naturalized in the United States, where it is also cultivated for medicinal purposes. It grows usually in clusters along the roadsides, or in waste grounds, and is found most abundantly near old settlements. It flowers in June and July. The whole plant, especially at this period, exhales a fetid odor, compared by some to that of mice, by others to that of the urine of cats; and narcotic effects result from breathing for a long time air loaded with the effluvia. The plant varies in narcotic power according to the weather and climate, being most active in hot and dry seasons and in warm countries. The hemlock of Greece, Italy, and Spain is said to be much more energetic than that of the north of Europe. As a general rule, those plants are most active which grow in a sunny exposure. The term *cicuta*, which has often been applied to this plant, belongs to a different genus. The leaves and fruit are officinal.

The proper season for gathering the leaves is when the plant is in flower; and Dr. Fothergill asserts, from experiment, that they are most active about the time when the flowers begin to fade. The footstalks* should be rejected, and the leaflets quickly dried, either in the hot sun, on tin plates before a fire, or by a stove-heat not exceeding 120° F. They should be kept in boxes or tin cases, excluded from the air and light, by exposure to which they lose their fine green color, and become deteriorated. The same end is answered by pulverizing them, and preserving the powder in opaque and well-stopped bottles. But little reliance can be placed on the dried leaves; as, even when possessed of a strong odor and a fine green color, they may be destitute of the narcotic principle. When rubbed with caustic potassa they should exhale the odor of conine. The fruit retains its activity much longer than the leaves. Dr. Christison found them to have sustained no diminution of power after having been kept eight years. Hirtz inferred from experiment that extract of the seeds was ten times stronger than that of the leaves. Commercial conium oc-

* Dr. Manlius Smith, of Manlius, N. Y., has demonstrated that the footstalks are almost destitute of the active alkaline principle. (*Ann. de Thérap.*, 1873, p. 39.)

casionally contains other umbelliferous plants, or it may be almost wholly composed of such plants, and even anise has been used as an adulteration to the fruit. The presence of such impurities is to be recognised by physical examination.

Properties. The dried leaves of the hemlock have a strong, heavy, narcotic odor, less disagreeable than that of the recent plant. Their taste is bitterish and nauseous; their color a dark green, which is retained in the powder. A slight degree of acrimony possessed by the fresh leaves is said to be dissipated by drying. The seeds have a yellowish gray color, a feeble odor, and a bitterish taste. Their form has already been described. Water distilled from the fresh leaves has the odor of hemlock, and a nauseous taste, but does not produce narcotic effects. The decoction has little taste, and the extract resulting from its evaporation is nearly inert. From these facts it is inferable that the active principle, as it exists in the plant, is not volatile at 100° C. (212° F.), and, if soluble in water, is injured by a boiling heat. Alcohol and ether take up the narcotic properties of the leaves; and the ethereal extract, which is of a rich dark green color, is stated by Dr. A. T. Thomson to have the smell and taste of the plant in perfection, and in the dose of half a grain to produce headache and vertigo. Upon destructive distillation, the leaves yield a very poisonous empyreumatic oil. Schrader found in the juice of the leaves, resin, extractive, gum, albumen, a green fecula, and various saline substances. Brandes obtained from the plant a very odorous oil, albumen, resin, coloring matter, and salts.

Geiger was the first who obtained the active principle in a separate state, and proved it to be alkaline. It appears that there are two volatile substances in hemlock; one of them an *oil*, which is in very small quantity, and has never been chemically studied; it is obtained by simple distillation. The volatile alkaloid, *conine*, is the active principle. As it exists in the plant in combination with an acid, it is not readily volatilized; but when alkali is previously added, it freely comes over with the distillate. The acid of conium Peschier believed to be peculiar, and named *conic acid*. Other observers claim that it is *malic acid*. Geiger obtained conine by the following process. He distilled fresh hemlock with caustic potassa and water, neutralized with sulphuric acid the alkaline liquid which came over, evaporated this liquid to the consistence of syrup, added anhydrous alcohol so long as a precipitate of sulphate of ammonium was afforded, separated this salt by filtration, distilled off the alcohol, mixed the residue with a strong solution of caustic potassa, and distilled anew. The conine passed over with the water, from which it separated, floating on the surface in the form of a yellowish oil. According to Dr. Christison, an easier process is to distil cautiously a mixture of a strong solution of potassa and the alcoholic extract of the unripe fruit. Dr. J. Schorm suggests an improvement in the process, which yields a purer conine, in *Ber. d. Deutsch. Chem. Ges.*, 1881, p. 1765; also *N. R.*, 1881, Dec. As obtained by the above process, conine is in the state of a hydrate, containing one-fourth of its weight of water and a little ammonia. From the former, it may be freed by chloride of calcium; from the latter, by exposing it under an exhausted receiver, till it ceases to emit bubbles of gas.

The fresh leaves or seeds should be employed in the preparation of conine; as the alkaloid undergoes decomposition by time and exposure. The seeds contain most of this principle; but even in these it exists in very small proportion. From 6 pounds of the fresh and 9 of the dried seeds, Geiger obtained about an ounce of conine; while from 100 pounds of the fresh herb he got only a drachm, and from the dried leaves none. Christison recommends the full-grown fruit while yet green, and states that 8 pounds will yield half an ounce of hydrate of conine, and contains much more. In relation to the relative strength of different parts of the plant, Dr. Manlius Smith, of New York, gives, as the result of a series of carefully conducted experiments, that the unripe fruit of the conium is far preferable to the dried leaves, and is even stronger than the full-grown fruit, that it may be dried without serious injury, and that a very active preparation may be made from it. He also found that full-grown fruit, collected in August, and dried in the dark, retained its activity unimpaired for several years. This would appear to contradict in some measure previous opinions of the injurious effects of time. (*P. J. Tr.*, Feb. 1869, pp. 491–2.)

Conine, $C_8H_{17}N$, has been thoroughly studied by Hofmann (1881), who established the correct formula as given, instead of $C_8H_{15}N$, as it was formerly assumed, and Ladenburg (1886), who effected its synthesis from *allyl pyridine* by reduction with sodium in alcoholic solution: $C_5H_4(C_3H_5)N + 8H = C_5H_{10}(C_3H_7)N$. This reaction gives normal *propyl piperidine*, which by the crystallization of its tartrate splits into *conine* (dextro-rotatory) and a very similar lævo-rotatory conine, just as racemic acid splits into dextro-rotatory and lævo-rotatory tartaric acid.

CONINE is in the form of a yellowish oily liquid, of sp. gr. 0·87 to 0·89, of a very acrid taste, and a strong penetrating odor, compared to that of the urine of mice, and recalling the smell of fresh hemlock, though not identical with it. In volatility it resembles the essential oils, readily rising with the vapor of boiling water, but when unmixed, requiring for ebullition a temperature of 170° C. (338° F.). It is freely soluble in alcohol, ether, the fixed and volatile oils, and slightly so in water. It unites with about one-fourth of its weight of water to form a hydrate. It reddens turmeric, and neutralizes the acids, forming with them soluble salts, some of which are crystallizable. With tannic acid it forms an insoluble compound. Like ammonia, it occasions a white cloud when approached by a rod moistened with hydrochloric acid; and the resulting hydrochlorate, contrary to previous statements, is asserted by Prof. Wertheim to be crystallizable, and not in the least deliquescent. The statement of Wertheim as to the crystallization of the hydrochlorate has been confirmed by Geo. C. Close, who prepared it by directly uniting its constituents and evaporating its solution by means of a water-bath. The salt crystallized from the solution. He did not succeed in obtaining crystallizable salts with sulphuric, citric, or oxalic acids. (*A. J. P.*, 1869, p. 62.) It coagulates albumen, and precipitates the salts of aluminium, copper, zinc, manganese, and iron. It also precipitates nitrate of silver, but in excess redissolves the precipitate. Most of its salts are decomposed by evaporation. When exposed to the air, it speedily assumes a deep brown color, and is ultimately converted into a resinous matter, and into ammonia which escapes. Under the influence of heat this change takes place with much greater rapidity. The presence of conine may be detected in an extract, or other preparation of hemlock, by rubbing it with potassa, which instantly develops its peculiar odor.* It is a most energetic poison; one drop of it injected into the eye of a rabbit killing the animal in nine minutes, and three drops killing a stout cat in a minute and a half when similarly applied. Locally the alkaloid appears to act as an irritant.

Methylconine. From a communication by Drs. A. von Planta and Aug. Kekulé to the *Annal. der Chem. und Pharm.* (lxxxix., s. 129–156), it would appear that commercial conine consists most commonly of at least two homologous bases; one being the proper *conine* ($C_8H_{17}N$), which contains one atom of hydrogen capable of being replaced by radicals, and the other, named *methylconine*, $C_8H_{16}(CH_3)N$, in which the methyl group CH_3 has been substituted for the replaceable H atom of conine. In relation to the modes of separating these alkaloids and their distinctive properties, we must content ourselves with referring to the original paper.

Conhydrine. Prof. T. Wertheim also found a new alkaloid mixed with the conine obtained by distillation from fresh hemlock flowers. It is crystallizable, fusible below 100° C. (212° F.), and volatilizable at a higher temperature, diffusing the peculiar odor of conine, or one very much like it. Water dissolves it considerably, ether and alcohol freely; and the solution has a strong alkaline reaction. Its formula is given as $C_8H_{17}NO$. When distilled with anhydrous phosphoric oxide it splits into conine and one molecule of water. (*A. J. P.*, xxix. 321.) It may be separated from conine by exposing the mixed alkaloids to a freezing mixture, expressing, and then repeatedly crystallizing from ether. (*Gmelin*, xiii. 169.)

Paraconine. Conine was supposed to have been artificially produced by Hugo

* Orfila gives the following additional chemical characters of conine. Heated in a capsule, it forms white vapors, *having a strong smell of celery and of the urine of mice.* Weak tincture of iodine gives a white precipitate, becoming olive with excess of the tincture. *Pure concentrated sulphuric acid does not alter it;* but when the mixture is heated, it becomes first brown, then blood-red, and finally black. *Nitric acid imparts a topaz color,* not changed by heat. The chlorides of platinum and of gold give yellow precipitates, and corrosive sublimate a white one. Permanganate of potassium is immediately decolorized. *Neutral acetate of lead gives no precipitate,* nor does the subacetate. The parts of this note in italics indicate the means of distinguishing this alkaloid from nicotina. (See *P. J. Tr.*, xi. 89.)

Schiff. From the reaction of *butyric aldehyd* with an alcoholic solution of ammonia, he obtained two bases, one of which, *dibutyraldine*, yielded on distillation, first a neutral oily substance, and afterwards a strong alkaline base, which proved to have all the physiological properties of natural conine, but was optically inactive, while true conine is right rotatory. Since the change in the formula of true conine it will be seen that the base *paraconine*, which is $C_8H_{15}N$, is not even isomeric with conine.

Medical Properties and Uses. Hemlock is supposed to be the narcotic used by the Athenians to destroy the life of condemned individuals, and by which Socrates and Phocion died. It was also used by the ancients as a medicine, but fell into entire neglect, and did not again come into notice till the time of Störck, by whom it was much employed and extravagantly praised. Anodyne, soporific, antispasmodic, antaphrodisiac, deobstruent, and diuretic properties have been ascribed to it. It was highly recommended by Störck as a remedy in schirrus and cancerous ulcers, and has since been employed in all kinds of chronic enlargements, and in diseases most numerous and most diverse.

Modern research has, however, greatly limited the use of the medicine, rendering its possession of alterative properties more than doubtful. When taken internally in sufficient dose it produces very profound muscular weakness, associated it may be with vertigo and disordered vision. After toxic doses the muscular prostration is extreme, the eyelids droop from weakness, the voice is suppressed, the pupils dilated, the light almost lost, consciousness is usually preserved to the last; and life finally is extinguished without struggle. In some cases there have been convulsive movements, and violent cardiac palpitation has been noted. The chief action of the poison is upon the motor nerves, which it paralyzes; the efferent or sensitive nerves are also affected, but to a much less extent. Conium probably exerts no direct influence upon the cerebral centres, but there is some reason for believing that it is a spinal depressant. At present conium is rarely employed by the general practitioner, except in spasmodic affections, such as chorea and hooping-cough. Probably the most frequent use of it is by alienists for the production of calm in maniacal excitement.

The powdered leaves and the inspissated juice are the preparations which have been most employed; but the juice of the fresh leaves is much used in England, and the fluid extract of the U. S. Pharmacopœia, made from the fruit, is the best of all preparations. The powdered leaves may be given in the dose of three or four grains (0·20–0·26 Gm.) twice a day, gradually increased till the occurrence of slight vertigo or nausea indicates that it has taken effect. To maintain a given impression, it is necessary to increase the dose even more rapidly than is customary with most other narcotics; as the system becomes very speedily habituated to its influence. In some instances, the quantity administered in one day has been augmented to more than two ounces. The strength of the preparations of hemlock is exceedingly unequal; and caution is therefore necessary, when the medicine is given in very large quantities, to employ the same parcel, or, if a change be made, to commence with the new parcel in small doses, so as to obviate any danger which might result from its greater power. Unpleasant consequences have followed a neglect of this precaution. There are also an officinal tincture, a fluid extract, an abstract, and an alcoholic extract, all of which, when properly made, are considered efficient preparations. The fresh juice of the plant has been recommended by Hufeland in the dose of from twelve to forty drops (0·72–2·5 C.c.). The expressed juice of the fresh plant, with a little alcohol for its preservation, recently introduced into the Pharmacopœias, is one of the most reliable forms in which the leaves can be used. The powdered seeds should be given in a dose considerably smaller than that of the leaves.* The fresh leaves are sometimes used externally as an anodyne cataplasm; and the extract, and an ointment prepared from the leaves,

* The root, while containing a small proportion of conine, is too feeble, according to the experiments of Dr. John Harley, of London, to be used practically with advantage. Dr. Harley has found in the root three new proximate principles, one a very bitter resin which he names *conamarine*, and the two others, crystallizable bodies, named, respectively, *rhizoconin* and *rhizoconicin*. They are all neutral, and so far as known medicinally inert. (See *P. J. Tr.*, Aug. 1867.)

are applied to the same purpose. A plaster made from the extract has also been employed.*

Conine acts precisely as does hemlock, and may be used for the same purposes. The dose is from one-fourth to one-half a drop (0·15 to 0·30 C.c.). A solution of one part in one hundred of very dilute alcohol has been used with advantage in certain cases of scrofulous ophthalmia with photophobia, applied several times daily by friction about the eyelids. (*Journ. de Pharm.*, 3e sér., xix. 219.) Prof. Mauthner, of Vienna, recommends it especially in the spasmodic contraction of the orbicularis oculi in scrofulous children, using a solution containing half a grain of conine in a drachm of almond oil, which he applies by a pencil to the eyelids twice or thrice daily. As a collyrium, from one to three drops may be added to six drachms of pure water, and two drachms of mucilage of quince seeds, the whole being very carefully strained.

The hydrochlorate of conine has been recommended for exhibition by Mr. G. C. Close, as preferable to the uncombined alkaloid. From half a grain he experienced no sensible effects; but a grain produced the characteristic symptoms of conine in an even unpleasant degree. These doses are probably dangerous, and not more than a fourth of a grain (0·015 Gm.) should be given as a commencing dose. (*A. J. P.*, 1869, p. 62.) According to Mourrut, one of the best crystallizable salts of conine is the *bromhydrate.* Dr. Harley has prepared an acid *benzoate of conine* by adding two mols. of the acid to one of the base, and found the resulting salt effectual in the dose of half a grain. (*P. J. Tr.*, Jan. 1871, p. 585.) Most of the conine of the market, however, is somewhat impure; it is accompanied by a brown oily body, which adheres to the crystals with great persistence: pure conine is colorless. The alkaloid is treated with aqueous bromhydric acid, which causes, especially with the brown variety of conine, an elevation of temperature, and a disengagement of white fumes of the odor of conine; the mixture then turns green, and finally blackish red. The crystals, which form after some time, may be obtained quite colorless by repeated crystallizations. They are colorless prismatic needles, soluble in water and alcohol, less so in ether and chloroform, inodorous and almost tasteless, and are not deliquescent. They should be kept in the dark, otherwise they assume a red tint. The salt has been used by various practitioners with great success, in the treatment of hooping-cough, in doses of about one-twelfth of a grain (·005 Gm.), if necessary, every hour, for a child three years of age; or one-thirtieth of a grain (·002 Gm.) for a child of one year; or one-sixth of a grain (·01 Gm.) for adults. In sciatica it has been employed hypodermically in quantities of one-twelfth of a grain (.005 Gm.) with good results. (*Répert. de Pharm.*, 1876, p. 369; *N. R.*, 1876, 1879, pp. 18, 178.)

Though fatal to some animals, hemlock is eaten with impunity by others, as horses, goats, and sheep. The best method of relieving its poisonous effects is the speedy evacuation of the stomach.†

* The following formula of Planche has been approved by the Society of Pharmacy, of Paris. Take of extract of hemlock 90 parts, of purified elemi 20 parts, of white wax 10 parts. Melt the resin and wax with a gentle heat, and incorporate the extract with the mixture. (*Journ. de Pharm.*, Juillet, 1862, p. 46.)

† Dr. Harley's experiments on the relative value of the different preparations of conium are based upon their physiological effects. The results obtained were as follows. 1. The Extractum Conii, *B. P.*, and Succus Conii, *B. P.*—20 grains of the extract equalled 2 fluidrachms of the juice (10 gr. to fʒj). 4. Succus Conii, *B. P.*; Tincture of the green fruit (London ℥v in ℥xx);—four drachms of the juice equalled fifty minims of the tincture (ʒiv to ♏50). 11. Different preparations of Succus, *B. P.*, prepared by different persons,—Buckle's (the plant yielding 75 per cent. of juice) and Hanbury's (the plant yielding 35 per cent. of juice);—nine drachms of Buckle's equalled three drachms of Hanbury's—(ʒix to ʒiij). 12. Extract of green fruit, Tincture of green fruit, and Succus, *B. P.*—Three grains of the extract equalled four fluidrachms of the Tincture, and four drachms of Succus (gr. iij of extract=fʒiv of Tincture, and ʒiv of Succus). 14. Of *Squibb's fluid extract* 50 minims equal of the *Tinct.* of the *green fruit*, London, ʒiss; of the Succus Conii, *B. P.*, ʒv; of the Tincture of the fresh plant, ʒiiiss to ʒiv; and of the Tincture of the dry plant, f℥j. 15. Of Squibb's fluid extract ʒj equals of pale Succus ʒvi, of dark Succus ʒij; of Tincture of the green fruit ʒiss; of Tincture of the fresh plant ʒiv; Neutral Benzoate of Conine, gr. ⅔. 18. Of Succus Conii, *B. P.* (Buckle's), ʒvj=Benzoate of Conine, gr. ⅓. The author draws the following conclusions from his experiments. The green fruit, as the basis of Tinctures and Extracts, is decidedly superior to any other part of the plant; and the spirituous extract of the green fruit should be substituted for the almost worthless Extract of the Br. Pharm. The variable strength of the Succus is an objection. (*P. J. Tr.*, Jan. 1871, p. 585.)

Off. Prep. Abstractum Conii; Extractum Conii Alcoholicum; Extractum Conii Fluidum; Tinctura Conii.
Off. Prep. Br. Tinctura Conii.
Off. Prep. of the Leaves. Br. Extractum Conii; Succus Conii.

COPAIBA. *U. S., Br.* *Copaiva.* [*Balsam of Copaiba.*]

(CO-PĀ'BA.)

"The oleoresin of Copaifera Langsdorffii, Desfontaines, and of other species of *Copaifera.* (*Nat. Ord.* Leguminosæ, Papilionaceæ.)" *U. S.* "The oleo-resin obtained by cutting deeply or boring into the trunk of Copaifera Langsdorffii, *Desf.*; and other species of Copaifera, *Linn.*" *Br.*

Balsamum Copaiva, *P.G.*; Balsam Copaiba, Balsam Capivi; Copahu, Oleo-résine (Baume) de Copahu, *Fr.*; Copaiva; Copaiva-Balsam, *G.*; Balsamo di Copaiba, *It.*; Balsamo de Copayva, *Sp.*

Gen. Ch. Calyx none. *Petals* four. *Legume* ovate. *Seed* one, with an ovate arillus. *Willd.*

Copaiba was first noticed in a work published by Purchas, in England, in 1625. The next reference to it was by Cristoval d'Acuña, in 1638. In 1648, Marcgrav and Piso gave a detailed account of the tree which produces it, and the methods of gathering it. Jacquin in 1763 described a species of Copaifera, growing in Martinique, which he named *C. officinalis.* As this was believed to be the same plant with the one observed by Marcgrav in Brazil, it was adopted in the Pharmacopœias; but their identity was denied; and Desfontaines proposed for Jacquin's species the title of *C. Jacquini*, in honor of that botanist. It is now known that many species of Copaifera exist in Brazil and other parts of South America; and all of them, according to Martius, yield copaiba. Besides *C. officinalis* or *C. Jacquini*, the following are described by Hayne:—*C. Guianensis, C. Langsdorffii, C. coriacea, C. Beyrichii, C. Martii, C. bijuga, C. nitida, C. laxa, C. cordifolia. C. Jussieui, C. Sellowii, C. oblongifolia*, and *C. multijuga.* Hayne believed that *C. bijuga* was the plant seen by Marcgrav and Piso. The four species to which in the Pharmacographia the production of copaiba is especially attributed are *C. officinalis*, L., *C. Guianensis*, Desf., *C. coriacea*, Mart., and the *C. Langsdorffii.*

C. officinalis is a native of Venezuela, and grows in the province of Carthagena, mingled with the trees which afford the balsam of Tolu. It grows also in some of the West India islands, particularly Trinidad and Martinique. Though recognized in former editions of the U. S. Pharmacopœia as a source of copaiba, it probably yields little of that now in use. According to Hayne (x. t. 17 f. c.), the species from which most of the copaiba of commerce is derived is *C. multijuga*, growing in the province of Para. It was recognized by the U. S. P. 1870; but Bentham, after examining the only specimens extant, asserts it not to be a Copaifera at all. It is probable that *C. Guianensis*, which inhabits the neighboring territory of Guiana, especially in the vicinity of the Rio Negro, affords also considerable quantities; and *C. Langsdorffii* and *C. coriacea*, which are natives of São Paulo, are thought to yield most of the juice collected in the latter province. *C. nitida*, inhabiting the province of Minas-Geraes, probably also contributes to the commercial supplies, through Rio Janeiro.

The juice is obtained by making a square chamber in the stems of the trees reaching to the very centre; and the operation is said to be repeated several times in the same season. A single tree is said to yield about eighty-four English Imperial pints. As it flows from the wound, it is clear, colorless, and very thin, but soon acquires a thicker consistence, and a yellowish tinge. It is most largely collected in the provinces of Para and Maranham, in Brazil, and is brought to this country from the port of Para, in small casks or barrels. Large quantities of it come from Maracaybo, in Venezuela, and from other ports on the Caribbean Sea, whence it is brought in casks, demijohns, cans, jugs, etc. The drug is also exported from Angostura, Cayenne, Rio Janeiro, and some of the West India islands.

Properties. Copaiba is a clear, transparent liquid, usually of the consistence of olive oil, of a pale yellow color, a peculiar not unpleasant odor, and a bitterish, hot, nauseous taste. Its sp. gr. varies ordinarily from 0·950 to 1·000, but has been known to be as low as 0·916. (Procter, *A. J. P.*, xxii. 292.)* It is insoluble in water, but entirely soluble in absolute alcohol, ether, and the fixed and volatile oils. Strong alkaline solutions dissolve it perfectly; but the resulting solution becomes turbid when largely diluted with water. With the alkalies and alkaline earths it forms saponaceous compounds, in which the resin of the copaiba acts the part of an acid. It dissolves magnesia, especially with the aid of heat, and even disengages carbonic acid from the carbonate of that earth. If triturated with a sixteenth of its weight of magnesia and set aside, it gradually assumes a solid consistence; and a similar change is produced with hydrate of lime. (See *Pilulæ Copaibæ.*) Its essential constituents are volatile oil and resin, with at times small quantities of acids. As it contains no benzoic acid, it cannot with propriety retain its old title of *balsam of copaiva.* The substances which it most closely resembles, both in composition and properties, are the turpentines. (See *Oleum Copaibæ.*)

"A transparent or translucent, more or less viscid liquid, of a color varying from pale yellow to brownish-yellow; having a peculiar, aromatic odor and a persistently bitter and acrid taste. Sp. gr. 0·940–0·993. It is readily soluble in absolute alcohol. It is not fluorescent, and when heated to 130° C. (266° F.), does not become gelatinous. When subjected to heat, it does not evolve the odor of turpentine, and after distilling off the volatile oil the residue, when cool, should be hard and friable (abs. of fixed oils). The essential oil distilled off from the oleoresin, when rectified, should not begin to boil below 200° C. (392° F.). On adding 1 drop of Copaiba to 19 drops of disulphide of carbon and shaking the mixture with 1 drop of a cold mixture of equal parts of sulphuric and nitric acids, it should not acquire a purplish-red or violet color (abs. of gurjun balsam)." *U. S.*

The *resinous* mass which remains after the distillation of the oil is hard, brittle, translucent, greenish brown, and nearly destitute of smell and taste. By mixing it with the oil in proper proportion, we may obtain a liquid identical or nearly so with the original juice. This resinous mass is of an acid character, and yields a series of amorphous salts. It may be obtained pure by exposing a mixture of 9 parts of copaiba and 2 parts of aqueous ammonia (sp. gr. 0·95) to a temperature of 10° C. In this way crystals of *copaivic acid*, $C_{20}H_{30}O_2$, are obtained. This acid agrees with the *abietic acid* of colophony in composition, but not in properties.

Copaivic acid is readily soluble in alcohol, and especially in warmed copaiba itself; much less in ether. When recrystallized from alcohol, copaivic acid fuses at 116°–117° C. (241°–242·6° F.). (*A. J. P.*, 1879, p. 305.) An analogous substance, *oxycopaivic acid*, $C_{20}H_{28}O_3$, was found in 1841 by H. von Fehling in Para copaiba; and Strauss in 1865 extracted *metacopaivic acid*, $C_{22}H_{34}O_4$, from Maracaibo copaiba.

Copaivic acid forms crystallizable salt with alkalies, and the *copaiviate of sodium*, $NaC_{20}H_{29}O_2$, made by combining equivalent quantities of the acid and soda, is claimed by Zlamál and Roquette to be more efficient than any other preparation of copaiba. A *miscible copaiba* proposed by Groves was made by treating copaiba with a saturated solution of carbonate of potassium. It resembled ordinary copaiba in appearance and consistence, but was alkaline, and when shaken with water, instead of floating on the surface readily formed a white emulsion, more or less stable according to the degree of dilution. (*P. J. Tr.*, ix. 195.)

Copaiba, upon exposure to the air, acquires a deeper color, a thicker consistence, and greater density, and, if spread out upon an extended surface, ultimately becomes dry and brittle. This change is owing partly to the volatilization, partly to the oxidation of the essential oil. As it is the soft resin that results from the oxidation of the oil, it follows that the proportion of this resin increases with age. Considerable

* The variety of copaiba found by Prof. Procter to have this low sp. gr. was supposed to be from Para. It was of a light straw color, very fluid, and possessed of the pure copaiba odor. It contained 80 per cent. of volatile oil and 20 of resin, and was not affected by recently calcined magnesia. It appears to be the same with a variety described by Dr. L. Posselt in the *Chemical Gazette* for May 1, 1849. The view of Prof. Procter that it is the product of young trees, in which the juice has not become fully elaborated, is highly probable. As the virtues of copaiba depend mainly on the oil, this variety should be more efficacious than the copaiba in common use.

diversity must, therefore, exist in the drug, both in physical properties and the properties of its ingredients, according to its age and degree of exposure. Similar differences also exist in the copaiba procured from different sources. Thus, that of the *West Indies*, when compared with the *Brazilian*, which is the variety above described, and in common use, is of a thicker consistence, of a deeper or darker yellow color, less transparent, and of a less agreeable, more terebinthinate odor; and specimens obtained from the ports of Venezuela or Colombia were found, upon examination by M. Vigne, to differ from each other not only in physical properties, but also in their chemical relations. (*Journ. de Pharm.*, N. S., i. 52.) The same is true, as observed by M. Buignet, in their action on polarized light, in which they differ not only in degree, but sometimes also even in direction. (*Journ. de Pharm.*, Oct. 1861, pp. 266–7.) It is not impossible that differences may exist in the juice according to the circumstances of its collection. The species of Copaifera from which the juice is collected, as well as the age of the tree, its position, and the season of collection, must also have influence over the product. It is highly probable that the resinous matter results from oxidation of the oil in the cells of the plant, and that the less elaborated the juice may be, the larger proportion it will contain of the oil. It is said that a volatile oil flows abundantly from a tree near Bogota, which is employed to adulterate the copaiba collected in that vicinity and shipped from Maracaibo and other neighboring ports.

Adulterations. Copaiba is said to be frequently adulterated.* The fixed oils are the most frequent addition, especially castor oil, which, in consequence of its solubility in alcohol, cannot, like the others, be detected by the agency of that fluid. Various plans have been proposed for detecting the presence of castor oil. The simplest is to boil a drachm of the copaiba in a pint of water, till the liquid is wholly evaporated. If the copaiba contain a fixed oil, the residue will be more or less soft, according to the quantity present; otherwise it will be hard. Another mode, proposed by M. Planche, consists in shaking together in a bottle one part of solution of ammonia of the sp. gr. 0·9212 (22° Baumé) with two and a half parts of copaiba, at a temperature of from 50° to 60° F. The mixture, at first cloudy, quickly becomes transparent if the copaiba is pure, but remains more or less opaque if it is adulterated with castor oil. According to J. E. Simon, however, a variety of genuine copaiba occurs in commerce in which this test fails (*A. J. P.*, xvi. 236); and it does not apply to the variety containing 80 per cent. of volatile oil, described by Prof. Procter. (See note, p. 490.) Carbonate of magnesium, caustic potassa, and sulphuric acid have also been proposed as tests. In the late Edinburgh Pharmacopœia, it was stated that copaiba "dissolves a fourth part of its weight of carbonate of magnesium, with the aid of a gentle heat, and continues translucent." The presence of a small proportion of any fixed oil renders the mixture opaque. One part of potassa dissolved in two of water forms a clear solution with nine parts of pure copaiba, and the liquid continues clear when moderately diluted with water or alcohol; but the presence of one-sixth of fixed oil in the copaiba occasions more or less opacity in the liquid, and half the quantity causes the precipitation of white flakes in a few hours. (*Stolze.*) Turpentine, which is said to be sometimes added to copaiba, may be detected by its smell, especially if the copaiba be heated. According to Mr. Redwood, most of the proposed tests of the purity of copaiba are liable to fallacy; and the best measure of its activity is the quantity of volatile oil it affords by distillation. Castor oil, Venice turpentine, linseed oil, or Gurjun Balsam may be detected by means of petroleum benzin, which makes a clear solution with pure copaiba, but if either of the substances mentioned be present a milky mixture, which soon settles into two layers, is formed, the copaiba solution being on top (*A. J. P.*, July, 1873; *Proc. A. P. A.*, xxiv. 191; xxvi. 286). Prof. Maisch has found that *ten* volumes of benzin, instead of *three* as proposed by Prof. Wayne, must be added to one of copaiba to get the best results from this test. Indeed,

* Some years since a substance was imported into New York, under the name of *red copaiba*, which had not a single character of the genuine drug. It was of a thick, semifluid consistence, not unlike that of balsam of Tolu, as it often reaches us, a brown color similar to that of the same balsam, though darker, and an unpleasant yet somewhat aromatic odor, recalling that of liquidambar, but less agreeable. Its origin is unknown.

it has been shown that pure copaiba will sometimes show turbidity when mixed with benzin. (*A. J. P.*, 1877, p. 131.) Hager recommends the use of absolute alcohol, which he says completely dissolves, without turbidity, all the varieties of copaiba except the Para, whose solution on standing clears itself by the deposition of a few white flakes. J. M. Fulton asserts that some pure copaibas are not entirely dissolved by absolute alcohol. (*A. J. P.*, 1877.)

Medical Properties and Uses. Copaiba is gently stimulant, diuretic, laxative, and in very large doses often actively purgative. It produces, when swallowed, a sense of heat in the throat and stomach, and extends an irritant action, not only throughout the alimentary canal, but also to the urinary passages, and in fact, in a greater or less degree, to all the mucous membranes, for which it appears to have a strong affinity. The urine acquires a peculiar odor during its use, and its smell may be detected in the breath. It sometimes occasions an eruption upon the skin, resembling that of measles, and attended with disagreeable itching and tingling. A case has been recently recorded, in which an acute attack of pemphigus over the whole body attended its use. (*N. Y. Med. Journ.*, Jan. 1873, p. 416.) Nausea and vomiting, painful purgation, strangury, and bloody urine, and a general state of fever are caused by excessive doses. As a remedy it has been found most efficient in diseases of the mucous membranes, particularly those of a chronic character. Thus, it is given with occasional advantage in leucorrhœa, gleet, chronic dysentery, and diarrhœa, painful hemorrhoidal affections, and chronic bronchitis, and has even been used in diphtheria and pseudo-membranous croup. By the late Dr. La Roche, of Philadelphia, it was highly recommended in catarrh and chronic irritation of the bladder. (*Am. Journ. of Med. Sci.*, xiv. 13.) It has been given in psoriasis and dropsy, and is said to be used as a vermifuge in Brazil. The complaint, however, in which it is most employed is gonorrhœa. It should not be administered in the first stages, when the inflammation is severe and acute, nor is it applicable to very chronic, indolent forms of the disorder, such as gleet. It was formerly much esteemed as a vulnerary, and as an application to ulcers; but it is now seldom used externally. Dr. Ruschenberger recommends it locally in chilblains. (*Med. Examiner*, i. 77.) Prof. Marchal, of Strasburg, has employed it with great success in gonorrhœa and leucorrhœa, injecting an emulsion made with 5 parts of copaiba, 8 of gum arabic, and 100 of water, or applying it smeared on catheters or tampons.

The dose of copaiba is from twenty drops to a fluidrachm (1·25–3·75 C.c.) three times a day, or a smaller quantity repeated more frequently. It may be given dropped on sugar, but in this form is often so exceedingly offensive as to render some concealment of its nauseous qualities necessary. A less disagreeable form is that of emulsion, prepared by rubbing the copaiba first with mucilage or the yolk of an egg, and sugar, and afterwards with some aromatic water, as that of mint or cinnamon. The *volatile oil*, which is officinal, may be given in the dose of ten or fifteen drops, in emulsion, or, as is almost universally preferred, in capsules.

Both the volatile oil and resin are eliminated by the kidneys in an altered condition: if to the urine of a person taking the drug nitric acid be added, a precipitate is thrown down, which may be mistaken for albumen. The volatile oil is more active than is the resin, which is not, however, inert. Dr. Wilks, of Guy's Hospital, London, speaks of the resin with great confidence as a hydragogue diuretic in obstinate dropsy, given in the dose of fifteen or twenty grains three times a day.

Velpeau has found the best effects from copaiba in the form of enema. He gives two drachms made into an emulsion with the yolk of an egg, twenty or thirty drops of laudanum, and eight fluidounces of water. Dr. E. Langlebert recommends a distilled water of copaiba internally, in the dose of one or two fluidounces (30–60 C.c.) three or four times a day, and as a vehicle in urethral injections.

Off. Prep. Massa Copaibæ. *Off. Prep. Br.* Oleum Copaibæ.

CORIANDRUM. *U. S.* *Coriander.*

(CŌ-RI-ĂN′DRŬM.)

"The fruit of Coriandrum sativum. Linné. (*Nat. Ord.* Umbelliferæ, Cœlospermæ.)" *U. S.* "The dried ripe fruit of Coriandrum sativum." *Br.*

Coriandri Fructus, *Br.;* Coriander Fruit; Fructus Coriandri, *P.G.;* Coriandre, *Fr.;* Koriander, *G.;* Coriandro, *It.;* Cilantro, *Sp.*

Gen. Ch. Corolla radiate. *Petals* inflex-emarginate. *Universal involucre* one-leafed. *Partial involucres* halved. *Fruit* spherical. *Willd.*

Coriandrum sativum. Willd. *Sp. Plant.* i. 1448; Woodv. *Med. Bot.* p. 137, t. 53. This is an annual plant, with an erect, round, smooth, branching stem, rising about two feet, and furnished with compound leaves, of which the upper are thrice ternate, with linear pointed leaflets, the lower pinnate, with the pinnæ cut into irregular serrated lobes like those of parsley. The flowers are white or rose-colored, and in compound terminal umbels; the fruit globular, and composed of two concave hemispherical portions.

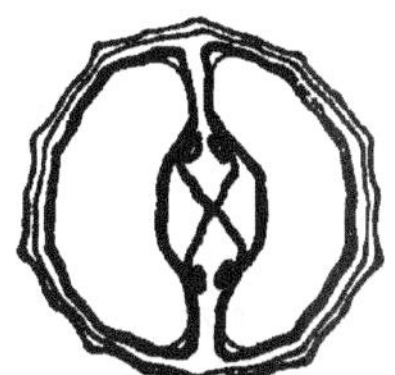
Transverse section, magnified.

C. sativum is a native of Italy, but at present grows wild in most parts of Europe, having become naturalized in consequence of its extended cultivation. The flowers appear in June, and the fruit ripens in August. It is a singular fact, that all parts of the fresh plant are extremely fetid when bruised, while the fruit becomes fragrant by drying. This is the officinal portion. It is brought to us from Europe.

The fruit of the coriander is globular, about an eighth of an inch in diameter, obscurely ten-ribbed, with minute indications of secondary ribs in the furrows, of a grayish or brownish yellow color, and separable into the two mericarps (half-fruits), which are only bound together by the membranous pericarp. Each half-fruit is provided with two oil-tubes on the conjoining face. The whole fruit has the persistent calyx at its base, and is sometimes surmounted by the adhering conical style. Coriander is thus described by the U. S. Pharm. "Globular; about one-sixth of an inch (4 mm.) in diameter; crowned with the calyx-teeth; brownish-yellow, with slight, longitudinal ridges; the two mericarps cohering, enclosing a lenticular cavity, and each furnished on the face with two oil-tubes; odor and taste agreeably aromatic." *U. S.* The aromatic smell and taste depend on a *volatile oil,* which may be obtained separate by distillation, and is said to belong to the camphene family. One pound of the seeds yields forty-two grains of the oil. (*Zeller.*) It is colorless or pale yellow, with an agreeable odor of coriander, a mild aromatic taste, and a sp. gr. varying from 0·859 to 0·871. It has the composition $C_{10}H_{18}O$, and is therefore isomeric with borneol. It is one of the most permanent of the volatile oils, resisting oxidation for a long time. The virtues of the fruit are imparted to alcohol by maceration, and less readily to water.

Medical Properties and Uses. Coriander has, in a moderate degree, the ordinary medicinal virtues of the aromatics. It is almost exclusively employed in combination with other medicines, either to cover their taste, to render them acceptable to the stomach, or to correct their griping qualities. It was well known to the ancients. The dose is from a scruple to a drachm (1·3–3·9 Gm.).

Off. Prep. Confectio Sennæ.

Off. Prep. Br. Confectio Sennæ; Oleum Coriandri; Syrupus Rhei; Tinctura Rhei; Tinctura Sennæ.

CORNUS. *U. S.* *Cornus.* [*Dogwood.*]

(CŎR'NŬS.)

"The bark of the root of Cornus Florida. Linné. (*Nat. Ord.* Cornaceæ.)" *U. S.*

Écorce de Cornouiller à grandes Fleurs, *Fr.;* Grossblüthige Cornelrinde, *G.*

Gen. Ch. Flowers perfect or diœcious. *Calyx* minutely four-toothed. *Petals* four, oblong, spreading. *Stamens* four. *Filaments* slender. *Style* slender. *Stigma* terminal, flat, or capitate. *Drupe* small, with a two-celled and two-seeded stone. *Gray's Manual.*

Cornus Florida. Willd. *Sp. Plant.* i. 661; Bigelow, *Am. Med. Bot.* ii. 73; Barton, *Med. Bot.* i. 44. This is a small indigenous tree, usually about fifteen or twenty feet in height, though sometimes not less than thirty or thirty-five feet. It is of slow growth; and the stem, which generally attains a diameter of four or five inches, is compact, and covered with a brownish bark, the epidermis of which is minutely divided by numerous superficial cracks or fissures. The branches are spreading, and regularly disposed, sometimes opposite, sometimes in fours nearly in the form of crosses. The leaves are opposite, oval, about three inches long, pointed, dark green and sulcated on the upper surface, glaucous or whitish beneath, and marked with strong parallel veins. Towards the close of summer they are speckled with black spots, and on the approach of cold weather become red. The proper flowers are small, yellowish, and collected in heads, which are surrounded by a large conspicuous involucre, consisting of four white obcordate leaves, having the notch at their summit tinged with red or purple. This involucre constitutes the chief beauty of the tree, and is commonly called the flower. The calyx is four-toothed, and the corolla composed of four obtuse reflexed petals. The fruit is an oval drupe, of a vivid glossy redness, containing a two-celled and two-seeded nucleus. The drupes are usually associated together to the number of three or four, and remain on the tree till after the early frosts. They ripen in September. The dogwood is found in all parts of the United States, from Massachusetts to the Mississippi and the Gulf of Mexico, but is most abundant in the Middle States. In the month of May it is clothed with a profusion of large white blossom-clusters, which render it one of the most conspicuous ornaments of the American forests. The bark is the officinal portion, and is derived for use both from the stem and the branches, and from the root. That from the root is preferred.

As brought into market, the bark is in pieces of various size, usually more or less rolled, sometimes invested with a fawn-colored epidermis, sometimes partially or wholly deprived of it, of a reddish gray color, very brittle, and affording, when pulverized, a grayish powder tinged with red. "In curved pieces of various sizes, about one-eighth of an inch (3 mm.) thick; deprived of the furrowed, brown-gray, corky layer; outer and inner surface pale-reddish, or light reddish-brown, striate; transverse and longitudinal fracture short, whitish, with brown, yellow striæ; inodorous; astringent and bitter." *U. S.* The odor of dogwood is feeble, its taste bitter, astringent, and slightly aromatic. Water and alcohol extract its virtues. From the experiments of Dr. Walker and Mr. James Cockburn (*A. J. P.*, vii. 109), it appears to contain bitter extractive, gum, resin, tannin, gallic acid, fixed oil, wax, red coloring matter, lignin, and salts of potassa and iron. Mr. Cockburn also obtained a crystallized substance, without taste, the characters of which, however, were not sufficiently investigated to authorize an opinion as to its nature. A peculiar bitter principle, for which the name of *cornine* was proposed, was announced as an ingredient by Mr. Carpenter; but his results have not been confirmed. Prof. John M. Maisch appears subsequently to have obtained the bitter principle pure in solution, but, in consequence of its extreme facility of decomposition, did not succeed in isolating it. Geiger (*Ann. Ch. und Pharm.*, xiv. 206) first obtained the bitter principle *cornin*, or *cornic acid*, in white, silky, bitter needles, readily soluble in water and alcohol, little in ether, colored dark by alkalies. It is neutral and is not precipitated by infusion of nutgalls, but is precipitated by acetate of lead and by silver solutions. A. G. Frey (*A. J. P*, 1879, p. 390) also obtained *cornin* in pure white crystals out of alcohol. The flowers of *C. Florida* have the same bitter taste as the bark, and, though not officinal, are sometimes employed for the same purposes.*

* Two other indigenous dogwoods were formerly recognized in the U. S. secondary list. *C. circinata* is a shrub from six to ten feet high, with warty branches, large, roundish, pointed leaves, waved on their edges and downy beneath, and white flowers disposed in depressed cymes. The fruit is blue. The plant is a native of the United States, extending from Canada to Virginia, and growing on hill-sides and the banks of rivers. It flowers in June and July. The bark, when dried, is in quills of a whitish or ash color, and affords a powder resembling that of ipecacuanha. Its taste is bitter, astringent, and aromatic. In chemical composition, so far as this has been ascertained, it is analogous to *Cornus Florida*.

C. sericea is usually six or eight feet in height, with numerous erect stems, which are covered with a shining reddish bark, and send out opposite spreading branches. The young shoots are more or less pubescent. The leaves are opposite, petiolate, ovate, pointed, entire, and on the under surface covered with soft brownish hairs. The flowers are small, white, and disposed in terminal cymes, which are depressed and woolly. The fruit consists of globular, berry-formed drupes, of a cerulean blue color, and collected in bunches. The bark of both of these species is said to be of equal medical value with that of *C. Florida*.

Medical Properties and Uses. *Cornus Florida* is tonic and astringent. By Dr. Walker it was found, when taken internally, to increase the force and frequency of the pulse, and the heat of the body. It is thought to possess remedial properties analogous to those of Peruvian bark, for which it has occasionally been successfully substituted in the treatment of intermittent fevers; but the introduction of sulphate of quinine into use has nearly banished this, as well as many other substitutes for cinchona, from regular practice. The dogwood has also been employed in low fevers, and other complaints for which Peruvian bark is usually prescribed.

It may be given in powder, decoction, or extract. The dose of the powder is from a scruple to a drachm (1·3–3·9 Gm.), repeated, in cases of intermittent fever, so that from one to two ounces may be taken in the interval between the paroxysms. The decoction was officinal in 1870. The dried bark is said to be preferable to the fresh; as it possesses all the activity of the latter, without being so liable to offend the stomach and bowels. An extract might probably be used with advantage in intermittents in large doses.

Off. Prep. Extractum Cornûs Fluidum.

CREASOTUM. *U. S., Br.* *Creasote.*

(CRĒ-A-SŌ'TŬM.)

"A product of the distillation of wood-tar." *U. S., Br.*

Kreosotum, *P.G.;* Créosote, *Fr.;* Kreosot, *G.*

This is a substance discovered in 1830 by Reichenbach in the products of the distillation of wood. This distillation of wood yields products very analogous to one fraction of the coal-tar obtained by the destructive distillation of bituminous coal. This fraction is the heavy oil of coal-tar, which comes over between 165° C. (329° F.) and 200° C. (392° F.): it is often called "*coal-tar creasote,*" and contains a group of phenols, including carbolic acid, or common *phenol*, C_6H_6O, boiling at 182° C. (359·6 F.), *cresylic acid*, or *cresol*, C_7H_8O, boiling at 198° C. (388·4 F.), and *xylenol*, or *dimethyl phenol*, $C_8H_{10}O$, boiling at 211° C. (411·8° F.).

"Wood-tar creasote," on the other hand, is chiefly composed of the following phenols. *Guiacol*, or *oxycresol*, $C_7H_8O_2$, boiling at 200° C. (392 F.), *creasol*, $C_8H_{10}O_2$, boiling at 217° C. (422·6° F.), *methyl-creasol*, $C_9H_{12}O_2$, boiling at 214° C. (417° F.) to 218° C. (424·4° F.), and *phlorol*, $C_8H_{10}O_1$, boiling at 219° C. (426·2 F.). (See also *Allen's Commerc. Org. Analysis*, p. 306.)

Preparation. Creasote is obtained either from wood-tar or from crude pyroligneous acid. When wood-tar is used, it is distilled until it has attained the consistence of pitch. The distilled liquid divides itself into three layers, an aqueous between two oily layers. The inferior oily layer, which alone contains the creasote, is separated, and saturated with carbonate of sodium to remove acetic acid. The liquid is allowed to rest, and the new oil which separates is decanted from it. This oil is distilled, and yields products lighter than water, and a liquid heavier. The latter alone is preserved, and, after having been agitated repeatedly with weak phosphoric acid to neutralize ammonia, is allowed to remain at rest for some time. It is next washed as long as acidity is removed, and then distilled with a fresh portion of weak phosphoric acid; care being taken to cohobate from time to time. The oily liquid thus rectified is colorless, and contains much creasote, but also a portion of *eupion* or light oil distillate. To separate the latter, the liquid is mixed with a solution of caustic soda of the density 1·12, which dissolves the creasote, but not the eupion. The eupion, which floats above from its levity, is then separated; and the alkaline solution of the creasote is exposed to the air, until it becomes brown in consequence of the decomposition of a foreign matter, and is then saturated with sulphuric acid. This sets free the creasote, which is decanted, and again distilled. The treatment by solution of soda, sulphuric acid, etc., is to be repeated until the creasote no longer becomes brown by exposure to the air, but only slightly reddish. It is then dissolved in a stronger solution of soda, and distilled again, and finally redistilled for the last time, rejecting the first portion which comes over on account of its containing much water, collecting the next portion, and avoiding to push the distillation too far. The product collected in this distillation is creasote.

When creasote is extracted from pyroligneous acid, the first step is to dissolve sulphate of sodium in it to saturation. The oil which separates and floats above is decanted, and, having been allowed to remain at rest for a few days, is saturated by carbonate of potassium with the assistance of heat, and distilled with water. The oleaginous liquid obtained is of a pale yellow color, and is to be treated with phosphoric acid, etc., as above detailed, in relation to the treatment of the corresponding oil obtained from wood-tar.

Properties. Creasote, when pure, is a colorless oleaginous liquid, of the consistence of oil of almonds, slightly greasy to the touch, volatilizable by heat, and having a caustic, burning taste, and a penetrating, disagreeable odor, like that of smoked meat, and analogous to, yet different from, that of phenol. As met with in the shops, it has frequently a brownish tinge. It burns with a sooty flame. Applied in a concentrated state to the skin, it corrugates and then destroys the cuticle, causing a white spot. On paper it leaves a greasy stain, which disappears in a few hours, or in ten minutes if heated to 100° C. (212° F.). Its sp. gr. is 1·057 at 55° (*Gorup-Besanez*), 1·035–1·085 (*U. S.*), 1·071 (*Br.*). It boils at about 203° C. (397° F.), and remains fluid at —27° C. (—17°F.). It is a non-conductor of electricity, and refracts light strongly. It is devoid of acid or alkaline reaction. Mixed with water, it forms two solutions; one consisting of one part of creasote and about eighty of water, the other, of one part of water and ten of creasote. (*Berzelius.*) It dissolves a large proportion of iodine and phosphorus, and a considerable amount of sulphur, especially when assisted by heat.

The Pharmacopœia describes creasote as "an almost colorless or yellowish, strongly refractive, oily liquid, turning to reddish-yellow or brown by exposure to light, having a penetrating, smoky odor, a burning, caustic taste and a neutral reaction. Sp. gr. 1·035–1·085. It begins to boil near 200° C. (392° F.), and most of it distils over between 205° and 220° C. (401°–428° F.). When cooled to —20° C. (—4°F.) it becomes thick, but does not solidify. It is inflammable, burning with a luminous, smoky flame. Creasote is soluble in about 80 parts of water at 15° C. (59° F.) to a somewhat turbid liquid, and in 12 parts of boiling water; it dissolves, in all proportions, in absolute alcohol, ether, chloroform, benzin, disulphide of carbon, or acetic acid. When applied to the skin, it produces a white stain. Creasote does not coagulate albumen or collodion (difference from carbolic acid). If 1 volume of Creasote be mixed with 1 volume of glycerin, a nearly clear mixture will result, from which the Creasote will be separated by the addition of 1 or more volumes of water. On adding to 10 C.c. of a 1 per cent. aqueous solution of Creasote, 1 drop of test-solution of ferric chloride, the liquid acquires a violet-blue tint, which rapidly changes to greenish and brown, with formation, usually, of a brown precipitate (diff. from carbolic acid)." *U. S.*

Creasote instantly dissolves ammonia, and retains it with great force. Strong nitric and sulphuric acids decompose it; the former giving rise to reddish vapors, the latter to a red color, which becomes black on the addition of more of the acid. Dilute nitric acid converts it into a brown resin, which, treated with ammonia, and then dissolved in boiling alcohol, gives, by evaporation, certain salts of ammonia, two of which contain new acids, discovered by Laurent. Hydrochloric acid produces no change in it. "Dropped on white filtering paper and exposed to a temperature of 212° F. (100° C.), it leaves no translucent stain. It turns the plane of polarization of a ray of polarized light to the right. It is not solidified by the cold produced by a mixture of hydrochloric acid and sulphate of sodium." *Br.* Mr. Morson, of London, who has long been a manufacturer of creasote, complains of the discredit into which it has fallen in consequence of the substitution for it in commerce, of carbolic acid; while he says that the directions of the Pharmacopœia for the distinction of the two are insufficient, and gives a test, discovered by his son Mr. Thos. Morson, which is at once simple and satisfactory. It consists in the solvent power of glycerin over carbolic acid, which is dissolved by it in all proportions, while pure creasote is insoluble or nearly so; and, consequently, if any liquid, assumed to be creasote, dissolves largely in glycerin, it probably consists in the whole, or in large part, of carbolic acid. (*P. J. Tr.*, May, 1872, p. 921.) Subsequent experiments appear to show that this test succeeds best with Morson's creasote; and beech-wood creasote, although pure, sometimes mixes with glycerin without turbidity. A still better test, according to Mr. John A. Clark, is an alcoholic solution of perchloride of iron (*Tr. Ferri Perchlor.* B. Ph.), which with an alcoholic solution of creasote produces a deep greenish blue color, but with carbolic acid a light brown. (*A. J. P.*, June, 1873, p. 269.) Creasote dissolves a large number of metallic salts, and reduces some of them to the metallic state; as, for example, nitrate and acetate of silver. *Froehde's reagent* (a solution of 1 part of molybdic acid in 100 parts of sulphuric acid) is recommended by E. W. Davy as a distinguishing test for carbolic acid. (*P. J. Tr.*, 1878, p. 1022.) A drop or two of the doubtful liquid is to be agitated with two fluidrachms of distilled water, the whole filtered, and a drop or two of the test-solution added. Pure creasote gives a brown or reddish brown reaction on standing or slight warming, passing to a light yellowish brown; with carbolic acid, the brown passing to a maroon soon develops a more or less intense purple.

Of all the properties of creasote, the most remarkable is its power of preserving meat. It is this property which has suggested its name, derived from κρεάς, *flesh*, and σώζω, *I preserve.*

Impurities and Adulterations. Creasote is apt to contain eupion, and is sometimes adulterated with rectified oil of tar, and the fixed and volatile oils. All these substances are detected by strong acetic acid, which dissolves the creasote, and leaves them behind, floating above the creasote solution. Creasote, however, from beech-wood tar, is only partially dissolved by hot acetic acid of ordinary strength. Fixed oils are also discovered by a stain on paper not discharged by heat. Any trace of the matter which produces the brownish tinge is detected by the liquid becoming discolored by exposure to sunshine.

Commercial creasote almost always contains carbolic and cresylic acids, from coal-tar; and indeed, much of what is sold for creasote is nothing more than impure carbolic acid. (See *Acidum Carbolicum.*) It has been already stated that this acid strongly resembles creasote; and this resemblance probably extends also to their therapeutical effects; so that the substitution is less to be regretted than might otherwise be the case. But, as the effects of the two on the system may not be identical, it is highly desirable to be able to distinguish between them. Tests for this purpose have been given above, and, with those quoted from the Pharmacopœia, are sufficient for the purpose.

Medical Properties, etc. The influence of creasote upon the animal economy has never been carefully studied, but is probably identical with that of carbolic acid. It is never used in medicine except for its local action. Applied in this way it is a powerful paralysant of nerve-tissue, and hence is frequently employed with great advantage in cases of nausea, vomiting, or diarrhœa dependent upon excessive irritability, without acute inflammation, of the gastric or intestinal mucous membrane; it has also been successfully used in nausea and vomiting of pregnancy or hysteria, in cholera morbus, cholera infantum, lienteric diarrhœa, typhoid fever, and even in dysentery. When in these cases there is a tendency to fermentation of the contents of the stomach or bowels, creasote is especially valuable, and may often be combined advantageously with an alkali or chalk. Externally creasote has been employed for exactly the same diseases as has carbolic acid. Indeed, the latter remedy, on account of its superior cheapness, has almost entirely supplanted it.

The skin diseases to the treatment of which creasote has been supposed to be best suited are those of a scaly character. In burns its efficacy has been insisted on, especially in those attended with excessive suppuration and fungous granulations. In chilblains also it is stated to be a useful application. Mixed with four parts of lard, it is said to have proved very serviceable in erysipelas. When applied to wounds it acts as a hæmostatic, stopping the capillary hemorrhage, but possessing no power to arrest the bleeding from large vessels. Accordingly, creasote water has been applied locally in menorrhagia, and to arrest uterine hemorrhage and the bleeding from leech-bites. The ulcers, in the treatment of which it has been found most useful, are those of an indolent and gangrenous character, in which its several properties of escharotic, stimulant, and antiseptic are usefully brought into play. In all these cases, should the remedy cause irritation, it must be suspended, or alternated with emollient and soothing applications. Injected into fistulous ulcers, it proves a useful resource, by exciting the callous surfaces and disposing them to unite.

Wherever there are foul ulcers, gangrenous surfaces, or inflamed serous, mucous, or glandular tissues giving rise to fetid discharges, creasote may be substituted for carbolic acid; as examples, may be mentioned fetid leucorrhœa, puerperal metritis, fetid otorrhœa, putrid or diphtheritic sore throat, chronic empyema. The strength of the application may vary from that of pure creasote to a single drop to the fluidounce of water, according to the delicacy of the part and the severity of the disease. On account of its local anæsthetic and antiseptic influence, it is much employed by dentists for the obtunding of sensitive dentine and as an ingredient of pastes for the destruction of nerves. One or two drops of the pure substance must be carefully introduced into the hollow of the tooth, on a little cotton, avoiding contact with the tongue or cheek. To render it effectual, the hollow of the tooth must be well cleansed before it is applied. A mixture of 15 parts of creasote and 10 of collodion is said to have a jelly-like consistence, and to be usefully applied to carious teeth, which it protects from the air; but, as pure creasote does not coagulate collodion, this remark applies properly to the impure carbolic acid, before stated to be commonly sold under the same name.

Under the name of VAPOR CREASOTI (*Inhalation of Creasote*), the British Pharmacopœia directs a preparation consisting of 12 minims of creasote and 8 fluidounces of boiling water, which are to be mixed in an inhaling apparatus, so arranged that the air shall be made to pass through the solution and then inhaled It may be used in chronic inflammation of the air-passages.

The internal dose of creasote is one to three minims (0·6–0·18 C.c.), administered in pill, mixture, or solution. In an overdose, it acts as a poison, producing giddiness, obscurity of vision, depressed action of the heart, convulsions, and coma. Whether the soluble sulphates would be antidotal to it, as to carbolic acid, is uncertain, but there is no other available antidote. The medical treatment consists in the evacuation of the poison, and the administration of ammonia and other stimulants.

The addition of three or four drops of creasote to a pint of ink effectually prevents it from becoming mouldy. Dr. Christison finds that creasote water is as good a preservative of some anatomical preparations as spirit, with the advantage of not hardening the parts. It is probably to creasote that the antiseptic properties of wood-smoke and of pyroligneous acid are owing.

Off. Prep. Aqua Creasoti.

Off. Prep. Br. Mistura Creasoti; Unguentum Creasoti; Vapor Creasoti.

CRETA. *Br.* *Chalk.*

$Ca\,CO_3$; 100. (CRĒ'TA.) $Ca\,O, CO_2$; 50.

"Native friable carbonate of lime." *Br.*

Craie, *Fr.*; Kreide, *G.*; Creta, *It.*; Greda, *Sp.*, *Port.*

Carbonate of calcium, in the extended meaning of the term, is the most abundant of simple minerals, constituting, according to its state of aggregation and other peculiarities, the different varieties of calcareous spar, common and shell limestone, marble, marl, and chalk. It occurs also in the animal kingdom, forming the principal part of shells, and a small proportion of the bones of the higher orders of animals. It is present in small quantity in most natural waters, being held in solution by the carbonic acid which they contain. In the waters of limestone districts it is a very common impregnation, and causes purging in those not accustomed to their use. In all such cases, boiling the water, by expelling the carbonic acid, causes the carbonate to be deposited. It has been shown, however, that carbonate of calcium is itself in a slight degree soluble in water; so that a small proportion remains in limestone water which has been long exposed to boiling. Hofmann estimated the quantity remaining in solution at thirty-four milligrammes in a litre. That the carbonate is not held in solution by free carbonic acid is shown by the fact that lime-water causes no precipitation. (*Journ. de Pharm. et de Chim.*, 4e sér., iii. 147.) Besides being officinal in the state of chalk, carbonate of calcium is also ordered as it exists in marble and oyster-shell, and as obtained by precipitation. (See *Marmor*, *Testa*, and *Calcii Carbonas Præcipitata.*) In the present article we shall confine our observations to chalk. This occurs abundantly in the south of England and the north of France. It exists massive in beds, and very frequently contains nodules of flint, and fossil remains of land and marine animals. Until recently it was not known to exist in the United States; but Prof. F. V. Hayden states that chalk-beds identical with those of Europe extend for 400 miles along the Missouri River in Dakota.

Properties. Chalk is an insipid, inodorous, insoluble, opaque, soft solid, generally white, but grayish white when impure. It is rough to the touch, easily pulverized, and breaks with an earthy fracture. It soils the fingers, yields a white trace when drawn across an unyielding surface, and when applied to the tongue adheres slightly. Its sp. gr. varies from 2·3 to 2·6. It is never a perfectly pure carbonate of calcium, but contains, besides gritty silicious particles, small portions of alumina and ferric oxide. If pure, it is entirely soluble in hydrochloric acid; but usually a little silica is left. If this solution is not precipitated by ammonia, it is free from alumina and iron. Like all carbonates, it effervesces with acids. Though insoluble in water, it dissolves in an excess of carbonic acid.

Chalk, on account of the gritty particles which it contains, is unfit for medicinal use until it has undergone levigation, when it is called *prepared chalk*. (See *Creta Præparata.*)

Off. Prep. Creta Præparata.

CRETA PRÆPARATA. *U. S., Br.* *Prepared Chalk.*

(CRĒ'TA PRÆ-PA-RĀ'TA—prē-pa-rā'ta.)

"Native, friable Carbonate of Calcium [$CaCO_3$; 100.—CaO,CO_2; 50], freed from most of its impurities by elutriation." *U. S.*

Craie préparée, *Fr.;* Präparirte Kreide, *G.*

Below will be found the process officinal in the Pharmacopœia of 1870.*

The Br. Pharmacopœia has abandoned its former process, and is now content with defining the medicine to be "chalk freed from most of its impurities by elutriation, and afterwards dried in small masses, which are usually of a conical form."

The object of the above process is to reduce chalk to a very fine powder. The mineral, previously pulverized, should be rubbed with a little water upon a porphyry slab, by means of a muller of the same material. Having been thus very minutely divided, it is agitated with water, which upon standing a short time deposits the coarser particles, and, being then poured off, slowly lets fall the remainder in an impalpable state. The former part of the process is called *levigation*, the latter *elutriation*. The soft mass which remains after the decanting of the clear liquor is made to fall upon an absorbent surface in small portions, which when dried have a conical shape.† Practically, prepared chalk is generally made on the large scale from *whiting* by the manufacturer. (See *P. J. Tr.*, vii. 146.)†

No directions are given now in the Pharmacopœia for its preparation; it is thus described. "A white, amorphous powder, generally agglutinated in form of small cones, permanent in the air, odorless and tasteless, and insoluble in water or alcohol. It is soluble in hydrochloric, nitric or acetic acid with copious effervescence, and without leaving more than a trifling residue. By exposure to a red heat, the salt loses carbonic acid gas, and the residue has an alkaline reaction. A neutral solution of the salt in acetic acid yields, with test-solution of oxalate of ammonium, a white precipitate soluble in hydrochloric, but insoluble in acetic acid. Another portion of the same solution should yield no precipitate with test-solution of sulphate of

* "Take of Chalk *a convenient quantity*. Add a little water to the chalk, and rub it into fine powder. Throw this into a large vessel nearly full of water, stir briskly, and, after a short interval, decant the supernatant liquor, while yet turbid, into another vessel. Treat the coarser particles of the Chalk, remaining in the first vessel, in a similar manner, and add the turbid liquid to that previously decanted. Lastly, set the liquor by that the powder may subside, and, having poured off the water, dry the powder." *U. S.* 1870.

† Mr. F. Harris Alcock found some very handsome specimens of "prepared chalk" in the English market to contain 67·016 per cent. of calcium sulphate. (*P. J. Tr.*, 1883, p. 1015.)

calcium (abs. of barium, strontium). On adding to another portion of the solution, first, chloride of ammonium, then carbonate of ammonium and water of ammonia in slight excess, and gently warming, the filtrate separated from the resulting precipitate should not be rendered more than faintly turbid by test-solution of phosphate of sodium (limit of magnesium). Another portion of the solution should not assume more than a slightly bluish tint with a few drops of test-solution of ferrocyanide of potassium (limit of iron)." *U. S.*

Medical Properties and Uses. This is the only form in which chalk is used in medicine. It is an excellent antacid; and, as the salts which it forms in the stomach and bowels, if not astringent, are at least not purgative, it is admirably adapted to diarrhœa accompanied with acidity. It is also sometimes used in acidity of stomach attending dyspepsia and gout, when a laxative effect is to be avoided; is one of the best antidotes for oxalic acid; and has been recommended in rachitis. In scrofulous affections it may sometimes do good by forming soluble salts with acid in the primæ viæ, and thus finding an entrance into the blood-vessels. It is frequently employed as an application to burns and ulcers, which it moderately stimulates, while it absorbs the ichorous discharge, and thus prevents it from irritating the diseased surface, or the sound skin. It is given internally in the form of powder, or suspended in water by the intervention of gum arabic and sugar. (See *Mistura Cretæ.*) It is better fitted for the chalk mixture than the precipitated carbonate of calcium, in consequence of its more impalpable character and greater powers of adhesion. The dose is from ten to forty grains (0·65–2·6 Gm.) or more.

Off. Prep. Hydrargyrum cum Cretâ; Trochisci Cretæ; Pulvis Cretæ Compositus.

Off. Prep. Br. Hydrargyrum cum Creta; Mistura Cretæ; Pulvis Cretæ Aromaticus; Pulvis Cretæ Aromaticus cum Opio.

CROCUS. *U. S., Br.* *Saffron.*

(CRŌ'CŬS.)

"The stigmas of Crocus sativus. Linné. (*Nat. Ord.* Iridaceæ.)" *U. S.* "The dried stigmas, and top of the style, of Crocus sativus." *Br.*

Safran, *Fr., G.;* Zafferano, *It.;* Azafran, *Sp.*

Gen. Ch. *Corolla* six-parted, equal. *Stigmas* convoluted. *Willd.*

Crocus sativus. Willd. *Sp. Plant.* i. 194; Woodv. *Med. Bot.* p. 763, t. 259. The common cultivated saffron is a perennial plant, with a rounded and depressed bulb or cormus, from which the flower rises a little above the ground, upon a long, slender, white, and succulent tube. The flower is large, of a beautiful lilac or bluish purple color, and appears in September or October. The leaves are radical, linear, slightly revolute, dark green upon their upper surface with a white longitudinal furrow in the centre, paler underneath with a prominent flattened midrib, and enclosed at their base, together with the tube of the corolla, in a membranous sheath, from which they emerge soon after the appearance of the flower. The style hangs out on one side between the two segments of the corolla, and terminates in three long convoluted stigmas, which are of a rich orange color, highly odorous, rolled in at the edges, and notched at the summit. These stigmas are the officinal part of the plant. The stigmas of the *Crocus orientalis* are used in the East.

C. sativus, or *autumnal crocus*, is believed to be a native of Greece and Asia Minor, where it has been cultivated from the earliest ages. It is, however, unknown in a wild state, and, as the French plant does not produce seed, Chappellier claims that it is a hybrid. (*Bull. Soc. Bot. de France*, xx.) More recently, however, Chappellier has found that the ordinary crocus, as grown in France, is readily fertilized by the Grecian variety, and it is most probable that the species is a distinct one. There are three main varieties of it, the French, the Grecian, and the Chinese. The first of these is superior in color and flavor, the second in the amount of yield, whilst the third is said to unite these qualities. Saffron is also cultivated for medicinal use in Sicily, Spain, France, England, and other temperate countries of Europe. Large quantities of saffron are raised in Egypt, Persia, and Cashmere, whence it is sent to India. Much of the drug reaches the market of Constantinople from the neighborhood of Tiflis and the Caucasus. We cultivate the plant in this country chiefly as a garden flower, although some of the drug of very fine quality has been produced in Pennsylvania. It is liable to two diseases, which interfere with its culture; one dependent on a parasitic fungus which attaches itself to the bulb, the other called by the cultivators in France *tacon*, by which the bulb is converted into a blackish powder. (*Journ. de Pharm.*, xviii. 41.)

In England the flowers appear in October, and the leaves continue green through the winter; but the plant does not ripen its seed, and is propagated by offsets from the bulb. These are planted in grounds prepared for the purpose, and are arranged either in rows or in small patches at certain distances. The flowers are gathered soon after they show themselves, as the period of flowering is very short. The stigmas, or summits of the pistils, together with a portion of the style, are separated from the remainder of the flower, and carefully dried by artificial heat, or in the sun. During this process, they are sometimes made to assume the form of a cake by pressure; but the finest saffron is that which has been dried loosely. The two forms are distinguished by the names of *cake-saffron* and *hay-saffron*. Five pounds of the fresh stigmas are said to yield one pound of the dried.

The English saffron, formerly most highly esteemed in this country, has disappeared from our market. What may be sold under the name is probably derived from other sources. Much of the drug is imported from Gibraltar, packed in canisters. Parcels of it are also brought from Trieste and other ports of the Mediterranean. The Spanish saffron is generally considered the best in the United States, although most European writers in materia medica give the preference to the French saffron. Genuine *cake saffron* is at present seldom found in commerce. The better grades of Spanish saffron are known as *Valencia* saffron, whilst *Alicante* saffron is said by Prof. Maisch to contain scarcely more than 50 per cent. of genuine saffron. According to Landerer, the stigmas of several other species besides those of *C. sativus* are gathered and sold as saffron in Greece and Turkey.*

Properties. Saffron has a peculiar, sweetish, aromatic odor, a warm, pungent, bitter taste, and a rich deep orange color, which it imparts to the saliva when chewed. The stigmas of which it consists are an inch or more in length, expanded and notched at the upper extremity, and narrowing towards the lower, where they terminate in a slender, capillary, yellowish portion, forming a part of the style. They are thus described by the U. S. Pharmacopœia. "Separate, or three, attached to the top of the style, about an inch and a quarter (3 cm.) long, flattish-tubular, almost thread-like, broader and notched above; orange-brown; odor strong, peculiar, aromatic; taste bitterish and aromatic. When chewed it tinges the saliva deep orange-yellow. Saffron should not be mixed with the yellow styles. When pressed between filtering-paper it should not leave an oily stain. When soaked in water it colors the liquid

* At the International Exhibition, in London, in the year 1862, Dr. Geo. B. Wood noticed a specimen of saffron from the island of Ceylon, closely resembling that of the *Crocus sativus*. It consisted of the stigmas of the *Crocus orientalis*.

According to Mr. Charles A. Heinitsh, until within a few years, saffron was cultivated to a considerable extent in Lancaster County, Pa. The plant requires a rich soil, which should be deeply dug and heavily manured. The bulbs are planted in August, eight inches apart, and the growing plant should be kept free from weeds. The flowering period begins about the middle of September, and continues till the beginning of October. The flowers are picked early in the morning, and the stigmas separated and dried in the shade. This is done every day during the period of flowering. He thinks the cultivation can be profitably conducted. A plot of 72 square feet will produce 9000 stigmas, weighing 420 grains, or from 33 to 36 lbs. to the acre. (*A. J. P.*, 1867, p. 38.)

In the Apennines the bulbs, which have been left in the ground during the winter without protection, are removed in August, are planted again in September in rows, and four weeks later the collection of the flowers is begun. (See *Arch. d. Pharm.*, Aug. 1885.) For an account of the cultivation in England, see *P. J. Tr.*, June, 1887.

M. Monthus, an experienced cultivator in France, prefers a dry calcareous soil; plants the bulbs 3 or 4 inches deep; after the harvest in October manures the ground; and renews the planting every three years. He thus prevents the diseases peculiar to the plant.

M. Monthus recommends the *petals* of the flower as applicable to the same purposes as the stigmas, having found them to be possessed of aromatic properties. They demand no peculiar caution in drying; but to preserve them it is necessary to exclude light and moisture. Acids redden them with extreme facility, and alkalies turn them green. He therefore recommends a tincture to be made from them, as a substitute for syrup of violets. He prepares the tincture by macerating 10 parts of the dried flowers in 100 parts of alcohol of 40°, for 48 hours. A longer maceration would destroy the color. Paper may be stained with the tincture, and kept green or red, the former for acids, the latter for alkalies. (*Journ. de Pharm.*, Juillet, 1867, p. 54.)

orange-yellow, and should not deposit any pulverulent mineral matter, nor show the presence of organic substances differing in shape from that described." *U. S.* Analyzed by Vogel and Bouillon-Lagrange, it afforded 65 per cent. of a peculiar extractive matter, and 7·5 of an odorous volatile oil, together with wax, gum, albumen, saline matter, water, and lignin. The extractive was named *polychroïte*, from the changes of color which it undergoes by the action of reagents. Weiss (Wiggers and Husemann, *Jahresbericht*, 1868, p. 35) showed that *polychroïte* was a glucoside, from the decomposition of which resulted an additional coloring matter of the saffron, to which he applied the name *crocin*. For the preparation of polychroïte according to Weiss, saffron is extracted with ether, by which fat, wax, and essential oil were removed; and it was then exhausted with water. From the aqueous solution, gummy matters and some inorganic salts were precipitated by strong alcohol. After the separation of these substances polychroïte was precipitated by addition of ether. Thus obtained, it is an orange-red, viscid, deliquescent substance, which dried over sulphuric acid becomes brittle and of a fine ruby-red color. Kayser has (*Ber. der Chem. Ges.*, 1884, p. 2228) made a thorough investigation of the coloring matter of the saffron. He calls it *crocin*, and gives it the formula $C_{44}H_{70}O_{28}$. He obtained it after purification as a pure yellow powder, easily soluble in water and dilute alcohol, slightly soluble only in absolute alcohol. Concentrated sulphuric acid gives a deep blue color, which turns violet, then cherry-red, and finally brown. It is easily decomposed by lime or baryta water into *crocetin* and a right rotating sugar which Kayser calls *crocose*. The crocetin is a clear red powder, not soluble in water, but easily soluble in alcohol and ether. Its solution in alkalies shows an orange-yellow color, from which solution acids separate it again in orange-colored flocks. Its formula is $C_{34}H_{46}O_{9}$. Kayser also found a bitter principle, to which he gave the name *picrocrocin* or *saffron bitter*, and the formula $C_{38}H_{66}O_{17}$. It is to the essential oil, which, according to M. Henry, is present to the amount of 10 per cent., that the medicine owes its activity. It may be partially separated by distillation. It is yellow, of a hot, acrid, bitterish taste, and heavier than water, in which it is slightly soluble.

Adulterations. The high price of this medicine gives rise to frequent adulterations. Water is said to be very often added in order to increase its weight. Oil or glycerin is also added for the same purpose, or to improve the appearance. In some specimens the dyed corolla of the crocus with the attached stamens is abundant. Sometimes the flowers of other plants, particularly *Carthamus tinctorius* or safflower, *Calendula officinalis* or officinal marigold, and *arnica*, are fraudulently mixed with the genuine stigmas. They may be known by their shape, which is rendered obvious by throwing a portion of the suspected mass into hot water, which causes them to expand. (See *Carthamus*.) A specimen of this adulteration has been introduced into the American market, by the name of *African saffron*. (Maisch, *A. J. P.*, March, 1872, p. 110.) Other adulterations are the fibres of dried beef, the stamens of the Crocus distinguishable by their yellow color, the stigmas previously exhausted in the preparation of the infusion or tincture, and various mineral substances easily detected upon close examination. The flowers of a Brazilian plant, named *Fuminella*, have, according to M. J. L. Soubeiran, been employed for the adulteration of saffron. They may be detected by shaking gently but repeatedly a large pinch of the suspected saffron over a piece of paper. The flowers of Fuminella, being smaller and heavier, separate and fall, and may be seen to consist of very short fragments, with a color like that of saffron, but a rusty tint which the latter does not possess. (*Journ. de Pharm.*, Avril, 1855, p. 267.) J. Müller recommends concentrated sulphuric acid as the most certain test of saffron. It instantly changes the color of pure saffron to indigo blue. (*Chem. Gaz.*, May, 1845, p. 197.)

A very successful adulteration which has been largely practised appears to consist of yellow-colored chalk or sulphate of barium, made into a thin paste probably with honey, and attached to the stigmas, sometimes isolated, sometimes in groups of five or six, enveloping them almost completely. If this saffron be kept in a dry place, and often handled, the paste becomes partly broken up, and the colored powder spreads itself in the mass and the envelope. The chalk can at once be detected by shaking the suspected saffron with water, and treating the precipitated powder with hydrochloric acid, when effervescence will occur. A less than the ordinary brightness of color in the saffron should lead to suspicion of this adulteration. Much can be told as to the purity of saffron by agitating the suspected flowers in distilled water; if the drug be pure the liquid will remain clear, assuming a fine pure yellow tint; the saffron also will retain its red color for hours. Another excellent plan is to scatter a pinch of the flowers upon the surface of warm water, when the stigmas should spread out and display their proper form. Minute fragments of Red Saunders, which are often added to saffron, may be separated by agitating with water. (For an elaborate discussion of adulteration, see *A. J. P.*, 1885, p. 487.)

Attention has been called to a product of the Cape of Good Hope, named *Cape saffron*, which has a remarkable resemblance to genuine saffron, having a similar odor, and yielding a similar color to water, though the flowers themselves are differently colored. It is the flower of a small plant very abundant at the Cape, belonging to the family of *Scrophulariaceæ*, and is said by Dr. Pappé, of Cape Town, to possess medical virtues closely resembling those of true saffron. The flowers have been used successfully in the convulsions of children. (*P. J. Tr.*, vi. 462, 1865.)

Choice of Saffron. Saffron should not be very moist, nor very dry, nor easily pulverized; nor should it emit an offensive smell when thrown upon live coals. The freshest is the best, and that which is less than a year old should, if possible, be selected. It should possess in a high degree the characteristic properties of color, taste, and smell. When agitated with water it should color it bright yellow, and it should not effervesce in the presence of a dilute acid. If it do not color the fingers when rubbed between them, or if it have an oily feel, or a musty flavor, or a black, yellow, or whitish color, it should be rejected. In the purchase of this medicine in cakes, those should be selected which are close, tough, and firm in tearing; and care should be taken to avoid *cakes of safflower*.

As its activity depends, partly at least, on a volatile ingredient, saffron should be kept in well-stopped vessels. Some recommend that it should be enclosed in a bladder, and introduced into a tin case.

Medical Properties and Uses. Saffron was formerly considered highly stimulant, antispasmodic, and even narcotic. It was thought also to act powerfully on the uterine system, promoting menstruation. The ancients employed it extensively, both as a medicine and condiment, under the name of *crocus*. It was also highly esteemed by the Arabians, and enjoyed considerable reputation among the physicians of modern Europe, till within a comparatively recent period. On the continent it is still much used as a stimulant and emmenagogue. But the experiments of Dr. Alexander have proved it to possess little activity; and in Great Britain and the United States it is seldom prescribed. In domestic practice saffron tea is occasionally used in exanthematous diseases, to promote the eruption. At present it is chiefly used to impart color and flavor. The dose is from ten to thirty grains (0·65–1·95 Gm.).*

Off. Prep. Tinctura Croci.

Off. Prep. Br. Decoctum Aloës Compositum; Pilulæ Aloës et Myrrhæ; Pulvis Cretæ Aromaticus; Tinctura Cinchonæ Composita; Tinctura Croci; Tinctura Opii Ammoniata; Tinctura Rhei.

CUBEBA. *U. S., Br.* *Cubeba.* [*Cubeb.*]

(CŪ-BĒ′BA.)

"The unripe fruit of Cubeba officinalis. Miquel. (*Nat. Ord.* Piperaceæ.)" *U. S.*
"The dried, unripe, full-grown fruit of Piper cubeba, *Linn. fil.*" *Br.*†

* *Syrupus Croci.* A *Syrup of Saffron* is sometimes called for, and would seem to be an appropriate preparation. The following formula is recommended by Mr. Geo. W. Kennedy, of Pottsville, as producing excellent results. Take of saffron ℥ss, glycerin ℥ij, water ℥vi. Macerate for a week, filter into a pint bottle, and add sufficient water through the filter to make ℥viij: then add 14 avoird. oz. of sugar, and dissolve without heat, frequently shaking. (*A. J. P.*, Feb. 1871, p. 54.)

† The fruit of the *Piper Afzelii* of Lindley, *Cubeba Clusii* of Miquel, figured in the *P. J. Tr.* (xiv. 201), is known in commerce as *African Cubebs*, *Ashantee Pepper*, *Guinea pepper*, or *African black pepper*. It was formerly taken to Europe in considerable quantities by the Portuguese, but has been superseded by the more agreeable products of the East Indies. The fruit is one-third smaller

Cubebs, Cubebæ, *P.G.;* Fructus (s. Baccæ) Cubebæ, Piper Caudatum; Cubebe, Cubèbe poivre à Queue, *Fr.;* Kubeben, *G.;* Cubebe, *It.;* Cubebas, *Sp.;* Kebabeh, *Ar.*

Gen. Ch. Calyx none. *Corolla* none. *Berry* one-seeded. *Willd.*

Cubebæ officinalis. Miquel.—*Piper Cubeba.* Willd. *Sp. Plant.* i. 159; Woodv. *Med. Bot.*, 3d ed., v. 95. This is a climbing perennial plant, with a smooth, flexuous, jointed stem, and entire, petiolate, oblong or ovate-oblong, acuminate leaves, rounded or obliquely cordate at the base, strongly nerved, coriaceous, and very smooth. The flowers are diœcious and in spikes, with peduncles about as long as the petioles. The fruit is a globose, pedicelled berry.

This species of Piper is a native of Java, Penang, and probably other parts of the East Indies. It is extensively grown in the coffee plantations, supported by the trees which are used for shade, and has been introduced into Ceylon. The dried unripe fruit is the officinal portion.

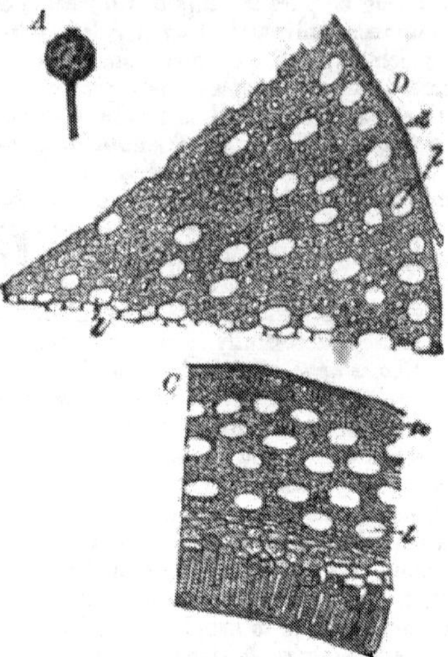

Cubeb fruit. *A*, fruit itself, natural size; *C*, segment of the fruit magnified; *tz*, ring of stony wall-cells; *l*, oil-cells; *D*, section of the seed; *l*, oil-tubes; *d*, epidermis.

Properties. Cubebs are round, about the size of a small pea, of a blackish or grayish brown color, and furnished with a short stalk, which is continuous with raised veins that run over the surface of the berry, and embrace it like a net-work. The shell is hard, almost ligneous, and contains within it a single loose seed,

than the officinal cubebs, is more compact, and has a taste more analogous to that of ordinary black pepper. Dr. Stenhouse has also shown that it is chemically more analogous to black pepper than to cubebs, as it contains piperine and not cubebin. (*Ibid.*, xiv. 364.) A variety of cubebs from the Dutch East Indies differs essentially from genuine cubebs in being somewhat larger, with less distinct veins and somewhat flattened footstalks, of a less agreeable odor, and a less hot and pungent taste. It has been ascribed to *Piper anisatum.* (See *A. J. P.*, xxxv. 511.) This is probably the cubebs referred by Flückiger and Hanbury to *P. crassipes*, and described by them as larger than the ordinary cubebs, much shrivelled, with a pedestal one and a half times to twice as long as the berry, of a very bitter taste and odor, different from that of cubebs. The subject of false cubebs has recently increased in importance from the appearance in the London markets in considerable quantities of a false cubebs, and the production thereby of marked symptoms of gastro-intestinal irritation. Examined by Wm. Kirby (*P. J. Tr.*, vol. xv.), this importation conforms to the description of *P. crassipes* by Flückiger and Hanbury except in the stalk not being so long and the taste not very bitter. Mr. Kirby says it resembles the fruit of the *Piper sylvestra.* Microscopically it is distinguished from other cubebs in having ten rows of cells in the endocarp instead of four, and about fourteen instead of eleven or twelve woody bundles (the last character is of very doubtful constancy). The berries of *Daphnidium Cubeba* have also been sold in London recently as cubebs; they resemble the true cubebs in general appearance, but differ in possessing a more agreeable flavor and in the seed readily splitting into two oily cotyledons with a superior radicle, indicating its lauraceous character. Even in powder the *Daphnidium Cubeba* is to be recognized from a species of piper by the absence of small angular starch granules. Mr. E. M. Holmes and Mr. E. D. Gravill (*P. J. Tr.*, vol. xv.) give the following tests, which may be available in detecting powdered false cubebs. After being crushed, the genuine cubebs gives on a porcelain slab with concentrated sulphuric acid a deep crimson with a distinct carmine tint in it. *P. crassipes* strikes a reddish-brown color, *Daphnidium Cubeba* a yellowish-brown color. Iodine gives with a decoction of genuine cubebs a pure blue tint, and with spurious cubebs a dull purple tint. One cubic centimetre of the tincture of true cubebs treated with ten cubic centimetres of strong sulphuric acid (sp. gr. 1·843) develops a deep violet color, the false cubebs similarly treated a deep red-brown. On diluting these mixtures with four fluidounces of distilled water and allowing them to stand, the true cubebs becomes opalescent and changes to a deep blue, the false becomes opalescent and changes to a dirty yellow. In applying these tests to adulterated cubebs, the color developed will, of course, be dependent upon the amount and character of the adulteration. It is probable that from time to time the fruits of several non-officinal pipers find their way into the market. A product with the name of *African cubebs* has been sent to London from Cape Coast Castle, in Africa, which is the fruit of a plant belonging to the *Xanthoxylaceæ*, probably either a *Toddalia* or *Vepris.* According to Prof. Archer, it is simply aromatic and stimulant, without any of the special virtues of cubebs. (*P. J. Tr.*, March, 1865, p. 463.)

covered with a blackish coat, and internally white and oleaginous. "Globular, about one-sixth of an inch (4 mm.) in diameter, contracted at the base into a stipe nearly a quarter of an inch (6 mm.) long, reticulately wrinkled, blackish gray, internally whitish and hollow; odor strong, spicy; taste aromatic and pungent. Cubeb should not be mixed with the nearly inodorous rachis or stalks." *U. S.* The odor of the berry is agreeably aromatic; the taste warm, bitterish, and camphorous, leaving in the mouth a peculiar sensation of coolness, like that produced by oil of peppermint. The pericarp of the cubeb berry consists of three layers, the exterior of which is composed of an interrupted row of small, thick-walled cubical cells, arranged in irregular groups of three or four. The middle layer of the pericarp is composed of loose, undeveloped tissue, interspersed with large oil-cells, and contains quantities of starch and sometimes groups of needle-shaped crystals. The inner layer is free from starch, and is formed of four rows of parenchymatous cells. At the junction of the inner and middle layer there are usually ten to twelve distinct woody bundles, chiefly composed of narrow spiral vessels along with a few dotted vessels. The testa consists of one row of large, thick-walled cells. The perisperm is surrounded by red membrane, formed of rather large cells, and is composed of angular parenchymatous cells containing starch and oil. On allowing thin sections to stand in glycerin for a few weeks crystals are formed both in the pericarp and in the perisperm. (*P. J. Tr.*, vol. xv. 653.) The powder is dark colored and of an oily aspect. The most obvious constituent of cubebs is the volatile oil, the proportion of which yielded by the drug varies from 4 to 13 per cent. It is, as shown by Oglialoro, a mixture of an oil $C_{10}H_{16}$, boiling at 158°–163° C. (316·4°–325·4° F.), which is present in very small amount, and two oils of the formula $C_{15}H_{24}$, boiling at 272°–265° C. (503·6°–509° F.). One of these is strongly lævogyrate, and yields a crystallized compound, $C_{15}H_{24}.2HCl$, melting at 118° C., while the other is less lævogyrate, and does not combine with HCl.

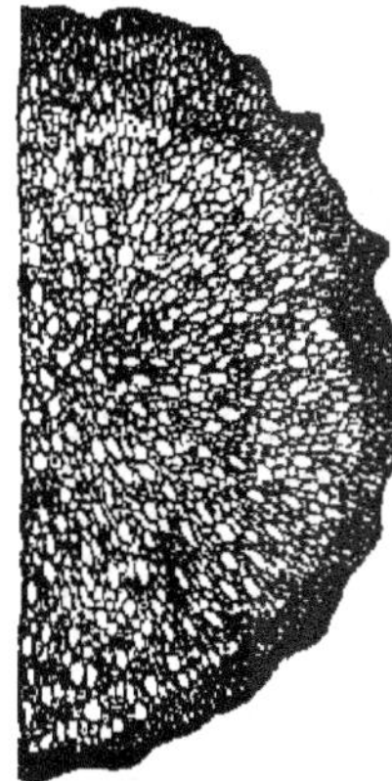
Transverse section.

The oil distilled from old cubebs on cooling at length deposits large transparent inodorous octohedra of *camphor of cubebs*, $C_{15}H_{26}O$. E. Schmidt (1873) found that this camphor melts at 66·5° C.; simply by standing over sulphuric acid, more rapidly on heating, it gave up water and passed into that fraction of cubeb oil which boils at 260° C., of which it is, therefore, simply the hydrate. Another constituent of cubebs is *cubebin*. This is an inodorous substance, crystallizing in small needles or scales, melting at 125° C. (257° F.), having a bitter taste in alcoholic solution; it dissolves freely in boiling alcohol, but deposits on cooling, and is abundantly soluble in chloroform. Its composition, according to Weidel (1877), is $C_{10}H_{10}O_3$. Fused with caustic potash it yields proto-catechuic acid. The resin extracted from cubebs consists of an indifferent portion, nearly 3 per cent., and of *cubebic acid*, $C_{13}H_{14}O_7$, amounting to about 1 per cent. (*Pharmacographia*, 2d ed., p. 587.)

According to MM. Capitaine and Soubeiran, *cubebin* is best obtained by expressing cubebs from which the oil has been distilled, preparing from them an alcoholic extract, treating this with a solution of potassa, washing the residue with water, and purifying it by repeated crystallizations in alcohol. It bears a close resemblance to piperine, but materially differs from it in composition, as it contains no nitrogen. (*Journ. de Pharm.*, xxv. 355.) In the officinal oleoresin of cubebs a deposit takes place consisting chiefly of cubebin, which may be obtained by washing the deposit with a small quantity of cold alcohol to remove adhering resin and oil, and then dissolving repeatedly in boiling alcohol, and crystallizing until the product is white.* The volatile oil is officinal. (See *Oleum Cubebæ.*) By practical trial Bernatzike has satisfied himself that the peculiar virtues of cubebs, as a remedy in gonor-

* Prof. E. Schaer calls attention to the similarity in reaction between cubebin and veratrine, aconitine, morphine, and digitalin. (*Archiv d. Pharm.*, 1887, p. 531.)

rhœa, depend not on the cubebin or the volatile oil, but on the cubebic acid. (See *Am. Journ. of Med. Sci.*, October, 1867, p. 534.) When the ethereal extract of cubebs is deprived of its volatile oil by evaporation on a water-bath, and of cubebin and wax by deposition, a soft resin is left, the *cubebic acid* of Bernatsike, in which, according to Mr. F. V. Heydenreich, who experimented with it as a physiological agent, the diuretic properties reside; the cubebin being without apparent effect, and the volatile oil, though stimulant and carminative, having no diuretic action. The soft resin, which was of the consistence of honey, of a dark olive-green color, and some remaining odor of cubebs, when taken in the dose of ten grains every two hours, for six hours, acted as a laxative, and gave the urine a peculiar odor, without increasing its quantity; but in the dose of a drachm, once repeated at an interval of three hours, while it produced the same effects as the smaller dose, considerably augmented the urine. In still larger doses it produced decided irritation of the urinary passages. (*A. J. P.*, Jan. 1868.) Mr. Heydenreich's experiments are confirmatory of Bernatsike's conclusion as to the peculiar active principles of cubebs. Cubebs gradually deteriorate by age, and in powder become rapidly weaker, in consequence of the escape of their volatile oil. They should be kept whole, and pulverized when dispensed. The powder is said to be sometimes adulterated with that of pimento.

Medical Properties and Uses. Cubebs are generally stimulant, with a special direction to the urinary organs. In considerable quantities they excite the circulation, increase the heat of the body, and sometimes occasion headache and giddiness. At the same time they frequently produce an augmented flow of the urine, to which they impart a peculiar odor. Among their effects are also occasionally nausea and moderate purging; and they are said to cause a sense of coolness in the rectum during the passage of the fæces. We have no evidence that they were known to the ancients. They were probably first brought into Europe by the Arabians, and were formerly employed for similar purposes with black pepper; but they were found much less powerful and fell into disuse. In India they have long been used in gonorrhœa and gleet, and as a grateful stomachic and carminative in disorders of the digestive organs, and are at present very frequently given both in this country and in Europe in gonorrhœa, after the subsidence of the first active inflammatory symptoms. They have been given also in leucorrhœa, cystirrhœa, the urethritis of women and female children, abscess of the prostate gland, piles, chronic bronchial inflammation, and, with great asserted advantage, in connection with copaiba, in pseudo-membranous croup, and diphtheritic affections of the fauces. In connection with copaiba they have been especially recommended in affections of the neck of the bladder and the prostatic portion of the urethra. They are best administered in powder, of which the dose in gonorrhœa is from one to three drachms (3·9–11·65 Gm.) three or four times a day. For other affections, the dose is sometimes reduced to ten grains (0·65 Gm.). The volatile oil may be substituted, in the dose of ten or twelve drops (0·6–0·72 C.c.), suspended in water by means of sugar; though, if the experiments of Bernatsike and Heydenreich are to be relied on, the oil is much less efficient than the soft resin as a remedy in gonorrhœa, and in diseases of the urinary passages generally. An ethereal extract is directed by the U. S. Pharmacopœia, and considerably used; and, as it contains the soft resin or cubebic acid, it is no doubt a very efficient preparation. (See *Oleoresina Cubebæ.*) An infusion, made in the proportion of an ounce of cubebs to a pint of water, has been employed as an injection in discharges from the vagina, with asserted advantage.

Off. Prep. Extractum Cubebæ Fluidum; Oleoresina Cubebæ; Tinctura Cubebæ.

Off. Prep. Br. Oleoresina Cubebæ; Oleum Cubebæ; Tinctura Cubebæ.

CUPRI ACETAS. *U. S.* *Acetate of Copper.*

$Cu(C_2H_3O_2)_2.H_2O$; 199·2. (CŪ'PRĪ A-CĒ'TĂS.) $CuO, C_4H_3O_3.HO$; 99·6.

Crystallized Verdigris, Crystals of Venus; Verdet, Cristaux de Vénus, *Fr.*; Essigsaures Kupfer, *G.*

This salt is now substituted for the impure subacetate of copper, formerly officinal. It may be prepared by dissolving verdigris in acetic acid, or by precipitating a concentrated solution of acetate of lead with sulphate of copper. It is the normal cupric acetate, as distinguished from the other basic salts.

Properties. "Deep green, prismatic crystals, yielding a bright green powder, efflorescent on exposure to air, odorless, having a nauseating, metallic taste and an acid reaction. Soluble in 15 parts of water and in 135 parts of alcohol at 15° C. (59° F.), in five parts of boiling water and in 14 parts of boiling alcohol. When heated above 100° C. (212° F.), the salt loses its water of crystallization, and at a temperature above 200° C. (392° F.), it is gradually decomposed. The aqueous solution of the salt has a bluish green color, which is rendered deep blue by an excess of ammonia. On heating the salt with sulphuric acid, acetous vapors are evolved. If the aqueous solution of the salt be treated with hydrosulphuric acid until all the copper is precipitated, the filtrate should leave no residue on evaporation (alkalies, alkaline earths and iron). If the aqueous solution be heated to boiling with solution of soda in excess, it will yield a filtrate which should not be clouded by hydrosulphuric acid (abs. of lead, zinc)." *U. S.* As its source is principally verdigris, it will be proper to consider this now.

VERDIGRIS (*Impure Subacetate of Copper*, U. S. 1870; *Aerugo*, P.G.; *Viride Æris, Subacetas cupricus; Verdigris; Ærugo*, Lat.; *Acetate de Cuivre brut, Vert-de-gris, Acétate basique de Cuivre, Verd-et-gris*, Fr.; *Grünspan, Spangrün, Basisches essigsaures Kupfer* (*Kupferoxyd*), G.; *Verde rame*, It.; *Cardenillo*, Sp.) is prepared in large quantities in the south of France, more particularly in the neighborhood of Montpellier. It is also manufactured in Great Britain and Sweden. In France the process is conducted in the following manner. Sheets of copper are stratified with the residue of the grape after the expression of the juice in making wine, and are allowed to remain in this state for a month or six weeks. At the end of this time the plates are found coated with a considerable quantity of verdigris. This is scraped off, and the plates are then replaced as at first, to be further acted on. The scrapings thus obtained form a paste, which is afterwards well beaten with wooden mallets, and packed in oblong leathern sacks, about ten inches in length by eight in breadth, in which it is dried in the sun, until the loaf of verdigris, as it is called, attains the proper degree of hardness. The rationale of the process is easily understood. The juice of the grape refuse undergoes the acetous fermentation, and the acetic acid attacking the copper forms the subacetate. In England a purer verdigris is prepared by alternating copper plates with pieces of woollen cloth, steeped in pyroligneous acid.

Verdigris comes to this country exclusively from France, being imported principally from Bordeaux and Marseilles. The leathern packages in which it is put up, called sacks of verdigris, weigh generally from twenty-five to thirty pounds, and arrive in casks, each containing from thirty to forty sacks.

Properties. Verdigris is in masses of a pale green color, and composed of a multitude of minute silky crystals. Sometimes, however, it occurs of a bright blue color. Its taste is coppery. It is insoluble in alcohol, and, by the action of water, a portion of it is resolved into the neutral acetate which dissolves, and the trisacetate which remains behind in the form of a dark green powder, gradually becoming black. It is hence evident that, when verdigris is prepared by levigation with water, it is altered in its nature. When verdigris is acted on by sulphuric acid, it is decomposed, vapors of acetic acid being evolved, easily recognized by their vinegar odor. It is soluble almost entirely in ammonia, and dissolves in hydrochloric and dilute sulphuric acid, with the exception of impurities, which should not exceed 5 per cent. When of good quality, it has a lively green color, is free from black or white spots, and is dry and difficult to break. The green rust, called in popular language verdigris, which copper vessels are apt to contract when not kept clean, is a carbonate of copper, and should not be confounded with true verdigris.

Composition. Verdigris, apart from its impurities, is a variable mixture of the basic acetates of copper. The *blue* variety has approximately the composition $(C_2H_3O_2)_2Cu,Cu(OH)_2 + 5H_2O$. When treated with water it is gradually decomposed into two parts according to the reaction: $3(Cu(C_2H_3O_2)_2, Cu(OH)_2 = Cu(C_2H_3O_2)_2 + 2Cu(OH)_2$ and $2Cu(C_2H_3O_2)_2 + Cu(OH)_2$. The latter of these products constitutes the *green* variety of verdigris. (Flückiger, *Pharm. Chem.*, p. 758.)

Medical Properties. The local and general action of verdigris upon the animal economy and the treatment of its poisoning are the same as those of the sulphate of copper. It is never used internally.*

CUPRI SULPHAS. *U.S., Br. Sulphate of Copper.*

$Cu\,SO_4.\,5H_2O$; 249·2. (CŪ'PRĪ SŬL'PHĂS.) $Cu\,O,\,SO_3.\,5HO$; 124·6.

"May be obtained by heating sulphuric acid and copper together, dissolving the soluble product in hot water, and evaporating the solution until crystallization takes place on cooling." *Br.*

Cuprum Sulfuricum, *P.G.;* Kupfersulfat, Cuprum Vitriolatum, Blue Vitriol, Roman Vitriol, Blue Stone; Sulfate de Cuivre, Vitriol bleu, Couperose bleu, *Fr.;* Schwefelsaures Kupfer, Kupfervitriol, Blauervitriol, Blauer Galitzenstein, *G.;* Rame solfato, Vitriolo di Rame, *It.;* Sulfato de Cobre, Vitriolo azul, *Sp.*

Preparation, etc. Sulphate of copper occasionally exists in nature, in solution in the water which flows through copper-mines. In this case the salt is procured by merely evaporating the waters which naturally contain it. Another method of obtaining it is to roast the native sulphide in a reverberatory furnace, whereby it is made to pass, by absorbing oxygen, into the state of sulphate. The roasted mass is lixiviated, and the solution obtained evaporated that crystals may form. The salt, procured by either of these methods, contains a little ferric sulphate, from which it may be freed by adding either an excess of cuprous oxide, which precipitates the sesquioxide of iron, or recently precipitated subcarbonate of copper, which causes the deposition of the iron as a carbonate. (*A. J. P.*, xxxiv. 507.) A third method consists in wetting, and then sprinkling with sulphur, sheets of copper, which are next heated to redness, and while hot plunged into water. The same operation is repeated until the sheets are entirely corroded. At first a sulphide of the metal is formed, which, by the action of heat and air, gradually passes into the state of sulphate. This is dissolved by the water, and obtained in crystals by evaporation. A fourth method is to dissolve copper scales to saturation in sulphuric acid, contained in a wooden vessel, lined with sheet lead. The scales consist of metallic copper, mixed with oxide, and are produced in the process for annealing sheet copper. Sometimes sulphate of copper is obtained in pursuing one of the methods for separating silver from gold. The silver is dissolved by boiling the alloy in sulphuric acid. The sulphate of silver formed is then decomposed by the immersion of copper plates in its solution, with the effect of forming sulphate of copper and precipitating the silver.

In the U. S. Pharmacopœia, sulphate of copper is presumed to be obtained pure from the manufacturer; the British suggests the method in which it may be prepared, without entering into the details of the process. The German Pharmacopœia has two kinds officinal, *Cuprum Sulfuricum*, which corresponds with the former *Cuprum Sulfuricum Purum*, and *Cuprum Sulfuricum Crudum*, or commercial sulphate.

Properties. Sulphate of copper has a rich deep blue color, and a strong metallic styptic taste. It reddens vegetable blues, and crystallizes in "large, translucent, deep blue, triclinic crystals, efflorescent, odorless, having a nauseous, metallic taste and an acid reaction. Soluble in 2·6 parts of water at 15° C. (59° F.), in 0·5 part of boiling water, and insoluble in alcohol. When heated to 100° C. (212° F.), the salt gradually loses 28·9 per cent. of its weight. At a temperature of about 230°

* *Linimentum Æruginis, Mel Ægyptiacum, Unguentum Ægyptiacum.* This is an old preparation, formerly officinal in Great Britain. The following is the process for it given in the old *London* Pharmacopœia. "Take of Verdigris (Subacetate of Copper), in powder, *an ounce;* Vinegar *seven fluidounces;* Honey *fourteen ounces.* Dissolve the Verdigris in the Vinegar, and strain through linen; then gradually add the Honey, and boil down to a proper consistence." The ounces used here are troyounces. It sometimes happens during the boiling of the acetic solution of the verdigris, that a red deposit rapidly forms, consisting of the red or suboxide of copper (cuprous oxide); and that at the end of the process, little or none of the metallic salt remains in the preparation. This happens especially when granular honey is employed. (Harley, *P. J. Tr.*, xi. 357.) The change is owing to the decomposition of the cupric oxide by the grape sugar of the honey, converting it into cuprous oxide. The inference is that, in making the preparation, so as to fulfil the objects of the original prescription, simple syrup should be used. It was formerly employed, either undiluted, or mixed with some mild ointment, to destroy fungous granulations, or to repress their growth. In the latter state, it acts as a stimulant to flabby, indolent, and ill-conditioned ulcers: and, largely diluted with water, it has been used as a gargle in venereal ulcerations of the mouth and throat. It is sometimes also applied undiluted, by means of a camel's-hair brush.

C. (446° F.) it becomes anhydrous, and at a red heat it is decomposed, evolving sulphurous vapors and finally leaving black cupric oxide. The aqueous solution of the salt has a pale blue color, which is rendered deep blue by an excess of ammonia. With test-solution of chloride of barium it yields a white precipitate insoluble in hydrochloric acid. If a little hydrochloric and some diluted sulphuric acid be added to a 5 per cent. aqueous solution of the salt, and this be treated with hydrosulphuric acid until the copper is completely precipitated, the filtrate should leave no residue on evaporation (foreign metals, alkalies, and alkaline earths)." *U. S.* When heated, sulphate of copper first melts in its water of crystallization, and then dries and becomes white. If the heat be increased, it next undergoes the igneous fusion, and finally, at a high temperature, loses its acid, cupric oxide being left. Four of the molecules of water of crystallization can be driven off at 100° C. (212° F.); but the fifth only goes off at a temperature of from 220° C. (428° F.) to 240° C. (464° F.), when the anhydrous salt remains. Potassa, soda, and ammonia throw down from it a bluish white precipitate of hydrated cupric oxide, which is immediately dissolved by an excess of the last-mentioned alkali, forming a rich deep blue solution, called *aqua sappharina*. It is decomposed by the alkaline carbonates, and by borax, acetate and subacetate of lead, acetate of iron, nitrate of silver, corrosive chloride of mercury, tartrate of potassium, and chloride of calcium; and it is precipitated by all astringent vegetable infusions. If it becomes very green on the surface by the action of the air, it contains sesquioxide of iron. This oxide may also be detected by ammonia, which will throw it down along with the oxide of copper, without taking it up when added in excess. When sulphate of copper is obtained from the *dipping liquid* of manufacturers of brass or German silver ware, it is always contaminated with sulphate of zinc, as pointed out by Mr. S. Piesse. This liquid is at first a mixture of sulphuric and nitric acids, but becomes, at last, nearly saturated with copper. When zinc is present in sulphate of copper, it will be taken up by solution of potassa, added in excess, from which it may be thrown down, in white flocks, by a solution of bicarbonated alkali.

Medical Properties and Uses. Sulphate of copper is irritant or mildly escharotic; and when in dilute solution, stimulant and astringent. At one time it was given in epilepsy and other nervous diseases; but at present it is never used internally, except for its influence upon the gastro-intestinal mucous membrane. In chronic diarrhœa with ulceration it is often a useful remedy. In doses of 5 grains it acts as a powerful, prompt emetic, without causing general depression or much nausea; hence it is preferred in narcotic poisoning, to dislodge false membrane or foreign bodies from the larynx and œsophagus, and for other similar purposes. Externally it is employed in solution as a stimulant to ill-conditioned ulcers, as an escharotic for destroying warts, fungous granulations, and callous edges, and as a styptic to bleeding surfaces. It is found, in not a few instances, to promote the cicatrisation of ulcers, and is not unfrequently employed, with that view, as a wash for chancres. The preparation called *cuprum aluminatum* (*lapis divinus—pierre divine*) is made, according to the French Codex, by mixing, in powder, three ounces, each, of sulphate of copper, nitrate of potassium, and alum, heating the mixture in a crucible, so as to produce watery fusion, then mixing in a drachm of powdered camphor, and, finally, pouring out the whole on an oiled stone to congeal. The mass, when cold, is broken into pieces, and kept in a well-stopped bottle. It is often desirable to employ sulphate of copper, as a caustic, in the form of pencil. Its tendency to effloresce interferes with its use in this way in the pure state. M. Llovet recommends for the purpose a mixture of one part of potassa-alum and two of sulphate of copper, which are to be first powdered, and then gradually melted together in a porcelain vessel, and poured into moulds made of bronze. (*Gaz. des Hôp.*, Juillet 28, 1863.) Another mode of preparing *pencils of sulphate of copper* is to rub briskly together four parts of that salt and one of borax, and to mould the plastic mass which results into the desired form. (*A. J. P.*, March, 1864, p. 106.) The best form is that of an elongated cone, made by selecting suitable crystals, and turning them in a lathe until the desired form is secured; or they may be made by filing the crystals into nearly the proper shape, and finishing with sand-paper.

The dose of sulphate of copper, as an astringent or tonic, is a quarter of a grain (0·016 Gm.), gradually increased; as an emetic, five grains (0 13–0·33 Gm.), repeated in fifteen minutes if necessary, but not oftener than once. As a stimulant wash, the solution may be made of the strength of two, four, or eight grains to the fluid-ounce of water. Orfila cautions against giving large doses of this salt as an emetic in cases of poisoning; as it is apt, from its poisonous effects, to increase the mischief when not expelled by vomiting. Upon the whole, such is the activity of sulphate of copper, that it should always be exhibited with caution. For its effects as a poison, see *Cuprum*.

CUPRUM. *Br.* Copper.

Cu; 63·2. (CŪ'PRŬM.) Cu; 31·6.

"Fine Copper wire, about No. 25 wire gauge, or about 0·02 inch." *Br.*

Cupreum Filum; Fil de Cuivre, Cuivre, *Fr.;* Kupfer, Kupferdraht, *G.;* Rame, *It.;* Cobre, *Sp.*

This metal is very generally diffused in nature, and exists principally in four states: as native copper, as an oxide, as a sulphide, and as a salt. Its principal native salts are the sulphate, carbonate, arseniate, and phosphate. In the United States it occurs in various localities, but especially in the neighborhood of Lake Superior, in East Tennessee, and in Montana. The principal copper-mines of Europe are those of the Pyrenees in France, Cornwall in England, and Fahlun in Sweden. The total production of copper in the United States during 1885 was 170,962,607 lbs.; in 1886, 161,235,381 lbs.; and in 1887, 181,170,524 lbs. These figures include copper manufactured from imported pyrites, of which 3,750,000 lbs. were made in 1887. The copper consumption of the United States for 1887 was estimated at 100,000,000 lbs. The copper production of the world for 1884 was estimated at 208,313 tons. The largest production was from the United States, and then Chili, the two countries together contributing more than half of the entire amount.

Properties. Copper is a brilliant, sonorous metal, of a reddish color, and very ductile, malleable, and tenacious. It has a slightly nauseous taste, and emits a disagreeable smell when rubbed. Its texture is granular, and its fracture hackly. Its sp. gr. is 8·92 to 8·95, and its fusing point 1398° C. (2538° F.) according to Daniell, being intermediate between the fusing points of silver and gold. Its atomic weight is 63·5, or, according to other determinations, 63·2. Exposed to the air it undergoes a slight tarnish. Its combinations are numerous and important. With oxygen it forms two well-characterized oxides, a red suboxide, better known as *cuprous* oxide, Cu_2O, and a black oxide, known as *cupric* oxide, CuO. While a cuprous chloride, iodide, and sulphide are known, it is the cupric oxide chiefly that unites with the common acids to form cupric salts. With metals copper forms numerous alloys, of which that with zinc, called brass, and that with tin, called bronze, are the most useful.

Characteristics. Copper is recognized by its color, and the effects of tests on the solution of its nitrate. This solution, with potassa, soda, and ammonia, yields a blue precipitate, soluble in excess of the latter alkali, with which it forms a deep azure blue liquid. Ferrocyanide of potassium occasions a brown precipitate of ferrocyanide of copper; and a bright plate of iron, immersed in the solution, immediately becomes covered with a film of metallic copper. The ferrocyanide of potassium is a very delicate test for minute portions of copper in solution. Another test, proposed by M. Verguin, is to precipitate the copper in the metallic state on platinum by electro-chemical action. For this purpose a drop of the liquid to be examined is placed on a slip of platinum foil, and a slip of bright iron is brought in contact with the platinum and the liquid. If copper be present it will be instantly precipitated on the surface of the platinum.

Action on the Animal Economy. Copper, in its pure state, is perfectly inert, but in combination it is highly deleterious. Nevertheless a minute portion of the metal has been found in the human body. According to Millon, copper, when it exists in the blood, is, like the iron, attached to the red corpuscles. To bring the copper into a state favorable for ready detection, he advises that the blood, as it escapes from a vein, be received in about three times its bulk of water, and the mixture poured into a bottle of chlorine and agitated. The whole, upon being rapidly filtered, furnishes a liquid in which copper is readily detected. Wackenroder found copper in the blood of man, but does not consider it a constant and normal constituent. He also detected this metal in the blood of domestic animals living on a mixed diet, but not in their blood when nourished on vegetable food only. (*Chem. Gaz.*, May 1, 1854.) It has been found in the feathers of certain birds, as of a grass-green paroquet from Australia, which is said to frequent districts of the country where copper is found. (*Ibid.*, Oct. 24, 1873, p. 212.) The soluble combinations of copper, when taken in poisonous doses, produce a coppery taste in the mouth; nausea and vomiting; violent pain in the stomach and bowels; frequent black and bloody stools; small, irregular, sharp, and frequent pulse; faintings; burning thirst; difficulty of breathing; cold sweats; paucity of urine, and burning pain in voiding it; violent headache; cramps, convulsions, and finally death. The best antidote is the ferrocyanide of potassium, given freely, which forms, with the poison, the very insoluble ferrocyanide of copper. Soap and alkalies are also antidotal. Before the antidote can be procured, large quantities should be given of milk, and white of eggs mixed with water, which act favorably by forming the caseate and albuminate of copper; but these compounds should be evacuated as soon as possible by vomiting and purging. Should vomiting not take place, the stomach-pump may be employed. The symptoms of slow poisoning by copper are, according to Dr. Corrigan, of Dublin, a cachectic appearance, emaciation, loss of muscular strength, colicky pains, cough without physical signs, and retraction of the gum, with a persistent purple edge, quite distinct from the blue edge produced by lead. (*Braithwaite's Retrospect*, Am. ed., xxx. 303.) But there is much doubt whether these symptoms can be produced by the metal. (See H. C. Wood's Therapeutics.)

Dr. Horsley has detected sulphate of copper in bread and flour used in London, and presumes that it was added with the view of improving the appearance of the flour. (*Chem. News*, No. 63, p. 111, and No. 65, p. 142.)

In medico-legal examinations, where cupreous poisoning is suspected, Orfila recommends that the viscera be boiled in distilled water for an hour, and that the matter obtained by evaporating the filtered decoction to dryness be carbonized by nitric acid. The carbonized product will contain the copper. By proceeding in this way, there is no risk of obtaining the copper which may happen to pre-exist in the animal tissues. This method of search is preferable to that of examining the contents of the stomach and intestines, from which copper may be absent; while it may have penetrated the different organs by absorption, especially the abdominal viscera.

Vessels of copper which are not coated with tin should not be used in pharmaceutical or culinary operations; for, although the metal uncombined is inert, yet the risk is great that the vessels may be acted on and a poisonous salt formed.

CUSPARIÆ CORTEX. *Br.* *Cusparia Bark.*

(CŬS-PĀ'RĮ-Æ CŎR'TĔX.)

"The dried bark of Galipea Cusparia." *Br.* (*Nat. Ord.* Rutaceæ.)

Angustura, *U.S.* 1870; Angusture, *Fr.*; Angusturarinde, *G.*; Corteccia dell' Angustura, *It.*; Cortesa de Angostura, *Sp.*

This bark was formerly officinal in the U. S. Pharmacopœia of 1870 under the name of Angustura, but it was dropped at the last revision.

The subject of Angustura bark, in its botanical relations, has been involved in some confusion. The drug was at first supposed to be derived from a species of Magnolia, and was referred by some to *Magnolia glauca* of this country. Humboldt and Bonpland were the first to throw light upon its true source. When at Angostura, a South American city on the Orinoco, they received specimens of the foliage of the plant from which the bark was obtained; and afterwards believed that they had found the same plant in a tree growing in the vicinity of Cumana. This latter they had the opportunity of personally inspecting, and were therefore enabled to describe accurately. Unable to attach it to any known genus, they erected it into a new one with the title of *Cusparia*, a name of Indian origin, to which they added the specific appellation of *febrifuga*. On their authority, *Cusparia febrifuga* was generally believed to be the true source of the medicine, and was recognized as such by the London College. A specimen having in the mean time been sent by them to Willdenow, the name of *Bonplandia* was imposed on the new genus by that celebrated botanist; and it was subsequently adopted by Humboldt and Bonpland themselves, in their great work on equinoctial plants. Hence the title of *Bonplandia trifoliata*, by which the tree is described in many works on Materia Medica. De Candolle, however, having found in the description all the characters of the genus *Galipea* of Aublet, rejected both these titles, and substituted that of *Galipea Cusparia*, which was adopted by the London College, and has been retained in the British Pharmacopœia. But, after all these commutations, it appears from the researches of Dr. Hancock, who resided for several months in the country of the Angustura bark tree, that it is doubtful whether the plant described by Humboldt and Bonpland is that which yields the medicine, and is not another species of the same genus. Among other striking differences between them is that of their size; the tree described by Humboldt and Bonpland being at least sixty feet high, while that from which the bark is obtained is never more than twenty feet. Hancock proposed for the latter the title of *Galipea officinalis*, which was adopted in the U. S. P. 1870.

Gen. Ch. *Corolla* inferior, irregular, four or five cleft, hypocrateriform. *Stamens* four; two sterile. *Loudon's Encyc.*

Galipea officinalis. Hancock, *Trans. Lond. Medico-Bot. Soc.*—*Galipea Cusparia.* St. Hilaire, *B. & T.* 43. This is a small tree, irregularly branched, rising to the medium height of twelve or fifteen feet, with an erect stem from three to five inches in diameter, and covered with a smooth gray bark. The leaves are alternate, petiolate, and composed of three leaflets, which are oblong, pointed at each extremity, from six to ten inches in length, from two to four in breadth, and supported upon the common petiole by short leaf-stalks. They are very smooth and glossy, of a vivid green color, marked occasionally with small whitish round spots, and when fresh, of a strong odor resembling that of tobacco. The flowers are numerous, white, arranged in axillary and terminal peduncled racemes, and of a peculiar unpleasant odor. The fruit consists of five bivalve capsules, of which two or three are commonly abortive. The seeds, two of which are contained in each capsule, one often abortive, are round, black, and of the size of a pea. The tree grows abundantly on the mountains of Carony, between the 7th and 8th degrees of N. latitude, and is well known in the missions, near the Orinoco, upwards of 200 miles from the ocean. It flourishes at the height of from six hundred to one thousand feet above the level of the sea. Its elegant white blossoms, which appear in vast profusion in August and September, add greatly to the beauty of the scenery.

The bark is generally brought from the West Indies, packed in casks; but, according to Mr. Brande, the original package, as it comes from Angostura, consists of the leaves of a species of palm, surrounded by a net-work of sticks.

Properties. The pieces are of various lengths, for the most part slightly curved, rarely quilled, sometimes nearly flat, from half a line to a line or more in thickness, pared away towards the edges, covered externally with a light yellowish gray or whitish wrinkled epidermis, easily scraped by the nail, and internally of a yellowish fawn color. They are very fragile, breaking with a short, resinous fracture, and yield, on being pulverized, a pale yellow powder; but when macerated for a short time in water, swell up to two or three times their original thickness and become soft and tenacious, and may be cut into strips with scissors. The cut surface usually exhibits under the microscope numerous white points or minute lines. *Br.* Oxalate of calcium raphides are abundant in the bark, but the most characteristic peculiarity are numerous cells, a little larger than the other parenchymatous cells and completely filled with oil or a yellowish resin.* The smell of Angustura bark is peculiar and disagreeable when fresh, but becomes fainter with age; the taste is bitter and slightly aromatic, leaving a sense of pungency at the end of the tongue. According to Fischer, it contains volatile oil, bitter extractive, a hard and bitter resin, a soft resin, a substance analogous to caoutchouc, gum, lignin, and various salts. Oberlin and Schlagdenhauffen (1878) found in the bitter extractive an alkaloid *angosturine*, $C_{10}H_{40}NO_{14}$, which

* For an elaborate microscopical study of the bark, see *Journ. de Pharm.*, xxviii. 280.

melts at 85° C., is crystallizable, and is turned red by pure sulphuric acid, and green by sulphuric acid with admixture of nitric acid. The volatile oil, which may be obtained by distillation with water, is of a pale yellowish color, lighter than water, of an acrid taste, and with the odor of the bark. Its formula is given as $C_{18}H_{24}O$ by Dr. C. Herzog, who states that its boiling point is 266·1° C. (511° F.), probably one of the highest of the volatile oils. (*Chem. Gaz.*, May 15, 1858.) *Cusparin* is the name given by Saladin to a principle, deposited in tetrahedral crystals, when an infusion of the bark is treated with absolute alcohol, at common temperatures, and allowed to evaporate spontaneously. It is neutral, fusible at a gentle heat, by which it loses 23·09 per cent. of its weight, soluble in 200 parts of cold and 100 parts of boiling water, soluble in the concentrated acids and in the alkalies, and precipitated by the infusion of galls. (*Journ. de Pharm.*, xxii. 662.)

Dr. A. T. Thomson states that precipitates are produced with the infusion by the solutions of sulphate of iron, tartrate of antimony and potassium, sulphate of copper, acetate and subacetate of lead, bichloride of mercury, nitrate of silver, and pure potassa; by nitric and sulphuric acids; and by the infusions of galls and yellow cinchona; but how far these substances are medicinally incompatible with the bark, it would be difficult to determine.

False Angustura. Under this title, European writers describe a bark which was introduced on the continent mixed with true Angustura bark, and, being possessed of poisonous properties, produced in some instances unpleasant effects, when dispensed by mistake for that medicine. It is distinguished by its greater thickness, hardness, weight, and compactness; by its resinous fracture; by the appearance of its epidermis, which is sometimes covered with a ferruginous efflorescence, sometimes is yellowish gray, and marked with prominent white spots; by the brownish color and smoothness of its internal surface, which is not, like that of the genuine bark, separable into laminæ; by the white slightly yellow powder which it yields; by its total want of odor, and its intense tenacious bitterness. When steeped in water, it does not become soft, like the true Angustura. Analyzed by Pelletier and Caventou, it was found to contain a peculiar alkaline principle which they called *brucine*, and upon which its poisonous operation depends. (See *Nux Vomica.*) In consequence of the presence of this principle, a drop of nitric acid upon the internal surface of the bark produces a deep red spot. The same acid, applied to the external surface, renders it emerald-green. In true Angustura bark, a dull red color is produced by the acid on both surfaces. The *false Angustura* was at first supposed to be derived from *Brucea antidysenterica*, but at present is ascribed to *Strychnos Nux Vomica*, the bark of which, according to Dr. O'Shaughnessy, exactly corresponds with the description of false Angustura, and like it contains brucia.

Brazilian Angustura Bark, the product of *Esenbeckia febrifuga*, consists of slightly curved pieces 8 to 10 inches long, about $\frac{1}{16}$ of an inch in thickness, of a persistently bitter taste. The outer surface is usually ashen gray, and always marked with longitudinal red or black spots on a yellow ground; the inner surface is reddish, with paler, distinct, elongated fibres. On maceration the bark does not swell. (Oberlin and Schlagdenhauffen, *Journ. de Pharm.*, xxviii. 242.)

Medical Properties and Uses. Angustura bark had been long used by the natives of the countries where it grows, before it became known elsewhere. From the continent its employment extended to the West Indies, where it acquired considerable reputation, and about eighty years since it was introduced into Europe. Its operation is that of a stimulant tonic. In large doses it also evacuates the stomach and bowels, and is often employed for this purpose in South America. It is said to be peculiarly efficacious in bilious diarrhœas and dysenteries, and has been recommended in dyspepsia and other diseases requiring a tonic treatment. The testimony, however, of practitioners in Europe and the United States is not strongly in its favor; and it is probably better adapted to tropical diseases than to those of temperate climates. Hancock employed it extensively in the malignant bilious intermittent fevers, dysenteries, and dropsies of Angustura and Demerara, and speaks in strong terms of its efficacy in these complaints. He used it in the form of fermented infusion, as recommended by the native practitioners.

It may be given in powder, infusion, tincture, or extract. The dose in substance is from ten to thirty grains (0·65–1·95 Gm.). In larger quantities it is apt to produce nausea. From five to fifteen grains (0·33–1 Gm.) is the dose of the extract, which, however, according to Dr. Hancock, is inferior to the powder or infusion. To obviate nausea, it is frequently combined with aromatics.

Off. Prep. Br. Infusum Cuspariæ.

CYDONIUM. *U.S.* *Cydonium.* [*Quince Seed.*]

(CȲ-DŌ′NĮ-ŬM.)

"The seed of Cydonia vulgaris. Persoon. (*Nat. Ord.* Rosaceæ, Pomeæ.)" *U. S.*

Semen Cydoniæ, *P.G.*; Semences (Pépins) des Coing, Semences de Coing, *Fr.*; Quittenkerne, Quittensamen, *G.*; Semi di Cotogno, *It.*; Semiente de Membrillo, *Sp.*

The quince-tree has been separated from the genus *Pyrus*, and erected into a new one called *Cydonia*, which differs in the circumstance that the cells of its fruit contain many seeds, instead of two only as in Pyrus.

Gen. Ch. Calyx five-parted, with leafy divisions. *Apple* closed, many-seeded. *Testa* mucilaginous. *Loudon's Encyc.*

Cydonia vulgaris. Persoon, *Enchir.* ii. 40.—*Pyrus Cydonia.* Willd. *Sp. Plant.* ii. 1020; Woodv. *Med. Bot.* p. 505, t. 182. The common quince-tree is characterized as a species by its downy deciduous leaves. It is supposed to be a native of Crete, but grows wild in Austria, on the banks of the Danube. It is abundantly cultivated in this country. The fruit is about the size of a pear, yellow, downy, of an agreeable odor, and a rough, astringent, acidulous taste; and in each of its five cells contains from eight to fourteen seeds. Though not eaten raw, it forms a very pleasant confection; and a syrup prepared from it may be used as a grateful addition to drinks in sickness, especially in looseness of the bowels, which it is supposed to restrain by its astringency. The seeds are the officinal portion.

They are ovate, angled, reddish brown externally, white within, inodorous, and nearly insipid, being slightly bitter when long chewed. Their coriaceous envelope abounds in mucilage, which is extracted by boiling water. "About a quarter of an inch (6 mm.) long, oval or oblong, triangularly compressed, brown, covered with a whitish, mucilaginous epithelium, causing the seeds of each cell to adhere. With water the seeds swell up, and form a mucilaginous mass. The unbroken seeds have an insipid taste." *U. S.* Two drachms of the seeds will render a pint of water thick and ropy. (*A. J. P.*, 1876, p. 35.) It has been proposed to evaporate the decoction to dryness, and powder the residue. Three grains of this powder form a sufficiently consistent mucilage with an ounce of water. According to M. Garot, one part communicates to a thousand parts of water a semi-syrupy consistence. (*Journ. de Pharm.*, 3e sér., iii. 298.) Dr. Pereira considers the mucilage as peculiar, and proposes to call it *cydonin.* It differs from arabin in not yielding a precipitate with silicate of potassium, and from bassorin and cerasin in being soluble in water both hot and cold. Tollens and Kirchner (*Ann. d. Chemie*, clxxv. 205–226) assign to it the formula $C_{18}H_{28}O_{14}$, regarding it as a compound of gum, $C_{12}H_{20}O_{10}$, and cellulose, $C_6H_{10}O_5$, less one molecule of water.

Medical Properties, etc. Quince mucilage may be used for the same purposes as other mucilaginous liquids. It is preferred as a local application in conjunctival ophthalmia, but in this country is less used than the infusion of sassafras pith.

Off. Prep. Mucilago Cydonii, *U. S.*

CYPRIPEDIUM. *U.S.* *Cypripedium.* [*Ladies' Slipper.*]

(ÇȲP-RĮ-PĒ′DĮ-ŬM.)

"The rhizome and rootlets of Cypripedium pubescens, Willdenow, and of Cypripedium parviflorum, Salisbury. (*Nat. Ord.* Orchidaceæ.)" *U. S.*

Rhizoma Cypripedii; Ladies' Slipper Root; Racine de Cypripède jaune, Valériane américaine, *Fr.*; Gelbfrauenschuh-Wurzel, *G.*

Gen. Ch. Sepals spreading; the two anterior generally united into one under the lip. *Petals* similar but usually narrower, spreading. *Lip* a large inflated sac, somewhat slipper-shaped. *Column* short, three-lobed; the lateral lobes bearing an anther under each, the middle dilated and petal-like. *Gray.*

Under the common name of *ladies' slipper*, or *moccasin plant*, several species of Cypripedium inhabit the woods in different parts of the United States. They are small plants, with large, many-nerved, plaited leaves, sheathing at the base, and large often beautiful flowers, of a shape not unlike the Indian moccasin, whence they derive one of their common names. Their generic name of Cypripedium (*Κύπρις*, Venus, and *πόδιον*, sock) had a similar origin. Several of them have been used by American physicians, the root being the part employed. Dr. R. P. Stevens, of Ceres, Pennsylvania, says of them, that he has found the *C. spectabile* and *C. acaule*, especially when growing in dark swamps, to be possessed of narcotic properties, and to be less safe than the *C. parviflorum*, which is gently stimulant with a tendency to the nervous system, and is quite equal to valerian. He has employed it advantageously in hysteria, and in the pains of the joints following scarlet fever. (*N. Y. Journ. of Med.*, iv. 359.) Dr. E. Ives considers *C. pubescens, spectabile*, and *humile* identical in their effects, but *C. pubescens* the most powerful. (*Trans. of Amer. Med. Assoc.*, iii. 312.) The roots of the two species *C. pubescens* and *C. parviflorum* are indiscriminately kept in the shops and sold by the same name.

Cypripedium pubescens. Willd. *Sp. Plant.* iv. 142. The *yellow ladies' slipper*, as this plant is called from the color of its flowers, has a simple often flexuous, pubescent, leafy stem, from one to two feet high. The leaves are pubescent, ovate-lanceolate, acuminate, narrowing at the base, about four or five inches long by two in breadth, alternate, sessile, and sheathing. The flower is usually solitary and terminal; with four divisions of the perianth, the two outer cohering nearly to the apex, the inner longer, narrower, undulatory or twisted, and the lip an inch or two in length, swelling sac-like, and of a yellow color. The fruit is an oblong capsule, tapering at each end, recurved, pubescent, and peduncled. The plant is indigenous, growing abundantly in rich, moist woods throughout the United States.

Cypripedium parviflorum. (Salisbury.) *Common Ladies' Slipper. Small-flowered Ladies' Slipper.* This is a perennial plant with a leafy stem, a foot or two in height, and comparatively small yellowish green flowers, appearing in May. The specific character of the flower, which is that also of the plant, is, that the lobe of the style is triangular and acute; the outer petals are oblong-ovate and acuminate; the inner linear and contorted; the lips shorter than the petals and compressed. This species grows extensively through the United States south of the Potomac, east and west of the Alleghanies, and in several of the Northern States, particularly New York, Michigan, Connecticut, and Vermont. In Pennsylvania, especially near Philadelphia, it does not appear to prevail, and it is not mentioned in Darlington's *Flora Cestrica* as among the plants of Chester County.

The root, in both species, is the officinal portion. This consists of a rhizome, from two to four inches long, with numerous rootlets attached. "Horizontal, bent, four inches (10 cm.) or less, long; about one-eighth of an inch (3 mm.) thick; on the upper side beset with numerous, circular, cup-shaped scars; closely covered below with simple, wiry rootlets varying from four to twenty inches (10 to 50 cm.) in length; brittle, dark brown, or orange brown; fracture short, white; odor faint but heavy; taste sweetish, bitter and somewhat pungent." *U. S.* Prof. Maisch gives a distinctive description of the roots of the two species, of which the following is a condensed account. Of *C. pubescens* the rhizome is almost horizontal, in its greatest length nearly four inches, slightly bent with a shallow downward curve, from $\frac{1}{8}$ to $\frac{3}{16}$ of an inch thick, with numerous deeply concave scars left by the stems, having fully the width of the rhizome. The rootlets are numerous, several inches in length, sometimes even nine inches or more, about $\frac{1}{12}$ of an inch thick, without branches, somewhat undulate, and, though attached to the rhizome on all sides, are abruptly turned downward, owing to its horizontal position in the ground. Their color is yellowish brown, becoming much darker on drying, which causes longitudinal wrinkles. The cortical part of both species is colored blue by iodine. The rhizome of *C. parviflorum* is altogether different from the former, being bent nearly at right angles, three or four times, each section about $\frac{3}{4}$ of an inch long; and the whole length, while only about two inches in a straight line, from end to end, is yet actually three inches along the course of the rhizome. This is about $\frac{1}{8}$ of an inch thick, and has stem-scars, about the same in width, with about three in each bend. The rootlets, which are attached to all sides of the rhizome, are numerous, four to six inches long, less undular than those of *C. pubescens*, and of a brighter color, being a decided orange brown when fresh, and changing little on drying. (*A. J. P.*, 1872, p. 297.)

The roots of the Cypripedia are sometimes mixed, as brought into the market, with those of *Hydrastis Canadensis*, from the plants occasionally growing in close contiguity. (See *Hydrastis.*) Roots of seneka have also been noticed in specimens of Cypripedium; but there can be no difficulty in distinguishing them.

Properties. Cypripedium has a somewhat aromatic odor which diminishes by time, and a bitter, sweetish, peculiar, and in the end somewhat pungent taste. It yields its virtues to water and alcohol. The root has been analyzed by Mr. Henry C. Blair, who found it to contain a volatile oil, a volatile acid, tannic and gallic acids, two resins, gum, glucose, starch, and lignin. (*A. J. P.*, 1866, p. 494.) The so-called eclectics prepare what they improperly call *cypripedin* by precipitating with water a concentrated tincture of the root. The substance thus obtained is complex, and has no claim to the name given it, which ought to be reserved for the active principle when discovered. It is probable that the virtues of the root reside in a volatile oil and bitter principle.

Medical Uses. Cypripedium appears to be a gentle nervous stimulant or antispasmodic, and has been used for the same purposes as valerian, though less powerful. Dr. E. Ives, of New Haven, Conn., has employed the remedy in a variety of nervous diseases with advantage, and has known it even to cure epilepsy. The other complaints mentioned by him are hypochondriasis, neuralgia, and morbid sensitiveness of the nervous system generally, and especially of the eye. The medicine may be used in powder, infusion, or tincture. The dose of the powder given by Dr. Ives was fifteen grains (1 Gm.) three times a day. The oleoresin, obtained by precipitating the tincture, has been given in doses varying from half a grain to three grains (0·03–0·20 Gm.).

Off. Prep. Extractum Cypripedii Fluidum.

DECOCTA. *Decoctions.*

(DE-CŎC′TA.)

Décoctions, *Fr.;* **Abkochungen,** *G.*

Decoctions are solutions of vegetable principles, obtained by *boiling* the substances containing these principles in water. Vegetables generally yield their soluble ingredients more readily, and in larger proportion, to water maintained at the point of ebullition, than to the same liquid at a lower temperature. Hence decoction is occasionally preferred to infusion as a mode of extracting the virtues of plants, when the call for the remedy is urgent, and the greatest possible activity in the preparation is desirable. The process should be conducted in a covered vessel, so as to confine the vapor over the surface of the liquid, and thus prevent the access of atmospheric air, which sometimes exerts an injurious agency upon the active principle. The boiling, moreover, should not, as a general rule, be long continued; as the ingredients of the vegetable are apt to react on each other, and thus lose, to a greater or less extent, their original character. The substance submitted to decoction should if dry be either powdered or well bruised, if fresh, should be sliced, so that it may present an extensive surface to the action of the solvent; and previous maceration for some time in water is occasionally useful by overcoming the cohesion of the vegetable fibre. Should the physician not happen to prescribe this preliminary comminution, the pharmacist should not omit it.

All vegetable substances are not proper objects for decoction. In many, the active principle is volatile at a boiling heat, in others, it undergoes some change unfavorable to its activity, and in a third set is associated with inefficient or nauseous principles, which, though insoluble or but slightly soluble in cool water, are abundantly extracted by that liquid at the boiling temperature, and thus encumber, if they do not positively injure, the preparation. In all these instances, infusion is preferable to decoction. Besides, by the latter process, more matter is often dissolved than the water can retain, so that upon cooling a precipitation takes place, and the liquid is rendered turbid.

and this constitutes the greatest objection to this class of preparations. When the active principle is thus dissolved in excess, the decoction should always be strained while hot; so that the matter which separates on cooling may be mixed again with the fluid by agitation at the time of administering the remedy.

In compound decoctions, the ingredients may be advantageously added at different periods of the process, according to the length of boiling requisite for extracting their virtues; and, should one of them owe its activity to a volatile principle, the proper plan is, at the close of the process, to pour upon it the boiling decoction, and allow the liquor to cool in a covered vessel.

As a general rule, glass or earthenware vessels should be preferred; as those made of metal are sometimes corroded by the ingredients of the decoction, which thus become contaminated. Vessels of clean cast-iron or common tin, or of block tin, are preferable to those of copper, brass, or zinc; but iron pots should not be used when astringent vegetables are concerned.

Decoctions, from the mutual reaction of their constituents, as well as from the influence of the air, are apt to spoil in a short time. Hence they should be prepared only when wanted for use, and should not be kept, in warm weather, for a longer period than forty-eight hours.

The tendency of modern medicine and pharmacy has been decidedly against the employment of decoctions; the nauseous taste, bulky dose, repulsive appearance, and non-permanent character have been powerful reasons for causing their retirement, whilst the use of tinctures and fluid extracts has largely increased. In the recent revision of the U. S. Pharmacopœia the number of officinal decoctions was reduced to two, and a general formula appended for the guidance of the pharmacist, as follows.

General Formula for Decoctions. "An ordinary Decoction, the strength of which is not directed by the physician, nor specified by the Pharmacopœia, shall be prepared by the following formula: Take of the Substance, coarsely comminuted, *ten parts*; Water, *a sufficient quantity*, To make *one hundred parts.* Put the Substance into a suitable vessel, provided with a cover, pour upon it *one hundred* (100) *parts* of cold Water, cover it well, and boil for fifteen minutes; then let it cool to about 45° C. (113° F.), strain the liquid, and pass through the strainer enough cold Water to make the product weight *one hundred* (100) *parts.*

"*Caution.* The strength of Decoctions of energetic or powerful substances should be specially prescribed by the physician." *U. S.* The decoctions which were officinal in 1870 but dropped at the last revision are: *Decoction of Pipsissewa, Yellow Cinchona, Red Cinchona, Dogwood, Bittersweet, Logwood, Barley, Oak Bark, Seneka, and Uva Ursi.* With the exception of decoction of barley, these were all made by boiling a troyounce of the drug with a pint of water for fifteen minutes, straining, and adding sufficient water through the strainer to make the decoction measure a pint. If the physician orders a decoction of either of the above now, without specifying the strength, it must be made by the *general formula*, which will make the new decoctions about one and a half times as strong as the decoctions of U. S. P. 1870.

DECOCTUM ALOES COMPOSITUM. *Br.* *Compound Decoction of Aloes.*

(DE-CŎC'TUM ĂL'O-ĒS COM-PŎS'I-TŬM.)

Tisane (Décocté) d'Aloès composée, *Fr.;* Zusammengesetztes Aloedecoct, *G.*

"Take of Extract of Socotrine Aloes *half an ounce* [av.]; Myrrh, Saffron, Carbonate of Potassium, of each, *quarter of an ounce* [av.]; Extract of Liquorice *two ounces* [av.]; Compound Tincture of Cardamoms *fifteen fluidounces* [Imp. meas.]; Distilled Water a sufficiency to make *fifty fluidounces* [Imp. meas.]. Reduce the Extract of Aloes and the Myrrh to coarse powder, and put them together with the Carbonate of Potassium and Extract of Liquorice into a suitable covered vessel with a pint of Distilled Water; boil gently for five minutes, then add the Saffron. Let the vessel with its contents cool, then add the Tincture of Cardamoms, and, covering the vessel closely, allow the ingredients to macerate for two hours; finally, strain through flannel, pouring as much Distilled Water over the contents of the strainer as will make the strained product measure *fifty fluidounces*. This preparation should be kept in vessels from which air is excluded as far as possible." *Br.*

This is essentially the former process of the British Colleges. The direction is properly given to rub the aloes, myrrh, and carbonate of potassium together before the addition of the other ingredients. The effect of the alkaline carbonate is, by combining with the resin of the myrrh, and the insoluble portion (apotheme of *Berzelius*) of the aloes, to render them more soluble in water, while the liquorice assists in the suspension of the portion not actually dissolved. The tincture of cardamom is useful not only by its cordial property, but also by preventing spontaneous decomposition. This decoction is said not to filter clear when first made, but, if kept for some time, to deposit insoluble matter, and then to become bright and clear on filtering. (*P. J. Tr.*, xiv. 491.)

Long boiling impairs the purgative property of aloes; and the same effect is thought to be produced, to a certain extent, by the alkalies, which certainly qualify its operation, and render it less apt to irritate the rectum. This decoction, therefore, is milder as a cathartic than aloes itself: it is also more tonic and cordial, from the presence of the myrrh, saffron, and cardamom, and derives antacid properties from the carbonate of potassium. It is given as a gentle cathartic, tonic, and emmenagogue, and is especially useful in dyspepsia, habitual constipation, and those complicated cases in which suppressed or retained menstruation is connected with enfeebled digestion and a languid state of the bowels. The dose is from a half to two fluidounces (15–60 C.c.). The decoction should not be combined in prescription with acids, acidulous salts, or other bodies incompatible with the alkaline carbonate.

DECOCTUM CETRARIÆ. *U. S., Br.* *Decoction of Cetraria. Decoction of Iceland Moss.*

(DE-CŎC'TUM CE-TRĀ'RI-Æ.)

Tisane (Décocté) de Lichen d'Islande, *Fr.;* Islandisch-Moos-Absud (Decoct), *G.*

"Cetraria, *five parts* [or one ounce av.]; Water, *a sufficient quantity*, To make *one hundred parts* [or twenty fluidounces]. Cover the Cetraria, in a suitable vessel, with *forty parts* [or half a pint] of cold Water, express after half an hour, and throw away the liquid. Then boil the Cetraria with *one hundred parts* [or twenty fluidounces] of Water for half an hour, strain, and add enough cold Water, through the strainer, to make the product weigh *one hundred parts* [or measure twenty fluidounces]." *U. S.*

"Take of Iceland Moss *one ounce* [avoirdupois]; Distilled Water *one pint* [Imperial measure]. Wash the Moss in cold water, to remove impurities; boil it with the Distilled Water for ten minutes in a covered vessel, and strain, with gentle pressure, while hot; then pour Distilled Water over the contents of the strainer until the strained product measures a pint [Imp. meas.]." *Br.*

This is one of the two decoctions retained in the present U. S. Pharmacopœia. It is stronger than the one officinal in 1870. At present there is 5 per cent. of Iceland moss used in the preparation, where there was formerly but about 3 per cent. It is now of the same strength as the British.

The directions of the U. S. Pharmacopœia of 1850 were to boil *half an ounce* of the Moss with *a pint and a half* of Water down to a pint, and to strain with compression; and this process is preferable when the object is to extract not only the bitter principle, but also the whole of the demulcent and nutritive matter. As the bitter principle is dissolved along with the starch-like matter of the moss, this decoction unites an unpleasant flavor to its demulcent properties; but the plan which has been proposed of first extracting the bitterness by maceration in water, or a very weak solution of an alkaline carbonate, and afterwards preparing the decoction, is inadmissible; as the peculiar virtues which distinguish the medicine from the ordinary demulcents are thus entirely lost. (See *Cetraria*.) A pint (472 C.c.) of the decoction may be taken during the day.*

* *Decoctum Chimaphilæ.* U. S. 1870. *Decoction of Pipsissewa.* "Take of Pipsissewa, bruised, *a troyounce;* Water *a sufficient quantity*. Boil the Pipsissewa in a pint of Water for fifteen minutes,

DECOCTUM CINCHONÆ. *Br.* *Decoction of Cinchona.*

(DE-CŎC'TUM CĬN-CHŌ'NÆ FLĀ'VÆ.)

Decoctum Chinæ Regiæ; Tisane (Décocté) de Quinquina jaune, *Fr.;* Königschina-Absud, *G.*

"Take of Red Cinchona Bark, in No. 20 powder, *one ounce and a quarter* [avoirdupois]; Distilled Water *one pint* [Imperial measure]. Boil for ten minutes in a covered vessel. Strain the decoction, when cold, and pour as much distilled water over the contents of the strainer as will make the strained product measure one pint [Imp. meas.]" *Br.** Dose, one to two fluidounces (30–60 C.c.).

DECOCTUM GRANATI RADICIS. *Br.* *Decoction of Pomegranate Root.*

(DE-CŎC'TUM GRA-NĀ'TĪ RA-DĪ'CĬS.)

Decoctum Corticis Radicis Granati; Tisane (Décocté) d'Écorce de la Racine de Grenadier, *Fr.;* Granatwurzel-Rinden-Absud, *G.*

"Take of Pomegranate Root Bark, sliced, *two ounces* [avoirdupois]; Distilled Water *two pints* [Imperial measure]. Boil down to a pint [Imp. meas.], and strain, making the strained product up to a pint [Imp. meas.], if necessary, by pouring distilled water over the contents of the strainer." *Br.* Dose, two to four fluidounces (60–120 C.c.).

For the uses and dose of this decoction, see *Granati Radicis Cortex.*

DECOCTUM HÆMATOXYLI. *Br.* *Decoction of Logwood.*

(DE-CŎC'TUM HÆ-MA-TŎX'Y-LĪ—hē-mą-tŏk'sį-lī.)

Tisane (Décocté) de Boise de Campêche, *Fr.;* Blauholtz-Absud, *G.*

"Take of Logwood, in chips, *one ounce* [avoirdupois]; Cinnamon Bark, bruised, *fifty-five grains;* Distilled Water *one pint* [Imperial measure]. Boil the Logwood in the Water for ten minutes in a covered vessel, adding the Cinnamon towards the end. Strain the decoction, and pour as much distilled water over the contents of the strainer as will make the strained product measure a pint [Imp. meas.]." *Br.*

We prefer the old U. S. formula, which ordered an ounce of the logwood to be boiled with two pints down to a pint, and doubt much whether the wood is exhausted by a boiling of ten or fifteen minutes. The cinnamon of the Br. formula is in general a very suitable addition; but there might be circumstances under which it would be better omitted; and in this case, as in others, any addition to the simple decoction might be left to the judgment of the prescriber.

strain, and add sufficient Water, through the strainer, to make the decoction measure a pint." *U. S.* 1870. This decoction is in every way inferior to the fluid extract. One pint (472 C.c.) of it may be given in the course of twenty-four hours.

* *Decoctum Cinchonæ Flavæ.* U. S. 1870. *Decoction of Yellow Cinchona.* "Take of Yellow Cinchona, bruised, *a troyounce;* Water *a sufficient quantity.* Boil the Yellow Cinchona in a pint of Water for fifteen minutes, strain, and add sufficient Water, through the strainer, to make the decoction measure a pint." *U. S.* 1870.

Decoctum Cinchonæ Rubræ. U. S. 1870. *Decoction of Red Cinchona. Decoction of Red Bark.* "Take of Red Cinchona, bruised, *a troyounce;* Water *a sufficient quantity.* Boil the Red Cinchona in a pint of Water for fifteen minutes, strain, and add sufficient Water, through the strainer, to make the decoction measure a pint." *U. S.* 1870.

These decoctions have been very appropriately dropped from the Pharmacopœia. Although capable, no doubt, of impressing the system, they are very ineligible preparations.

The dose of the decoction is two fluidounces (60 C.c.), to be repeated more or less frequently according to circumstances. Two drachms of orange peel, added to the decoction while still boiling hot, improve its flavor, and render it more acceptable to the stomach.

Decoctum Cornûs Floridæ. U. S. 1870. *Decoction of Dogwood.* "Take of Dogwood, bruised, *a troyounce;* Water *a sufficient quantity.* Boil the Dogwood in a pint of Water for fifteen minutes, strain, and add sufficient Water, through the strainer, to make the decoction measure a pint." *U. S.* 1870. This decoction has been proposed as a substitute for that of Peruvian bark; but, though possessed of analogous properties, it is much inferior in efficacy, and is not likely to be extensively employed so long as the Peruvian tonic is attainable. The dose is two fluidounces (60 C.c.).

Decoctum Dulcamaræ. U. S. 1870. *Decoction of Bittersweet.* "Take of Bittersweet, bruised, *a troyounce;* Water *a sufficient quantity.* Boil the Bittersweet in a pint of Water for fifteen minutes, strain, and add sufficient Water, through the strainer, to make the decoction measure a pint." *U. S.* 1870. This is a good preparation of bittersweet if it is absolutely necessary to use an aqueous menstruum. The properties and uses of this decoction may be found under the head of *Dulcamara.* The dose is from one to two fluidounces (30–60 C.c.) three or four times a day, or more frequently.

This is an excellent astringent in diarrhœa, particularly in that form of it which succeeds the cholera infantum of this climate, or occurs as an original complaint in children during summer. The dose for an adult is two fluidounces (60 C.c.), for a child about two years old, two or three fluidrachms (7·5–11·25 C.c.), repeated several times a day. A little bruised cinnamon may often be added with advantage at the end of the boiling, as directed in the British process.

DECOCTUM HORDEI. *Br.* *Decoction of Barley.*

(DĘ-CŎC'TŲM HŎR'DĘ-Ī.)

Tisane d'Orge perlé, *Fr.;* Gerstenschleim, *G.*

"Take of Pearl Barley *two ounces* [avoirdupois]; Distilled Water *one pint and a half* [Imperial measure]. Wash the Barley in cold water, and reject the washings; boil the washed barley with the Distilled Water for twenty minutes, in a covered vessel, and strain. The product is about one pint." *Br.*

Barley water, as this decoction is usually called, is much employed as a nutritive drink in febrile and inflammatory complaints, and, from the total absence of irritating properties, is peculiarly adapted to cases in which the gastric or intestinal mucous membrane is inflamed. As the stomach of those for whom it is directed is often exceedingly delicate, and apt to revolt against anything having the slightest unpleasantness of flavor, it is important that the decoction should be properly made; and, though the office of preparing it generally falls to nurses, yet the introduction of the process into the Pharmacopœia is not without advantage; as a formula is thus ever before the physician, by which he may give his directions, with the certainty, if obeyed, of having a good preparation. The object of the washing with cold water, is completely to remove any mustiness, or other disagreeable flavor, which the barley may have acquired from exposure. Dose, one to four fluidounces (30–120 C.c.).

DECOCTUM PAPAVERIS. *Br.* *Decoction of Poppy.*

(DĘ-CŎC'TŲM PĄ-PĀ'VĘ-RĬS.)

Tisane de Pavot, *Fr.;* Mohnkapseln-Absud, *G.*

"Take of Poppy Capsules, bruised, *two ounces* [avoirdupois]; Distilled Water *a pint and a half* [Imperial measure]. Boil for ten minutes in a covered vessel, then strain, and pour as much distilled water over the contents of the strainer as will make the strained product measure a pint [Imp. meas.]." *Br.*

This decoction is used as an anodyne fomentation in painful tumors, and in superficial cutaneous inflammation or excoriation. It is recommended not to reject the seeds, as their oil, suspended in the water by the mucilage of the capsules, adds to the emollient virtues of the preparation.

DECOCTUM PAREIRÆ. *Br.* *Decoction of Pareira.*

(DĘ-CŎC'TŲM PĄ-REI'RÆ—pę-rā'rē.)

Tisane de Pareira Brava, *Fr.;* Pareirawurzel-Absud, Grieswurzel-Absud, *G.*

"Take of Pareira Root, in No. 20 powder, *one ounce and a quarter* [avoirdupois]; Distilled Water *one pint* [Imperial measure]. Boil for fifteen minutes in a covered vessel, then strain, and pour as much distilled water over the contents of the strainer as will make the strained product measure a pint [Imp. meas.]." *Br.*

This is apt to remain turbid after straining, but, if allowed to stand, gradually deposits insoluble matter, and then can be filtered perfectly clear. (*P. J. Tr.*, xiv. 491.) The dose is from one to two fluidounces (30–60 C.c.) three or four times a day.

DECOCTUM QUERCUS. *Br.* *Decoction of Oak Bark.*

(DĘ-CŎC'TŲM QUĔR'CŬS—kwĕr'kŭs.)

Tisane (Décocté) d'Écorce de Chêne, *Fr.;* Eichenrinden-Absud, *G.*

"Take of Oak Bark, bruised, *one ounce and a quarter* [avoirdupois]; Distilled Water *one pint* [Imperial measure]. Boil for ten minutes in a covered vessel, then strain, and pour as much distilled water over the contents of the strainer as will make the strained product measure a pint [Imp. meas.]." *Br.**

This decoction contains the tannin, bitter principle, and gallic acid of oak bark. It affords precipitates with the decoction of Peruvian bark and other substances containing vegetable alkaloids, with solution of gelatin, and with most metallic salts, particularly those of iron. Alkaline solutions diminish or destroy its astringency. Its uses have been already detailed. The dose is two fluidounces (60 C.c.), frequently repeated.

DECOCTUM SARSÆ. *Br.* *Decoction of Sarsaparilla.*

(DĔ-CŎC'TŬM SĂR'SÆ—sâr'sē.)

Tisane de Salsepareille, *Fr.;* Sarsaparilla-Absud, *G.*

"Take of Jamaica Sarsaparilla, cut transversely, *two ounces and a half* [avoirdupois]; Boiling Distilled Water *one pint and a half* [Imperial measure]. Digest the Sarsaparilla in the Water for an hour; boil for ten minutes in a covered vessel, cool, and strain, pouring distilled water, if required, over the contents of the strainer, or otherwise making the strained product measure a pint [Imp. meas.]." *Br.*

An idea was long entertained that the virtues of sarsaparilla resided in its fecula, the extraction of which was, therefore, the main object of the decoction. Hence the long boiling formerly ordered by the London and Edinburgh Colleges. But this opinion is now admitted to have been erroneous. The activity of the root is believed to depend upon one or more acrid principles, soluble to a certain extent in water, cold or hot, and either volatilized, or rendered inert by chemical change, at the temperature of 100° C. (212° F.). This fact appears to be demonstrated by the experiments of Pope,† Hancock,‡ Soubeiran,§ Beral, and others. Soubeiran macerated one portion of bruised sarsaparilla in cold water for twenty-four hours; infused another portion in boiling water, and digested with a moderate heat for two hours; boiled a third portion bruised, and a fourth unbruised, in water for two hours; and in each instance used the same relative quantities. Testing these various preparations by the taste, he found the cold and hot infusions scarcely different in this respect; and both possessed of a stronger odor and more acrid taste than the decoctions, of which that prepared with the bruised root was the strongest. From these facts the inference is obvious, that the best method of imparting the virtues of sarsaparilla to water is either by cold or hot infusion. Digestion for some hours in water maintained at a temperature of 82·2° C. (180° F.), or somewhat less, in a covered vessel, has strong testimony in its favor. Percolation in a displacement apparatus, if properly conducted, is a convenient and no doubt efficient mode of exhausting the root, so far as water will effect that object. Decoction is the worst method; and the longer it is continued, the weaker will be the preparation. For these reasons the decoction of sarsaparilla has not been officinal in the U. S. Pharmacopœia since 1840. The unsplit root is ordered in the British Pharmacopœia from the conviction, probably, that the internal amylaceous part is inert; but there can be no doubt that the drug yields its virtues more readily when well bruised or otherwise comminuted than in the natural state. Precipitates are produced by various substances with this decoction; but it has not been ascertained how far such substances interfere with its activity. Those which merely throw down the fecula do not injure the preparation.

By this preparation it is possible to administer sarsaparilla in the form of decoction, without combination with other medicines, as in the Compound Decoction.

The decoction of sarsaparilla may be administered in the dose of four or six fluidounces (120–180 C.c.) four times a day.

* *Decoctum Quercûs Albæ.* U. S. 1870. *Decoction of White-oak Bark.* "Take of White-oak Bark, bruised, *a troyounce;* Water *a sufficient quantity.* Boil the White-oak Bark in a pint of Water for fifteen minutes, strain, and add sufficient Water, through the strainer, to make the decoction measure a pint." *U. S.* 1870.

† Trans. of the Medico-Chirurg. Society of London, vol. xii. p. 344.

‡ Trans. of the Medico-Botan. Society of London. See also Journ. of the Phila. Coll. of Pharm., vol. i. p. 295. The observations of Dr. Hancock are entitled to much credit, as he practised long in South America, in the neighborhood of the best sarsaparilla regions.

§ Journ. de Pharmacie, tom. xvi. p. 38.

DECOCTUM SARSAPARILLÆ COMPOSITUM. *U.S. Compound Decoction of Sarsaparilla.*

(DE-CŎC'TŬM SĂR-SA-PA-RĬL'LÆ CŎM-PŎS'I-TŬM.)

Decoctum Sarsæ Compositum, *Br.;* Tisane (Apozème) sudorifique, Décocté de Salsepareille composé, *Fr.;* Zusammengesetztes Sarsaparilla-Decoct, *G.*

"Sarsaparilla, cut and bruised, *ten parts* [or five ounces av.]; Sassafras, in No. 20 powder, *two parts* [or one ounce av.]; Guaiacum Wood, rasped, *two parts* [or one ounce av.]; Glycyrrhiza, bruised, *two parts* [or one ounce av.]; Mezereum, cut and bruised, *one part* [or half an ounce av.]; Water, *a sufficient quantity,* To make *one hundred parts* [or three pints]. Boil the Sarsaparilla and Guaiacum Wood for half an hour in a suitable vessel with *one hundred parts* [or three pints] of Water; then add the Sassafras, Glycyrrhiza, and Mezereum, cover the vessel well and macerate for two hours; finally strain, and add enough cold Water, through the strainer, to make the product weigh *one hundred parts* [or measure three pints]." *U. S.*

"Take of Jamaica Sarsaparilla, cut transversely, *two ounces and a half;* Sassafras Root, in chips, Guaiacum Wood turnings, Dried Liquorice Root, bruised, each *a quarter of an ounce;* Mezereon Bark, *one-eighth of an ounce;* Boiling Distilled Water *one pint and a half* [Imperial measure]. Digest the solid ingredients in the Water for an hour; then boil for ten minutes in a covered vessel; cool and strain, pouring distilled water, if required, over the contents of the strainer, or otherwise making the strained product measure a pint [Imp. meas.]." *Br.* The ounce employed in this process is the avoirdupois ounce.

This decoction is an imitation of the celebrated *Lisbon diet drink.* The sarsaparilla and mezereon are the active ingredients; the guaiacum wood imparting scarcely any of its virtues, and the sassafras and liquorice serving little other purpose than to communicate a pleasant flavor. An improvement was made in the present U. S. formula in directing the sassafras, glycyrrhiza, and mezereum to be added, after the boiling of the ligneous drugs has been completed. Compound Decoction of Sarsaparilla now contains a little more sarsaparilla, sassafras, guaiacum wood, and glycyrrhiza than the U. S. formula of 1870, but nearly double the quantity of mezereum: as the latter has been believed by many to be the only active substance in this weak preparation, the increase in quantity was judicious.

If prepared with good sarsaparilla, and with a due regard to the practical rules which may now be considered as established, the decoction may be used with advantage as a gentle diaphoretic and alterative in secondary syphilis, either alone, or as an adjuvant to a mercurial course; also in certain scrofulous and other depraved conditions of the system, in chronic rheumatism, and in various obstinate cutaneous affections. The dose is from four to six fluidounces (120–180 C.c.) three or four times a day. The patient during its use should wear flannel next the skin, and avoid unnecessary exposure to changes of temperature.*

* The *Decoction of Zittmann* (Decoctum Zittmanni) is a preparation of Sarsaparilla much used in Germany, for similar purposes with our compound decoction of sarsaparilla; and, as it has attracted some attention in this country as a remedy in obstinate ulcerative affections, we give the formula of the German Pharmacopœia, which is generally followed in its preparation. *Decoctum Sarsaparillæ Compositum Fortius,* P. G. [*Zittmann's Stronger Decoction.*] *Stärkeres Zittmann'sches Decoct.*—"Take of sarsaparilla root, cut, *one hundred parts;* pour upon it common water, *two thousand six hundred parts;* digest for twenty-four hours; then add of sugar powdered, alum powdered, each, *six parts,* and heat them in a covered vessel, in a steam bath, for three hours, stirring frequently. Towards the end of the boiling, add of anise bruised, fennel seed bruised, each, *four parts;* senna cut, *twenty-four parts;* liquorice root cut, *twelve parts.* Strain by expression, and set aside for a short time. The clear decanted liquid should be *two thousand five hundred parts.* When not otherwise directed, a colature of two thousand five hundred grammes is divided into eight portions.

"N.B.—When Decoctum Zitmanni is prescribed, it is prepared in a similar manner, except that to the sugar and alum are added of mild chloride of mercury, *four parts;* cinnabar (red sulphide of mercury), *one part,* enclosed in a linen bag." *P. G.*

Decoctum Sarsaparillæ Compositum Mitius, P. G. [*Zittmann's Milder Decoction.*] *Milderes Zittmann'sches Decoct.*—"Take the residue of the stronger decoction and sarsaparilla root, cut, *fifty parts;* pour upon them common water, *two thousand six hundred parts,* and expose to the heat of a steam bath for three hours in a covered vessel, stirring frequently. Towards the end of the operation add of lemon peel, cassia bark, small cardamoms, liquorice root, each, cut and bruised, *three parts.* Strain by expression, and set aside for a short time. The clear decanted liquid should be *two thousand five hundred parts.* When not otherwise directed, a colature of two thousand

DECOCTUM SCOPARII. *Br.* *Decoction of Broom.*

(DE-CŎC'TUM SCO-PĀ'RI-Ī.)

Tisane de Genêt à Balais, *Fr.;* Besenginster-Absud, *G.*

"Take of Broom-tops, dried, *one ounce* [avoirdupois]; Distilled Water *one pint* [Imperial measure]. Boil for ten minutes in a covered vessel, then strain, and pour as much distilled water over the contents of the strainer as will make the strained product measure a pint [Imp. meas.]." *Br.*

This decoction is a useful diuretic in dropsy. From half a pint to a pint (236–472 C.c.) may be taken during the day, in doses of from two to four fluidounces (60–120 C.c.).*

DECOCTUM TARAXACI. *Br.* *Decoction of Dandelion.*

(DE-CŎC'TUM TĂ-RĂX'Ă-CĪ—tă-răk'să-sī.)

Tisane de Pissenlit, *Fr.;* Löwenzahnwurzel-Absud, *G.*

"Take of Dried Dandelion Root, sliced and bruised, *one ounce* [avoirdupois]; Distilled Water *one pint* [Imperial measure]. Boil for ten minutes in a covered vessel, then strain, and pour as much distilled water over the contents of the strainer as will make the strained product measure a pint [Imp. meas.]." *Br.*

Dose, two fluidounces (60 C.c.) two or three times a day. (See *Taraxacum.*)

DIGITALIS. *U.S.* *Digitalis.* [*Foxglove.*]†

(DĬG-Ĭ-TĀ'LĬS.)

"The leaves of Digitalis purpurea, Linné (*Nat. Ord.* Scrophulariaceæ), collected from plants of the second year's growth." *U. S.* "The dried leaf of Digitalis purpurea, Purple Foxglove, collected from wild British plants of the second year's growth, when about two-thirds of the flowers are expanded, and carefully dried." *Br.*

Digitalis Folia, *Br.;* Digitalis Leaf; Folia Digitalis, *P. G.;* Digitalis Leaves, Foxglove Leaves, Feuilles de Digitale pourprée (de grande Digitale), Digitale pourprée, Doigtier, *Fr.;* Purpurrother Fingerhut, Fingerhutkraut, *G.;* Digitale purpurea, *It.;* Dedalera, *Sp.*

Gen. Ch. *Calyx* five-parted. *Corolla* bell-shaped, five-cleft, ventricose. *Capsule* ovate, two-celled. *Willd.*

Digitalis purpurea. Willd. *Sp. Plant.* iii. 383; Woodv. *Med. Bot.* p. 218, t. 78. The foxglove is a beautiful plant, with a biennial or perennial fibrous root, which, in the first year, sends forth large tufted leaves, and in the following summer, a single erect, downy, and leafy stem, rising from two to five feet, and terminating in an elegant spike of purple flowers. The lower leaves are ovate, pointed, about eight inches in length and three in breadth, and stand upon short, winged footstalks; the upper are alternate, sparse, and lanceolate; both are obtusely serrate, and have wrinkled velvety surfaces, of which the upper is of a fine deep green, the under paler and more downy. The flowers are numerous, and attached to the upper part of the stem by short peduncles, in such a manner as generally to hang down upon one side. At the base of each peduncle is a floral leaf, which is sessile, ovate, and pointed. The calyx is divided into five segments, of which the uppermost is narrower than the others. The corolla is monopetalous, bell-form, swelling on the lower side, irregularly divided at the margin into short obtuse lobes, and in shape and size not unlike the end of the finger of a glove, a circumstance which has suggested most of the names by which the plant is designated in different languages. Its mouth is guarded by long soft hairs. Externally, it is in general of a bright purple; internally, is sprinkled

five hundred grammes is divided into eight portions." *P. G.* Mercury was detected by Wiggers in this decoction in very small proportion. It should not be prepared in metallic vessels, lest the mercurial in solution should be decomposed. The decoction may be drunk freely.

* *Decoctum Senegæ.* U.S. 1870. *Decoction of Seneka.* "Take of Seneka, bruised, a *troyounce;* Water *a sufficient quantity.* Boil the Seneka in a pint of Water for fifteen minutes, strain, and add sufficient Water, through the strainer, to make the decoction measure a pint." *U. S.* 1870.

This is one of the decoctions in which experience has shown that long boiling impairs the activity of the medicine. It is customary to add to the seneka in decoction an equal weight of liquorice root, which serves to cover its taste, and in some measure to obtund its acrimony. The virtues and practical application of seneka will be treated of under *Senega.* The dose of the decoction is about *two fluidounces* (60 C.c.) three or four times a day, or a tablespoonful every two or three hours.

† Foxglove is a corruption of Folksglove, Folk being an old English synonyme of Fairies.

with black spots upon a white ground. There is a variety with white flowers. The filaments are white, curved, and surmounted by large yellow anthers. The style is simple, and supports a bifid stigma. The seeds are numerous, very small, grayish brown, and contained in a pyramidal two-celled capsule.

The foxglove grows wild in the temperate parts of Europe, where it flowers in the middle of summer. In this country it is cultivated both for ornament and for medical use. The leaves are the part generally employed. Much care is requisite in selecting, preparing, and preserving them, in order to insure their activity. They should be gathered in the second year, immediately before or during the period of efflorescence, and those only chosen which are full-grown and perfectly fresh (*Geiger*); but the observations of F. Schneider would lead to the conclusion that they are much stronger when not gathered before the latter part of summer, or the beginning of autumn. (*A. J. P.*, 1870, p. 221.) It is said that those plants are preferable which grow spontaneously in elevated places, exposed to the sun. (*Duncan.*) As the leafstalk and midrib are comparatively inactive, they may be rejected. Withering recommends that the leaves should be dried either in the sunshine, or by a gentle heat before the fire; and care should be taken to keep them separate while drying. Pereira states that a more common, and, in his opinion, a preferable mode, is to dry them in a basket, in a dark place in a drying stove. It is probably owing, in part, to the want of proper attention in preparing digitalis for the market, that it is so often inefficient. Much of the medicine kept in our shops is obtained from the Shakers,* and is in oblong compact masses, into which the leaves have been compressed. In some of these cakes the digitalis is of good quality; but we have seen others in which it was quite the reverse, and some which were mouldy in the interior; and, upon the whole, we cannot but consider this mode of preparing the drug as objectionable. The dried leaves should be kept in tin canisters, well closed so as to exclude light and moisture; or they may be pulverized, and the powder preserved in well-stopped and opaque bottles. As foxglove deteriorates by time, it should be frequently renewed, as often, if possible, as once a year. Its quality must be judged of by the degree in which it possesses the characteristic properties of color, smell, and especially taste. It is said to be sometimes adulterated; but if it be bought in leaf, there can be little difficulty, to one acquainted with the characters of the genuine leaves, in detecting the sophistication.

The seeds contain more of the active principle than the leaves, are less apt to suffer in drying, and keep better, but are little used. So far as the relative strength of these two parts can be determined from that of their alcoholic extracts, it would appear, from the experiments of Prof. Hirtz, that the seeds are ten times stronger than the leaves. (See *A. J. P.*, xxxiii. 414.)

Properties. Foxglove is without smell in the recent state, but acquires a faint narcotic odor when dried. The color of the dried leaf is a dull pale green, modified by the whitish down upon the under surface; that of the powder is a fine deep green. "From four to twelve inches (10 to 30 cm.) long, ovate-oblong, narrowed into a petiole; crenate, downy; dull green and wrinkled above; paler and reticulate beneath; midrib near the base broad; odor faint, tea-like; taste bitter, nauseous." *U. S.* Digitalis yields its virtues both to water and alcohol. It contains, besides active principles, a volatile oil, a fatty matter, a red coloring substance analogous to extractive, chlorophyll, albumen, starch, sugar, gum, lignin, and salts of potassa and lime, among which, according to Rein and Hasse, is superoxalate of potassium. M. Morin, of Geneva, has discovered in the leaves two acids; one fixed, called *digitalic acid*, the other volatile and resembling valerianic acid, which he proposes to name *antirrhinic acid*. (*P. J. Tr.*, vii. 294.) Dr. Morries obtained a narcotic empyreumatic oil by the destructive distillation of the leaves.

Under the name of *digitalin*† there have long been in commerce two distinct sub-

* A portion of the Shakers' digitalis, purchased in the market, with parcels from England and Germany, being chemically examined by Dr. S. P. Duffield, of Detroit, with the view of determining the relative powers of the several varieties as measured by their yield of digitalin, was found superior to the others, the English giving 63·60 grains to the pound, the German 56·50 grains, and the American 65·01 grains. (*A. J. P.*, 1869, p. 57.)

† *French digitalin* may be prepared according to the following process, which was formerly recommended by the British Pharmacopœia:

"Take of Digitalis Leaf, in coarse powder, *forty ounces* [avoirdupois]; Rectified Spirit, Distilled

stances obtained from digitalis, both of them of the nature of extracts rather than of organic principles. The *French* digitalin was that originally prepared by Homolle. It is a whitish powder, of a neutral reaction, soluble in 2000 parts of cold and in 1000 parts of hot water. It is this digitalin which was formerly recognized by the U. S. and Br. Pharmacopœias. The so-called *German* digitalin is distinguished from the French by being, in great part or entirely, freely soluble in water.

In 1871, M. Nativelle received from the French Academy the prize of Orfila for the discovery of the active principle of digitalis, which he had obtained in fine crystals. The method of preparation, as finally improved and modified by himself, and published in the *Journ. de Pharm.*, xx. 1874, p. 81, and a process which has the advantage of being far shorter and more readily carried out, devised by M. Tanret (*Ibid.*, Oct. 1875), will be found on p. 1143, 14th ed., U. S. Dispensatory.

Crystallized digitalin occurs in granular radiating masses of acicular crystals, or in brilliant acicular crystals. The characteristic reactions of it are stated by Tanret to be, the yellowish green color which it strikes with hydrochloric acid; the brown or rose color, according to the amount of digitalin, developed by concentrated sulphuric acid; and the violet color, which is produced in its solution in dilute sulphuric acid when a drop of bromine-water or, better still, some of the vapor of bromine is added. According to Nativelle, it is insoluble in water, very soluble in chloroform, soluble in 12 parts of cold and in 6 parts of boiling alcohol of 90 per cent. When heated to 100° C. (212° F.), it softens and becomes elastic; heated on platinum foil, it fuses without coloring, and evaporates in white vapor. Solution of chloral dissolves it readily. Hydrochloric acid dissolves it with emerald-green color; sulphuric acid with green color, changing to clear red on treatment with bromine, but turning green again on addition of water. According to Flückiger, it is also dissolved by warm concentrated phosphoric acid with intensely green color. The formula of Nativelle's digitalin is $C_{25}H_{40}O_{15}$. Nativelle's *digitalin* appears to be a glucoside, as diluted sulphuric acid decomposes it with the formation of *digitaliretin* and glucose. According to Ch. Blaquart (*L'Union Pharmaceutique*, Nov. 1872), ten per cent. of it can readily be obtained from the crude drug. Besides digitalin, M. Nativelle obtained a crystallizable but inert substance, to which he gave the name of *digitin*.

The relation of Nativelle's crystallized digitalin to digitalis and the amorphous digitalin has given rise to considerable controversy. The French commission affirmed that it acted similarly to digitalin, but was much stronger. M. Gubler, M. Vulpian, and M. Blaquart have separately arrived at a different result from this; they found

Water, Acetic Acid, Purified Animal Charcoal, Solution of Ammonia, Tannic Acid, Oxide of Lead in fine powder, Pure Ether, of each, *a sufficiency*. Digest the Digitalis with a gallon [Imperial measure] of the Spirit for twenty-four hours at a temperature of 120°; then put them into a percolator, and, when the tincture has ceased to drop, pour a gallon [Imp. meas.] of Spirit on the contents of the percolator, and allow it slowly to percolate through. Distil off the greater part of the Spirit from the tincture, and evaporate the remainder over a water-bath until the whole of the alcohol has been dissipated. Mix the residual extract with five [fluid]ounces of Distilled Water to which half an ounce [avoird.] of Acetic Acid has been previously added, and digest the solution thus formed with a quarter of an ounce of Purified Animal Charcoal; then filter, and dilute the filtrate with Distilled Water until it measures a pint [Imp. meas.]. Add Solution of Ammonia nearly to neutralization, and afterwards add one hundred and sixty grains of Tannic Acid dissolved in three [fluid]ounces of Distilled Water. Wash the precipitate that will be formed with a little Distilled Water; mix it with a small quantity of the Spirit and a quarter of an ounce of the Oxide of Lead, and rub them together in a mortar. Place the mixture in a flask, and add to it four [fluid]ounces of the Spirit; raise the temperature to 160°, and keep it at this heat for about an hour. Then add a quarter of an ounce of Purified Animal Charcoal; put it on a filter, and from the filtrate carefully drive off the Spirit by the heat of a water-bath. Lastly, wash the residue repeatedly with Pure Ether." According to the method of Walz (Husemann, *Die Pflanzenstoffe*, p. 900), *German digitalin* is prepared by extracting under pressure one part of digitalis with eight parts of alcohol, evaporating, digesting the residue with successive portions of water so long as they acquire a bitter taste, uniting the liquids, and treating them with litharge and acetate of lead until a portion filtered for testing is no longer precipitated by acetate of lead. Sulphuric acid is added to the filtrate to precipitate the lead, and, after filtration, neutralized with ammonia, and the liquid precipitated by tannic acid. The precipitate, having been well washed and pressed, is rubbed up with freshly precipitated oxide of lead, the mass boiled with alcohol, and, after the lead has been separated by precipitation with sulphuric acid, and most of the alcohol distilled off, the residue is allowed to slowly evaporate, the crude digitalin being left behind.

the crystallized digitalin no stronger—sometimes even weaker—than the amorphous French preparation. However this may be, it is plain that Nativelle's digitalin cannot be the sole or even the chief principle of digitalis, since he found it in the residue left as exhausted and inert in the preparation of French digitalin. Further, there is abundant proof that the French digitalin is a powerful preparation, and, if it contain no crystallised digitalin, the latter is not the sole or even the chief active principle of digitalis. Dr. Roucher (*Les Mondes*, Juillet, 1872) affirms that Nativelle's digitalin is a complex body, and O. Schmiedeberg (*Archiv für Exper. Pathologie und Pharmak.*, Bd. iii. p. 19; *P. J. Tr.*, 1875, p. 741) confirms this. The latter author has examined the constitution of digitalis very carefully, and found that there are four principles in it: *digitonin*, $C_{31}H_{52}O_{17}$, a substance allied to saponin, which constitutes the bulk of the German or soluble digitalin; *digitalin*, $(C_5H_8O_2)x$, which constitutes the greater part of the French or soluble digitalin; *digitalein;* and *digitoxin*, the most active of all the substances. These principles readily break up into a number of derivatives; hence the various principles which have been obtained from digitalis by investigators.

According to Schmiedeberg (*loc. cit.*), the digitalin of Nativelle is a mixture of digitalin with digitoxin, a second base. The pure *digitalin*, according to Schmiedeberg, forms soft, colorless, uncrystallizable granules. These are easily soluble in alcohol, slightly so in ether or chloroform, and almost insoluble in water. It is a glucoside, yielding glucose and digitaliretin.

For the extraction of *digitoxin* Schmiedeberg precipitates the extract obtained with the 50 per cent. alcohol by the aid of lead acetate, evaporates the filtrate, and, washing the separated residue with weak soda solution, dries it and extracts with chloroform.

Some yellowish matter is removed with benzin, and the crude digitoxin purified by crystallization from warm alcohol of 80 per cent., adding a little charcoal. The yellowish crystals so obtained must be washed with carbonate of soda, ether, or benzin, and then recrystallized from warm absolute alcohol containing a little chloroform. The formula of digitoxin, according to Schmiedeberg, is $C_{21}H_{32}O_7$. It is not a glucoside, but in alcoholic solution it is decomposed by dilute acids, and then affords *toxiresin*, an uncrystallizable substance, which may easily be separated on account of its ready solubility in ether; it appears to be produced also if digitoxin is maintained for some time in the state of fusion at about 240° C. (464° F.). "Toxiresin proved to be a very powerful poison, acting energetically upon the heart and muscles of frogs. The very specific action of foxglove is due not exclusively, however, to digitoxin."

The above résumé of our present knowledge clearly shows that the chemistry of digitalis cannot be considered as settled; but it also clearly shows that no digitalin represents digitalis. Moreover, the digitalin * of commerce varies almost indefinitely, and we do not think it ought to be used at all in practical medicine.

Medical Properties and Uses. Experiments upon the lower animals, confirmed by clinical observation, have shown that digitalis acts primarily and with most force upon the circulation, producing a great rise in the arterial pressure, followed, in poisoning, by a no less marked fall, which, however, does not take place at all after moderate doses. The increased blood force is partly due to increased cardiac action and partly to vaso-motor spasm. Upon the heart, digitalis acts by stimulating the peripheral ends of the inhibitory nerves and also the cardiac muscle. By the first influence it produces prolongation of the diastole; by the second, an increased putting forth of power in the systole. The work done by the heart under the influence of the drug is much beyond normal. After a toxic dose the systolic irritation overbalances the diastolic stimulation, and the pulse becomes dichrotic, because the diastole is interrupted by an abortive systole. Finally, the apex of the heart never dilates, diastole is continually interrupted by systolic contractions, and the aortic system remains

* According to E. Merck, there occur in commerce: *German digitalin*, composed of digitalein with some digitonin and digitalin; soluble in water and alcohol; *Nativelle's crystallised digitalin*, consisting chiefly of digitoxin; *Homolle's amorphous digitalin*, or *digitalin* of the French and Belgium Pharmacopœias, nearly insoluble in water, consisting of digitalin with some digitoxin; *Merck's crystallised digitalin*, composed of d.gitin; *digitoxin*, occurring in concentrically grouped needles

empty, because the left ventricle never relaxes sufficiently to receive blood. The final cessation of the heart's action is not due to paralysis, but to spasm, the heart ceasing not in diastole but in systole.

This résumé of our knowledge of the physiological action clearly shadows forth the proper use of the drug. It is indicated when the heart is weak, not absolutely, but relatively weak, or, in other words, when the work required of the heart is greater than its power. When digitalis is administered in ordinary doses, it produces at first no distinct effect; but if the dose be repeated, after a time the pulse becomes less frequent. The pauses between the beats are longer than before, and the individual beat is longer, fuller, and stronger, indicating that the heart is acting with more force than normal. When the reduction of the pulse-rate has commenced, it is apt to continue for some days, and even to increase for a time, although the use of the remedy be intermitted, slowness and permanency of action being characteristic of digitalis. In some cases, gastric disturbance, and even nausea, vomiting, and diarrhœa, are produced by therapeutic doses of the drug. If sufficient of the remedy has been taken into the system, the pulse may fall to 35 or 40 a minute, still preserving the peculiarity of a distinctly dichrotic beat. Now, a very peculiar phenomenon may often be witnessed. Whilst the patient is quiet in the horizontal position the pulse is very slow and strong, but when he rises to his feet it becomes at once rapid, irregular, small, and feeble, and even hobbling.

During the milder operation of digitalis there may be some sense of cerebral disturbance, brow-tightness, and even a confusion of thought and giddiness. After toxic doses the symptoms are severe; a feeble, scarcely perceptible pulse, nausea and vomiting, stupor or delirium, cold sweats, extreme prostration of strength, hiccough, convulsions, and syncope have in several cases preceded the fatal issue.

The dilated heart is of course a weak heart, and simple cardiac dilatation is one of the strongest indications for the use of digitalis, whilst cardiac hypertrophy is a contraindication. It must not be forgotten, however, that in valvular disease of the heart, the heart, although stronger than normal, may be relatively weak, because the leakage at the diseased valve requires more power to overcome its effect than even the increased strength of the cardiac muscle is able for. Hypertrophy exists, but is not sufficient to be compensatory. In all forms of valvular lesion, when the hypertrophy is not compensatory, digitalis is very useful. It is also to be employed (hypodermically) in sudden cardiac exhaustion from any cause.

Dropsy is very frequently the result of a general venous repletion, which also interferes with the function of the kidneys. Under these circumstances digitalis is a favorite remedy, and also acts as a decided diuretic. In these cases the result is in greater or less part due to the improvement of the circulation; but the drug has some tendency, even in health, to provoke diuresis. It is especially when it fails to do this that the so-called cumulative action is apt to be witnessed. After giving the drug for a long time without apparent effect, suddenly symptoms so severe as to be toxic are manifested. In aneurism, or when from any reason the coats of the vessels are thin or fragile, digitalis is contraindicated. We have seen a dilated aorta ruptured by the powerful blood-current produced by the drug.

Externally applied, digitalis sometimes acts speedily and powerfully as a diuretic, and has proved useful in dropsy. For this purpose the fresh leaves bruised, or the dried leaves made into a poultice, or flannels wet with the tincture, may be applied to the abdomen and on the inside of the thighs. Ch. Hoffman has shown by experiments on himself that the active matter of digitalis is capable of being absorbed through the skin, and that its effects on the system may be obtained by means of baths.* A case is recorded in which a cataplasm of the leaves applied to the abdomen for the relief of obstinate and dangerous suppression of urine, and repeated in six hours, brought on excessive diuresis, with a discharge amounting to probably

* M. Hoffman, during a period of 44 days, took 16 baths prepared with 300 litres of water and 250 grammes of digitalis leaves. After the third bath he began to feel the effects of the medicine; namely a peculiar uneasiness, and a reduction of the pulse 4 or 5 pulsations per minute; and this condition persisted several hours. At the eighth bath the uneasiness was increased, and the pulse decreased from 68 to 51. After the sixteenth bath, the pulse fell to 48. (*Journ. de Pharm. et de Chim.*, Juillet, 1867, p. 37.)

8 gallons in less than 24 hours, producing fatal exhaustion. (*Med. Times and Gaz.*, Jan. 1868, p. 86.)

Digitalis is administered in substance. The dose of the powder is one grain (0·065 Gm.), repeated twice or three times a day, and gradually increased till some effect is produced upon the head, stomach, pulse, or kidneys, when it should be omitted or reduced. The infusion and tincture are officinal preparations often resorted to. (See *Infusum Digitalis* and *Tinctura Digitalis*.) The extract has also been employed; and Orfila found it, whether prepared with water or with alcohol, more powerful than the powder. Enormous doses of this medicine have been given with asserted impunity; and, when they occasion full vomiting, it is possible that they may sometimes prove harmless; but, when the alarming effects sometimes experienced from comparatively moderate doses are considered, the practice must be condemned as exceedingly hazardous.

Digitalin has been used internally, but, for reasons assigned on p. 541, is a very ineligible preparation, and is of uncertain strength. The dose to begin with should not exceed the fiftieth or sixtieth of a grain (0·001 Gm.), and should not be carried beyond the twelfth (0·005 Gm.). It is much administered in the form of granules, made by saturating small globules of sugar with an alcoholic solution of digitalin. The granules of Homolle, which are commonly used in Europe, each contain a milligramme, or about the seventieth of a grain; equivalent, on the average, to perhaps a grain and a half of digitalis of medium strength. One of these globules may be given as a commencing dose. Forty of them taken with a view to suicide, though followed by copious vomiting, so that most of the poison was probably discharged, produced the most alarming prostration, with a pulse, weak, 46 to 48 in a minute, intermittent, and sometimes scarcely perceptible. The patient, however, ultimately recovered. (*Ann. de Thérap.*, 1858, p. 103.)

Off. Prep. Abstractum Digitalis; Extractum Digitalis; Extractum Digitalis Fluidum; Infusum Digitalis; Tinctura Digitalis.

Off. Prep. Br. Infusum Digitalis; Tinctura Digitalis.

DULCAMARA. *U.S.* *Dulcamara.* [*Bittersweet.*]

(DŬL-CĄ-MĀ'RĄ.)

"The young branches of Solanum Dulcamara. Linné. (*Nat. Ord.* Solanaceæ.)" *U. S.*

Stipites Dulcamaræ, *P.G.;* Tiges de Douce-amère (de Nevrelle grimpante), Douce-amère, *Fr.;* Bittersüss, Bittersüss-Stengel, Alpranken, *G.;* Dulcamara, *It., Sp.*

Gen. Ch. Corolla wheel-shaped. *Anthers* somewhat coalescing, opening by two pores at the apex. *Berry* two-celled. *Willd.*

This genus includes numerous species, of which several have been used in medicine. Besides *S. Dulcamara*, which is the only officinal species, a few others merit notice. 1. *Solanum nigrum*, the *common garden* or *black nightshade*, is an annual plant from one to two feet high, with an unarmed herbaceous stem, ovate, angular-dentate leaves, and white or pale violet flowers, arranged in peduncled nodding umbel-like racemes, and followed by clusters of spherical black berries, about the size of peas. There are numerous varieties of this species, one of which is a native of the United States. The leaves are the part employed. They are said to produce diaphoresis, sometimes diuresis and moderate purging, and in large doses nausea and giddiness. As a medicine they have been used in cancerous, scrofulous, and scorbutic diseases, and other painful ulcerous affections, being given internally, and applied at the same time to the parts affected in the form of poultice, ointment, or decoction. A grain of the dried leaves may be given every night, and gradually increased to ten or twelve grains, or till some sensible effect is experienced. The medicine, however, is scarcely used at present. By some persons the poisonous properties ascribed to the common nightshade are doubted. M. Dunal, of Montpellier, states, as the result of numerous experiments, that the berries are not poisonous to man or the inferior animals; and the leaves are said to be consumed in large quantities in the Isles of France and Bourbon as food, having been previously boiled in water. In the latter case, the active principle of the plant must have been extracted by decoction. 2. The leaves, stalks, and unripe berries of *Solanum tuberosum*, or the *common potato*, are asserted to be narcotic; and an extract prepared from the leaves has been employed in cough and spasmodic affections, in which it is said to act like opium. (*Geiger.*) Dr. Latham, of London, found the extract to produce favorable effects in protracted cough, chronic rheumatism, angina pectoris, cancer of the uterus, etc. On the other hand, Dr. Worsham, of Philadelphia, found the extract, in the quantity of nearly one hundred grains, to cause no sensible effect. (*Phila. Journ. of the Med. and Phys. Sciences*, vi. 22.) We can reconcile these opposite statements only upon the supposition that the properties of the plant vary with the season, or with the place and circumstances of culture. Dr. Julius Otto found *solanine* in the germs of the potato. He was induced to make the investigation by observing that cattle were destroyed by feeding on the residue of germinating potatoes, used for the manufacture of brandy. A case of death in a girl of fourteen, from eating the unripe fruit of the potato, is recorded in the *British Med. Journ.* for Sept. 3, 1859. The prominent symptoms were partial stupor, speechlessness, jactitation, hurried breathing, lividness of the skin, cold sweats, very frequent and feeble pulse, and a constant spitting through the closed teeth of viscid frothy phlegm. Death occurred on the second day. C. Haaf has found the same alkaloid in old potatoes which had begun to germinate, in the proportion of 0·16 in 500 parts; and in very young potatoes, deprived of their coating, precisely the same quantity. Fully ripe potatoes, which had not begun to sprout, gave a negative result. (*Neues Repert. für Pharm.*, 1864, p. 559.) 3. The well-known *tomato*, so much used as a vegetable at the table, and so advantageous through its nutritive, laxative, and antiscorbutic properties, is the fruit of a species of Solanum, denominated *S. Lycopersicum*. The juice of the fruit is free from solanine, but contains several acids. Mr. T. D. McElhenie demonstrated the presence of citric, malic, and oxalic acids. (See *A. J. P.*, 1872, p. 198.) The seeds probably contain the alkaloid, as their alcoholic extract has a bitter, pungent taste. (See *A. J. P.*, xxxiv. 519.) Solanine has been obtained from the leaves and herbaceous part of the plant generally, by Mr. Geo. W. Kennedy. (*P. J. Tr.*, 1873, p. 606.) An infusion of the leaves is strongly recommended by M. Stanislaus Martin as a diuretic. (*Am. J. of Med. Sci.*, 1873, p. 246.) 4. Several instances of poisoning are on record from the fruit of *S. pseudocapsicum*, or *Jerusalem cherry*, which, from its resemblance to the common cherry, is liable to be eaten by children. 5. In the *Edin. Med. Journ.* (1867, p. 398) several cases are recorded by Dr. Manners, of Jamaica, W. I., of poisoning by the *susumber berries*, of which one proved fatal, and several others recovered, probably in consequence of the early evacuation of the stomach by a mustard emetic. The symptoms recorded were anxious countenance, dilated pupil, cold skin, and difficult articulation. The fatal case was not seen by Dr. Manners till after death. The susumber berries are the fruit of a species of Solanum, denominated by Lunnan, in his "Hortus Jamaicensis," *S. bacciferum*, of which there are two varieties, one relatively innocent, as its fruit is habitually used by the natives, the other poisonous, as would be inferred from the cases here noticed. 6.

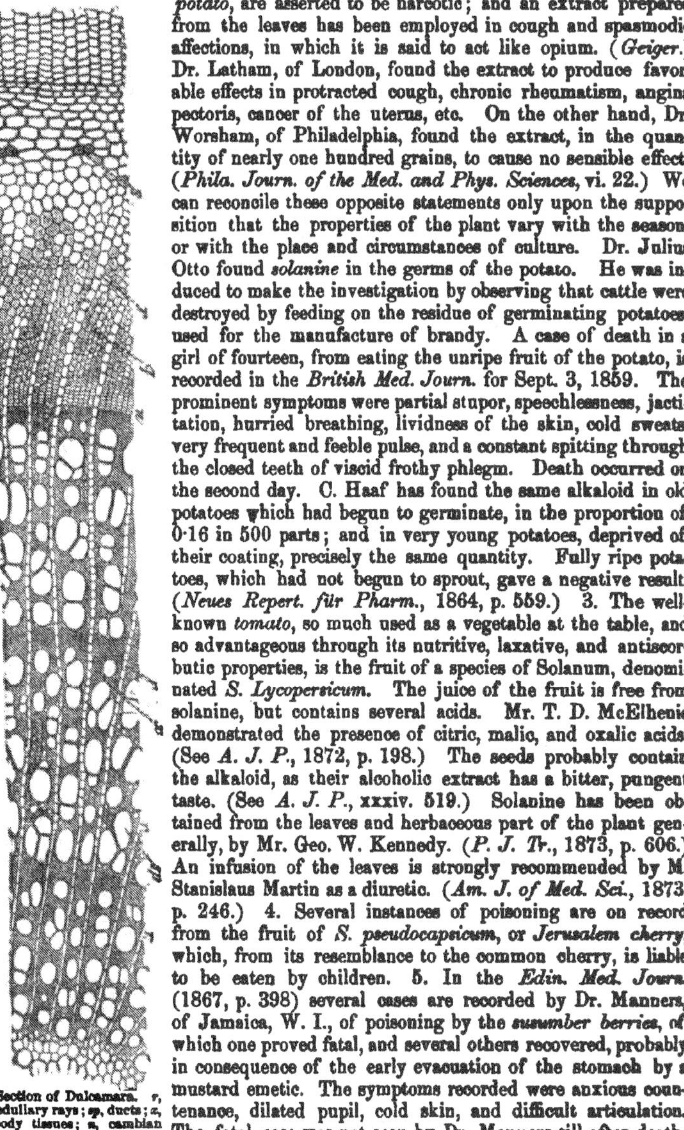

Section of Dulcamara. *r*, Medullary rays; *sp*, ducts; *x*, woody tissues; *n*, cambian layer; *q*, bast-tissue; *s*, bast-cells.

The *Solanum paniculatum*, called *jerubeba* in Brazil, is said to be largely used in South America, in affections of the liver and spleen, catarrh of the bladder, anæmia, and amenorrhœa. The leaves, fruit, and root are employed, externally in the form of a plaster, internally in the form of syrup, wine, and extract. (*London Lancet*, 1866, p. 158.)

Solanum Dulcamara. Willd. *Sp. Plant.* i. 1028; Woodv. *Med. Bot.* p. 237, t. 84; Bigelow, *Am. Med. Bot.* i. 169. The *bittersweet* or *woody nightshade* is a climbing shrub, with a slender, roundish, branching, woody stem, which, in favorable situations, rises six or eight feet in height. The leaves are alternate, petiolate, ovate, pointed, veined, soft, smooth, and of a dull green color. Many near the top of the stem are furnished with lateral projections at their base, giving them a hastate form. Some have the projection only on one side. Most of them are quite entire, some cordate at the base. The flowers are disposed in elegant clusters, somewhat analogous to cymes, and standing opposite to the leaves. The calyx is very small, purplish, and divided into five blunt, persistent segments. The corolla is wheel-shaped, with five pointed, reflected segments, which are of a violet blue color, with a darker purple vein running longitudinally through their centre, and two shining greenish spots at the base of each. The filaments are very short, and support large, erect, lemon-yellow anthers, which cohere in the form of a cone around the style. The berries are of an oval shape and a bright scarlet color, and continue to hang in beautiful bunches after the leaves have fallen.

This plant is common to Europe and North America. In the United States it extends from New England to Ohio, and is in bloom from June to August. The root and stalk have medicinal properties, though the latter only is officinal. A case, however, of death caused by the use of the berries by a child has been recorded. (See *P. J. Tr.*, 1861, p. 436.) Bittersweet should be gathered in autumn, after the fall of the leaf; and the extreme twigs should be selected. That grown in high and dry situations is said to be the best.

The dried twigs, as brought to the shops, are of various lengths, cylindrical, about as thick as a goose-quill, externally wrinkled, and of a grayish ash color, consisting of a thin bark, an interior ligneous portion, and a central pith. They are inodorous, though the stalk in the recent state emits, when bruised, a peculiar, rather nauseous smell. Their taste, which is at first bitter and afterwards sweetish, has given origin to the name of the plant. "About a quarter of an inch (6 mm.) or less, thick, cylindrical, somewhat angular, longitudinally striate, more or less warty, usually hollow in the centre, cut into short sections. The thin bark is externally pale greenish, or light greenish brown, marked with alternate leaf-scars, and internally green; the greenish or yellowish wood forms one or two concentric rings. Odor slight; taste bitter, afterwards sweet." *U. S.* Boiling water extracts all their virtues. These are supposed to depend, at least in part, upon an alkaloid called *solanine* or *solania*, which was originally discovered by M. Desfosses, of Besançon, in the berries of *Solanum nigrum*, and has subsequently been found in the stalks, leaves, and berries of *S. Dulcamara* and *S. tuberosum.** Winckler (1841) first observed that the alkaloid of dulcamara stems can be obtained only in an amorphous state, and that it behaves to platinic and mercuric chlorides differently from the solanine of potatoes. Moitessier (1856) confirmed this observation, and obtained only amorphous salts of the solanine of bittersweet. Zwenger and Kind on the one hand, and O. Gmelin on the

* Solanine is most conveniently obtained from the sprouts of the common potato. The following is Wackenroder's process for extracting it. The sprouts, collected in the beginning of June, and pressed down in a suitable vessel by means of pebbles, are macerated for twelve or eighteen hours in water enough to cover them, previously acidulated with sulphuric acid, so as to have a strongly acid reaction during the maceration. They are then expressed by the hand; and the liquor, with the addition of fresh portions of sulphuric acid, is added twice successively, as at first, to fresh portions of sprouts, and in like manner separated by expression. After standing for some days it is filtered and treated with powdered hydrate of lime in slight excess. The precipitate which forms is separated by straining, dried in a warm air, and boiled several times with alcohol. The alcoholic solution, having been filtered while hot, will, upon cooling, deposit the solanine in flocculent crystals. An additional quantity of the alkaloid may be obtained by evaporating the mother-liquor to one-quarter, and then allowing it to cool. The whole residuary liquor will assume a gelatinous consistence, and, upon being dried, will leave the solanine in the form of a translucent, horny, amorphous mass. (*Pharm. Centralb.*. 1848, p. 174.)

other (1859 and 1858), found that solanine, $C_{43}H_{69}NO_{16}$ (or $C_{42}H_{87}NO_{15}$, according to Hilger, 1879), is a compound of sugar and a peculiar crystallizable alkaloid, *solanidine*, $C_{25}H_{39}NO$. The latter, under the influence of strong hydrochloric acid, gives up water, and is converted into the amorphous and basic compound *solanicine.* Wittstein (1852) supposed another alkaloid, *dulcamarine*, to be present, but Geissler (1875) showed that this substance was a glucoside, and not an alkaloid, yielding on decomposition with dilute acids *dulcamaretin* and sugar. He assigned the formula $C_{22}H_{34}O_{10}$ to dulcamarine, and $C_{16}H_{26}O_{6}$ to dulcamaretin. (Flückiger, *Pharmacographia*, 2d ed., p. 451.) *Solanine* is in the form of a white opaque powder, or of delicate acicular crystals, somewhat like those of sulphate of quinine, though finer and shorter. It is inodorous, of a bitter taste, fusible at a little above 100° C. (212° F.), scarcely soluble in water, soluble in alcohol and ether, and capable of neutralizing the acids. It is distinguished by the deep brown, or brownish yellow color which iodine imparts to its solution, and by its reaction with sulphuric acid, which becomes first reddish yellow, then purplish violet, then brown, and lastly, again colorless, with the deposition of a brown powder.* In regard to the physiological action of solanine, the statements of the earlier and later observers are at such variance that they must have worked with different substances. J. Otto found one grain sufficient to kill a rabbit in six hours; whilst Dr. Gaignard found five grains insufficient. The symptoms produced by solanine are said to be spasmodic labored respiration, dilatation of the pupils, intense dyspnœa, convulsions, paraplegia. There seems to be no reason for believing that the alkaloid will be of any value in practical medicine. (Consult *B. & F. Med.-Chir. Rev.*, July, 1854, Am. ed., p. 189; *Arch. Gén. de Méd.*, Mars, 1859, p. 360; *Bull. Gén. de Thérap.*, July 15, 1887.) Besides solanine, the stalks of *S. Dulcamara* contain, according to Pfaff, a peculiar principle to which he gave the name of *picroglycion*, indicative of the taste, at once bitter and sweet, which it is said to possess. This was obtained by Blitz, in the following manner. The watery extract was treated with alcohol, the tincture evaporated, the residue dissolved in water, the solution precipitated with subacetate of lead, the excess of this salt decomposed by sulphuretted hydrogen, the liquor then evaporated to dryness, and the residue treated with acetic ether, which yielded the principle in small isolated crystals by spontaneous evaporation. Pfaff found also in dulcamara a vegeto-animal substance, gummy extractive, gluten, green wax, resin, benzoic acid, starch, lignin, and various salts of lime.

Medical Properties and Uses. Dulcamara possesses feeble narcotic properties, with the power of increasing the secretions, particularly those of the kidneys and skin. We have observed, in several instances, when the system was under its influence, a dark purplish color of the face and hands, and at the same time considerable languor of the circulation. Its narcotic effects do not become obvious unless when it is taken in large quantities. In overdoses it produces nausea, vomiting, faintness, vertigo, and convulsive muscular movements. A case is recorded in Casper's *Wochenschrift*, in which a man took, in one forenoon, from three to four quarts of a decoction made from a peck of the stalks, and was attacked with pain in the joints, numbness of the limbs, dryness of the mouth, and palsy of the tongue, with consciousness unimpaired, the pulse quiet, but small and rather hard, and the skin cool. The symptoms disappeared under the use of stimulants. (*Lond. Med. Gaz.*, 1850, p. 548.) Dulcamara has been recommended in various diseases, but is now chiefly employed in the treatment of cutaneous eruptions, particularly those of a scaly character, as lepra, psoriasis, and pityriasis. In these complaints it is often beneficial, especially in combination with minute doses of the antimonials. Its influence upon the secretions is insufficient to account for its favorable effects. Perhaps they may be ascribed to its sedative influence on the capillary circulation. It is said to have been beneficially employed in chronic rheumatism and chronic catarrh. Antaphrodisiac properties have been ascribed to it. We have seen it apparently useful in

* The following reaction is proposed as a test for solanine. Equal measures of concentrated sulphuric acid and alcohol are mixed. A trace of solanine added to the mixture, while warm, produces a rose-red color; larger quantities, a cherry-red color, which disappears after five or six hours, and the intensity of which is not affected by the presence of morphine even in large quantities. (*A. J. P.*, 1873, p. 484.)

mania connected with strong venereal propensities. The usual form of administration is that of decoction, of which two fluidounces may be taken four times a day, and gradually increased till some slight disorder of the head indicates the activity of the medicine. A fluid extract is officinal. The dose of the extract is from five to ten grains (0·33–0·65 Gm.), of the fluid extract thirty minims to a fluidrachm (1·9–3·75 C.c.). That of the powder would be from thirty grains to a drachm (1·95–3·9 Gm.). In cutaneous affections, a strong decoction is often applied to the skin at the same time that the medicine is taken internally.

Off. Prep. Extractum Dulcamaræ Fluidum.

ELATERINUM. *U. S.* *Elaterin.*

$C_{20}H_{28}O_5$; 348. (ĔL-A-TĒ-RĪ'NŬM.) $C_{40}H_{28}O_{10}$; 348.

"A neutral principle extracted from Elaterium, a substance deposited by the juice of the fruit of Ecbalium Elaterium. A. Richard. (*Nat. Ord.* Cucurbitaceæ.)" *U. S.* "The active principle of Elaterium. It may be obtained by exhausting elaterium with chloroform, adding ether to the chloroformic solution, collecting the precipitate, washing the latter with ether, and purifying by recrystallization in chloroform." *Br.*

This preparation was introduced into the Pharmacopœias on account of the well-known variability in quality of commercial elaterium. (See *Elaterium.*) Care must be taken to examine the elaterin, which is itself liable to be adulterated. It is in "small, colorless, shining, hexagonal scales or prisms, permanent in the air, odorless, having a bitter, somewhat acrid taste, and a neutral reaction. Insoluble in water; soluble in 125 parts of alcohol at 15° C. (59° F.); in 2 parts of boiling alcohol, in 290 parts of ether, and also in solutions of the alkalies, from which it is precipitated by supersaturating with an acid. When heated to 200° C. (392° F.), the crystals turn yellow and melt; on ignition they are wholly dissipated. A solution of Elaterin in cold, concentrated sulphuric acid assumes a yellow color gradually changing to red. The alcoholic solution should not be precipitated by tannic acid nor by salts of mercury or of platinum (abs. of, and difference from alkaloids)." *U. S.* "With melted carbolic acid it yields a solution which, on the addition of sulphuric acid, acquires a crimson color, rapidly changing to scarlet." *Br.* Ernst Johannson (*Inaug. Dis.*, Dorpat, 1884) gives the following reaction for elaterin besides those mentioned in the Pharmacopœia. In all of them elaterin is held in alcoholic solution. Froehde's reagent gives a green color passing into brown which fades away. Vanadinsulphuric acid with the fortieth of a milligramme produced a splendid blue color passing into a clear green, finally into reddish brown. After mixing with selenic acid and an addition of sulphuric acid, in a few minutes a red-brown color develops, which is not so deep as that which is produced by sulphuric acid. Kohler's reaction is made by dissolving elaterin in a few drops of concentrated hydrochloric acid, evaporating the acid in a water-bath, washing the white, amorphous residue with boiling water, and adding some concentrated sulphuric acid, when an amaranth-red color develops. By means of these reactions Johannson has been able to find elaterin in large quantities in the fæces of animals poisoned by it, but no trace either in the blood or urine or any part of the organism. It may be procured by evaporating an alcoholic tincture of elaterium to the consistence of thin oil, and throwing the residue while yet warm into a weak boiling solution of potassa. The potassa holds the green resin in solution, and the elaterin crystallizes as the liquor cools. Mr. Hennell obtained it by treating with ether the alcoholic extract procured by the spontaneous evaporation of the tincture. This consists of elaterin and the green resin, the latter of which, being much more soluble in ether than the former, is completely extracted by this fluid, leaving the elaterin pure. But, as elaterin is also slightly soluble in ether, a portion of this principle is wasted by Mr. Hennell's method. By evaporating the ethereal solution, the green resin is obtained separate. Mr. Hennell says that this was found to possess the purgative property of elaterium, as it acted powerfully in a dose less than one-third of a grain. But the effect was probably owing to the presence of a portion of elaterin which had been dissolved.

by the ether. Flückiger prefers to exhaust elaterium with chloroform, and add to the percolate ether, which precipitates elaterin. The precipitate may be dissolved in chloroform and recrystallized.

Medical Properties. The late Dr. Duncan, of Edinburgh, ascertained that elaterin produced, in the quantity of $\frac{1}{12}$ or $\frac{1}{16}$ of a grain (0·005 or ·004 Gm.), all the effects of a dose of elaterium. These doses are, however, probably too large, and it would scarcely be safe to commence with more than $\frac{1}{20}$ of a grain (0·003 Gm.); the doses of the Br. Ph. are from $\frac{1}{40}$ to $\frac{1}{10}$ of a grain.

Mr. Morries obtained 26 per cent. from the best British elaterium, 15 per cent. from the worst, and only 5 or 6 per cent. from the French; while a portion, procured according to the directions of the London College, yielded to Mr. Hennell upwards of 40 per cent. The Br. Pharmacopœia directs that the proportion of elaterin should not be less than 20 per cent. Experiments by Mr. John Williams satisfactorily prove that the fruit, exhausted of the free juice from which elaterium is obtained, contains very little if any elaterin, certainly not enough to compensate for the cost of its extraction. (*Chem. News*, 1860, p. 124.)

Off. Prep. Trituratio Elaterini. *Off. Prep. Br.* Pulvis Elaterini Compositus.

ELATERIUM. *Br.* *Elaterium.*

(ĔL-Ą-TĒ'RĮ-ŬM.)

"A sediment from the juice of the Squirting Cucumber fruit." *Br.*

The British Pharmacopœia recognizes the fruit under the name of *Ecbalii Fructus, Squirting Cucumber Fruit*, and defines it as the fruit, very nearly ripe, of Ecbalium Elaterium, from plants cultivated in Britain.

Extractum Elaterii; Elaterium, Elaterion, *Fr.;* Elaterium, *G.;* Elaterio, *It., Sp.*

Gen. Ch. MALE. *Calyx* five-cleft. *Corolla* five-parted. *Filaments* three. FEMALE. *Calyx* five-cleft. *Corolla* five-parted. *Style* trifid. *Gourd* bursting elastically. *Willd.*

Momordica Elaterium. Willd. *Sp. Plant.* iv. 605; Woodv. *Med. Bot.* p. 192, t. 72.—*Ecbalium agreste.* Richard; Lindley, *Med. and Œcon. Bot.* p. 95.—*Ecbalium officinarum.* Br.—*Ecbalium Elaterium.* French Codex, 1837. The *wild* or *squirting cucumber* is a perennial plant, with a large fleshy root, from which rise several round, thick, rough stems, branching and trailing like the common cucumber, but without tendrils. The leaves are petiolate, large, rough, irregularly cordate, and of a grayish green color. The flowers are yellow, and proceed from the axils of the leaves. The fruit has the shape of a small oval cucumber, about an inch and a half long, an inch thick, of a greenish or grayish color, and covered with stiff hairs or prickles. When fully ripe, it separates from the peduncle, and throws out its juice and seeds with considerable force through an opening at the base, where it was attached to the footstalk. The name of squirting cucumber was derived from this circumstance, and the scientific and officinal title is supposed to have had a similar origin; though some authors maintain that the term *elaterium* was applied to the medicine rather from the mode of its operation upon the bowels, than from the projectile property of the fruit.*

This species of Momordica is a native of the south of Europe, and is cultivated in Great Britain, where, however, it perishes in the winter. Elaterium is the substance spontaneously deposited by the juice of the fruit, when separated and allowed to stand. From the experiments of Dr. Clutterbuck, it has been supposed that only the free juice about the seeds, which is obtained without expression, affords the product. The substance of the fruit itself, the seeds, as well as other parts of the plant, have been thought to be nearly or quite inert. From the statements made by Mr. Bell (see note below), these opinions must probably be somewhat modified; but there is no doubt that strong expression injures the product. When the fruit is sliced and placed upon a sieve, a perfectly limpid and colorless juice flows out, which soon becomes turbid, and in the course of a few hours begins to deposit a sediment. This, when collected and carefully dried, is very light and pulverulent, of a yellowish white color, slightly tinged with green. It is the genuine elaterium, and was found by

* From the Greek ἐλαύνω, I drive, or ἐλατήρ, driver. The word *elaterium* was used by Hippocrates to signify any active purge. Dioscorides applied it to the medicine of which we are treating.

Clutterbuck to purge violently in the dose of one-eighth of a grain. But the quantity contained in the fruit is very small. Clutterbuck obtained only six grains from forty cucumbers. Commercial elaterium is often a weaker medicine, owing in part, perhaps, to adulteration, but much more to the mode in which it is prepared. In order to increase the product, the juice of the fruit is often expressed with great force; and there is reason to believe that it is sometimes evaporated so as to form an extract, instead of being allowed to deposit the active matter. The French elaterium is prepared by expressing the juice, clarifying it by rest and filtration, and then evaporating to a suitable consistence. As the liquid remaining after the deposition of the sediment is comparatively inert, it will be perceived that the preparation of the French Codex must be relatively feeble. The following are the directions of the British Pharmacopœia. "Cut the fruit lengthwise, and lightly press out the juice. Strain it through a hair sieve, and set aside to deposit. Carefully pour off the supernatant liquor; pour the sediment on a linen filter, and dry it on porous tiles, in a warm place. The decanted fluid may deposit a second portion of sediment, which can be dried in the same way." The latter portion deposited is of a lighter color. (*Pereira.*) The slight pressure directed is necessary for the separation of the juice from the somewhat immature fruit employed. The perfectly ripe fruit is not used; as, in consequence of its disposition to part with its contents, it cannot be carried to market. In the British Pharmacopœia, the former name of Extractum Elaterii of the London College has been very properly abandoned; as the preparation is in no correct sense of the word an extract. Elaterium is brought chiefly from England; but it is probable that a portion of the elaterium, of which Dr. Pereira speaks as coming from Malta, reaches our market also.*

Properties. The *best elaterium* is in thin flat or slightly curled cakes or fragments, often bearing the impression of the muslin upon which it was dried, of a greenish gray color becoming yellowish by exposure, of a feeble odor, and a bitter somewhat acrid taste. It is pulverulent and inflammable, and so light that it swims when thrown upon water. When of *inferior quality*, it is sometimes dark-colored, much curled, and rather hard, breaking with difficulty, or presenting a resinous fracture. The *Maltese elaterium* is in larger pieces, of a pale color, sometimes without the least tinge of green, destitute of odor, soft, and friable, and not unfrequently gives evidence of having been mixed with chalk or starch. It sinks in water. "Does not effervesce with acids; boiled with water and the cooled mixture treated with iodine, affords little or no blue color; yields half its weight to boiling rectified spirit. Treated by the method described for 'Elaterin,' it should yield twenty-five per cent., or not less than twenty per cent. of that substance." *Br.*

Dr. Clutterbuck first observed that the activity of elaterium resided in the por-

* The following notice of the cultivation of the elaterium plant, and the preparation of the drug at Mitcham, in Surrey, England, condensed from a paper by Mr. Jacob Bell in the *P. J. Tr.* for October, 1850, may have some interest for the American reader. The seeds are sown in March, and the seedlings planted in June. In luxuriant plants the stem sometimes acquires an extraordinary breadth. In one instance, though not thicker than the forefinger where it issued from the earth, it was in its broadest part four inches wide and half an inch thick. A wet season interferes with the productiveness of the plant. At the spontaneous separation of the fruit, it throws out its juice sometimes to the distance of twenty yards; and hazard of injury to the eyes is incurred by walking among the plants at their period of maturity. A bushel of the fruit weighs 40 pounds, and the price varies from 7 to 10 shillings sterling. In the manufacture of elaterium, which begins early in September, the fruit, having been washed, if necessary, to cleanse it from earthy matters, is sliced longitudinally into halves, and then submitted to expression, wrapped in a hempen cloth, in a common screw-press. Considerable force is used in the expression. The juice is then strained through hair, cypress, or wire sieves, and set aside for deposition. The deposit usually takes place in three or four hours. When this part of the process is completed, the supernatant liquor is carefully poured off, the deposit is placed on calico cloths resting on hair sieves, and allowed to drain for about twelve hours, after which it is removed by a knife, spread over small cloths, and dried on canvas frames in the drying stove. About half an ounce of fine elaterium is obtained from a bushel of fruit. Some obtain more; but the product is inferior, in consequence of the use of too much force in the expression. Good elaterium has a pale pea-green tint; that of inferior quality is of a duller hue. The juice expelled in bursting is said to undergo very little change in the air, while that expressed from the ripe fruit immediately afterwards becomes milky, and deposits elaterium. The recently burst fruit, therefore, is nearly if not quite as good for the preparation of the drug as that collected before perfect maturity. For a paper on the cultivation of the elaterium plant at Hitchin, Herts, England, see *A. J. P.*, 1860, p. 163; at Market Deeping, *P. J. Tr.*, Sept. 1881, p. 239.

tion of it soluble in alcohol and not in water. This fact was afterward confirmed by Dr. Paris, who found that the alcoholic extract, treated with boiling distilled water, and afterwards dried, had the property of purging in minute doses, while the remaining portion of the elaterium was inactive. The subsequent experiments of Mr. Hennell, of London, and Mr. Morries, of Edinburgh, which were nearly simultaneous, demonstrated the existence of a crystallizable matter in elaterium, which is the active principle, and has been named *elaterin.** (See *Elaterinum.*) According to Mr. Hennell, 100 parts of elaterium contain 44 of elaterin, 17 of a green resin (*chlorophyll*), 6 of starch, 27 of lignin, and 6 of saline matters. The alcoholic extract which Dr. Paris called *elatin* is probably a mixture of elaterin and the green resin or chlorophyll.†

Walz (1859) found in the juice of the fruits and herb of *Ecballium*, as well as in that of *Cucumis Prophetarum*, L., a second crystallizable bitter principle, *prophetin*, and the amorphous substances *ecballin* or *elateric acid*, *hydro-elaterin*, and *elateride*, all of which require further examination.

Choice of Elaterium. The inequality of elaterium depends probably more on diversities in the mode of preparation than on adulteration. Sometimes, however, it is greatly sophisticated; and large quantities are said to have been imported into this country, consisting mainly of chalk, and colored green artificially. (B. Canavan, *N. Y. Journ. of Pharm.*, iii. 385.) It should possess the sensible properties above indicated as characterizing good elaterium, should not effervesce

* H. W. Jones and F. Ransom detail an improved method of assaying elaterium in the *Year-Book of Pharmacy*, 1886, p. 442; it is as follows: "Macerate 1 gramme of finely powdered elaterium with chloroform in a covered dish for a few hours, then transfer to a miniature glass percolator (*e.g.*, the barrel of a small glass syringe) plugged with cotton, and wash with chloroform, allowing about 10 C.c. to pass through the marc after the menstruum has begun to pass in a colorless condition. Place the percolate in a small dish, and evaporate off the chloroform at a gentle heat. Treat the residue with a small quantity of pure, absolute ether, and transfer to a small percolator or funnel, plugged with cotton. Wash with pure ether until at least 10 C.c. have passed through colorless, and reserve the ethereal washings. Redissolve the elaterin, so obtained, by passing chloroform through it whilst still in the funnel or percolator, and evaporate the chloroformic solution once more to dryness in a small dish. Treat the residue so obtained with ether, exactly as before. Allow the united ethereal washings to evaporate spontaneously until the bulk is reduced to about 3 C.c. Transfer this liquid to a small cylinder (*e.g.*, a 10 C.c. measure), and allow the separated elaterin to deposit. Carefully decant the colored supernatant liquid, add 4 C.c. of pure ether to the residue, and again decant after deposition has taken place. Finally dissolve the elaterin in the cylinder with the aid of chloroform, and wash out the larger amount previously collected in the funnel with the same solvent. Unite the chloroformic solutions, evaporate in a tared dish, dry on the water-bath, and weigh."

† *Chlorophyll.* The substance to which Pelletier gave this name, under the impression that it was a peculiar proximate principle, was subsequently supposed by that chemist to be a mixture of wax and a green fixed oil. (*Journ. de Pharm.*, xix. 109.) Afterwards, M. Frémy succeeded, by the joint action of a menstruum composed of two parts of ether and one of hydrochloric acid diluted with a little water, in separating chlorophyll into two coloring principles, one yellow and the other blue; the former being dissolved by the ether, and the latter by the hydrochloric acid. The yellow, M. Frémy proposed to name *phylloxanthin*, the blue *phyllocyanin*. (*Ibid.*, Avril, 1860.)

Phylloxanthin is neutral, insoluble in water, soluble in alcohol and ether, and crystallizable, sometimes in yellow plates, sometimes in reddish prisms, resembling bichromate of potassium, and possessing dyeing powers analogous to those of chromic acid.

Phyllocyanic acid is soluble in water, alcohol, and ether, giving to these an olive-like color, with bronze-red or violet reflections. All its salts are brown or green; but only the alkaline are soluble in water. This acid dissolves in sulphuric and hydrochloric acid, giving rise to solutions which, according to their strength, are green, reddish, violet, or beautifully blue. This M. Frémy considers the important fact of the investigation, as it explains the various tints which chlorophyll offers in vegetation.

According to Filhol, chlorophyll in alcoholic solution is decomposed by hydrochloric acid into four distinct coloring matters: one, rich in nitrogen, brown, and insoluble in alcohol; one, free from nitrogen, yellow, and soluble in alcohol; one blue, which forms on adding an excess of hydrochloric acid, and a yellow compound separated from this latter by ether.

Stokes also makes chlorophyll to be a mixture of four coloring substances optically different. Of these two are green and two yellow. The green colors fluoresce strongly with red tint; the yellow colors, on the contrary, do not show any fluorescence.

It follows, from all that has been said, that chlorophyll is an immediate proximate principle, of great mobility, which undergoes diversified changes of color in the progress of vegetation, and other changes, such as have been mentioned, under the influence of different reagents. (*Journ. de Pharm. et de Chim.*, 4e sér., ii. 185, 1865.)

An interesting fact in relation to chlorophyll is the part it plays in vegetable growth. By its presence in the vegetable cells, carbon is assimilated through the agency of light; while, in its absence, light alone is not able to effect such assimilation. (*Chem. News*, 1872, p. 132.)

with acids, and should yield from one-sixth to one-fourth of elaterin. (See *Elaterinum.*)

Medical Properties and Uses. Elaterium is a powerful hydragogue cathartic, and in a large dose generally excites nausea and vomiting. If too freely administered, it operates with great violence both upon the stomach and bowels, producing inflammation of these organs, which has in some instances eventuated fatally. It also increases the flow of urine. The fruit was employed by the ancients, and is recommended in the writings of Dioscorides as a remedy in mania and melancholy. Sydenham and his contemporaries considered elaterium highly useful in dropsy; but, in consequence of some fatal results from its incautious employment, it fell into disrepute, and was generally neglected till again brought into notice by Dr. Ferriar. It is now considered one of the most efficient hydragogue cathartics in the treatment of dropsical diseases, in which it has sometimes proved successful after all other remedies have failed. The full dose of commercial elaterium, as formerly found in commerce, was often from one to two grains (0·065 to 0·13 Gm.); but, as the quality has greatly improved, this dose might now be much too large, and the best plan is to give it in the dose of a sixth to a quarter of a grain (0·01 to 0·016 Gm.), repeated every hour till it operates, and increased if necessary. It should be observed that these doses are inapplicable to the very old and feeble and those prostrated by disease. A case is recorded in which two-fifths of a grain proved fatal by excessive purging in an old lady of 70 years, in the last stage of liver and heart disease, complicated with dropsy; a result which a very little consideration would have anticipated. (*A. J. P.*, 1868, p. 373.) The dose of Clutterbuck's elaterium is the eighth of a grain (·008 Gm.), that of elaterin is from the twentieth to the sixteenth of a grain (0·003 to 0·004 Gm.). One grain may be dissolved in a fluidounce of alcohol with four drops of nitric acid, and from 25 to 30 minims may be given diluted with water, but the granule affords a preferable method.

ELEMI. *Br.* *Manila Elemi.*

(ĔL′Ē-MĪ.)

"A concrete, resinous exudation, the botanical source of which is undetermined but is sometimes referred to Canarium commune, *Linn.*" *Br.* (*Nat. Ord.* Terebintaceæ, *Juss.*)

Résine élemi. *Fr.;* Oelbaumharz, Elemi, *G.;* Elemi, *It.;* Goma de Limon, *Sp.*

Gen. Ch. *Calyx* four-toothed. *Petals* four, oblong. *Stigma* four-cornered. *Berry* drupaceous. *Willd.*

Some botanists separate from this genus the species which have their fruit in the form of a capsule instead of a nut, and associate them together in a distinct genus with the name of *Icica.* This is recognized by De Candolle.

Most of the trees belonging to these two genera yield, when wounded, a resinous juice analogous to the turpentines. It is not improbable that the drug, usually known by the name of *elemi,* is derived from several different trees. That known to the ancients is said to have been obtained from Ethiopia, and all the elemi of commerce was originally brought from the Levant. The tree which afforded it was not accurately known, but was supposed to be a species of Amyris. At present the drug is said to be derived from three sources, namely, Brazil, Mexico, and Manilla. The Brazilian is believed to be the product of a plant mentioned by Marcgrav under the name of *icicariba,* and called by De Candolle *Icica Icicariba.* It is a lofty tree, with pinnate leaves, consisting of three or five pointed, perforated leaflets, smooth on their upper surface and woolly beneath. It is erroneously stated in some works to be a native of Carolina. The elemi is obtained by incisions into the trees, through which the juice flows and concretes upon the bark. The Mexican is said by Dr. Royle to be obtained from a species of Elaphrium, which that author has described from dried specimens, and proposes to name *E. elemiferum.* (*Mat. Med.*, Am. ed., p. 339.) The Manilla elemi is conjecturally referred to *Canarium commune.* (*Ibid.*, p. 340.)

Elemi is in masses of various consistence, sometimes solid and heavy like wax, sometimes light and porous; unctuous to the touch; diaphanous; of diversified colors, generally greenish with intermingled points of white or yellow, sometimes greenish white with brown stains, sometimes yellow like sulphur; fragile and friable when cold; softening by the heat of the hand; of a terebinthinate somewhat aromatic odor, diminishing with age, and resembling to some extent that of lemon and fennel; of a warm, slightly bitter, disagreeable taste; entirely soluble, with the exception of impurities, in boiling alcohol; and affording a volatile oil by distillation. "Moistened with rectified spirit, it breaks up into small particles, which, when examined by the microscope, are seen partly to consist of acicular crystals." *Br.* A variety examined by M. Bonastre was found to consist of 60 parts of resin, 24 of a resinous matter soluble in boiling alcohol, but deposited when the liquid cools, 12·5 of volatile oil, 2 of extractive, and 1·5 of acid and impurities. M. Baup found the resin to be of two kinds, one amorphous, the other crystallizable; the latter of which, as obtained from West India elemi, he proposes to call *elemin*, and considers identical with the crystallizable resin *amyrin*, obtained from Manila elemi. (*Journ. de Pharm.*, 3e sér., xx. 331.) Elemi is sometimes adulterated with colophony and turpentine. Dr. Emil Mannkoff obtained from Brazilian elemi about 6 per cent. of a colorless volatile oil, insoluble in water, but easily dissolved both by alcohol and ether, of a not unpleasant odor, and a somewhat acrid and bitter taste. (*B. & F. Medico-Chir. Rev.*, July, 1859, p. 170.) Prof. Flückiger obtained as much as 10 per cent. of essential oil from Manila elemi. He found it to be a fragrant, colorless, neutral oil of sp. gr. 0·861 at 15° C. (59° F.), and strongly dextrogyrate. Deville, on the other hand, obtained an oil equally strongly lævogyrate. Flückiger thus sums up the constituents of elemi: essential oil $C_{10}H_{16}$; *amyrin* $2(C_{10}H_{16}) + H_2O$; amorphous resin $2(C_{10}H_{16}) + 2H_2O$; *bryoidin* $2(C_{10}H_{16}) + 3H_2O$; *elemic acid* and bitter extractive.

Medical Properties and Uses. Elemi has properties analogous to those of the turpentines, but is exclusively applied to external use. In the United States it is rarely employed even in this way. In the pharmacy of Europe it enters into the composition of numerous plasters and ointments. We are told that it is occasionally brought to this country in small fragments mixed with the coarser kinds of gum arabic from the Levant and India.

Off. Prep. Br. Unguentum Elemi.

ELIXIRIA. *Elixirs.*

(ĔL-IX-IR'I-Ă—ĕl-ĭk-sĭr'ĕ-ă.)

Elixirs as they are known in modern American pharmacy are aromatic, sweetened, spirituous preparations, containing small quantities of active medicinal substances. They differ greatly from the liquids formerly termed elixirs, from the fact that the first object sought for in the modern elixir is an agreeable taste, and usually this is attained only by such sacrifices as to render the effect of the medicine almost *nil*, whilst the principal activity is due to the alcohol, which has proved in many cases very injurious. These considerations have heretofore prevented an official recognition of elixirs, and the present Pharmacopœia recognises but one, *i.e.*, elixir of orange, which has been introduced merely as a vehicle. Owing to their extensive use by practitioners all over our country, it becomes necessary to notice some of the most important in this commentary, and in the 15th edition of the Dispensatory a number of formulas for elixirs were inserted here; but, owing to the extensive list now to be found in the National Formulary, and as these will have a semi-official standing, it was deemed best to group them all together under their proper titles in Part II.; *q. v.*

ELIXIR AURANTII. *U.S.* *Elixir of Orange.* [*Simple Elixir.*]

(Ē-LĬX'IR ĂU-RĂN'TI-Ī—ĕ-lĭk'sur ăw-răn'shē-ī.)

"Oil of Orange Peel, *one part* [or two and a half fluidrachms]; Cotton, *two parts* [or half an ounce av.]; Sugar, in coarse powder, *one hundred parts* [or twenty-five ounces av.]; Alcohol, Water, each, *a sufficient quantity*, To make *three hundred parts* [about four pints]. Mix Alcohol and Water in the proportion of *one part* [or one pint] of Alcohol to *three parts* [or two and a half pints] of Water. Add the Oil of Orange to the Cotton, in small portions at a time, distributing it thoroughly by picking the Cotton apart after each addition; then pack tightly in a conical percolator, and gradually pour on the mixture of Alcohol and Water, until *two hundred parts* [or three and a quarter pints] of filtered liquid are obtained. In this liquid dissolve the Sugar by agitation, without heat, and strain." *U. S.*

This is a new officinal preparation. Its introduction grew out of the necessity for some official action, which would enable pharmacists to readily furnish elixirs when called for by an extemporaneous or speedy process. The elixir of orange is, of course, merely a base or vehicle, and in many cases the medicinal substance may be simply dissolved in the elixir. It may be necessary to add some insoluble, inert powder, like precipitated chalk, carbonate of magnesium, etc., to the liquid before filtering, in order to obtain a perfectly transparent elixir, and it is customary in many parts of the country to color the preparation with cochineal or caramel. (See Part II. for formulas for various elixirs.)

EMPLASTRA. *Plasters.*

(EM-PLĂS'TRA.)

Emplâtres, *Fr.;* Pflaster, *G.*

Plasters are solid compounds intended for external application, adhesive at the temperature of the human body, and of such a consistence as to render the aid of heat necessary in spreading them. Most of them have as their basis a compound of olive oil and litharge, constituting the Emplastrum Plumbi of the Pharmacopœias. Others owe their consistence and adhesiveness to resinous substances, or to a mixture of these with wax and fats.

In the preparation of the plasters, care is requisite that the heat employed be not sufficiently elevated to produce decomposition, nor so long continued as to drive off any volatile ingredient upon which the virtues of the preparation may in any degree depend. After having been prepared, they are usually shaped into cylindrical rolls, and wrapped in paper to exclude the air. Plasters should be firm at ordinary temperatures, should spread easily when heated, and, after being spread, should remain soft, pliable, and adhesive, without melting, at the heat of the human body. When long kept, they are apt to change color and to become hard and brittle; and, as this alteration is most observable upon their surface, it must depend chiefly upon the action of the air, which should therefore be as much as possible excluded. The defect may usually be remedied by melting the plaster with a moderate heat, and adding a sufficient quantity of oil to give it the due consistence.

Plasters are prepared for use by spreading them upon leather, linen, or muslin, according to the particular purposes they are intended to answer. Leather is most convenient when the application is made to the sound skin, linen or muslin when the plaster is used as a dressing to ulcerated or abraded surfaces, or with the view of bringing and retaining together the sides of wounds. The leather usually preferred is white sheep-skin, or the kind known commercially as "hemlock splits." A margin about a quarter or half an inch broad should usually be left uncovered, in order to facilitate the removal of the plaster, and to prevent the clothing in contact with its edges from being soiled. An accurate outline may be obtained by pasting upon the leather a piece of paper, so cut as to leave in the centre a vacant space of the required dimensions, and removing the paper when no longer needed. The same object may often be accomplished by employing two narrow rulers of sheet tin graduated in inches, and so shaped that each of them may form two sides of a rectangle. These may be applied in such a manner as to enclose within them any given rectangular space, and may be fixed by weights upon the leather, or preferably adjusted by set-screws, while the plaster is spread. For any other shape, as in the instance of plasters for the breast, pieces of tin may be employed having a vacuity within, corresponding to the required outline. The spreading of the plaster is most conveniently accomplished by the use of a spatula or plaster iron. This may be heated by means of a spirit lamp. Care must be taken that the instrument be not so hot as to discolor or decompose the plaster; and special care is requisite in the case of those plasters which contain a volatile ingredient. A sufficient portion of the plaster should first be melted by the heated instrument, and, having been received on a piece of coarse stiff paper, or in a shallow tin tray open on one side, should, when nearly cool, be transferred to the leather, and applied quickly and evenly over its surface. By this plan the melted plaster is prevented from penetrating the leather, as it is apt to do when applied too hot. Before removing the paper from the edge of the plaster, if this has become so hard as to crack, the iron should be drawn over the line of junction. When linen or muslin is used, and the dimensions of the portion to be spread are large, as is often the case with adhesive plaster, the best plan is to pass the cloth "on which the plaster has been laid through a machine, formed of a spatula fixed by screws at a proper distance from a plate of polished steel." A machine for spreading plasters is described by M. Hérent in the *Journ. de Pharm.* (3e ser., ii. 403).* (See also *N. R.*, 1879, p. 337.)

The spreading of plasters has become to a great extent a lost art to the pharmacist of this country, owing to the introduction of machine-spread plasters, which contain india rubber in the adhesive composition. These are reasonably permanent, and do not require the application of heat. When made by reliable manufacturers they are in many cases to be preferred, but, unfortunately, the introduction of immense quantities of worthless plasters by unscrupulous makers has caused many practitioners to direct these to be spread by the pharmacist from officinal plaster. The perforation or "porousing" of plasters is usually accomplished on a large scale by expensive apparatus. Prof. J. P. Remington has devised an inexpensive apparatus whereby the apothecary can perforate those spread by himself. (*A. J. P.*, 1878, p. 171.)† Dr. J. J. Edmondson read a paper before the Pennsylvania Pharm. As-

* It has been customary with apothecaries to employ an apparatus, such as that figured on the opposite page, for spreading quantities of plasters. An oblong rectangular block of hard wood (*a e*) has its upper surface (*c*) slightly convex. To this is attached by a movable joint (at *r*) a sheet-iron frame (*b*), with an opening (*n*) of the dimensions of the plaster to be spread, and clasps (*d*) at the other end, by which this may be fixed to the block. Another portion of the apparatus is a sheet-iron or tin frame (*m*), by which the leather is cut out, and the margin marked. The leather thus prepared is laid on the convex surface of the block (*c*); the sheet-iron frame is brought down on it evenly (as at *h i*); the plaster, previously melted, but not too hot, is poured on the leather in the centre, and, by means of an iron instrument (*g*) previously heated by a spirit lamp, is spread uniformly over the surface, the thickness being regulated by the frame against which the iron is pressed. Any excess of plaster is thus pressed over upon the frame. The point of a sharp instrument (*l*) is then

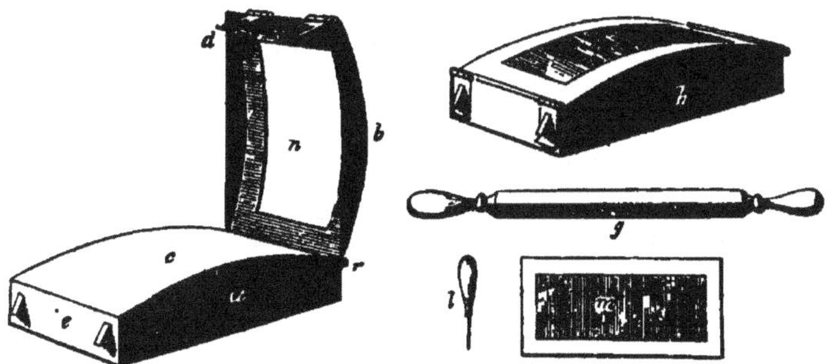

drawn along the interior edge of the frame so as to separate the plaster from it, after which the clasps are unfastened and the plaster removed.

† *Emplastrum Aconiti. Aconite Plaster.* (Emplâtre d'Aconit, *Fr.;* Aconit-Pflaster, *G.*) "Take of Aconite Root, in fine powder, *sixteen troyounces;* Alcohol, Resin Plaster, each, *a sufficient quantity.* Moisten the Aconite Root with six fluidounces of Alcohol, and pack it in a conical percolator. Cover the surface with a disk of paper, and pour upon it ten fluidounces of Alcohol. When the liquid begins to drop, cork the percolator, and, having closely covered it to prevent evaporation, set it aside in a moderately warm place for four days. Then remove the cork, and gradually pour on Alcohol until two pints of tincture have been obtained or the Aconite Root is exhausted. Distil off a pint and a half of alcohol, and evaporate the residue to a soft uniform extract by means of a water-bath. Add to this sufficient Resin Plaster, previously melted, to make the mixture weigh sixteen troyounces, and then mix them thoroughly." *U. S.* 1870.

This plaster was introduced into the Pharmacopœia of 1870. The formula is a modification of that proposed by Prof. Procter. (*A. J. P.*, xxv. 202.) Aconite Plaster may be used whenever it is desired to produce a very powerful local anodyne effect.

sociation in 1887 giving the process for manufacturing rubber-mass plasters as carried on by Johnson and Johnson, of New York. It is as follows: The ingredients employed are—Rubber, two parts; Burgundy Pitch, one part; Gum Olibanum, one part. This may vary with some special plasters, but they constitute the component parts of the mass used for the majority.

The crude rubber is at first steeped in hot water to cleanse and soften it, then the rubber is passed through the washer and crusher, where it is subjected to severe pressure between two corrugated rolls, eight inches in diameter and one foot wide, while a stream of water falling continually washes it thoroughly, and it comes out in sheets somewhat softened.

After these sheets are dried, which requires a number of days, they are passed through the grinder, where they are crushed between two smooth rollers, fourteen inches in diameter and thirty-six inches across. This thoroughly softens the rubber and makes it plastic, so that it can be readily worked up with the other ingredients. The principal operation, the mixing, then takes place.

The medication must be carefully combined, and the whole manipulation so managed that the plaster will be uniform, so that age or varying temperature shall not affect it.

This operation is performed by means of rollers, sixteen inches in diameter, arranged so that one revolves at twice the speed of the other. Between these large rollers the mass is passed with whatever medication is required: *e g.*, when a belladonna mass is to be made, a certain amount of the stock mass is taken and of extract of belladonna in proportions corresponding to the formula in the Pharmacopœia. These are repeatedly passed through the rollers until the extract of belladonna is thoroughly mixed with the mass, care being taken to keep the temperature from rising high enough to decompose or affect the atropine. The spreading is also done by rollers, into which the thoroughly-mixed mass is fed at the same time that the cloth is fed, the thickness of the plasters being governed by adjusting screws on the side of the machine.

The rubber base is pliable, adhesive, will not become too hard or too soft, will yield up the medication to the absorbents of the skin, and will retain its properties indefinitely.

EMPLASTRUM AMMONIACI. *U.S.* *Ammoniac Plaster.*

(ĔM-PLĂS'TRŬM ĂM-MO-NĪ'Ă-CĪ.)

Emplâtre de Gomme Ammoniaque, Emplâtre fondant (résolutif), ***Fr.;*** **Ammoniak-Pflaster,** ***G.***

"Ammoniac, *one hundred parts* [or five ounces av.]; Diluted Acetic Acid, *one hundred and forty parts* [or half a pint]. Digest the Ammoniac in the Diluted Acetic Acid, in a suitable vessel, avoiding contact with metals, until it is entirely emulsionized; then strain and evaporate the strained liquid, by means of a water-bath, stirring constantly, until a small portion, taken from the vessel, hardens on cooling." *U.S.*

This plaster has been omitted in the British Pharmacopœia.

As ammoniac is not usually kept purified in our shops, the straining of the solution in the diluted acid is directed, as the most convenient method of separating impurities. Dr. Duncan remarked that the plaster, prepared in iron vessels, "acquires an unpleasant dark color, from being impregnated with iron, whereas, when prepared in a glass or earthenware vessel, it has a yellowish white color, and more pleasant appearance." Care should also be used to avoid iron spatulas in its preparation, as the acetic acid acts on that metal, and discolors the plaster. The use of a moderate heat will facilitate the action of the diluted acid; and at best it is a thick creamy mass that is obtained, which requires the aid of the hand to strain it properly.

Medical Properties. The ammoniac plaster is stimulant, and is applied over scrofulous tumors and chronic swellings of the joints, to promote their resolution. It often produces a papular eruption, and sometimes occasions considerable inflammation of the skin.

EMPLASTRUM AMMONIACI CUM HYDRARGYRO. *U.S., Br.*
Ammoniac Plaster with Mercury.

(ĔM-PLĂS'TRŬM ĂM-MO-NĪ'A-CĪ CŬM HȲ-DRĂR'GY-RŌ.)

Emplâtre de Gomme Ammoniaque mercuriel, *Fr.;* Quecksilber- und Ammoniak-Pflaster, *G.*

"Ammoniac, *seven hundred and twenty parts* [or thirteen ounces av.]; Mercury, *one hundred and eighty parts* [or three and one-quarter ounces av.]; Olive Oil, *eight parts* [or sixty grains]; Sublimed Sulphur, *one part* [or eight grains]; Diluted Acetic Acid, *one thousand parts* [or seventeen fluidounces]; Lead Plaster, *a sufficient quantity,* To make *one thousand parts* [or eighteen ounces av.]. Digest the Ammoniac in the Diluted Acetic Acid, in a suitable vessel, avoiding contact with metals, until it is entirely emulsionized; then strain, and evaporate the strained liquid by means of a water-bath, stirring constantly, until a small portion, taken from the vessel, hardens on cooling. Heat the Olive Oil, and gradually add the Sulphur, stirring constantly until they unite; then add the Mercury, and triturate until globules of the metal cease to be visible. Next add, gradually the Ammoniac, while yet hot; and finally, having added enough Lead Plaster, previously melted by means of a water-bath, to make the mixture weigh *one thousand parts* [or eighteen ounces av.], mix the whole thoroughly." *U. S.*

"Take of Ammoniacum *twelve ounces* [avoirdupois]; Mercury *three ounces* [avoird.]; Olive Oil *fifty-six grains;* Sublimed Sulphur *eight grains.* Heat the Oil, and add the Sulphur to it gradually, stirring till they unite. With this mixture triturate the Mercury until globules are no longer visible; and, lastly, add the Ammoniacum, previously liquefied, mixing the whole carefully." *Br.*

The finished preparation does not differ materially from that produced by the formula of the last Pharmacopœia. The use of diluted acetic acid to facilitate the straining of the ammoniac is an improvement over the water formerly used. The use of lead plaster to bring up the weight is needless, in our opinion.

The only use of the sulphur is to aid in the extinguishment of the mercury; as the compound formed by it with the metal is probably inert. When ammoniac not previously prepared is used, as it is not fusible by heat, it must be brought to the proper consistence by softening it in a small quantity of hot water, straining, and evaporating.

Medical Properties and Uses. This plaster unites with the stimulant power of the ammoniac the specific properties of the mercury, which is sometimes absorbed in sufficient quantity to affect the gums. It is used as a discutient in enlargement of the glands, tumefaction of the joints, nodes, and other indolent swellings, especially when dependent on a venereal taint. It is also sometimes applied over the liver in chronic hepatitis.*

EMPLASTRUM ARNICÆ. *U. S.* *Arnica Plaster.*

(ĔM-PLĂS'TRŬM ÄR'NI-ÇÆ—ăr'nĭ-sē.)

Emplâtre d'Arnique, *Fr.;* Arnicapflaster, *G.*

"Extract of Arnica Root, *fifty parts* [or four ounces av.]; Resin Plaster, *one hundred parts* [or eight ounces av.]. Add the Extract to the Plaster, previously melted by means of a water-bath, and mix them thoroughly." *U. S.*

These ingredients incorporate readily, and form a good plaster. The preparation was introduced into the Pharmacopœia, to enable the apothecary to meet the demand for a convenient preparation of arnica for external use. It is supposed to be useful in sprains and bruises, and sometimes probably acts beneficially by its stimulant properties in chronic rheumatism and other chronic external inflammations.

* *Emplastrum Antimonii. Antimonial Plaster.* (Emplastrum Stibiatum, s. Antimoniale; Emplâtre (Poix) émétisée, Emplâtre antimonial, *Fr.;* Brechweinstein-Pflaster, *G.*) "Take of Tartrate of Antimony and Potassium, in fine powder, *a troyounce;* Burgundy Pitch *four troyounces.* Melt the Pitch by means of a water-bath, and strain; then add the powder, and stir them well together until the mixture thickens on cooling." *U. S.* 1870.

This is a useful formula, although no longer officinal. It affords one of the most convenient methods of obtaining the local pustulating effects of tartar emetic. For its effects and uses, see *Antimonii et Potassii Tartras.*

EMPLASTRUM ASAFŒTIDÆ. *U. S.* *Asafetida Plaster.*

(ĔM-PLĂS'TRUM ĂS-Ą-FŒT'Į-DÆ—ăs-ę-fĕt'ĭ-dȧ.)

Emplastrum Assafœtidæ, Emplastrum Fœtidum; Emplâtre d'Asafétide, Emplâtretfétide (antihystérique), *Fr.;* Stinkasant-Pflaster, *G.*

"Asafetida, *thirty-five parts* [or thirteen ounces av.]; Lead Plaster, *thirty-five parts* [or thirteen ounces av.]; Galbanum, *fifteen parts* [or five and a half ounces av.]; Yellow Wax, *fifteen parts* [or five and a half ounces av.]; Alcohol, *one hundred and twenty parts* [or three pints]. Digest the Asafetida and Galbanum with the Alcohol on a water-bath, separate the liquid portion, while hot, from the coarser impurities by straining, and evaporate it to the consistence of honey; then add the Lead Plaster and the Wax, previously melted together, stir the mixture well, and evaporate to the proper consistence." *U. S.*

This plaster has been omitted in the British Pharmacopœia.

The directions of the U. S. Pharmacopœia indicate the mode in which the gum-resins may be brought to the liquid state before being incorporated with the other ingredients. Galbanum melts sufficiently by the aid of heat to admit of being strained; but this is not the case with asafetida, which must be prepared by dissolving it in a small quantity of hot water or alcohol, straining, and evaporating to the consistence of honey; and even galbanum may be most conveniently treated in the same way. Formerly these gum-resins were ordered merely to be melted and strained.

This plaster may be advantageously applied over the stomach or abdomen, in cases of hysteria attended with flatulence, and to the chest or between the shoulders in hooping-cough.

EMPLASTRUM BELLADONNÆ. *U. S., Br.* *Belladonna Plaster.*

(ĔM-PLĂS'TRUM BĔL-LĄ-DŎN'NÆ.)

Emplâtre de Belladone, *F.;* Belladonna-Pflaster, *G.*

"Belladonna Root, in No. 60 powder, *one hundred parts* [or 16 ounces av.]; Alcohol, Resin Plaster, each, *a sufficient quantity,* To make *one hundred parts.* Moisten the powder with *forty parts* [or 7 fluidounces] of Alcohol, and pack it firmly in a cylindrical percolator; then add enough Alcohol to saturate the powder and leave a stratum above it. When the liquid begins to drop from the percolator, close the lower orifice, and, having closely covered the percolator, macerate for forty-eight hours. Then allow the percolation to proceed, gradually adding Alcohol, until the Belladonna Root is exhausted. Reserve the first *ninety parts* [or 14 fluidounces] of the percolate; evaporate the remainder at a temperature not exceeding 50° C. (122° F.), to *ten parts* [or 2 fluidounces]; mix this with the reserved portion, and evaporate at or below the above-mentioned temperature to a soft uniform extract. Add to this enough Resin Plaster, previously melted, to make the whole weigh *one hundred parts* [or 16 ounces av.], and mix thoroughly." *U.S.*

"Take of Alcoholic Extract of Belladonna *four ounces* [av.]; Resin Plaster, Soap Plaster, of each, *eight ounces* [av.]. Melt the plasters by the heat of a water-bath, then add the extract, and mix the whole thoroughly together." *Br.*

This preparation was formerly prepared, in both Pharmacopœias, with the extract made from the inspissated juice of the leaves; but in the last edition of the U. S. and Br. Pharmacopœias an alcoholic extract of the root was substituted with the effect of rendering the plaster easier to be spread and more adhesive, and the officinal preparation is now of a light yellowish brown color, without a shade of green. It is a useful anodyne application in neuralgic and rheumatic pains, and in dysmenorrhœa. We have seen the constitutional effects of belladonna result from its external use. Mr. T. W. Worthington proposes a formula for making belladonna plaster with caoutchouc in the *A. J. P.*, xliii. 153. (See page 555.) Machine-spread belladonna plaster can be found in the market, which was admitted by a representative of the manufacturer to contain no extract of belladonna whatever, and to be purely factitious. In deference to popular prejudice, most machine-spread belladonna plasters have a dark green color.

EMPLASTRUM CALEFACIENS. *Br.* *Warming Plaster.* [*Warm Plaster.*]

(EM-PLĂS'TRUM CĂL-E-FĀ'CI-ENS—kăl-e-fā'she-enz.)

See *Emplastrum Picis cum Cantharide.* U. S.

EMPLASTRUM CANTHARIDIS. *Br.* *Cantharides Plaster.* *Blistering Plaster.*

(EM-PLĂS'TRUM CAN-THĂR'I-DĬS.)

See *Ceratum Cantharidis.* U. S.

EMPLASTRUM CAPSICI. *U. S.* *Capsicum Plaster.*

(EM-PLĂS'TRUM CĂP'SI-CĪ.)

"Resin Plaster, Oleoresin of Capsicum, each, *a sufficient quantity.* Melt the Resin Plaster at a gentle heat, spread a thin and even layer of it upon muslin, and allow it to cool. Then having cut off a piece of the required size, apply a thin coating of Oleoresin of Capsicum, by means of a brush, leaving a narrow, blank margin along the edges. A space of four inches, or ten centimeters square, should contain four grains, or twenty-five centigrammes, of Oleoresin of Capsicum." *U. S.*

This is a new officinal. It is a convenient way of obtaining the rubefacient effects of capsicum; of course the practice will be for the pharmacist to employ machine adhesive plaster as the base; although, with a little experience, very good work can be done by hand.

EMPLASTRUM FERRI. *U. S.* *Iron Plaster.* [*Strengthening Plaster.*]

(EM-PLĂS'TRUM FĔR'RĪ.)

Emplastrum Roborans, *Br.* 1867; Chalybeate Plaster; Emplastrum Ferratum, s. Martiale; Emplâtre d'Oxyde rouge de Fer, Emplâtre de Canet, *Fr.*; Eisenpflaster, Stärkendes Pflaster, *G.*

"Hydrated Oxide of Iron, dried at a temperature not exceeding 80° C. (176° F.), *ten parts* [or one ounce av.]; Canada Turpentine, *ten parts* [or one ounce av.]; Burgundy Pitch, *ten parts* [or one ounce av.]; Lead Plaster, *seventy parts* [or seven ounces av.], To make *one hundred parts* [or ten ounces av.]. Melt the Lead Plaster, Canada Turpentine, and Burgundy Pitch by means of a water-bath; then add the Oxide of Iron, and stir constantly until the mixture thickens on cooling." *U. S.*

"Take of Peroxide of Iron, in fine powder, *one ounce;* Burgundy Pitch *two ounces;* Lead Plaster *eight ounces.* Add the Peroxide of Iron to the Burgundy Pitch and Lead Plaster, previously melted together, and stir the mixture constantly till it stiffens on cooling." *Br.*

This preparation differs from that officinal in 1870 in the substitution of hydrated oxide of iron for the subcarbonate, and of Canada turpentine for a portion of the Burgundy pitch. This latter change is of questionable utility, the object being to render the plaster more adhesive and flexible. It will probably be found too soft now, and the Canada turpentine irritant. The same end could have been accomplished, if desired, by the addition of olive oil. The use of hydrated oxide of iron in the place of the subcarbonate is an improvement, and in this respect the plaster is in accord with the British formula.

This preparation has enjoyed some popular celebrity, under the impression that it strengthens the parts to which it is applied; whence it has derived the name of strengthening plaster. It is used in those conditions of the loins, larger muscles, and joints which, though usually ascribed to debility, are in fact most frequently dependent on rheumatic or other chronic inflammatory affections, and, if relieved by the plaster, are so in consequence of the gentle excitation produced by it in the vessels of the skin, or of the exclusion of the air. It may also, in some instances, give relief by affording mechanical support; but neither in this nor in any other respect can it be deemed very efficient, because the ingredients composing it have no useful properties that are capable of being taken up by the absorbents.

EMPLASTRUM GALBANI. *U. S., Br.* *Galbanum Plaster.*

(ĔM-PLĂS'TRŬM GĂL'BA-NĪ.)

Emplastrum Galbani Compositum, *U. S.* 1870; **Emplastrum Lithargyri (vel Plumbi) Compositum, Emplastrum Diachylon Compositum; Emplâtre de Galbanum,** *Fr.;* **Mutterharz-Pflaster, Gummipflaster, Zugpflaster,** *G.*

"Galbanum, *sixteen parts* [or eight ounces av.]; Turpentine, *two parts* [or one ounce av.]; Burgundy Pitch, *six parts* [or three ounces av.]; Lead Plaster, *seventy-six parts* [or thirty-eight ounces av.], To make *one hundred parts* [or fifty ounces av.]. To the Galbanum and Turpentine, previously melted together and strained, add, first, the Burgundy Pitch, then the Lead Plaster, melted over a gentle fire, and mix the whole thoroughly." *U. S.*

"Take of Galbanum, Ammoniacum, Yellow Wax, of each, *one ounce;* Lead Plaster, *eight ounces.* Melt the Galbanum and Ammoniacum together, and strain. Then add them to the Lead Plaster and Wax, also previously melted together, and mix the whole thoroughly." *Br.*

This is the Compound Galbanum Plaster of the U. S. Pharm. 1870, the title having been changed, with the trifling alteration of 4 per cent. increase of lead plaster.

In the British process the galbanum and ammoniac are best prepared by dissolving them in a small quantity of hot water or diluted alcohol, straining the solution, and evaporating it to the proper consistence for mixing with the other ingredients.

Before being employed in this process, the galbanum should be purified, as it often contains foreign matters which must injure the plaster. It may be freed from these by melting it with a little water or diluted alcohol, straining, and evaporating to the due consistence.

This plaster acts as an excellent local stimulant in chronic scrofulous enlargements of the glands and joints. We have employed the compound plaster in obstinate cases of this kind, which, after having resisted general and local depletion, blistering, and other measures, have yielded under its use. As a discutient it is also employed in the induration which sometimes remains after the discharge of abscesses. It is said to have been useful in rickets, applied over the whole lumbar region, and has been recommended in chronic gouty and rheumatic articular affections. It should not be used in the discussion of tumors in which any considerable inflammation exists.

EMPLASTRUM HYDRARGYRI. *U. S., Br.* *Mercurial Plaster.*

(ĔM-PLĂS'TRŬM HȲ-DRĂR'GY-RĪ.)

Emplastrum Mercuriale; Emplâtre mercuriel, *Fr.;* **Quecksilber-Pflaster,** *G.*

"Mercury, *thirty parts* [or three ounces av.]; Olive Oil, *ten parts* [or one ounce av.]; Resin, *ten parts* [or one ounce av.]; Lead Plaster, *fifty parts* [or five ounces av.], To make *one hundred parts* [or ten ounces av.]. Melt the Olive Oil and Resin together, and, when the mixture has become cool, rub the Mercury with it until globules of the metal cease to be visible. Then gradually add the Lead Plaster, previously melted, and mix the whole thoroughly." *U. S.*

"Take of Mercury *three ounces;* Olive Oil *fifty-six grains;* Sublimed Sulphur *eight grains;* Lead Plaster *six ounces.* Heat the Oil and add the Sulphur to it gradually, stirring until they unite; with this mixture triturate the Mercury until globules are no longer visible, then add the Lead Plaster, previously liquefied, and mix the whole thoroughly." *Br.* The ounce employed in this process is the avoirdupois ounce.

The present officinal process differs from that of the U. S. Pharm. 1870 in employing about 9 per cent. less of lead plaster. The quantity of mercury is thus slightly increased, there being now 30 per cent. where there was formerly 27·3 per cent. The British preparation is stronger, containing nearly 50 per cent.

The U. S. and former British processes may be considered identical in their results. The sulphuretted oil which was employed in the process of the London College to facilitate the extinguishment of the mercury was abandoned in the first British Pharmacopœia, as just in proportion to the increased facility of the process it lessened the efficacy of the resulting plaster; sulphide of mercury being wholly inert. Nevertheless, the Br. Pharmacopœia has in its last revision retained the old London formula. Mr. Thomas Blunt has found it almost impossible to divide the mercury sufficiently by trituration with oil and resin, and the resulting plaster was so crumbly that it could not be formed into rolls; but by substituting a weight of Venice turpentine equal to that of the oil and resin combined, he found it to answer completely. An objection, however, to the turpentine is, that it might render the plaster too irritant for susceptible skins. (*P. J. Tr.*, 1864, p. 56.)

This plaster is employed to produce the local effects of mercury upon venereal buboes, nodes, and other chronic tumefactions of the bones or soft parts, dependent on a syphilitic taint. In these cases it sometimes acts as a powerful discutient. It is frequently also applied to the side in chronic hepatitis or splenitis. In peculiarly susceptible persons it occasionally affects the gums.

From observations made in France by M. Serres and others, it appears that the mercurial plaster of the Codex (*Emplastrum de Vigo cum Mercurio*) has the power, when applied over the eruption of smallpox, before the end of the third day from its first appearance, to check its progress, and prevent suppuration and pitting. This operation of the plaster, so far from being attended with an increase of the general symptoms, seems to relieve them in proportion to the diminution of the local affection. It is also thought that the course of the disease is favorably modified when the mercurial impression is produced upon the system. That the local effect is not ascribable to the mere exclusion of the air is proved by the fact that the use of lead plaster was not followed by the same results. It is probable that other mercurial preparations would answer the same purpose; and the common mercurial ointment has, in our own hands, proved effectual in rendering the eruption upon the face to a considerable extent abortive, in one bad case of smallpox. But, as the most successful results were obtained with the plaster above mentioned, we give the formula of the French Codex for its preparation.

Emplastrum de Vigo cum Mercurio. "Take of simple plaster [lead plaster] *forty ounces;* yellow wax *two ounces;* resin *two ounces;* ammoniac, bdellium, olibanum, and myrrh, each, *five drachms;* saffron *three drachms;* mercury *twelve ounces;* turpentine [common European] *two ounces;* liquid storax *six ounces;* oil of lavender *two drachms.* Powder the gum-resins and saffron, and rub the mercury with the storax and turpentine in an iron mortar until completely extinguished. Melt the plaster with the wax and resin, and add to the mixture the powders and volatile oil. When the plaster shall have been cooled, but while it is yet liquid, add the mercurial mixture, and incorporate the whole thoroughly." This should be spread upon leather or linen cloths, and applied so as to effectually cover the part to be protected.

EMPLASTRUM ICHTHYOCOLLÆ. *U. S.* *Isinglass Plaster.* [*Court Plaster.*]

(ĔM-PLĂS'TRŲM ĬÇH-THȲ-Ǫ-CŎL'LÆ.)

"Isinglass, *ten parts* [or one hundred and fifty-five grains]; Alcohol, *forty parts* [or one and three-fourths fluidounces]; Glycerin, *one part* [or twelve minims]; Water, Tincture of Benzoin, each, *a sufficient quantity.* Dissolve the Isinglass in a sufficient quantity of hot Water to make the solution weigh *one hundred and twenty parts* [or measure four fluidounces]. Spread one-half of this in successive layers, upon taffeta (stretched on a level surface), by means of a brush, waiting after each application until the layer is dry. Mix the second half of the Isinglass solution with the Alcohol and Glycerin, and apply it in the same manner. Then reverse the taffeta, coat it on the back with Tincture of Benzoin and allow it to become perfectly dry. Cut the plaster in pieces of suitable length and preserve them in well-closed vessels. Substituting *gramme* (15·5 *grains*) for *part*, the above quantities are sufficient to cover a piece of taffeta *fifteen inches* (*thirty-eight cm.*) square." *U. S.*

This is a new officinal preparation. Although it will probably be seldom made by the pharmacist, the introduction of a formula will be of service by indicating the manner in which isinglass plaster can be made by those who desire to furnish a good preparation. The addition of glycerin prevents it from becoming brittle, and the tincture of benzoin is intended to render it water-proof. This it only partially accomplishes. Castor oil and weak collodion have been used instead with better results. (See *Court Plaster*, Part II.)

EMPLASTRUM OPII. *U. S., Br.* *Opium Plaster.*

(ĔM-PLĂS'TRŬM Ō'PĬ-Ī.)

Emplastrum Opiatum, *P. G.;* Emplastrum Cephalicum, s. Odontalgicum; Emplâtre d'Opium, Emplâtre céphalique (temporal, odontalgique, calmant), *Fr.;* Opiumpflaster, Hauptpflaster, *G.*

"Extract of Opium, *six parts* [or one ounce av.]; Burgundy Pitch, *eighteen parts* [or three ounces av.]; Lead Plaster, *seventy-six parts* [or twelve and one-half ounces av.]; Water, *eight parts* [or one and a half fluidounces], To make *one hundred parts* [or seventeen ounces av.]. Rub the Extract of Opium with the Water, until uniformly soft, and add it to the Burgundy Pitch and Lead Plaster, melted together by means of a water-bath; then continue the heat for a short time, stirring constantly, until the moisture is evaporated." *U. S.*

"Take of Opium, in the finest powder, *one ounce;* Resin Plaster *nine ounces.* Melt the Resin Plaster by means of a water-bath; then add the Opium by degrees, and mix thoroughly." *Br.*

We decidedly prefer the extract of opium, as employed in the present U. S. process, to the opium itself of the British formula. It not only forms a better plaster, but, being soluble, is more likely to produce the anodyne effect desired, by being brought by the perspiration to the liquid state necessary for its absorption. The use of water in the former process is also an advantage, as it enables the opium to be more thoroughly incorporated with the other ingredients; but care should be taken that the moisture be well evaporated.

The opium plaster is intended to relieve rheumatic and other pains in the parts to which it is applied.

EMPLASTRUM PICIS. *Br.* *Pitch Plaster.*

(ĔM-PLĂS'TRŬM PĬ'CĬS.)

"Take of Burgundy Pitch *twenty-six ounces;* Common Frankincense [Terebinthina, U. S.] *thirteen ounces;* Resin, Yellow Wax, of each, *four ounces and a half;* Expressed Oil of Nutmeg *one ounce;* Olive Oil, Water, of each, *two fluidounces.* Add the Oils and the Water to the Frankincense, Burgundy Pitch, Resin, and Wax, previously melted together; then, constantly stirring, evaporate to a proper consistence." *Br.* The ounce used in this process is the avoirdupois ounce, and the fluidounce that of the Imperial measure.

This is a rubefacient plaster, applicable to catarrhal and other pectoral affections, chronic inflammation of the liver, and rheumatic pains in the joints and muscles. It often keeps up a serous discharge, which requires that it should be frequently renewed. The irritation which it sometimes excites is so great as to render its removal necessary.

EMPLASTRUM PICIS BURGUNDICÆ. *U. S.* *Burgundy Pitch Plaster.*

(ĔM-PLĂS'TRŬM PĬ'CĬS BŬR-GŬN'DĬ-ÇÆ.)

Emplastrum Picatum, *F. P.;* Emplâtre de Poix de Bourgogne, *Fr.;* Burgunder Pech-Pflaster, *G.*

"Burgundy Pitch, *ninety parts* [or nine ounces av.]; Yellow Wax, *ten parts* [or one ounce av.], To make *one hundred parts* [or ten ounces av.]. Melt them together, strain the mixture, and stir constantly until it thickens on cooling." *U. S.*

In the present revision of the Pharmacopœia the quantity of wax has been diminished 3 per cent. in this plaster. This is undoubtedly a step in the wrong direction; it was done to round up the formula, but it would have made a better plaster if 15 per cent. of wax had been directed instead of 10, whilst the addition of 5 per cent. of olive oil would have still further improved it. The object of the wax is to give a proper consistence to the Burgundy pitch, and to prevent its great tendency to become brittle. M. Lavigne proposes to obviate the tendency of Burgundy pitch plaster to crack by incorporating with it caoutchouc, in the following method. Dissolve 35 parts, by weight, of caoutchouc, in small pieces, in 13 parts of oil of petroleum in a close vessel. Melt together 300 parts of Burgundy pitch and 25 parts of white wax. Warm the solution of caoutchouc in a suitable vessel, and add gradually, with constant stirring, the melted pitch and wax, and finally incorporate thoroughly with the mass 3 parts of glycerin. (*Journ. de Pharm.*, 4e sér., ix. 131.)

EMPLASTRUM PICIS CANADENSIS. *U.S.* *Canada Pitch Plaster.* [*Hemlock Pitch Plaster.*]

(ĔM-PLĂS'TRŬM PĪ'CĬS CĂN-Ą-DĔN'SĮS.)

Hemlock Plaster; Emplâtre de Poix de Canada, *Fr.*; Canadapech-Pflaster, *G.*

"Canada Pitch, *ninety parts* [or nine ounces av.]; Yellow Wax, *ten parts* [or one ounce av.], To make *one hundred parts* [or ten ounces av.]. Melt them together, strain the mixture, and stir constantly until it thickens on cooling." *U. S.*

The yellow wax, in this preparation, answers the same purpose as in the Burgundy Pitch Plaster, and is even more necessary, in order to give the proper consistence to the Canada Pitch. As in the case of Burgundy Pitch Plaster, 15 per cent. of wax would have been preferable to 10. (See *Emplastrum Picis Burgundicæ.*)

EMPLASTRUM PICIS CUM CANTHARIDE. *U.S.* *Pitch Plaster with Cantharides.* [*Warming Plaster.*]

(ĔM-PLĂS'TRŬM PĪ'CĬS CŬM CĄN-THĂR'Į-DĒ.)

Emplastrum Calefaciens, *Br.*; Emplâtre de Poix cantharidé, *Fr.*; Pechpflaster mit Canthariden, *G.*

"Burgundy Pitch, *ninety-two parts* [or twenty-three ounces av.]; Cerate of Cantharides, *eight parts* [or two ounces av.], To make *one hundred parts* [or twenty-five ounces av.]. Heat the Cerate as nearly as possible to 100° C. (212° F.) on a water-bath, and, having continued the heat for fifteen minutes, strain it through a close strainer which will retain the Cantharides. To the strained liquid add the Pitch, melt them together by means of a water-bath, and, having removed the vessel, stir the mixture constantly until it thickens on cooling." *U. S.*

"Take of Cantharides, in coarse powder, Expressed Oil of Nutmeg, Yellow Wax, Resin, of each, *four ounces* [avoir.]; Resin Plaster *three pounds and a quarter* [avoir.]; Soap Plaster *two pounds* [avoir.]; Boiling Water *one pint* [Imperial measure]. Infuse the Cantharides in the Boiling Water for six hours; squeeze strongly through calico, and evaporate the expressed liquid by a water-bath, till reduced to one-third. Then add the other ingredients, and melt in a water-bath, stirring well until the whole is thoroughly mixed." *Br.*

This Plaster is an excellent rubefacient, more active than Burgundy pitch, yet in general not sufficiently so to produce vesication. As prepared by the former U. S. process, it occasionally blistered; and the proportion of cantharides has, therefore, been considerably diminished in the present formula. This is unfortunate; for, while such a reduction may render the plaster insufficiently active in most cases, it does not entirely obviate the objection; as the smallest proportion of flies, or even the Burgundy pitch alone, would vesicate in certain persons. In whatever mode, therefore, this plaster may be prepared, it cannot always answer the expectations which may be entertained; and the only plan, when the skin of any individual has been found to be very susceptible, is to accommodate the proportions to the particular circumstances of the case. Much, however, may be accomplished by care in the preparation of the plaster, towards obviating its tendency to blister. If the flies of the *Ceratum Cantharidis* have been coarsely pulverized, the larger particles, coming in contact with the skin, will exert upon the particular part to which they may be applied their full vesicatory effect, while if reduced to a very fine powder they would be more thoroughly enveloped in the other ingredients, and thus have their strength much diluted. Hence the cerate, when used as an ingredient of the warming plaster, should contain the cantharides as minutely divided as possible; and, if that usually kept is not in the proper state, a portion should be prepared for this particular purpose. The plan of keeping the cerate used in this preparation, for a considerable time, at the temperature of 100° C. (212° F.), and then straining it so as to separate the flies is a good one, but it would be better yet to substitute cerate *of the extract* of cantharides for the cerate of cantharides. (See *Ceratum Cantharidis.*) The mode frequently pursued of preparing the warming plaster by simply sprinkling a very small proportion of powdered flies upon the surface of Burgundy pitch is altogether objectionable.

It has been objected to the U. S. plaster that it is apt to be too soft in hot weather. Mr. G. C. Close, ascribing this inconvenience to the proportion of lard in the cerate employed, proposes to obviate it by substituting Burgundy pitch plaster for Burgundy pitch, and powdered cantharides for the cerate, and offers a formula in compliance with this suggestion. (See *A. J. P.*, 1867, p. 20; from *Proc. A. P. A.*, 1866.)

The warming plaster is employed in chronic rheumatism, and in chronic internal diseases attended with inflammation or an inflammatory tendency; such as catarrh, asthma, pertussis, phthisis, hepatitis, and the sequelæ of pleurisy and pneumonia.

EMPLASTRUM PLUMBI. *U.S., Br. Lead Plaster.* [*Diachylon Plaster.*]

(EM-PLĂS'TRUM PLŬM'BĪ.)

Emplastrum Lithargyri, *Br.* 1864; Emplastrum Lithargyri Simplex, *P.G.;* Emplastrum Simplex, *F.P.;* Emplastrum Diachylon Simplex, Emplastrum Album Coctum; Litharge Plaster, Emplâtre simple, Emplâtre de Plomb (de Litharge), *Fr.;* Emplastrum Cerussæ, Froschlaichpflaster, Bleipflaster, Diachylon-Pflaster, *G.*

"Oxide of Lead, in very fine powder, *thirty-two parts* [or thirty-two ounces av.]; Olive Oil, *sixty parts* [or sixty-three fluidounces]; Water, *a sufficient quantity.* Rub the Oxide of Lead with about one-half of the Olive Oil, and add the mixture to the remainder of the Oil, contained in a suitable vessel of a capacity equal to three times the bulk of the ingredients. Then add *ten parts* [or ten fluidounces] of boiling Water, and boil the whole together until a homogeneous plaster is formed, adding, from time to time, during the process, a little Water, as that first added is consumed." *U. S.*

"Lead Plaster is white, pliable, and tenacious, free from greasiness or stickiness. It should be entirely soluble in warm oil of turpentine (abs. of uncombined oxide of lead)." *U. S.*

"Take of Oxide of Lead, in fine powder *five pounds;* Olive Oil *ten pounds;* Water *five pounds.* Boil all the ingredients together gently by the heat of a steam-bath, and keep them simmering for four or five hours, stirring constantly, until the product acquires a proper consistence for a plaster, and adding more water during the process if necessary." *Br.* The weights used in this process are avoirdupois.

The importance of this plaster, as the basis of most of the others, requires a somewhat detailed account of the principles and manner of its preparation.

It was formerly thought that the oil and oxide of lead entered into direct union, and that the presence of water was necessary only to regulate the temperature and prevent the materials from being decomposed by heat. The discovery, however, was afterwards made, that this liquid was essential to the process; and that the oil and oxide alone, though maintained at a temperature of 220° F., would not combine; while the addition of water, under these circumstances, would produce their immediate union. It was now supposed that the oil was capable of combining only with the hydrated oxide of lead, and that the use of the water was to bring the oxide into that state; and, in support of this opinion, the fact was advanced that the hydrated oxide of lead and oil would form a plaster, when heated together without any free water. But, since the general reception of Chevreul's views in relation to oils, and their combinations with alkalies and other metallic oxides, the former opinions have been abandoned; and it is now admitted that the preparation of the lead plaster affords a genuine example of saponification, as explained by that chemist. A reaction takes place between the oil and water, resulting in the development of *glycerin,* and of two acid bodies, *oleic* and *palmitic acids,* to which, when animal fat is employed instead of olive oil, a third is added, namely *stearic acid.* The plaster is formed by a union of these acids with the oxide, and, prepared according to the directions of the Pharmacopœias, is in fact an oleo-palmitate of lead, and if the olive oil contained stearin it would be an oleo-stearo-palmitate of lead. The glycerin remains dissolved in the water, or mechanically mixed with the plaster. That such is the correct view of the nature of this compound is evinced by the fact that, if the oxide of lead be separated from the plaster by digestion at a moderate heat in very dilute nitric acid, the fatty matter which remains will unite with litharge with the greatest facility, without the intervention of water. According to the modern chemical views, the fixed or fatty oils are compounds of the free fatty acids mentioned and the radical *glyceryl.* When boiled with the oxide of lead and water, the fatty acids combine with the metallic oxide to form the plaster, and the glyceryl unites with the liberated hydrogen and becomes glycerin.

The reaction for olein and lead oxide is as follows: $\underset{\text{olein}}{2C_3H_5(C_{18}H_{33}O_2)_3} + \underset{\text{litharge}}{3PbO} + \underset{\text{water}}{3H_2O} = \underset{\text{lead oleate}}{3Pb(C_{18}H_{33}O_2)_2} + \underset{\text{glycerin}}{2C_3H_5(OH)_3}$. The radical glyceryl ($C_3H_5$) is a triad, and combines with three groups of a fatty acid or three groups of hydroxyl (OH).

Other oleaginous substances and other metallic oxides are susceptible of the same combination, and some of them form compounds having the consistence of a plaster; but, according to M. Henry, of Paris, no oily matter except animal fat can properly be substituted for olive oil, and no metallic oxide, not even one of the other oxides of lead, for litharge. He ascertained, moreover, that the English litharge is preferable for the formation of lead plaster to the German. From more recent experiments of Soubeiran, it appears that massicot or even minium may be substituted for litharge, and a plaster of good consistence be obtained; but that a much longer time is required for completing the process than when the officinal formula is followed. Owing to the necessity for its partial deoxidation the use of minium requires a longer continuance of the process than when massicot is employed. According to M. Davallon, Professor in the School of Medicine and Pharmacy at Lyons, it is important that the olive oil employed should be pure; for when adulterated, as it frequently is, it yields an imperfect product. Mr. N. S. Thomas prepared a good plaster by substituting lard for olive oil, in the proportion of eight pounds of lard to five of litharge (*A. J. P.*, xix. 175); and we are told that it is a common practice, in this country, to make lead plaster with a mixture of lard oil and olive oil. Mueller uses equal parts of lard, olive oil, and litharge, having previously heated the litharge, until a small sample causes no effervescence when dropped into nitric acid, showing the absence of carbonate. (*Pharm. Ztg.*, 1879, p. 70; *A. J. P.*, 1879, p. 190.) It is said that the English plaster-makers rarely follow the Br. Pharm. direction, preferring the recipe of the old London Pharmacopœia, which contains more litharge and yields a much firmer and less adhesive product.* (*P. J. Tr.*, 3d ser., v. 701, 716.)

Lead plaster has also been prepared by double decomposition between soap and acetate or subacetate of lead; but the results have not been so advantageous as to lead to the general adoption of this process. (See *A. J. P.*, ix. 727, and *Journ. de Pharm.*, xxiii. 163 and 322.) †

Preparation. The vessel in which the lead plaster is prepared should be of such a size that the materials will not occupy more than two-thirds of its capacity. The oil should be first introduced, and the litharge then sprinkled in by means of a sieve, the mixture being constantly stirred with a spatula. The particles of the oxide are thus prevented from coalescing in small masses, which the oil would not

* *Schwarze's Mutterpflaster, Emplastrum Fuscum* of the German Pharmacopœia, is made by boiling 64 parts of olive oil with 32 parts of very finely powdered red lead in a copper kettle until the mass is of a dark brown color, and then adding 16 parts of yellow wax.

Emplastrum Fuscum Camphoratum is the same, with the addition of 1 per cent. of camphor.

† M. de Mussey, physician of the hospital *de la Pitié*, having witnessed inconveniences from lead plaster in consequence of the absorption of the lead, substituted for it a plaster with a basis of oxide of zinc, which he has found to answer very well in practice. It cannot be made by direct combination of the oxide; and it is necessary to have recourse to the method of double decomposition. Solutions of white olive oil soap and of sulphate of zinc being mixed, a copious precipitate takes place of oleo-palmitate of zinc, which, after being washed and dried, may be combined with resins, oil, and wax, to give it the necessary consistence. (*Journ. de Pharm.*, xxvii. 100.)

easily penetrate, and which would therefore delay the process. While the water exerts an important chemical agency in the changes which occur, it is also useful by preventing too high a temperature, which would decompose the oil, and cause the reduction of the oxide. The waste must, therefore, be supplied by fresh additions as directed in the process; and the water added for this purpose should be previously heated, as otherwise it would not only delay the operation, but by producing explosion might endanger the operator. During the continuance of the boiling, the material should be constantly stirred, and the spatula should be repeatedly passed along the bottom of the vessel, from side to side, so as to prevent any of the oxide, which is disposed by its greater density to sink to the bottom, from remaining in that situation. The materials swell up considerably, in consequence partly of the vaporization of the water, partly of the escape of carbonic acid gas, which is liberated by the oily acids from some carbonate of lead usually contained in the litharge. The process should not be continued longer than is sufficient to produce complete union of the ingredients, and this may be known by the color and consistence of the mass. The color of the litharge gradually becomes paler, and at length almost white when the plaster is fully formed. The consistence increases with the progress of the boiling, and is sufficiently thick, when a portion of the plaster, taken out and allowed to cool upon the end of a spatula, or thrown into cold water, becomes solid, without adhering in this state to the fingers. The portion thus solidified should not present, when broken, any red points, which would indicate the presence of a portion of uncombined litharge. When the plaster is formed, it should be removed from the fire, and after a short time cold water should be poured upon it. Portions should then be detached from the mass, and, having been well kneaded under water, in order to separate the viscid solution of glycerin contained in the interior, should be formed into cylindrical rolls, and wrapped in paper. Such at least has been the course of proceeding usually recommended. But M. Davallon maintains that the presence of glycerin in the plaster is useful by keeping it in a plastic state, and that washing and kneading are injurious, the former by removing the glycerin, the latter by introducing particles of air and moisture into the mass, which is thus rendered more disposed to rancidity. (*A. J. P.*, xv. 274; from *Journ. de Chim. Méd.*) By employing steam heat in the preparation of this plaster, the risk of burning it is avoided. For a good arrangement for this purpose, see *Mohr and Redwood's Pharmacy*, edited by Prof. Procter, p. 420. Bernbeck found that lead plaster could be preserved from hardening and oxidation if kept in air-tight canisters. (*Pharm. Zeitung*, 1881, p. 589.)

Mr. C. Lewis Diehl found it almost impossible, in following the U. S. directions of 1860, to obtain a plaster wholly free from uncombined litharge. He obviated the difficulty by first rubbing the sifted litharge with about half its weight of oil, then stirring the mixture with the remainder of the oil, in a tinned copper kettle, adding the water, and heating to 212° F. until a uniform plaster was formed. (*A. J. P.*, 1867, p. 385.)

Kremel states that when lead plaster is made from oleic acid, the product is almost entirely soluble in ether; when made with olive oil or lard, it contains stearate and palmitate of lead, and thus a larger proportion is insoluble in ether. (*Archiv d. Pharm.*, 1887, p. 405.)

Medical Properties and Uses. This plaster, which has long been known under the name of *diachylon*, is used as an application to excoriated surfaces, and to slight wounds, which it serves to protect from the action of the air. It may also be beneficial by the sedative influence of the lead which enters into its composition. A case is on record in which lead colic resulted from its long-continued application to a large ulcer of the leg. (*Am. Journ. of Med. Sci.*, xxiii. 246.) Dr. J. M. Bigelow reports a case of excessive sweating of the feet, which he cured by putting the patient in bed for thirteen days and keeping the feet enveloped in strips of lead plaster. (*N. R.*, Oct. 1875.) Its chief use is in the preparation of other plasters.*

* *Logan's Plaster.* Take of Litharge, Carbonate of Lead, each, *a pound;* Castile Soap, *twelve ounces;* Butter (fresh) *four ounces;* Olive Oil *two and a half pints;* Mastic, in powder, *two drachms.* It is to be understood that the pound and ounce are of the avoirdupois weight. Having mixed

Off. Prep. Emplastrum Ammoniaci cum Hydrargyro; Emplastrum Asafœtidæ; Emplastrum Ferri; Emplastrum Galbani; Emplastrum Hydrargyri; Emplastrum Opii; Emplastrum Resinæ; Emplastrum Saponis; Unguentum Diachylon.

Off. Prep. Br. Emplastrum Ferri; Emplastrum Galbani; Emplastrum Hydrargyri; Emplastrum Plumbi Iodidi; Emplastrum Resinæ; Emplastrum Saponis.

EMPLASTRUM PLUMBI IODIDI. *Br. Iodide of Lead Plaster.*

(ĔM-PLĂS'TRŬM PLŬM'BĪ Ī-ŎD'Ĭ-DĪ.)

Emplâtre d'Iodure de Plomb, *Fr.;* Jodblei-Pflaster, *G.*

"Take of Iodide of Lead *two ounces*; Lead Plaster *one pound;* Resin *two ounces.* Add the Iodide of Lead, in fine powder, to the Plaster and Resin previously melted at as low a temperature as possible, and mix them intimately." *Br.*

This is a local discutient plaster, which may also be used with other means to affect the system. (See *Plumbi Iodidum.*)

EMPLASTRUM RESINÆ. *U. S., Br. Resin Plaster.* [*Adhesive Plaster.*]

(ĔM-PLĂS'TRŬM RĘ-SĪ'NÆ.)

Emplastrum Adhesivum, *P.G.;* Emplâtre résineux (adhésif), *Fr.;* Heftpflaster, *G.*

"Resin, in fine powder, *fourteen parts* [or seven ounces av.]; Lead Plaster, *eighty parts* [or forty ounces av.]; Yellow Wax, *six parts* [or three ounces av.], To make *one hundred parts* [or fifty ounces av.]. To the Lead Plaster and Wax, melted together over a gentle fire, add the Resin, and mix them." *U. S.*

"Take of Resin *four ounces;* Lead Plaster *two pounds;* Curd Soap *two ounces.* To the Lead Plaster, previously melted at a low temperature, add the Resin and Soap, first liquefied, and stir them until they are thoroughly mixed." *Br.* The weights here referred to are the avoirdupois.

The alteration from the previous officinal formula is the addition of yellow wax, which is an improvement, rendering the plaster somewhat less irritating without diminishing its adhesive properties.

Resin plaster differs from the lead plaster in being more adhesive and somewhat more stimulating. It is the common adhesive plaster of commerce, and is much employed for retaining the sides of wounds in contact, and for dressing ulcers according to the method of Baynton, by which the edges are drawn towards each other, and a firm support is given to the granulations. As prepared by the Dublin College it contained soap, which gave it greater pliability, and rendered it less liable to crack in cold weather, without impairing its adhesiveness; and the process of that College has been adopted in the British Pharmacopœia. It is usually spread upon muslin; and the spreading is best accomplished, on a large scale, by means of a machine, as described in the general observations upon plasters. It is kept ready spread by the pharmacist; but, as the plaster becomes less adhesive by long exposure to the air, the supply should be frequently renewed. When the skin is very delicate, it occasionally excites some irritation, and, under these circumstances, a plaster may be

the Soap, Oil, and Butter, add the Litharge, and boil the mixture gently, constantly stirring, for an hour and a half, or until it shall assume a pale brown color; then increase the heat somewhat, and continue to boil, until a portion of the liquid, dropped on a smooth board, is found not to adhere to it on cooling; then remove it from the fire, and mix the Mastic with it. Logan's plaster has long been in popular use in Philadelphia, and is yet employed by regular practitioners as a protective and discutient application.

Plaster of Carbonate of Lead. This was originally introduced into our Pharmacopœia as a substitute for *Mahy's plaster,* at one time much employed in some parts of the United States; but was omitted in the edition of 1840. It is a good application to surfaces inflamed or excoriated by friction, and may be resorted to with advantage in those troublesome cases of cutaneous irritation, and even ulceration, which are apt to occur upon the back and hips during long-continued confinement to one position. We give the process as contained in the Pharmacopœia of 1830. "Take of Carbonate of Lead *a pound;* Olive Oil *two pints;* Yellow Wax *four ounces;* Lead Plaster *a pound and a half;* Florentine Orris, in powder, *nine ounces.* Boil together the Oil and Carbonate of Lead, adding a little water, and constantly stirring, till they are thoroughly incorporated; then add the Wax and Plaster, and, when these are melted, sprinkle in the Orris, and mix the whole together." By this process a good plaster may be prepared, rather too soft at first, but soon acquiring the proper consistence.

substituted containing a smaller proportion of resin. That originally employed by Baynton contained only six drachms of resin to the pound of lead plaster. To obviate the same evil, M. Herpin recommends the addition of tannate of lead, the proportion of which, when adhesiveness is required in the plaster, should not exceed one-twentieth, but, under other circumstances, may be increased to one-twelfth. (*Bull. de Thérap.*, xlviii. 155.)

In order to render the plaster more adhesive, and less brittle in cold weather, it is customary with many manufacturers to employ a considerable proportion of Burgundy pitch or turpentine in its preparation; but these additions are objectionable, as they greatly increase the liability of the plaster to irritate the skin, and thus materially interfere with the purposes for which the preparation was chiefly intended.*

Off. Prep. Emplastrum Arnicæ; Emplastrum Belladonnæ; Emplastrum Capsici.

Off. Prep. Br. Emplastrum Belladonnæ; Emplastrum Calefaciens; Emplastrum Opii.

EMPLASTRUM SAPONIS. *U. S., Br.* *Soap Plaster.*

(ĔM-PLĂS'TRŬM SĄ-PŌ'NĬS.)

Emplastrum Saponatum, *P.G.;* Emplastrum cum Sapone, *F.P.;* Emplâtre de Savon, *Fr.;* Seifenpflaster, *G.*

"Soap, dried and in coarse powder, *ten parts* [or one ounce av.]; Lead Plaster, *ninety parts* [or nine ounces av.]; Water *a sufficient quantity.* Rub the Soap with Water until brought to a semi-liquid state; then mix it with the Lead Plaster, previously melted, and evaporate to the proper consistence." *U. S.*

"Take of Curd Soap *six ounces;* Lead Plaster *two pounds and a quarter;* Resin *one ounce.* To the Lead Plaster, melted at a low temperature, add the Soap and the Resin, first liquefied; then, constantly stirring, evaporate to a proper consistence." *Br.* The avoirdupois weights are used in this process.

The present U. S. formula is an improvement upon that of a former edition of the Pharmacopœia. By directing the soap to be in powder instead of sliced, it may be more thoroughly incorporated with the plaster. Greater plasticity is accomplished, in some degree, in the British process by the resin. In preparing the U. S. plaster, Mr. C. Lewis Diehl has found some difficulty in rubbing the soap up perfectly and rapidly with the water, and has, therefore, adopted the plan of first rubbing the soap with its weight of water, then straining the mixture through coarse muslin, and lastly reducing the residue with a proportionate quantity of water, before stirring the whole into the melted plaster. (*A. J. P.*, 1867, p. 386.)

Soap plaster is considered discutient, and is sometimes used as an application to tumors, where a dressing is required. Somewhat softer in its character, the soap cerate, formerly officinal, may be found useful.

Off. Prep. Br. Emplastrum Belladonnæ; Emplastrum Calefaciens.

EMPLASTRUM SAPONIS FUSCUM. *Brown Soap Plaster.* [*Emplastrum Cerati Saponis.*]

(ĔM-PLĂS'TRŬM SĄ-PŌ'NĬS FŬS'CŬM.)

Soap Cerate Plaster; Emplâtre de Savon saturné, *Fr.;* Seifencerat-Pflaster, *G.*

"Take of Curd Soap, in powder, *ten ounces* [avoirdupois]; Yellow Wax *twelve and a half ounces* [avoir.]; Olive Oil *one pint* [Imperial measure]; Oxide of Lead *fifteen ounces* [avoir.]; Vinegar *one gallon* [Imp. meas.]. Boil the Vinegar and Oxide of Lead together, by the heat of a steam-bath, constantly stirring them until the Oxide has combined with the Acid; then add the Soap and boil again until most of the moisture is evaporated; finally, add the Wax and Oil melted together, and stir the whole continuously, maintaining the heat until by the evaporation of

* An adhesive plaster, exempt from oxide of lead, is prepared by Pettenkofer. It consists of calcareous soap incorporated with turpentine and suet, and may be prepared in the following manner. A solution of soap is decomposed by a solution of chloride of calcium. The precipitate, having been expressed and dried, is powdered with half its weight of turpentine dried by heat; and the mixture is melted, along with an eighth part of suet, in boiling water. The mixture is boiled until the mass melts into a homogeneous fluid, when it is worked by the hand, in the ordinary manner, in cold water. Should portions of the calcareous soap not melt, they should be separated by straining through flannel. (*Journ. de Pharm.*, 3e sér., x. 358.)

the remaining moisture the product has acquired the proper consistence for a plaster." *Br.*

This is the old *Ceratum Saponis Compositum* of the London College, the name of which has been changed in the British Pharmacopœia, because, the former class of Cerates having been abandoned, it was necessary to put the preparation into another class with a different title. It is not strictly a plaster, as this term is understood in American pharmacy; for heat is not required to spread it, it being applied to the leather or cloth by means of a spatula, like our Cerates, to which it properly belongs. Indeed, it is essentially the same preparation as the *Ceratum Saponis* of the U. S. P. 1870,* consisting, like that, of soap plaster with wax and olive oil, though made differently, and containing some acetate of sodium, as an incidental result of the process. In the British formula, subacetate of lead is first formed by the boiling of litharge or oxide of lead with vinegar; and the subacetate is then converted, by double decomposition with hard soap, into a compound of the oxide of lead and the fatty acids of the soap, and acetate of sodium, which, with some glycerin formed in the process, remains as an ingredient of the lead plaster. The process is completed by incorporating this with the melted wax and oil, thus in fact converting the preparation into a cerate. (See *Ceratum Saponis.*)

ENEMATA. *Clysters.*

(Ĕ-NĔM'Ă-TĂ.)

These can scarcely be considered proper objects for officinal direction; but, having been introduced into the former British Pharmacopœias, and retained in the present, the plan of this work requires that they should be noticed. They are substances in the liquid form, intended to be thrown up the rectum, with the view either of evacuating the bowels, of producing the peculiar impression of a remedy upon the lower portion of the alimentary canal and neighboring organs, or of acting on the system generally through the medium of the surface to which they are applied. They are usually employed to assist the action of remedies taken by the mouth, or to supply their place when the stomach rejects them or is insensible to their impression. Sometimes they are preferably used when the seat of the disorder is in the rectum or its vicinity. As a general rule, three times as much of any remedy is required to produce a given impression by enema, as when taken into the stomach; but this rule should be acted on with caution, as the relative susceptibilities of the stomach and rectum are not the same in all individuals; and, with regard to all very active remedies, the best plan is to administer less than the stated proportion. Attention should also be paid to the fact that, by the frequent use of a medicine, the susceptibility of the stomach may be in some measure exhausted, without a proportionate diminution of that of the rectum.

When the object is to evacuate the bowels, the quantity of liquid administered should be considerable; for an adult, from ten fluidounces to a pint; for a child of eight or ten years, half that quantity; for an infant within the year, from one to three fluidounces. Much larger quantities of mild liquids may sometimes be given with safety and advantage; as the bowels will occasionally feel the stimulus of distention, when insensible to irritating impressions.

When the design is to produce the peculiar impression of the remedy upon the neighboring parts, or on the system, it is usually desirable that the enema should be retained, and the vehicle should therefore be bland, and as small in quantity as is compatible with convenient administration. A solution of starch, flaxseed tea, or other mucilaginous fluid should be selected, and the quantity should seldom exceed two or three fluidounces. In every case, the patient should be instructed to resist any immediate disposition to discharge the injected fluid; and his efforts to retain it should be assisted, if necessary, by pressure with a warm folded towel upon the fun-

* *Ceratum Saponis.* U. S. 1870. *Soap Cerate.* (Cérat de Savon, *Fr.;* Seifencerat, *G.*) "Take of Soap Plaster *two troyounces;* White Wax *two troyounces and a half;* Olive Oil *four troyounces.* Melt together the Plaster and Wax, add the Oil, and, after continuing the heat a short time, stir the mixture until cool." *U. S.* 1870.

Soap cerate is thought to be cooling and sedative, and is used in scrofulous swellings and other instances of chronic external inflammation.

dament. The best instrument for administering enemata is a rubber bulb and tube syringe.

ENEMA ALOES. *Br.* *Enema of Aloes.*

(ĔN'Ḛ-MA̡ ĂL'Ō-ĒS.)

"Take of Aloes *forty grains;* Carbonate of Potassium *fifteen grains;* Mucilage of Starch *ten fluidounces.* Mix and rub together." *Br.*

This is intended as a formula for the use of aloes in cases of ascarides in the rectum, and of amenorrhœa attended with constipation.

ENEMA ASAFŒTIDÆ. *Br.* *Enema of Asafetida.*

(ĔN'Ḛ-MA̡ ĂS-A̡-FŒT'Ị-DÆ—ăs-ą-fĕt'ị-dą.)

Enema Fœtidum; Fetid Enema.

"Take of Asafetida *thirty grains;* Distilled Water *four fluidounces.* Rub the Asafetida in a mortar with the Water added gradually, so as to form an emulsion." *Br.*

This is carminative and antispasmodic as well as laxative. In the former Br. Pharmacopœia it was directed to be made by mixing the tincture and Distilled Water; and, in commenting on it, we stated that we should prefer a preparation consisting of the gum-resin rubbed up with water; as the alcohol of the tincture might in some instances prove injurious. In the present formula this plan has been adopted. The whole quantity directed may be administered at once.

ENEMA MAGNESII SULPHATIS. *Br.* *Enema of Sulphate of Magnesium.*

(ĔN'Ḛ-MA̡ MĂG-NĒ'ṢỊ-Ī SŬL-PHĀ'TĬS.)

Enema Catharticum; Cathartic Clyster.

"Take of Sulphate of Magnesium *one ounce* [avoirdupois]; Olive Oil *one fluidounce;* Mucilage of Starch *fifteen fluidounces.* Dissolve the Sulphate of Magnesium in the Mucilage of Starch, add the Oil, and mix." *Br.*

The laxative enema, most commonly employed in this country, consists of a tablespoonful of common salt, two tablespoonfuls of lard or olive oil, the same quantity of molasses, and a pint of warm water. It has the advantage of consisting of materials which are always at hand in families, and is in all respects equal to the officinal preparation.

ENEMA OPII. *Br.* *Enema of Opium.*

(ĔN'Ḛ-MA̡ Ō'PỊ-Ī.)

Enema Opii vel Anodynum; Anodyne Enema.

"Take of Tincture of Opium *half a fluidrachm;* Mucilage of Starch *two fluidounces.* Mix." *Br.*

This formula is unobjectionable. Every one in the habit of prescribing opium in this way, must have seen a much greater effect produced by a certain amount of laudanum injected into the rectum than by one-third of the quantity swallowed. The fluidrachm contains at least one hundred drops of laudanum of the ordinary size, and not less than one hundred and twenty as they are often formed. From twenty to twenty-five drops are usually considered a medium dose by the mouth; so that sixty drops, equivalent to about thirty minims, are abundantly sufficient by enema. As the object is that the enema should remain in the rectum, the smaller the quantity of the vehicle the better; and a mucilaginous fluid is preferable to water, as it involves the tincture, and prevents the irritation of the alcohol before the opium begins to take effect. The ordinary anodyne enema, employed in this country, consists of about sixty drops of laudanum and one or two fluidounces of flaxseed tea or solution of starch, conforming precisely with the present British formula.

This is an admirable remedy in obstinate vomiting, strangury from blisters, painful affections of the kidneys, bladder, and uterus, and in the tenesmus of dysentery. It may also frequently be employed to produce the effects of opium upon the system, when circumstances prevent the administration of that medicine by the mouth.

ENEMA TEREBINTHINÆ. *Br.* *Enema of Turpentine.*

(ĔN'Ę-MA TĔR-Ę-BĬN'THI-NÆ.)

"Take of Oil of Turpentine *one fluidounce;* Mucilage of Starch *fifteen fluidounces.* Mix." *Br.*

For the dose of this preparation, see *Oleum Terebinthinæ.*

ERGOTA. *U.S., Br.* *Ergot.* [*Ergot of Rye.*]

(ĔR'GO-TA.)

"The sclerotium of Claviceps purpurea, Tulasne (*Nat. Ord.* Fungi), replacing the grain of Secale cereale, Linné. (*Nat. Ord.* Graminaceæ.)" *U. S.* "The sclerotium of Claviceps purpurea, *Tulasne*, produced within the pales and replacing the grain of Secale cereale." *Br.*

Secale Cornutum, *P.G.;* Secale Clavatum, Mater Secalis, Clavus Secalinus; Spurred Rye; Ergot, Seigle ergoté (noir), Blé cornu, *Fr.;* Mutterkorn, Kornmutter, Lapfenkorn, *G.*

"Ergot should be preserved in a dry place, and should not be kept longer than a year." *U. S.*

In all the Graminaceæ, or grass tribe, and in some of the Cyperaceæ, the place of the seeds is sometimes occupied by a morbid growth, which, from its resemblance to the spur of a cock, has received the name of *ergot*, adopted from the French. This product is most frequent in the rye, *Secale cereale*, and from that grain was adopted in the first edition of the U. S. Pharmacopœia, under the name of *secale cornutum*, or *spurred rye.* In the edition of 1840 the name was changed to *ergota.* It is probable that this morbid growth has similar properties from whatever plant derived; and the fact has been proved in relation to the ergot of wheat. (See *Am. Journ. of Med. Sci.*, N. S., xxxii. 479.) Indeed, in a case reported by Dr. D. L. McGugin (*Iowa Med. Journ.*, iv. 93), this variety of ergot is said to have succeeded promptly, when that of rye, previously tried, had failed.* A short thick ergot, produced upon the wild rice of Minnesota, is said to be used as an abortifacient and during labor by the Indian women.†

M. Leperdriel, Jr., of Montpellier, in France, affirms that the *ergot of wheat* is destitute of the poisonous properties of that of rye, and is less liable to change. The former point is, to say the least, very uncertain. Prof. Bentley, of London, found that of two specimens, one of the ergot of rye, the other of wheat, which had been kept under similar circumstances for ten years, the former was quite destroyed, while the latter was apparently unchanged. Ergot is rarer in wheat than in rye; and in the head of the former there is generally but one and very rarely more than two of the diseased grains. It is produced usually in wheat in wet seasons, and on that side of the head most exposed to the dampness. It is shorter and much thicker than the ergot of rye, being about half an inch long and three-quarters of an inch or more in circumference, and cleft into two or three divisions. In color and smell it resembles the spurred rye. (*P. J. Tr.*, March and April, 1863.)

The very beautiful and praiseworthy investigations of M. Tulasne have shown that ergot is not the diseased grain of the rye, but is the *sclerotium* of a fungus, the *Claviceps purpurea*, Tulasne. This fungus has three stages in its life-history. The development of the *sphacelia*, or first stage, commences with that of

* For the various views that have been held in regard to the nature of ergot, see 15th edition U. S. D.; the sketch is omitted here, as being solely of historic interest.

† There is, indeed, reason for believing that this ergot is specifically identical with the officinal one, since Tulasne has cultivated the dissimilar sclerotia obtained from twelve species of grasses, and found the fructification in each case identical with that of the ergot of rye. Moreover, from time to time of late years epidemics of abortion in cows have been reported as produced by the use of various ergots. This is a strong indication that all the ergots are similar in medical properties. The ergot of *diss*, an Algerian reed, *Ampelodesmos tenax*, has appeared in commerce to some extent. It is, when small, slightly curved, but when long (6–9 centimetres) it takes a spiral turn from right to left, the longitudinal furrows being present on the inner face. It is thinner, dryer, and more brittle than the ergot of rye, and has been used for the preparation of an ergotine or extract closely resembling the officinal one, but said to be of a clearer red or brown color. M. Lallemand claims that the ergot of diss is twice as strong as the ergot of rye, and states that it is abundant and readily collected. It is also stated to be less hygroscopic and less apt to be attacked by acari than is the officinal article. (*P. J. Tr.*, xvi. 684, 1886.)

the pistil, which serves as a soil for it. The ovary of the rye consists of a cellular membrane of two coats, the outer of which has a thick parenchyma, white and gorged with juice; the inner is very delicate and green. The sphacelia, when it takes possession of the ovary, identifies itself with the outer parenchyma, and in some measure replaces it, being as it were borne by the inner membrane. It rapidly increases, taking the form of the ovary, and almost obliterating its cavity. The ovule is either entirely wanting, or may be seen, on a careful examination, in an imperfect form. For some time the parasite is represented entirely by the sphacelia, which is an oblong, fungous mass, almost homogeneous, soft and tender, marked on its surface by numerous sinuous furrows, and having within many irregular cavities, which, as well as the outer coat, are uniformly covered with linear parallel cells. From the summits of these peripheric cells, internal as well as external, issue oval corpuscles, from ·005 to ·007 mm. in length, which spread upon neighboring objects, and especially the glumes of the flowers they inhabit. They are a kind of reproductive cells, called conidia, which are produced by many fungi, long before the perfect plant is developed. M. Tulasne calls them "*spermatie.*" In the early stage, the sphacelia respects the top of the ovary and the stigmas attached. The stamens often abort; but the filaments and anthers may sometimes be seen buried in the tissue of the sphacelia, and altered by its action. Sometimes the ovule is not completely aborted, but it is certainly never developed into a monster grain. In all ergotized plants, the pistils and stigmas, when they remain, are often covered with a mouldiness, consisting of spores and entangled filaments, which end by covering the parts with an abundant ashy or sooty powder. This is a different fungus, and was confounded by Mr. Quekett with the ergot plant. It is found as well in the non-ergotized as in the ergotized flowers, and in those of plants which do not bear ergot. At a somewhat advanced period of the development of the sphacelia, there exudes, especially from the summit, a very adhesive juice, which spreads over that structure, bearing along with it an immense number of the seedlets or "*spermaties.*" This leaves on the surface when dry an oily appearance, and afterwards the spots, where it remains, become brownish or blackish. But this exudation does not appear until the sphacelia has ceased to constitute the whole plant.

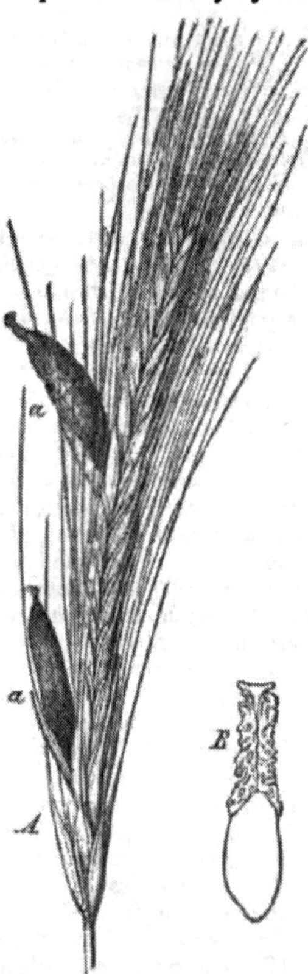

Ergot. *A*, head of rye with ergot (*a*) growing in it; *B*, young ergot, showing the growing sclerotium carrying upon its top the old diseased ovary. (After Berg.)

At the base of the sphacelia is produced a compact body, violet black without and white within, which is the ergot in a rudimentary state. With this commences the second stage in the development of the fungus. The young ergot is everywhere invested by the tissue of the sphacelia (which Tulasne calls also *spermagonia*, from its office); but, as it increases, it seems to be placed below the spermatopherous apparatus, and raises it steadily out of the floral bracts which concealed it, ending by supporting it wholly at its summit. Sometimes it carries with it the atrophied ovary, which still shows the hairs that crowned it, and some remains of the stigmas. It results that the ergot, which is technically the *sclerotium* of the fungus, remains for some time concealed in the sphacelia, so that this seems to constitute the whole plant. But, when the function belonging to this has been fulfilled, it begins to become dry, and is much deformed. The ergot, on the contrary, increases in all directions, and soon appears above the glume. As it augments, the thin coating which it has received from the spermatopherous tissue, especially below, gradually becomes thinner, and seems to disappear; so that its surface, instead of being uniformly violet black, is only here and there covered with the remains of the tissue, or by a deposit of the conidia or "*spermatie.*" Nevertheless, the sphacelia, deformed, shrunken, and worn away by rains and other causes, remains long at the top of the ergot, along with the abortive ovary, etc., and may even continue to adhere when the ergot is detached from the plant. The time required for the full development of the sphacelia and the ergot or sclerotium varies. In an example under the observation of M. Tulasne, at least a month elapsed after the appearance of the sphacelia, before the growth was completed.

Ergot has absolutely nothing in common with normal grain. The anatomical structure and all the physical characters of ergot are those of the mushrooms, or rather of a sclerotic mycelium. The parenchyma, which is whitish, dry, and brittle, consists in all its parts of irregular, globular, or polyhedric thick-walled cells, intimately united, and filled with a limpid oil, but feebly colored by iodine. The superficial utricles, which alone are colored, have an outer wall thicker than the inner, and the color of these is what gives its characteristic hue to ergot. Not the least trace of starch is to be detected.

If ergot be planted in a suitable soil, evidences of germination are seen in about three months. Little globular prominences appear on its surface, and gradually enlarge, and raise themselves upon cylindrical stems, and finally become perfect pilei or fruiting fungi, and produce elongated, rod-like spores in flask-shaped cavities, which open by a little pore. These little fungi belong to the genus *Sphæria.* As they increase, the interior of the ergot becomes exhausted, by contributing to their growth. Falling to the ground, in its natural course, the ergot in the soil germinates, and produces pilei, the spores of which, carried up with the juices of rye, become lodged in the ovary, where they begin the course of life and progress which has been delineated. Different grains are probably infested with different species of Claviceps; but there is no reason to think that any other species is concerned in the product of any officinal variety of ergot. (*Annales des Sciences Naturelles*, 3e sér., xx. 5, 1853.)

The ergot usually projects out of the glume or husk beyond the ordinary outline of the spike or ear. In some spikes the place of the seeds is wholly occupied by the ergot, in others only two or three spurs are observed. It is said to be much more energetic when collected before than after harvest. Rye has generally been thought to be most subject to the disease in poor and wet soils, and in rainy seasons; and intense heat succeeding continued rains has been said to favor its development, especially if these circumstances occur at the time the flower is forming. It is now, however, asserted that moisture has little or nothing to do with its production. It should not be collected until some days after it has begun to form; as, according to M. Bonjean, if gathered on the first day, it does not possess the poisonous properties which it exhibits when taken on the sixth day. (See *P. J. Tr.*, Jan. 1842.)

Properties. Ergot is in solid, brittle yet somewhat flexible grains, from a third of an inch to an inch and a half long, from half a line to three lines in thickness, cylindrical or obscurely triangular, tapering towards each end, obtuse at the extremities, usually curved like the spur of a cock, marked with one or two longitudinal furrows, often irregularly cracked or fissured, of a violet brown color and often somewhat glaucous externally, yellowish white or violet white within, of an unpleasant smell when in mass resembling that of putrid fish, and of a taste which is at first scarcely perceptible, but ultimately disagreeable and slightly acrid. "Somewhat fusiform, obtusely triangular, usually curved, about one inch (25 mm.) long, and one-eighth of an inch (3 mm.) thick; three-furrowed, obtuse at both ends, purplish black, internally whitish, with some purplish striæ, breaking with a short fracture; odor peculiar, heavy, increased by trituration with solution of potassa; taste oily and disagreeable." *U. S.* Ergot yields its virtues to water and alcohol. The aqueous infusion or decoction is claret-colored, and has an acid reaction. It is precipitated by acetate and subacetate of lead, nitrate of silver, and tincture of galls, but affords with iodine no evidence of the presence of starch. Long boiling impairs the virtues of the medicine.

Ergot has been analyzed by Vauquelin, Winckler, Wiggers, Wright, Legrip, Wenzell, Tanret, Dragendorff, and several others. Dr. Wright supposed the virtues of ergot to reside in the fixed oil, which he therefore recommended as a substitute for the medicine. The *oil of ergot*, when obtained from grains recently collected, is, according to Dr. Wright, often quite free from color; but, as usually prepared, it is reddish brown. It has a disagreeable, somewhat acrid taste, is lighter than water, and is soluble in alcohol and alkaline solutions. It is prepared by forming an ethereal tincture of ergot by the process of displacement, and evaporating the ether with a gentle heat. It may be more cheaply prepared by substituting benzin for ether. Experience has shown that, though the oil thus prepared with ether may have produced effects analogous to those of ergot, they were to be ascribed rather to some principle extracted along with the oil by the menstruum than to the oil itself; for, when procured by expression, this has been found to be inactive; although Prof. Procter has ascertained that it contains a little *secalin*, one at least of the active principles of ergot, which may be separated from it by washing with acidulated water. According to Mr. T. R. Baker, the oil has a taste and smell similar to those of castor oil, with which it also agrees in ultimate composition, and yields analogous results in saponification. (*A. J. P.*, xxiv. 101–2.) Dr. T. C. Herrmann investigated specially the chemical constitution of the oil of ergot. As obtained by means of ether, it was brownish yellow, of an aromatic smell and acrid taste, viscid, of the sp. gr. 0·9249, and without the drying property. It consists of 22·703 per cent. of palmitic acid, 69·205 of oleic acid, and 8·091 of glycerin. (*N. R.*, 1872, p. 238; from *Buchner's Repertorium*, 1871, p. 283.) The *sugar of ergot* was found by Mitscherlich to be peculiar, and was named by him *mycose*. He described it as crystallizable, very soluble in water, almost insoluble in cold but dissolved by about 100 parts of boiling alcohol, quite insoluble in ether, and without the action of glucose on the salts of copper. Its formula is $C_{12}H_{22}O_{11} + 2H_2O$, allying it to cane sugar, and possibly making it identical with *trehalose*.

According to Wenzell (*A. J. P.*, May, 1864), ergot of rye contains two peculiar alkaloids, which he designates *ecboline* and *ergotine*, and claims to be the active principles of the drug. The two bases of ergot are, according to Wenzell, combined with *ergotic acid*, the existence of which has been further admitted by Ganser. It is said to be a volatile body yielding crystallizable salts.

A crystallized, colorless alkaloid, *ergotinine*, $C_{35}H_{40}N_4O_6$, has been isolated (1877–78) by Tanret. He obtained it to the amount of 0·04 per cent., some amorphous ergotinine, moreover, being present. The solutions of ergotinine turn greenish and red very soon; they are fluorescent. Sulphuric acid imparts to it a red, violet, and finally a blue hue.

Dragendorff and several of his pupils since 1875 have isolated the following *amorphous* principles of the drug: 1, *sclerotic acid*, said to be a very active substance, used chiefly in subcutaneous injections; about 4 per cent. of colorless acid may be obtained from good ergot of rye; 2, *scleromucin*, a mucilaginous matter which may be precipitated by alcohol from aqueous extracts of the drug; 3, *sclererythrin*, the red coloring matter probably allied to anthrachinon and the coloring substances of madder, chiefly to purpurin; 4, *scleroiodin*, a bluish black powder soluble in alkalies; 5, *fusco-sclerotinic acid;* 6, *picrosclerotine*, apparently a highly poisonous alkaloid; lastly, 7, *scleroxanthin*, $C_7H_7O_3 + H_2O$, and 8, *sclerocrystallin*, $C_7H_7O_3$, have been obtained in crystals; their alcoholic solution is but little colored, yet assumes a violet hue on addition of ferric chloride.

Tanret also observed in ergot of rye a volatile *camphoraceous* substance.

When ergot or its alcoholic extract is treated with an alkali, it yields as products of the decomposition of the albuminoid matters ammonia or ammonia bases, according to Ludwig and Stahl, *methylamine;* according to others, *trimethylamine*. Wenzell states that phosphate of trimethylamine is present in an aqueous extract of ergot, but Ganser ascertained that no such base pre-exists in ergot. Flückiger found that the crystals which abound in the extract after it has been kept for some time are an acid phosphate of sodium and ammonium with a small proportion of sulphate.

We quote from Dilg's summary of "the active constituents of ergot" (*A. J. P.*, 1878, p. 335) Dragendorff's process for the two most active constituents of ergot, *sclerotic* or *sclerotinic acid* and *scleromucin.* "Digest ergot, previously exhausted by ether and absolute alcohol, with water, dialyse, evaporate the dialysate to a syrupy consistence, and treat with sufficient alcohol to obtain a mixture containing 40 to 45 per cent. alcohol, which precipitates the potassium phosphate, while more alcohol added until the strength is increased to 75 or 80 per cent., precipitates the salts of sclerotic acid, which are soluble in dilute but insoluble in stronger alcohol, and leave about 19 per cent. of ash.

"The filtrate, upon which alcohol has no further effect, produces with ether a slight precipitate, which after a few days' standing forms a syrupy, brown mass, which has scarcely any medicinal virtue. The filtrate from this precipitate, in which the reactions still distinctly indicate the presence of Wenzell's alkaloids, after evaporating the ether and alcohol, does *not* produce the specific action of ergot.

"The dark liquid remaining on the dialysator, when mixed with sufficient alcohol to bring it to 45–50 per cent., precipitates the *scleromucin*, which while moist forms a mucilaginous solution with water, but after drying is only partially soluble, differing in this respect from sclerotic acid, which is soluble, in all proportions, before and after drying.

"*Sclerotic acid* is obtained in a nearly pure state by kneading the mixed sclerotates as obtained above, with 80 per cent. alcohol, and afterwards dissolving them in 40 per cent. alcohol; the solution is mixed with an excess of hydrochloric acid, and after several hours precipitated with absolute alcohol, whereby the ash is reduced to about 3 per cent., and consists mainly of some silica, magnesia, and phosphates of iron and potassium. The acid is not a glucoside, and yields no precipitates with the reagents for alkaloids, except with phosphomolybdic acid a yellow, and with tannin a nearly colorless one. Sclerotic acid is obtained as a yellowish brown, tasteless and inodorous substance, which has a very slight acid reaction, and is hygroscopic without being deliquescent. It is very well adapted for subcutaneous applications, in doses of 0·03–0·045 Gm.

"*Scleromucin* is darker in color, slightly hygroscopic, gummy, inodorous and tasteless; yields 26·8 per cent. of ash, and, like sclerotic acid, contains nitrogen, is not a glucoside, and is precipitated by tannin and phosphomolybdic acid.

"Good ergot yields about 4 to 4½ per cent. of sclerotic acid, and about 2 to 3 per cent. of scleromucin."

For an improved process for making sclerotic acid, by Podwissotzky, see *N. R.*, 1883, p. 271.

Kobert (*Pharm. Centralhalle*, 1884, p. 607; All, *Das Mutter Korns*, Leipzig, 1884) found three physiologically active principles: 1st, *ergotic acid*, which he considers the principal constituent of the sclerotic acid of Dragendorff and Podwissotzky, and which is isolated by precipitation with ammoniacal subacetate of lead; 2d, *sphacelic acid*, which can be isolated by taking advantage of the insolubility of the free acid in water and its solubility in alcohol; 3d, the alkaloid *cornutine*, which is not identical with the crystalline or with the amorphous ergotinine of Tanret; it is readily soluble in alcohol, and is obtained from an alkaline aqueous solution by agitation with ether. This alkaloid is said to be very poisonous. Dr. Kobert's conclusions have been questioned by Tanret (*P. J. Tr.*, 1885, p. 889), but the former reaffirms his statements and believes that ergotinine is worthless, and that the activity of fresh ergot is due to sphacelic acid and cornutine as above described: the important fact, however, is noted that these latter principles entirely lose their properties on keeping; he therefore proposes that they be made into pills and coated to protect them. (*Archiv d. Pharm.*, 1886, p. 597.)

The odor of ergot is no doubt owing to the liberation of its volatile alkaloid, probably in consequence of a slow decomposition of the native salt. A method of detecting ergot in a mixed powder, rye flour for example, is thus afforded. If, on the addition of solution of potassa, the odor of ergot be perceived, its presence is sufficiently proved.

Ergot, when perfectly dry and kept in well-stopped bottles, will retain its virtues for a considerable time; but, exposed to air and moisture, it speedily undergoes chemical change and deteriorates. M. Gobley kept for more than ten years, perfectly sound, some ergot which he had selected from the year's harvest, carefully sifted, wiped with linen, then exposed to a heat of from 50° to 60° C. for three or four hours, and finally put into small boxes, holding each about 30 Gm. (a troyounce), previously heated with the ergot, and finally closed air-tight with pitch. (*Journ. de Pharm.*, Mar. 1873, p. 216.) It is, moreover, apt to be attacked by a minute worm, which consumes the interior of the grain, leaving merely the exterior shell and an excrementitious powder. This insect is sometimes found in the ergot before removal from the plant. In the state of powder, the medicine still more readily deteriorates; but Prof. Dragendorff believes that the decay is due to oxidization of the fatty principles of the ergot, and can be prevented by depriving the ergot of its oil before powdering. (*A. P. S.*, xxv.) This has since been confirmed by Zschiesing, who preserved ergot for two years, and Bombelon, who kept ergot in good condition for nine years, by previously removing the fixed oil with ether (*Phar. Zeitung*, No. 49, p. 51; *A. J. P.*, 1881, p. 457.) It is best, as a general rule, to renew it every year or two. M. Viel recommends that it should be well dried at a gentle heat, and incorporated with double its weight of loaf sugar, by means of which, if protected from moisture, it will retain its virtues for many years. According to M. Zanon, the same result is obtained by stratifying it with well washed and perfectly dried sand, in a bottle from which air and light are excluded. Camphor and powdered benzoin are said to prevent injury from worms.

Medical Properties and Uses. Given in small doses to men or non-pregnant women, ergot produces no obvious effect. In the quantity of half a drachm or a drachm it may occasion nausea or vomiting, but in order to produce very distinct symptoms enormous doses must be taken. We have given the fluid extract in doses of three ounces, daily, for one or more weeks without perceiving any marked effect. In some cases, after very large doses, the pulse is distinctly reduced in frequency, and Dr. Hardy has noted that the fœtal cardiac pulsations are rendered infrequent by it. But one instance of fatal poisoning has occurred, except when abortion has been produced. A case is recorded in which ergot produced great prostration, with an almost absent pulse, paleness and coldness of the surface, partial palsy, with pricking of the limbs, and great restlessness, without stupor or delirium. (*Gazette Med. de Paris*, Juillet 25, 1857.) The symptoms in another case, recorded by Dr. Oldright, were very similar to those just detailed. The most characteristic is the intense coldness of the surface, which has also been noted in the lower animals. In the fatal case narrated by Dr. Pratschke, uneasiness in the head, oppression of stomach, diarrhœa, urgent thirst, burning pains in the feet, tetanic spasms, violent convulsions, and death ensued upon eating freely of ergotized grain. (*Lond. Med. Gaz.*, Oct. 1850, p. 579.)

The long-continued and free use of ergot is highly dangerous, even when no immediate effects are perceptible. Fatal epidemics in different parts of the continent of Europe, particularly in certain provinces of France, have long been ascribed to the use of bread made from rye contaminated with this fungus.* Dry gangrene, typhus fever, and disorder of the nervous system attended with convulsions, are the forms of disease which have followed the use of this unwholesome food. It is true that ergot has been denied to be the cause; but accurate investigations, made by competent men upon the spot where the epidemics have prevailed, together with the results of experiments made upon inferior animals,† leave no room for reasonable doubt that at least the gangrenous affection alluded to has resulted from it.

Upon the lower animals ergot acts as upon man. Besides its influence upon the uterus, the most important physiological action of the drug is upon the vaso-motor nervous system. It has been abundantly proved that in full therapeutic dose it

* Dr. Hofmann states that $\frac{1}{10}$ per cent. of ergot can be detected in bread by macerating 30 grains of coarsely grated bread in 40 grains of ether and 20 drops of diluted sulphuric acid for 24 hours, straining, shaking with solution of bicarbonate of sodium and allowing to stand, when the solution separates and is of a violet color. (See also *N. R.*, 1888, p. 465.)

† An epidemic among sheep was caused by eating ergotized grain. (See *P. J. Tr.*, x. 195.)

raises remarkably the arterial pressure by producing a general vaso-motor spasm. This spasm is almost certainly the result of a stimulation of the vaso-motor nerve centres, but there are still some authorities who believe that the drug acts peripherally upon the muscular coats of the vessels or upon the nerves connected therewith.

On the continent of Europe, in Germany, France, and Italy, ergot has long been empirically employed by midwives for promoting the contraction of the uterus; and its German name of *mutterkorn* implies a popular acquaintance with its peculiar powers. But the attention of the medical profession was first called to it by Dr. Stearns, of Saratoga County, N. Y., in the eleventh volume of the *New York Medical Repository*, 1807. In its operation upon the pregnant uterus, it produces a constant unremitting contraction and rigidity, rather than that alternation of spasmodic effort and relaxation which is observable in the natural process of labor. Hence, unless the os uteri and external parts are sufficiently relaxed, the medicine is apt to produce injury to the fœtus by the incessant pressure which it maintains; and the death of the child is thought not unfrequently to have resulted from its injudicious employment. The cases to which it is thought to be especially adapted are those of lingering labor, when the os uteri is sufficiently dilated and the external parts sufficiently relaxed, when no mechanical impediment is offered to the passage of the child, and the delay is ascribable solely to want of energy in the uterus. Other cases are those in which the death of the fœtus has been ascertained, and when great exhaustion or dangerous constitutional irritation imperiously calls for speedy delivery. The medicine may also be given to promote the expulsion of the placenta, to restrain inordinate hemorrhage after delivery, and to hasten the discharge of the fœtus in protracted cases of abortion. In women subject to dangerous flooding, a dose of ergot given immediately before delivery is said to have the happiest effects. Ergot is also much used to cause the expulsion of coagula of blood, polypi, and hydatids from the uterine cavity, and even a number of successful cases of its employment for the destruction by strangulation of fibroid tumors of the uterus have been reported. In uterine hemorrhage, unconnected with pregnancy, the medicine is very useful; and it is probably the most used and most efficient of all remedies in pulmonary and other similar internal hemorrhages. Its action in these cases is no doubt the result of the contracting power it has over the smaller vessels. This action of ergot upon the blood-vessels suggests its employment in those cases in which there is local or general dilatation of the blood-vessels. It has been used in pulmonic congestion with apparent good results, and it has been highly lauded in the first stages of pneumonia by several clinicians, especially by Dr. J. E. Kelly (*Med. Register*, 1887, vol. x.), as giving immediate relief when injected hypodermically in low forms of pulmonary hyperæmia such as occurs in typhoid fevers. It will probably also be found of service as a vaso-motor stimulant in surgical shock, and has been used with asserted good results against cerebral congestion following injuries to the head, also in spinal congestion. In cases of apoplexy, by increasing the blood-pressure its tendency will be to do harm rather than good. The best preparation of ergot for internal administration, except when an immediate influence is desired, is the officinal solid extract given in capsules. The fluid extract is perhaps absorbed a little more quickly, but it is much more apt to sicken the stomach. The dose of the solid extract is 5 to 30 grains (0·33–1·95 Gm.); of the fluid, half a fluidrachm to two fluidrachms (3·9–7·8 C.c.).

In hemorrhoids, and in varicose veins of the leg, it has been injected into the diseased tissue with success, but probably acts only by producing a severe local inflammation.

Under the name of Bonjean's *ergotine*, a purified extract is sometimes used in the dose of from five to ten grains (0·33–0·65 Gm.). It is made by exhausting ergot with water, evaporating to the consistence of syrup, precipitating the albumen, gum, etc., by a large excess of alcohol, decanting the clear liquid, and evaporating to the consistence of a soft extract.

When promptness and certainty of action are required, ergot may be used hypodermically. Solutions of extract of ergot are very prone to undergo speedy decomposition, and, as such altered solutions are very irritating, it is important that solutions for hypodermic use be made freshly, especially as the experiments of M. Engelmann (*Deutsch. Med. Wochen.*, Sept. 30, 1886) have shown that the addition of ordinary antiseptic agents to such solutions, unless in very large amount, simply delays decomposition, and that the changes may be far advanced although the preparations seem to the eye unaltered. Notwithstanding all possible precautions, the hypodermic injections of ergot have a tendency to produce local inflammations and abscesses, but the danger may be reduced to a minimum by absolute obedience to the following directions: Extract of ergot, five grains, should be dissolved in twenty minims of recently boiled water, and two or three drops of glycerin and half a drop of carbolic acid be added. This solution should be filtered, to remove any solid particles, and then at once be thrown deeply into the cellular tissues.

Dujardin-Beaumetz gives the dose of Tanret's crystallised ergotine for hypodermic use as 5 milligrammes ($\frac{7}{100}$ grain). (*Bull. Thérap.*, xciv. 236.) Sclerotic acid does not represent ergot, as was, so far as concerns the commercial article, shown by experiments made in the laboratory of the University of Pennsylvania; indeed, the research of Nikitin, who claims that it is the active principle, affords abundant evidence that it is not so. (*Lond. Med. Record*, 1879, p. 21.)

Off. Prep. Extractum Ergotæ Fluidum; Extractum Ergotæ; Vinum Ergotæ.

Off. Prep. Br. Extractum Ergotæ Liquidum; Infusum Ergotæ; Tinctura Ergotæ.

ERYTHROXYLON, *U.S.* *Erythroxylon.* [*Coca.*]

(ĔR-Y̆-THRŎX'Y̆-LON.)

"The leaves of Erythroxylon Coca. Lamarck. (*Nat. Ord.* Erythroxylaceæ.)" *U.S.*

Feuilles de Coca, *Fr.;* Cocablätter, *G.*

Gen. Ch. *Calyx* five-parted, at the base five-angular. *Styles*, three, distinct to the base and not united into one. *De Candolle*, *Prodromus*, i. 573.

E. coca. Lam. *B. & T.* i. 40. Leaves ovate, areolate, membranaceous, branches squamous, pedicels lateral, aggregated in twos or threes, a little longer than the flower. *De C.*

Although it grows wild in various parts of South America, the coca shrub is largely cultivated for the sake of its leaves. The plant, which is propagated from the seed in nurseries, begins to yield in eighteen months, and continues productive for half a century. The leaves, when mature, are carefully picked by hand so as to avoid breaking them or injuring the young buds, are slowly dried in the sun, and then packed in bags (*cestos*) holding from twenty-five to one hundred and fifty pounds each. They were in general use among the natives of Peru at the time of the conquest, and have continued to be much employed to the present time. It is affirmed that nearly ten million dollars' worth, or forty million pounds, are annually produced; some plantations yielding three or four harvests a year. For details as to method of cultivation, etc., see *Therap. Gazette*, Jan. 1886.

Properties. The leaves resemble in size and shape those of tea, being oval-oblong, pointed, two inches or more in length by somewhat over an inch in their greatest breadth, and furnished with short delicate footstalks; but they are not, like the tea-leaves, dentate, and are distinguished from most other leaves by a slightly curved line on each side of the midrib, running from the base to the apex. These lines are not ribs but curves, which have been produced by the peculiar folding of the leaf in the bud. Good specimens are perfectly flat, of a fine green color; brown leaves should always be rejected as inferior. They have an agreeable odor resembling that of tea, and a peculiar taste, which, in decoction, becomes bitter and astringent. "Oval or obovate-oblong, two to three inches (50 to 75 mm.) long, short-petiolate, entire, rather obtuse or emarginate at the apex, reticulate on both sides, with a prominent midrib, and, on each side of it, a curved line running from base to apex; odor slight and tea-like; taste somewhat aromatic and bitter." *U. S.*

Chemical Constitution. In 1853, Wackenroder demonstrated the existence of tannic acid in coca leaves; and in 1859, M. Stanislas Martin found in them a peculiar bitter principle, resin, tannin, an aromatic principle, extractive, chlorophyll, a substance analogous to theine, and salts of lime. Previous to this (1855) Gardeke had isolated the crystalline alkaloid and given it the name of *erythroxyline.* Dr. Albert Niemann, of Goslar, made the first thorough investigation of the leaves, and gave to the alkaloid the name it now usually bears of *cocaine.* The following was his process. The leaves were exhausted with 85 per cent. alcohol acidulated with 2 per cent. of sulphuric acid; the tincture was treated with milk of lime and filtered; the filtrate was neutralized with sulphuric acid, and the alcohol distilled off. The syrupy residue was treated with water to separate resin, and then precipitated by carbonate of sodium. The deposited matter was exhausted by ether, and the ethereal solution, after most of the ether had been distilled, was allowed to evaporate spontaneously. The cocaine was thus obtained in colorless crystals, mixed with a yellowish brown matter of a disagreeable odor, which was separated by washing with cold alcohol. Dr. Squibb's process for cocaine and its hydrochlorate is as follows: Coarsely ground coca leaves are repercolated with an aqueous five per cent. solution of sulphuric acid, and a very dense, slightly acid percolate is obtained; this is thoroughly agitated with pure coal oil and an excess of sodium carbonate; the liberated alkaloid is retained by the coal oil, and is nearly free from coloring matter; the oily solution is then agitated with acidulated water, and again precipitated by sodium carbonate in the presence of ether. The ethereal solution of cocaine is treated with diluted hydrochloric acid fractionally, and the nearly colorless solutions of cocaine hydrochlorate are cautiously evaporated in shallow porcelain pans almost to dryness. The product is in the form of a white, crystalline, granular powder, and it is a nearly pure anhydrous salt. (*Ephemeris*, 1887, p. 906.) Pure cocaine is in colorless transparent prisms, inodorous, of a bitterish taste, soluble in 704 parts of cold water, more soluble in alcohol, and freely so in ether. The solution has an alkaline reaction, and a bitterish taste, leaving a peculiar numbness on the tongue, followed by a sensation of cold. The alkaloid melts at 97·7° C. (208° F.), and on cooling congeals into a transparent mass, which gradually becomes crystalline. Heated above this point it changes color, and is decomposed. It is inflammable, burning with a bright flame, and leaving charcoal. With the acids it forms soluble and crystallizable salts, which are more bitter than the alkaloid itself. The formula is $C_{17}H_{21}NO_4$. Dr. Niemann also obtained wax, a variety of tannic acid (*coca-tannic acid*), and a concrete volatile odorous substance. (See *A. J. P.*, 1861, p. 122.) A volatile alkaloid, *hygrine*, first noticed by Maclagan, but named by Lossen, is a thick, pale yellow, oily liquid, having a strong alkaline reaction, burning taste, and the odor of trimethylamine. Its existence has, however, been doubted. M. Lossen has examined cocaine, and ascertained that, when heated with hydrochloric acid, it splits into benzoic acid, methyl alcohol, and a new base which he calls *ecgonine*, of which the formula is $C_9H_{15}NO_3$. The mutability of cocaine with acids explains why the attempts to extract the alkaloid with acid liquids have failed. M. Lossen therefore recommends the omission of acid in operating on the leaves, and proposes the following modification of Niemann's plan. An infusion is first made; this is precipitated with acetate of lead; the lead is removed by sulphate of sodium; the liquid is concentrated, carbonate of sodium added, and the whole shaken with ether. The ether extracts the alkaloid, and yields it in a crude state by evaporation. It is then purified as in the process of Dr. Niemann. (*Journ. de Pharm.*, Juin, 1862, p. 522.) The tannin of coca leaves strikes a green-black with ferric salts, and has received the name of *coca-tannic acid.* For methods of assaying coca leaves, see Lyons, *Chicago Pharmacist*, 1885, Sept.; Squibb, *Ephemeris*, 1887, p. 912; Prescott, *Organic Analysis*, pp. 178, 179.

The alkaloid cocaine acts upon the lower animals much as does theine. It tetanizes frogs, or in overwhelming doses paralyses the sensory nerves and the posterior columns. Rabbits and dogs are killed by it through paralysis of the respiratory centres. In proper doses it elevates arterial pressure by an action upon the vaso-motor centres and the cardiac-motor system. (*I. Ott.*)

Medical Properties. As a nerve stimulant, coca has been used immemorially by the Peruvian and Bolivian natives. In 1853, Dr. Weddell stated that it produces a gently excitant effect, with an indisposition to sleep; in these respects resembling tea and coffee; also, that it will support the strength for a considerable time in the absence of food; but does not supply the place of nutriment, and probably, in this respect also, acts like the two substances referred to. The Indians, while chewing it, mixed with some alkaline substance, as the ashes of certain plants, or lime, pass whole days in travelling or working without food. It is, however, clearly proven that these leaves do not take the place of nutriment, but simply put off the sense of fatigue and hunger, the Indian making up at his evening meal for the day's abstinence. It is probable that they prevent hunger simply by their local benumbing influence upon the nerves of the stomach. Their moderate habitual use does not seem to be injurious, but the habit is said readily to grow upon the person, and finally the inveterate excessive coca-chewer can be recognized by his uncertain step, general apathy, sunken eyes surrounded by deep purple aureoles, his trembling lips, green and crusted teeth, and excessively fetid breath, with peculiar blackness about the corners of the mouth. An incurable insomnia is apt to be developed, emaciation becomes extreme, dropsy appears, and even death results in a condition of general marasmus. When coca is taken in a single large dose it produces a condition of peculiar physical beatitude and calm, followed by a sensation of excessive power, which is affirmed to be accompanied by a real increase of physical ability. Dr. Montegazza took in the course of two hours about 900 grains of the coca leaf, with the result of great increase in the number of the heart-beats, and a condition of intoxication resembling that produced by hasheesh. He was possessed by a feeling of intense joyousness, while a succession of visions and phantasmagoria, most brilliant in form and color, trooped rapidly before his eyes. He then passed into a condition of delirious excitement, which was succeeded by a deep sleep that lasted three hours. The symptoms which are described as produced by coca in the natives of Bolivia and Peru are so different from those commonly caused by cocaine itself as to suggest that the alkaloid does not completely represent the crude leaf. Five grains of cocaine have been in several cases taken by the mouth or hypodermically, the result being nausea, disturbance of vision, incoherence of speech, severe sweating, with fall of bodily temperature, dilatation of the pupils, marked disturbance of respiration with evidences of asphyxia, feeble pulse, and finally other symptoms of collapse. In a case in which 22 grains were taken in a glass of beer, the man shortly afterwards went to sleep, and awoke after some hours with great abdominal pains, dryness in the mouth, excessive weakness, and vertigo. There was also suppression of urine for twenty-four hours, but the patient finally recovered. The experiments upon the lower animals show that whilst cocaine is a feeble toxic agent, it will, in sufficient amount, produce death through arrest of respiration by paralysis of the respiratory centres. The influence of the alkaloid upon the circulation seems to be entirely subservient to its action on the respiration, and there is so much conflict of evidence as to the exact action of the drug upon the heart and vaso-motor system that at present it is not possible to reach definite conclusions. The most susceptible portion of the nervous system to the action of cocaine is the cerebrum, and the delirious excitement which in man is so prominent after the taking of large doses of coca is said to be almost equally pronounced in the dog. The researches of various physiologists indicate that the drug has also influence upon the spinal cord and the nerve-trunks, it having special power over the sensory side of the cord and the sensory nerves.

The stimulant effect which coca appears to exert upon the cerebrum has led to its extensive use in melancholia, neurasthenia, hysteria, and allied disorders. The results obtained, however, have not been what was expected. Almost all clinicians agree that in melancholia no good whatever is achieved, and that in neurasthenia and hysteria the drug, unless given in small doses, acts deleteriously, although in some cases the fluid extract of coca or a coca wine seems to be of service for a time in stimulating the digestion, and to some slight extent the general nervous system.

The chief use of cocaine in practical medicine is for its local effects. When brought in contact with a mucous membrane or with an exposed surface it produces a peculiar pallor, followed in a few moments by complete loss of sensitiveness. When the mucous membrane is extremely sensitive, as in the conjunctiva, a burning pain is at first produced, but this soon subsides, and leaves a condition in which the part may be cut or burnt without the patient being conscious of it. All mucous membranes are permeable to cocaine solutions, which will, however, not penetrate through the skin. When brought in contact with the nerve-trunks or endings, cocaine rapidly produces paralysis of sensation. When the circumstances are favorable, solutions of cocaine are extremely useful in allaying pain, as in hemorrhoidal inflammations, superficial cancerous or other painful ulcerations, but they are especially employed for surgical purposes. In surgical operations about the eye, nose, and mouth, unless the cutting is to be too deep and extensive, a simple application of the solution once or twice by means of a camel's-hair brush is sufficient for the purposes of the surgeon. Even deeper operations, such as the removal of tumors, the opening of felons, and the amputation of fingers, may be rendered painless by hypodermic injections of cocaine solution, provided the part is so situated that with a band or other contrivance the circulation in it can be temporarily restrained.

When applied to the eye the solution of cocaine acts as a rapid and powerful mydriatic: the dilatation produced is affirmed to be even greater than that which can be caused by atropine, although it can be at any time readily overcome by eserine. The maximum dilatation is usually reached (4 per cent. solution) in one hour, and maintained for three or four hours, and recovered from in about twenty-four hours. The intraocular pressure is not increased, so that there is no danger, as with atropine, of producing a glaucoma. The accommodation is partially but not entirely paralyzed.

The dose of coca is from one-half to one drachm (1·95–3·9 Gm.). If given in infusion the leaves should be swallowed, as it is by no means certain that they yield their virtues to water. The fluid extract is now officinal, and is a very eligible preparation; a *tincture of coca*, made in the proportion of one part in five of diluted alcohol, and *a wine of coca*, one in ten, would also be efficient. The *elixir of coca*, as usually found, is too weak to be of much value. (See Part II.)

Off. Prep. Extractum Erythroxyli Fluidum.

ESSENTIÆ. *Br. Essences.*

(ĚS-SĔN'TĮ-Æ—ęs-sĕn'shę-ē.)

Essenzen, *G.;* Alcoolés concentrés, *Fr.*

Under this name two preparations have been admitted to the British Pharmacopœia. They correspond with the class of officinal Spirits (see *Spiritus*) in every particular except strength, the Essences having about three times the strength of the Spirits, both being solutions of volatile substances in alcohol.

ESSENTIA ANISI. *Essence of Anise.*

(ĚS-SĔN'TĮ-Ą Ą-NĪ'SĪ—ęs-sĕn'shę-ą.)

"Take of Oil of Anise *one fluidounce;* Rectified Spirit *four fluidounces.* Mix. The medical properties of this essence are those of the oil of anise. Dose, 10 to 20 minims" (0·65–1·3 C.c.).

ESSENTIA MENTHÆ PIPERITÆ. *Essence of Peppermint.*

(ĚS-SĔN'TĮ-Ą MĔN'THÆ PĪ-PĘ-RĪ'TÆ—ęs-sĕn'shę ą.)

"Take of Oil of Peppermint *one fluidounce;* Rectified Spirit *four fluidounces.* Mix. The medical properties of this essence are those of the oil of peppermint. Dose, 10 to 20 minims" (0·65–1·3 C.c.).

EUCALYPTUS. *U. S. Eucalyptus.*

(EŪ-CĄ-LЎP'TŲS—yū-ką-lĭp'tųs.)

"The leaves of Eucalyptus globulus, Labillardière (*Nat. Ord.* Myrtaceæ), collected from rather old trees." *U. S.*

Eucalyptus Leaves; Feuilles d'Eucalyptus, *Fr.;* Eucalyptus-Blätter, *G.*

Gen. Ch. Calyx obovate or globose cupulæform, the tube persistent, the limb deciduous, dehiscing by a circular irregular line from the operculiform base. *Stamens* free. *Capsule* 4 loculate or by abortion 3 loculate, dehiscent at the apex, many-seeded. *De Candolle, Prodromus,* iii. 220.

The genus Eucalyptus affords one of the most characteristic features of the Australian and Tasmanian landscapes. There are about one hundred and thirty-five described species, all evergreens, and most of them large trees, popularly known as *Gum trees*, *Woolly butts*, *Iron barks*, etc.* The most important of them is the *E. globulus*.

E. globulus. Labill. *B. & T.* ii. 109. The young operculum conical, the length of the four-sided cupule, the adult depressed and mucronate in the middle; axillary peduncles very short, one-flowered; leaves alternate, lanceolate, subfalcate.

This is one of the largest known trees, attaining sometimes a height of 300 or even 350 feet, with a smooth, ash-colored bark; leaves a foot in length, and varying, according to age, from a glaucous white to a bluish green color; and large pinkish white axillary flowers, sometimes single, sometimes in clusters. Although its wood is very resinous, hard, and durable, the tree is remarkable for the rapidity of its growth, reaching, under favorable circumstances, fifty feet of height in five or six years. It flourishes best in valleys having a rich, moist soil, and has very largely been naturalized in semi-tropical countries, partly on account of its economic value, but chiefly because of the reputation it enjoys as a means of overcoming malaria. It does not seem to require great heat for its perfection, but is exceedingly sensitive to frost. Large forests of it have been planted in Algeria and Southern Europe, and its culture is spreading to California, Florida, and other of our Southern States. Its sanitary powers appear to be established, numerous notoriously miasmatic stations and districts having been rendered healthful by its growth. It is not probable that the destruction of the miasma is due so much to emanations from the tree as to the fact that it evaporates water so rapidly from its innumerable large leaves as to drain the swamps and marshes in which it is planted.† It is possible, however, that the large amount of volatile oil which must escape from it has some effect, and it is even affirmed (*A. J. P.*, 1875, p. 423) that the parasitic phylloxera will not attack grape-vines growing near it.

The eucalyptus trees afford a number of products besides the officinal oil. The eucalyptus oil of commerce is, indeed, composed chiefly of the oils of *E. amygdalina* and *E. dumosa*, which yield a very much larger product than does the officinal species. The oils of *E. piperita* and *E. hæmastoma* have a peppermint odor, and that of *E. citriodora* a citron-like odor, whilst oil of *E. Staigeriana* exactly resembles the oil of verbena; it is probable that these oils will soon come into commerce for the purposes of the perfumer. The gum resins are collected from many species, the most important for medicinal use being that produced by the *E. rostata*, which is a mucilaginous astringent said to be used as a substitute for kino. (See *P. J. Tr.*, vol. xvi.)

Properties. The leaves are the officinal portion of the plant: they are "petiolate, lanceolately scythe-shaped, from six to twelve inches (15 to 30 cm.) long, rounded below, tapering above, entire, leathery, gray-green, glandular, feather-veined between the midrib and marginal veins; odor strongly camphoraceous; taste pungently aromatic, somewhat bitter and astringent." *U. S.*

In March, 1870, M. Cloez (*Journ. de Pharm.*, 4e sér., xii. 201) reported an elaborate chemical study of the Eucalyptus leaves, and his results have been substantially confirmed by Debray (*De l'Eucalyptus Globulus*, Paris, 1872), M. Rabuteau (*Mém. de l'Académie*, Nov. 1872), and by Mr. Broughton (*P. J. Tr.*, 3d ser., iii. 463). M. Cloez found, besides chlorophyll, resin, tannin, and inert substances, an essential oil, upon which the virtues of the drug appear to depend. Of this oil, the fresh leaves afforded 2·75 parts per hundred, the recently dried leaves 6 parts; leaves which had been kept some time yielded a much smaller percentage. In the distillation, the oil for a time comes over freely at from 170° C. (338° F.) to 178° C. (352·4° F.); subsequently another portion of oil distils at 188° C. (370·4° F.) to

* Descriptions and accurate figures of most of this species may be found in Baron Ferd. von Mueller's *Descriptive Notes of the Eucalypts of Australia*, London and Melbourne, 1882.

† Dr. Bonavia, of the Lucknow Horticultural Gardens, has denied the value of the *Eucalyptus globulus*, because in his district the moisture and heat combined kill the trees. This, however, seems to us simply to show that India is too hot for the *Eucalyptus globulus*, and not that the species is unavailing for use in more moderate climates. Dr. Bonavia further states that the *E. citriodora* does well in India.

190° C. (374° F.), and finally a very minute portion does not volatilize until the temperature reaches 200° C (392° F.). M. Cloez believes the oil to be composed of two camphors, differing in their volatility. The bulk of the oil yielded is the portion first distilled; to this Cloez has given the name of *eucalyptol.* To obtain it pure a redistillation from caustic potash or chloride of calcium is necessary. It is very liquid, nearly colorless, with a strong, aromatic camphoraceous odor, polarizes to the right, is slightly soluble in water, but very soluble in alcohol, and has the formula $C_{12}H_{20}O$. Nitric acid produces with it a crystallizable acid; by the action of phosphoric anhydride (*Journ. de Pharm.*, 4e sér., xii. 204) it is converted into *eucalyptene*, $C_{10}H_{18}$, a substance allied to cymene, and *eucalyptolen.*

The presence of *cymol*, $C_{10}H_{14}$, was asserted by Faust and Homeyer (1874), but its presence in the oil of *Eucalyptus globulus* is denied by H. Schulz (1881), who made a careful study of this variety.

C. Jahns (*A. J. P.*, 1885, p. 237) gives the formula $C_{10}H_{18}O$ to eucalyptol, and considers it to be identical with cajuputol.

According to M. Duquesnel, the oil is adulterated—with alcohol, to be detected by means of fuchsin, which is insoluble in the pure oil but soluble in that containing even a very small percentage of alcohol; with fixed oil, to be detected by boiling with water, when the fixed oil remains on the surface; with essential oil of copaiba or turpentine, to be detected by means of the boiling point, that of eucalyptol being 170° C. (338° F.), that of oil of turpentine 155° C. (311° F.), that of oil of copaiba 260° C. (500° F.). (*Journ. de Pharm.*, 4e sér., xvi. 45.) It is affirmed that much of the oil from *E. amygdalina* does not yield *eucalyptol.* (*A. J. P.*, 1879, p. 303.)

Medical Properties. Eucalyptus was originally recommended as a remedy in intermittent fever, but experience has failed to establish its value as an antiperiodic. Whatever medical virtues it possesses beyond astringency reside in the volatile oil. This when applied locally acts as a powerful irritant. When taken internally in doses from 20 to 30 drops, it causes increased rapidity of pulse and general excitation, with restlessness and increased venereal appetite, usually followed by a feeling of calmness and repose, ending in sleep. In some cases, disturbance of the bowels, fever, constitutional disturbance, and even symptoms of cerebral congestion have been produced. In animals small doses produce the same effect as in man, and after large doses symptoms of general depression are manifested by falling of the arterial pressure, progressive diminution of temperature, muscular weakness deepening into paralysis, loss of sensibility, irregular respiration, and finally death from failure of respiration. Upon man, when taken in sufficient quantity, the oil exerts a similar influence. In a case noted by M. Gimbert, 80 drops of the oil produced in an old man a feeling of great internal heat, followed by almost complete loss of power and of feeling in the limbs; and after 75 drops Prof. Binz noted somewhat similar phenomena. The palsy produced by toxic doses is due to a direct action upon the spinal cord. Taken internally it is eliminated by the breath, to which it imparts its odor, and also in a condition of oxidation by the kidneys, to the secretion of which it gives a strong smell of violets. M. Gimbert found that in rabbits it augmented to a marvellous extent the excretion of urea. As a stimulating narcotic the oil of eucalyptus has been used with asserted success in migraine and other forms of neuralgia. As an antispasmodic it has been highly lauded in asthma. In this affection it is best given by inhalation. Cigarettes may be made by rolling up the dried leaves, or the vapor from boiling water containing the oil may be inhaled. In chronic or subacute bronchitis it may often be employed with advantage, especially where there is a tendency to spasm. In subacute or chronic inflammation of the genito-urinary organs it is said to exert a very happy influence. The experiments of Binz and of Gimbert have shown that it acts very positively upon the infusoria and other low forms of life. Gimbert even claims superiority for it as an antiseptic over carbolic acid. Externally it may be used in chronic skin affections and ulcerations when a stimulant antiseptic application is indicated. Various formulas have been published for tinctures, fluid extracts, etc., of the leaves, but the oil is now officinal, and is much the best form for internal administration. It should be given in doses of 10 to 15 drops (0·5 to 0·72 C.c.) on sugar or in a sweetened emulsion.

Off. Prep. Extractum Eucalypti Fluidum, *U. S.*

EUONYMUS. *U. S.* *Euonymus.* [*Wahoo.*]

(EU-ŎN'Y-MUS—yū-ŏn'ẹ-mŭs.)

"The bark of Euonymus atropurpureus. Jacquin. (*Nat. Ord.* Celastraceæ.)" *U. S.*

Gen. Ch. *Flowers* perfect. *Sepals* 4 or 5, united at the base, forming a short and flat calyx. *Petals* 4–5, rounded, spreading. *Stamens* very short, inserted on the edge or face of a broad and flat 4–5 angled disk, which coheres with the calyx and is stretched over the ovary, adhering to it more or less. *Style* short or none. *Pod* 3–5 lobed, with 1–3 seeds in each cell in a red arillus.

Euonymus Atropurpureus. Willd. *Sp. Plant.* i. 1132; Gray's *Manual*, p. 81; figured in Griffith's *Med. Bot.*, p. 219. The plant has been named variously *wahoo*, *spindle-tree*, and *burning-bush.* It is a tall, erect shrub, with quadrangular branchlets, and opposite, petiolate, oval-oblong, pointed, serrate leaves. The flowers, which stand in loose cymes on axillary peduncles, are small and dark purple, with sepals and petals commonly in fours. The capsule or pod is smooth and deeply lobed. The plant is indigenous, growing throughout the Northern and Western States, and sometimes cultivated for the beauty of its crimson fruit.

The plants belonging to this genus are shrubs or small trees, presenting in the autumn a striking appearance from the rich red color of their fruit, which has obtained for them the name of *burning-bush.* *E. Americanus* and *E. Europæus* have been cultivated in gardens as ornamental plants. Two or more of the species have been used in medicine. Their properties are probably similar, if not identical. Grundner, who experimented with the fruit of *E. Europæus*, found it to have no other effect than that of a diuretic. (*Pharm. Centralbl.*, 1847, p. 873.) An oil expressed from the seeds is used in Europe for the destruction of vermin in the hair, and sometimes also as an application to old sores. (*Ibid.*, 1851, p. 641.) Dr. Griffith says that the seeds of this and other species are purgative and emetic, and that the leaves are poisonous to sheep and other animals feeding on them. He states also that the inner bark of *E. tingens* is beautifully yellow, and used in India for dyeing, and in diseases of the eye. (*Med. Bot.*, p. 220.) It is probable that much of the wahoo of our drug-stores has been obtained from *E. Americanus*, which is distinguished from *E. atropurpureus* by its rough, warty, depressed pods, and almost sessile, thickish leaves.

Properties. The dried bark is in thin pieces, whitish with a darker grayish epidermis, brittle, of a feeble, peculiar, not disagreeable odor, and a bitterish slightly sweetish taste, and somewhat pungent after-taste. "In quilled or curved pieces, about one-twelfth of an inch (2 mm.) thick; outer surface ash-gray, with blackish patches, detached in thin and small scales; inner surface whitish or slightly tawny, smooth; fracture smooth, whitish, the inner layers tangentially striate; nearly inodorous; taste sweetish, somewhat bitter and acrid." *U. S.* It imparts its virtues to water and alcohol. Analyzed by Mr. Wm. T. Wentzell, it was found to contain a bitter principle which he named *euonymin*, asparagin, a soft resin, a crystallizable resin, a yellow resin, a brown resin, fixed oil, wax, starch, albumen, glucose, pectin, and various salts of organic and inorganic acids. Euonymin was obtained by agitating with chloroform a tincture made with diluted alcohol, separating the chloroformic solution and allowing it to evaporate spontaneously, treating the residue with ether, dissolving what was left in alcohol, adding acetate of lead to the solution, filtering, precipitating the lead with hydrosulphuric acid, and evaporating. The euonymin obtained was uncrystallizable, intensely bitter, soluble in water and alcohol, and neuter in its reactions. It was abundantly precipitated from its solution by subacetate of lead and phospho-molybdic acid. (*A. J. P.*, 1862, p. 387.) Mr. W. P. Clothier found the bark to yield no volatile oil on distillation. According to the same writer, if a concentrated tincture be poured into water, a dark yellow substance will be thrown down, containing resin and fixed oil, which is the euonymin of the eclectics, very improperly so named, as, though it contains a portion of the active principle, it is a very complex substance. Mr. Clothier found it to purge actively without griping. (*Ibid.*, 1861, p. 491.) Kubel has discovered in the fresh inner bark of *E. Europæus* a saccharine, crystallizable substance, closely resembling mannit, but differing in its crystalline form, and its melting point. He calls it *euonymite*. (*Journ. de Pharm.*, Dec. 1862, p. 523.)

For an examination of commercial *euonymin* (the eclectic resinoid) by Paul Thibault, see *N. R.*, 1883, p. 294.

Medical Properties and Uses. About twenty years since, this bark was introduced into notice in Philadelphia, as a remedy for dropsy, under the name of Wahoo,* by Mr. George W. Carpenter, who had obtained a knowledge of its virtues in the Western States. In some cases it acts as a mild cathartic, but at other times it fails to produce purgation. We have also seen distinct evidences of an irritant influence upon the gastro-intestinal mucous membrane. Cholagogue properties have been ascribed to it, and probably with correctness, as in the experiments of Prof. Rutherford it was found to act most powerfully in causing hepatic secretion in dogs, and in some clinical studies we have made it seemed to have a similar action on man. The fluid extract of it is an efficient preparation, and may be given in doses, as a purgative, of one to two fluidrachms (3·75–7·5 C.c.); as a laxative, of half a fluidrachm to one fluidrachm (1·9–3·75 C.c.).

Off. Prep. Extractum Euonymi, *U. S.*

EUPATORIUM. *U. S.* *Eupatorium.* [*Thoroughwort.*]

(EŪ-PA-TŌ′RI-ŬM—yū-pa-tō′rĭ-ŭm.)

"The leaves and flowering tops of Eupatorium perfoliatum. Linné. (*Nat. Ord.* Compositæ.)" *U. S.*

Herba Eupatorii Perfoliati; Boneset, Indian Sage; Herbe d'Eupatoire perfoliée, Herbe à Fièvre, Herbe parfaite, *Fr.*; Durchwachsener Wasserhanf, *G.*

Gen. Ch. *Calyx* simple or imbricate, oblong. *Style* long and semi-bifid. *Receptacle* naked. *Pappus* pilose, or more commonly scabrous. *Seed* smooth and glandular, quinquestriate. *Nuttall.*

Of this numerous genus, comprising not less than thirty species within the limits of the United States, most of which probably possess analogous medical properties, *E. perfoliatum* alone now holds a place in our national Pharmacopœia, *E. purpureum* and *E. teucrifolium* having been discarded at the revision of 1840. They merit, however, a brief notice, if only from their former officinal rank.

Eupatorium purpureum, or *gravel root*, is a perennial herbaceous plant, with a purple stem, five or six feet in height, and furnished with ovate-lanceolate, serrate, rugously veined, slightly scabrous, petiolate leaves, placed four or five together in the form of whorls. The flowers are purple, and consist of numerous florets contained in an eight-leaved calyx. It grows in swamps and other low grounds, from Canada to Virginia, and flowers in August and September. The root has, according to Dr. Bigelow, a bitter aromatic and astringent taste, and is said to be diuretic. Its vulgar name of gravel root indicates the popular estimation of its virtues.

Eupatorium teucrifolium (Willd. *Sp. Plant.* iii. 1753), *E. pilosum* (Walt. *Flor. Car.* 199), *E. verbenæfolium* (Mich. *Flor. Am.* ii. 98), commonly called *wild horehound*, is also an indigenous perennial, with an herbaceous stem, which is about two feet high, and supports sessile, distinct, ovate, acute, scabrous leaves, of which the lower are coarsely serrate at the base, the uppermost entire. The flowers are small, white, composed of five florets within each calyx, and arranged in the form of a corymb. The plant grows in low wet places from New England to Georgia, and abounds in the Southern States. It is in flower from August to November. The whole herb is used. In sensible properties it corresponds with *E. perfoliatum*, though less bitter and disagreeable, and has been used for similar purposes and in like manner. *E. incarnatum* and *E. aromaticum* are said to contain an aromatic principle similar to if not identical with coumarin, obtained by Guibourt from *Coumarouna odorata*, or Tonka bean. (See *P. J. Tr.*, Oct. 1874, 303.) *E. Cannabinum*, of Europe, the root of which was formerly used as a purgative, and *E. Aya-Pana*, of Brazil, the leaves of which at one time enjoyed a very high reputation, have fallen into neglect. The *aya-pana* is an aromatic bitter, like *E. perfoliatum*, but weaker,

* The name of Wahoo or Waahoo (pronounced *wawhoo*) was given to it by the Indians. The same name has also been applied to *Ulmus alata*, of the Southern States, and has thus led to mistakes.

and is said to be still occasionally met with in European commerce. (*A. J. P.*, 1887, 154.) *E. villosum* is used in Jamaica, under the name of *bitter-bush*, in the preparation of beer, as a tonic, and as a stimulant in low zymotic diseases. (*P. J. Tr.*, Oct. 1866; *A. J. P.*, 1887, 155.) *E. collinum* is included in the Mexican Pharmacopœia.

Eupatorium perfoliatum. Willd. *Sp. Plant.* iii. 1761; Bigelow, *Am. Med. Bot.* i. 33; Barton, *Med. Bot.* ii. 125. *Thoroughwort*, or *boneset*, is an indigenous perennial plant, with numerous herbaceous stems, which are erect, round, hairy, from two to five feet high, simple below, and trichotomously branched near the summit. "Leaves opposite, united at base, lanceolate, from four to six inches (10 to 15 cm.) long, tapering, crenately serrate, rugosely veined, rough above, downy and resinous-dotted beneath; flower-heads corymbed, numerous, with an oblong involucre of lance-linear scales, and with from ten to fifteen white florets, having a bristly pappus in a single row." *U. S.* The leaves serve to distinguish the species at the first glance. They may be considered either as perforated by the stem, *perfoliate*, or as consisting each of two leaves, joined at the base, *connate*. In the latter point of view, they are opposite and in pairs, which decussate each other at regular distances upon the stem; in other words, the direction of each pair is at right angles with that of the pair immediately above or beneath it. They are narrow in proportion to their length, broadest at the base where they coalesce, gradually tapering to a point, serrate, much wrinkled, paler on the under than on the upper surface, and beset with whitish hairs, which give them a grayish green color. The uppermost pairs are sessile, not joined at the base. The flowers are white, numerous, supported on hairy peduncles, in dense corymbs, forming a flattened summit. The calyx, which is cylindrical and composed of imbricated, lanceolate, hairy scales, encloses from twelve to fifteen tubular florets, having their border divided into five spreading segments. The anthers are five, black, and united into a tube, through which the bifid filiform style projects.

This species of Eupatorium inhabits meadows, the banks of streams, and other moist places, growing generally in bunches, and abounding in almost all parts of the United States. It flowers from the middle of summer to the end of October. All parts of it are active; but the herb only is officinal.

It has a faint odor, and a strongly bitter, somewhat peculiar taste. The virtues of the plant are readily imparted to water and alcohol. Mr. W. Peterson found it to contain a peculiar bitter principle, chlorophyll, resin, a crystalline matter of undetermined character, gum, tannin, yellow coloring matter, extractive, lignin, and salts. (*A. J. P.*, xxiii. 210.) Mr. Bickley found also albumen, gallic acid, and signs of volatile oil. (*Ibid.*, xxvi. 495.) Dr. Peter Collier, chemist of the Department of Agriculture, recently submitted it to analysis, finding 18·84 per cent. of bitter extractive, which he considers the constituent of medicinal importance, 2·87 per cent. of an indifferent crystalline substance, obtained from the alcoholic extract, and traces only of a volatile oil. (*Ibid.*, 1879, p. 342.)

George Latin (*A. J. P.*, Aug. 1880) found a glucoside, *eupatorin*, and a crystallizable body of the nature of a wax. O. F. Dana, Jr., obtained 3·80 per cent. of extract with benzin; 4·60 per cent. with ether; 33·80 per cent. with alcohol; 24·80 per cent. with water; 5·80 per cent. with alkali. (*A. J. P.*, 1887, p. 229.)

Medical Properties and Uses. Thoroughwort is tonic, diaphoretic, and in large doses emetic and aperient, and was at one time employed as an antiperiodic. The medicine has also been used as a tonic and diaphoretic in remittent and typhoid fevers. Given in warm infusion, so as to produce vomiting or copious perspiration, at the commencement of catarrh, of influenza, or of that form of muscular rheumatism known as a general cold, it will sometimes abort the attack. As a tonic it is given with advantage in dyspepsia, general debility, and other cases in which the simple bitters are employed. Dr. H. S. Wilkins has found the infusion useful in the expulsion of tapeworm. (*A. J. P.*, 1874, p. 295.)

With a view to its tonic effects, it is best administered in substance, or cold infusion. The dose of the powder is twenty or thirty grains (1·3–1·95 Gm.), that of the infusion a fluidounce (30 C.c.) frequently repeated. (See *Infusum Eupatorii.*)

The aqueous extract has been used with advantage. When the diaphoretic operation is required in addition to the tonic, the infusion should be administered warm, and the patient remain covered in bed. As an emetic and cathartic, a strong decoction, prepared by boiling an ounce with three half pints of water to a pint, may be given in doses of from four fluidounces to a half-pint (118 to 236 C.c.), or more.

Off. Prep. Extractum Eupatorii Fluidum.

EXTRACTA. *Extracts.*

(EX-TRĂC'TA.)

Extraits, *Fr.*; Extrakte, *G.*

Extracts, as the term is employed in the Pharmacopœias, are solid preparations, resulting from the evaporation of the solutions of vegetable principles, obtained either by exposing a dried drug to the action of a solvent, or by expressing the juice from a fresh plant. A distinction was formerly made between those prepared from the infusions, decoctions, or tinctures, and those from the expressed juices of plants, the former being called *Extracta*, the latter *Succi Spissati*; but the distinction has been generally abandoned. There is no such essential difference between these two sets of preparations as to require that they should be separately classed; and something is gained in the simplicity of nomenclature, as well as of arrangement, which results from their union. We shall consider them under the same head, taking care, however, to detail distinctly whatever is peculiar in the mode of preparing each.

The composition of extracts varies with the nature of the vegetable, the character of the solvent, and the mode of preparation. The object is generally to obtain as much of the active principle of the plant, with as little of the inert matter as possible; though sometimes it may be desirable to separate two active ingredients from each other, when their effects upon the system are materially different; and this may be accomplished by employing a menstruum which, while it dissolves one, leaves the other untouched. The proximate principles most commonly present in extracts are gum, sugar, starch, tannin, extractive, coloring matter, salts, and the peculiar principles of plants; to which, when a spirituous solvent is employed, may usually be added resinous substances, fatty matter, and frequently more or less essential oil; gum and starch being excluded when the menstruum is pure alcohol. Of these substances, as well as of others which, being soluble, are sometimes necessarily present in extracts, we have taken occasion to treat under various heads in this commentary. There is one, however, which, from its supposed almost uniform presence in this class of preparations, and from the influence it is thought to exert upon their character, deserves particular consideration in this place. We allude to *extractive*, or, as it is sometimes called, *extractive matter*.

It has long been observed that in most vegetables there is a substance, soluble both in water and alcohol, which, in the preparation of extracts, undergoes chemical change during the process of evaporation, imparting to the liquid, even if originally limpid, first a greenish, then a yellowish brown, and ultimately a deep brown color, and becoming itself insoluble. This substance, originally called *saponaceous matter* by Scheele, afterwards received the more expressive name of *extractive*, derived from its frequent presence in extracts. Its existence as a distinct principle is denied, or at least doubted, by some chemists, who consider the phenomena supposed to result from its presence, as depending upon the mutual reaction of other principles; and, in relation to Peruvian bark, it appears to have been proved that the insoluble matter which forms during its decoction in water is a compound of starch and tannin. A similar compound must also be formed in other cases when these two principles coexist; but they are not always present in the same vegetable, nor can all the changes which have been attributed to extractive be accounted for by their union, even when they are present; so that, until further light is shed on the subject, it is best to admit the existence of a distinct class of substances, which, though not the same in all plants, possess sufficient identity of character to be entitled, like sugars, resins, etc., to a generic name. The most important property of extractive is its disposition to pass, by the influence of atmospheric air at a high temperature, into an insoluble substance. If a vegetable infusion or decoction be evaporated in the open air to the consistence of an extract, then diluted, filtered, and again evaporated, and the process repeated so long as any insoluble matter is formed, the whole of the extractive will be separated from the liquid, while the other ingredients may remain. If chlorine be passed through an infusion or decoction, a similar precipitate is formed with much greater rapidity. The change is usually ascribed to the absorption of oxygen by the extractive, which has, therefore, been called, in its altered condition, oxidized extractive; but De Saussure ascertained that, though oxygen is absorbed during the process, an equal measure of carbonic acid gas is given out, and the oxygen and hydrogen of the extractive unite to form water in such a manner as to leave the principle richer in carbon than it was originally. The name of oxidized extractive is, therefore, obviously incorrect; and Berzelius proposed to substitute for it that of *apotheme*, synonymous with deposit. According to Berzelius, apotheme is not completely insoluble in water, but imparts a slight color to that liquid when cold, and is rather more soluble in boiling water, which becomes turbid upon cooling. It is still more soluble in alcohol, and is freely dissolved by solutions of the alkalies and alkaline carbonates, from which it is precipitated by acids. It has a great tendency, when precipitated from solutions, to unite with other principles, and to carry them along with it; thus acquiring properties somewhat different according to the source from which it is obtained. In this way, also, even when the extractive of a plant is itself medicinally inert, its conversion into apotheme may be injurious by causing a precipitation of a portion of the active principle; and, in practical pharmaceutical operations, this change should always, if possible, be avoided. With these preliminary views, we shall proceed to the consideration of the practical rules necessary to be observed in the preparation of extracts. We shall treat of the subject under the several heads of, 1, the extraction of the soluble principles from the plant; 2, the method of conducting the evaporation; 3, the proper condition of extracts, the changes they are liable to undergo, and the best method of preserving them.

1. *Extraction of the Soluble Principles.*

There are two distinct modes of obtaining, in a liquid state, the principles which we wish to extract; 1, by expression alone; 2, by the agency of a solvent, with or without expression.

1. **By Expression.** This method is applicable to recent vegetables. All plants cannot be usefully treated in this way, as many have too little juice to afford an appreciable quantity upon pressure, and of the succulent a considerable portion do not yield all their active principles with their juice. Succulent fruits, and various acrid and narcotic plants, are proper subjects for this treatment. The plants should be operated upon, if possible, immediately after collection. Mr. Battley, of London, recommended that, if not entirely fresh, they should be revived by the immersion of the stalks in water for twelve or eighteen hours, and those only used which recover their freshness by this management. They should then be cut into pieces, and bruised in a stone mortar till brought to a pulpy consistence. When the plant is not very succulent, it is necessary to add a little water during this part of the process, in order to dilute the juice. After sufficient contusion, the pulp is introduced into a linen or canvas bag, and the liquid parts expressed. Mr. Brande states that light pressure only should be employed; as the extract is thus procured greener, of a less glutinous or viscid consistence, and, in his opinion, more active than when considerable force is used in the expression. (*Practice of Pharmacy.*) The juice thus obtained is opaque and usually green, in consequence of the presence of green wax or chlorophyll, and of a portion of the undissolved vegetable fibre in minute division. By heating the juice to about 71·1° C. (160° F.) the albumen contained in it coagulates, and, involving the chlorophyll and vegetable fibre, forms a greenish precipitate. If the liquid is now filtered, it becomes limpid and nearly colorless, and is prepared for evaporation. The clarification, however, is not absolutely necessary, and is generally neglected. Sometimes the precipitate carries with it a considerable portion of the active principle; in which case it should be subsequently incorporated with the

juice, when reduced by evaporation to the consistence of syrup.* Ether added to the expressed juices of plants enables them to be kept long without injurious change. M. Lepage, of Gisors, France, has kept the juice of belladonna in this way more than ten years, and found it, at the end of that time, to yield an extract, identical in physical, chemical, and physiological properties with that obtained from the fresh juice. If this fact is found to be of general applicability, it will be of considerable importance, as enabling the pharmaceutist to supply himself, at pleasure, with extracts to be relied on, without reference to the season.

2. By Solution. The active principles of dried vegetables can be extracted only by means of a liquid solvent. The menstruum usually employed is either water or alcohol, or a mixture of the two. Water, on account of its cheapness, is always preferred, when circumstances do not strongly call for the use of alcohol. It has the advantage, moreover, that it may be assisted in its action, if necessary, by a higher degree of heat than the latter. Pump water is often unfit for the purpose, in consequence of the quantity of its saline matter, which, in some instances, may exert an unfavorable influence on the active principle, and must always be left in the extract. Rain, river, or distilled water should be preferred. Alcohol is employed when the principles to be extracted are insoluble, or but slightly soluble in water, as in the case of the resins; when it is desirable to avoid in the extract inert substances, such as gum and starch, which are dissolved by water and not by alcohol; when the heat required to evaporate the aqueous solution would dissipate or decompose the active ingredients of the plant, as the volatile oils and the active principle of sarsaparilla; when the reaction of the water itself upon the vegetable principles is injurious; and, finally, when the nature of the substance to be exhausted requires so long a maceration in water as to endanger spontaneous decomposition. The watery solution requires to be soon evaporated, as this fluid rather promotes than counteracts chemical changes; while an alcoholic tincture may be preserved unaltered for an indefinite period. An addition of alcohol to water is sufficient to answer some of the purposes for which the former is preferable; and the employment of both fluids is essential, when the virtues of the plant reside in two or more principles, all of which are not soluble in either of these menstrua. In this case it is usually better to submit the vegetable to the action of the two fluids successively, than of both united. Extracts obtained by the agency of water are called *watery* or *aqueous extracts;* those by means of alcohol, undiluted or diluted, *alcoholic* or *spirituous extracts.* Sometimes the term *hydro-alcoholic* is applied to extracts obtained by the joint agency of alcohol and water.

The method of preparing the solution is not a matter of indifference. The vegetable should be thoroughly bruised, or reduced to a coarse powder, so as to allow the access of the solvent to all its parts, and yet not so finely pulverized as to prevent a ready precipitation of the undissolved and inactive portion. When water is employed, it has been customary to boil the medicine for a considerable time, and if the first portion of liquid does not completely exhaust it, to repeat the operation with successive portions, till the whole of the active matter is extracted. This may be known by the sensible properties of the liquid, and by its influence upon reagents. But the boiling temperature produces the decomposition of many vegetable principles, or at least so modifies them as to render them inert; and the extracts prepared by decoction are usually less efficient than those made with a less degree of heat. From numerous experiments upon extracts, Orfila concluded that their virtues were less in proportion to the heat employed. It has, therefore, been recommended to substitute for decoction the process of maceration, digestion, or hot infusion; in the first of which the liquid acts without heat, in the second is assisted by a moderately increased temperature sustained for a considerable time, and in the third is poured boiling hot upon the vegetable matter, and allowed to stand for a short period in a covered vessel. When the active principles are readily soluble in cold water, *maceration* is often preferable to the other modes, as starch, which is inert, is thus left behind; but in many instances the preparation would spoil before the extraction would be completed. By *digestion*, though the solvent power of water is moderately

* See the process for inspissated juices under Extractum Aconiti, *Br.*, page 603.

increased, the advantage is often more than counterbalanced by the increased disposition to spontaneous decomposition. *Hot infusion*, therefore, is to be preferred where the vegetable does not readily yield its virtues to cold water. It has the advantage, moreover, in the case of albuminous substances, that the albumen is coagulated, and thus prevented from increasing the bulk of the extract, without adding to its virtues. A convenient mode of performing this process, is to introduce the solid material into a vessel with an opening near the bottom temporarily closed, or into a funnel with its mouth loosely stopped, then to pour on the boiling water, and, having allowed it to remain a sufficient length of time, to draw it off through the opening. This operation may be repeated till the water comes away without any obvious impregnation. It is always desirable to obtain the solution in the first place as concentrated as possible, so as to prevent the necessity of long-continued evaporation, which injures the extract. It is better, therefore, to incur the risk, both when decoction and infusion are employed, of leaving a portion of the active matter behind, than to obtain a very weak solution. When successive portions of water are employed, those which are least impregnated should be brought by evaporation to the strength of that first obtained before being mixed with it, as the latter thus escapes unnecessary exposure to heat.

Sometimes the filtering of a turbid infusion or decoction, before evaporation, causes the resulting extract to keep better, by removing substances which, besides undergoing decomposition themselves, may act as a ferment, and thus occasion the decomposition of the active matter of the extract.

When alcohol is employed as a menstruum, the vegetable should be macerated in it for one or two weeks, and care should be taken that the tincture be as nearly saturated as possible. The extraction may be hastened by substituting digestion for maceration; as the moderate heat employed, while it facilitates the action of the alcohol, has in this case no effect in promoting decomposition, and the influence of the atmospheric air may be excluded by performing the process in close vessels. When alcohol and water are both used, it is best, as a general rule, to exhaust the vegetable with each separately, as the two menstrua require different modes of treatment. In whichever of these modes the extraction is effected, it requires the assistance of occasional agitation; and, when the vegetable matter is very porous, and absorbs a large quantity of the solvent, expression must be resorted to.

Acetic acid has been introduced into use as a menstruum in the preparation of extracts. It is supposed to be a better solvent of the active principles of certain substances than either water or alcohol alone. According to Girolamo Ferrari, the acrid narcotics, such as aconite, hemlock, hyoscyamus, and stramonium, yield much stronger extracts with distilled vinegar than with water, and still stronger with alcohol to which strong acetic acid has been added. (*Journ. de Pharm.*, 3e sér., i. 239.) This acid is used in the preparation of the acetic extract of colchicum.

Ether also is now used to a considerable extent in the preparation of certain extracts. Having the property of dissolving volatile oil and resin, and of evaporating at a temperature insufficient to volatilise the oil, it is admirably adapted for the preparation of extracts from those substances, the virtues of which reside in the two principles referred to. An ethereal tincture is first prepared by the process of percolation or displacement, and the ether is then either allowed to escape by spontaneous evaporation, or is distilled off at a very moderate heat. The oleoresinous extracts thus obtained are usually of a thick fluid or semi-fluid consistence. Several of them are now ranked among the officinal preparations, in the U. S. Pharmacopœia, under the title of *Oleoresins*.

The process of *percolation* or *displacement* has in this country been very advantageously applied to the preparation of extracts, both with water and spirituous menstrua. It has the following great advantages: 1, that it enables the soluble principles to be sufficiently extracted by cold water, thereby avoiding the injury resulting from heat in decoction and hot infusion; 2, that it effects the extraction much more quickly than can be done by maceration, thereby not only saving time, but also obviating the risk of spontaneous decomposition; and, 3, that it affords the opportunity of obtaining highly concentrated solutions, thus diminishing the injurious effects of the subsequent evaporation. While thus advantageous, it is less liable in this particular case than in others to the objection of yielding imperfect results if not well performed; for, though an inexpert or careless operator may incur loss by an incomplete exhaustion of the substance acted on, and the extract may be deficient in quantity, it may still be of the intended strength and quality, which is not the case with infusions or tinctures unskilfully prepared upon this plan. In the U. S. Pharmacopœia, all the extracts to which the process is applicable are prepared by percolation, and with merely sufficient previous maceration or digestion to thoroughly soften the extractive. In the British Pharmacopœia, the process is applied, as it were, hesitatingly to a portion of the extracts, and withheld in others to which it seems equally appropriate. The first requisite in performing the process of percolation is to have the drug reduced to the proper degree of fineness. The U. S. Pharmacopœia gives the following directions on the subject.

Fineness of Powder. "The fineness of powder is expressed, in the Pharmacopœia, either by descriptive words (generally so in the case of brittle or easily pulverizable substances), or in terms expressing the number of meshes to a linear inch, in the sieve.

"These different forms of expression correspond to each other as follows:

A *very fine* powder	should pass through a sieve having 80 or more meshes to the linear inch	= No. 80 powder.
A *fine* powder	should pass through a sieve having 60 meshes to the linear inch	= No. 60 powder.
A *moderately fine* powder	should pass through a sieve having 50 meshes to the linear inch	= No. 50 powder.
A *moderately coarse* powder	should pass through a sieve having 40 meshes to the linear inch	= No. 40 powder.
A *coarse* powder	should pass through a sieve having 20 meshes to the linear inch	= No. 20 powder.

"In certain cases, powders of a different degree of fineness (*e.g.*, No. 30, No. 12) are directed to be taken." *U. S.*

Percolation. The officinal directions for this process are as follows. "The process of percolation, or displacement, directed in this Pharmacopœia, consists in subjecting a substance or substances, in powder, contained in a vessel called a percolator, to the solvent action of successive portions of menstruum in such a manner that the liquid, as it traverses the powder in its descent to the recipient, shall be charged with the soluble portion of it, and pass from the percolator free from insoluble matter.

"When the process is successfully conducted, the first portion of the liquid, or percolate, passing through the percolator will be nearly saturated with the soluble constituents of the substance treated; and if the quantity of menstruum be sufficient for its exhaustion, the last portion will be destitute of color, odor, and taste, other than that possessed by the menstruum itself.

"The percolator most suitable for the quantities contemplated by this Pharmacopœia should be nearly cylindrical, or slightly conical, with a funnel-shaped termination at the smaller end. The neck of this funnel-end should be rather short, and should gradually and regularly become narrower toward the orifice, so that a perforated cork, bearing a short glass tube, may be tightly wedged into it from within until the end of the cork is flush with its outer edge. The glass tube, which must not protrude above the inner surface of the cork, should extend from one and one-eighth to one and one-half inch (3 to 4 cm.) beyond the outer surface of the cork, and should be provided with a closely-fitting rubber tube, at least one-fourth longer than the percolator itself, and ending in another short glass tube, whereby the rubber tube may be so suspended that its orifice shall be above the surface of the menstruum in the percolator, a rubber band holding it in position.

"The dimensions of such a percolator, conveniently holding five hundred grammes of powdered material, are preferably the following: Length of body, fourteen inches (36 cm.); length of neck, two inches (5 cm.); internal diameter at top, four inches (10 cm.); internal diameter at beginning of funnel-shaped end, two and one-half inches (6·5 cm.); internal diameter of the neck, one-half inch (12 mm.), gradually reduced at the end to one-fifth of an inch (1 cm.). It is best, constructed of glass, but, unless otherwise directed, may be constructed of a different material.

"The percolator is prepared for percolation by gently pressing a small tuft of cotton into the space of the neck above the cork, and a small layer of clean and dry sand is then poured upon the surface of the cotton to hold it in place.

"The powdered substance to be percolated (which must be uniformly of the fineness directed in the formula, and should be perfectly air-dry before it is weighed) is put into a basin, the specified quantity of menstruum is poured on, and it is thoroughly stirred with a spatula, or other suitable instrument, until it appears uniformly moistened. The moist powder is then passed through a coarse sieve—No. 40 powders and those that are finer requiring a No. 20 sieve, whilst No. 30 powders require a No. 15 sieve for this purpose. Powders of a less degree of fineness usually do not require this additional treatment after the moistening. The moist powder is now transferred to a sheet of thick paper and the whole quantity poured from it into the percolator. It is then shaken down lightly and allowed to remain in that condition for a period varying from fifteen minutes to several hours, unless otherwise directed; after which the powder is pressed, by the aid of a plunger of suitable dimensions, more or less firmly, in proportion to the character of the powdered substance and the alcoholic strength of the menstruum; strongly alcoholic menstrua, as a rule, permitting firmer packing of the powder than the weaker. The percolator is now placed in position for percolation, and, the rubber tube having been fastened at a suitable height, the surface of the powder is covered by an accurately-fitting disk of filtering paper, or other suitable material, and a sufficient quantity of the menstruum poured on through a funnel reaching nearly to the surface of the paper. If these conditions are accurately observed, the menstruum will penetrate the powder equally, until it has passed into the rubber tube and has reached, in this, the height corresponding to its level in the percolator, which is now closely covered to prevent evaporation, and the apparatus allowed to stand at rest for the time specified in the formula.

"To begin percolation, the rubber tube is lowered and its glass end introduced into the neck of a bottle previously marked for the quantity of liquid to be percolated, if the percolate is to be measured, or of a tared bottle, if the percolate is to be weighed; and by raising or lowering this recipient, the rapidity of percolation may be increased or lessened as may be desirable, observing, however, that the rate of percolation, unless the quantity of material taken in operation is largely in excess of the pharmacopœial quantities, shall not exceed the limit of ten to thirty drops in a minute. A layer of menstruum must constantly be maintained above the powder, so as to prevent the access of air to its interstices, until all has been added, or the requisite quantity of percolate has been obtained. This is conveniently accomplished, if the space above the powder will admit of it, by inverting a bottle containing the entire quantity of menstruum over the percolator in such a manner that its mouth may dip beneath the surface of the liquid, the bottle being of such shape that its shoulder will serve as a cover for the percolator.

"When the dregs of a tincture or similar preparation are to be subjected to percolation, after maceration with all or with the greater portion of the menstruum, the liquid portion should be drained off as completely as possible, the solid portion packed in a percolator, as before described, and the liquid poured on, until all has passed from the surface, when immediately a sufficient quantity of the original menstruum should be poured on to displace the absorbed liquid, until the prescribed quantity has been obtained.

"*Modification of the above Process.* Authority is given to employ, in the case of Fluid Extracts, where it is applicable, the process of Repercolation, without change of the initial menstruum." *U. S.*

For an account of Dr. Squibb's process of *Repercolation*, see *Extracta Fluida.*

Some prefer the mode of expression to that of displacement. This also is applicable both to watery and alcoholic menstrua. The substance to be acted upon is mixed with the menstruum, cold or hot according to circumstances; and the mixture is allowed to stand from twelve to twenty-four hours. The liquid part is then filtered off, and the remainder submitted to strong pressure, in a linen bag, by means of a common screw press, or other convenient instrument. Another portion of the menstruum may then be added, and pressure again applied, and, if the substance is not sufficiently exhausted, the same operation may be performed a third time. Frequently only a single expression is required, and very seldom a third. The quantity of menstruum added must vary with the solubility of the principles to be extracted. According to Mohr, the method of expression has the advantages over that of displacement, that it yields solutions of more uniform concentration, that it does not require the materials to be so carefully powdered, or otherwise so skilfully managed, in order to insure favorable results, and finally that it occupies less time.

2. *Mode of Conducting the Evaporation.*

In evaporating the solutions obtained in the modes above described, attention should always be paid to the fact that the extractive matter is constantly becoming insoluble at high temperatures with the access of air, and that other chemical changes are going on, sometimes not less injurious than this, while the volatile principles are expelled with the vapor. The operator should, therefore, observe two rules: 1, to conduct the evaporation at as low a temperature as is consistent with other objects; 2, to exclude atmospheric air as much as possible, and, when this cannot be accomplished, to expose the liquid the shortest possible time to its action. According to Berzelius, the injurious influence of atmospheric air is much greater at the boiling point of water than at a less heat, even allowing for the longer exposure in the latter case; and therefore a slow evaporation at a moderate heat is preferable to the more rapid effects of ebullition. Bearing these principles in mind, we shall proceed to examine the different modes in practice. First, however, it is proper to observe that decoctions generally let fall upon cooling a portion of insoluble matter; and it is a question whether this should be rejected, or retained so as to form a part of the extract. Though it is undoubtedly in many instances inert, as in that of the insoluble tannate of starch formed during the decoction of certain vegetable substances, yet, as it frequently also contains a portion of the active principle which a boiling saturated solution necessarily deposits on cooling, and as it is difficult to decide with certainty when it is active and when otherwise, the safest plan, as a general rule, is to allow it to remain.

The method of evaporation formerly resorted to in the case of aqueous solutions is rapid boiling over a fire. The more quickly the process is conducted, the better, provided the liquid is to be brought to the boiling point; for the temperature cannot exceed this, and the length of exposure is diminished. But, where this method is employed, it should never be continued till the completion of the evaporation; for when most of the water has escaped, the temperature can no longer be kept down to the boiling point, and the extract is burnt. The caution, therefore, should always be observed of removing the preparation from the fire before it has attained the consistence of thick syrup, and completing the evaporation, either by means of a water-bath, or in shallow vessels at a moderate heat. When large quantities of liquid are to be evaporated, it is best to divide them into portions and evaporate each separately; for, as each portion requires less time for evaporation than the whole, it will thus be a shorter time exposed to heat. (*Mohr.*) But the mode of evaporation by boiling is always objectionable, and should be employed only in cases where the principles of the plant are so fixed and unchangeable as to authorise their extraction by decoction.

Evaporation by means of the water-bath, from the commencement of the process, is safer than the plan just mentioned, as it obviates all danger of burning the extract; but, as the heat is not supplied directly from the fire, the volatilization of the water cannot go on so rapidly, and the temperature being nearly the same, when the water-bath is kept boiling, there is greater risk of injurious action from the air. The liquid should be stirred during the process. The use of the steam-bath has become very general in this country; as it requires a smaller consumption of fuel, and the heat imparted to the liquid, while sufficient to evaporate it, is less than 100° C. (212° F.). The apparatus consists of an ordinary boiler, containing water, the vapor of which is conducted through a pipe into the evaporating vessels, communicating with each other by means of iron steam pipes. These vessels have the form of an ordinary copper basin, to the inside of which is riveted a shallow tinned copper evaporating basin, intended to contain the liquid to be evaporated. The vapor from the boiler circulates between these vessels, and the water into which it condenses is allowed to escape through a steam valve attached to the bottom of each vessel. The liquid to be evaporated is first distributed in two or three basins, but, when considerably concentrated, is transferred to a single one, where it is stirred towards the close of the process to hasten the evaporation. The heat applied to the liquid can be easily regulated by the steam valves. An incidental advantage of this apparatus is, that it may be made to afford a large supply of distilled water.

As the heat capable of being applied by a boiling water-bath to the evaporating liquid does not exceed 93·3° C. (200° F.), while that by steam can, by a moderate pressure, be increased to the boiling point or beyond it, the evaporation by the latter agency may be much more rapid than by the former, when the pressure is from ten to twenty pounds to the square inch; so that there is a temptation to raise the heat to a degree seriously injurious to the product. Evaporation, therefore, by steam heat always requires caution, while the water-bath is much less liable to be abused. In this respect, the latter method has the advantage.

A good plan of evaporation, though slow, is to place the liquid in a broad, shallow vessel, exposed in a stove or drying room to a temperature of about 100° F., or a little higher, taking care that the air have free access in order to facilitate the evaporation. This mode is particularly applicable to those cases in which maceration or infusion is preferred to decoction for extracting the active principles. Berzelius says that we may thus usually obtain the extract in the form of a yellowish transparent mass, while extracts prepared in the ordinary way are almost black, and are opaque even in very thin layers. Even when the liquid is boiled at first, the process may often be advantageously completed in this manner. It has been proposed to effect the evaporation at the common temperature, by directing a strong current of air, by means of a pair of smith's bellows, over the surface of the liquid; and, in reference to substances which are injured by heat and not by atmospheric air, the plan will be found useful.

Plans have been proposed and carried into execution for performing evaporation without the admission of atmospheric air. The apparatus for *evaporation in vacuo*, now largely used by manufacturing pharmacists, is well calculated to meet this object, at the same time that, by removing the atmospheric pressure, it enables the water to rise in vapor more rapidly, and at a comparatively low temperature. The method of Barry consists in distilling the liquid into a large receiver, from which the air has been expelled by steam, and in which the vapor is condensed by cold water applied to the surface of the receiver, so as to maintain a partial vacuum. Prof. Redwood modified this process by keeping an air-pump in action during the evaporation, thus removing not only the air, but the vapor as fast as it forms, and maintaining a more complete vacuum than can be done by the condensation of the vapor alone. (*Journ. de Pharm.*, 3e sér., i. 231.)*

* A very ingenious apparatus for evaporating in vacuo on a small scale has been invented by Prof. A. B. Prescott (*A. J. P.*, xlii. 349). Two vessels are required: a small one, for evaporation; a large one, which is best made of copper, and should be so arranged as to be readily heated or refrigerated at will. The two are to be connected by glass tubing, through rubber corks, and into the cork of the evaporating dish is to be set a short straight glass tube with a piece of rubber tubing fitted to it so that it can be tightly closed with a glass rod at will. An ounce or two of

A convenient plan of excluding the air, though it does not at the same time meet the object of reducing the degree of heat, is to distil off the water in close vessels. Berzelius says that this is the best mode of concentration next to that *in vacuo*. Care, however, must be taken that the fire be not too long applied, lest the extract should be burnt. The process should, therefore, be completed by means of the water-bath.

In the concentration of alcoholic solutions, distillation should always be performed; as not only is the atmospheric air thus excluded, but the alcohol is recovered, if not absolutely pure, certainly fit for the purpose to which it was originally applied. Here also the water-bath should be employed, to obviate any possible risk of injury from the fire. When the decoction or infusion and the tincture of the same vegetable have been made separately, they should be separately evaporated to the consistence of syrup, and then mixed together, while they are of such a consistence as to incorporate without difficulty. The object of this separate evaporation is, that the spirituous extract may not be exposed to the degree of heat, or lengthened action of the air, which is necessary in the ordinary mode of concentrating the infusion or decoction.

In every instance, care should be taken to prevent any portion of the extract from becoming dry and hard on the sides of the evaporating vessel, as in this state it will not readily incorporate with the remaining mass. The heat, therefore, should be applied to the bottom and not to the sides of the vessel.

3. *Condition and Preservation of Extracts.*

Extracts are prepared of two different degrees of consistence: soft so that they may be readily made into pills, and hard that they may be pulverized. (See *Abstracta.*) The soft extracts always contain a notable percentage of water; in the case of belladonna and hyoscyamus, this has been found by Mr. Chas. Ekin to be about 20 per cent., and in that of conium 25 per cent. (*P. J. Tr.*, iv. 391.)* In astringent extracts, the evaporation should be carried to dryness. Those obtained from the expressed juices of plants are apt to attract moisture from the air, in consequence of the deliquescent nature of the salts existing in the juice. They are thus rendered softer, and more liable to become mouldy upon the surface. Others, especially such as contain much chlorophyll, harden by time, in consequence of the escape of their moisture; and it not unfrequently happens that small crystals of saline matter are formed in their substance. Most extracts, especially those containing nitrogenous principles, are capable, when left to themselves, of producing nitrates. Prof. John Attfield, of London, has made a chemical examination of the crystals found in numerous extracts, and ascertained that, in a large number, they consisted of chloride of potassium, and, in a comparatively few, of the nitrate

water having been put in the receiver, and the material in the evaporating vessel, a gentle heat is, by means of water, applied to the evaporating vessel, but a strong heat to the receiver. The water in this latter boils furiously, and the vapor escapes through the opened tube in the evaporating vessel. When the water is exhausted the tube is closed and the receiver refrigerated. Of course a vacuum results, and is maintained by the continuous condensation of vapor in the receiver.

* *Yield of Extracts when made by the Officinal Process.* Mr. Francis J. Lammer, Jr., prepared the following extracts according to the direction of the U. S. Pharmacopœia, and determined the percentage yield of the finished product as follows:

Extractum.	Per cent.	Extractum.	Per cent.	Extractum.	Per cent.
Aconiti	12·766	Digitalis	25·5	Malti	44·72
Aloes aquosum	91·54	Euonymi	18·31	Mezerei	7·1
Arnicæ radicis	19·53	Gentianæ	44·6	Nucis vomicæ	6·17
Belladonnæ alcoh	32·23	Glycyrrhizæ purum	25·32	Opii	49·6
Cannabis indicæ	16·56	Hæmatoxyli	5·3	Physostigmatis	6·2
Cinchonæ	26·4	Hyoscyami alcoh	16·64	Podophylli	8·31
Colchici radicis	23·2	Iridis	8·9	Quassiæ	2·24
Colocynthidis	15·135	Juglandis	16·82	Rhei	25·66
" comp	95·77	Krameriæ	8·4	Stramonii	14·62
Conii alcohol	10·73	Leptandræ	15·97	Taraxaci	11·3

A. J. P., 1886, p. 537.

of potassium.* The air, moreover, exercises an unfavorable chemical influence over the softer extracts, which are enfeebled, and ultimately become nearly inert, by the same changes which they undergo more rapidly in the liquid state at an elevated temperature. If an extract be dissolved in water, and the liquid be saturated with common salt or any other very soluble salt of difficult decomposition, the greater part of it will be precipitated, in consequence of the insolubility of this class of substances in saline solutions. The precipitate may be again dissolved in pure water.

At the last revision of the U. S. Pharmacopœia it was not deemed advisable to introduce powdered extracts, containing sugar of milk and standardized, under the name of powdered extracts, for fear that they would be prescribed under the impression that they were 20 or 25 per cent. stronger than the pilular extract, having lost that much moisture. They were therefore given a distinctive name, *Abstracts.* (See *Abstracta.*) There are, however, at present (1882) many powdered extracts in the market, claiming to be of the same strength as the pilular extract, having merely the moisture replaced by some dry inert powder. It is to be feared that in most cases the evaporation of the remaining traces of moisture is accomplished at such a high temperature as seriously to injure the activity of the extract. It is quite common to perceive an empyreumatic odor about them.

Extracts, in order that they may keep well, should be placed in glazed earthenware, glass, or porcelain jars, and completely protected from the access of the air. This may be effected by covering their surface with a layer of melted wax, or with a piece of paper moistened with strong spirit, then closing the mouth of the vessel with a cork, spreading wax or rosin over this, and covering the whole with leather, or a piece of bladder. (*Duncan.*) The dry extracts, being less liable to be affected by atmospheric oxygen, do not require so much care. The application of alcohol to the surface has a tendency to prevent mouldiness. A method of protecting extracts from the action of the air, frequently resorted to, is to cover them closely with oiled bladder; but this, though better than to leave them uncovered, is not entirely effectual. Should the extract become too moist, it may be dried by means of a water-bath; should it, on the contrary, be too dry, the proper consistence may be restored by softening it in the same manner, and incorporating with it a little distilled water. Martin (1880) proposes to preserve extracts in a soft condition by surrounding the vessel containing the extract by another of larger diameter, which is furnished with a tight cover, the space between the two vessels being filled with crystallized sulphate of sodium, which gradually parts with its water of crystallization and prevents the extract from becoming hard and dry.

When extracts which are too soft are subjected to a moderate temperature, fermentation may set in, and E. Cocardas describes the various forms of "Penicillium-ferment" which grow in such extracts, and concludes that the ferment causes them to undergo changes similar to those affected by heat, viz., the absorption of oxygen and disengagement of carbon dioxide. (*P. J. Tr.*, 1886, p. 590.)

Some extracts when powdered have a tendency to cohere again. According to Geiseler, this may be obviated by the addition of sugar of milk or powdered liquorice-root; two or three parts of the former and one part of the latter to one of the extract being sufficient for the purpose. (*Pharm. Centralb.*, 1850, p. 238.) Mohr recommends the following plan of drying and preserving extracts. Take equal parts of powdered liquorice-root and of the extract, rub them well together in a mortar, put the resulting paste into an earthen vessel with a flat bottom, place this in another of iron, a little deeper, containing chloride of calcium thoroughly dried by heat insufficient to melt it; then enclose the whole with a cover fitted to the iron vessel, and allow them to stand for a day or more. When the mixture is quite dry, powder it, and add so much of the powdered root as to make the weight double that of the original extract. (*Ibid.*, p. 119.) This process has been substantially adopted in the new German Pharmacopœia (1882). The old process of using

* Thus, chloride of potassium was detected in the extracts of belladonna, hemlock, sarsaparilla (compound), colchicum seeds, stramonium seeds, and aconite; nitrate of potassium in extracts of belladonna, hyoscyamus, and lettuce; and sulphate of sodium in extract of stramonium seeds. (*P. J. Tr.*, March, 1862, p. 448.)

dextrin as a diluent was found very objectionable, principally on account of the tendency of the extracts to reabsorb moisture. Four parts of extract are now mixed with three parts of finely powdered liquorice-root, and dried in a porcelain capsule at 40°–50° C. (104°–122° F.) until the mixture ceases to lose weight. The mass is then rubbed to powder, and sufficient powdered liquorice-root added to make the whole weigh eight parts, or double the weight of extract used. In our opinion this method is not so good as that adopted for abstracts. The German powdered extracts are always half the strength of the extracts, no relation whatever with the drug is established, and the variations in the yield of extract from different drugs has been repeatedly shown to be great. Kirchmann proposes exsiccated sodium sulphate as a diluent instead of dextrin, liquorice-root, etc. (*Phar. Zeitung*, 1881, p. 116.) W. Stromeyer has found sugar to answer very well as an addition to too moist narcotic extracts. It is necessary, however, that the extract be not exposed to a heat of over 112° F., else it remains soft. (*A. J. P.*, 1872, pp. 300, 353.)

The plan of incorporating a little glycerin with extracts has been adopted in the formulas of the present U. S. Pharmacopœia. By its unchangeable liquid character it keeps the extract soft, so that it can be readily made into pills, and exercises also a favorable influence through its chemical properties. It is preferable to add a definite weight of the glycerin to the pilular extract. If added to the menstruum, owing to the variation in the yield of extracts from plants, some samples would be too soft, and at another time, in the case of a large yield of extract, the quantity of glycerin would be insignificant.

Extracts from recent plants should be prepared at the season when the plant is medicinally most active; and a good rule is to prepare them once a year.*

EXTRACTA FLUIDA. *Fluid Extracts.*

(EX-TRĂC′TA FLŬ′I-DA.)

Extracta Liquida, *Br.*; Extraits liquides, *Fr.*; Flüssige Extrakte, *G.*

These were first introduced into the U. S. Pharmacopœia of 1850, as a distinct class of preparations; the fluid extract of sarsaparilla being the only one previously directed, either in our own officinal code, or by the British Colleges. Since then they have increased so rapidly in favor that at the present time seventy-seven are officinal, and in addition large quantities of non-officinal fluid extracts are annually produced. They are now perhaps the most important class of liquid preparations in use. Their distinctive character is the concentration of the active ingredients of medicinal substances into a small bulk, in the liquid form, a cubic centimetre or fluigramme of any one of them now representing a gramme of the crude drug. Independently of the greater convenience of administration, the advantage of this class of preparations is that, the evaporation not being carried so far as in the ordinary extracts, the active principles are less liable to be injured by heat. Formerly the main difficulty, in relation to them, was the liability of substances in the liquid state to undergo spontaneous decomposition. In the Pharmacopœia of 1850 this was counteracted by means of sugar and of alcohol, but in 1865 (*A. J. P.*, 1865, p. 50) Mr. Alfred B. Taylor proposed the use of glycerin, and in the revision of the Pharmacopœia for 1870 his suggestion was adopted. Glycerin, while it exerts a powerful preservative influence, possesses the very valuable property of dissolving matters which were deposited by some of the fluid extracts when made with sugar, as in the old officinal recipes. Consequently these fluid extracts were much clearer

* M. Lepage, of Gisors, gives the following method of testing the quality of the narcotic extracts, and determining whether they contain any of the alkaloids to which they owe their efficiency. Take a gramme (15·5 grs.) of the extract, dissolve it in twice its weight of distilled water, introduce the solution into a test-tube, and add from 25 to 30 centigrammes (4 or 5 grs.) of powdered bicarbonate of potassium. When effervescence has ceased, add to the mixture 5 or 6 times its bulk of pure ether, cork the tube, and shake briskly three times in 2 or 3 minutes. Then let the mixture rest; and, when the ether has become transparent, decant, and allow it to evaporate spontaneously. Dissolve the residue in 6 or 8 grammes (f℥iss to f℥ij) of water, acidulated with a drop or two of hydrochloric acid. If the extract be good, the solution will be rendered very turbid by a few drops of a solution of the double iodide of mercury and potassium, and will give a flocculent precipitate with solution of tannic acid. (*Journ. de Pharm.*, Mai, 1863, p. 362.) The test is applicable to the extracts of aconite, belladonna, hyoscyamus, and conium.

and more elegant preparations than were the old ones. Subsequent experience with these fluid extracts has shown that the use of glycerin should be circumscribed, and that it was employed too freely in the formulas of the fluid extracts of the last Pharmacopœia. The solvent powers of glycerin are so great that the fluid extracts were frequently loaded with many inert principles, which it dissolved, giving them a dense, rich appearance without increasing their activity. As the primary object of fluid extracts is concentration, suitable menstrua should in each case be selected with the single object of dissolving and retaining permanently the active constituents of the drug. In order to do this, many experiments are necessary to determine which is the most suitable menstruum, and each drug must be separately and individually studied. Whilst the formulas for the fluid extracts in the U. S. Pharmacopœia of 1880 show a great improvement in this respect over all others, ten years' experience will demonstrate the necessity of further changes. The relative strength adopted at the last revision differs from that formerly used, and will doubtless elicit considerable criticism. An exception is made here to the usual rule followed in the Pharmacopœia of constructing all formulas in parts by weight. Although there is no difficulty in making fluid extracts of such strength that one troyounce should represent one troyounce of the drug, the Committee of Revision believed it to be better to substitute measure for weight here, not only on account of the greater convenience of measuring the reserved portion, but also because of there being less variation in strength from the fluid extracts of 1870.

The present fluid extracts are just *five per cent. weaker* than those formerly officinal, and are based upon the theory that from a given weight of drug an amount of fluid extract shall be made equal in measure to the bulk of the same weight of distilled water; in other words, the relation of gramme to cubic centimetre.* Many will prefer to use weights and measures that they have been accustomed to; in such cases, to make 20 *fluidounces* of fluid extract 19 *troyounces* of drug will be required, whilst if avoirdupois weight is preferred, which it doubtless will be, the most convenient relation to recollect will be that 50 *avoirdupois ounces* are required to make 48 *fluidounces*, or *three pints* of fluid extract. The general formula for the preparation of fluid extracts does not differ materially from that formerly officinal; the length of time required for maceration has been judiciously reduced, whilst the quantity reserved has been generally slightly increased, although the formulas are not uniform in this respect. The fact cannot escape observation, that there has been a close study of the solubilities, physical properties, and individuality of each drug, whilst uniformity amongst the formulas has not been sought for, so much as the best method of producing the fluid extract. The general formula may be expressed as follows. 100 Gm. of the powdered drug is moistened with a certain quantity of menstruum, packed in a suitable percolator, and enough menstruum added to saturate the powder and leave a stratum above it; the lower orifice of the percolator is closed when the liquid begins to drop, and the percolator is closely covered to prevent evaporation and permit maceration for a specified time; additional menstruum is poured on and percolation continued until the drug is exhausted. Usually from seven- to nine-tenths of the first portion of the percolate is reserved, and the remainder evaporated to a soft extract; this is to be dissolved in the reserved portion, and enough menstruum added to make the fluid extract measure 100 C.c. The precipitation experienced heretofore when the evaporated weak percolate was added to the reserved portion is considerably diminished by causing the former to be evaporated to a soft extract. This precipitation, formerly noticed more particularly in alcoholic fluid extracts, was due to the greater volatility of the alcohol in the weak percolates, which, when evaporated, left the residue to a great extent

* The following table shows the relation of the crude drug to the fluid extract when made by the process of the U. S. Pharmacopœias of 1880 and 1870:

Weight of Drug.	*Measure of Fluid Extract.*	
	Pharm. 1880.	Pharm. 1870.
100 grammes of drug make	100 C.c.	94·9 C.c.
100 troyounces of drug make	105·3 fluidounces.	100 fluidounces.
100 avoirdupois ounces of drug make	96 fluidounces.	91·1 fluidounces.

aqueous; when this was added to the strongly alcoholic reserved portion, a precipitation of resinous and frequently active matter took place, which necessitated the storing of the fluid extract until precipitation ceased, and subsequent filtration. This is almost altogether avoided by evaporating to a soft extract, and the loss of activity through precipitation thus greatly diminished.

A useful distillatory apparatus has been contrived by Prof. Jos. P. Remington for recovering alcohol from weak percolates, and for general pharmaceutical uses. The still shown in the cut is the new form. It is made of tinned copper, the still body holding about three gallons; the condenser has seven straight tubes surrounded with the cold water introduced by a rubber tube from a hydrant or bucket of water placed higher than the still, and carried off as it becomes warmed by another tube as indicated by the arrows. By the siphon arrangement shown in the cut, it is possible to feed the still from a reservoir, whilst distillation is in progress, thus using a three-gallon still where a much larger one would have been necessary. The joints are carefully ground, and troublesome lutes and water-joints are entirely superseded. The condenser having straight tubes, instead of a spiral one, is easily cleaned, and is powerful enough to condense a gallon of alcohol in thirty minutes.

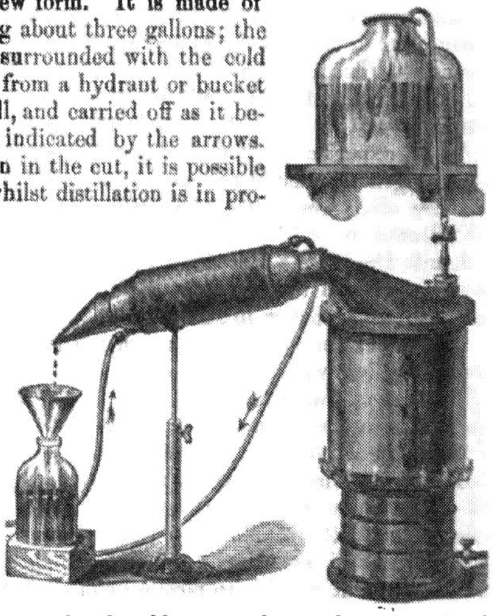

The still may be set into a kettle partly filled with water and thus used as a water-bath, or a shallow tinned-copper dish with flat rim, which accompanies the still, may be placed between the two brass ring bands and clamped securely. (*A. J. P.*, May, 1879.)

For valuable papers on percolation and fluid extracts, by Prof. Procter, Dr. Squibb, Alonzo Robbins, and others, see *Proc. A. P. A.*, 1859, p. 265; 1863, p. 222; *A. J. P.*, 1878, pp. 209, 329; 1873, pp. 85, 189.

Several methods have been suggested for preparing fluid extracts more economically. The most important is the plan of repercolation, as proposed by Dr. E. R. Squibb, to this class of preparations as well as to the dry extracts.

Repercolation. In consequence of the existing high price of alcohol, it is important to adopt some plan by which, while the ends aimed at are attained, the consumption of the menstruum used in percolation may be diminished. This object has been accomplished, to a considerable extent, by Dr. E. R. Squibb, of Brooklyn, N. Y., by a modification of the process of percolation to which he has given the name at the head of the present paragraph. As defined by the author, repercolation consists in the successive application of the same percolating menstruum to fresh portions of the substance to be percolated. The result is that the same menstruum, acting repeatedly on unexhausted portions of the substance, becomes concentrated to the greatest possible extent; so that much of the menstruum is saved, while subsequent evaporation is avoided, which is itself an object of great importance in the preparation of extracts. It is obvious that repercolation is not applicable to the preparation of infusions, decoctions, tinctures, etc., in which the object in general is less a high degree of concentration than precision in the strength of the preparation, and consequently in the dose. It is to the extracts and fluid extracts that the process is peculiarly adapted, and there now remains no doubt whatever of the great value of the improvement. One of its disadvantages is that the substance treated is less completely exhausted than when the proceeding is inverted, and fresh portions of menstruum are made to act on the same material until the latter is deprived of all its soluble matter. But the loss in this way is trifling, compared with the gain when a menstruum as high-priced as alcohol is at the present time, is employed. Another practical disadvantage is the inconvenience of keeping the weak percolates, as these have to be labelled, numbered, and stored away for use until the same operation is repeated. In deciding when to adopt it, the operator will of course be influenced by the relative value of the drug and the menstruum. In order to secure the most favorable results in repercolation, certain methods of proceeding are advisable in various steps of the process, differing with the character of the substance to be acted on; and these can be determined only by a careful study, confirmed by repeated experiment. Dr. Squibb uses repercolation exclusively on the large scale in the manufacture of extracts and fluid extracts, and has applied it especially to the preparation of fluid extract of cinchona; and since his first paper, which was reproduced in the 14th revision of the U. S. Dispensatory, p. 1164, he has introduced several improvements, which are intended to make the process useful to the apothecary in his every-day work. By presenting in a note below an abstract of his plan of proceeding in this case, with the accompanying explanations, we can more forcibly impress on the mind of the pharmaceutical student the lessons applicable to the case than by a general description.*

* *Dr. Squibb's Process for Extract of Cinchona by Repercolation,* revised and improved (1878): "Take of Yellow Cinchona, in powder No. 50, 32 parts; Stronger Alcohol, sp. gr. ·819, 2 parts; Glycerin, sp. gr. 1·250, 1 part; Water, 2 parts, or a sufficient quantity of menstruum.

"Weigh the Stronger Alcohol, Glycerin, and Water in succession, in any convenient quantity at a time, into a tared bottle, and mix them thoroughly for a menstruum.

"Moisten 8 parts of the Cinchona with 8 parts of the menstruum, by thoroughly mixing them, and allow the mixture to stand 8 hours in a closely covered vessel. Then pass the moist powder through a No. 8 sieve, and pack it firmly in a percolator. Pour menstruum on top until the mass is filled with liquid and a stratum remains on top unabsorbed; cover the percolator closely and macerate for 48 hours. Then arrange the percolator for an automatic supply of menstruum, and start the percolation at such a rate as to give 1 part of percolate in about 4 hours. Reserve the first 6 parts of percolate and continue the percolation until the Cinchona is exhausted, separating the percolate received after the reserved portion into fractions of about 8 parts each.

"Moisten a second portion of 8 parts of the Cinchona with 8 parts of the weak percolate,—the first portion that was obtained next after the reserved percolate,—and allow the moist powder to stand for 8 hours in a vessel closely covered. Then pack it moderately in a percolator, and supply the percolator automatically with the remaining fractions of the weak percolate in the order in which they were received, and finally with fresh menstruum until the Cinchona is exhausted. Percolate in the same manner and at the same rate as with the first portion of Cinchona, and, reserving 8 parts of the first percolate, separate the weaker percolate into fractions of about 8 parts each.

"Percolate the third and fourth portions of 8 parts each of the Cinchona in the same way as the second portion.

"Finally mix the four reserved percolates together to make 30 parts of finished fluid extract; and having corked, labelled, and numbered the bottles containing the fractions of weak percolate, set them away until the process for Cinchona is to be resumed.

"When this fluid extract is to be again made, repeat the process as with the second portion, and reserve 8 parts of the first percolate as finished fluid extract from each 8 parts of Cinchona from that time forward so long as the fractions of weak percolate are carried forward with which to commence each operation."

Dr. Squibb draws the following deductions, which, although they have reference to the fluid extracts of the U. S. P. 1870, yet they apply in some respects to the new officinal preparation:

"First, that the present formulas and processes for percolation (U.S. 1870) are so defective that the relation to the drug which they profess is not practically accurate either as to quality or quantity, and therefore that a better process is greatly needed.

"Second, that the process by repercolation, though it has some grave disadvantages, and is liable to defects in practice, yet gives far better results both in quality and quantity of product; while it is not difficult in practice except by comparison with the delusive simplicity of the former processes; and therefore that repercolation is better adapted to pharmacopœial uses as a model or standard process than any which has yet been tried.

"Third, that repercolation may be used on a scale as small as 4 or 8 ounces, by great care and skill, but is not very successful with less than an avoirdupois pound of material for each percolation.

"Fourth, that powders for percolation should not be finer than No. 60 for hard compact substances, nor coarser than No. 40 for more loose and spongy substances,—with a few special exceptions.

"Fifth, that the menstruum should be so adjusted as to dissolve out the medicinal principles with the least practicable disturbance of their natural relations to each other and to the extractive matters whereby they are rendered soluble and permanent. Next that the menstruum should contain the smallest practicable proportion of alcohol; and glycerin only when absolutely necessary, as in Cinchonas. By repercolation the exhaustion is never less than 90 per cent. and perhaps rarely more than 97 per cent. of the total soluble matter.

"Sixth, that the powder be moistened with as much liquid as it can be made to hold and yet pass through a No. 8 sieve; that it be not tightly packed; and that it be well macerated before starting the percolation.

"Seventh, that the rate of percolation be uniform and very slow. At first, for the reserved portion, the percolate in 24 hours should not exceed the weight of the powder; nor need the rate be

The plan of Mr. N. Spencer Thomas consists in exposing the substance to be acted on to successive expressions, by means of a press, with the menstruum divided

slower than to obtain the weight of the powder in 48 hours, although as a general rule the slower the rate the better the results. After the reserved portion the rate may be increased gradually so that the last portion be received in about 6 hours. The separate portions of weak percolate should not exceed the weight of the powder.

"Eighth, that a good practical exhaustion requires—as a general rule—for the first percolation, with fresh menstruum, that the total percolates should weigh 3·5 times the weight of the powder. That for the second percolation or first repercolation, the weight should be 4·5 times that of the powder. And for all subsequent repercolations the weight should be 5, 6, or 7 times that of the powder, according to the nature of the substance percolated, and the skill and care with which the process is managed.

"Ninth, that the relation of weight for weight, instead of minim for grain, should be established under proper controlling conditions: but that, unless properly guarded in the quality and moisture of the drug used, the new relation is liable to be even more inaccurate than the old, because, the poorer the quality of the drug the less dense will be the percolates, and the greater will be the volume for the prescribed weight, and this involves the serious difficulty that, when the fluid extract is made by weight but administered by measure, the poorer the drug from which it was made, the smaller, as well as the weaker, the dose will be.

"Tenth, that some good practical method of comparing fluid extracts by a standard is very much needed; and that for such drugs as Cinchona, a method of arithmetical dilution would be easy and practical if well worked out."

Dr. Squibb has devised an ingenious siphon percolator whereby the rapidity of the flow of the percolate may be controlled.

The accompanying illustration shows a convenient way of applying the principles involved in the siphon percolator to the glass percolator in common use. The cut is so plain and so easily

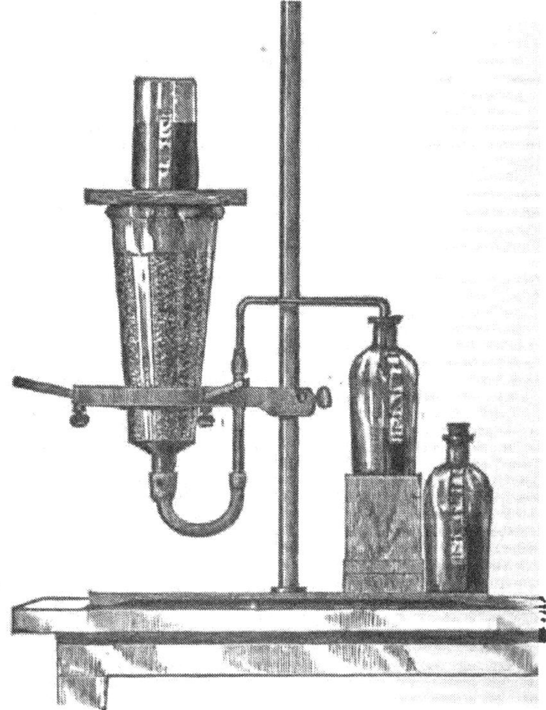

Scale, one-sixth of the actual linear size.

understood that it needs but little explanation. The percolator is shown in the position of having been stopped for the night lest the receiving bottle should be filled beyond the proper mark. The siphon here is made in two parts, one end of the upper part being telescoped within a larger piece

into different portions; so that fresh portions of liquid are brought to act on the same solid body in different stages of exhaustion; and then mixing the expressed liquids. The due proportion between the weight of the medicine and the bulk of the ultimate fluid extract is secured by regulating the measure of the last-added portion of menstruum, which, in the process as described by Mr. Thomas, is the third. Whatever may be the advantages of this method, and it is not without its recommendations, it is liable to the objections of loss of alcohol through exposure during expression, and of being patented. (*A. J. P.*, 1866, p. 219.)

Another method of limiting the quantity of alcohol used, has been proposed by Mr. S. P. Duffield, of Detroit. It consists in macerating, for from six to ten days, the medicine to be acted on, previously deprived, by means of a vacuum apparatus, of all the air, and of all readily volatilizable matter contained in its pores, with a certain volume of the menstruum, which is forced through a tube into the vacuum pan by atmospheric pressure, and thus brought into the most intimate contact with all parts of the powder. The process is completed by submitting the mass thus impregnated to hydraulic pressure, and, after allowing the liquid to settle in glass carboys, drawing off the clear liquid into bottles. It is only by experience that the value of this process can be determined. (*Ibid.*, Jan. 1869, p. 2.) It is obviously inapplicable to substances whose virtues depend in any considerable degree upon readily volatilizable constituents. Mr. Campbell (*A. J. P.*, xlii. 17) has proposed a method for doing away with the use of heat, which, however, although in some cases it may do well, cannot be relied upon for the complete exhaustion of all drugs. In carrying it out, mix with sixteen troyounces of the powder four to six fluidounces of the menstruum (usually alcohol), and pack it in a glass funnel moderately but uniformly tight, a piece of sponge having previously been put in the beak of the funnel; then cover the surface of the powder with a disk of paper, and pour on twelve fluidounces of menstruum. When the sponge becomes saturated, cork tightly the beak of the funnel, and set the whole aside for four days, at the end of which time the percolation may be allowed to proceed. Mr. James W. Mill has called attention to the advantage of separating the powder into fine and coarse parts by means of sieves and packing the finer powder at the bottom.

H. Biroth (*Pharmacist*, April, 1877) proposes the method which he terms "*insuccation*," for making non-alcoholic fluid extracts; the advantages claimed for it are simplicity and economy. Sixteen troyounces of the drug, cut, crushed, or whole, are placed in a stone jar or tin percolator. Eight fluidounces of glycerin mixed with

of glass tubing, and the junction made tight by a short section of rubber tubing through which the smaller tube is free to slide. During maceration, or when the percolation is arrested, the upper part of the siphon is drawn up until the liquid will no longer flow over into the bottle, and the height at which this column of liquid ceases to flow over is a measure of the comparative density of the liquid within and without. As seen in the cut, the liquid will not flow over into the bottle although the column is several inches short of the height of the liquid in the percolator. But as exhaustion progresses and the liquid in this column becomes less dense, its counterbalancing height becomes greater, until finally, when the powder is exhausted and the liquid within and without is of the same density, the column rises to the level of the liquid within the percolator, minus the friction and capillarity. When the percolation is to be started, the siphon is simply pushed down through the rubber until the liquid flows over, and then the rate is established by carefully raising or lowering the siphon. This sliding joint for varying the length of this column of liquid at will being understood, the other details are plain enough, whilst the charging and the general management are the same as in the smaller and larger percolators.

The powder, moistened with great care and uniformity, is packed loosely, firmly, or very firmly, according to its nature or condition, with the square end of a stick, say ·8 inch = 2 mm. diameter. As a rule, the largest practicable proportion of liquid should be used in moistening the powder, because then the powder occupies the smallest space in the percolator, requires the loosest packing, and is saturated for the maceration by the smallest additional quantity of liquid, and therefore gives the most concentrated first percolate for the reserve, and secures the most rapid exhaustion by the smallest quantity of liquid. A disk of filtering paper is placed on the surface of the powder, of such size that the edge is reflected up against the glass. A disk of board, card-board, or better of thick sheet rubber, with a central hole 1·5 inches = 37 mm. in diameter, is used for a cover. A stratum of liquid, maintained at a uniform thickness of ·25 inch = 6 mm., should cover the powder from first to last, so that it may not drain and contract, or admit air; and this is best maintained by an inverted bottle of the supply liquid, as shown in the cut. The length of the neck and mouth of such bottle may be conveniently elongated when needed, so as to regulate the depth of the stratum of liquid above the powder, by stretching over it a short section of rubber tubing in the manner shown in the cut.

four pints of boiling water are poured upon the drug and allowed to "insuocate," or macerate, for twenty-four hours, the liquid poured off, and the residue treated with four pints more of boiling water as before. The decanted liquors are mixed, strained, and evaporated by means of a water-bath to one pint and filtered. It is obvious that this process is adapted to a very limited number of drugs, and it is equally certain that the resulting preparation is not entitled to the name of fluid extract, as it is understood in this country; boiling water and glycerin are not effective as general solvents for thoroughly exhausting many drugs; a better name would be "concentrated infusions."

Prof. J. U. Lloyd proposes to recover the alcohol which remains absorbed by the residue after percolation by mixing the wet residues with an equal bulk or less of dry sawdust, and then percolating this with water. (*A. J. P.*, June, 1877.)

Wm. M. Thomson, of Philadelphia, has lately devised a very complete method of preparing fluid extracts on a large scale; the principles of his process are maceration and percolation *in vacuo*, and although the principles which have been applied have been long known, and similar apparatus used by Duffield and others, there are many useful practical points which merit a notice in detail. The percolators are egg-shaped, and made of tinned copper; they are capable of being tightly covered, and communicate by means of stopcocks above and below, and iron and stout rubber tubing, with a very efficient double-acting air-pump. The moistened powder is packed tightly in the percolator, and the cover securely bolted on. The stopcock in the cover is now opened, which communicates with the air-pump and a partial vacuum created in the space above the moistened drug; the stopcock is now closed and another stopcock in the cover opened, which communicates by a tube with the reservoir containing the menstruum. The menstruum, of course, quickly penetrates the powder, taking the place of the interstitial air, and when the powder is saturated, it is permitted to macerate *in vacuo* a sufficient length of time. To start percolation, a receiver is connected with the beak of the percolator, and, the air being exhausted from it, the percolate at once makes its appearance. When the flow slackens, if desired, air may be forced by the pump in the space above the powder, and the receiver again exhausted below. In this way it can be seen that entire control of these powerful physical forces may be secured. The advantages are very apparent in preventing the loss of volatile principles and alcohol, whilst protecting from chemical change caused by exposure to the air. It is quite possible to make many officinal fluid extracts without recourse to subsequent evaporation of weak percolate. For a cut of this apparatus, see *A. J. P.*, 1882, p. 237; or *Amer. Pharmacist*, 1882, p. 11.

In order to carry out the strictly alphabetical arrangement now adopted in the U. S. Pharmacopœia, it will be necessary in this commentary to deviate from the plan heretofore used of treating of the Extracts and Fluid Extracts in separate classes. Whilst the wisdom of adopting this course on the part of the Committee of Revision of the Pharmacopœia may be open to question, it is obviously the duty of the commentator to follow the authority.

☞ IMPORTANT. As before noted, the quantity of drug selected for the practical alternative formula is in the case of fluid extracts *fifty avoirdupois ounces*, the end product being *three pints;* the relative proportions of the various menstrua, ingredients, etc., are of course retained, and in each case are preceded by the word "or," and the alternative quantities always enclosed in brackets.

EXTRACTUM ACONITI. *U.S., Br.* *Extract of Aconite.*

(EX-TRĂC'TUM ĂC-O-NĪ'TĪ.)

Extract of Aconite Root; Extrait de Racine d'Aconit, *Fr.;* Eisenhutknollen-Extrakt, *G.*

"Aconite, in No. 60 powder, *one hundred parts* [or sixteen ounces av.]; Tartaric Acid, *one part* [or seventy grains]; Glycerin, Alcohol, each, *a sufficient quantity*. Moisten the powder with *forty parts* [or seven and a half fluidounces] of Alcohol in which the Tartaric Acid has previously been dissolved, and pack it firmly in a cylindrical glass percolator; then add enough Alcohol to saturate the powder and leave a stratum above it. When the liquid begins to drop from the percolator, close the lower orifice, and, having closely covered the percolator, macerate for forty-eight hours. Then allow the percolation to proceed, gradually adding Alcohol, until *three hundred parts* [or three and a half pints] of tincture are obtained, or the Aconite is exhausted. Reserve the first *ninety parts* [or fifteen and a half fluidounces] of the percolate, evaporate the remainder in a porcelain capsule, at a temperature not exceeding 50° C. (122° F.), to *ten parts* [or one and a half fluidounces], add the reserved portion, and evaporate at or below the above-mentioned temperature, until an extract of a pilular consistence remains. Lastly, weigh the Extract and thoroughly incorporate with it, while still warm, *five per cent.* of Glycerin." *U. S.*

"Take of the fresh Leaves and Flowering Tops of Aconite *one hundred and twelve pounds* [avoirdupois]. Bruise in a stone mortar, and press out the juice; heat it gradually to 130° F. (54°·4 C.), and separate the green coloring matter by a calico filter. Heat the strained liquor to 200° F. (93°·3 C.) to coagulate the albumen, and again filter. Evaporate the filtrate by a water-bath to the consistence of a thin syrup; then add to it the green coloring matter previously separated and passed through a hair-sieve, and stirring the whole together assiduously, continue the evaporation at a temperature not exceeding 140° F. (60° C.), until the extract is of a suitable consistence for forming pills." *Br.*

The extract from the fresh leaves of aconite was abandoned in the U. S. Pharmacopœia in 1870 in favor of one made by means of alcohol from the dried plant, probably because the plant was not generally cultivated in this country. But the *present preparation is very much stronger* than either; aconite root having been substituted for the leaves, which are no longer officinal, and alcohol for diluted alcohol as a menstruum. It is greatly to be regretted that the title of this Extract is not Extractum Aconiti Radicis; there will be likely to be three extracts of Aconite in use, of varying strengths,—*i.e.*, the present officinal alcoholic extract made from the root, the former hydro-alcoholic extract made from the leaves, and the English extract made from the fresh leaves. When serious changes are made in powerful preparations, great care should be taken to draw as much attention to the alteration as possible. The use of tartaric acid is in accordance with the views of Duquesnel and C. R. Alder Wright. (See *Abstractum Aconiti.*) The exhaustion of the aconite in the U. S. process is indicated by the absence of its peculiar taste in the liquid which passes. To save the alcohol at the low temperature at which the evaporation is directed, would require the aid of a vacuum apparatus. The attempt to save the alcohol by ordinary distillation would imply an elevation of the heat above that officinally ordered, and thus endanger the decomposition of the active principle of the aconite; and views of economy should never be allowed to interfere with the efficiency of medicines. It will be perceived that, in the British process, not the leaves only but the flowering tops also are used, as experience has shown that these are at least equally efficient. The process consists essentially in the evaporation of the expressed juice; and the product, therefore, ranks with inspissated juices.

In relation to the preparation of this extract, as well as of all others derived from the expressed juices of narcotic plants, the following summary of the plan pursued by Mr. Battley, an experienced apothecary of London, may be of service. Having passed the expressed juice through a fine hair sieve, he places it immediately upon the fire. Before it boils, a quantity of green matter rises to the surface, which in some plants is very abundant. This is removed by a perforated tin dish, and preserved. It ceases to appear soon after the liquid begins to boil. The boiling is continued till rather more than half the fluid has been evaporated, when the decoction is poured into a conical pan and allowed to cool. An abundant dark green precipitate forms, from which the supernatant liquid is poured off; and this, having been reduced one-half by a second boiling, is again allowed to stand. The precipitate which now falls is less green than the first. The remaining fluid is once more placed over the fire, and allowed to boil till it assumes the consistence of syrup, when it is removed. The matter at first collected by skimming, together with that precipitated, is now incorporated with it, and the whole placed in a metallic pan, and by means of a water-bath evaporated to the consistence of an extract. In the latter part of the process, care is necessary to prevent the extract from hardening on the sides of the vessel, as it thus loses its fine green color, and becomes proportionately feeble.

The superiority of this plan over a continuous boiling is, that the portions of active matter which are deposited at different stages of the process are subjected for a shorter time to heat than if allowed to remain in the liquor, and are consequently less deteriorated. The matter which coagulates before the fluid boils is chiefly albumen, embracing portions of chlorophyll and of the undissolved vegetable fibre. It might probably be thrown away without diminishing the virtues of the extract; but as chlorophyll, though itself inactive, has often associated with it a portion of the active principle, it is the most economical plan to incorporate it with the other matters, and, besides, its presence in the mass is said to render it easier to be worked into pills. Mr. Brande states that one cwt. of fresh aconite yields about five pounds of extract. According to Geiger, one pound yields an ounce and a half. For a method of assaying Extract of Aconite by Beckhurts, see *Pharm. Era*, 1887, p. 447.

In the process of the British Pharmacopœia, it will be perceived that a discrimination is made between the chlorophyll and albumen; the former, which coagulates at 54·4° C. (130° F.), being at first separated in order to prevent the continuous action of heat upon it, and afterwards added to the extract; the latter, coagulating at 93·3° C. (200° F.), is separated and rejected. The rejection of the albumen is altogether advisable, as it is not only inert, but renders the extract more liable to decomposition. The chlorophyll is retained for the reasons stated in the preceding paragraph, and also to give a greenish color to the extract, which has come to be associated in general opinion with its goodness of quality.

If made from recently dried leaves, which have not yet been impaired by time, the extract officinal in 1870 was a good preparation of aconite; and it was believed to be more powerful, and to keep better, than the inspissated juice. According to Prof. Schroff, of Vienna, it had four times the strength of that preparation. The dose is half a grain or a grain (0·03 to 0·065 Gm.), to be gradually increased if necessary. The alcoholic extract of U. S. P. 1880 is stronger, and may be given in the dose of one-sixth or one-quarter of a grain (0·01 to 0·016 Gm.), to be gradually increased until its effects are experienced; and it would be well to specify on prescription (*U. S. P.*, 1880) when that preparation is desired.

When properly prepared, the British extract has a greenish brown color, with a disagreeable narcotic odor, and the acrid taste of the plant. It may be given in the dose of one or two grains (0·065 to 0·13 Gm.), night and morning, to be gradually increased till the system is affected. Twenty grains (1·3 Gm.) or more have been given in the course of a day.

EXTRACTUM ACONITI FLUIDUM. *U. S. Fluid Extract of Aconite.*

(ĔX-TRĂC'TŬM ĂC-Ọ-NĪ'TĪ FLŪ'Ị-DŬM.)

Fluid Extract of Aconite Root; Extrait liquide de Racine d'Aconit, *Fr.;* Flüssiges Eisenhutknollen-Extrakt, *G.*

"Aconite, in No. 60 powder, *one hundred grammes* [or fifty ounces av.]; Tartaric Acid, *one gramme* [or half an ounce av.]; Alcohol, *a sufficient quantity*, To make *one hundred cubic centimeters* [or three pints]. Moisten the powder with *forty grammes* [or twenty-three fluidounces] of Alcohol in which the Tartaric Acid has previously been dissolved, and pack it firmly in a cylindrical glass percolator; then add enough Alcohol to saturate the powder and leave a stratum above it. When the liquid begins to drop from the percolator, close the lower orifice, and, having closely covered the percolator, macerate for forty-eight hours. Then allow the percolation to proceed, gradually adding Alcohol, until the Aconite is exhausted. Reserve the first *ninety cubic centimeters* [or forty-three fluidounces] of the percolate, and evaporate the remainder in a porcelain capsule, at a temperature not exceeding 50° C. (122° F.), to a soft extract; dissolve this in the reserved portion, and add enough Alcohol to make the Fluid Extract measure *one hundred cubic centimeters* [or three pints]." *U. S.*

This is a new officinal preparation of Aconite-root; it will be found useful as a basis for making the other preparations of Aconite—the abstract, plaster, extract, tincture, or liniment. This fluid extract is of a bright deep reddish brown color;

it may be given internally in doses of one-half to one minim (0·03 to 0·06 C.c.), but on account of its very powerful character should always be used with caution, beginning with the smallest dose. It will doubtless be frequently employed as an addition to liniments for obtaining the peculiar effects of aconite.

EXTRACTUM ALOES AQUOSUM. *U. S.* *Aqueous Extract of Aloes.*

(EX-TRĂC'TŬM ĂL'O-ĒS A-QUŌ'SŬM—ą-kwō'sŭm.)

Extrait d'Aloès, *Fr.*; Aloe-Extrakt, *G.*

"Aloes, *one hundred parts* [or sixteen ounces av.]; Boiling Distilled Water, *one thousand parts* [or ten pints]. Mix the Aloes with the Water in a suitable vessel, stirring constantly, until the particles of Aloes are thoroughly disintegrated, and let the mixture stand for twelve hours; then pour off the clear liquor, strain the residue, mix the liquids, and evaporate to dryness by means of a water or steam bath." *U. S.*

This is a new officinal, and the process is based upon the British formulas for extract of Barbadoes aloes and Socotrine aloes, which are treated of in the two articles following this. With a purified aloes officinal, the necessity for this preparation is not obvious. An extract made with cold distilled water is officinal in the German Pharmacopœia, as is also the vitriolated extract, "*Extractum Aloes Acido Sulfurico Correctum*," made by suspending eight parts of extract of aloes in thirty-two parts of distilled water, adding drop by drop one part of pure sulphuric acid, and evaporating in a porcelain vessel to dryness; the dose is from two to ten grains (0·13–0·65 Gm.).

EXTRACTUM ALOES BARBADENSIS. *Br.* *Extract of Barbadoes Aloes.*

(EX-TRĂC'TŬM ĂL'O-ĒS BĂR-BA-DĔN'SIS.)

Extrait d'Aloès de Barbades, *Fr.*; Barbadoes Aloe-Extrakt, *G.*

"Take of Barbadoes Aloes, in small fragments, *one pound* [avoirdupois]; Boiling Distilled Water *one gallon* [Imperial measure.] Add the Aloes to the Water, and stir well until they are thoroughly mixed. Set aside for twelve hours; then pour off the clear liquid, strain the remainder, and evaporate the mixed liquors by a current of warm air to dryness." *Br.*

The revised direction, to evaporate "by a current of warm air" instead of by a water-bath, is in accordance with the views of Robert Aiken, who believes that prolonged exposure to heat converts the extractive into inert resinous matter. (*P. J. Tr.*, 1882, p. 501.) The dose of this extract is two to six grains (0·13–0·4 Gm.).

EXTRACTUM ALOES SOCOTRINÆ. *Br.* *Extract of Socotrine Aloes.*

(EX-TRĂC'TŬM ĂL'O-ĒS SŎC-O-TRĪ'NÆ.)

Extrait d'Aloès sucotrin, *Fr.*; Socotora Aloe-Extrakt, *G.*

This is prepared precisely as the Extract of Barbadoes Aloes.

The object of these processes is to separate from Aloes the resinoid matter, the *apotheme* of Berzelius, which is supposed to irritate the bowels, without possessing purgative properties; but the truth appears to be that, when deprived of a small portion of adhering extractive, this matter is quite inert. It cannot, therefore, injuriously affect the virtues of the medicine; and, as it exists in comparatively small proportion, and during the process a part of the extractive becomes insoluble, the preparation may be considered as at best unnecessary. The dose of the purified aloes is from two to ten grains (0·13 to 0·65 Gm.).*

Off. Prep. Br. Decoctum Aloes Compositum; Extractum Colocynthidis Compositum.

* *Glycerate of Aloes. Glycerole of Aloes.* Under the latter name, M. Chausit brought to the notice of the profession a preparation consisting of an alcoholic extract of aloes dissolved in glycerin. Mr. Haselden prepared this in the following method. Macerating half an ounce of aloes in four fluidounces of alcohol until dissolved, he filtered the tincture through bibulous paper, evaporated it to the consistence of molasses, and, while it was still warm, added enough glycerin to make four fluidounces. Finding that the aloes was wholly dissolved, with the exception of a little

EXTRACTUM ANTHEMIDIS. *Br.* *Extract of Chamomile.*

(ĘX-TRĂC'TŲM ĄN-THĔM'Į-DĬS.)

Extrait de Camomille romaine, *Fr.;* Extractum Chamomillæ Romanæ; Römisch-Kamillen-Extrakt, *G.*

"Take of Chamomile Flowers *one pound* [avoirdupois]; Oil of Chamomile *fifteen minims;* Distilled Water *one gallon* [Imperial measure]. Boil the Chamomile with the Water until the volume is reduced to one-half, then strain, press, and filter. Evaporate the liquor by a water-bath until the extract is of a suitable consistence for forming pills, adding the Oil of Chamomile at the end of the process." *Br.*

According to Mr. Brande, one cwt. of dried chamomile flowers affords upon an average 48 pounds of extract.

This extract has a deep brown color, with the bitter taste and aroma of chamomile. It much better represents the chamomile than did the old Edinburgh extract, which, being obtained by decoction and inspissation, contained none of the volatile oil of the plant. In the present British process, care is taken not only to avoid boiling, but also to supply any possible loss of oil during the cautious evaporation, by the addition of a small portion near the close of the process. The extract may be given for the same purpose as the flowers, but is most used as a vehicle for other tonics in the pilular form. The dose is from two to ten grains (0·13 to 0·65 Gm.). An extract may be prepared having the peculiar flavor as well as bitterness of chamomile, by macerating the flowers in water, and evaporating the infusion *in vacuo.*

EXTRACTUM ARNICÆ RADICIS. *U.S.* *Extract of Arnica Root.*

(ĘX-TRĂC'TŲM ÄR'NĮ-ÇÆ RĄ-DĪ'CĬS.)

Extrait de Racine d'Arnique, *Fr.;* Arnika-Extrakt, *G.*

"Arnica Root, in No. 60 powder, *one hundred parts* [or sixteen ounces av.]; Glycerin, Diluted Alcohol, each, *a sufficient quantity.* Moisten the powder with *forty parts* [or six and a half fluidounces] of Diluted Alcohol, and pack it firmly in a cylindrical percolator; then add enough Diluted Alcohol to saturate the powder and leave a stratum above it. When the liquid begins to drop from the percolator, close the lower orifice, and, having closely covered the percolator, macerate for twenty-four hours. Then allow the percolation to proceed, gradually adding Diluted Alcohol, until *three hundred parts* [or three pints] of tincture are obtained, or the Arnica Root is exhausted. Reserve the first *ninety parts* [or fourteen fluidounces] of the percolate; evaporate the remainder to *ten parts* [or two fluidounces] at a temperature not exceeding 50° C. (122° F.), mix the residue with the reserved portion, and evaporate at or below the above-mentioned temperature to a pilular consistence. Lastly, weigh the Extract and thoroughly incorporate with it, while still warm, *five per cent.* of Glycerin." *U.S.*

This extract differs from the extract formerly officinal, in being made from the root in place of the flowers; it very well represents the virtues of arnica, and is a convenient form for its administration. The dose is from three to five grains (0·20 to 0·33 Gm.). But the chief employment of the extract is in the preparation of the plaster. (See *Emplastrum Arnicæ.*)

EXTRACTUM ARNICÆ RADICIS FLUIDUM. *U.S.* *Fluid Extract of Arnica Root.*

(ĘX-TRĂC'TŲM ÄR'NĮ-ÇÆ RĄ-DĪ'CĬS FLŪ'Į-DŬM.)

Extrait liquide de Racine d'Arnique. *Fr.;* Flüssiges Arnicawurzel-Extrakt, *G.*

"Arnica Root, in No. 60 powder, *one hundred grammes* [or fifty ounces av.];

impurity, he concluded that the spirit might very well be dispensed with, and the aloes used directly in the process. Accordingly he proposes to substitute the following method. Mix well in a mortar half an ounce of Socotrine aloes, in fine powder, and four fluidounces of glycerin; transfer the mixture to a bottle, and agitate occasionally for several days; if the aloes be not now dissolved, heat for fifteen minutes by a water-bath, and strain through linen to separate impurities. The resulting liquid is of a bright mahogany color, and of the consistence of glycerin. The preparation has been recommended as an external remedy in lichen agrius and the excoriations of eczema, applied by means of a camel's-hair brush. (*P. J. Tr.*, 1859, p. 322.) For the mode of preparing *a fluid extract of aloes* with the aid of glycerin, by Prof. Procter, see *Proc. A. P. A.*, 1863, p. 240.

Diluted Alcohol, *a sufficient quantity*, To make *one hundred cubic centimeters* [or three pints]. Moisten the powder with *forty grammes* [or twenty fluidounces] of Diluted Alcohol, and pack it firmly in a cylindrical percolator; then add enough Diluted Alcohol to saturate the powder and leave a stratum above it. When the liquid begins to drop from the percolator, close the lower orifice, and, having closely covered the percolator, macerate for forty-eight hours. Then allow the percolation to proceed, gradually adding Diluted Alcohol, until the Arnica Root is exhausted. Reserve the first *ninety cubic centimeters* [or forty-three fluidounces] of the percolate, and evaporate the remainder, at a temperature not exceeding 50° C. (122° F.), to a soft extract; dissolve this in the reserved portion, and add enough Diluted Alcohol to make the Fluid Extract measure *one hundred cubic centimeters* [or three pints]." *U. S.*

This is one of the new officinal fluid extracts; it is of a clear, reddish brown color, possessing little odor, and having an acrid taste. It well represents the virtues of the root, and will probably be used as a basis for preparing the extract when wanted for the plaster. The dose, if desired for internal administration, would be from five to ten minims (0·3–0·6 C.c.).

EXTRACTUM AROMATICUM FLUIDUM. *U. S.* *Aromatic Fluid Extract.*

(EX-TRĂC′TUM ĂR-O-MĂT′I-CŬM FLŪ′I-DŬM.)

Extrait liquide aromatique, *Fr.;* **Flüssiges Aromatisches Extrakt,** *G.*

"Aromatic Powder, *one hundred grammes* [or fifty ounces av.]; Alcohol, *a sufficient quantity*, To make *one hundred cubic centimeters* [or three pints]. Moisten the powder with *thirty-five grammes* [or twenty fluidounces] of Alcohol, and pack it firmly in a cylindrical percolator; then add enough Alcohol to saturate the powder and leave a stratum above it. When the liquid begins to drop from the percolator, close the lower orifice, and, having closely covered the percolator, macerate for forty-eight hours. Then allow the percolation to proceed, gradually adding Alcohol, until the Aromatic Powder is exhausted. Reserve the first *eighty-five cubic centimeters* [or forty fluidounces] of the percolate, and evaporate the remainder to a soft extract; dissolve this in the reserved portion, and add enough Alcohol to make the Fluid Extract measure *one hundred cubic centimeters* [or three pints]." *U. S.*

This is another new officinal fluid extract; it is an excellent aromatic in concentrated form, and will be found very useful not only as an addition to liquids when an aromatic is desired, but its concentrated form will permit its use in small quantities with dry powders like pepsin, subnitrate of bismuth, etc., when desired for administration. It will probably be rarely used alone, but may be given in the dose of ten to twenty minims (0·6–1·25 C.c.), diluted with water, or dropped on sugar.

EXTRACTUM AURANTII AMARI FLUIDUM. *U. S.* *Fluid Extract of Bitter Orange Peel.*

(EX-TRĂC′TUM ÂU-RĂN′TI-Ī A-MĀ′RĪ FLŪ′I-DŬM—âw-răn′shē-ī.)

Extrait liquide d'Écorce d'Oranges amères, *Fr.;* **Flüssiges Pomeranzenschale-Extrakt,** *G.*

"Bitter Orange Peel, in No. 40 powder, *one hundred grammes* [or fifty ounces av.]; Alcohol, Water, each, *a sufficient quantity*, To make *one hundred cubic centimeters* [or three pints]. Mix *two parts* of Alcohol with *one part* of Water [or four and a half pints of alcohol and two pints of water], and, having moistened the powder with *thirty-five grammes* [or nineteen fluidounces] of the mixture, pack it moderately in a conical percolator; then add enough of the menstruum to saturate the powder and leave a stratum above it. When the liquid begins to drop from the percolator, close the lower orifice, and, having closely covered the percolator, macerate for forty-eight hours. Then allow the percolation to proceed, gradually adding menstruum, until the Orange Peel is exhausted. Reserve the first *eighty cubic centimeters* [or thirty-eight fluidounces] of the percolate, and evaporate the remainder, at a temperature not exceeding 50° C. (122° F.), to a soft extract; dissolve this in the reserved portion, and add enough menstruum to make the Fluid Extract measure *one hundred cubic centimeters* [or three pints]." *U. S.*

This is another new officinal fluid extract; it will be found useful as a tonic; the bitter orange peel having very little oil present in its dry condition, there is necessarily very little agreeable orange flavor to the fluid extract. Monroe Bond recommends a *Fluid Extract of Sweet Orange Peel*, made with a menstruum of seven parts of alcohol and one of glycerin. (*A. J. P.*, 1873, p. 482.) It is simply a concentrated pure bitter tonic, and may be given in doses of fifteen to thirty minims (0·9–1·9 C.c.).

EXTRACTUM BELÆ LIQUIDUM. *Br.* *Liquid Extract of Bael.*

(ĔX-TRĂC'TŬM BĒ'LÆ LĬQ'-UĬ-DŬM—lĭk'wĭ-dŭm.)

Extrait liquide de Bael, *Fr.;* Flüssiges Bael-Extrakt, *G.*

"Take of Bael Fruit *one pound* [avoirdupois]; Distilled Water *twelve pints* [Imperial measure]; Rectified Spirit *three fluidounces*. Macerate the Bael for twelve hours in one-third of the Water; pour off the clear liquor; repeat the maceration a second and third time for one hour in the remaining two-thirds of the Water; press the marc; and filter the mixed liquors through flannel. Evaporate to thirteen fluidounces; and, when cold, add the Rectified Spirit." *Br.*

This is an officinal of the British Pharmacopœia, of which very little is known in the United States. It is one of the forms in which the India remedy bael is employed, and the reader is referred to the article on that subject. Each fluidounce of the extract represents an avoirdupois ounce of the medicine, and the dose is from one to two fluidrachms (3·75–7·5 C.c.).

EXTRACTUM BELLADONNÆ. *Br.* *Extract of Belladonna*

(ĔX-TRĂC'TŬM BĔL-LA-DŎN'NÆ.)

Extrait de Belladone, *Fr.;* Tollkirschen-Extrakt, *G.*

This extract made from the fresh leaves was formerly recognized by the U. S. Pharmacopœia, but was very properly abandoned in the last revision. It has been supplanted of late years by the alcoholic extract, which has been proved to be much more reliable.

The British Pharmacopœia takes the "fresh leaves and young branches of Belladonna," and prepares the Extract from them in the same manner precisely as Extract of Aconite. (See *Extractum Aconiti.*)

The U. S. Pharmacopœia of 1870 directed the extract to be prepared from the leaves of the plant, the British from the leaves and young branches. The latter direction was probably based on experiments by Mr. Squire, of London, who found that an extract prepared from the soft herbaceous parts of the plant generally, including leaves, flowers, and young stalks, not only has a better consistence, and is less apt to become mouldy by keeping, than that made from the leaves exclusively, but is more effectual in the same quality. (*P. J. Tr.*, 1861, p. 300.) There is little doubt of the accuracy of these results. It is probable that these remarks are as applicable to other extracts prepared from fresh leaves as to that of belladonna, at least in relation to perennial plants.

From the experiments of MM. Solon and Soubeiran, it appears that, in relation to this extract, the insoluble matter separated from the expressed juice by filtering, and that coagulated by heat, are nearly if not quite inert; so that advantage results from clarifying the juice by these means before evaporating it. So far as the albumen is concerned, there can be no doubt of the accuracy of this statement; but it is questionable whether the same remark is applicable to the chlorophyll which first separates, and which is reserved in the British process. (See *Extractum Aconiti.*) Mr. Brande states that one cwt. of fresh belladonna yields from 4 to 6 pounds of extract. According to M. Recluz, nearly ten parts may be obtained from one hundred. The best extract is brought chiefly from England; but Mr. Alfred Jones has found that it may be prepared of equally good quality from the plant grown in the United States. (*A. J. P.*, xxiv. 108.) It has usually a dark brown color, a slightly narcotic not unpleasant odor, a bitterish taste, and a soft consistence which it long retains. Asparagin has been found in this extract. (*Journ. de Pharm.*, xxi. 178.)

Its medical properties and uses have been detailed under the head of Belladonna.

The dose of the extract is uncertain on account of its variable strength. The best plan is to begin with one-quarter or one-half of a grain (0·016 or 0·03 Gm.), repeated two or three times a day, and gradually to increase the dose till the effects of the medicine are experienced. To a child two years old not more than one-twelfth of a grain (0·005 Gm.) should be administered at first.

EXTRACTUM BELLADONNÆ ALCOHOLICUM. *U. S., Br.*

Alcoholic Extract of Belladonna.

(ĔX-TRĂC'TŬM BĔL-LA-DŎN'NÆ ĂL-CO-HŎL'I-CŬM.)

Extrait de Belladone alcoolique, *Fr.;* Spirituöses Tollkirschen-Extrakt, *G.*

"Belladonna Leaves, in No. 60 powder, *one hundred parts* [or sixteen ounces av.]; Alcohol, *two hundred parts* [or two pints and four fluidounces]; Water, *one hundred parts* [or one pint]; Glycerin, Diluted Alcohol, each, *a sufficient quantity.* Mix the Alcohol and Water, and, having moistened the powder with *forty parts* [or seven fluidounces] of the mixture, pack it firmly in a cylindrical percolator, then add enough of the menstruum to saturate the powder and leave a stratum above it. When the liquid begins to drop from the percolator, close the lower orifice, and, having closely covered the percolator, macerate for forty-eight hours. Then allow the percolation to proceed, gradually adding, first, the remainder of the menstruum, and then Diluted Alcohol, until *three hundred parts* [or three pints] of tincture are obtained, or the Belladonna Leaves are exhausted. Reserve the first *ninety parts* [or fourteen fluidounces] of the percolate, evaporate the remainder, at a temperature not exceeding 50° C. (122° F.), to *ten parts* [or two fluidounces]; mix the residue with the reserved portion, and evaporate at or below the above-mentioned temperature to a pilular consistence. Lastly, weigh the Extract, and thoroughly incorporate with it, while still warm, *five per cent.* of Glycerin." *U. S.*

"Take of Belladonna Root, in No. 20 powder, *one pound* [av.]; Rectified Spirit, Distilled Water, of each, *a sufficiency.* Mix the Belladonna with *two pints* [Imp. meas.] of the Spirit, and macerate in a closed vessel for forty-eight hours; then transfer to a percolator, and when the fluid ceases to pass, continue the percolation with water until *two pints* [Imp. meas.] of liquid have been collected. Evaporate the percolated liquid by a water-bath until the extract has acquired a suitable consistence." *Br.* The British Pharmacopœia introduced in the 1885 revision for the first time an alcoholic extract of belladonna, but it differs from the U. S. extract in being made from the root instead of the leaves; this would render the British extract the stronger of the two. The absence of chlorophyll in an extract made from the root would make ointments, cerates, plasters, etc., made from it deficient in the characteristic green color so much prized, and would probably lead to its rejection for a time, but there can be no question of the greater uniformity in strength of the root.* For a method of assaying Extract of Belladonna, by Beckurts, see *Pharm. Era*, 1887, p. 447.

* *Standard Extract of Belladonna.* This preparation has been proposed by Prof. Dunston and Ransom as a type of a class of standardized solid extracts having a definite alkaloidal strength; whilst resembling an extract, it has the advantage over it of being based upon a certain percentage of alkaloid instead of that of representing a given amount of a variable drug. "Take of belladonna root, in No. 20 powder, 1 pound; rectified spirit, 48 fluidounces; distilled water, 12 fluidounces. Mix the spirit with the water. Macerate the belladonna in 2 pints of this mixture for forty-eight hours, agitating occasionally; then transfer to a percolator, and when the fluid ceases to pass continue the percolation with the remainder of the diluted spirit. Afterwards subject the contents of the percolator to pressure, filter the product, mix the liquids, and measure the exact volume of the mixture (a). Estimate the alkaloidal nature of this solution by the following method. Evaporate 50 C.c. of the liquid over a water-bath with a gentle heat until all the alcohol is dispelled. Dissolve the extract thus obtained in about 5 C.c. of warm distilled water, acidulated with a few drops of diluted hydrochloric acid; filter, if necessary, through a small fragment of cotton-wool; pour into a stoppered glass separator, and add ammonia until the solution is distinctly alkaline. Agitate for a few minutes with 5 C.c. of chloroform, separate, and again wash the aqueous liquid with 3 C.c. of chloroform. Agitate the mixed chloroformic solutions with 5 C.c. of diluted hydrochloric acid, separate, again wash with 3 C.c of the diluted acid, mix the acid solutions, render alkaline with ammonia, and agitate with 5 C.c. of chloroform. After separation wash the alkaline solution with 3 C.c. of chloroform, mix the chloroformic solutions, evaporate in a dish of known weight, and dry the residue, which should be nearly colorless at a temperature of 200° F. (93° C.). The weight of the residue thus obtained multiplied by 2 will give the parts by weight of the alka-

The formula for this extract does not differ essentially from that officinal in the former revision; it is a good preparation, and is officinal in the French Codex. It is much used externally. Thus, in rigidity of the os uteri, it is applied at intervals to the neck of the uterus, mixed with simple ointment in the proportion of one drachm to an ounce; but care must be taken not to affect the system too powerfully; and the preparation, therefore, should be used in a small quantity at first. In irritability of the bladder, chordee, spasm of the urethra, and painful constriction of the rectum, it may either be rubbed in the form of ointment upon the perineum, along the urethra, etc., or may be used in the form of enema; but care is requisite not to introduce it too freely into the bowel. It is sometimes smeared upon the bougie, mixed with oil, in the treatment of stricture of the urethra. In the form of ointment it has been beneficially employed in phimosis and paraphimosis, and in that of plaster or ointment, in local neuralgic or rheumatic pains. (See *Emplastrum Belladonnæ.*) For internal use, the dose to begin with is one-fourth of a grain (0·016 Gm.).

Off. Prep. Unguentum Belladonnæ.

Off. Prep. Br. Emplastrum Belladonnæ; Unguentum Belladonnæ.

EXTRACTUM BELLADONNÆ FLUIDUM. *U.S.* *Fluid Extract of Belladonna.*

(EX-TRĂC'TUM BĔL-LA-DŎN'NÆ FLŪ'I-DŬM.)

Extrait liquide de Racine de Belladone, *Fr.;* Flüssiges Tollkirschenwurzel-Extrakt, *G.*

"Belladonna Root, in No. 60 powder, *one hundred grammes* [or fifty ounces av.]; Alcohol, *a sufficient quantity,* To make *one hundred cubic centimeters* [or three pints]. Moisten the powder with *thirty-five grammes* [or twenty fluidounces] of Alcohol, and pack it firmly in a cylindrical percolator; then add enough Alcohol to saturate the powder and leave a stratum above it. When the liquid begins to drop from the percolator, close the lower orifice, and, having closely covered the percolator, macerate for forty-eight hours. Then allow the percolation to proceed, gradually adding Alcohol, until the Belladonna Root is exhausted. Reserve the first *ninety cubic centimeters* [or forty-three fluidounces] of the percolate, and evaporate the remainder, at a temperature not exceeding 50° C. (122° F.), to a soft extract; dissolve this in the reserved portion, and add enough Alcohol to make the Fluid Extract measure *one hundred cubic centimeters* [or three pints]." *U. S.*

This fluid extract was formerly officinal under the name of *Extractum Belladonnæ Radicis Fluidum,* and it is to be regretted that this name was not continued, as both the root and leaves of the plant are officinal, and it had become an established custom, when the part of this plant was not specified, to understand that the leaf was wanted. We now have the extract made from the leaves and the fluid extract made from the root, yet called respectively extract and fluid extract of belladonna. The fluid extract of the root is a good preparation, of reddish brown color, very different in appearance from the fluid extract of the leaves which is often seen in the market, and which is of a deep green color. It may be given internally in doses of one or two minims (0·06–0·12 C.c.).

Off. Prep. Linimentum Belladonnæ.

EXTRACTUM BRAYERÆ FLUIDUM. *U.S.* *Fluid Extract of Brayera.*

(EX-TRĂC'TUM BRĀY-E'RÆ FLŪ'I-DŬM.)

Fluid Extract of Kousso; Extrait liquide de Kousso, *Fr.;* Flüssiges Kosso-Extrakt, *G.*

"Brayera, in No. 40 powder, *one hundred grammes* [or fifty ounces av.]; Alco-

loids in 100 fluid parts of the liquid. The exact volume of the liquid being known, and the strength having been thus ascertained, the total amount of alkaloid present therein can be calculated. Evaporate to dryness over a water-bath, and add sufficient sugar of milk to make the mixed product exactly fifty times the weight of the total alkaloid found to have been present in the liquid (a), allowing for that quantity which was used for the estimation. Mix intimately, powder as quickly as possible in a dry atmosphere, and transfer at once to a well-stoppered bottle. This extract will contain 2 per cent. of total alkaloid." (*P. J. Tr.,* 1887, p. 844.)

hol, a *sufficient quantity*. To make *one hundred cubic centimeters* [or three pints]. Moisten the powder with *forty grammes* [or twenty-three fluidounces] of Alcohol, and pack it firmly in a cylindrical percolator; then add enough Alcohol to saturate the powder and leave a stratum above it. When the liquid begins to drop from the percolator, close the lower orifice, and, having closely covered the percolator, macerate for forty-eight hours. Then allow the percolation to proceed, gradually adding Alcohol, until the Brayera is exhausted. Reserve the first *ninety cubic centimeters* [or forty-three fluidounces] of the percolate; by means of a water-bath, distil off the Alcohol from the remainder, and evaporate the residue to a soft extract; dissolve this in the reserved portion, and add enough Alcohol to make the Fluid Extract measure *one hundred cubic centimeters* [or three pints]." *U. S.*

This is a new officinal fluid extract, and, although possessing a very disagreeable bitter taste, well represents the activity of kousso; the bitter resinous principle upon which the anthelmintic virtues are now believed to depend is readily extracted by alcohol. This preparation should be of a dark green color; the objection to it is the large dose and the considerable quantity of strong alcohol which the patient gets; as it is best to give the remedy fasting, the stimulating action of the alcohol would be apt to be apparent. The dose is from a half to one fluidounce (15–30 C.c.). An extract made by evaporating the fluid extract spontaneously would be a good preparation, and the objection to the alcohol could be thus overcome.

EXTRACTUM BUCHU FLUIDUM. *U. S.* *Fluid Extract of Buchu.*

(ĔX-TRĂC'TŬM BŪ'CHŪ FLŪ'Ĭ-DŬM—bū'kū.)

Extrait liquide de Bucco, *Fr.*; Flüssiges Bucco-Extrakt, *G.*

"Buchu, in No. 60 powder, *one hundred grammes* [or fifty ounces av.]; Alcohol, Water, each, *a sufficient quantity*, To make *one hundred cubic centimeters* [or three pints]. Mix *two parts* of Alcohol with *one part* of Water [or four and a half pints of alcohol and two pints of water], and, having moistened the powder with *thirty grammes* [or one pint] of the mixture, pack it firmly in a cylindrical percolator, then add enough of the menstruum to saturate the powder and leave a stratum above it. When the liquid begins to drop from the percolator, close the lower orifice, and, having closely covered the percolator, macerate for forty-eight hours. Then allow the percolation to proceed, gradually adding menstruum, until the Buchu is exhausted. Reserve the first *eighty-five cubic centimeters* [or forty fluidounces] of the percolate, and evaporate the remainder to a soft extract; dissolve this in the reserved portion, and add enough menstruum to make the Fluid Extract measure *one hundred cubic centimeters* [or three pints]." *U. S.*

This fluid extract has been greatly improved by lessening the alcoholic strength of the menstruum. After having ordered a stronger alcoholic menstruum for twenty years, the Pharmacopœia now adopts the menstruum originally suggested by Prof. I. J. Grahame as long ago as 1859. (See *A. J. P.*, 1859, p. 349.) It has been abundantly proved by experience that the weaker menstruum effectually exhausts buchu of its virtues, whilst there is no doubt of its superiority when the fluid extract is an ingredient in an aqueous mixture.

In consequence of the peculiar structure of the leaves, it is somewhat difficult to powder them in a mortar, and it will be convenient to resort to a mill for the purpose. As the most active ingredient of buchu is volatile, the direction in the formula to set aside the first portion of tincture obtained, which is a highly concentrated solution, is peculiarly important; for, if it were subjected to evaporation, much of the volatile oil would necessarily escape. The tincture subsequently obtained probably contains a large proportion of the fixed ingredients of the leaves, and will, therefore, allow of concentration without material loss.

This fluid extract is clear, greenish black, and possessed in a high degree of the sensible properties of the leaves. It acquires the odor of mint when long kept, showing that some change takes place in its volatile oil. This fluid extract affords the best means at our command for the exhibition of buchu. It is often combined with Liquor Potassæ with excellent results. The dose is thirty minims to a fluidrachm (1·9–3·8 C.c.), to be given diluted with water three to five times a day.

EXTRACTUM CALAMI FLUIDUM. *U.S.* *Fluid Extract of Calamus.*

(ĔX-TRĂC'TŬM CĂL'A-MĪ FLŪ'I-DŬM.)

Extrait liquide d'Acore vrai, *Fr.;* Flüssiges Kalmuswurzel-Extrakt, *G.*

"Calamus, in No. 60 powder, *one hundred grammes* [or fifty ounces av.]; Alcohol, *a sufficient quantity*, To make *one hundred cubic centimeters* [or three pints]. Moisten the powder with *thirty-five grammes* [or twenty fluidounces] of Alcohol, and pack it firmly in a cylindrical percolator; then add enough Alcohol to saturate the powder and leave a stratum above it. When the liquid begins to drop from the percolator, close the lower orifice, and, having closely covered the percolator, macerate for forty-eight hours. Then allow the percolation to proceed, gradually adding Alcohol, until the Calamus is exhausted. Reserve the first *ninety cubic centimeters* [or forty-three fluidounces] of the percolate, and evaporate the remainder to a soft extract; dissolve this in the reserved portion, and add enough Alcohol to make the Fluid Extract measure *one hundred cubic centimeters* [or three pints]." *U. S.*

This is a new officinal fluid extract, which has been introduced with the view of bringing into use an excellent indigenous aromatic stimulant. It will probably be most frequently used in combination with tonics in dyspepsia and gastric disorders to relieve flatulence, etc. The dose is from five to fifteen minims (0·3–0·9 C.c.).

EXTRACTUM CALUMBÆ. *Br.* *Extract of Calumba.*

(ĔX-TRĂC'TŬM CA-LŬM'BÆ.)

Extractum Colombo, *P. G.;* Extrait de Colombo, *Fr.;* Kolombo-Extrakt, *G.*

"Take of Calumba Root, cut small, *one pound* [avoirdupois]; Proof Spirit *four pints* [Imperial measure]. Macerate the Calumba with *two pints* [Imp. meas.] of the Proof Spirit for twelve hours, strain and press. Macerate again with the same quantity of Proof Spirit, strain and press as before. Mix and filter the liquors, recover the spirit by distillation, and evaporate the residue by the heat of a water-bath until the extract is of a suitable consistence for forming pills." *Br.*

The views expressed in this commentary (15th revision, p. 595) have been adopted, and the aqueous extract of calumba of the former Br. Pharmacopœia has very properly been abandoned, the present hydro-alcoholic one taking its place. It is to be regretted, however, that percolation was not selected as the process in preference to maceration. The extract may be given in the dose of from five to fifteen grains (0·33–1 Gm.) three times a day. It is an efficient preparation for tonic pills.

EXTRACTUM CALUMBÆ FLUIDUM. *U. S.* *Fluid Extract of Calumba.*

(ĔX-TRĂC'TŬM CA-LŬM'BÆ FLŪ'I-DŬM.)

Extrait liquide de Colombo, *Fr.;* Flüssiges Kolombo-Extrakt, *G.*

"Calumba, in No. 20 powder, *one hundred grammes* [or fifty ounces av.]; Diluted Alcohol, *a sufficient quantity*, To make *one hundred cubic centimeters* [or three pints]. Moisten the powder with *thirty grammes* [or fifteen and a half fluidounces] of Diluted Alcohol, and pack it firmly in a cylindrical percolator; then add enough Diluted Alcohol to saturate the powder and leave a stratum above it. When the liquid begins to drop from the percolator, close the lower orifice, and, having closely covered the percolator, macerate for forty-eight hours. Then allow the percolation to proceed, gradually adding Diluted Alcohol, until the Calumba is exhausted. Reserve the first *seventy cubic centimeters* [or thirty-four fluidounces] of the percolate; by means of a water-bath, distil off the Alcohol from the remainder, and evaporate the residue to a soft extract; dissolve this in the reserved portion, and add enough Diluted Alcohol to make the Fluid Extract measure *one hundred cubic centimeters* [or three pints]." *U. S.*

The formula for fluid extract of calumba of U. S. Pharm. 1870 was faulty, in directing the root to be in fine powder: the large quantity of mucilage present swelled under the influence of the menstruum, and frequently prevented the passage of the percolate; indeed, the powder will probably still be found to give trouble, as there will be some difficulty in thoroughly exhausting it; it should be slowly percolated. This extract is a dark brown liquid, of an intense and purely bitter taste. The absence of tannin makes it a very desirable tonic, in combination with chalybeates. The dose is from fifteen to thirty minims (0·9–1·9 C.c.).

EXTRACTUM CANNABIS INDICÆ. *U. S., Br.* *Extract of Indian Hemp. Extract of Indian Cannabis.*

(ĘX-TRĂC'TŲM CĂN'NĄ-BĬS ĬN'DI-ÇÆ.)

Extrait de Chanvre indien, *Fr.;* Indischer Hanf-Extrakt, *G.*

"Indian Cannabis, in No. 20 powder, *one hundred parts* [or sixteen ounces av.]; Alcohol, *a sufficient quantity.* Moisten the powder with *thirty parts* [or seven fluidounces] of Alcohol, and pack it firmly in a cylindrical percolator; then add enough Alcohol to saturate the powder and leave a stratum above it. When the liquid begins to drop from the percolator, close the lower orifice, and, having closely covered the percolator, macerate for forty-eight hours. Then allow the percolation to proceed, gradually adding Alcohol until *three hundred parts* [or three and a half pints] of tincture are obtained, or the Cannabis is exhausted. By means of a water-bath, distil off the Alcohol from the tincture, and, having placed the residue in a porcelain capsule, evaporate it, on a water-bath, to a pilular consistence." *U. S.*

"Take of Indian Hemp, in coarse powder, *one pound* [avoirdupois]; Rectified Spirit *four pints* [Imperial measure]. Macerate the Hemp in the Spirit for seven days, and press out the tincture. Distil off the greater part of the Spirit, and evaporate what remains by a water-bath to the consistence of a soft extract." *Br.*

It will be noticed that the English name of the drug has been changed in the U. S. Pharmacopœia to Indian Cannabis to prevent its being mistaken for the root of *Apocynum Cannabinum*, which is also called Indian Hemp. Several mistakes have occurred through this unfortunate confusion of nomenclature.

Although there is some difference in the details of the two processes, the preparations of the U. S. and Br. Pharmacopœias are practically identical. The preparation varies exceedingly in strength, so that it is wisest to commence with a small dose, one-quarter of a grain (Gm. 0·016), and rapidly increase the amount given until some effect is produced.

Prof. Procter investigated the subject of the tests for the purified extract or resin, and came to the following conclusions. Its peculiar odor when moderately heated, its indifference to alkalies, and its solubility in alcohol, ether, chloroform, benzol, and oil of turpentine, are characteristic though not entirely distinctive properties. The best test, he found, was nitric acid (sp. gr. 1·38), which acts slowly when cold, but with heat rapidly, evolving red fumes, and converting the resin into an orange-red resinoid substance, which, when washed and dried, closely resembles gamboge in color. (*Proc. A. P. A.*, 1864.) The dose of an active preparation is a quarter of a grain (0·016 Gm.).

Off. Prep. Br. Tinctura Cannabis Indicæ.

EXTRACTUM CANNABIS INDICÆ FLUIDUM. *U. S.* *Fluid Extract of Indian Cannabis.*

(ĘX-TRĂC'TŲM CĂN'NĄ-BĬS ĬN'DI-ÇÆ FLŪ'I-DŬM.)

Extrait liquide de Chanvre indien, *Fr.;* Flüssiges Indischer Hanf-Extrakt, *G.*

"Indian Cannabis, in No. 20 powder, *one hundred grammes* [or fifty ounces av.]; Alcohol, *a sufficient quantity,* To make *one hundred cubic centimeters* [or three pints]. Moisten the powder with *thirty grammes* [or seventeen fluidounces] of Alcohol, and pack it firmly in a cylindrical percolator; then add enough Alcohol to saturate the powder and leave a stratum above it. When the liquid begins to drop from the percolator, close the lower orifice, and, having closely covered the percolator, macerate for forty-eight hours. Then allow the percolation to proceed, gradually adding Alcohol, until the Indian Cannabis is exhausted. Reserve the first *ninety cubic centimeters* [or forty-three fluidounces] of the percolate; by means of a water-bath distil off the alcohol from the remainder, and evaporate the residue to a soft extract;

dissolve this in the reserved portion, and add enough Alcohol to make the Fluid Extract measure *one hundred cubic centimeters* [or three pints]." *U. S.*

This is another new officinal fluid extract. It has come into use because of its convenience, and probably on account of the impression that heat injures the activity of the drug, and that the extract owes its inactivity sometimes to the influence of heat. The fluid extract is of a dark green color, having the characteristic peculiar odor of the drug. The dose is one-half to one minim (0·03 to 0·06 C.c.).

EXTRACTUM CAPSICI FLUIDUM. *U. S.* *Fluid Extract of Capsicum.*

(EX-TRĂC'TUM CĂP'SI-CI FLŪ'I-DŬM.)

Extrait liquide de Capsique, *Fr.;* Flüssiges Spanischer Pfeffer-Extrakt, *G.*

"Capsicum, in No. 60 powder, *one hundred grammes* [or fifty ounces av.]; Alcohol, *a sufficient quantity,* To make *one hundred cubic centimeters* [or three pints]. Moisten the powder with *fifty grammes* [or twenty-nine fluidounces] of Alcohol, and pack it firmly in a cylindrical percolator; then add enough Alcohol to saturate the powder and leave a stratum above it. When the liquid begins to drop from the percolator, close the lower orifice, and, having closely covered the percolator, macerate for forty-eight hours. Then allow the percolation to proceed, gradually adding Alcohol, until the Capsicum is exhausted. Reserve the first *ninety cubic centimeters* [or forty-three fluidounces] of the percolate, and evaporate the remainder to a soft extract; dissolve this in the reserved portion, and add enough Alcohol to make the Fluid Extract measure *one hundred cubic centimeters* [or three pints]." *U. S.*

The necessity for an officinal fluid extract of capsicum is not apparent. The oleoresin and tincture are preparations which are well known and established, and why three liquid preparations of this very active drug are needed is not apparent. It will probably be rarely necessary to administer it internally. The dose is one-half to one minim (0·03 to 0·06 C.c.).

EXTRACTUM CASCARÆ SAGRADÆ. *Br.* *Extract of Cascara Sagrada.*

(EX-TRĂC'TUM CĂS'CA-RÆ SA-GRĂ'DÆ.)

Extractum Rhamni Purshiani.

"Take of Cascara Sagrada, in No. 40 powder, *one pound* [av.]; Proof Spirit, Distilled Water, of each, *a sufficiency.* Mix the Cascara with *two pints* [Imp. meas.] of the Spirit, and macerate in a closed vessel for forty-eight hours, then transfer to a percolator, and when the fluid ceases to pass, continue the percolation with water until *three pints* [Imp. meas.] of liquid have been collected, or the Cascara is exhausted. Evaporate the percolated liquid by a water-bath until the extract has acquired a suitable consistence." *Br.*

The selection of the title is not above criticism; the title of the bark is "Rhamni Purshiani Cortex," and the extract should without doubt be termed "Extractum Rhamni Purshiani." If the name "Extractum Cascaræ Sagradæ" be preferred, then the title of the drug should be made to correspond.

This is a new preparation, which well represents the virtues of the bark, and furnishes a good means of administering this purgative in pilular form. Dose, two to eight grains. (0·13–0·52 Gm.).

EXTRACTUM CASCARÆ SAGRADÆ LIQUIDUM. *Br.* *Liquid Extract of Cascara Sagrada.*

(EX-TRĂC'TUM CĂS'CA-RÆ SA-GRĂ'DÆ LIQ'UI-DŬM—lik'we-dŭm.)

Extractum Rhamni Purshiani Liquidum.

"Take of Cascara Sagrada, in coarse powder, *one pound* [av.]; Rectified Spirit *four fluidounces* [Imp. meas.]; Distilled Water *a sufficiency.* Boil the bark in three or four successive quantities of the water until exhausted. Evaporate the strained liquors by a water-bath, to *twelve fluidounces* [Imp. meas.]; when cold add the spirit, allow the mixture to remain for some hours, then filter, and make up to the volume of *sixteen fluidounces* [Imp. meas.] with distilled water." *Br.*

This is a new liquid extract, and the remarks in the previous article on the subject of the title apply equally well to this preparation. Simple percolation could be substituted with advantage for the tedious manipulation of making four decoctions: straining them, then evaporating, adding alcohol, and filtering again. The process employed for making fluid extract of frangula, page 631, could be used effectively here. Dose one-half to two fluidrachms (1·9–7·5 C.c.).

EXTRACTUM CASTANEÆ FLUIDUM. *U.S.* *Fluid Extract of Castanea.*

(ĔX-TRĂC'TŬM CĂS-TĀ'NĒ-Æ FLŪ'Ĭ-DŬM.)

Extrait liquide de Feuilles de Châtaignier, *Fr.;* Flüssiges Kastanienblätter-Extrakt, *G.*

"Castanea, in No. 30 powder, *one hundred grammes* [or fifty ounces av.]; Alcohol, Water, each, *a sufficient quantity,* To make *one hundred cubic centimeters* [or three pints]. Pour *five hundred cubic centimeters* [or fifteen pints] of Boiling Water upon the powder, allow it to macerate for two hours, then express the liquid, transfer the residue to a percolator, and pour Water upon it until the powder is exhausted. Evaporate the united liquids, on a water-bath, to *two hundred cubic centimeters* [or six pints], let cool, and add *sixty cubic centimeters* [or twenty-nine fluidounces] of Alcohol. When the insoluble matter has subsided, separate the clear liquid, filter the remainder, evaporate the united liquids to *eighty cubic centimeters* [or thirty-eight fluidounces], allow to cool, and add enough Alcohol to make the Fluid Extract measure *one hundred cubic centimeters* [or three pints]." *U. S.*

This fluid extract has acquired some reputation in the treatment of hooping-cough, and it has been shown that the efficacy largely depends upon the mucilaginous principle found in the leaves. The object of the special process is to obtain and retain this principle, and it will be observed that the preparation is an aqueous fluid extract with only sufficient alcohol to preserve it. It is a thick reddish brown liquid, having an astringent taste. The dose is one to two fluidrachms (3·75–7·5 C.c.).

EXTRACTUM CHIMAPHILÆ FLUIDUM. *U.S.* *Fluid Extract of Chimaphila.*

(ĔX-TRĂC'TŬM CHĬ-MĂPH'Ĭ-LÆ FLŪ'Ĭ-DŬM.)

Extrait liquide de Pyrole ombellée, *Fr.;* Flüssiges Doldenblüthiges Harnkraut-Extrakt, *G.*

"Chimaphila, in No. 30 powder, *one hundred grammes* [or fifty ounces av.]; Glycerin, *ten grammes* [three and three-quarter fluidounces]; Diluted Alcohol, *a sufficient quantity,* To make *one hundred cubic centimeters* [or three pints]. Mix the Glycerin with *ninety grammes* [or forty-six and a half fluidounces] of Diluted Alcohol. Moisten the powder with *forty grammes* [or twenty fluidounces] of the mixture, and pack it firmly in a cylindrical percolator; then add enough of the menstruum to saturate the powder and leave a stratum above it. When the liquid begins to drop from the percolator, close the lower orifice, and, having closely covered the percolator, macerate for forty-eight hours. Then allow the percolation to proceed, gradually adding, first, the remainder of the menstruum, and afterward, Diluted Alcohol, until the Chimaphila is exhausted. Reserve the first *seventy cubic centimeters* [or thirty-four fluidounces] of the percolate, and evaporate the remainder to a soft extract; dissolve this in the reserved portion, and add enough Diluted Alcohol to make the Fluid Extract measure *one hundred cubic centimeters* [or three pints]." *U. S.*

The quantity of glycerin has been greatly reduced in the formula for this fluid extract, in accordance with the views expressed in the general article on Fluid Extracts. The advantage of using a comparatively small proportion of glycerin in fluid extracts of drugs containing tannin is well established. This is a rather thick dark brownish green fluid extract, and may be given in the dose of a fluidrachm (3·75 C.c.).

EXTRACTUM CHIRATÆ FLUIDUM. *U. S.* *Fluid Extract of Chirata.*

(EX-TRĂC′TŬM CHI-RĀ′TÆ FLŪ′I-DŬM.)

Extrait liquide de Chiretta, *Fr.;* Flüssiges Chiretta-Extrakt, *G.*

"Chirata, in No. 30 powder, *one hundred grammes* [or fifty ounces av.]; Glycerin, *ten grammes* [three and three-quarter fluidounces]; Diluted Alcohol, *a sufficient quantity,* To make *one hundred cubic centimeters* [or three pints]. Mix the Glycerin with *ninety grammes* [or forty-six and a half fluidounces] of Diluted Alcohol. Moisten the powder with *thirty-five grammes* [or eighteen fluidounces] of the mixture, and pack it firmly in a cylindrical percolator; then add enough of the menstruum to saturate the powder and leave a stratum above it. When the liquid begins to drop from the percolator, close the lower orifice, and, having closely covered the percolator, macerate for forty-eight hours. Then allow the percolation to proceed, gradually adding, first, the remainder of the menstruum, and afterward, Diluted Alcohol, until the Chirata is exhausted. Reserve the first *eighty-five cubic centimeters* [or forty fluidounces] of the percolate; by means of a water-bath, distil off the Alcohol from the remainder, and evaporate the residue to a soft extract; dissolve this in the reserved portion, and add enough Diluted Alcohol to make the Fluid Extract measure *one hundred cubic centimeters* [or three pints]." *U. S.*

This is a useful addition to the list of fluid extracts. The necessity for the use of Glycerin is, however, not apparent, although the amount is insufficient to be harmful. This extract is a clear, reddish brown liquid, of an intensely bitter taste. The dose is half a fluidrachm (1·9 C.c.).

EXTRACTUM CIMICIFUGÆ FLUIDUM. *U.S.* *Fluid Extract of Cimicifuga.*

(EX-TRĂC′TŬM CĬM-I-CĬF′Ū-GÆ FLŪ′I-DŬM.)

Extractum Cimicifugæ Liquidum, *Br.;* Liquid Extract of Cimicifuga; Extrait liquide d'Actée à Grappes, *Fr.;* Flüssiges Cimicifuga-Extrakt, *G.*

"Cimicifuga, in No. 60 powder, *one hundred grammes* [or fifty ounces av.]; Alcohol, *a sufficient quantity,* To make *one hundred cubic centimeters* [or three pints]. Moisten the powder with *twenty-five grammes* [or fourteen and a half fluidounces] of Alcohol, and pack it firmly in a cylindrical percolator; then add enough Alcohol to saturate the powder and leave a stratum above it. When the liquid begins to drop from the percolator, close the lower orifice, and, having closely covered the percolator, macerate for forty-eight hours. Then allow the percolation to proceed, gradually adding Alcohol, until the Cimicifuga is exhausted. Reserve the first *ninety cubic centimeters* [or forty-three fluidounces] of the percolate, and evaporate the remainder to a soft extract; dissolve this in the reserved portion, and add enough Alcohol to make the Fluid Extract measure *one hundred cubic centimeters* [or three pints.]" *U. S.*

"Take of Cimicifuga, in No. 60 powder, *twenty ounces* [av.]; Rectified Spirit *a sufficiency.* Mix the Cimicifuga with *two pints* [Imp. meas.] of the Spirit, and macerate in a closed vessel for forty-eight hours; then transfer to a percolator, and when the fluid ceases to pass continue the percolation with more spirit until the cimicifuga is exhausted. Reserve the first *fifteen fluidounces* [Imp. meas.] of the percolate, and evaporate the remainder by a water-bath to the consistence of a soft extract; dissolve this in the reserved portion, and make up the volume to *twenty fluidounces* [Imp. meas.] by the addition of more spirit." *Br.*

This formula does not differ essentially from that of the U. S. Pharm. 1870. The British preparation has been modelled after that of the United States. There probably cannot be two opinions about the menstruum, although it has been asserted that a good fluid extract can be made with a menstruum of three parts alcohol and one part water. The probabilities are, however, that a portion of the resinous principle would precipitate on standing. This fluid extract is of a deep reddish brown color, and thoroughly represents the drug. The dose is from thirty minims to one fluidrachm (1·9 to 3·75 C.c.).

EXTRACTUM CINCHONÆ. *U.S.* *Extract of Cinchona.*

(EX-TRĂC'TUM CIN-CHŌ'NÆ.)

Extractum Chinæ; Extrait de Quinquina jaune, *Fr.;* China-Extrakt, *G.*

"Yellow Cinchona, in No. 60 powder, *one hundred parts* [or sixteen ounces av.]; Alcohol, *three hundred parts* [or three and a half pints]; Water, *one hundred parts* [or one pint]; Glycerin, Diluted Alcohol, each, *a sufficient quantity.* Mix the Alcohol and Water, and, having moistened the powder with *thirty-five parts* [or six fluidounces] of the mixture, pack it firmly in a cylindrical percolator; then add enough of the menstruum to saturate the powder and leave a stratum above it. When the liquid begins to drop from the percolator, close the lower orifice, and, having closely covered the percolator, macerate for forty-eight hours. Then allow the percolation to proceed, gradually adding, first, the remainder of the menstruum, and then Diluted Alcohol, until *four hundred parts* [or four and a half pints] of tincture are obtained, or the Cinchona is exhausted. By means of a water-bath, distil off the Alcohol from the tincture, and, having placed the residue in a porcelain capsule, evaporate it on a water-bath, to a pilular consistence. Lastly, weigh the Extract, and thoroughly incorporate with it, while still warm, *five per cent.* of Glycerin." *U.S.*

The yellow or Calisaya bark is selected for this preparation, as it can usually be relied on as efficient. By this process all the virtues of the bark are extracted. In the officinal formula of 1870 the alcohol and water were used separately; the parts soluble in alcohol being first taken up, and afterwards those in water. This proceeding had the advantage that no more heat was necessary to evaporate the tincture than the alcoholic menstruum required; while, if the two liquids were mixed, it would be necessarily subjected to a longer continuance if not a higher degree of heat; and the advantage was the greater as most of the active matter was extracted in the first percolation with alcohol. The present officinal process is an excellent one, and if proper care be taken in executing the process, both in relation to the percolation and the avoidance of too high a temperature, the extract will fully represent the virtues of the bark.

The former extracts of cinchona of the British Colleges are all omitted in the new British Pharmacopœia, which directs in their place a fluid extract, under the name of *Extractum Cinchonæ Liquidum* (which see).

A very good extract of bark was formerly prepared, in Philadelphia, by macerating cinchona for a considerable length of time in a large proportion of water, and slowly evaporating the infusion, by a very moderate heat, in large shallow dishes placed upon the top of a stove. Many years ago Dr. Geo. B. Wood found ten grains of this extract equivalent to nearly a drachm of powdered cinchona.

Medical Uses. The extract of Peruvian bark is at present much less employed than before the discovery of quinine. It is still, however, occasionally prescribed as a tonic in combination with other medicines; and, as it possesses, when properly prepared with a spirituous menstruum, almost all the active principles as they exist in the bark itself, it may be used in preference to the sulphate of quinine, whenever it is supposed that the latter is incapable of exerting all the curative influence of cinchona. We are led to believe, however, that, on account of the high price of Calisaya bark, much of the extract now in the market is prepared from inferior varieties. The dose is from ten to thirty grains (0·65–1·95 Gm.), equivalent to about a drachm (3·9 Gm.) of the powdered bark.

EXTRACTUM CINCHONÆ FLUIDUM. *U.S.* *Fluid Extract of Cinchona.*

(EX-TRĂC'TUM CIN-CHŌ'NÆ FLŪ'I-DŬM.)

Extractum Cinchonæ Liquidum, *Br.;* Liquid Extract of Cinchona; Extractum Chinæ Calisayæ Fluidum; Extrait liquide de Quinquina jaune, *Fr.;* Flüssiges Kalisayarinden-Extrakt, *G.*

"Yellow Cinchona, in No. 60 powder, *one hundred grammes* [or fifty ounces av.]; Glycerin, *twenty-five grammes* [or nine and a half fluidounces]; Alcohol, Water, each, *a sufficient quantity,* To make *one hundred cubic centimeters* [or three pints].

Mix the Glycerin with *seventy-five grammes* [or forty-four fluidounces] of Alcohol. Moisten the powder with *thirty-five grammes* [or eighteen fluidounces] of the mixture, pack it firmly in a cylindrical percolator, and pour on the remainder of the menstruum. When the liquid begins to drop from the percolator, close the lower orifice, and, having closely covered the percolator, macerate for forty-eight hours. Then allow the percolation to proceed, and, when the liquid in the percolator has disappeared from the surface, gradually pour on a mixture of Alcohol and Water, made in the proportion of *three parts* [or three and a half pints] of Alcohol to *one part* [or one pint] of Water, and continue the percolation until the Cinchona is exhausted. Reserve the first *seventy-five cubic centimeters* [or thirty-six fluidounces] of the percolate, and evaporate the remainder to a soft extract; dissolve this in the reserved portion, and add enough of a mixture of Alcohol and Water, using the same proportions as before, to make the Fluid Extract measure *one hundred cubic centimeters* [or three pints]." *U. S.*

"Take of Red Cinchona Bark, in No. 60 powder, *twenty ounces* [av.], Hydrochloric Acid *five fluidrachms* [Imp. meas.]; Glycerine *two and a half fluidounces* [Imp. meas.]; Rectified Spirit, Distilled Water, of each, *a sufficiency*. Mix the Bark with *five pints* [Imp. meas.] of the water to which the Acid and Glycerine have been added, and macerate in a covered vessel for forty-eight hours, stirring frequently; then transfer to a percolator, and when the fluid ceases to pass, and the contents of the percolator have been properly packed, continue the percolation with water until *fifteen pints* [Imp. meas.] of liquid have passed, or that which is passing has ceased to give a precipitate on the addition to it of an excess of solution of soda. Evaporate the percolated liquid in a porcelain or enamelled iron vessel at a temperature not exceeding 180° F. (82°·2 C.) until it is reduced to *twenty fluidounces* [Imp. meas.].

"Put *fifty fluidgrains* of this liquid (*a*) with *half an ounce* [Imp. meas.] of distilled water into a stoppered glass separator capable of holding *four fluidounces* [Imp. meas.]; add to this *one fluidounce* [Imp. meas.] of Benzolated Amylic Alcohol,* and *half a fluidounce* [Imp. meas.] of Solution of Soda, shake them together thoroughly and repeatedly, then allow them to remain at rest until the spirituous solution of the alkaloids shall have separated and formed a distinct stratum over the dark-colored alkaline solution of the other constituents of the extract. Run off the latter by the stopcock, add a little more distilled water to wash away any still adhering alkaline solution from the separator and its contents, and having run off this as before, as completely as possible, decant the spirituous solution into a small porcelain or glass dish the weight of which is known. Evaporate by the heat of a water-bath until a perfectly dry residue is left. The weight now of the dish and its contents, after deducting the known weight of the dish, will give that of the alkaloids, and this multiplied by 2 will give the parts by weight of the alkaloids in 100 fluid parts of the liquid (*a*).

"Having thus ascertained the alkaloidal strength of the liquid (*a*), every fluid part of it containing *five grains* of total alkaloids is first to be brought to the volume of *eighty-five grains* by evaporation, or if necessary by dilution with water, then 12·5 *fluidgrains* of rectified spirit are to be added, and the final adjustment of the volume to 100 *fluidgrains* is to be effected by the addition of distilled water. The finished liquid extract will thus contain *five grains* of the alkaloids of the bark in every 100 *fluidgrains*." *Br.*

Of these two formulas, the first is decidedly preferable. It is based upon that of Mr. Alfred B. Taylor, of Philadelphia. (*A. J. P.*, Jan. 1865.) The British Pharmacopœia uses acidulated water with glycerin as the solvent, while it adds alcohol to the liquid to preserve it. In the U. S. process a mixture of alcohol and glycerin is used as the menstruum. Now, it is well known that cinchona bark cannot be exhausted by the British solvent; and, though by its use as a menstruum the resin and cinchonic red are mainly left behind, so also is a considerable proportion of the alkaloids. By using alcohol, the U. S. Pharmacopœia extracts all the virtues of the bark, though it may also take up some of the resin and cinchonic red. The process of the British Pharmacopœia yields a preparation which would be more appropriately

* Made by mixing together three measures of benzol and one measure of amylic alcohol.

termed an "alkaloidal solution of cinchona." The U. S. fluid extract, like others of its class, is a preparation which represents all of the soluble active constituents of cinchona; the British liquid extract, although an improvement on the former process, is simply a "preserved infusion" made by prolonged evaporation; the improvement consists in the addition of acid to the menstruum and the assaying of a portion of the evaporated percolate by the process similar to that adopted by the British Pharmacopœia for cinchona and making the finished product contain 5 per cent. of mixed alkaloids; thus any imperfections in the manipulation are overcome by the check of the assay; but it is doubtful whether a better preparation, and one involving much less complication, could not be made by dissolving definite quantities of the commercial alkaloids in a mixture of water, alcohol, acid, and glycerin. In this there would be the advantage of knowing the exact proportion of each constituent.* The U. S. fluid extract of cinchona is a moderately thin, dark reddish brown, translucent fluid, of a bitter, astringent taste. The dose equivalent to a drachm (3·9 Gm.) of the bark is one fluidrachm (3·75 C.c.); and to produce an antiperiodic effect, at least two fluidounces (60 C.c.) should be taken between the paroxysms. The dose of the British liquid extract is given as five to ten minims (0·3–0·6 C.c.).

EXTRACTUM COCÆ LIQUIDUM. *Br.* *Liquid Extract of Coca.*

(EX-TRĂC'TUM CŌ'CÆ LĬQ'UI-DŬM—lik'we-dŭm.)

See *Extractum Erythroxyli Fluidum.*

EXTRACTUM COLCHICI. *Br.* *Extract of Colchicum.*

(EX-TRĂC'TUM CŎL'CHI-CĪ—kŏl'ki-sī.)

Extrait de Colchique, *Fr.;* Zeitlosen-Extrakt, *G.*

"Take of Fresh Colchicum Corms, deprived of their coats, *seven pounds* [avoir.]. Crush the Corms; press out the juice; allow the feculence to subside, and heat the clear liquor to 212° F. (100° C.); then strain through flannel, and evaporate by a water-bath, at a temperature not exceeding 160° F. (71°·1 C.), until the extract is of a suitable consistence for forming pills." *Br.*

There scarcely seems to be occasion for both this and the following extract. The dose is one or two grains (0·065–0·13 Gm.).

In Great Britain a preparation called *preserved juice of colchicum* is given in the dose of five minims (0·3 C.c.) or more. It is made by expressing the fresh bulb, allowing the juice to stand for forty-eight hours that the feculent matter may subside, then adding one-quarter of its bulk of alcohol, allowing it again to stand for a short period, and ultimately filtering.

EXTRACTUM COLCHICI RADICIS. *U.S.* *Extract of Colchicum Root.*

(EX-TRĂC'TUM CŎL'CHI-CĪ RA-DĪ'CĬS—kŏl'ki-sī.)

Extractum Colchici Aceticum, *Br.;* Acetic Extract of Colchicum; Extrait de Colchique acétique, *Fr.;* Zeitlosen Essigextrakt, *G.*

"Colchicum Root, in No. 60 powder, *one hundred parts* [or sixteen ounces av.]; Acetic Acid, *thirty-five parts* [or five and a half fluidounces]; Water, *a sufficient quantity.* Mix the Acetic Acid with *one hundred and fifty parts* [or twenty-three fluidounces] of Water, and, having moistened the powder with *fifty parts* [or seven and a half fluidounces] of the mixture, pack it moderately in a cylindrical glass percolator; then add enough menstruum to saturate the powder and leave a stratum above it. When the liquid begins to drop from the percolator, close the lower orifice, and, having closely covered the percolator, macerate for forty-eight hours. Then allow the percolation to proceed, gradually adding, first, the remainder of the

* *Liquid Extract of Cinchona* (simplified). Take of Quinine 75 grains, Cinchonidine 35 grains, Cinchonine 20 grains, Hydrochloric Acid 40 minims, Glycerin 5 fluidrachms, Alcohol 1 fluidrachm. Dissolve the alkaloids in the alcohol and glycerin mixed with 5 fluidounces of water, add the acid, agitate until dissolved, and add sufficient water to make 6 fluidounces. If the color and flavor of the bark are desired, add 60 grains of Red Cinchona in powder to the solution, allow it to stand 24 hours, then filter.

menstruum, and then Water, until the Colchicum Root is exhausted. Evaporate the percolate, in a porcelain vessel, by means of a water-bath, at a temperature not exceeding 80° C. (176° F.), to a pilular consistence." *U. S.*

"Take of Fresh Colchicum Corms, deprived of their coats, *seven pounds* [av.]; Acetic Acid *six fluidounces* [Imp. meas.]. Crush the corms, add the Acetic Acid, and press out the juice; allow the feculence to subside, and heat the clear liquor to 212° F. (100° C.); then strain through flannel, and evaporate by a water-bath at a temperature not exceeding 160° F. (71°·1 C.) to the consistence of a soft extract." *Br.*

As the fresh colchicum bulb is rarely to be had in this country, the U. S. Pharmacopœia employs the dried bulb; and its process, if properly conducted, will afford a very efficient extract. In our opinion it would be preferable to add the whole of the menstruum specified, to the powdered colchicum root, and satisfy its tendency to swell at once, instead of using the small quantity directed to moisten. The swelling of the powder will frequently cause an entire stoppage of the percolation and necessitate the repacking of the percolator. Some inconveniences are experienced in preparing the extract, according to the British process, from the recent bulb by expression, which would seem to render the U. S. process under all circumstances preferable. (*P. J. Tr.*, xiii. 62.)

The use of the acetic acid, in this preparation, is to render more soluble the alkaloid upon which the virtues of meadow-saffron are thought to depend. The acetic extract of colchicum is highly commended by Sir C. Scudamore, who prefers it made by evaporating, to the consistence of honey, a saturated acetic infusion of the dried bulb. (*Lond. Med. Gazette*, Dec. 10, 1841.) The dose of the extract is one or two grains (0·065–0·13 Gm.), to be repeated two or three times a day, and increased if necessary.

EXTRACTUM COLCHICI RADICIS FLUIDUM. *U. S.* *Fluid Extract of Colchicum Root.*

(ĔX-TRĂC'TŬM CŎL'ĈHĬ-CĪ RĂ-DĪ'CĬS FLŪ'Ĭ-DŬM.)

Extrait liquide de Bulbe de Colchique, *Fr.*; Flüssiges Zeitlosenknollen-Extrakt, *G.*

"Colchicum Root, in No. 60 powder, *one hundred grammes* [or fifty ounces av.]; Alcohol, Water, each, *a sufficient quantity*, To make *one hundred cubic centimeters* [or three pints]. Mix *two parts* [or four and a half pints] of Alcohol with *one part* [or two pints] of Water, and, having moistened the powder with *thirty-five grammes* [or twenty fluidounces] of the mixture, pack it moderately in a cylindrical percolator; then add enough of the menstruum to saturate the powder and leave a stratum above it. When the liquid begins to drop from the percolator, close the lower orifice, and, having closely covered the percolator, macerate for forty-eight hours. Then allow the percolation to proceed, gradually adding menstruum, until the Colchicum Root is exhausted. Reserve the first *eighty-five cubic centimeters* [or forty fluidounces] of the percolate, and evaporate the remainder to a soft extract; dissolve this in the reserved portion, and add enough menstruum to make the Fluid Extract measure *one hundred cubic centimeters* [or three pints]." *U. S.*

This fluid extract is not essentially different from that formerly officinal. The principal difference is in the disuse of glycerin, which solvent there is certainly no advantage in retaining. The present menstruum will thoroughly exhaust the root, and this fluid extract is now a good preparation. It is of a reddish brown color and bitter taste. The dose is from two to eight minims (0·12–0·5 C.c.).

EXTRACTUM COLCHICI SEMINIS FLUIDUM. *U. S.* *Fluid Extract of Colchicum Seed.*

(ĔX-TRĂC'TŬM CŎL'ĈHĬ-CĪ SĔM'Ĭ-NĬS FLŪ'Ĭ-DŬM.)

Extrait liquide de Semences de Colchique, *Fr.*; Flüssiges Zeitlosensamen-Extrakt, *G.*

"Colchicum Seed, in No. 30 powder, *one hundred grammes* [or fifty ounces av.]; Alcohol, Water, each, *a sufficient quantity*, To make *one hundred cubic centimeters* [or three pints]. Mix *two parts* [or four and a half pints] of Alcohol with *one part* [or two pints] of Water, and, having moistened the powder with *thirty grammes* [or seventeen fluidounces] of the mixture, pack it firmly in a cylindrical percolator;

then add enough menstruum to saturate the powder and leave a stratum above it. When the liquid begins to drop from the percolator, close the lower orifice, and, having closely covered the percolator, macerate for forty-eight hours. Then allow the percolation to proceed, gradually adding menstruum, until the Colchicum Seed is exhausted. Reserve the first *eighty-five cubic centimeters* [or forty fluidounces] of the percolate, and evaporate the remainder to a soft extract; dissolve this in the reserved portion, and add enough menstruum to make the Fluid Extract measure *one hundred cubic centimeters* [or three pints]." *U. S.*

The use of glycerin in this fluid extract (U. S. P. 1870) was even more objectionable than in that of the root, as the fixed oil contained in the seeds was always thrown out of solution, and was usually found floating on the fluid extract, rendering the preparation unsightly. L. I. Morris (*A. J. P.*, 1881, p. 7) believes that it is unnecessary to grind the colchicum seeds, and that if the whole seeds are digested with diluted alcohol at 80° C. (176 F.) the colchicine is easily extracted.

Considering that we had one tincture, two wines, and two extracts of Colchicum, all efficient preparations requiring small doses, these additions to our pharmacy might have been spared, unless some peculiar advantage could have been gained from them. They are, however, well made, and no doubt concentrate the virtues of colchicum, and have a limited use. The dose is from two to eight minims (0·12–0·5 C.c.).

EXTRACTUM COLOCYNTHIDIS. *U.S. Extract of Colocynth.*

(ĔX-TRĂC′TŬM CŎL-Ō-CȲN′THĬ-DĬS.)

Extrait de Coloquinte, *Fr.;* Koloquinten-Extrakt, *G.*

"Colocynth, dried and freed from the seeds, *one hundred parts* [or sixteen ounces av.]; Diluted Alcohol, *a sufficient quantity*. Reduce the Colocynth to a coarse powder by grinding or bruising, macerate it in *two hundred and fifty parts* [or forty-one fluidounces] of Diluted Alcohol for four days, with occasional stirring; then express strongly, and strain through flannel. Pack the residue, previously broken up with the hands, firmly in a cylindrical percolator, cover it with the strainer, and gradually pour Diluted Alcohol upon it until the tincture and expressed liquid, mixed together, weigh *five hundred parts* [or measure five pints]. Having recovered from the mixture *three hundred parts* [or three and a half pints] of Alcohol by distillation, evaporate the residue to dryness, by means of a water-bath. Lastly, reduce the dry mass to powder. Extract of Colocynth should be kept in well-stopped bottles." *U. S.*

Colocynth should be deprived of its seeds, as directed by the U. S. Pharmacopœia, before being submitted to the action of the menstruum. Dr. Duncan found half a pound of colocynth to contain 2770 grains of seeds, which, boiled by themselves, yielded almost nothing to water. Dr. Squibb found selected fruits to yield from 25·8 to 34 per cent. of medullary part; and this, when well exhausted by diluted alcohol, to yield 60·7 to 60·8 per cent. of dry extract; while from the whole fruit, including pulp and seeds, from 15·69 to 20·6 per cent. was obtained, according to the degree of dryness. (*A. J. P.*, 1857, p. 98.) Boiling water extracts so much pectic acid and mucilage from colocynth, that the decoction or hot infusion gelatinises on cooling; and the extract made by means of it is loaded with inert matter, and, besides, is apt to become mouldy, or so tough and hard as to resist trituration and formation into pills. Hence the London College, following in this respect the French Codex, directed, in the last edition of its Pharmacopœia, maceration with cold water; but diluted alcohol has been found to be a much better menstruum, and has been adopted in the U. S. process; while in the British Pharmacopœia the simple extract has been discarded altogether. The chief, if not exclusive, use of the alcoholic extract is in the preparation of the compound extract.

This preparation should never be substituted by an extract prepared with a more aqueous menstruum, because water extracts a large quantity of mucilaginous and inert matter. Commercial extract of colocynth may be often found in the market made with an aqueous menstruum.

Off. Prep. Extractum Colocynthidis Compositum.

EXTRACTUM COLOCYNTHIDIS COMPOSITUM. *U. S., Br.*
Compound Extract of Colocynth.

(EX-TRĂC'TUM CŎL-O-CȲN'THI-DĬS CŎM-PŎS'I-TŬM.)

Extrait de Coloquinte composé, *Fr.;* Zusammengesetztes Koloquinten-Extrakt, *G.*

"Extract of Colocynth, *sixteen parts* [or eight ounces av.]; Aloes, *fifty parts* [or twenty-five ounces av.]; Cardamom, in No. 60 powder, *six parts* [or three ounces av.]; Resin of Scammony, in fine powder, *fourteen parts* [or seven ounces av.]; Soap, dried and in coarse powder, *fourteen parts* [or seven ounces av.]; Alcohol, *ten parts* [or six fluidounces]. Heat the Aloes, on a water-bath, until it is completely melted; then add the Alcohol, and, having stirred the mixture thoroughly, strain it through a fine sieve, which has just been dipped into boiling water. To the strained mixture, contained in a suitable vessel, add the Soap, Extract of Colocynth, and Resin of Scammony, and heat the mixture at a temperature not exceeding 120° C. (248° F.), until it is perfectly homogeneous, and a thread taken from the mass becomes brittle when cool. Then withdraw the heat, thoroughly incorporate the Cardamom with the mixture, and cover the vessel until the contents are cold. Finally, reduce the product to a fine powder. Compound Extract of Colocynth should be kept in well-stopped bottles." *U. S.*

"Take of Colocynth Pulp *six ounces;* Extract of Socotrine Aloes *twelve ounces;* Resin of Scammony *four ounces;* Curd Soap, in powder, *three ounces;* Cardamom Seeds, in the finest powder, *one ounce;* Proof Spirit *one gallon* [Imperial measure]. Macerate the Colocynth in the Spirit for four days; press out the tincture, and distil off the Spirit; then add the Aloes, Scammony, and Soap, and evaporate by a water-bath until the extract is of a suitable consistence for forming pills, adding the Cardamoms towards the end of the process." *Br.* The ounce employed in this process is the avoirdupois.

The U. S. formula of 1870 differed from that of 1850, in taking the extract of colocynth already prepared, instead of directing its preparation from the colocynth, and in substituting resin of scammony for the scammony itself. This provision insures uniformity of result so far as the colocynth is concerned; whereas by the old formula this was impossible, owing to the variable quality of the colocynth employed, unless an unusual amount of care was taken in its selection. The second change contributes to the same result of uniformity; because the resin of scammony is very nearly of equable strength, while scammony is notoriously otherwise; and it has the additional advantage of yielding a stronger extract, as the resin is much more energetic in an equal dose than the crude drug as ordinarily found in the market. The object of the soap in this formula is to improve the consistence of the mass, which, when hardened by time, it renders more soluble in the liquors of the stomach. It may possibly also serve the purpose of qualifying the action of the aloes. In the U. S. process the extract is in the form of powder, which is very convenient for admixture with other substances; while, if given uncombined, it may be readily made into pills by suitable additions. The alternative of using the scammony or its resin, in the first British formula, which appeared to us very objectionable, has been abandoned in the present edition, and the resin only directed. It was objected to the U. S. compound extract of 1860, that it is apt to gripe in consequence of deficiency in the proportion of the aromatic ingredient, and the addition of some aromatic oil, as oil of cloves, was recommended; but this was remedied in the revision of 1870 by increasing the proportion of cardamom. The plan of having the powders simply mixed is liable to the objection, that the mixture is not apt to be so thoroughly effected as to obtain a uniform result; and hence the present Pharmacopœia adopted Dr. Squibb's suggestion, to melt together all the ingredients unpowdered, except the cardamom, add a little alcohol, and, when the mixture is thoroughly made, to stir in the powdered aromatic, and finally to reduce the whole to a fine powder. The active principle of the cardamom (the volatile oil) is thus not dissipated, but absorbed by the other ingredients, and one of the objections to the British process is avoided—*i.e.*, the necessity for directing cardamom in "the finest" powder,—the previous desiccation of the cardamom, a requisite if a fine powder is desired, being very wasteful of the volatile oil.

This extract is an energetic and safe cathartic, possessing the activity of its three purgative ingredients, with comparatively little of the drastic character of the colocynth and scammony. It may be still further and advantageously modified by combination with rhubarb, jalap, calomel, etc., with one or more of which it is often united in prescription. In such combination it is much employed whenever an active cathartic is desirable, particularly in the commencement of fevers and febrile complaints, in congestion of the liver or portal system, and in obstinate constipation. In small doses it is an excellent laxative in that state of habitual costiveness, depending on a want of the due irritability of the bowels, which often occurs in old people. The dose is from five to thirty grains (0·33–1·95 Gm.), according to the effect to be produced, and the susceptibility of the bowels. A very eligible combination is the compound cathartic pill of the U. S. Pharmacopœia. We are informed that much of the extract sold in this country is made with inferior scammony and aloes, and an insufficient proportion of colocynth, so that it is comparatively inert. Compound extract of colocynth should be looked on with suspicion when cheap, and the pharmacist should always prepare it for himself.

Off. Prep. Pilulæ Catharticæ Compositæ.

EXTRACTUM CONII. *Br.* *Extract of Hemlock.*

(ĔX-TRĂC'TŬM CŎ-NĪ'Ī.)

Extract of Hemlock; Extrait de Ciguë, *Fr.;* Schierlings-Extrakt, *G.*

Owing to the great variability in the quality of this extract, it was very properly abandoned in the last revision of the U. S. Pharmacopœia in favor of the abstract or an alcoholic extract of conium fruit. (See next article.)

The directions of the British Pharmacopœia for this extract are precisely the same as those for the extract of aconite, the fresh leaves and young branches of conium being used.

The most important point in the preparation of this extract is to evaporate the juice without an undue degree of heat. At a temperature of 100° C. (212° F.), or upwards, its active principle undergoes rapid decomposition, being converted into resinous matter and ammonia. This is detected by the operator by the ammoniacal odor mixed with that which is peculiar to the plant. The juice always to a certain extent undergoes this decomposition when evaporated over a fire, and is not exempt from it even when the heat is regulated by a water-bath. Hence the propriety of the directions in the British Pharmacopœia. An excellent plan in the evaporation is to conduct it first in a vacuum, and afterwards in shallow vessels with a current of air at common temperatures. By the direction to heat the juice to the boiling point, or 93·3° C. (200° F.) (*Br.*), and then to filter, whereby the inert albumen is coagulated, and, with the equally inert chlorophyll and vegetable fibre, is separated from the liquid before evaporation, the extract is procured in a more concentrated state, and, besides, deprived of substances which might favor its decomposition. Long-continued exposure to the air is productive of the same result as too much heat, so that old extracts are frequently destitute of activity. (*Journ. de Pharm.*, xxii. 416.) No one of the extracts is more variable in its qualities than this. The season at which the herb is collected, the place and circumstances of its growth, the method of preparing the extract, are all points of importance, and are all too frequently neglected. (See *Conii Folia.*) In this country the process has often been carelessly conducted; and large quantities of an extract, prepared by boiling the plant in water and evaporating the decoction, have been sold as the genuine drug. The apothecary should always prepare the extract himself, or procure it from persons in whom he can have confidence. That imported from London has usually been considered the best; but the new officinal *Abstract* made from the fruit or seed is greatly to be preferred. It is not improbable that, as suggested by Professor Procter, the addition of a portion of acetic acid to the juice, before evaporation, might tend to fix the conine, and enable it better to resist the influence of heat, than in its native combination. The activity of any specimen of the extract may be in some measure judged of by rubbing it with potassa, which, disengaging the conine and rendering it volatile, gives rise to the peculiar mouse-like odor of that principle. If no odor be evolved under these circumstances, the extract may be deemed inert.

The extract of hemlock prepared without separating the chlorophyll has a fresh olive or green color. It should have a strong narcotic, somewhat fetid odor, and a bitterish saline taste. According to Brande, from three to five pounds are obtained from one cwt. of the leaves. M. Reclus got rather more than an ounce from sixteen ounces. Of the medical properties and application of this extract, we have spoken under the head of Conium. The dose is two grains (0·13 Gm.), two, three, or four times a day, to be gradually increased till evidences of its action upon the system are afforded. It may be administered in pill or solution.

Off. Prep. Br. Pilula Conii Composita.

EXTRACTUM CONII ALCOHOLICUM. *U. S.* *Alcoholic Extract of Conium.*

(ĔX-TRĂC'TŬM CO-NĪ'Ī ĂL-CO-HŎL'Ĭ-CŬM.)

Alcoholic Extract of Hemlock; Extrait alcoolique de Ciguë, *Fr.;* Spirituöses Schierlings-Extrakt, *G.*

"Conium (Fruit), in No. 40 powder, *one hundred parts* [or sixteen ounces av.]; Diluted Hydrochloric Acid, *three parts* [or three fluidrachms]; Glycerin, Diluted Alcohol, each, *a sufficient quantity*. Moisten the powder with *thirty parts* [four and a half fluidounces] of Diluted Alcohol, and pack it firmly in a cylindrical percolator; then add enough Diluted Alcohol to saturate the powder and leave a stratum above it. When the liquid begins to drop from the percolator, close the lower orifice, and, having closely covered the percolator, macerate for forty-eight hours. Then allow the percolation to proceed, gradually adding Diluted Alcohol, until *three hundred parts* [three pints] of tincture are obtained, or until the Conium is exhausted. Reserve the first *ninety parts* [or fourteen fluidounces] of the percolate, add the Diluted Hydrochloric Acid to the remainder, and evaporate it at a temperature not exceeding 50° C. (122° F.), to *ten parts* [or one and a half fluidounces]; mix this with the reserved portion, in a porcelain capsule, and evaporate at or below the before-mentioned temperature, to a pilular consistence. Lastly, weigh the Extract, and thoroughly incorporate with it, while still warm, *five per cent.* of Glycerin." *U. S.*

This preparation is not identical with the preparation formerly officinal under the above title, the very important change of substituting the fruit for the leaves having been made. As the preparation has thus been made considerably stronger, it is our opinion that the word "Fructus" should have been inserted in the title to draw attention to this fact. In the event of accident, the Committee of Revision might properly be severely censured. The change itself is undoubtedly a good one, and the improvement was needed; if carefully made, the extract is now reliable. The addition of hydrochloric acid is an important one, as the volatile alkaloid is thereby rendered more stable by being in combination. The dose to begin with is one-half to one grain (0·03–0·065 Gm.), to be increased if necessary.

EXTRACTUM CONII FLUIDUM. *U. S.* *Fluid Extract of Conium.*

(ĔX-TRĂC'TŬM CO-NĪ'Ī FLŪ'Ĭ-DŬM.)

Extractum Conii Fructus Fluidum, *U. S.* 1870; Fluid Extract of Conium Seed; Extrait liquide de Fruit de Ciguë, *Fr.;* Flüssiges Schierlingsfrucht-Extrakt, *G.*

"Conium (Fruit), in No. 40 powder, *one hundred grammes* [or fifty ounces av.]; Diluted Hydrochloric Acid, *three grammes* [or one and a half fluidounces]; Diluted Alcohol, *a sufficient quantity*, To make *one hundred cubic centimeters* [or three pints]. Moisten the powder with *thirty grammes* [or fifteen and a half fluidounces] of Diluted Alcohol, and pack it firmly in a cylindrical percolator; then add enough Diluted Alcohol to saturate the powder and leave a stratum above it. When the liquid begins to drop from the percolator, close the lower orifice, and, having closely covered the percolator, macerate for forty-eight hours. Then allow the percolation to proceed, gradually adding Diluted Alcohol, until the Conium is exhausted. Reserve the first *ninety cubic centimeters* [or forty-three fluidounces] of the percolate, and, having added the Diluted Hydrochloric Acid to the remainder, evaporate it, at a temperature not exceeding 50° C. (122° F.), to a soft extract; dissolve this in the reserved portion, and add enough Diluted Alcohol to make the Fluid Extract measure *one hundred cubic centimeters* [or three pints]." *U. S.*

The fluid extract of conium of the U. S. Pharmacopœia of 1860 was prepared from the leaves, and was, therefore, of necessity a very uncertain, if not for the most part inert, preparation. The alkaloid conine is contained in very unequal proportions in the fresh leaves, and is so very volatile and destructible that in the dried leaves it may be altogether wanting. Dr. Wm. Manlius Smith (*A. J. P.*, xl. 459), as the result of an elaborate investigation, found that the immature fruits of conium are not only richer in the alkaloids than are the leaves, but are less variable in the proportion they contain, and have the conine in them in such form that drying does not dissipate it. The superiority of the fluid extract of conium seed over the same preparation of the leaves was shown by Dr. Smith, and has been since abundantly confirmed by experience. The revisers of the Pharmacopœia of 1870 acted very wisely in abandoning the old for the new preparation. The reservation of the first tincture is important, because it probably contains all or nearly all of the active principle, so that little or none of this is lost during the evaporation. In the present formula, a still greater improvement was made by abandoning glycerin as a portion of the officinal menstruum. The present fluid extract is a brownish green dark liquid having the mouse-urine odor and emitting a still stronger conium smell on the addition of potassa; any sample which fails to do this should be rejected as wanting in the alkaloid. Dr. Smith found sixteen minims (1 C.c.) of a fluid extract of the seed prepared by Dr. Squibb to produce violent symptoms. Dr. L. Wheeler, however, took thirty minims (1·9 C.c.) without experiencing any result. (*Boston Med. and Surg. Journ.*, June, 1870.) Dangerous results have followed from the administration of much smaller doses, and it would seem hardly safe to commence with a dose of more than five minims (0·3 C.c.), to be increased until a feeling of general weakness or some other manifest effect is produced.

EXTRACTUM CORNUS FLUIDUM. *U. S.* *Fluid Extract of Cornus.*

(EX-TRĂC'TUM CŎR'NUS FLU'I-DŬM.)

Extractum Cornûs Floridæ Fluidum, *U. S.* 1870; Fluid Extract of Dogwood; Extrait liquide de Cornouiller à grandes Fleurs, *Fr.;* Flüssiges Kornelrinden-Extrakt, *G.*

"Cornus, in No. 60 powder, *one hundred grammes* [or fifty ounces av.]; Glycerin, *twenty grammes* [or seven and a half fluidounces]; Diluted Alcohol, *a sufficient quantity*, To make *one hundred cubic centimeters* [or three pints]. Mix the Glycerin with *eighty grammes* [or forty-one fluidounces] of Diluted Alcohol. Moisten the powder with *thirty grammes* [or fifteen fluidounces] of the mixture, and pack it firmly in a cylindrical percolator; then add enough of the menstruum to saturate the powder and leave a stratum above it. When the liquid begins to drop from the percolator, close the lower orifice, and, having closely covered the percolator, macerate for forty-eight hours. Then allow the percolation to proceed, gradually adding, first, the remainder of the menstruum, and afterward, Diluted Alcohol, until the Cornus is exhausted. Reserve the first *eighty-five cubic centimeters* [or forty fluidounces] of the percolate, and evaporate the remainder to a soft extract; dissolve this in the reserved portion, and add enough Diluted Alcohol to make the Fluid Extract measure *one hundred cubic centimeters* [or three pints]." *U. S.*

This preparation was improved at the late revision by greatly reducing the proportion of glycerin in the menstruum; the fluid extract, without doubt, represents whatever virtues the crude drug may contain, but it was scarcely worth introduction into the Pharmacopœia. The dose is half a fluidrachm (1·9 C.c.).

EXTRACTUM CUBEBÆ FLUIDUM. *U. S.* *Fluid Extract of Cubeb.*

(EX-TRĂC'TUM CŪ-BĒ'BÆ FLU'I-DŬM.)

Extrait liquide de Cubèbe, *Fr.;* Flüssiges Cubeben-Extrakt, *G.*

"Cubeb, in No. 60 powder, *one hundred grammes* [or fifty ounces av.]; Alcohol, *a sufficient quantity,* To make *one hundred cubic centimeters* [or three pints]. Moisten the powder with *twenty-five grammes* [or fourteen and a half fluidounces] of Alcohol, and pack it firmly in a cylindrical percolator; then add enough Alcohol to saturate the powder and leave a stratum above it. When the liquid begins to drop from the percolator, close the lower orifice, and, having closely covered the percolator, macerate for forty-eight hours. Then allow the percolation to proceed, gradually adding Alcohol, until the Cubeb is exhausted. Reserve the first *ninety cubic centimeters* [forty-three fluidounces] of the percolate, and evaporate the remainder to a soft extract; dissolve this in the reserved portion, and add enough Alcohol to make the Fluid Extract measure *one hundred cubic centimeters* [or three pints]." *U. S.*

Notwithstanding the fact that the oleoresin of cubeb thoroughly represents in a concentrated liquid form all of the virtue of this drug, the alcoholic fluid extract is a useful preparation; it permits the administration of cubeb in aqueous or hydro-alcoholic mixtures where the oleoresin would not be admissible except in emulsion. It is a dark olive, translucent fluid, with the sensible properties of the drug. It may be given in doses of from ten to forty minims (0·6–2·5 C.c.).

EXTRACTUM CYPRIPEDII FLUIDUM. *U. S.* *Fluid Extract of Cypripedium.*

(ĔX-TRĂC'TŬM ÇȲP-RĮ-PĒ'DĮ-Ī FLŪ'Į-DŬM.)

Extrait liquide de Cypripède jaune, *Fr.;* Flüssiges Gelbfrauenschuh-Extrakt, *G.*

"Cypripedium, in No. 60 powder, *one hundred grammes* [or fifty ounces av.]; Alcohol *a sufficient quantity,* To make *one hundred cubic centimeters* [or three pints]. Moisten the powder with *thirty-five grammes* [or twenty fluidounces] of Alcohol, and pack it firmly in a cylindrical percolator; then add enough Alcohol to saturate the powder and leave the stratum above it. When the liquid begins to drop from the percolator, close the lower orifice, and, having closely covered the percolator, macerate for forty-eight hours. Then allow the percolation to proceed, gradually adding Alcohol, until the Cypripedium is exhausted. Reserve the first *eighty-five cubic centimeters* [or forty fluidounces] of the percolate, and evaporate the remainder to a soft extract; dissolve this in the reserved portion, and add enough Alcohol to make the Fluid Extract measure *one hundred cubic centimeters* [or three pints]." *U. S.*

This is one of the new officinal fluid extracts; it well represents the drug, although its use is at present very limited. It is very dark reddish brown in color, and may be given in doses of fifteen minims (0·9 C.c.).

EXTRACTUM DIGITALIS, *U. S.* *Extract of Digitalis.*

(ĔX-TRĂC'TŬM DĬǤ-Į-TĀ'LĬS.)

Extrait alcoolique de Digitale, *Fr.;* Fingerhut-Extrakt, *G.*

"Digitalis, recently dried and in No. 60 powder, *one hundred parts* [or sixteen ounces av.]; Alcohol, *two hundred parts* [or two and a quarter pints]; Water, *one hundred parts* [or one pint]; Glycerin, Diluted Alcohol, each, *a sufficient quantity.* Mix the Alcohol and Water, and, having moistened the powder with *forty parts* [or six fluidounces] of the mixture, pack it firmly in a cylindrical percolator; then add enough of the menstruum to saturate the powder and leave a stratum above it. When the liquid begins to drop from the percolator, close the lower orifice, and, having closely covered the percolator, macerate for forty-eight hours. Then allow the percolation to proceed, gradually adding, first, the remainder of the menstruum, and then, Diluted Alcohol, until *three hundred parts* [or three pints] of tincture are obtained, or the Digitalis is exhausted. By means of a water-bath, distil off the alcohol from the tincture, and, having placed the residue in a porcelain capsule, evaporate it on a water-bath, to a pilular consistence. Lastly, weigh the Extract, and thoroughly incorporate with it, while still warm, *five per cent.* of Glycerin." *U. S.*

This was a new officinal of the U. S. Pharmacopœia of 1860, though less needed than many others; because the dose of digitalis itself is small, and nothing is gained on the point of equability of strength, as the really active part of digitalis constitutes but a small proportion even of the extract, and might be altogether wanting without observably affecting the bulk. The same caution is used, in preparing this extract, against the injurious effects of heat as in the instance of the extract of conium. The extract now officinal does not differ essentially from that of U. S. P. 1870, with this exception, that instead of percolating first with alcohol and then with diluted alcohol, a menstruum of two parts alcohol and one part water is now used, finishing with diluted alcohol. The alcoholic extract of digitalis contains all the virtues and may be used for all the purposes of the powdered leaves. According to Messrs. Vielguth and Nentwich, the amount of alcoholic extract obtained from dried digitalis by cold displacement is 27·1 per cent. (See *A. J. P.*, May, 1859, p. 237.) The dose, therefore, of this extract to begin with should not exceed one-fourth of a grain (·016 Gm.).

EXTRACTUM DIGITALIS FLUIDUM. *U. S.* *Fluid Extract of Digitalis.*

(EX-TRĂC′TUM DĬG-I-TĀ′LĬS FLŪ′I-DŬM.)

Extrait liquide de Digitale, *Fr.;* Flüssiges Fingerhut-Extrakt, *G.*

"Digitalis, recently dried and in No. 60 powder, *one hundred grammes* [or fifty ounces av.]; Alcohol, Water, each, *a sufficient quantity*, To make *one hundred cubic centimeters* [or three pints]. Mix *three parts* [or three and a half pints] of Alcohol with *one part* [or one pint] of Water, and, having moistened the powder with *thirty-five grammes* [or twenty fluidounces] of the mixture, pack it firmly in a cylindrical percolator; then add enough of the menstruum to saturate the powder and leave a stratum above it. When the liquid begins to drop from the percolator, close the lower orifice, and, having closely covered the percolator, macerate for forty-eight hours. Then allow the percolation to proceed, gradually adding menstruum, until the Digitalis is exhausted. Reserve the first *eighty-five cubic centimeters* [or forty fluidounces] of the percolate, and evaporate the remainder to a soft extract; dissolve this in the reserved portion, and add enough menstruum to make the Fluid Extract measure *one hundred cubic centimeters* [or three pints]." *U. S.*

Glycerin was abandoned at the last revision, and there certainly was no necessity for its use. The present highly spirituous menstruum is well suited to the drug, although it could be made more aqueous without detriment, and without danger of precipitation. This fluid extract is dark, greenish black in color, and represents the drug thoroughly. The dose is one to two minims (0·06–0·12 C.c.).

EXTRACTUM DULCAMARÆ FLUIDUM. *U. S.* *Fluid Extract of Dulcamara.*

(EX-TRĂC′TUM DŬL-CA-MĀ′RÆ FLŪ′I-DŬM.)

Extrait liquide de Douce-Amère, *Fr.;* Flüssiges Bittersüss-Extrakt, *G.*

"Dulcamara, in No. 60 powder, *one hundred grammes* [or fifty ounces av.]; Diluted Alcohol, *a sufficient quantity*, To make *one hundred cubic centimeters* [or three pints]. Moisten the powder with *forty grammes* [twenty fluidounces] of Diluted Alcohol, and pack it firmly in a cylindrical percolator; then add enough Diluted Alcohol to saturate the powder and leave a stratum above it. When the liquid begins to drop from the percolator, close the lower orifice, and, having closely covered the percolator, macerate for forty-eight hours. Then allow the percolation to proceed, gradually adding Diluted Alcohol, until the Dulcamara is exhausted. Reserve the first *eighty cubic centimeters* [or thirty-eight fluidounces] of the percolate, and evaporate the remainder to a soft extract; dissolve this in the reserved portion, and add enough Diluted Alcohol to make the Fluid Extract measure *one hundred cubic centimeters* [or three pints]." *U. S.*

The present formula differs from that of U. S. P. 1870 in the absence of glycerin. This fluid extract is a rather thick, dark brown liquid. The dose is from thirty minims to a fluidrachm (1·9–3·75 C.c.), three or four times a day, gradually increased if necessary.

EXTRACTUM ERGOTÆ. *U. S.* *Extract of Ergot.*

(ĔX-TRĂC'TŬM ĔR-GŌ'TÆ.)

Ergotinum, *Br.;* Ergotin; Extrait de Seigle ergoté, *Fr.;* Mutterkornextrakt, *G.*

"Purified extract of Ergot, commonly called Ergotin, Ergotine, or Bonjean's Ergotine." *Br.*

"Fluid Extract of Ergot, *five hundred parts* [or sixteen ounces av.], To make *one hundred parts* [or three ounces and eighty-eight grains av.]. Evaporate the Fluid Extract of Ergot in a porcelain capsule, by means of a water-bath, at a temperature not exceeding 50° C. (122° F.), constantly stirring, until it is reduced to *one hundred parts* [or three ounces and eighty-eight grains av.]." *U. S.*

"Take of Liquid Extract of Ergot, Rectified Spirit, of each, *four fluidounces.* Evaporate the Fluid Extract by a water-bath to a syrupy consistence, and when cold mix with the spirit. Let it stand for half an hour, then filter, and evaporate the filtered liquid to the consistence of a soft extract." *Br.*

This is a new officinal and a valuable addition to the list of extracts. It originated with Dr. E. R. Squibb, who, becoming dissatisfied with the so-called ergotins of the market, devised this simple process. (*Proc. A. P. A.*, 1873, p. 644.) The present preparation leaves little to be desired. The original formula made an extract slightly weaker; it was one-sixth of the weight of the fluid extract, instead of one-fifth, as it is now in the officinal formula; the acid present in the fluid extract was acetic, instead of hydrochloric as at present: these changes are, however, trifling. The British preparation is modelled upon the process of Bonjean's for ergotine, and being made from liquid extract of ergot, a process of purification is necessary, due to the fact that the aqueous menstruum of the liquid extract takes up albumen, gum, and inert constituents from the ergot, and these must be precipitated by alcohol. The U. S. menstruum, being almost of the strength of diluted alcohol, rejects a larger quantity of the inert substances, and hence precipitation with alcohol as directed by the British Pharmacopœia is unnecessary. This is much the best preparation of ergot, being the only one that should be used hypodermically, and much less apt to cause nausea when given by the mouth. For method of hypodermic use, see *Ergota.* It is also well adapted for suppositories, and has been applied topically to the os uteri, the desired dose being put on a dossil of absorbent cotton. Internally it is best given in gelatin capsules; although it may be made into pills, they soon flatten and lose their shape, unless combined with some inert powder. The dose is one-fifth that of the fluid extract or drug—*i.e.*, five grains to half a drachm (0·33–1·9 Gm.).

Off. Prep. Br. Injectio Ergotini Hypodermica.

EXTRACTUM ERGOTÆ FLUIDUM. *U. S.* *Fluid Extract of Ergot.*

(ĔX-TRĂC'TŬM ĔR-GŌ'TÆ FLŪ'Ĭ-DŬM.)

Extractum Ergotæ Liquidum, *Br.;* Liquid Extract of Ergot; Extrait liquide de Seigle ergoté, *Fr.;* Flüssiges Mutterkornextrakt, *G.*

"Ergot, recently ground and in No. 60 powder, *one hundred grammes* [or fifty ounces av.]; Diluted Hydrochloric Acid, *six grammes* [or three fluidounces]; Alcohol, Water, each, *a sufficient quantity*, To make *one hundred cubic centimeters* [or three pints]. Mix *three parts* [or two and a half pints] of Alcohol with *four parts* [or two and three-quarter pints] of Water, and, having moistened the powder with *thirty grammes* [or fifteen and a half fluidounces] of the mixture, pack it firmly in a cylindrical percolator; then add enough of the menstruum to saturate the powder and leave a stratum above it. When the liquid begins to drop from the percolator, close the lower orifice, and, having closely covered the percolator, macerate for forty-eight hours. Then allow the percolation to proceed, gradually adding menstruum, until the Ergot is exhausted. Reserve the first *eighty-five cubic centimeters* [or forty fluidounces] of the percolate, and, having added the Diluted Hydrochloric Acid to the remainder, evaporate to a soft extract; dissolve this in the reserved portion, and add enough menstruum to make the Fluid Extract measure *one hundred cubic centimeters* [or three pints]." *U. S.*

"Take of Ergot, crushed, *one pound* [av.]; Distilled Water *six pints* [Imp.

meas.]; Rectified Spirit *six fluidounces* [Imp. meas.]. Digest the Ergot in four pints of the Water for twelve hours. Draw off the infusion and repeat the digestion with the remainder of the water. Press out, strain, and evaporate the liquors by the heat of a water-bath to eleven fluidounces; when cold, add the Spirit. Allow it to stand for an hour to coagulate, then filter. The product should measure sixteen fluidounces." *Br.*

This fluid extract was first suggested by Mr. Jos. Laidley, of Richmond, Va.; but the process has since been much modified. The improvement first suggested by Prof. Procter, of adding an acid to the menstruum to fix the alkaloids, and the selection of the proper menstruum, placed this important preparation at once on a permanent footing; and his original formula, published in 1857, and made officinal in 1860, is now practically adopted in 1880, notwithstanding the numerous changes of views concerning the active constituents of ergot. Practical experience has shown that it is not only a reliable, but, if carefully made, a permanent preparation. The use of glycerin in the menstruum is of no benefit whatever, and it would render the fluid extract unfit for use as a basis for the extract now officinal; as an addition, diluted hydrochloric probably answers as well as acetic acid for fixing alkaloids, although, if Dragendorff's researches were thoroughly accepted, there would seem to be no need of it, as the alkaloids are not now believed to be the active principles. (See *Ergota.*) Diluted alcohol dissolves all the active matter of ergot, leaving its oil behind, and the tincture first obtained, holding most of the active principles, is reserved without concentration. In the British process the prolonged digestion and evaporation must act disadvantageously upon principles which are known to be very easily affected by heat and exposure.

The U. S. fluid extract of ergot is a clear, very dark reddish brown liquid, having the taste of ergot, but without its fishy odor, owing to the fixation of the trimethylamine, upon which that odor depends. On the addition, however, of solution of potassa, the odor is strongly developed, and the alkaloid escapes so largely that, if hydrochloric acid be held near it, a cloud of trimethylamine chloride will be perceived. This may be considered as a good test of the efficiency of the preparation; for, though the virtues of ergot do not depend on its volatile alkaloid, yet, if this be retained in the fluid extract, there can be little doubt that the other more fixed principles will be retained also. The preparation is an active one, but in large doses more apt to sicken the stomach than is the simple extract. The dose is from half a fluidrachm to half a fluidounce (1·9 to 15 C.c.).

Off. Prep. Extractum Ergotæ.

EXTRACTUM ERYTHROXYLI FLUIDUM. *U.S., Br.* *Fluid Extract of Erythroxylon.* [*Fluid Extract of Coca.*]

(ĔX-TRĂC′TŬM ĔR-Y̆-THRŎX′Y̆-LĪ FLŪ′Ĭ-DŬM.)

Extractum Cocæ Liquidum, *Br.;* Liquid Extract of Coca; Extrait liquide de Coca, *Fr.;* Flüssiges Cocablätter-Extrakt, *G.*

"Erythroxylon, in No. 40 powder, *one hundred grammes* [or fifty ounces av.]; Diluted Alcohol, *a sufficient quantity,* To make *one hundred cubic centimeters* [or three pints]. Moisten the powder with *forty-five grammes* [or twenty-three and a half fluidounces] of Diluted Alcohol, and pack it firmly in a cylindrical percolator; then add enough Diluted Alcohol to saturate the powder and leave a stratum above it. When the liquid begins to drop from the percolator, close the lower orifice, and, having closely covered the percolator, macerate for forty-eight hours. Then allow the percolation to proceed, gradually adding Diluted Alcohol, until the Erythroxylon is exhausted. Reserve the first *eighty cubic centimeters* [or thirty-eight fluidounces] of the percolate, and evaporate the remainder to a soft extract; dissolve this in the reserved portion, and add enough Diluted Alcohol to make the Fluid Extract measure *one hundred cubic centimeters* [or three pints]." *U. S.*

"Take of Coca, in No. 40 powder, *twenty ounces* [av.]; Proof Spirit *a sufficiency.* Mix the Coca with two pints [Imp. meas.] of the spirit, and macerate in a closed vessel for forty-eight hours; then transfer to a percolator, and when the fluid ceases to pass, continue the percolation with more of the spirit until the Coca is exhausted.

Reserve the first fifteen fluidounces [Imp. meas.] of the percolate, and evaporate the remainder by a water-bath to the consistence of a soft extract; dissolve this in the reserved portion, and make up the volume to twenty fluidounces [Imp. meas.] by the addition of more spirit." *Br.*

This new officinal fluid extract is one of the most useful of the preparations of coca. It is of a dark greenish brown color, of an agreeable tea-like taste, but with little odor. The dose is from twenty minims to a fluidrachm (1·25–3·75 C.c.).

EXTRACTUM EUCALYPTI FLUIDUM. *U. S.* *Fluid Extract of Eucalyptus.*

(ĔX-TRĂC'TŬM EŪ-CĂ-LȲP'TĪ FLŪ'Ĭ-DŬM—yū-ka-lip'tī.)

Extrait liquide d'Eucalyptus, *Fr.;* Flüssiges Eucalyptus-Extrakt, *G.*

"Eucalyptus, in No. 40 powder, *one hundred grammes* [or fifty ounces av.]; Alcohol, *a sufficient quantity,* To make *one hundred cubic centimeters* [or three pints]. Moisten the powder with *thirty-five grammes* [or twenty fluidounces] of Alcohol, and pack it firmly in a cylindrical percolator; then add enough Alcohol to saturate the powder and leave a stratum above it. When the liquid begins to drop from the percolator, close the lower orifice, and, having closely covered the percolator, macerate for forty-eight hours. Then allow the percolation to proceed, gradually adding Alcohol until the Eucalyptus is exhausted. Reserve the first *eighty-five cubic centimeters* [or forty fluidounces] of the percolate, and evaporate the remainder to a soft extract; dissolve this in the reserved portion, and add enough Alcohol to make the Fluid Extract measure *one hundred cubic centimeters* [or three pints]." *U. S.*

This is another of the new fluid extracts admitted to the Pharmacopœia at the last revision. It well represents the drug, and is of a dark greenish brown color, having the peculiar odor and taste of eucalyptus very strongly developed, but for administration is much inferior to the volatile oil. The dose is from five to ten minims (0·3–0·6 C.c.).

EXTRACTUM EUONYMI. *U. S.* *Extract of Euonymus.*

(ĔX-TRĂC'TŬM EŪ-ŎN'Ȳ-MĪ—yū-ŏn'ĭ-mī.)

Extrait de Fusain, *Fr.;* Spindelbaum-Extrakt, *G.*

"Euonymus, in No. 30 powder, *one hundred parts* [or sixteen ounces av.]; Glycerin, Diluted Alcohol, each, *a sufficient quantity.* Moisten the powder with *forty parts* [or six fluidounces] of Diluted Alcohol, and pack it firmly in a cylindrical percolator; then add enough Diluted Alcohol to saturate the powder and leave a stratum above it. When the liquid begins to drop from the percolator, close the lower orifice, and, having closely covered the percolator, macerate for forty-eight hours. Then allow the percolation to proceed, gradually adding Diluted Alcohol, until *three hundred parts* [or three pints] of tincture are obtained, or the Euonymus is exhausted. By means of a water-bath distil off the Alcohol from the tincture, and, having placed the residue in a porcelain capsule, evaporate it, on a water-bath, to a pilular consistence. Lastly, weigh the Extract, and thoroughly incorporate with it, while still warm, *five per cent.* of Glycerin." *U. S.*

This is a new extract introduced in the U. S. P. 1880, with the view of affording to practitioners a convenient method of administering wahoo. The dose is from one to three grains (0·065–0·20 Gm.).

EXTRACTUM EUPATORII FLUIDUM. *U. S.* *Fluid Extract of Eupatorium.*

(ĔX-TRĂC'TŬM EŪ-PĂ-TŌ'RĬ-Ī FLŪ'Ĭ-DŬM—yū-pa-tō'rē-ī.)

Extrait liquide d'Eupatoire, *Fr.;* Flüssiges Durchwachsener Wasserhanf-Extrakt, *G.*

"Eupatorium, in No. 40 powder, *one hundred grammes* [or fifty ounces av.]; Diluted Alcohol, *a sufficient quantity,* To make *one hundred cubic centimeters* [or three pints]. Moisten the powder with *forty grammes* [or twenty fluidounces] of

Diluted Alcohol, and pack it firmly in a cylindrical percolator; then add enough Diluted Alcohol to saturate the powder and leave a stratum above it. When the liquid begins to drop from the percolator, close the lower orifice, and, having closely covered the percolator, macerate for forty-eight hours. Then allow the percolation to proceed, gradually adding Diluted Alcohol, until the Eupatorium is exhausted. Reserve the first *eighty cubic centimeters* [or thirty-eight fluidounces] of the percolate, and evaporate the remainder to a soft extract; dissolve this in the reserved portion, and add enough Diluted Alcohol to make the Fluid Extract measure *one hundred cubic centimeters* [or three pints]." *U. S.*

This new officinal fluid extract will have but a limited use, although it well represents the drug, since boneset is chiefly employed in domestic medicine. It is of a dark greenish brown color, and the dose may be stated as from twenty minims to a fluidrachm (1·25–3·75 C.c.).

EXTRACTUM FILICIS LIQUIDUM. *Br.* *Liquid Extract of Male Fern.*

(ĔX-TRĂC'TŬM FĬL'Ĭ-CĬS LĬQ'UĬ-DŬM—lik'wĭ-dŭm.)

This, being properly an oleoresin, will be considered under the head of the *Oleoresinæ*, to which the reader is referred. See *Oleoresina Aspidii*, page 1027.

EXTRACTUM FRANGULÆ FLUIDUM. *U.S.* *Fluid Extract of Frangula.*

(ĔX-TRĂC'TŬM FRĂN'GŪ-LÆ FLŪ'Ĭ-DŬM.)

Extrait liquide de Bourdaine, *Fr.;* **Flüssiges Faulbaumrinde-Extrakt,** *G.*

"Frangula, in No. 40 powder, *one hundred grammes* [or fifty ounces av.]; Alcohol, Water, each, *a sufficient quantity*, To make *one hundred cubic centimeters* [or three pints]. Mix *one part* [or two and a quarter pints] of Alcohol with *two parts* [or four pints] of Water, and, having moistened the powder with *thirty-five grammes* [or seventeen fluidounces] of the mixture, pack it firmly in a cylindrical percolator; then add enough of the menstruum to saturate the powder and leave a stratum above it. When the liquid begins to drop from the percolator, close the lower orifice, and, having closely covered the percolator, macerate for forty-eight hours. Then allow the percolation to proceed, gradually adding menstruum, until the Frangula is exhausted. Reserve the first *eighty cubic centimeters* [or thirty-eight fluidounces] of the percolate, and evaporate the remainder to a soft extract; dissolve this in the reserved portion, and add enough menstruum to make the Fluid Extract measure *one hundred cubic centimeters* [or three pints]." *U. S.*

This is another new fluid extract which has been quite largely used in this country during the last ten years. It is intended to be a laxative, but it is frequently disappointing, as the drug is rarely to be obtained of uniform good quality. The fluid extract is of a dark reddish brown color. The dose is ten to twenty minims.

EXTRACTUM GELSEMII ALCOHOLICUM. *Br.* *Alcoholic Extract of Gelsemium.*

(ĔX-TRĂC'TŬM GĔL-SĒM'Ĭ-Ī ĂL-CO-HŎL'Ĭ-CŬM.)

"Take of Gelsemium, in No. 60 powder, *one pound* [av.]; Rectified Spirit, Distilled Water, of each, *a sufficiency*. Mix the Gelsemium with two pints [Imp. meas.] of the Spirit, and macerate in a closed vessel for forty-eight hours; then transfer to a percolator, and when the fluid ceases to pass, continue the percolation with water until two pints [Imp. meas.] of liquor have been collected. Evaporate the percolated liquor by a water-bath until the extract has acquired a suitable consistence." *Br.*

This is an excellent preparation of gelsemium, enabling the practitioner to give the drug in small quantities in pilular form. The dose given by the British Pharmacopœia is one-half to two grains (0·033–0·13 Gm.); the smaller quantity should be given as the commencing dose, and its effects very carefully watched. (See *Gelsemium.*)

EXTRACTUM GELSEMII FLUIDUM. *U. S.* *Fluid Extract of Gelsemium.*

(EX-TRĂC'TUM GEL-SEM'I-Ī FLŪ'I-DŬM.)

Extrait liquide de Jasmine jaune, *Fr.;* Flüssiges Gelber Jasmin-Extrakt, *G.*

"Gelsemium, in No. 60 powder, *one hundred grammes* [or fifty ounces av.]; Alcohol, *a sufficient quantity,* To make *one hundred cubic centimeters* [or three pints]. Moisten the powder with *thirty grammes* [or seventeen fluidounces] of Alcohol, and pack it firmly in a cylindrical percolator; then add enough Alcohol to saturate the powder and leave a stratum above it. When the liquid begins to drop from the percolator, close the lower orifice, and, having closely covered the percolator, macerate for forty-eight hours. Then allow the percolation to proceed, gradually adding Alcohol, until the Gelsemium is exhausted. Reserve the first *ninety cubic centimeters* [or forty-three fluidounces] of the percolate, and evaporate the remainder to a soft extract; dissolve this in the reserved portion, and add enough Alcohol to make the Fluid Extract measure *one hundred cubic centimeters* [or three pints]." *U. S.*

This is identical with the fluid extract formerly officinal, which has proved very useful. It is of a dark reddish brown color. The dose is from two to three minims (0·12–0·18 C.c.).

EXTRACTUM GENTIANÆ. *U. S., Br.* *Extract of Gentian.*

(EX-TRĂC'TUM GĔN-TI-Ā'NÆ—jĕn-she-ā'nē.)

Extrait de Gentiane, *Fr.;* Enzian-Extrakt, *G.*

"Gentian, in No. 20 powder, *one hundred parts* [or sixteen ounces av.]; Water, *a sufficient quantity.* Moisten the powder with *forty parts* [or six fluidounces] of Water, and let it macerate for twenty-four hours; then pack it in a conical percolator, and gradually pour Water upon it until the infusion passes but slightly imbued with the properties of the Gentian. Reduce the liquid to three-fourths of its weight by boiling, and strain; then, by means of a water-bath, evaporate to a pilular consistence." *U. S.*

"Take of Gentian Root, sliced, *one pound* [avoir.]; Boiling Distilled Water *one gallon* [Imp. measure]. Infuse the Gentian in the Water for two hours, boil for fifteen minutes; pour off, press, and strain. Then evaporate the liquor by a water-bath until the extract is of a suitable consistence for forming pills." *Br.*

The U. S. plan of percolation with cold water is admirably adapted to the extraction of the active matter of gentian, and even the British method of maceration with hot water is much better than the old plan of decoction. By the use of cold water, starch and pectic acid are left behind, while any albumen that may be taken up is disposed of by the subsequent boiling and straining.

The extract, however, may be advantageously made by macerating the root in two parts of water for thirty-six hours, then expressing in a powerful press, again macerating with additional water, and in like manner expressing, and evaporating the united expressed liquors. MM. Guibourt and Cadet de Vaux obtained by maceration in cold water an extract not only greater in amount, but more transparent, more bitter, and possessing more of the color and smell of the root than that prepared by decoction. Guibourt attributes this result to the circumstance that, as gentian contains little if any starch, it yields nothing to boiling which it will not also yield to cold water; while decoction favors the combination of a portion of the coloring matter with the lignin. But this opinion requires modification, now that it is understood that gentian contains pectic acid, which water will extract when boiling hot, but not when cold. Gentian, according to Brande, yields half its weight of extract by decoction.

As ordinarily procured, the extract of gentian has an agreeable odor, is very bitter, and of a dark brown color approaching to black, shining, and tenacious. It is frequently used as a tonic, in the form of pill, either alone or in connection with metallic preparations; but the practice of some pharmacists of using it indiscriminately as a pill excipient is very wrong and deserving of severe censure. The dose is from five to ten grains (0·33–0·65 Gm.).

EXTRACTUM GENTIANÆ FLUIDUM. *U. S.* *Fluid Extract of Gentian.*

(EX-TRĂC'TUM GĔN-TI-Ā'NÆ FLŪ'I-DŬM—jĕn-she-ā'nē.)

Extrait liquide de Gentiane, *Fr.;* Flüssiges Enzian-Extrakt, *G.*

"Gentian, in No. 30 powder, *one hundred grammes* [or fifty ounces av.]; Diluted Alcohol, *a sufficient quantity,* To make *one hundred cubic centimeters* [or three pints]. Moisten the powder with *thirty-five grammes* [or eighteen fluidounces] of Diluted Alcohol, and pack it firmly in a cylindrical percolator; then add enough Diluted Alcohol to saturate the powder and leave a stratum above it. When the liquid begins to drop from the percolator, close the lower orifice, and, having closely covered the percolator, macerate for forty-eight hours. Then allow the percolation to proceed, gradually adding Diluted Alcohol, until the Gentian is exhausted. Reserve the first *eighty cubic centimeters* [or thirty-eight fluidounces] of the percolate. By means of a water-bath, distil off the Alcohol from the remainder and evaporate the residue to a soft extract; dissolve this in the reserved portion, and add enough Diluted Alcohol to make the Fluid Extract measure *one hundred cubic centimeters* [or three pints]." *U. S.*

This is a translucent, reddish brown fluid, with the smell and taste of the root. It may be questionable whether it was needed, though it has the advantage that we may obtain from it the tonic effects of the drug with less alcohol than in an equivalent quantity of the tincture; and pharmaceutically it affords a convenient method of giving to mixtures the tonic properties of gentian when required. The dose is from ten to thirty minims (0·6–1·9 C.c.).

EXTRACTUM GERANII FLUIDUM. *U. S.* *Fluid Extract of Geranium.*

(EX-TRĂC'TUM GE-RĀ'NI-Ī FLŪ'I-DŬM.)

Extrait de Bec de Grue tacheté, *Fr.;* Flüssiges Fleckenstorchschnabel-Extrakt, *G.*

"Geranium, in No. 30 powder, *one hundred grammes* [or fifty ounces av.], Glycerin, *ten grammes* [or three and three-quarter fluidounces]; Diluted Alcohol, *a sufficient quantity,* To make *one hundred cubic centimeters* [or three pints]. Mix the Glycerin with *ninety grammes* [or forty-six and a half fluidounces] of Diluted Alcohol, and having moistened the powder with *thirty-five grammes* [or eighteen fluidounces] of the mixture, pack it firmly in a cylindrical percolator; then add enough of the menstruum to saturate the powder and leave a stratum above it. When the liquid begins to drop from the percolator, close the lower orifice, and, having closely covered the percolator, macerate for forty-eight hours. Then allow the percolation to proceed, gradually adding, first, the remainder of the menstruum, and afterward, Diluted Alcohol, until the Geranium is exhausted. Reserve the first *seventy cubic centimeters* [or thirty-four fluidounces] of the percolate, and evaporate the remainder to a soft extract; dissolve this in the reserved portion, and add enough Diluted Alcohol to make the Fluid Extract measure *one hundred cubic centimeters* [or three pints]." *U. S.*

The quantity of glycerin has been greatly diminished in this fluid extract, and the process is now unobjectionable. It is a dark reddish brown liquid, having little odor and a very astringent taste. The dose is from thirty minims to a fluidrachm (1·9–3·75 C.c.).

EXTRACTUM GLYCYRRHIZÆ. *U. S., Br.* *Extract of Glycyrrhiza.* [*Extract of Liquorice.*]

(EX-TRĂC'TUM GLY̆Ç-Y̆R-RHĪ'ZÆ—glis-ir-rī'zē.)

"The commercial extract of the root of Glycyrrhiza glabra. Linné. (*Nat. Ord.* Leguminosæ, Papilionaceæ.)" *U. S.*

Succus Liquiritiæ, *P. G.;* Liquorice, Licorice; Extrait de Réglisse, *Fr.;* Lakriz, Lakrizensaft, Süssholzsaft, *G.;* Sugo di Liquirisia, *It.;* Regaliza en Ballos, *Sp.*

Liquorice is an article of export from the north of Spain, particularly Catalonia, where it is obtained in the following manner. The roots of the *G. glabra,* having been dug up, thoroughly cleansed, and half dried by exposure to the air, are cut into small pieces, and boiled in water till the liquid is saturated. The decoction is then allowed to rest, and, after the dregs have subsided, is decanted, and evaporated to the proper consistence. The extract, thus prepared, is formed into rolls from five to six inches long by an inch in diameter, which are dried in the air, and wrapped in laurel leaves.

The British Pharmacopœia gives a process for making extract of liquorice. (See *Extractum Glycyrrhizæ Purum*, page 636.)

"In flattened cylindrical rolls, from six inches to six and three-quarter inches (150 to 175 mm.) long, and from five-eighths to one and one-sixteenth inch (15 to 30 mm.) thick; of a glossy black color. It breaks with a sharp, conchoidal, shining fracture, and has a very sweet, peculiar taste. Not less than 60 per cent. of it should be soluble in cold water." *U. S.*

Much liquorice is prepared in Calabria, according to M. Fée, from the *G. echinata*, which abounds in that country. The process is essentially the same as that just described, but conducted with greater care; and the Italian liquorice is purer and more valuable than the Spanish. It is in cylinders, generally somewhat smaller than the Spanish, and usually stamped with the manufacturer's brand. Most of the extract brought to this country comes from Messina and Catania in Sicily and Naples, from Seville and Saragossa in Spain, and from Smyrna in Turkey. Perhaps in no part of the world is more liquorice consumed than in this country, from four to five thousand tons having been imported annually before the war; but the article is now made on an extensive scale in this country, very successfully, with the best modern appliances, and of such good quality as to have almost driven the foreign article out of the market. The principal use of Extract of Liquorice is in the manufacture of chewing tobacco; that in the form of rolls as sold by the druggists being a comparatively small portion of the whole amount consumed.

Crude Liquorice, *Liquorice Paste*, or *Liquorice Mass*, as it is variously termed, is found in the market in cases ranging from two hundred and fifty to four hundred pounds, of a hard pilular consistence and, as its name implies, in a mass, which has been run into the case while hot and then allowed to cool.

The importation of liquorice root into the United States for the year 1887 amounted to 79,603,835 pounds, and was valued at $1,670,041.

Liquorice is usually in cylindrical rolls, somewhat flattened, and often covered with bay leaves. We have seen it in the London market in large cubical masses. When good, it is very black, dry, brittle, breaking with a shining fracture, of a very sweet, peculiar, slightly acrid or bitterish taste, and almost entirely soluble, when pure, in boiling water. Neumann obtained 460 parts of aqueous extract from 480 parts of Spanish liquorice. It is, however, considerably less soluble in cold water. It is often impure from accidental or fraudulent addition, or careless preparation. Starch, sand, the juice of prunes, etc., are sometimes added; and carbonaceous matter, and even particles of copper, are found in it, the latter arising from the boilers in which the decoction is evaporated. Four pounds of the extract have yielded two drachms and a half of metallic copper. (*Fée.*) In different commercial specimens examined by Chevallier, he found from 9 to 50 per cent. of insoluble matter. (*Journ. de Pharm.*, xxx. 429.) This is by no means, however, always impurity. In the preparation of the extract by decoction, a portion of matter originally insoluble, or rendered so by decoction, is taken up, and is, in fact, necessary to the proper constitution of the liquorice. When this is prepared with cold water, or even with hot water by simple displacement, the extract attracts moisture from the air, becomes soft, and loses the characteristic brittleness of the drug. The additional substances taken up in decoction serve to protect the extract against this change. M. Delondre has obtained the same result by using steam as the solvent. He prepares from the root an excellent liquorice, having all the requisite qualities of color, taste, and permanence, by passing steam, in suitable vessels, through the coarse powder of the root. The vapor thoroughly penetrates the powder, and is drawn off as it condenses. With about 500 lbs. of the root, this treatment is continued for 12 hours, and repeated at the end of 5 days. The liquors are collected, decanted, clarified with about 4 lbs. of gelatin, and quickly evaporated. After being put into the form of cylinders, the extract is kept for ten days in a drying room, at a temperature of 77°. (*Ibid.*, p. 433.) A bitter or empyreumatic taste is a sign of inferior quality in liquorice. As ordinarily found in commerce, it requires to be purified.* (See *Extractum Glycyrrhizæ Purum*; also, *Liquor Extracti Glycyrrhizæ*, Part II.)

Liquorice contains glycyrrhizin, $C_{24}H_{36}O_{9}$, a glucoside, partly free and partly in combination with ammonia, to which combination the characteristic sweet taste of liquorice is due. The glycyrrhizin when boiled with dilute acids decomposes into *glycyrrhetin*, $C_{18}H_{26}O_{4}$, and a fermentable sugar.

The *refined liquorice*, found in commerce in small cylindrical pieces not thicker than a pipe stem, is prepared by dissolving the impure extract in water without boiling, straining the solution, and evaporating. The object of this process is to separate not only the insoluble impurities, but also the acrid oleoresinous substance, which is extracted by long boiling from the liquorice root, and is necessarily mixed with the unrefined extract. It is customary to add, during the process, a portion of sugar, gum, flour, starch, or perhaps glue. These additions, or something equivalent, are necessary to obviate the deliquescent property of the pure liquorice. According to M. Delondre, 15 per cent. of gum is the proper proportion, when this substance is used; Dr. Geisler has found sugar of milk to lessen the disposition of the extract to absorb moisture; but he considers the best addition, on the whole, to be very finely powdered liquorice root, which should be used in the proportion of one part to 16 of the purified extract. (*A. J. P.*, xxviii. 225.) The preparation is sometimes attacked by small worms, probably in consequence of the farinaceous additions. Excellent liquorice is prepared in some parts of England, from the root cultivated in that country. The *Pontefract cakes* are small lozenges of liquorice made in the vicinity of Pomfret, England.

Medical Properties and Uses. Liquorice is a useful demulcent, much employed in cough mixtures, and frequently added to infusions or decoctions, in order to cover the taste or obtund the acrimony of the principal medicine. A piece of it held in the mouth and allowed slowly to dissolve, is often found to allay cough by sheathing the irritated membrane of the fauces. It is used in pharmacy to impart consistence to pills and troches, and to modify the taste of other medicines.

Off. Prep. Pilulæ Ferri Iodidi; Tinctura Aloes; Trochisci Cubebæ; Trochisci Glycyrrhizæ et Opii.

Off. Prep. Br. Confectio Sennæ; Decoctum Aloes Compositum; Tinctura Aloes; Trochisci Opii.

EXTRACTUM GLYCYRRHIZÆ FLUIDUM. *U.S.* *Fluid Extract of Glycyrrhiza.*

(ĔX-TRĂC'TŲM GLȲÇ-ȲR-RHĪ'ZÆ FLŪ'Į-DŬM.)

Extractum Glycyrrhizæ Liquidum, *Br.;* Liquid Extract of Liquorice; **Extrait liquide de Réglisse,** *Fr.;* Flüssiges Süssholz-Extrakt, *G.*

"Glycyrrhiza, in No. 40 powder, *one hundred grammes* [or fifty ounces av.];

* The following results of an examination of different brands of liquorice in the market in relation to the proportion of matters soluble and those insoluble in cold water contained in them respectively, by Mr. L. J. Schroeder, is published in the *A. J. P.* (1884, p. 311). Five hundred grains of each commercial extract were used.

Brand.	Residue.		Glycyrrhizin.		
	Weight.	Per cent.	Soluble.	Insoluble.	Total.
	Grains.				Grains.
1. M. & R.	180	36	38	5	43
2. Y. & S.	174	34·8	30	10	40
3. Dean	239	47·8	8	5	13
4. Royal	274	54·8	6	3	9
5. Corigliano	150	30	15	15	30
6. Guzzolini	132	26·4	10	7	17
7. P. & S.	125	25	10	11	21
8. S. C	130	26	...	13	13

It will be seen that the American exceeds all the other brands in the amount of the sweet principle.

Water of Ammonia, Diluted Alcohol, each, *a sufficient quantity*, To make *one hundred cubic centimeters* [or three pints]. Mix *three parts* [or three fluidounces] of Water of Ammonia with *ninety-seven parts* [or six and a quarter pints] of Diluted Alcohol, and, having moistened the powder with *thirty-five grammes* [or eighteen fluidounces] of the mixture, pack it firmly in a cylindrical glass percolator; then add enough of the menstruum to saturate the powder and leave a stratum above it. When the liquid begins to drop from the percolator, close the lower orifice, and, having closely covered the percolator, macerate for forty-eight hours. Then allow the percolation to proceed, gradually adding menstruum, until the Glycyrrhiza is exhausted. Reserve the first *seventy-five cubic centimeters* [or thirty-six fluidounces] of the percolate, and, having added *three grammes* [or one and a half fluidounces] of Water of Ammonia to the remainder, evaporate to a soft extract; dissolve this in the reserved portion, and add enough Diluted Alcohol to make the Fluid Extract measure *one hundred cubic centimeters* [or three pints]." *U. S.*

"Take of Liquorice Root, in No. 20 powder, *one pound* [av.]; Distilled Water, *four pints* [Imp. meas.]; Rectified Spirit, *a sufficiency*. Macerate the liquorice root with *two pints* [Imp. meas.] of the water for twelve hours, strain and press; again macerate the pressed marc with the remainder of the water for six hours, strain and press. Mix the strained liquors, heat them to 212° F. (100° C.), and strain through flannel; then evaporate by a water-bath until it has acquired, when cold, a specific gravity of 1·160; add to this one-sixth of its volume of rectified spirit; let the mixture stand for twelve hours, and filter." *Br.*

The fluid extract of U. S. Pharm. 1880 differs from that officinal in 1870 in the absence of glycerin in the menstruum, and the presence of water of ammonia. The addition of the ammonia to the menstruum was suggested by Prof. J. P. Remington. (See *Proc. A. P. A.*, 1878, p. 757.) The formula for the liquid extract of liquorice of the British Pharmacopœia has several inconvenient manipulative features about it, such as the repeated macerations and expressions, evaporating to a certain specific gravity, etc. This preparation is now very largely used as an adjuvant, and for disguising the bitter taste of quinine, which should be added to the preparation of liquorice just before the dose is taken. It is a very convenient form for using liquorice, the objection to the former fluid extracts of the root being the slight acridity and the presence of too much alcohol. The ammonia not only renders the glycyrrhizin soluble, and thus materially adds to the power and sweetness of the fluid extract, but the acridity is greatly lessened through its influence. It is a very dark reddish brown liquid, having the well-known sweet taste of liquorice. A *syrup of liquorice* may be made by adding two parts of fluid extract to fourteen of simple syrup. An aromatic elixir of liquorice is treated of under Elixirs. (See Part II.)

EXTRACTUM GLYCYRRHIZÆ PURUM. *U. S.* *Pure Extract of Glycyrrhiza.*

(ĔX-TRĂC'TŬM GLŸÇ-YR-RHĪ'ZÆ PŪ'RŬM.)

Extractum Glycyrrhizæ Depuratum, Succus Liquiritiæ Depuratus; Extrait de Réglisse pur, *Fr.*; **Reines Lakris,** *G.*

"Glycyrrhiza, in No. 20 powder, *one hundred parts* [or sixteen ounces av.]; Water of Ammonia, *fifteen parts* [or two and a half fluidounces]; Distilled Water, *a sufficient quantity*. Mix the Water of Ammonia with *three hundred parts* [or three pints] of Distilled Water, and, having moistened the powder with *one hundred parts* [or one pint] of the menstruum, let it macerate for twenty-four hours. Then pack it moderately in a cylindrical glass percolator, and gradually pour upon it, first, the remainder of the menstruum, and then, Distilled Water, until the Glycyrrhiza is exhausted. Lastly, by means of a water-bath, evaporate the infusion to a pilular consistence." *U. S.*

The British directions are to macerate *an avoirdupois pound* of liquorice root, in coarse powder, for twelve hours, in *two pints* of distilled water, strain and press; again to macerate the pressed marc with distilled water for six hours, strain and press; then to mix the strained liquors, heat to 212° F. (100° C.), strain through flannel; and finally evaporate, by means of a water-bath, to a proper consistence for forming pills. The object in heating the infusion to 212° is to coagulate the albumen, and thus exclude it from the extract.

The necessity for a pure extract of liquorice must be apparent to every pharmacist; the very variable quality of the commercial extract has frequently led to disappointment; the officinal process affords a preparation which is unexceptionable, the ammonia rendering the glycyrrhizin soluble, yet care must be taken in its evaporation, as it is very easily injured by too much heat, which gives it an empyreumatic taste, destroying at once its usefulness as an agreeable adjuvant.

Off. Prep. Mistura Glycyrrhizæ Composita.

EXTRACTUM GOSSYPII RADICIS FLUIDUM. *U. S.* *Fluid Extract of Cotton Root.*

(EX-TRĂC'TUM GOS-SÝP'I-I RA-DĬ'CIS FLŪ'I-DŬM.)

Extrait liquide d'Écorce de Cotonnier, *Fr.;* Flüssiges Baumwollenwurzel-Extrakt, *G.*

"Cotton Root, in No. 30 powder, *one hundred grammes* [or fifty ounces av.]; Glycerin, *thirty-five grammes* [or thirteen and a half fluidounces]; Alcohol, *a sufficient quantity*, To make *one hundred cubic centimeters* [or three pints]. Mix the Glycerin with *sixty-five grammes* [or thirty-eight fluidounces] of Alcohol, and, having moistened the powder with *fifty grammes* [or twenty-six fluidounces] of the mixture, pack it firmly in a cylindrical percolator, and pour on the remainder of the menstruum. When the liquid begins to drop from the percolator, close the lower orifice, and, having closely covered the percolator, macerate for forty-eight hours. Then allow the percolation to proceed, and, when the liquid in the percolator has disappeared from the surface, gradually pour on Alcohol, and continue the percolation until the Cotton Root is exhausted. Reserve the first *seventy cubic centimeters* [or thirty-three and a half fluidounces] of the percolate, and evaporate the remainder to a soft extract; dissolve this in the reserved portion, and add enough Alcohol to make the Fluid Extract measure *one hundred cubic centimeters* [or three pints]." *U. S.*

This is one of the fluid extracts which is improved by the use of glycerin; the menstruum here selected, it is believed, will prevent the gelatinization, which has been a troublesome objection to the fluid extract of the Pharmacopœia of 1870. Prof. J. U. Lloyd prefers a menstruum composed of ten fluidounces of alcohol and three fluidounces each of glycerin and water, and finishing the percolation with a mixture composed of ten fluidounces of alcohol and six fluidounces of water. It is a deep reddish liquid, and well represents the root. The dose is half a fluidrachm to a fluidrachm (1·9–3·75 C.c.).

EXTRACTUM GRINDELIÆ FLUIDUM. *U. S.* *Fluid Extract of Grindelia.*

(EX-TRĂC'TUM GRĬN-DĒ'LI-Æ FLŪ'I-DŬM.)

"Grindelia, in No. 30 powder, *one hundred grammes* [or fifty ounces av.]; Alcohol, Water, each, *a sufficient quantity*, To make *one hundred cubic centimeters* [or three pints]. Mix *three parts* [or three pints and six fluidounces] of Alcohol with *one part* [or one pint] of Water, and, having moistened the powder with *thirty grammes* [or seventeen and a half fluidounces] of the mixture, pack it firmly in a cylindrical percolator; then add enough menstruum to saturate the powder and leave a stratum above it. When the liquid begins to drop from the percolator, close the lower orifice, and, having closely covered the percolator, macerate for forty-eight hours. Then allow the percolation to proceed, gradually adding menstruum, until the Grindelia is exhausted. Reserve the first *eighty-five cubic centimeters* [or forty fluidounces] of the percolate, and evaporate the remainder to a soft extract; dissolve this in the reserved portion, and add enough menstruum to make the Fluid Extract measure *one hundred cubic centimeters* [or three pints]." *U. S.*

This is a new officinal fluid extract which well represents the drug; owing to the large quantity of resinous matter present it does not mix well with aqueous liquids.

It is a dark brown liquid having the peculiar odor of grindelia. The dose is half a fluidrachm to a fluidrachm (1·9–3·75 C.c.).

EXTRACTUM GUARANÆ FLUIDUM. *U. S.* *Fluid Extract of Guarana.*

(ĔX-TRĂC′TŲM GUĄ-RÄ′NÆ FLŪ′Į-DŬM—gwą-rä′nȧ.)

"Guarana, in No. 60 powder, *one hundred grammes* [or fifty ounces av.]; Alcohol, Water, each, *a sufficient quantity*, To make *one hundred cubic centimeters* [or three pints]. Mix *three parts* [or three pints and six fluidounces] of Alcohol with *one part* [or one pint] of Water, and, having moistened the powder with *twenty grammes* [or twelve fluidounces] of the mixture, pack it firmly in a cylindrical percolator; then add enough of the menstruum to saturate the powder and leave a stratum above it. When the liquid begins to drop from the percolator, close the lower orifice, and, having closely covered the percolator, macerate for forty-eight hours. Then allow the percolation to proceed, gradually adding menstruum, until the Guarana is exhausted. Reserve the first *eighty cubic centimeters* [or thirty-eight fluidounces] of the percolate. By means of a water-bath, distil off the Alcohol from the remainder, and evaporate the residue to a soft extract; dissolve this in the reserved portion, and add enough menstruum to make the Fluid Extract measure *one hundred cubic centimeters* [or three pints]." *U. S.*

This new officinal fluid extract is of doubtful utility. The powdered drug itself is portable, not unpleasant to the taste, and is efficient when given diffused in water; nothing is gained by making it into a fluid extract. The fluid extract is of a deep reddish brown color. The dose is one to two fluidrachms (3·75–7·5 C.c.).

EXTRACTUM HÆMATOXYLI. *U.S., Br.* *Extract of Hæmatoxylon.* [*Extract of Logwood.*]

(ĔX-TRĂC′TŲM HÆ-MĄ-TŎX′Y̨-LĪ—hē-mą-tŏk′sę-lī.)

Extractum Ligni Campechiani, *P. G.;* Extrait de Bois de Campêche, *Fr.;* Campecheholz-Extrakt, *G.*

"Hæmatoxylon, rasped, *one hundred parts* [or sixteen ounces av.]; Water, *one thousand parts* [or ten pints]. Macerate the Hæmatoxylon with the Water for forty-eight hours. Then boil (avoiding the use of metallic vessels) until one-half of the Water has evaporated; strain the decoction, while hot, and evaporate to dryness." *U. S.*

"Take of Logwood, in fine chips, *one pound* [avoirdupois]; Boiling Distilled Water *one gallon* [Imperial measure]. Infuse the Logwood in the Water for twenty-four hours, then boil down to one-half, strain, and evaporate to dryness by a water-bath, stirring with a wooden spatula. Iron vessels should not be used." *Br.*

This is one of the few instances in which decoction in the preparation of extracts is not considered objectionable. Iron vessels should not be employed in the process, in consequence of the presence of tannic acid. The evaporation should be carried so far that the extract may be dry and brittle when cold. About 20 lbs. of it are obtained from one cwt. of logwood. (*Brande.*) It is of a deep ruby color, and an astringent, sweetish taste, and has all the medical virtues of the wood. If given in pills, these should be recently made, as, when long kept, they are said to become so hard as sometimes to pass unchanged through the bowels. The extract, however, is best administered in solution. The dose is from ten to thirty grains (0·65–1·95 Gm.). This extract is said to be prepared largely in Yucatan and other parts of Mexico.

EXTRACTUM HAMAMELIDIS FLUIDUM. *U. S.* *Fluid Extract of Hamamelis.*

(ĔX-TRĂC′TŲM HĂM-Ą-MĔL′Į-DĬS FLŪ′Į-DŬM.)

"Hamamelis, in No. 40 powder, *one hundred grammes* [or fifty ounces av.]; Alcohol, Water, each, *a sufficient quantity*, To make *one hundred cubic centimeters* [or three pints]. Mix *one part* [or two and a quarter pints] of Alcohol with *two parts* [or four pints] of Water, and, having moistened the powder with *thirty-five grammes* [or eighteen fluidounces] of the mixture, pack it firmly in a cylindrical percolator; then add enough of the menstruum to saturate the powder and leave a stratum above it. When the liquid begins to drop from the percolator, close the lower orifice, and, having closely covered the percolator, macerate for forty-eight hours. Then allow the percolation to proceed, gradually adding menstruum, until the Hamamelis is exhausted. Reserve the first *eighty-five cubic centimeters* [or forty fluidounces] of the percolate, and evaporate the remainder to a soft extract; dissolve this in the reserved portion, and add enough menstruum to make the Fluid Extract measure *one hundred cubic centimeters* [or three pints]." *U. S.*

This is a new officinal fluid extract, which well represents the virtues of witch-hazel. It is a dark reddish brown color; the dose is half a fluidrachm (1·9 C.c.).

EXTRACTUM HYDRASTIS FLUIDUM. *U. S.* *Fluid Extract of Hydrastis.*

(ĔX-TRĂC'TŬM HȲ-DRĂS'TĬS FLŪ'Ĭ-DŬM.)

Extrait liquide de Hydrastis, *Fr.;* Flüssiges Hydrastis-Extrakt, *G.*

"Hydrastis, in No. 60 powder, *one hundred grammes* [or fifty ounces av.]; Alcohol, Water, each, *a sufficient quantity*, To make *one hundred cubic centimeters* [or three pints]. Mix *three parts* [or three pints and six fluidounces] of Alcohol with *one part* [or one pint] of Water, and, having moistened the powder with *thirty grammes* [or seventeen fluidounces] of the mixture, pack it firmly in a cylindrical percolator; then add enough of the menstruum to saturate the powder and leave a stratum above it. When the liquid begins to drop from the percolator, close the lower orifice, and, having closely covered the percolator, macerate for forty-eight hours. Then allow the percolation to proceed, gradually adding menstruum, until the Hydrastis is exhausted. Reserve the first *eighty-five cubic centimeters* [or forty fluidounces] of the percolate. By means of a water-bath, distil off the Alcohol from the remainder, and evaporate the residue to a soft extract; dissolve this in the reserved portion, and add enough menstruum to make the Fluid Extract measure *one hundred cubic centimeters* [or three pints]." *U. S.*

This preparation does not differ materially from that officinal in 1870. The small proportion of glycerin directed in the former process has been dropped; the present menstruum is slightly more alcoholic. The fluid extract thoroughly represents the drug, is of a deep brownish yellow color, and the dose is from one to two fluidrachms (3·75–7·5 C.c.).

EXTRACTUM HYOSCYAMI. *Br.* *Extract of Henbane.*

(ĔX-TRĂC'TŬM HȲ-ŎS-CȲ'Ă-MĪ.)

Extrait de Jusquiame, *Fr.;* Bilsenkraut-Extrakt, *G.*

The process of preparing this Extract from the fresh leaves is no longer officinal in U. S. P. (See *Alcoholic Extract of Hyoscyamus.*)

In the British Pharmacopœia this extract is prepared from "the fresh Leaves, flowering Tops, and young Branches of Henbane" in the same manner precisely as Extract of Aconite. (See *Extractum Aconiti.*)

MM. Solon and Soubeiran have shown that the insoluble matter separated from the expressed juice of henbane by filtering, and that coagulated by heat, are nearly if not quite inert; so that the juice may be usefully clarified before evaporation. (*A. J. P.*, viii. 228.) The retention of the chlorophyll, however, as provided for in the British formula, is thought to be advantageous. This kind of Extract of Henbane is chiefly derived from England. Mr. Brande says that one cwt. of the fresh herb affords between four and five pounds. M. Reclus obtained one part from sixteen.

The extract is of a dark olive color, of a narcotic rather unpleasant odor, and a bitterish, nauseous, slightly saline taste. It retains its softness for a long time, but at the end of three or four years becomes dry, and exhibits, when broken, small crystals of nitrate of potassium and chloride of sodium. (*Reclus.*) Like all the inspissated juices, it is of variable strength, according to its age, the care used in its preparation, and the character of the leaves. (See *Hyoscyamus.*)

Much depends on the choice of the leaves; and too little attention is paid to this point. In reference to the biennial plant, there seems to be no doubt that the leaves of the second year are much more efficacious than those of the first, and should, therefore, always be selected. It is stated under Hyoscyamus, that the leaves should be gathered soon after the plant has flowered. Mr. Charles Cracknell gives more particular directions. He thinks that the plant is in a fit state for collection only during a very short period, namely, when the flowers at the top are blown, but have not yet begun to fade, and the seed-vessels and seeds which have been formed are still soft and juicy. For other observations on the preparation of this extract, see a paper by Mr. Cracknell in *A. J. P.* (xxiii. 245).

An important contribution to our knowledge, as to the proper choice of the parts of this plant to be expressed, has been made by Mr. T. B. Groves, of England. Whatever may be the case with those plants, such as aconite, the roots of which are active, and in which the juice containing the active matter, on its way from the leaves to the root, might be supposed to exist in the young stems, this does not appear to be the case with the Hyoscyamus; and, accordingly, an extract obtained by inspissating the juice of the stems was found altogether inferior to another obtained in like manner from the leaves, being not only less in amount, but less bitter and odorous, and more saline, showing that it contained more of the ordinary salts of the plant, and less of its active matter. (*P. J. Tr.*, 1862, p. 376.)

In the use of the extract it is advisable to begin with a moderate dose, two or three grains (0·13–0·20 Gm.) for instance, and gradually to increase the quantity till some effect is experienced, and the degree of efficiency of the particular parcel employed is ascertained. It is usually given in pill. It is sometimes used externally for the same purpose as extract of belladonna.

Off. Prep. Br. Pilula Colocynthidis et Hyoscyami.

EXTRACTUM HYOSCYAMI ALCOHOLICUM. *U.S.* *Alcoholic Extract of Hyoscyamus.*

(ĔX-TRĂC'TŬM HȲ-ǪS-CȲ'Ą-MĪ ĂL-CǪ-HŎL'Į-CŬM.)

Extrait alcoolique de Jusquiame, *Fr.;* **Spirituöses Bilsenkraut-Extrakt,** *G.*

"Hyoscyamus, recently dried and in No. 60 powder, *one hundred parts* [or sixteen ounces av.]; Alcohol, *two hundred parts* [or two and a quarter pints]; Water, *one hundred parts* [or one pint]; Diluted Alcohol, *a sufficient quantity.* Mix the Alcohol and Water, and, having moistened the powder with *forty parts* [or six fluidounces] of the mixture, pack it firmly in a cylindrical percolator; then add enough of the menstruum to saturate the powder and leave a stratum above it. When the liquid begins to drop from the percolator, close the lower orifice, and, having closely covered the percolator, macerate for forty-eight hours. Then allow the percolation to proceed, gradually adding, first, the remainder of the menstruum, and then, Diluted Alcohol, until *three hundred parts* [or three pints] of tincture are obtained, or the Hyoscyamus is exhausted. Reserve the first *ninety parts* [or fourteen fluidounces] of the percolate, evaporate the remainder, at a temperature not exceeding 50° C. (122° F.), to *ten parts* [or one fluidounce]; mix this with the reserved portion, and evaporate, at or below the before-mentioned temperature, to a pilular consistence." *U. S.*

This is a much more reliable and active preparation than the inspissated juice, or, as it is usually termed, English extract. It is of a dark olive color, with the peculiar odor of hyoscyamus. The dose is from one to two grains (0·065–0·13 Gm.).

EXTRACTUM HYOSCYAMI FLUIDUM. *U.S.* *Fluid Extract of Hyoscyamus.*

(ĔX-TRĂC'TŬM HȲ-ǪS-CȲ'Ą-MĪ FLŪ'Į-DŬM.)

Extrait liquide de Jusquiame, *Fr.;* **Flüssiges Bilsenkraut-Extrakt,** *G.*

"Hyoscyamus, in No. 60 powder, *one hundred grammes* [or fifty ounces av.]; Alcohol, Water, each, *a sufficient quantity,* To make *one hundred cubic centimeters* [or three pints]. Mix *three parts* [or three pints and six fluidounces] of Alcohol, with *one part* [or one pint] of water, and, having moistened the powder with *forty grammes* [or twenty-three fluidounces] of the mixture, pack it firmly in a cylindrical percolator; then add enough of the menstruum to saturate the powder and leave a stratum above it. When the liquid begins to drop from the percolator, close the lower orifice, and, having closely covered the percolator, macerate for forty-eight hours. Then allow the percolation to proceed, gradually adding menstruum until the Hyoscyamus is exhausted. Reserve the first *ninety cubic centimeters* [or forty fluidounces] of the percolate, and evaporate the remainder, at a temperature not exceeding 50° C. (122° F.), to a soft extract; dissolve this in the reserved portion, and add enough menstruum to make the Fluid Extract measure *one hundred cubic centimeters* [or three pints]." *U. S.*

This fluid extract was improved in the last revision by abandoning the glycerin directed in the former process. It is of a very dark greenish brown color, and is given in the dose of five minims (0·3 C.c.) to commence with. For the medical properties, see *Hyoscyamus.*

EXTRACTUM IPECACUANHÆ FLUIDUM. *U.S. Fluid Extract of Ipecac.*

(EX-TRĂC'TŬM ĬP-E-CĂC-Ū-ĂN'HÆ FLŪ'I-DŬM—ĭp-e-kăk-yū-ăn'ē.)

Extrait liquide d'Ipécacuanha, *Fr.;* Flüssiges Ipecacuanha-Extrakt, *G.*

"Ipecac, in No. 80 powder, *one hundred grammes* [or fifty ounces av.]; Alcohol, Water, each, *a sufficient quantity,* To make *one hundred cubic centimeters* [or three pints]. Moisten the powder with *thirty-five grammes* [or twenty fluidounces] of Alcohol, and pack it firmly in a cylindrical percolator; then add enough Alcohol to saturate the powder and leave a stratum above it. When the liquid begins to drop from the percolator, close the lower orifice, and, having closely covered the percolator, macerate for forty-eight hours. Then allow the percolation to proceed until the Ipecac is exhausted. By means of a water-bath distil off the Alcohol from the tincture until the residue measures *fifty cubic centimeters* [or one and a half pints], and add to it *one hundred cubic centimeters* [or three pints] of Water. Evaporate the mixture to *seventy-five cubic centimeters* [or two and a quarter pints], and, when cool, filter. Wash the precipitate upon the filter, with Water, until the latter passes through tasteless, evaporate the filtrate and washings to *fifty cubic centimeters* [or one and a half pints], allow to cool, and add enough Alcohol to make the Fluid Extract measure *one hundred cubic centimeters* [or three pints]."

It is probable that a greater improvement will be noticed in this than in any of the other fluid extracts; indeed, the process of the Pharmacopœia of 1870 was almost inoperative; the preparation was turbid and unfit for its principal use, the making of syrup of ipecacuanha (*A. J. P.*, 1873, pp. 211, 481; 1876, p. 337; *N. R.*, 1880, p. 14),* because no provision was made for the separation of the apothegmatic substance which causes the turbidity. The present formula closely resembles that officinal in 1860; in our opinion, it would have been better to have directed the mixture to stand undisturbed forty-eight hours before filtering. This would have allowed sufficient time for the insoluble apothegmatic substances to thoroughly subside.

An interesting paper on the alkaloidal strength of Ipecac and its Fluid Extract, by H. W. Snow, will be found in *Pharm. Era*, 1887, p. 400.

This fluid extract is a thin, dark reddish brown, transparent liquid, of a bitterish slightly acrid taste, but without the nauseous flavor of the root. The emetic dose would be from fifteen to thirty minims (0·9–1·9 C.c.). It is a convenient preparation for adding to expectorant and diaphoretic mixtures, and is used officinally principally in preparing the syrup of ipecacuanha, with which it should mix without precipitation, or more than slight cloudiness.

Off. Prep. Syrupus Ipecacuanhæ; Tinctura Ipecacuanhæ et Opii; Vinum Ipecacuanhæ.

* *Fluid Extract of Ipecac.* R. Rother recommends alcohol for a menstruum and the use of magnesia, and the percolation of the finely-powdered ipecac upon what he calls the disc principle. (*Drug. Circ.*, 1886, p. 4.)

EXTRACTUM IRIDIS. *U. S.* *Extract of Iris.*

(ĔX-TRĂC'TŬM ĬR'Ĭ-DĬS.)

Extrait d'Iris varié, *Fr.;* Verschiedenfarbige Schwertlilie-Extrakt, *G.*

"Iris in No. 60 powder, *one hundred parts* [or sixteen ounces av.]; Alcohol, *two hundred and twenty-five parts* [or two and a half pints]; Water, *seventy-five parts* [or twelve fluidounces]; Diluted Alcohol, *a sufficient quantity.* Mix the Alcohol and Water, and, having moistened the powder with *forty parts* [or six and a half fluidounces] of the mixture, pack it firmly in a cylindrical percolator; then add enough menstruum to saturate the powder and leave a stratum above it. When the liquid begins to drop from the percolator, close the lower orifice, and, having closely covered the percolator, macerate for forty-eight hours. Then allow the percolation to proceed, gradually adding, first, the remainder of the menstruum, and then, Diluted Alcohol, until *three hundred parts* [or three pints] of tincture are obtained, or the Iris is exhausted. By means of a water-bath, distil off the Alcohol from the tincture, and, having placed the residue in a porcelain capsule, evaporate it, on a water-bath, to a pilular consistence." *U. S.*

This is a new officinal extract, which has been introduced to afford an opportunity of using blue flag in the pilular form. The drug appears to us to be too seldom used to merit this distinction. The dose is one to two grains (0·065 to 0·13 Gm.).

EXTRACTUM IRIDIS FLUIDUM. *U. S.* *Fluid Extract of Iris.*

(ĔX-TRĂC'TŬM ĬR'Ĭ-DĬS FLŪ'Ĭ-DŬM.)

Fluid Extract of Blue Flag; Extrait liquide d'Iris varié, *Fr.;* Flüssiges Verschiedenfarbige Schwertlilie-Extrakt, *G.*

"Iris, in No. 60 powder, *one hundred grammes* [or fifty ounces av.]; Alcohol, Water, each, *a sufficient quantity,* To make *one hundred cubic centimeters* [or three pints]. Mix *three parts* [or three pints and six fluidounces] of Alcohol with *one part* [or one pint] of Water, and, having moistened the powder with *forty grammes* [or twenty-three fluidounces] of the mixture, pack it firmly in a cylindrical percolator; then add enough of the menstruum to saturate the powder and leave a stratum above it. When the liquid begins to drop from the percolator, close the lower orifice, and, having closely covered the percolator, macerate for forty-eight hours. Then allow the percolation to proceed, gradually adding menstruum until the Iris is exhausted. Reserve the first *ninety cubic centimeters* [or forty fluidounces] of the percolate, and evaporate the remainder, on a water-bath, to a soft extract; dissolve this in the reserved portion, and add enough menstruum to make the Fluid Extract measure *one hundred cubic centimeters* [or three pints]." *U. S.*

This is a new officinal fluid extract. The menstruum used is practically the same as that employed in exhausting blue flag in making the extract, and it will no doubt make a representative fluid extract. The dose is five to ten minims (0·3 to 0·6 C.c.).

EXTRACTUM JABORANDI. *Br.* *Extract of Jaborandi.*

(ĔX-TRĂC'TŬM JĂB-Ọ-RĂN'DĪ.)

"Take of Jaborandi, in No. 40 powder, *one pound* [av.]; Proof Spirit, Distilled Water, of each, *a sufficiency.* Mix the Jaborandi with two pints [Imp. meas.] of the spirit, and macerate in a closed vessel for forty-eight hours; then transfer to a percolator, and when the fluid ceases to pass, continue the percolation with water until two pints [Imp. meas.] of liquid have been collected. Evaporate the percolated liquid until the extract has acquired a suitable consistence." *Br.*

This is a new preparation in the British Pharmacopœia, and a good one. It possesses the virtues of Pilocarpus, to which the reader is referred for the medical properties. The dose of the extract is given in the British Pharmacopœia as from two to ten grains (0·13–0·65 Gm.). The first quantity would be the best commencing dose.

Off. Prep. Br. Pilocarpinæ Nitras.

EXTRACTUM JALAPÆ. *Br.* *Extract of Jalap.*

(EX-TRĂC'TUM JA-LĀ'PÆ.)

Extrait de Jalap, *Fr.;* Jalapen-Extrakt, *G.*

"Take of Jalap, in coarse powder, *one pound* [avoirdupois]; Rectified Spirit *four pints* [Imperial measure]; Distilled Water *one gallon* [Imp. meas.]. Macerate the Jalap in the Spirit for seven days; press out the tincture, then filter, and distil off the Spirit, leaving a soft extract. Again macerate the residual Jalap in the Water for four hours, express, strain through flannel, and evaporate, by a water-bath, to a soft extract. Mix the two extracts, and evaporate, at a temperature not exceeding 140° F. (60° C.), until it has acquired a suitable consistence for forming pills." *Br.*

This extract has been replaced in the present U. S. Pharmacopœia by the abstract.

Jalap contains a considerable quantity of starch, which is extracted by decoction, but left behind by cold water; and, as this principle serves only to impede the filtration or straining, and augment the bulk of the extract, without adding to its virtues, cold water is very properly used in the process. The use both of alcohol and of water was deemed necessary, in order to extract all the medicinal qualities of the drug; and they are employed successively, under the impression that the previous removal of the resin by the former facilitates the action of the latter; but Mr. A. B. Taylor satisfactorily determined that the substance which water will extract from jalap, previously exhausted by alcohol, has no observable influence on the system; having taken 240 grains of the matter thus extracted without effect. (*Proc. A. P. A.*, 1864, p. 215.) And it was shown, moreover, that the aqueous extract of jalap is hygroscopic, and that it is the cause of the inconvenient hardening of the powdered extract. The substitution of dried sugar of milk for the inert, hygroscopic, aqueous extract is certainly an improvement. (See *Abstractum Jalapæ.*) The use of percolation, as directed by the U. S. Pharmacopœia of 1870, enabled the cold water to extract the soluble parts without the long maceration which would otherwise have been necessary. According to Cadet de Gassicourt, water at ordinary temperatures, and in the old mode, acts so slowly that fermentation takes place before the active matter is all dissolved. Hence, if the extract be prepared without percolation, the residuum, after the tincture has been decanted, should be digested with water at a heat of about 90° or 100° F., which, while it is insufficient for the solution of the starch, enables the solvent to take up the active matter with sufficient rapidity.

One cwt. of jalap affords, according to Mr. Brande, about fifty pounds of aqueous extract and fifteen of resin. The product of the former is somewhat less by infusion than by decoction; and the extract is proportionately stronger.

There is reason to believe, as we have been informed on good authority, that what is sold for extract of jalap is sometimes prepared from tubers which have been previously exhausted of their resin by alcohol; and a spurious substance has been offered in considerable quantities in our markets for extract of jalap, which Messrs. Chas. Bullock and Prof. Parrish proved to owe its purgative property to 42 per cent. of gamboge. (*A. J. P.*, 1862, p. 113.)

Extract of jalap is of a dark brown color, slightly translucent at the edges, and tenacious when not perfectly dry. It contains the resin and gummy extractive, and, consequently, has all the medical properties of the root; but it is not often exhibited alone, being chiefly used as an ingredient of purgative pills, for which it is adapted by its comparatively small bulk. It is most conveniently kept for use in the form of powder, which, however, is apt to attract moisture and to aggregate into a solid mass, unless carefully excluded from the air. The dose is from ten to twenty grains (0·65–1·3 Gm.), or rather more than half that of jalap.*

* *Fluid Extract of Jalap.* The following process has been proposed by Prof. Procter. Take of jalap, in coarse powder, ℥xvi; sugar, ℥viij; carbonate of potassium, ℥ss; alcohol, water, each, *q. s.* Add to the jalap one pint of a mixture consisting of two parts of alcohol and one of water, and set aside for twenty-four hours. Then put the mixture into a percolator, and pour on it diluted alcohol until half a gallon has passed. Evaporate the filtered liquid one-half, add the sugar

EXTRACTUM JUGLANDIS. *U. S.* *Extract of Juglans.*

(EX-TRĂC'TUM JUG-LĂN'DIS.)

Extrait d'Écorce de Noyer gris, *Fr.;* Butternussrinden-Extrakt, *G.;* Extract of Butternut.

"Juglans, in No. 30 powder, *one hundred parts* [or sixteen ounces av.]; Glycerin, Alcohol, each, *a sufficient quantity.* Moisten the powder with *forty parts* [or six fluidounces] of Alcohol, and pack it firmly in a cylindrical percolator; then add enough Alcohol to saturate the powder and leave a stratum above it. When the liquid begins to drop from the percolator, close the lower orifice, and, having closely covered the percolator, macerate for forty-eight hours. Then allow the percolation to proceed, gradually adding Alcohol, until *three hundred parts* [or three pints] of tincture are obtained, or the Juglans is exhausted. By means of a water-bath, distil off the Alcohol from the tincture, and, having placed the residue in a porcelain capsule, evaporate it, on a water-bath, to a pilular consistence. Lastly, weigh the Extract and thoroughly incorporate with it, while still warm, *five per cent.* of Glycerin." *U. S.*

This extract was formerly for the most part prepared by the country people, who are said to have used the bark of the branches, and even the branches themselves, instead of the inner bark of the root; and to have injured the preparation by too much heat. That it should have proved uncertain in the hands of many physicians is, therefore, not a matter of surprise. It should be prepared by the apothecary, and from the inner bark of the root gathered in May or June. Experiments made by B. F. Moise (*A. J. P.*, 1881, p. 153) prove that alcohol and diluted alcohol are better menstrua than water for the bark. Prof. Procter found an extract of the fresh bark prepared with diluted alcohol to have much more of the pungency of the bark than the officinal; on account of these results, the process for the extract was changed at the last revision, and alcohol substituted for water as a menstruum, with marked improvement.

The extract of butternut is of a black color, sweetish odor, and bitter astringent taste. In the dose of five or ten grains (0·33–0·65 Gm.), it acts as a mild cathartic, whilst in larger doses it is an active purge.

EXTRACTUM KRAMERIÆ. *U. S., Br.* *Extract of Krameria. Extract of Rhatany.*

(EX-TRĂC'TUM KRA-MĒ'RI-Æ.)

Extractum Ratanhæ, *P.G.;* Extrait de Ratanhia, *Fr.;* Ratanha-Extrakt, *G.*

"Krameria, in No. 40 powder, *one hundred parts* [or sixteen ounces av.]; Water, *a sufficient quantity.* Moisten the powder with *thirty parts* [or four and a half fluidounces] of Water, pack it in a conical glass percolator, and gradually pour Water upon it, until the infusion passes but slightly imbued with the astringency of the Krameria. Heat the liquid to the boiling point, strain, and, by means of a water-bath, at a temperature not exceeding 70° C. (158° F.), evaporate to dryness." *U. S.*

"Take of Rhatany Root, in No. 40 powder, *one pound* [avoirdupois]; Distilled Water *a sufficiency.* Macerate the Rhatany in a pint and a half [Imperial measure] of the Water for twenty-four hours; then pack in a percolator, and add more Distilled Water, until twelve pints [Imp. meas.] have been collected, or the Rhatany is exhausted. Evaporate the liquor by a water-bath to dryness." *Br.*

In selecting a plan for the preparation of this extract, it was undoubtedly wise to adopt the mode of displacement, with cold water as the menstruum. It is absolutely necessary to the success of the process, that the root should be well and uniformly comminuted; and the "No. 30 powder" of the U. S. Pharmacopœia is, therefore, preferable to the "coarse powder" of the British. The wood of the root yielded to Prof. Procter only 6·8 per cent. of extract, while the bark separated from the wood

and carbonate of potassium, and evaporate to 12 fluidounces. Put the liquid, while warm, into a pint bottle, add four fluidounces of alcohol, and mix. The carbonate of potassium renders the resin soluble in water, and probably favorably qualifies the irritating properties of the jalap. A fluidrachm of this extract would represent a drachm of jalap, so that the dose should be from 15 to 30 minims (0·9 to 1·9 C.c.). (*A. J. P.*, xxix. 108.)

yielded 33 per cent. As the wood is of difficult pulverization, the inference is obvious, that, in powdering the roots, the ligneous portion may be rejected with advantage. (*A. J. P.*, xiv. 270.) As a prolonged exposure of the infusion to the air is attended with the absorption of oxygen, and the production of insoluble apotheme, it is desirable that the evaporation should be conducted rapidly, or in a vacuum. There scarcely appears to be occasion, in the case of rhatany, for heating and filtering the infusion before evaporation, the only use of which is to get rid of albumen, which is not among the recognised ingredients of the root.

Very inferior extracts of rhatany are often sold. Such is the South American extract, which has been occasionally imported. As the product obtained by decoction is greater than that afforded by the officinal plan, the temptation to substitute the former is not always resisted, although it has been shown to contain nearly 50 per cent. of insoluble matter. Some druggists prepare the extract with an alcoholic menstruum, with a view to the greater product; but the extract thus prepared has from 20 to 30 per cent. less of the active principle than the officinal. A substance has been shown to us, said to have been imported as extract of rhatany from Europe, which was nearly tasteless, and was plausibly conjectured to be the dried coagulated matter of old tincture of kino. Indeed, we are informed that very little of the genuine extract, prepared according to the officinal directions, is to be found in the drug stores.

Extract of rhatany should have a reddish brown color, a smooth shining fracture, and a very astringent taste, and should be almost entirely soluble in water. Its virtues may be considered as in proportion to its solubility. It is much used for all the purposes for which the astringent extracts are employed. The dose is from ten to twenty grains (0·65–1·3 Gm.).

Off. Prep. Trochisci Krameriæ.

EXTRACTUM KRAMERIÆ FLUIDUM. *U.S.* *Fluid Extract of Krameria.*

(ĔX-TRĂC'TŬM KRĂ-MĒ'RĬ-Æ FLŪ'Ĭ-DŬM.)

Extrait liquide de Ratanhia, *Fr.;* Flüssiges Ratanha-Extrakt, *G.*

"Krameria, in No. 30 powder, *one hundred grammes* [or fifty ounces av.]; Glycerin, *twenty grammes* [or seven and a half fluidounces]; Diluted Alcohol, *a sufficient quantity*, To make *one hundred cubic centimeters* [or three pints]. Mix the Glycerin with *eighty grammes* [or forty-one fluidounces] of Diluted Alcohol, and, having moistened the powder with *forty grammes* [or twenty fluidounces] of the mixture, pack it firmly in a cylindrical glass percolator; then add enough of the menstruum to saturate the powder and leave a stratum above it. When the liquid begins to drop from the percolator, close the lower orifice, and, having closely covered the percolator, macerate for forty-eight hours. Then allow the percolation to proceed, gradually adding, first, the remainder of the menstruum, and afterward, Diluted Alcohol, until the Krameria is exhausted. Reserve the first *seventy cubic centimeters* [or thirty-three fluidounces] of the percolate, and evaporate the remainder to a soft extract; dissolve this in the reserved portion, and add enough Diluted Alcohol to make the Fluid Extract measure *one hundred cubic centimeters* [or three pints]." *U. S.*

This process does not differ essentially from that formerly officinal; the fluid extract well represents the root, and is of a deep red color and very astringent taste. The dose is from ten minims to a fluidrachm (0·6–3·75 C.c.).

Off. Prep. Syrupus Krameriæ.

EXTRACTUM LACTUCÆ. *Br.* *Extract of Lettuce.*

(ĔX-TRĂC'TŬM LĂC-TŪ'ÇÆ.)

Extractum Lactucæ Virosæ, *P.G.;* Thridacium; Extrait de Tiges de Laitue, Thridace, *Fr.;* Giftlattich-Extrakt, *G.*

In the British Pharmacopœia, this extract is prepared from "the Flowering Herb of Lettuce," in the same manner precisely as Extract of Aconite. (See *Ex-*

tractum Aconiti.) For the medical properties and uses of extract of lettuce the reader is referred to the article on Lactucarium. The dose is from five to fifteen grains (0·33–1 Gm.).

EXTRACTUM LACTUCARII FLUIDUM. *U.S.* *Fluid Extract of Lactucarium.*

(EX-TRĂC'TŬM LĂC-TŪ-CĀ'RĮ-Ī FLŪ'Į-DŬM.)

Extrait liquide de Tiges de Laitue (Thridace), *Fr.*; Flüssiges Giftlattich-Extrakt, *G.*

"Lactucarium, in coarse pieces, *one hundred grammes* [or twelve and a half ounces av.]; Ether, *one hundred grammes* [or one pint]; Alcohol, Water, each, *a sufficient quantity*, To make *one hundred cubic centimeters* [or twelve fluidounces]. Add the Lactucarium to the Ether contained in a tared flask having the capacity of *six hundred cubic centimeters* [or about four and a half pints], and let it macerate for twenty-four hours; then add *three hundred grammes* [or two and a quarter pints] of Water, and shake the mixture well. Fit a bent glass tube into the neck of the flask, and, having immersed the flask in hot water, recover the Ether by distillation. When all the Ether has distilled over, remove the tube, and, after thoroughly shaking the contents of the flask, continue the heat for half an hour. Let the mixture cool, add *one hundred grammes* [or fourteen and a half fluidounces] of Alcohol, and enough Water to make the whole mixture weigh *five hundred grammes* [or sixty-four ounces av.]; after maceration for twenty-four hours, with occasional agitation, express and filter the liquid. Return the dregs to the flask and macerate them with *two hundred grammes* [or twenty-eight fluidounces] of a mixture of Alcohol and Water made in the proportion of *one part* [or eight fluidounces] of Alcohol to *three parts* [or twenty fluidounces] of Water; repeat the maceration two or three times successively with fresh portions of the mixture, until the dregs are tasteless, or nearly so. Mix, and filter the liquids thus obtained, and concentrate them, by means of a water-bath (the first expressed liquid by itself), until the combined weight of the liquids is *sixty grammes* [or seven and a half ounces av.]; mix the liquids, add *forty grammes* [or six fluidounces] of Alcohol, and let the mixture cool in the evaporating vessel, stirring the mixture frequently, and during the intervals keeping the vessel well covered. When cool, add enough Alcohol to make the mixture weigh *one hundred grammes* [or twelve and a half ounces av.], transfer the liquid to a flask, and add enough Water to make the mixture measure *one hundred cubic centimeters* [or twelve fluidounces], using the Water so required to rinse the evaporating vessel. Shake the mixture occasionally, during several hours (and frequently, if a portion of the precipitate is found to be tenacious), and, when a uniform mixture results, set it aside for twenty-four hours, so that any precipitate formed may subside. Decant the clear liquid, transfer the precipitate to a filter, and, after thoroughly draining it into the decanted liquid, wash it with a mixture of Alcohol and Water made in the proportion of *three parts* [or ten fluiddrachms] of Alcohol to *four parts* [or eleven fluidrachms] of Water, until the washings pass tasteless. Concentrate the washings, by evaporation, to a syrupy consistence, mix with the decanted liquid, and add enough of the last-named mixture of Alcohol and Water to make the whole measure *one hundred cubic centimeters* [or twelve fluidounces]. Lastly, after twenty-four hours, having meanwhile shaken the Fluid Extract occasionally, filter it through paper." *U. S.*

This is a new officinal fluid extract, the process being that recommended by Prof. C. Lewis Diehl. Lactucarium is one of the most difficult substances to operate upon with the view of obtaining and retaining in a soluble form all of the active principles. In this process the object of the preliminary treatment with ether and water is to secure the fine division of the particles by dissolving the lactucerin and resin and to keep them from coalescing, through the presence of water. This pasty mass is subsequently treated with alcohol and water by repeated maceration with expression and decantation; taking care to wash the precipitate with alcohol and water in order thoroughly to retain all the soluble active ingredients; the washings are subsequently concentrated by evaporation, mixed with the decanted liquid, and brought up to the standard strength. Jos. L. Lemberger recommends the previous extraction of the lactucerin from the lactucarium by treatment with benzin; he then mixes the dried lactucarium with an equal bulk of clean sand, introduces it into a percolator, macerates, and afterward percolates with diluted alcohol, reserving the first fourth of the percolate, and continuing the percolation to exhaustion, and evaporating the weak percolate to three-fourths, as is usual in making fluid extracts. The object of these processes is to secure a fluid extract which will form with syrup a clear liquid and retain its efficiency. The dose would be five to thirty minims (0·3–1·9 C.c.).

Off. Prep. Syrupus Lactucarii.

EXTRACTUM LEPTANDRÆ. *U. S. Extract of Leptandra.*

(EX-TRĂC'TUM LEP-TĂN'DRÆ.)

Extract of Culver's Root; Extrait de Leptandra, *Fr.;* Leptandra-wurzel-Extrakt, *G.*

"Leptandra, in No. 40 powder, *one hundred parts* [or sixteen ounces av.]; Alcohol, *two hundred parts* [or two and a quarter pints]; Water, *one hundred parts* [or one pint]; Glycerin, Diluted Alcohol, each, *a sufficient quantity.* Mix the Alcohol and Water, and, having moistened the powder with *forty parts* [or six fluidounces] of the mixture, pack it firmly in a cylindrical percolator; then add enough of the menstruum to saturate the powder and leave a stratum above it. When the liquid begins to drop from the percolator, close the lower orifice, and, having closely covered the percolator, macerate for forty-eight hours. Then allow the percolation to proceed, gradually adding, first, the remainder of the menstruum, and then, Diluted Alcohol, until *three hundred parts* [or three pints] of tincture are obtained or the Leptandra is exhausted. By means of a water-bath, distil off the Alcohol from the tincture, and, having placed the residue in a porcelain capsule, evaporate it, on a water-bath, to a pilular consistence. Lastly, weigh the Extract, and thoroughly incorporate with it, while still warm, *five per cent.* of Glycerin." *U. S.*

This is a new officinal extract, which will furnish those practitioners who have been in the habit of prescribing the so-called *leptandrin,* with a preparation of uniform character. The dose is five to ten grains (0·33–0·65 Gm.)

EXTRACTUM LEPTANDRÆ FLUIDUM. *U. S. Fluid Extract of Leptandra.*

(EX-TRĂC'TUM LEP-TĂN'DRÆ FLŪ'I-DŬM.)

Fluid Extract of Culver's Root; Extrait liquide de Leptandra, *Fr.;* Flüssiges Leptandra-Extrakt, *G.*

"Leptandra, in No. 60 powder, *one hundred grammes* [or fifty ounces av.]; Glycerin, *fifteen grammes* [or five and a half fluidounces]; Diluted Alcohol, *a sufficient quantity,* To make *one hundred cubic centimeters* [or three pints]. Mix the Glycerin with *eighty-five grammes* [or forty-four fluidounces] of Diluted Alcohol, and, having moistened the powder with *forty grammes* [or twenty-three fluidounces] of the mixture, pack moderately in a cylindrical percolator; then add enough of the menstruum to saturate the powder and leave a stratum above it. When the liquid begins to drop from the percolator, close the lower orifice, and, having closely covered the percolator, macerate for forty-eight hours. Then allow the percolation to proceed, gradually adding first the remainder of the menstruum and afterward Diluted Alcohol, until the Leptandra is exhausted. Reserve the first *eighty cubic centimeters* [or thirty-eight fluidounces] of the percolate, and evaporate the remainder to a soft extract; dissolve this in the reserved portion, and add enough Diluted Alcohol to make the Fluid Extract measure *one hundred cubic centimeters* [or three pints]." *U. S.*

This is a new officinal fluid extract. It is of a reddish brown color, and is given in the dose of twenty minims to a fluidrachm (1·25–3·75 C.c).

EXTRACTUM LOBELIÆ FLUIDUM. *U. S. Fluid Extract of Lobelia.*

(EX-TRĂC'TUM LO-BĒ'LI-Æ FLŪ'I-DŬM.)

Extrait liquide de Lobélie enflée, *Fr.;* Flüssiges Lobelienkraut-Extrakt, *G.*

"Lobelia, in No. 60 powder, *one hundred grammes* [or fifty ounces av.]; Diluted

Alcohol, *a sufficient quantity*, To make *one hundred cubic centimeters* [or three pints]. Moisten the powder with *thirty-five grammes* [or eighteen fluidounces] of Diluted Alcohol, and pack it firmly in a cylindrical percolator; then add enough Diluted Alcohol to saturate the powder and leave a stratum above it. When the liquid begins to drop from the percolator, close the lower orifice, and, having closely covered the percolator, macerate for forty-eight hours. Then allow the percolation to proceed, gradually adding Diluted Alcohol, until the Lobelia is exhausted. Reserve the first *eighty-five cubic centimeters* [or forty fluidounces] of the percolate, and evaporate the remainder, at a temperature not exceeding 50° C. (122° F.), to a soft extract; dissolve this in the reserved portion, and add enough Diluted Alcohol to make the Fluid Extract measure *one hundred cubic centimeters* [or three pints]." *U. S.*

This is another new fluid extract. It is of a dark olive color, having the acrid taste of lobelia very marked. The dose as an expectorant is from one to five minims (0·06–0·3 C.c.); as an emetic, from ten to twenty minims (0·6–1·25 C.c.).

EXTRACTUM LUPULI. *Br.* *Extract of Hop.*

(EX-TRĂC'TŬM LŪ'PŪ-LĪ.)

Extractum Humuli; Extrait de Houblon, *Fr.*; Hopfenextrakt, *G.*

"Take of Hop *one pound* [avoirdupois]; Rectified Spirit *one pint and a half* [Imperial measure]; Distilled Water *one gallon* [Imp. meas.]. Macerate the Hop in the Spirit for seven days; press out the tincture, filter, and distil off the spirit, leaving a soft extract. Boil the residual Hop with the Water for one hour, press out the liquor, strain, and evaporate by a water-bath to the consistence of a soft extract. Mix the two extracts, and evaporate, at a temperature not exceeding 140° F. (60° C.), until it has acquired a suitable consistence for forming pills." *Br.*

This is a great improvement on the old Lond. and Ed. process by maceration with water and evaporation. Alcohol is necessary for the exhaustion of the hop, and very cautious evaporation, to preserve the aroma in the extract. But since the discovery of the fact that the active properties of hops reside chiefly in the lupulin, the extract has been to a great extent superseded by that substance in this country, and has been little used. Lupulin may be advantageously substituted for it in all cases in which it was formerly employed. Mr. Brande says that the average yield of one cwt. of hops is 40 lbs. of the extract. The dose is from ten to thirty grains (0·6–1·9 Gm.).

Under the inappropriate name of *humuline*, an extract has been prepared by first treating hops with alcohol and subsequently with water, evaporating the tincture and infusion separately, and mixing the products. (*P. J. Tr.*, xiii. 231.)

EXTRACTUM LUPULINÆ FLUIDUM. *U. S.* *Fluid Extract of Lupulin.*

(EX-TRĂC'TŬM LŪ-PŪ-LĪ'NÆ FLŪ'I-DŬM.)

Extrait liquide de Lupuline, *Fr.*; Flüssiges Lupulin-Extrakt, *G.*

"Lupulin, *one hundred grammes* [or fifty ounces av.]; Alcohol, *a sufficient quantity*, To make *one hundred cubic centimeters* [or three pints]. Moisten the Lupulin with *twenty grammes* [or twelve fluidounces] of Alcohol, and pack it firmly in a cylindrical percolator; then add enough Alcohol to saturate the Lupulin and leave a stratum above it. When the liquid begins to drop from the percolator, close the lower orifice, and, having closely covered the percolator, macerate for forty-eight hours. Then allow the percolation to proceed, gradually adding Alcohol, until the Lupulin is exhausted. Reserve the first *seventy cubic centimeters* [or thirty-three fluidounces] of the percolate, and evaporate the remainder to a soft extract; dissolve this in the reserved portion, and add enough Alcohol to make the Fluid Extract measure *one hundred cubic centimeters* [or three pints]." *U. S.*

This fluid extract is of a very dark brown color, having the odor and taste of hops very distinctly. Owing to its resinous character, it is not miscible with aqueous liquids, and if desired in combination, it is necessary to use gum arabic or other emulsifying agent. The dose is ten or fifteen minims (0·6–0·9 C.c.).

EXTRACTUM MALTI. *U.S.* *Extract of Malt.*

(EX-TRĂC'TUM MĂL'TĪ.)

Extrait de Malt d'Orge, *Fr.;* Gerstenmalz-Extrakt, *G.*

"Malt, in coarse powder, not finer than No. 12, *one hundred parts* [or eighty ounces av.]; Water, *a sufficient quantity.* Upon the powder, contained in a suitable vessel, pour *one hundred parts* [or five pints] of Water, and macerate for six hours. Then add *four hundred parts* [or twenty pints] of Water, heated to about 30° C. (86° F.), and digest for an hour at a temperature not exceeding 55° C. (131° F.). Strain the mixture with strong expression. Finally, by means of a water-bath, or vacuum apparatus, at a temperature not exceeding 55° C. (131° F.), evaporate the strained liquid rapidly to the consistence of thick honey.

"Keep the product in well-closed vessels, in a cool place." *U.S.*

Under the name of extract of malt, two distinct preparations have been put upon the market; the one being a very strong beer, the other an extract prepared from malt, and chiefly composed of dextrin and glucose, with some albumen and phosphates. The object of this officinal process is to obtain all of the soluble principles of malt in a permanent form. To secure this, strict attention to the details of the process is necessary. The changes effected in the starch granules of barley by the process of malting are described under *Hordeum* and *Maltum.* Good extract of malt should contain no starch, have the consistence of thick honey, a brown color, and should be free from empyreumatic taste. A great deal of commercial extract of malt is adulterated with glucose to a surprising extent.*

The officinal process does not differ materially from that of M. L. W. Jassoy (*Journ. de Pharm.*, 4e sér., xvi. 440), who recommends the following method. Macerate malt for three hours in its weight of cold water, then add four times its weight of water, and carefully raise the temperature to 65° C. during one hour. Filter, boil the residue with three parts of water for a quarter of an hour, remove from the fire, and allow to cool to 75° C., filter, and express the residue. Mix the liquids, maintain for some time at a temperature of 50° C., until the starch is converted into sugar. Reduce to one-third the volume by gentle boiling, allow to stand overnight, filter through a woollen strainer, and evaporate upon a water-bath to the consistence of an extract. A *dry extract of malt* is coming into extensive use as an infants' food, made by artificially drying the thick syrupy extract. It is in the form of straw-colored, coarse powder, and is given dissolved in milk or water. O. F. Romer and H. R. Randoll, of Brooklyn, have patented several improvements in the process of making extract of malt, namely: 1, the properly ground malt is treated with an alkaline solution, in order to neutralize the fatty acids which usually impart a bad taste to the product; 2, the extract is separated from the solid matters by pressing in press-cloths, whereby it is obtained as a clear liquid with scarcely any loss. (*N. R.*, 1880, p. 179.) Pharmaceutically, extract of malt has been used as an emulsifying agent; it makes a good basis for a cod-liver oil emulsion, for which purpose it is admirably adapted therapeutically. The dose is one to four drachms.

EXTRACTUM MATICO FLUIDUM. *U.S.* *Fluid Extract of Matico.*

(EX-TRĂC'TUM MA-TĪ'CŌ FLŪ'Ĭ-DŬM—ma-tē'kō.)

Extrait liquide de Matico, *Fr.;* Flüssiges Matico-Extrakt, *G.*

"Matico, in No. 40 powder, *one hundred grammes* [or fifty ounces av.]; Glycerin, *ten grammes* [or three and three-quarter fluidounces]; Alcohol, Water, each, *a sufficient quantity,* To make *one hundred cubic centimeters* [or three pints]. Mix the Glycerin with *seventy-five grammes* [or forty-four fluidounces] of Alcohol and *twenty-five grammes* [or twelve fluidounces] of Water, and, having moistened the powder with *thirty grammes* [or fifteen fluidounces] of the mixture, pack it firmly

* *Midzu-ame.* This is a thick semi-liquid substance, of the color and translucency of honey and a sweetish, insipid taste, which is manufactured in Japan, and is said to be used for the same purposes as malt extracts are in America. It is prepared from a mixture of barley malt and a very glutinous rice in water. This is allowed to stand for twelve hours in a moderate temperature, strained under pressure, and the liquid obtained is evaporated to a proper consistence over a slow fire. It is probably a preparation of glucose, with very little if any diastase in it.

in a cylindrical percolator; then add enough of the menstruum to saturate the powder and leave a stratum above it. When the liquid begins to drop from the percolator, close the lower orifice, and, having closely covered the percolator, macerate for forty-eight hours. Then allow the percolation to proceed, gradually adding, first, the remainder of the menstruum, and afterward, a mixture of Alcohol and Water, made in the proportion of *three parts* [or three and a half pints] of Alcohol to *one part* [or one pint] of Water, until the Matico is exhausted. Reserve the first *eighty-five cubic centimeters* [or forty fluidounces] of the percolate, and evaporate the remainder to a soft extract; dissolve this in the reserved portion, and add enough of a mixture of Alcohol and Water, using the same proportions as before, to make the Fluid Extract measure *one hundred cubic centimeters* [or three pints]." *U. S.*

This is probably the best liquid preparation of matico; the present formula does not differ materially from that of 1870. It is a greenish black liquid, which probably contains all of the virtues of matico, and affords an excellent form for internal administration. The dose is from a half to one fluidrachm (1·9–3·75 C.c.).

EXTRACTUM MEZEREI. *U. S.* *Extract of Mezereum.*

(ĔX-TRĂC'TŬM MĔ-ZĒ'RĔ-Ī.)

Extrait alcoolique de Mézéréon, *Fr.;* Spirituöses Seidelbast-Extrakt, *G.*

"Mezereum, in No. 30 powder, *one hundred parts* [or sixteen ounces av.]; Alcohol, *a sufficient quantity*. Moisten the powder with *forty parts* [or six fluidounces] of Alcohol, and pack it firmly in a cylindrical percolator; then add enough Alcohol to saturate the powder and leave a stratum above it. When the liquid begins to drop from the percolator, close the lower orifice, and, having closely covered the percolator, macerate for forty-eight hours. Then allow the percolation to proceed, gradually adding Alcohol, until *three hundred parts* [or three pints] of tincture are obtained, or the Mezereum is exhausted. Reserve the first *ninety parts* [or thirteen fluidounces] of the percolate; evaporate the remainder, at a temperature not exceeding 50° C. (122° F.), to *ten parts* [or two fluidounces]; mix this with the reserved portion, and evaporate at or below the before-mentioned temperature in a porcelain capsule, on a water-bath, to a pilular consistence." *U. S.*

This is a good preparation, yet differing from the ethereal extract of the British Pharmacopœia in not being quite so powerful. It is used as an irritant. (See next article.)

Off. Prep. Linimentum Sinapis Compositum, *U. S.*

EXTRACTUM MEZEREI ÆTHEREUM. *Br.* *Ethereal Extract of Mezereon.*

(ĔX-TRĂC'TŬM MĔ-ZĒ'RĔ-Ī Æ-THĒ'RĔ-ŬM—ē-thē'rē-ŭm.)

Extrait éthéré de Mézéréon (de Garou), *Fr.;* Ætherisches Seidelbast-Extrakt, *G.*

"Take of Mezereon Bark, cut small, *one pound* [avoirdupois]; Rectified Spirit *eight pints* [Imperial measure]; Ether *one pint* [Imp. meas.]. Macerate the Mezereon in six pints of the Spirit for three days, with frequent agitation; strain and press. To the residue of the Mezereon add the remainder of the Spirit, and again macerate for three days, with frequent agitation; strain and press. Mix and filter the strained liquors; recover the greater part of the Spirit by distillation, evaporate what remains to the consistence of a soft extract; put this into a stoppered bottle with the Ether, and macerate for twenty-four hours, shaking them frequently. Decant the ethereal solution; recover part of the Ether by distillation, and evaporate what remains to the consistence of a soft extract." *Br.*

This is the process of the present French Codex, with slight modifications, which do not affect the result. In the Codex the mezereon is exhausted by means of percolation, instead of by a double maceration; and in this respect the process is, we think, preferable, in the hands of a skilful operator. With those not experienced in percolation, it may be better to follow the British Pharmacopœia.

By the method of proceeding in the preparation of this extract the irritating properties of mezereon are concentrated in a small bulk; all the ingredients of the bark not soluble both in alcohol and in ether being excluded. For external use this is probably desirable; and the extract is therefore chiefly useful as an external irritant; for which purpose it is brought into the state of an ointment, as in the French "*pommade épispastique au garou*," or used in liniments, as in the British "*compound liniment of mustard.*" The French "pommade," which might properly be designated as *Unguentum Mezerei*, or *Ointment of Mezereon*, is prepared in the following manner.

"Take of Ethereal Extract of Mezereon *forty parts*; Lard *nine hundred parts*; White Wax *one hundred parts*; Alcohol *ninety parts*. Dissolve the Extract in the Alcohol, add the Lard and Wax, and heat moderately, with continual agitation, until the alcohol is evaporated. Pass through linen; pour into a pot, and shake until the ointment is partly cooled." (*Fr. Codex.*)

The object of this preparation is to act as an irritant agent, and especially as a dressing for issues and blistered surfaces to keep them open. For this purpose it is preferable to the ointment of cantharides, in all cases in which the latter is disposed to cause strangury.

Off. Prep. Br. Linimentum Sinapis Compositum.

EXTRACTUM MEZEREI FLUIDUM. *U.S.* *Fluid Extract of Mezereum.*

(EX-TRĂC'TUM ME-ZĒ'RE-Ī FLŪ'I-DŬM.)

Extrait liquide de Mésérĕon (de Garou) *Fr.*; Flüssiges Seidelbast-Extrakt, *G.*

"Mezereum, in No. 30 powder, *one hundred grammes* [or fifty ounces av.]; Alcohol, *a sufficient quantity*, To make *one hundred cubic centimeters* [or three pints]. Moisten the powder with *forty grammes* [or twenty-three fluidounces] of Alcohol, and pack it firmly in a cylindrical percolator; then add enough Alcohol to saturate the powder and leave a stratum above it. When the liquid begins to drop from the percolator, close the lower orifice, and, having closely covered the percolator, macerate for forty-eight hours. Then allow the percolation to proceed, gradually adding Alcohol, until the Mezereum is exhausted. Reserve the first *ninety cubic centimeters* [or forty-three fluidounces] of the percolate, and evaporate the remainder, at a temperature not exceeding 50° C. (122° F.), to a soft extract; dissolve this in the reserved portion, and add enough Alcohol to make the Fluid Extract measure *one hundred cubic centimeters* [or three pints]." *U. S.*

This fluid extract is identical with that formerly officinal. It is too acrid for internal administration; its principal use is as the active ingredient in the stimulating ointment of mezereon.

Off. Prep. Unguentum Mezerei.

EXTRACTUM NUCIS VOMICÆ. *U.S., Br.* *Extract of Nux Vomica.*

(EX-TRĂC'TUM NŪ'CIS VŎM'I-CÆ—vŏm'e-sē.)

Extractum Strychni Spirituosum, *P. G.*; Extractum Nucum Vomicarum Spirituosum (vel Alcoholicum); Extrait de Noix vomique, *Fr.*; Weingeistiges Krähenaugen-Extrakt, *G.*

"Nux Vomica, in No. 60 powder, *one hundred parts* [or sixteen ounces av.]; Alcohol, Water, each, *a sufficient quantity*. Mix Alcohol and Water in the proportion of *eight parts* [or four and a half pints] of Alcohol and *one part* [or half a pint] of Water, and, having moistened the powder with *one hundred parts* [or fifteen fluidounces] of the mixture, let it macerate in a closed vessel, in a warm place, for forty-eight hours. Then pack it in a cylindrical percolator, and gradually pour menstruum upon it, until the tincture passes but slightly imbued with bitterness. By means of a water-bath, distil off the Alcohol from the tincture, and, having placed the residue in a porcelain capsule, evaporate it, on a water-bath, to a pilular consistence." *U. S.*

"Take of Nux Vomica *one pound* [av.]; Rectified Spirit *sixty-four fluidounces* [Imp. meas.]; Distilled Water *sixteen fluidounces* [Imp. meas.]. Heat the previously split seeds to a temperature of 212° F. (100° C.) for three hours, and then reduce to a fine powder. Mix the spirit with the water, and make the powdered nux vomica into a paste with one pint of the mixture. Allow this to macerate for twelve hours, then transfer to a percolator, and add another pint of the mixture. When this has percolated, pour on the remainder of the diluted spirit in successive portions; press the marc, filter the expressed liquor, and add it to the percolated liquid.

"Take of this liquid one fluidounce, and estimate the amount of total alkaloid in the following way. Evaporate almost to dryness over a water-bath, dissolve the residue in two fluidrachms of chloroform and half a fluidounce of dilute sulphuric acid with an equal bulk of water; agitate and warm gently. When the liquors have separated, draw off the chloroform, and add to the acid liquor excess of solution of ammonia and half a fluidounce of chloroform; well agitate, gently warm, and, after the liquors have completely separated, transfer the chloroform to a weighed dish, evaporate over a water-bath, and dry for one hour at 212° F. (100° C.). Allow the residue of total alkaloid to cool, and then weigh.

"Take of the percolated liquid as much as contains 131¼ grains of total alkaloid, distil off the spirit, and evaporate over a water-bath until the extract weighs two ounces. This extract will contain fifteen per cent. of total alkaloid.

"*Test.* Ten grains of the extract when treated in the following manner should yield one grain and a half of total alkaloid. Dissolve the extract in half a fluidounce of water, heating gently if necessary, and add a drachm of carbonate of sodium previously dissolved in half a fluidounce of water and half a fluidounce of chloroform; agitate, warm gently, and separate the chloroform. Add to this half a fluidounce of dilute sulphuric acid with an equal bulk of water; again agitate, warm, and separate the acid liquor from the chloroform. To this acid liquor add now an excess of ammonia, and agitate with half a fluidounce of chloroform; when the liquors have separated, transfer the chloroform to a weighed dish, and evaporate the chloroform over a water-bath. Dry the residue for one hour, and weigh." *Br.*

The process of the British Pharmacopœia is that recommended by Profs. Dunstan and Short (*P. J. Tr.*, 1884, p. 623), and it probably represents the most successful effort to standardize officinal pharmaceutical preparations. The menstruum has been carefully selected so that the alkaloids shall be extracted and as much of the oil left in the residue as possible. In order to make a dry powdered extract it would be necessary to separate the fixed oil before assaying it, and then to make up the weight, if necessary, with sugar of milk or some inert, soluble powder. Of the advantages, aside from those of securing uniformity and safety, is the important one that the operator need not carry the percolation beyond the point where it ceases to be profitable (on account of the waste of alcohol), because the extract must be brought to a definite alkaloidal strength. Such an extract can be used with great advantage to make tincture of nux vomica of definite alkaloidal strength. For Beckurt's method of assaying nux vomica see *Pharm. Era*, 1887, p. 447.

In both the U. S. and Br. Pharmacopœias the nux vomica is directed in fine powder; but in the latter only are we told how to reduce it to that state. When the extract is kept in powder, it is apt to agglutinate into a tough mass. According to Zippel, this may be prevented by adding a little water before the close of the evaporation, and then continuing the evaporation to dryness.

The fixed oil which is found in this extract in the proportion of from 2 to 3 per cent. should be separated, shaken with a little alcohol to dissolve out the alkaloids taken up by the oil, and the solution evaporated and added to the extract. The abstract is to be preferred to the U. S. extract, which is an active preparation, though not always of uniform strength, owing to the variable proportion of strychnine in the nux vomica. M. Reclus obtained from sixteen ounces of nux vomica the average product of one ounce and a quarter. The dose of the extract is from half a grain to two grains (0·03–0·13 Gm.), to be repeated three times a day.

Off. Prep. Br. Tinctura Nucis Vomicæ.

EXTRACTUM NUCIS VOMICÆ FLUIDUM. *U.S.* *Fluid Extract of Nux Vomica.*

(ĔX-TRĂC'TŬM NŪ'CIS VŎM'Ĭ-ÇÆ FLŪ'Ĭ-DŬM.)

Extrait liquide de Noix Vomique, *Fr.;* Flüssiges Krähenaugen-Extrakt, *G.*

"Nux Vomica, in No. 60 powder, *one hundred grammes* [or fifty ounces av.];

Alcohol, Water, each, *a sufficient quantity*, To make *one hundred cubic centimeters* [or three pints]. Mix *eight parts* [or nine pints] of Alcohol with *one part* [or one pint] of Water, and, having moistened the powder with *one hundred cubic centimeters* [or three pints] of the mixture, let it macerate in a closed vessel, in a warm place, for forty-eight hours. Then pack it firmly in a cylindrical percolator, and gradually pour menstruum upon it, until the tincture passes but slightly imbued with bitterness. Reserve the first *ninety cubic centimeters* [or forty-three fluidounces] of the percolate. By means of a water-bath, distil off the Alcohol from the remainder, and evaporate the residue to a soft extract; dissolve this in the reserved portion, and add enough menstruum to make the Fluid Extract measure *one hundred cubic centimeters* [or three pints]." *U. S.*

This is a new officinal fluid extract; its usefulness is not very apparent. The drug is a difficult one to exhaust at best; the dose of the best known liquid preparation, the tincture, is small enough, and, in our opinion, there was no necessity for introducing a fluid extract which will, in the majority of cases, not thoroughly represent the drug. The dose is three to five minims (0·18 to 0·3 C.c.).

EXTRACTUM OPII. *U. S., Br.* *Extract of Opium.*

(ĔX-TRĂC'TŬM Ō'PĬ-Ī.)

Extrait d'Opium, Extrait thébaïque, *Fr.;* Opiumextrakt, *G.*

"Opium, *one hundred parts* [or sixteen ounces av.]; Water, *seven hundred and fifty parts* [or seven and a half pints]; Glycerin, *a sufficient quantity*. Cut the Opium into small pieces, let it macerate for twenty-four hours in *one hundred and fifty parts* [or one and a half pints] of the Water, and reduce it to a soft mass by trituration. Express the liquid from it, and treat the residue again in the same manner with *one hundred and fifty parts* [or one and a half pints] of the Water. Repeat the maceration and expression three times more, using a fresh portion of the Water each time. Having mixed the liquids, filter the mixture, and evaporate, by means of a water-bath, to a pilular consistence. Lastly, weigh the Extract and thoroughly incorporate with it, while still warm, *five per cent.* of Glycerin." *U. S.*

"Take of Opium *one pound* [avoirdupois]; Distilled Water *six pints* [Imperial measure]. Macerate the Opium in two pints of the water for twenty-four hours, and express the liquor. Thoroughly mix the residue of the Opium with two pints of Water, macerate again for twenty-four hours, and express. Repeat the operation a third time. Mix the liquors, strain through flannel, and evaporate by a water-bath to about half a pound [av.]." *Br.* "*Test.* Analysed as described under 'Opium,' this extract should yield about twenty per cent. of morphine."

The U. S. and Br. processes are essentially the same.

As purely aqueous preparations of opium have been found to agree better with certain individuals than opium alone or its alcoholic preparations, there is reason to believe that there are in the crude drug one or more principles, capable of causing nausea, headache, nervous disturbance, etc., which are insoluble in water, though extracted by alcohol or ether. (See *Opium Denarcotisatum.*) The aqueous extract of opium formerly officinal became hard and friable on keeping, and the addition of glycerin is now made to cause it to retain its pilular consistence. Some pharmacists prefer to evaporate the extract to dryness, and keep it in a powdered condition. If carefully evaporated by water-bath there can be no objection to this. M. Guibourt states that this extract, when kept, is apt to swell up, owing, as he at first supposed, to the fermentation of glucose; but he now ascribes the phenomenon to the change of meconic acid into the parameconic, with the escape of carbonic acid. (*Journ. de Pharm.*, Août, 1860, p. 138.)

Reclus obtained from sixteen ounces of opium an average product of nine ounces by hot water and six by cold; and the U. S. formula usually yields about seven and a half ounces from the same quantity. The dose of the extract of opium is half a grain to one grain (0·031–0·065 Gm.).

Off. Prep. Emplastrum Opii; Trochisci Glycyrrhizæ et Opii.

Off. Prep. Br. Extractum Opii Liquidum; Trochisci Opii; Vinum Opii.

EXTRACTUM OPII LIQUIDUM. *Br.* *Liquid Extract of Opium.*

(ĔX-TRĂC'TŨM Ō'PĪ-Ī LĬQ'UĪ-DŬM—lĭk'wę-dŭm.)

Extrait liquide d'Opium, *Fr.;* Flüssiges Opiumextrakt, *G.*

"Take of Extract of Opium *one ounce* [avoirdupois]; Distilled Water *sixteen fluidounces* [Imperial measure]; Rectified Spirit *four fluidounces* [Imp. meas.]. Macerate the Extract of Opium in the Water for an hour, stirring frequently; then add the Spirit, and filter. The product should measure *one pint* [Imp. meas.]." *Br.*

"It contains twenty-two grains of extract of opium, nearly, in one fluidounce. Sp. gr. from 0·985 to 0·995." "*Test.* Analyzed as described under 'Opium,' this liquid extract should yield about one per cent. of morphine." *Br.*

This is a good preparation, one which has long been needed, and in the absence of which from the Pharmacopœia empirical preparations have obtained a certain vogue. It is well known that in opium there are principles soluble in alcohol but not in water, which often produce various disagreeable effects, not experienced from the watery extract. What was wanted was a liquid preparation meeting this demand. All that was required was to make an aqueous solution of the watery extract, and to add something to preserve it. The British Pharmacopœia uses alcohol for the purpose, and in the original formula employed it in such proportion that an Imperial pint of the liquid should contain three fluidounces of the spirit, or between one-sixth and one-seventh by measure. But this amount of alcohol, according to Mr. Squire, is insufficient for its preservation, and should be doubled. In the present Pharmacopœia the spirit has been increased to four fluidounces, and the water diminished from seventeen to sixteen fluidounces; but even with this increase the spirit constitutes only one-fifth, which is considerably short of the proportion recommended by Mr. Squire. A preparation similar to the British was made some years since by Mr. Eugene Dupuy, of New York. (See *Opium.*) In the *Deodorized Tincture of Opium* of the U. S. Pharmacopœia, the advantages of the preparation have, we think, been still better secured. The dose of the liquid extract, equivalent to a grain of opium, would be about ten minims (0·6 C.c.).

EXTRACTUM PAPAVERIS. *Br.* *Extract of Poppies.*

(ĔX-TRĂC'TŨM PĄ-PĀ'VĘ-RĬS.)

Extrait de Pavot, *Fr.;* Mohnextrakt, *G.*

"Take of Poppy Capsules, freed from the seeds, and in No. 20 powder, *one pound* [avoirdupois]; Rectified Spirit *two ounces* [av.]. Boiling Distilled Water *a sufficiency.* Mix the Poppy Capsules with two pints [Imperial measure] of the Water, and infuse for twenty-four hours, stirring them frequently; then pack in a percolator, and, adding more of the Water, allow the liquor slowly to pass until about a gallon [Imp. meas.] has been collected, or until the residue is exhausted. Evaporate the liquor by a water-bath until it is reduced to a pint [Imp. meas.], and, when cold, add the Spirit. Let the mixture stand for twenty-four hours; then separate the clear liquor by filtration, and evaporate this by a water-bath, until the extract has acquired a suitable consistence for forming pills." *Br.*

The Extract of Poppy Capsules was an officinal of the Lond. and Edin. Colleges, but was abandoned in the formation of the first British Pharmacopœia. It has, however, been introduced into the last edition of that work, though with a process somewhat modified. It possesses the virtues of opium, but is inferior, and much less uniform in strength. The dose is from five to ten grains (0·33–0·65 Gm.).

EXTRACTUM PAREIRÆ. *Br.* *Extract of Pareira.*

(ĔX-TRĂC'TŨM PĄ-REI'RÆ—pę-rā'rē.)

Extrait de Pareira Brava, *Fr.;* Pareira-Extrakt, *G.*

"Take of Pareira Root, in No. 40 powder, *one pound* [avoirdupois]; Boiling Distilled Water *a sufficiency.* Digest the Pareira with a pint [Imp. meas.] of the Water for twenty-four hours, then pack in a percolator, and, adding more of the Water, allow the liquor slowly to pass until about a gallon [Imp. meas.] has been collected, or the Pareira is exhausted. Evaporate the liquor by a water-bath until the extract has acquired a suitable consistence for forming pills." *Br.*

This was formerly directed by the London and Edinburgh Colleges, was omitted in the first British Pharmacopœia, and has been adopted again in the last edition. By the formula of the London College, it was prepared by boiling the root in water, straining while hot, and then evaporating to dryness. The British Pharmacopœia more wisely exhausts the root by percolation, and evaporates by a water-bath, thus avoiding the bad effects of long-continued heat. The dose is from ten to thirty grains (0·65–1·95 Gm.).

Off. Prep. Br. Extractum Pareiræ Liquidum.

EXTRACTUM PAREIRÆ FLUIDUM. *U.S.* *Fluid Extract of Pareira.*

(EX-TRĂC'TUM PA-REI'RÆ FLŪ'I-DŬM—pa-rā'rē.)

Extractum Pareiræ Liquidum, *Br.;* **Liquid Extract of Pareira; Extrait liquide de Pareira Brava,** *Fr.;* **Flüssiges Pareira-Extrakt,** *G.*

"Pareira, in No. 40 powder, *one hundred grammes* [or fifty ounces]; Glycerin, *twenty grammes* [or seven and a half fluidounces]; Diluted Alcohol, *a sufficient quantity,* To make *one hundred cubic centimeters* [or three pints]. Mix the Glycerin with *eighty grammes* [or forty-one fluidounces] of Diluted Alcohol, and, having moistened the powder with *forty grammes* [or twenty fluidounces] of the mixture, pack it firmly in a cylindrical percolator; then add enough of the menstruum to saturate the powder and leave a stratum above it. When the liquid begins to drop from the percolator, close the lower orifice, and, having closely covered the percolator, macerate for forty-eight hours. Then allow the percolation to proceed, gradually adding, first, the remainder of the menstruum, and afterward, Diluted Alcohol, until the Pareira is exhausted. Reserve the first *eighty-five cubic centimeters* [or forty fluidounces] of the percolate. By means of a water-bath, distil off the Alcohol from the remainder, and evaporate the residue to a soft extract; dissolve this in the reserved portion, and add enough Diluted Alcohol to make the Fluid Extract measure *one hundred cubic centimeters* [or three pints]." *U. S.*

"Take of Extract of Pareira, Distilled Water, Rectified Spirit, of each, *a sufficiency.* Dissolve four parts of the extract in a sufficient quantity of a mixture of one fluid part of rectified spirit and three parts of water to form sixteen fluid parts of liquid extract. Filter, if necessary." *Br.*

The British preparation is a concentrated solution of the extract, preserved by adding somewhat less than one-fourth of its measure of alcohol, and is said to have all the virtues of the root. There must be considerable loss through the action of the heat in evaporating the extract, and again through precipitation, due to attempting to dissolve an aqueous extract in a hydro-alcoholic menstruum; an examination, however, would alone determine whether the precipitate, which is directed to be filtered out, is active. The American fluid extract is made with diluted alcohol and glycerin, is practically identical with that of 1870, and is undoubtedly the better preparation. The dose is one or two fluidrachms (3·75–7·5 C.c.).

EXTRACTUM PHYSOSTIGMATIS. *U.S., Br.* *Extract of Physostigma.*

(EX-TRĂC'TUM PHȲ-SO-STĬG'MA-TĬS.)

Extractum Fabæ Calabaricæ, *P.G.;* **Extract of Calabar Bean; Extrait de Fève de Calabar,** *Fr.;* **Kalabarbohnen-Extrakt,** *G.*

"Physostigma, in No. 40 powder, *one hundred parts* [or sixteen ounces av.]; Alcohol, *a sufficient quantity.* Moisten the powder with *forty parts* [or six fluidounces] of Alcohol, and pack it firmly in a cylindrical percolator; then add enough Alcohol to saturate the powder and leave a stratum above it. When the liquid begins to drop from the percolator, close the lower orifice, and, having closely covered the percolator, macerate for forty-eight hours. Then allow the percolation to proceed, gradually adding Alcohol, until *three hundred parts* [or three pints] of tincture are obtained, or the Physostigma is exhausted. Reserve the first *ninety parts* [or fourteen fluidounces] of the percolate; evaporate the remainder, at a temperature not exceeding 50° C. (122° F.), to *ten parts* [or two fluidounces], mix this with the reserved portion, and evaporate at or below the before-mentioned temperature in a porcelain capsule, on a water-bath, to a pilular consistence." *U. S.*

"Take of Calabar Bean, in No. 40 powder, *one pound* [avoirdupois]; Rectified Spirit *four pints* [Imperial measure]. Macerate the Bean for forty-eight hours with *one pint* [Imp. meas.] of the Spirit in a closed vessel, agitating occasionally, then transfer to a percolator, and, when the fluid ceases to pass, add the remainder of the Spirit so that it may slowly percolate through the powder. Subject the residue of the Bean to pressure, adding the expressed liquor to the product of the percolation; filter, distil off most of the Spirit, and evaporate what is left in the retort by a water-bath to the consistence of a soft extract." *Br.*

As alcohol is a much better solvent than water of the active principles of the bean, it is preferred in making the extract. For the uses of the extract, see *Physostigma*. The dose for internal use is from one-sixteenth to one-sixth of a grain (0·004–0·01 Gm.).

Off. Prep. Br. Physostigmina.

EXTRACTUM PILOCARPI FLUIDUM. *U. S.* *Fluid Extract of Pilocarpus.* [*Fluid Extract of Jaborandi.*]

(EX-TRĂC'TUM PĪ-LO-CĂR'PĪ FLŪ'I-DŬM.)

"Pilocarpus, in No. 40 powder, *one hundred grammes* [or fifty ounces av.]; Diluted Alcohol, *a sufficient quantity*, To make *one hundred cubic centimeters* [or three pints]. Moisten the powder with *thirty-five grammes* [or eighteen fluidounces] of Diluted Alcohol, and pack it firmly in a cylindrical percolator; then add enough Diluted Alcohol to saturate the powder and leave a stratum above it. When the liquid begins to drop from the percolator, close the lower orifice, and, having closely covered the percolator, macerate for forty-eight hours. Then allow the percolation to proceed, gradually adding Diluted Alcohol, until the Pilocarpus is exhausted. Reserve the first *eighty-five cubic centimeters* [or forty fluidounces] of the percolate, and evaporate the remainder, at a temperature not exceeding 50° C. (122° F.), to a soft extract; dissolve this in the reserved portion, and add enough Diluted Alcohol to make the Fluid Extract measure *one hundred cubic centimeters* [or three pints]." *U. S.*

This is undoubtedly the most valuable of the new officinal fluid extracts. It represents jaborandi leaves thoroughly. Of the liquid preparations, the infusion and tincture are both open to objection, the former on account of the bulkiness of the dose, and the latter from the amount of alcohol it contains. The dose of the fluid extract is fifteen minims to half a fluidrachm (0·9 to 1·9 C.c.).

EXTRACTUM PODOPHYLLI. *U. S.* *Extract of Podophyllum.*

(EX-TRĂC'TUM PŎD-O-PHȲL'LĪ.)

Extrait de Podophylle, *Fr.*; Fussblattwurzel-Extrakt, *G.*

"Podophyllum, in No. 60 powder, *one hundred parts* [or sixteen ounces av.]; Alcohol, Water, each, *a sufficient quantity*. Mix Alcohol and Water in the proportion of *three parts* [or three and a half pints] of Alcohol and *one part* [or one pint] of Water, and, having moistened the powder with *thirty parts* [or four and a half fluidounces] of the mixture, pack it firmly in a cylindrical percolator; then add enough of the menstruum to saturate the powder and leave a stratum above it. When the liquid begins to drop from the percolator, close the lower orifice, and, having closely covered the percolator, macerate for forty-eight hours. Then allow the percolation to proceed, gradually adding menstruum, until *five hundred parts* [or five pints] of tincture have passed. By means of a water-bath, distil off the Alcohol from the tincture, and evaporate the residue to a pilular consistence." *U. S.*

This is possessed of the purgative properties of the root, and may be given in the dose of from one to three grains (0·06–0·2 Gm.). From experiments made by Mr. John R. Lewis, it is probable that the alcoholic extract would be much more powerful as a purgative than the officinal preparation; but it does not follow that it would be more serviceable. (See *A. J. P.*, xix. 170.)

EXTRACTUM PODOPHYLLI FLUIDUM. *U. S.* *Fluid Extract of Podophyllum.*

(EX-TRĂC′TUM PŎD-O-PHȲL′LĪ FLŪ′I-DŬM.)

Extrait liquide de Podophylle, *Fr.;* Flüssiges Fussblattwurzel-Extrakt, *G.*

"Podophyllum, in No. 60 powder, *one hundred grammes* [or fifty ounces av.]; Alcohol, Water, each, *a sufficient quantity,* To make *one hundred cubic centimeters* [or three pints]. Mix *three parts* [or three and a half pints] of Alcohol with *one part* [or one pint] of Water, and, having moistened the powder with *thirty grammes* [or one pint] of the mixture, pack it firmly in a cylindrical percolator; then add enough of the menstruum to saturate the powder and leave a stratum above it. When the liquid begins to drop from the percolator, close the lower orifice, and, having closely covered the percolator, macerate for forty-eight hours. Then allow the percolation to proceed, gradually adding menstruum, until the Podophyllum is exhausted. Reserve the first *eighty-five cubic centimeters* [or forty fluidounces] of the percolate; by means of a water-bath, distil off the Alcohol from the remainder; dissolve the residue in the reserved portion, and add enough menstruum to make the Fluid Extract measure *one hundred cubic centimeters* [or three pints]." *U. S.*

This is another new officinal fluid extract. It well represents the root, but is of very little use. The dose is from five to fifteen minims (0·3 to 0·9 C.c.).

EXTRACTUM PRUNI VIRGINIANÆ FLUIDUM. *U. S.* *Fluid Extract of Wild Cherry.*

(EX-TRĂC′TUM PRŪ′NĪ VĬR-GĬN-I-Ā′NÆ FLŪ′I-DŬM.)

Extrait liquide de Cerisier de Virginie, *Fr.;* Flüssiges Wildkirschenrinden-Extrakt, *G.*

"Wild Cherry, in No. 20 powder, *one hundred grammes* [or fifty ounces av.]; Diluted Alcohol, Glycerin, Water, each, *a sufficient quantity,* To make *one hundred cubic centimeters* [or three pints]. Mix *two parts* [or seventeen fluidounces] of Water with *one part* [or seven fluidounces] of Glycerin, and, having moistened the powder with *fifty grammes* [or twenty-four fluidounces] of the mixture, pack it loosely in a cylindrical percolator, cover the latter well, and set it aside for forty-eight hours. Then pack the damp powder firmly in the percolator, and pour on enough Diluted Alcohol to saturate the powder and leave a stratum above it. When the liquid begins to drop from the percolator, close the lower orifice, and, having closely covered the percolator, macerate for forty-eight hours. Then allow the percolation to proceed, gradually adding Diluted Alcohol, until the Wild Cherry is exhausted. Reserve the first *eighty cubic centimeters* [or thirty-eight fluidounces] of the percolate and set it aside; collect the next *one hundred and twenty cubic centimeters* [or forty-eight fluidounces] separately, and evaporate to a thin syrup. By means of a water-bath, distil off the Alcohol from the remainder of the percolate and evaporate the residue to a thin syrup. Unite the two syrupy liquids, and evaporate them, on a water-bath, to a soft extract; dissolve this in the reserved portion, and add enough Diluted Alcohol to make the Fluid Extract measure *one hundred cubic centimeters* [or three pints]." *U. S.*

This preparation has been practically more troublesome than any of the other fluid extracts. We had first Prof. Procter's original process, then his modified one, in which almonds were used to supply emulsin to assist in the development of hydrocyanic acid. (See U. S. D., 15th edition, p. 637.) This was abandoned as too cumbersome in 1870, and we had the glycerin experiment. The fluid extract of 1870 deposited heavily soon after being made, and was immiscible with aqueous liquids without precipitation. These were fatal objections. The present formula is the result of much careful work on the part of the Committee, and it is believed to be an improvement over all its predecessors.* It is of a very dark wine color, of a

* *Fluid Extract of Wild Cherry* (Improved). This process is advocated by Mr. Cyrus M. Boger, who states that all of the hydrocyanic acid is developed, tannin is excluded as much as possible, and consequently precipitation is reduced to the lowest point. "Take of Ground Wild Cherry Bark, *ten troyounces;* Water and Alcohol, each, *ten fluidounces;* Glycerin, *four fluidrachms.* Moisten the bark with *ten fluidounces* of water and put loosely in the percolator, close tightly, and allow it to macerate sixty hours; then pack very firmly, mix the *ten fluidounces* of alcohol and *four* of glycerin and pour it upon the bark; now cork up the percolator tightly and macerate

rough astringent taste, with a decided odor and taste of hydrocyanic acid. The dose is thirty minims to a fluidrachm (1·9–3·75 C.c).

EXTRACTUM QUASSIÆ. *U.S., Br.* *Extract of Quassia.*

(EX-TRĂC'TUM QUAS'SI-Æ—kwŏsh'ṣ-ē.)

Extrait de Quassie (Bois amer), *Fr.;* Quassia-Extrakt, *G.*

"Quassia, in No. 20 powder, *one hundred parts* [or sixteen ounces av.]; Glycerin, Water, each, *a sufficient quantity.* Moisten the powder with *forty parts* [or six fluidounces] of Water, pack it firmly in a conical percolator, and gradually pour Water upon it until the infusion passes but slightly imbued with bitterness. Reduce the liquid to three-fourths of its weight, by boiling, and strain; then, by means of a water-bath, evaporate to a pilular consistence. Lastly, weigh the Extract, and thoroughly incorporate with it, while still warm, *five per cent.* of Glycerin." *U.S.*

"Take of Quassia Wood, rasped, *one pound* [avoirdupois]; Distilled Water, *a sufficiency.* Macerate the Quassia with eight fluidounces of the Water for twelve hours; then pack in a percolator, and, adding more of the Water, allow the liquor slowly to pass until the Quassia is exhausted. Evaporate the liquor; filter before it becomes too thick; and again evaporate by a water-bath until the extract is of a suitable consistence for forming pills." *Br.*

According to M. Recluz, sixteen ounces of quassia yield by infusion in water seven drachms of extract; by maceration in alcohol of 19° Baumé, two ounces five drachms and a half. The difference between these quantities is so great that we suspect some mistake in the Dictionnaire des Drogues, from which we quote, although it is known that alcohol yields a larger proportion of extractive than does water or a mixture of alcohol and water.

The extract of quassia is dark brown or black, and excessively bitter. It is apt to become dry and disposed to crumble by time. It concentrates a greater amount of tonic power within a given weight than any other extract of the simple bitters, and may, therefore, be given with great advantage in cases in which it is desirable to administer this class of substances in as small a bulk as possible. The dose is one to two grains (0·065 to 0·13 Gm.), to be given in pill. The alcoholic extract is a better preparation, and the yield is greater; but it is probably wisest to adhere to the aqueous extract, on account of its cheapness.

EXTRACTUM QUASSIÆ FLUIDUM. *U.S.* *Fluid Extract of Quassia.*

(EX-TRĂC'TUM QUAS'SI-Æ FLU'I-DUM—kwŏsh'ṣ-ē.)

Extrait liquide de Quassia, *Fr.;* Flüssiges Quassia-Extrakt, *G.*

"Quassia, in No. 60 powder, *one hundred grammes* [or fifty ounces av.]; Diluted Alcohol, *a sufficient quantity,* To make *one hundred cubic centimeters* [or three pints]. Moisten the powder with *forty grammes* [or twenty fluidounces] of Diluted Alcohol, and pack it firmly in a cylindrical percolator; then add enough Diluted Alcohol to saturate the powder and leave a stratum above it. When the liquid begins to drop from the percolator, close the lower orifice, and, having closely covered the percolator, macerate for forty-eight hours. Then allow the percolation to proceed, gradually adding Diluted Alcohol, until the Quassia is exhausted. Reserve the first *ninety cubic centimeters* [or forty-three fluidounces] of the percolate, and evaporate the remainder to a soft extract; dissolve this in the reserved portion, and add enough Diluted Alcohol to make the Fluid Extract measure *one hundred cubic centimeters* [or three pints]." *U.S.*

This is another new officinal fluid extract. It is exceedingly bitter, and will probably never be given by itself internally, but used to form the basis for infusions, mixtures, etc. The dose would be five to ten minims (0·3 to 0·6 C.c.).

twenty-four hours longer, at the expiration of this time remove the cork, and about *twelve fluidounces* of percolate will come through; water should now be poured on to force the other four fluidounces out, when the percolation should be stopped and the product will be finished." (*A. J. P.,* 1887, pp. 231, 232.

EXTRACTUM RHAMNI FRANGULÆ. *Br.* *Extract of Rhamnus Frangula.*

(EX-TRĂC'TŬM RHĂM'NĪ FRĂN'GŲ'LÆ.)

Extractum Frangulæ.

"Take of Rhamnus Frangula Bark, in No. 40 powder, *one pound* [av.]; Proof Spirit, Water, of each, *a sufficiency*. Mix the Rhamnus with two pints [Imp. meas.] of the Spirit, and macerate in a closed vessel for forty-eight hours; then transfer to a percolator, and when the fluid ceases to pass, continue the percolation with water until three pints [Imp. meas.] of liquor have been collected, or the Rhamnus is exhausted. Evaporate the percolated liquor by a water-bath until the extract has acquired suitable consistence." *Br.*

This is a new officinal extract in the British Pharmacopœia; it will no doubt be useful in some cases, although the bulkiness of the dose, which is given as fifteen to sixty grains (0·9–3·9 Gm.), would militate against its extended employment.

EXTRACTUM RHAMNI FRANGULÆ LIQUIDUM. *Br.* *Liquid Extract of Rhamnus Frangula.*

(EX-TRĂC'TŬM RHĂM'NĪ FRĂN'GŲ-LÆ LĬQ'UĮ-DŬM—lĭk'wę-dŭm.)

"Take of Rhamnus Frangula Bark, in coarse powder, *one pound* [av.]; Rectified Spirit *four fluidounces*; Distilled Water *a sufficiency*. Boil the Bark in three or four successive quantities of the water, until exhausted. Evaporate the liquors by the heat of a water-bath to twelve fluidounces [Imp. meas.]; when cold add the spirit, allow the mixture to remain for some hours, then filter, and make up to the volume of sixteen fluidounces [Imp. meas.] with distilled water." *Br.*

This is a new liquid extract of the British Pharmacopœia. It is questionable whether the full strength of the drug is thoroughly represented in this "preserved decoction." The dose is given as one to four fluidrachms (3·75–15 C.c.).

EXTRACTUM RHEI. *U.S., Br.* *Extract of Rhubarb.*

(EX-TRĂC'TŬM RHĒ'Ī—rē'ī.)

Extractum Rhei Alcoholicum; Extrait de Rhubarbe, *Fr.*; Rhubarber-Extrakt, *G.*

"Rhubarb, in No. 30 powder, *one hundred parts* [or sixteen ounces av.]; Alcohol, Water,* each, *a sufficient quantity*. Mix Alcohol and Water in the proportion of *three parts* [or three and a half pints] of Alcohol and *one part* [or one pint] of Water, and having moistened the powder with *forty parts* [or half a pint] of the mixture, pack it firmly in a conical percolator; then gradually pour the menstruum upon it until the tincture passes nearly tasteless. Reserve the first *one hundred parts* [or fifteen fluidounces] of the percolate, and set it aside in a warm place, until it is reduced by spontaneous evaporation to *fifty parts* [or eight ounces av.]. Evaporate the remainder of the percolate, in a porcelain vessel, by means of a water-bath, at a temperature not exceeding 70° C. (158° F.), to the consistence of syrup. Mix this with the reserved portion, and continue the evaporation until the mixture is reduced to a pilular consistence." *U. S.*

"Take of Rhubarb Root, in No. 40 powder, *one pound* [avoirdupois]; Proof Spirit, Distilled Water, of each, *a sufficiency*. Mix the Rhubarb with three pints [Imp. meas.] of the Spirit, and macerate in a closed vessel for forty-eight hours; then transfer to a percolator, and when the fluid ceases to pass, continue the percolation with water until five pints [Imp. meas.] of liquor have been collected, or the Rhubarb is exhausted. Evaporate the percolated liquor by a water-bath until the extract has acquired a suitable consistence for forming pills." *Br.*

The British extract is probably less active than the U. S. preparation, because the menstruum used to complete the former is more aqueous. Rhubarb yields all its active matter to water and alcohol; but, unless the evaporation is performed with great care and with a moderate heat, it is certain that the purgative principle is, to

* There is evidently an editorial oversight in the U. S. Pharm. 1880, in the insertion of the words after Alcohol of "*one hundred and twenty parts*," and the succeeding line, "Diluted Alcohol, *a sufficient quantity*." They have no connection with the succeeding directions.

a greater or less extent, injured or dissipated in the process; and the extract may thus become even less efficient than the root. Among other consequences which result from the boiling temperature, is the formation of a compound of the tannin and starch, which is insoluble in cold water, and upon its precipitation probably carries with it a portion of the purgative principle. There is, moreover, reason to believe that this principle is volatilizable by heat, and that a portion of it escapes with the vapor. When properly prepared, the extract has decidedly the peculiar odor of rhubarb. The dose of the extract is from five to ten grains (0·3–0·65 Gm.).

EXTRACTUM RHEI FLUIDUM. *U. S.* *Fluid Extract of Rhubarb.*

(EX-TRĂC'TUM RHĒ'Ī FLŬ'I-DŬM—rē'ī.)

Extrait liquide de Rhubarbe, *Fr.*; Flüssiges Rhubarber-Extrakt, *G.*

"Rhubarb, in No. 30 powder, *one hundred grammes* [or fifty ounces av.]; Alcohol, Water, each, *a sufficient quantity*, To make *one hundred cubic centimeters* [or three pints]. Mix *three parts* [or three and a half pints] of Alcohol with *one part* [or one pint] of Water, and, having moistened the powder with *forty grammes* [or one pint] of the mixture, pack it firmly in a conical percolator; then add enough of the menstruum to saturate the powder and leave a stratum above it. When the liquid begins to drop from the percolator, close the lower orifice, and, having closely covered the percolator, macerate for forty-eight hours. Then allow the percolation to proceed, gradually adding menstruum, until the Rhubarb is exhausted. Reserve the first *seventy-five cubic centimeters* [or thirty-six fluidounces] of the percolate, and evaporate the remainder, at a temperature not exceeding 70° C. (158° F.), to a soft extract; dissolve this in the reserved portion, and add enough menstruum to make the Fluid Extract measure *one hundred cubic centimeters* [or three pints]." *U. S.*

Although the process for the fluid extract of rhubarb of U. S. P. 1870 was an improvement on its predecessors, on the addition of water the fluid extract precipitated heavily, so that syrups or mixtures made with it were very unsightly. As the chief use of the fluid extract is in making such preparations, this is very unfortunate, and constitutes sufficient grounds for the abandonment of an officinal formula in favor of one which will exhaust the root of its purgative properties, and yet afford an extract that remains clear when water is added to it. Mr. Geo. Bille claims that all that is necessary is to exhaust the sixteen troyounces of rhubarb with cold water, evaporate, by means of a water-bath, to twelve fluidounces, and add four fluidounces of glycerin. The present process affords a fluid extract which thoroughly represents the root, but it has the same objection that the former preparation had, immiscibility with syrups and water, with loss of transparency. The dose for an adult may be twenty or thirty minims (1·25–1·9 C.c.) as a purgative, and from five to ten minims (0·3–0·6 C.c.) as a laxative.

Off. Prep. Mistura Rhei et Sodæ.

EXTRACTUM RHOIS GLABRÆ FLUIDUM. *U. S.* *Fluid Extract of Rhus Glabra.*

(EX-TRĂC'TUM RHŌ'ĬS GLĀ'BRÆ FLŬ'I-DŬM.)

Extrait liquide de Sumac, *Fr.*; Flüssiges Sumach-Extrakt, *G.*

"Rhus Glabra, in No. 40 powder, *one hundred grammes* [or fifty ounces av.]; Glycerin, *ten grammes* [or three and three-quarter fluidounces]; Diluted Alcohol, *a sufficient quantity*, To make *one hundred cubic centimeters* [or three pints]. Mix the Glycerin with *ninety grammes* [or forty-six and a half fluidounces] of Diluted Alcohol, and, having moistened the powder with *thirty-five grammes* [or eighteen fluidounces] of the mixture, pack it firmly in a cylindrical percolator; then add enough of the menstruum to saturate the powder and leave a stratum above it. When the liquid begins to drop from the percolator, close the lower orifice, and, having closely covered the percolator, macerate for forty-eight hours. Then allow the percolation to proceed, gradually adding, first, the remainder of the menstruum, and afterward, Diluted Alcohol, until the Rhus Glabra is exhausted. Reserve the first *eighty cubic centimeters* [or thirty-eight fluidounces] of the percolate, and evaporate the remainder to a soft extract; dissolve this in the reserved portion, and add enough Diluted Alcohol to make the Fluid Extract measure *one hundred cubic centimeters* [or three pints]." *U. S.*

This is a new officinal fluid extract. A formula for this preparation was proposed by Prof. J. P. Remington (*A. J. P.*, 1874, p. 7) which differs from that at present officinal, merely in containing a larger proportion of glycerin in the menstruum. Experience has shown that this is a valuable preparation of sumach berries, and is a useful addition to mouth and throat washes, gargles, etc.

EXTRACTUM ROSÆ FLUIDUM. *U. S.* *Fluid Extract of Rose.*

(ĔX-TRĂC'TŬM RŌ'ṢÆ FLŪ'Ĭ-DŬM.)

Extrait liquide de Rose rouge, *Fr.;* Flüssiges Essigrosenblätter-Extrakt, *G.*

"Red Rose, in No. 30 powder, *one hundred grammes* [or fifty ounces av.]; Glycerin, *ten grammes* [or three and three-quarter fluidounces]; Diluted Alcohol, *a sufficient quantity*, To make *one hundred cubic centimeters* [or three pints]. Mix the glycerin with *ninety grammes* [or forty-six and a half fluidounces] of Diluted Alcohol, and, having moistened the powder with *forty grammes* [or twenty fluidounces] of the mixture, pack it firmly in a cylindrical glass percolator; then add enough of the menstruum to saturate the powder and leave a stratum above it. When the liquid begins to drop from the percolator, close the lower orifice, and, having closely covered the percolator, macerate for forty-eight hours. Then allow the percolation to proceed, gradually adding, first, the remainder of the menstruum, and afterward, Diluted Alcohol, until the Red Rose is exhausted. Reserve the first *seventy-five cubic centimeters* [or thirty-six fluidounces] of the percolate, and evaporate the remainder to a soft extract; dissolve this in the reserved portion, and add enough Diluted Alcohol to make the Fluid Extract measure *one hundred cubic centimeters* [or three pints]." *U. S.*

This is another new officinal fluid extract, which will be found very useful as an adjuvant and elegant astringent. It is of a deep red color, with the agreeable flavor of rose. It may be given in the dose of one or two fluidrachms (3·75 or 7·5 C.c.).

EXTRACTUM RUBI FLUIDUM. *U. S.* *Fluid Extract of Rubus.*

(ĔX-TRĂC'TŬM RŪ'BĪ FLŪ'Ĭ-DŬM.)

Extrait liquide d'Écorce de Ronce, *Fr.;* Flüssiges Brombeerrinden-Extrakt, *G.*

"Rubus, in No. 60 powder, *one hundred grammes* [or fifty ounces av.]; Glycerin, *twenty grammes* [or seven and a half fluidounces]; Alcohol, Water, each, *a sufficient quantity*, To make *one hundred cubic centimeters* [or three pints]. Mix the Glycerin with *forty-five grammes* [or twenty-six fluidounces] of Alcohol and *thirty-five grammes* [or one pint] of Water, and, having moistened the powder with *thirty-five grammes* [or seventeen fluidounces] of the mixture, pack it firmly in a cylindrical percolator; then add enough of the menstruum to saturate the powder and leave a stratum above it. When the liquid begins to drop from the percolator, close the lower orifice, and, having closely covered the percolator, macerate for forty-eight hours. Then allow the percolation to proceed, gradually adding, first, the remainder of the menstruum, and afterward, a mixture of Alcohol and Water, made in the proportion of *nine parts* [or twenty-six fluidounces] of Alcohol to *seven parts* [or one pint] of Water, until the Rubus is exhausted. Reserve the first *seventy cubic centimeters* [or thirty-three fluidounces] of the percolate; by means of a water-bath, distil off the Alcohol from the remainder, and evaporate the residue to a soft extract; dissolve this in the reserved portion, and add enough of a mixture of Alcohol and Water, using the last-named proportions, to make the Fluid Extract measure *one hundred cubic centimeters* [or three pints]." *U. S.*

This fluid extract does not differ essentially from that formerly officinal. It is a very dark, reddish brown, translucent fluid, having the properties of the root in a marked degree. The dose is a half fluidrachm to a fluidrachm (1·9–3·75 C.c.).

Off. Prep. Syrupus Rubi.

EXTRACTUM RUMICIS FLUIDUM. *U.S.* *Fluid Extract of Rumex.*

(EX-TRĂC′TUM RŪ′MI-CĬS FLŬ′I-DŬM.)

Fluid Extract of Yellow Dock; Extrait liquide de Patience frisée, *Fr.;* Flüssiges Grindwurzel-Extrakt, *G.*

"Rumex, in No. 40 powder, *one hundred grammes* [or fifty ounces av.]; Diluted Alcohol, *a sufficient quantity,* To make *one hundred cubic centimeters* [or three pints]. Moisten the powder with *thirty-five grammes* [or eighteen fluidounces] of Diluted Alcohol, and pack it firmly in a cylindrical percolator; then add enough Diluted Alcohol to saturate the powder and leave a stratum above it. When the liquid begins to drop from the percolator, close the lower orifice, and, having closely covered the percolator, macerate for forty-eight hours. Then allow the percolation to proceed, gradually adding Diluted Alcohol, until the Rumex is exhausted. Reserve the first *eighty cubic centimeters* [or thirty-eight fluidounces] of the percolate, and evaporate the remainder to a soft extract; dissolve this in the reserved portion, and add enough Diluted Alcohol to make the Fluid Extract measure *one hundred cubic centimeters* [or three pints]." *U. S.*

A new officinal fluid extract having a dark yellowish brown color, and the peculiar odor and taste of rumex. The dose is a fluidrachm (3·75 C.c.).

EXTRACTUM SABINÆ FLUIDUM. *U.S.* *Fluid Extract of Savine.*

(EX-TRĂC′TUM SA-BĪ′NÆ FLŬ′I-DŬM.)

Extrait liquide de Sabine, *Fr.;* Flüssiges Sadebaum-Extrakt, *G.*

"Savine, in No. 40 powder, *one hundred grammes* [or fifty ounces av.]; Alcohol, *a sufficient quantity,* To make *one hundred cubic centimeters* [or three pints]. Moisten the powder with *twenty-five grammes* [or fifteen fluidounces] of Alcohol, and pack it firmly in a cylindrical percolator; then add enough Alcohol to saturate the powder and leave a stratum above it. When the liquid begins to drop from the percolator, close the lower orifice, and, having closely covered the percolator, macerate for forty-eight hours. Then allow the percolation to proceed, gradually adding Alcohol, until the Savine is exhausted. Reserve the first *ninety cubic centimeters* [or forty-three fluidounces] of the percolate, and evaporate the remainder to a soft extract; dissolve this in the reserved portion, and add enough Alcohol to make the Fluid Extract measure *one hundred cubic centimeters* [or three pints]." *U. S.*

This is identical with the fluid extract formerly officinal. It is a dark greenish black fluid, not mixing well with aqueous liquids without the use of an emulsifying agent. It is rarely given internally; the dose is three to eight minims (0·18–0·5 C.c.).

Off. Prep. Ceratum Sabinæ.

EXTRACTUM SANGUINARIÆ FLUIDUM. *U.S.* *Fluid Extract of Sanguinaria.*

(EX-TRĂC′TUM SĂN-GUI-NĀ′RI-Æ FLŬ′I-DŬM—săng-gwĭ-nā′rĭ-ē.)

Fluid Extract of Blood Root; Extrait liquide de Sanguinaire, *Fr.;* Flüssiges Blutwurzel-Extrakt, *G.*

"Sanguinaria, in No. 60 powder, *one hundred grammes* [or fifty ounces av.]; Alcohol, *a sufficient quantity,* To make *one hundred cubic centimeters* [or three pints]. Moisten the powder with *thirty grammes* [or seventeen fluidounces] of Alcohol, and pack it firmly in a cylindrical percolator; then add enough Alcohol to saturate the powder and leave a stratum above it. When the liquid begins to drop from the percolator, close the lower orifice, and, having closely covered the percolator, macerate for forty-eight hours. Then allow the percolation to proceed, gradually adding Alcohol, until the Sanguinaria is exhausted. Reserve the first *eighty-five cubic centimeters* [or forty fluidounces] of the percolate, and evaporate the remainder to a soft extract; dissolve this in the reserved portion, and add enough Alcohol to make the Fluid Extract measure *one hundred cubic centimeters* [or three pints]." *U. S.*

The liquid preparations of sanguinaria all have an unfortunate tendency to precipitate, and this new fluid extract will not prove an exception. It is of a very deep red color. The dose is three to five minims (0·18 to 0·3 C.c.).

EXTRACTUM SARSAPARILLÆ COMPOSITUM FLUIDUM.
U.S. Compound Fluid Extract of Sarsaparilla.

(EX-TRĂC'TUM SÄR-SA-PA-RĬL'LÆ COM-PŎS'I-TŬM FLŪ'I-DŬM.)

Extrait liquide de Salsepareille composé, *Fr.;* Zusammengesetztes flüssiges Sarsaparilla-Extrakt, *G.*

"Sarsaparilla, in No. 30 powder, *seventy-five grammes* [or thirty-seven and a half ounces av.]; Glycyrrhiza, in No. 30 powder, *twelve grammes* [or six ounces av.]; Sassafras Bark, in No. 30 powder, *ten grammes* [or five ounces av.]; Mezereum, in No. 30 powder, *three grammes* [or one and a half ounces av.]; Glycerin, *ten grammes* [or three and three-quarter fluidounces]; Alcohol, Water, each, *a sufficient quantity*, To make *one hundred cubic centimeters* [or three pints]. Mix the Glycerin with *thirty grammes* [or seventeen fluidounces] of Alcohol and *sixty grammes* [or thirty fluidounces] of Water, and, having moistened the mixed powders with *forty grammes* [or twenty fluidounces] of the mixture, pack it firmly in a cylindrical percolator; then add enough of the menstruum to saturate the powder and leave a stratum above it. When the liquid begins to drop from the percolator, close the lower orifice, and, having closely covered the percolator, macerate for forty-eight hours. Then allow the percolation to proceed, gradually adding, first, the remainder of the menstruum, and afterward, a mixture of Alcohol and Water, made in the proportion of *one part* [or two and a quarter pints] of Alcohol to *two parts* [or four pints] of Water, until the powder is exhausted. Reserve the first *eighty cubic centimeters* [or thirty-eight fluidounces] of the percolate, and evaporate the remainder to a soft extract; dissolve this in the reserved portion, and add enough of a mixture of Alcohol and Water, using the last-named proportions, to make the Fluid Extract measure *one hundred cubic centimeters* [or three pints]." *U. S.*

Everything depends in the process upon having the several ingredients equably powdered, mixing them well and duly moistening them, and then packing them properly in the percolator. The moistening of the mixed powders is more easily effected, as they are less disposed to form lumps than is the sarsaparilla powder alone. The preparation is intended to represent, in a concentrated state, the compound decoction of sarsaparilla, having all its ingredients with the exception of the guaiacum wood, which probably adds little to the efficacy of the decoction. It was originally proposed by Wm. Hodgson, Jr. (*Journ. of the Phila. Col. of Pharm.*, ii. 285); and the officinal process differs from his mainly in the omission of the guaiacum wood, the resin of which, separating during the evaporation, somewhat embarrassed the process, without adding to the virtues of the extract. The dose is from thirty minims to a fluidrachm (1·9–3·75 C.c.), three or four times a day.

EXTRACTUM SARSAPARILLÆ FLUIDUM. *U.S. Fluid Extract of Sarsaparilla.*

(EX-TRĂC'TUM SÄR-SA-PA-RĬL'LÆ FLŪ'I-DŬM.)

Extractum Sarsæ Liquidum, *Br.;* Liquid Extract of Sarsaparilla; Liquor Sarsæ; Extrait liquide de Salsepareille, *Fr.;* Flüssiges Sarsaparilla-Extrakt, *G.*

"Sarsaparilla, in No. 30 powder, *one hundred grammes* [or fifty ounces av.]; Glycerin, *ten grammes* [or three and three-quarter fluidounces]; Alcohol, Water, each, *a sufficient quantity*, To make *one hundred cubic centimeters* [or three pints]. Mix the Glycerin with *thirty grammes* [or seventeen fluidounces] of Alcohol and *sixty grammes* [or thirty fluidounces] of Water, and, having moistened the powder with *forty grammes* [or twenty fluidounces] of the mixture, pack it firmly in a cylindrical percolator; then add enough of the menstruum to saturate the powder and leave a stratum above it. When the liquid begins to drop from the percolator, close the lower orifice, and, having closely covered the percolator, macerate for forty-eight hours. Then allow the percolation to proceed, gradually adding, first, the remainder of the menstruum, and afterward, a mixture of Alcohol and Water, made in the proportion of *one part* [or two and a quarter pints] of Alcohol to *two parts* [or four pints] of Water, until the Sarsaparilla is exhausted. Reserve the first *eighty cubic centimeters* [or thirty-eight fluidounces] of the percolate, and evaporate the remainder to a soft extract; dissolve this in the reserved portion, and add enough of a mixture of Alcohol and Water, using the last-named proportions, to make the Fluid Extract measure *one hundred cubic centimeters* [or three pints]." *U. S.*

"Take of Jamaica Sarsaparilla, in No. 40 powder, *forty ounces* [av.]; Proof Spirit *two pints* [Imp. meas.]; Sugar *five ounces* [av.]; Distilled Water *twelve pints* [Imp. meas.]. Mix the Sarsaparilla with the Spirit, and macerate in a closed vessel for ten days; then press out twenty fluidounces [Imp. meas.] of liquor, and set this aside. Mix the pressed residue with the water, and macerate at 160° F. (71°·1 C.) for sixteen hours, then strain and press out the liquid, dissolve the sugar in this and evaporate in a water-bath to about eighteen fluidounces [Imp. meas.]. Mix the two liquids, and make up the volume to forty fluidounces [Imp. meas.], by the addition of distilled water." *Br.*

Of these two processes, that of the U. S. Pharmacopœia, except in respect to the high price of alcohol, is greatly preferable; and this objection will be in great measure obviated by recovering the alcohol, which can be done by using a distillatory apparatus in the evaporation. There can be no doubt that Sarsaparilla is more thoroughly exhausted when submitted, in the state of powder, to percolation with a mixture of diluted alcohol and glycerin, than it can be by maceration and subsequent digestion of the whole root in water, even though continued for twelve hours. The non-use of heat in the U. S. process is also a great advantage; and the glycerin is preferable as a preservative to alcohol alone. There is some difficulty in properly mixing the powder with the menstruum, as it is apt to agglutinate in lumps; but this can be obviated by suitable manipulation, and a uniformly moistened mass obtained. The introduction of a simple fluid extract of sarsaparilla into our Pharmacopœia was judicious; as it enables the physician to associate this medicine with others at his pleasure, and in such proportions as he may deem expedient. He may rely upon the efficiency of the preparation, if made with sufficient care and skill, and from good parcels of the root. The U. S. fluid extract is a somewhat thickish, scarcely translucent liquid, of a very dark reddish brown color, and of a sweetish and a slightly, though persistently, acrid taste. The dose is from thirty to sixty minims (1·9–3·75 C.c.), equivalent to the same number of grains of sarsaparilla in substance. The dose of the British preparation is stated in the Pharmacopœia to be from two to four fluidrachms (7·5–15 C.c.).

EXTRACTUM SCILLÆ FLUIDUM. *U. S.* *Fluid Extract of Squill.*

(ĔX-TRĂC'TŬM SCĬL'LÆ FLŪ'Ĭ-DŬM—sĭl'lē.)

Extrait liquide de Scille, *Fr.*; Flüssiges Meerzwiebel-Extrakt, *G.*

"Squill, in No. 20 powder, *one hundred grammes* [or fifty ounces av.]; Alcohol, *a sufficient quantity*, To make *one hundred cubic centimeters* [or three pints]. Moisten the powder with *twenty grammes* [or twelve fluidounces] of Alcohol, and pack it in a cylindrical percolator; then add enough Alcohol to saturate the powder and leave a stratum above it. When the liquid begins to drop from the percolator, close the lower orifice, and, having closely covered the percolator, macerate for forty-eight hours. Then allow the percolation to proceed, gradually adding Alcohol, until the Squill is exhausted. Reserve the first *seventy-five cubic centimeters* [or thirty-six fluidounces] of the percolate, and evaporate the remainder to a soft extract; dissolve this in the reserved portion, and add enough Alcohol to make the Fluid Extract measure *one hundred cubic centimeters* [or three pints]." *U. S.*

This fluid extract differs from the one formerly officinal in containing no glycerin in the menstruum. It is a beautifully clear dark red liquid, which is especially useful for combining with stimulant expectorants, such as carbonate of ammonium, which are incompatible with the officinal syrup of squill. Prof. J. U. Lloyd recommends diluted acetic acid for a menstruum, and that this fluid extract should be made half strength,—*i.e.*, 2 C.c. represent 1 Gm. (See *Am. Drug.*, 1886, p. 202.) The dose of the officinal fluid extract as an expectorant is two to three minims (0·12 to 0·18 C.c.).

EXTRACTUM SCUTELLARIÆ FLUIDUM. *U.S.* *Fluid Extract of Scutellaria.*

(ĔX-TRĂC'TŬM SCŪ-TĔL-LĀ'RĪ-Æ FLŪ'Ĭ-DŬM.)

Fluid Extract of Skullcap; Extrait liquide de Scutellaire, *Fr.;* Flüssiges Helmkraut-Extrakt, *G.*

"Scutellaria, in No. 40 powder, *one hundred grammes* [or fifty ounces av.]; Alcohol, Water, each, *a sufficient quantity,* To make *one hundred cubic centimeters* [or three pints]. Mix *one part* [or two and a quarter pints] of Alcohol with *two parts* [or four pints] of Water, and, having moistened the powder with *thirty-five grammes* [or one pint] of the mixture, pack it firmly in a cylindrical percolator; then add enough of the menstruum to saturate the powder and leave a stratum above it. When the liquid begins to drop from the percolator, close the lower orifice, and, having closely covered the percolator, macerate for forty-eight hours. Then allow the percolation to proceed, gradually adding menstruum, until the Scutellaria is exhausted. Reserve the first *eighty cubic centimeters* [or thirty-eight fluidounces] of the percolate, and evaporate the remainder to a soft extract; dissolve this in the reserved portion, and add enough menstruum to make the Fluid Extract measure *one hundred cubic centimeters* [or three pints]." *U.S.*

A new fluid extract in the Pharmacopœia, but thoroughly representing the activity of Scutellaria. It is of a dark greenish brown color, and is given in the dose of one-half to one fluidrachm (1·9 to 3·75 C.c.).

EXTRACTUM SENEGÆ FLUIDUM. *U.S.* *Fluid Extract of Senega.*

(ĔX-TRĂC'TŬM SĔN'Ĕ-GÆ FLŪ'Ĭ-DŬM.)

Extrait liquide de Polygale de Virginie, Extrait liquide de Sénéca, *Fr;* Flüssiges Senega-Extrakt, *G.*

"Senega, in No. 40 powder, *one hundred grammes* [or fifty ounces av.]; Water of Ammonia, *two grammes* [or one fluidounce]; Alcohol, Water, each, *a sufficient quantity,* To make *one hundred cubic centimeters* [or three pints]. Mix *two parts* [or four and a half pints] of Alcohol with *one part* [or two pints] of Water, and, having moistened the powder with *forty-five grammes* [or twenty-six fluidounces] of the mixture, pack it firmly in a cylindrical percolator; then add enough of the menstruum to saturate the powder and leave a stratum above it. When the liquid begins to drop from the percolator, close the lower orifice, and, having closely covered the percolator, macerate for forty-eight hours. Then allow the percolation to proceed, gradually adding menstruum, until the Senega is exhausted. Reserve the first *eighty-five cubic centimeters* [or forty fluidounces] of the percolate, and evaporate the remainder to a soft extract; dissolve this in the reserved portion, and add, first, the Water of Ammonia, and afterward, enough menstruum to make the Fluid Extract measure *one hundred cubic centimeters* [or three pints]." *U.S.*

Fluid Extract of Senega was very frequently the cause of annoyance to the pharmacist through gelatinization. This was due to the presence of pectinous bodies in the root. The addition of an alkali to the menstruum effectually prevents this, and in this respect the present preparation is a great improvement over the former one. It is a blackish brown moderately thin liquid, which may be used for the same purposes as the crude drug, in doses of from one to five minims (0·06–0·3 C.c.).

For other processes for this fluid extract, by Clay W. Holmes and Prof. P. W. Bedford, see *N. R.*, 1883, pp. 195, 196.

Off. Prep. Syrupus Senegæ.

EXTRACTUM SENNÆ FLUIDUM. *U.S.* *Fluid Extract of Senna.*

(ĔX-TRĂC'TŬM SĔN'NÆ FLŪ'Ĭ-DŬM.)

Extrait liquide de Séné, *Fr.;* Flüssiges Senna-Extrakt, *G.*

"Senna, in No. 30 powder, *one hundred grammes* [or fifty ounces av.]; Alcohol, Water, each, *a sufficient quantity,* To make *one hundred cubic centimeters* [or three pints]. Mix *three parts* [or three pints and six fluidounces] of Alcohol with *four parts* [or four pints] of Water, and, having moistened the powder with *forty grammes* [or twenty fluidounces] of the mixture, pack it firmly in a cylindrical percolator; then add enough of the menstruum to saturate the powder and leave a stratum above it. When the liquid begins to drop from the percolator, close the lower orifice, and, having closely covered the percolator, macerate for forty-eight hours. Then allow the percolation to proceed, gradually adding menstruum, until the Senna is exhausted. Reserve the first *eighty cubic centimeters* [or thirty-eight fluidounces] of the percolate, and evaporate the remainder to a soft extract; dissolve this in the reserved portion, and add enough menstruum to make the Fluid Extract measure *one hundred cubic centimeters* [or three pints]." *U. S.*

The officinal fluid extract of senna of 1870 differed materially from that of the Pharmacopœias of 1850 and 1860, containing neither sugar, oil of fennel, nor Hoffmann's anodyne. It was deemed better to leave to the prescriber the choice of the volatile oil, and to depend for the preservation of the fluid extract upon the glycerin and what might remain of the alcohol after the evaporation. The present officinal fluid extract is again very different from that of 1870, which contained 50 per cent. of glycerin. There is no glycerin in the menstruum now, and there really seems no occasion for its use. The fluid extract is a dark, blackish, thickish, and somewhat turbid liquid, with a strong flavor of senna. The dose is from one to four fluidrachms (3·75–15 C.c.) for an adult. In consequence of its griping tendency, it should be mixed with one of the volatile oils, as of fennel, anise, or caraway, in the proportion of about two minims (0·12 C.c.) to the fluidounce (30 C.c.). It is well adapted for exhibition with saline cathartics, such as Epsom salt or cream of tartar, which also obviate its griping. In this case not more than one-half of the full dose of the fluid extract should be given at once.

EXTRACTUM SERPENTARIÆ FLUIDUM. *U. S.* *Fluid Extract of Serpentaria.*

(EX-TRĂC'TUM SĔR-PEN-TĀ'RI-Æ FLŪ'I-DŬM.)

Fluid Extract of Virginia Snake Root; Extrait liquide de Serpentaire, *Fr.*; Flüssiges Schlangenwurz-Extrakt, *G.*

"Serpentaria, in No. 60 powder, *one hundred grammes* [or fifty ounces av.]; Alcohol, Water, each, *a sufficient quantity*, To make *one hundred cubic centimeters* [or three pints]. Mix *three parts* [or three pints and six fluidounces] of Alcohol with *one part* [or one pint] of Water, and, having moistened the powder with *thirty grammes* [or seventeen fluidounces] of the mixture, pack it firmly in a cylindrical percolator; then add enough of the menstruum to saturate the powder and leave a stratum above it. When the liquid begins to drop from the percolator, close the lower orifice, and, having closely covered the percolator, macerate for forty-eight hours. Then allow the percolation to proceed, gradually adding menstruum, until the Serpentaria is exhausted. Reserve the first *ninety cubic centimeters* [or forty-three fluidounces] of the percolate, and evaporate the remainder to a soft extract; dissolve this in the reserved portion, and add enough menstruum to make the Fluid Extract measure *one hundred cubic centimeters* [or three pints]." *U. S.*

This, though simply a concentrated tincture, is a good preparation, containing the virtues of the root within a small bulk. The fluid extract of serpentaria originated with Mr. J. C. Savery, whose formula was published in the eleventh edition of the U. S. Dispensatory (page 713). It was afterwards modified by Mr. A. B. Taylor (*A. J. P.*, xxv. 206). In the present preparation the alcoholic strength of menstruum is slightly less than that of the fluid extract of U. S. P. 1870. The fluid extract is thin, reddish brown, and transparent, with the peculiar bitterness of the root in perfection, but its odor less obviously. The dose is twenty or thirty minims (1·25 or 1·9 C.c.), to be frequently repeated.

EXTRACTUM SPIGELIÆ FLUIDUM. *U. S.* *Fluid Extract of Spigelia.*

(EX-TRĂC'TUM SPI-GĒ'LI-Æ FLŪ'I-DŬM.)

Fluid Extract of Pink Root; Extrait liquide de Spigélie, *Fr.*; Flüssiges Spigelien-Extrakt, *G.*

"Spigelia, in No. 60 powder, *one hundred grammes* [or fifty ounces av.]; Diluted Alcohol, *a sufficient quantity*, To make *one hundred cubic centimeters* [or three pints]. Moisten the powder with *thirty grammes* [or fifteen fluidounces] of Diluted

Alcohol, and pack it firmly in a cylindrical percolator; then add enough Diluted Alcohol to saturate the powder and leave a stratum above it. When the liquid begins to drop from the percolator, close the lower orifice, and, having closely covered the percolator, macerate for forty-eight hours. Then allow the percolation to proceed, gradually adding Diluted Alcohol, until the Spigelia is exhausted. Reserve the first *eighty-five cubic centimeters* [or forty fluidounces] of the percolate, and evaporate the remainder to a soft extract; dissolve this in the reserved portion, and add enough Diluted Alcohol to make the Fluid Extract measure *one hundred cubic centimeters* [or three pints]." *U. S.*

This preparation differs from that formerly officinal in having no glycerin in the menstruum; the U. S. P. 1870 fluid extract had 50 per cent.

The fluid extract of spigelia is a dark brown, translucent liquid, with the flavor of the root. The dose of it is one or two fluidrachms (3·75–7·5 C.c.) for an adult, from ten to twenty minims (0·6–1·25 C.c.) for a child two or three years old, to be repeated morning and evening for three or four days, and then followed by a brisk cathartic. It is, however, most used in connection with the fluid extract of senna; the fluid extract of spigelia and senna formerly officinal being an excellent combination, which should not have been dropped from the Pharmacopœia.*

EXTRACTUM STILLINGIÆ FLUIDUM. *U.S.* *Fluid Extract of Stillingia.*

(EX-TRĂC'TUM STIL-LĬN'GI-Æ FLŪ'I-DŬM.)

Extrait liquide de Stillingie, *Fr.;* Flüssiges Stillingia-Extrakt, *G.*

"Stillingia, in No. 40 powder, *one hundred grammes* [or fifty ounces av.]; Diluted Alcohol, *a sufficient quantity,* To make *one hundred cubic centimeters* [or three pints]. Moisten the powder with *thirty grammes* [or fifteen fluidounces] of Diluted Alcohol, and pack it firmly in a cylindrical percolator; then add enough Diluted Alcohol to saturate the powder and leave a stratum above it. When the liquid begins to drop from the percolator, close the lower orifice, and, having closely covered the percolator, macerate for forty-eight hours. Then allow the percolation to proceed, gradually adding Diluted Alcohol, until the Stillingia is exhausted. Reserve the first *eighty-five cubic centimeters* [or forty fluidounces] of the percolate, and evaporate the remainder to a soft extract; dissolve this in the reserved portion, and add enough Diluted Alcohol to make the Fluid Extract measure *one hundred cubic centimeters* [or three pints]." *U. S.*

The glycerin in the menstruum has been abandoned in the last revision of the formula for this fluid extract, which is of a dark reddish brown color: and the dose is from fifteen to forty-five minims (0·9–2·8 C.c.).

EXTRACTUM STRAMONII. *U.S., Br.* *Extract of Stramonium.*

(EX-TRĂC'TUM STRA-MŌ'NI-Ī.)

Extractum Stramonii Seminis, *U. S.* 1870; Extract of Stramonium Seed; Extrait de Semences de Stramoine, *Fr.;* Stechapfelsamen-Extrakt, *G.*

"Stramonium Seed, in No. 40 powder, *one hundred parts* [or sixteen ounces av.]; Diluted Alcohol, *a sufficient quantity.* Moisten the powder with *thirty parts* [or five fluidounces] of Diluted Alcohol, and pack it firmly in a cylindrical percolator; then add enough Diluted Alcohol to saturate the powder and leave a stratum above it. When the liquid begins to drop from the percolator, close the lower orifice, and, having closely covered the percolator, macerate for forty-eight hours. Then allow the percolation to proceed, gradually adding Diluted Alcohol, until *three hundred parts* [or three pints] of tincture are obtained, or the Stramonium Seed is exhausted.

* *Extractum Spigeliæ et Sennæ Fluidum,* U. S. 1870. *Fluid Extract of Spigelia and Senna.* "Take of Fluid Extract of Spigelia *ten fluidounces;* Fluid Extract of Senna *six fluidounces;* Oil of Anise, Oil of Caraway, each, *twenty minims.* Mix the Fluid Extracts, and dissolve the Oils in the mixture." *U. S.*

It combines the cathartic property of senna with the anthelmintic virtues of pinkroot, and is a very good vermifuge, being generally acceptable to the stomach, and not offensive to the taste. The dose is from two fluidrachms to half a fluidounce (7·5–15 C.c.) for an adult, from thirty minims to a fluidrachm (1·9–3·75 C.c.) for a child two years old.

Reserve the first *ninety parts* [or fourteen fluidounces] of the percolate, evaporate the remainder, at a temperature not exceeding 50° C. (122 F.), to *ten parts* [or two fluidounces], mix the residue with the reserved portion in a porcelain capsule, and, by means of a water-bath, evaporate, at or below the before-mentioned temperature, to a pilular consistence." *U. S.*

"Take of Stramonium Seeds, in coarse powder, *one pound* [avoirdupois]; Ether *one pint* [Imperial measure], or *a sufficiency;* Distilled Water, Proof Spirit, of each, *a sufficiency.* Shake the Ether in a bottle with half a pint of the Water, and after separation decant the Ether. Pack the Stramonium in a percolator, and free it from its oil by passing the washed Ether slowly through it. Having removed and rejected the ethereal solution, pour the Spirit over the residue of the Stramonium in the percolator and allow it to pass through slowly until the powder is exhausted. Distil off most of the Spirit from the tincture, and evaporate the residue by a water-bath until the extract has acquired a suitable consistence for forming pills." *Br.*

This preparation was omitted from the U. S. Pharmacopœia of 1860, but, in accordance with suggestions made in the U. S. Dispensatory, was reinstated at the revision of 1870. It is an excellent preparation, not only stronger, but more uniform, and therefore more to be relied on than any other officinal extract of stramonium. As the seeds yield their virtues more freely to spirit than to water alone, the Pharmacopœias have very properly adopted diluted alcohol as the menstruum. The use of the ether is to separate inert fatty matter, and consequently to make the extract stronger than when prepared according to the Br. process of 1864, in which ether was not used; and the ether is washed, in order to separate any alcohol contained in it, which might dissolve the active matter. According to the table of Reclus, sixteen ounces of the seed afford two ounces and two drachms of extract by maceration in diluted alcohol, and one ounce and a half by decoction. The dose to begin with is the quarter or half of a grain (0·016–0·03 Gm.), twice a day, to be gradually increased.

Off. Prep. Unguentum Stramonii.

EXTRACTUM STRAMONII FLUIDUM. *U. S.* *Fluid Extract of Stramonium.*

(EX-TRĂC'TUM STRA-MŌ'NI-I FLŪ'I-DŬM.)

Extrait liquide de Semences de Stramoine, *Fr.;* Flüssiges Stechapfelsamen-Extrakt, *G.*

"Stramonium Seed, in No. 40 powder, *one hundred grammes* [or fifty ounces av.]; Alcohol, Water, each, *a sufficient quantity,* To make *one hundred cubic centimeters* [or three pints]. Mix *three parts* [or three pints and six fluidounces] of Alcohol with *one part* [or one pint] of Water, and, having moistened the powder with *twenty grammes* [or twelve fluidounces] of the mixture, pack it firmly in a cylindrical percolator; then add enough of the menstruum to saturate the powder and leave a stratum above it. When the liquid begins to drop from the percolator, close the lower orifice, and, having closely covered the percolator, macerate for forty-eight hours. Then allow the percolation to proceed, gradually adding menstruum, until the Stramonium Seed is exhausted. Reserve the first *ninety cubic centimeters* [or forty-three fluidounces] of the percolate, and evaporate the remainder, at a temperature not exceeding 50° C. (122° F.), to a soft extract; dissolve this in the reserved portion, and add enough menstruum to make the Fluid Extract measure *one hundred cubic centimeters* [or three pints]." *U. S.*

This is a new officinal fluid extract. The menstruum is well adapted for thoroughly exhausting the seed. It is of a dark brown color, and the dose is one to two minims (0·06 to 0·12 C.c.).

EXTRACTUM TARAXACI. *U. S., Br.* *Extract of Taraxacum.*

(EX-TRĂC'TUM TA-RĂX'A-CĪ.)

Extract of Dandelion; Extrait de Dent-de-Lion, *Fr.;* Löwenzahn-Extrakt, *G.*

"Fresh Taraxacum, gathered in September, *a convenient quantity;* Water, *a sufficient quantity.* Slice the Taraxacum, and bruise it in a stone mortar, sprinkling on it a little Water, until reduced to a pulp; then express and strain the juice, and evaporate it in a vacuum-apparatus, or in a shallow porcelain dish, by means of a water-bath, to a pilular consistence." *U. S.*

"Take of Fresh Dandelion Root *four pounds* [avoirdupois]. Crush the Root; press out the juice, and allow it to deposit; heat the clear liquor to 212° F. (100° C.), and maintain the temperature for ten minutes; then strain, and evaporate by a water-bath, at a temperature not exceeding 160° F. (71°·1 C.), until the extract has acquired a suitable consistence for forming pills." *Br.*

This extract is undoubtedly stronger, prepared from the root alone than from the whole plant. It is important that the root should be collected at the right season. The juice expressed from it in the spring is thin, watery, and of a feeble flavor; in the latter part of the summer, and in autumn, thick, opaque, cream-colored, very bitter, and abundant, amounting to one-third or one-half its weight. It may be collected in August, and afterwards until severe frost. According to Mr. Squire, frost has the effect of diminishing the bitterness and increasing the sweetness of the root. An extract prepared by inspissating the juice, as in the present U. S. and Br. processes, is much more efficient than that prepared in the old way by decoction. The inspissation should be effected by exposing the juice in shallow vessels to a current of warm dry air, or by evaporation in a vacuum, and should not be unnecessarily protracted. Long exposure, during evaporation, changes the bitterness of the juice into sweetness, which is a sign of inferiority. In the British process, it is wisely directed that, before the evaporation of the juice, it shall be exposed for a short time to a heat sufficient to coagulate the albumen, which is then separated and rejected as useless, and indeed injurious by favoring decomposition. As often found in the shops, the extract is dark-colored, sweet, and in all probability nearly inert. Mr. Houlton took more than an ounce of it in a day, without any sensible effect. (*P. J. Tr.*, i. 421.) When prepared from the root and leaves together, it has a greenish color. Mr. Brande states that one cwt. of the fresh root affords from twenty to twenty-five pounds of extract by decoction in water. The expressed juice yields from 11 to 25 per cent. of extract, the greatest product being obtained in November, and the least in April and May. This extract deteriorates by keeping, and should, therefore, be renewed annually. It is conveniently given in an aromatic water. The dose is from a scruple to a drachm (1·3–3·95 Gm.) three times a day.

EXTRACTUM TARAXACI FLUIDUM. *U. S.* *Fluid Extract of Taraxacum.*

(EX-TRĂC'TŬM TA-RĂX'A-CĪ FLŪ'I-DŬM.)

Extractum Taraxaci Liquidum, *Br.;* Liquid Extract of Dandelion; Fluid Extract of Dandelion; Extrait liquide de Pissenlit, *Fr.;* Flüssiges Löwenzahn Extrakt, *G.*

"Taraxacum, in No. 30 powder, *one hundred grammes* [or fifty ounces av.]; Alcohol, Water, each, *a sufficient quantity*, To make *one hundred cubic centimeters* [or three pints]. Mix *two parts* [or four and a half pints] of Alcohol with *three parts* [or six pints] of Water, and, having moistened the powder with *thirty grammes* [or seventeen fluidounces] of the mixture, pack it firmly in a cylindrical percolator; then add enough of the menstruum to saturate the powder and leave a stratum above it. When the liquid begins to drop from the percolator, close the lower orifice, and, having closely covered the percolator, macerate for forty-eight hours. Then allow the percolation to proceed, gradully adding menstruum, until the Taraxacum is exhausted. Reserve the first *eighty-five cubic centimeters* [or forty fluidounces] of the percolate; by means of a water-bath, distil off the Alcohol from the remainder, and evaporate the residue to a soft extract; dissolve this in the reserved portion, and add enough menstruum to make the Fluid Extract measure *one hundred cubic centimeters* [or three pints]." *U. S.*

"Take of Dry Dandelion Root, in No. 20 powder, *forty ounces* [av.]; Proof Spirit *four pints* [Imp. meas.]; Distilled Water *a sufficiency*. Mix the Dandelion with the Spirit, and macerate in a closed vessel for forty-eight hours; then press out twenty fluidounces [Imp. meas.] of liquid, and set this aside. Mix the pressed residue with the water, and again macerate for forty-eight hours; press out and strain the liquid;

evaporate this by a water-bath to about eighteen fluidounces [Imp. meas.]. Mix the two liquids, and make up the volume to forty fluidounces [Imp. meas.] by the addition of distilled water." *Br.*

The activity of this preparation depends more upon the proper selection of the root than anything else. The process of exhausting the drug is not difficult, and one of the best tests of this fluid extract is its bitter taste. It is a blackish, moderately thick liquid, which may be given in doses of from one to three fluidrachms (3·75–11·25 C.c.). It is said to be an excellent vehicle for quinine.

EXTRACTUM TRITICI FLUIDUM. *U. S.* *Fluid Extract of Triticum.*

(EX-TRĂC'TUM TRĬT'I-CĪ FLŪ'I-DŬM.)

Fluid Extract of Couch-grass Root; Extrait liquide de petit Chiendent, *Fr.;* Flüssiges Queckenwurzel-Extrakt, *G.*

"Triticum, finely cut, *one hundred grammes* [or fifty ounces av.]; Alcohol, Water, each, *a sufficient quantity*, To make *one hundred cubic centimeters* [or three pints]. Pack the Triticum in a cylindrical percolator, and pour Boiling Water upon it until it is exhausted. Evaporate the percolate to *eighty cubic centimeters* [or thirty-eight fluidounces], and, having added to it *twenty cubic centimeters* [or ten fluidounces] of Alcohol, mix well and set it aside for forty-eight hours. Then filter the liquid and add to the filtrate enough of a mixture composed of *four parts* [or four fluidounces] of Water and *one part* [or one and one-eighth fluidounces] of Alcohol to make the Fluid Extract measure *one hundred cubic centimeters* [or three pints]." *U.S.*

This is a new officinal fluid extract, and it is a valuable preparation. The German Pharmacopœia directs an *Extractum Graminis*, made by digesting 1 part of Triticum with 6 parts of hot water, for six hours, straining, evaporating to a syrup; mixing 1 part of this extract with 4 parts of cold distilled water, filtering, and evaporating to an extract. The fluid extract is preferable, as the excessive use of heat is avoided. The dose is from three to six fluidrachms (11·25–22·5 C.c.).

EXTRACTUM UVÆ URSI FLUIDUM. *U. S.* *Fluid Extract of Uva Ursi.*

(EX-TRĂC'TUM Ū'VÆ ŪR'SĪ FLŪ'I-DŬM.)

Extrait liquide de Busserole, *Fr.;* Flüssiges Bärentraubenblätter-Extrakt, *G.*

"Uva Ursi, in No. 30 powder, *one hundred grammes* [or fifty ounces av.]; Glycerin, *ten grammes* [or three and three-quarter fluidounces]; Diluted Alcohol, *a sufficient quantity*, To make *one hundred cubic centimeters* [or three pints]. Mix the Glycerin with *ninety grammes* [or forty-six fluidounces] of Diluted Alcohol, and, having moistened the powder with *thirty-five grammes* [or eighteen fluidounces] of the mixture, pack it firmly in a cylindrical percolator; then add enough of the menstruum to saturate the powder and leave a stratum above it. When the liquid begins to drop from the percolator, close the lower orifice, and, having closely covered the percolator, macerate for forty-eight hours. Then allow the percolation to proceed, gradually adding, first, the remainder of the menstruum, and afterward, Diluted Alcohol, until the Uva Ursi is exhausted. Reserve the first *seventy cubic centimeters* [or thirty-three fluidounces] of the percolate, and evaporate the remainder to a soft extract; dissolve this in the reserved portion, and add enough Diluted Alcohol to make the Fluid Extract measure *one hundred cubic centimeters* [or three pints]." *U.S.*

This preparation has been improved by diminishing the glycerin. It is a thickish, black liquid, of a sweet, bitterish, astringent, but not very disagreeable taste. The dose is from thirty minims to a fluidrachm (1·9–3·75 C.c.), three times a day.

EXTRACTUM VALERIANÆ FLUIDUM. *U. S.* *Fluid Extract of Valerian.*

(EX-TRĂC'TUM VA-LĒ-RI-Ā'NÆ FLŪ'I-DŬM.)

Extrait liquide de Valériane, *Fr.;* Flüssiges Baldrian-Extrakt, *G.*

"Valerian, in No. 60 powder, *one hundred grammes* [or fifty ounces av.]; Alcohol, Water, each, *a sufficient quantity*, To make *one hundred cubic centimeters* [or three pints]. Mix *two parts* [or four and a half pints] of Alcohol with *one part* [or two pints] of Water, and, having moistened the powder with *thirty grammes* [or seventeen fluidounces] of the mixture, pack it firmly in a cylindrical percolator; then add enough of the menstruum to saturate the powder and leave a stratum above it. When the liquid begins to drop from the percolator, close the lower orifice, and, having closely covered the percolator, macerate for forty-eight hours. Then allow the percolation to proceed, gradually adding menstruum, until the Valerian is exhausted. Reserve the first *eighty-five cubic centimeters* [or forty fluidounces] of the percolate, and evaporate the remainder to a soft extract; dissolve this in the reserved portion, and add enough menstruum to make the Fluid Extract measure *one hundred cubic centimeters* [or three pints]." *U. S.*

This is a concentrated tincture, strong both in alcohol and the virtues of valerian. It is probable that all or nearly all the volatile ingredients of the root are extracted by the reserved portion which first passes, and which, not being exposed to evaporation, loses none of the volatile oil and acid that have been dissolved; while the soluble matter subsequently extracted, consisting chiefly of the fixed principles, will not be dissipated by the concentration ordered. The fluid extract may, therefore, be considered as fully representing the virtues of the root. The formula is, with some modification, that of Prof. Grahame (*A. J. P.*, xxi. 379). The preparation is a dark brownish red liquid, transparent in thin layers, with the smell and taste of valerian. The dose is about a fluidrachm (3·75 C.c.).

EXTRACTUM VERATRI VIRIDIS FLUIDUM. *U. S.* *Fluid Extract of Veratrum Viride.*

(EX-TRĂC'TUM VE-RĀ'TRĪ VĬR'I-DĬS FLŪ'I-DŬM.)

Extrait liquide de Vératre américain, *Fr.;* Flüssiges Grüngermerwurz-Extrakt, *G.*

"Veratrum Viride, in No. 60 powder, *one hundred grammes* [or fifty ounces av.]; Alcohol, *a sufficient quantity*, To make *one hundred cubic centimeters* [or three pints]. Moisten the powder with *thirty grammes* [or seventeen fluidounces] of Alcohol, and pack it firmly in a cylindrical percolator; then add enough Alcohol to saturate the powder and leave a stratum above it. When the liquid begins to drop from the percolator, close the lower orifice, and, having closely covered the percolator, macerate for forty-eight hours. Then allow the percolation to proceed, gradually adding Alcohol, until the Veratrum Viride is exhausted. Reserve the first *ninety cubic centimeters* [or forty-three fluidounces] of the percolate, and evaporate the remainder to a soft extract; dissolve this in the reserved portion, and add enough Alcohol to make the Fluid Extract measure *one hundred cubic centimeters* [or three pints]." *U. S.*

It may be doubted whether this fluid extract is among those demanded by the wants of the profession. We have already a tincture, which, supposing none of the virtues of the medicine to be lost in preparing the fluid extract, will be at least half as strong, and at all events is quite strong enough. It is true that the proportion of alcohol is somewhat less in the fluid extract; but, in so powerful a preparation, this is of little consequence. The tincture itself purports to be saturated; and, though it is probable that, by the concentration of the alcoholic solution, more of the active matter is held by it in the same measure of alcohol than by the tincture, the necessity of multiplying the number of preparations of a powerful drug where the dose is small is not apparent. It would be injudicious to prescribe more of it, as a commencing dose, than from one to two minims (0·06–0·12 C.c.).

EXTRACTUM VIBURNI FLUIDUM. *U. S.* *Fluid Extract of Viburnum.*

(EX-TRĂC'TUM VI-BŬR'NĪ FLŪ'I-DŬM.)

Fluid Extract of Black Haw: Extrait liquide de Viburné, *Fr.*

"Viburnum, in No. 60 powder, *one hundred grammes* [or fifty ounces av.]; Alcohol, Water, each, *a sufficient quantity*, To make *one hundred cubic centimeters* [or three pints]. Mix *two parts* [or four and a half pints] of Alcohol with *one part* [or two pints] of Water, and, having moistened the powder with *thirty grammes* [or seventeen fluidounces] of the mixture, pack it moderately in a cylindrical percolator; then add enough of the menstruum to saturate the powder and leave a stratum above it. When the liquid begins to drop from the percolator, close the lower orifice, and, having closely covered the percolator, macerate for forty-eight hours. Then allow the percolation to proceed, gradually adding menstruum, until the Viburnum is exhausted. Reserve the first *eighty-five cubic centimeters* [or forty fluidounces] of the percolate, and evaporate the remainder to a soft extract; dissolve this in the reserved portion, and add enough menstruum to make the Fluid Extract measure *one hundred cubic centimeters* [or three pints]." *U. S.*

This is a new officinal fluid extract, which well represents the drug. It is of a dark reddish brown color. The dose is one-half to one fluidrachm (1·9–3·75 C.c.).

EXTRACTUM XANTHOXYLI FLUIDUM. *U. S.* *Fluid Extract of Xanthoxylum.*

(EX-TRĂC'TUM XAN-THŎX'Y-LĪ FLŪ'I-DŬM—zan-thŏk'se-lī.)

Fluid Extract of Prickly Ash; Extrait liquide de Frêne épineux, *Fr.*; Flüssiges Zahnwehholz-Extrakt, *G.*

"Xanthoxylum, in No. 40 powder, *one hundred grammes* [or fifty ounces av.]; Alcohol, *a sufficient quantity*, To make *one hundred cubic centimeters* [or three pints]. Moisten the powder with *twenty-five grammes* [or fourteen fluidounces] of Alcohol, and pack it firmly in a cylindrical percolator; then add enough Alcohol to saturate the powder and leave a stratum above it. When the liquid begins to drop from the percolator, close the lower orifice, and, having closely covered the percolator, macerate for forty-eight hours. Then allow the percolation to proceed, gradually adding Alcohol, until the Xanthoxylum is exhausted. Reserve the first *ninety cubic centimeters* [or forty-three fluidounces] of the percolate, and evaporate the remainder to a soft extract; dissolve this in the reserved portion, and add enough Alcohol to make the Fluid Extract measure *one hundred cubic centimeters* [or three pints]." *U. S.*

This new officinal fluid extract thoroughly represents the virtues of the drug. The dose is one-half to one fluidrachm (1·9–3·75 C.c.).

EXTRACTUM ZINGIBERIS FLUIDUM. *U. S.* *Fluid Extract of Ginger.*

(EX-TRĂC'TUM ZIN-ǦIB'E-RĬS FLŪ'I-DŬM.)

Extrait liquide de Gingembre, *Fr.*; Flüssiges Ingwer-Extrakt, *G.*

"Ginger, in No. 40 powder, *one hundred grammes* [or fifty ounces av.]; Alcohol, *a sufficient quantity*, To make *one hundred cubic centimeters* [or three pints]. Moisten the powder with *twenty-five grammes* [or fourteen fluidounces] of Alcohol, and pack it firmly in a cylindrical percolator; then add enough Alcohol to saturate the powder and leave a stratum above it. When the liquid begins to drop from the percolator, close the lower orifice, and, having closely covered the percolator, macerate for forty-eight hours. Then allow the percolation to proceed, gradually adding Alcohol, until the Ginger is exhausted. Reserve the first *ninety cubic centimeters* [or forty-three fluidounces] of the percolate, and evaporate the remainder to a soft extract; dissolve this in the reserved portion, and add enough Alcohol to make the Fluid Extract measure *one hundred cubic centimeters* [or three pints]." *U. S.*

The fluid extract of ginger is a highly concentrated alcoholic solution of the active principles of ginger. It is transparent, and of a reddish color. The dose is from ten to twenty minims (0·6–1·25 C.c.).

Off. Prep. Syrupus Zingiberis, *U. S.*

FARINA TRITICI. *Br.* *Wheaten Flour.*

(FA-RĪ'NA TRĬT'I-CĪ.)

Wheat Flour; Farine de Froment, *Fr.*; Weizenmehl, *G.*; Farina di Frumento, *It.*; Flor del Trigo, Acemite, *Sp.*

"The grain of wheat, Triticum sativum, ground and sifted." *Br.* *Nat. Ord.* Graminaceæ.

Gen. Ch. *Calyx* two-valved, solitary, transverse, many-flowered, on a flexuose, toothed receptacle. *Rees's Cyclopædia.*

Triticum hybernum. Willd. *Sp. Plant.* i. 477.—*T. vulgare*, var. *β. hybernum.* Kunth, *Gramin.* 438. The *common winter wheat* has a fibrous root and one or more erect, round, smooth, jointed, stems, which rise from three to five feet in height, and are furnished with linear, pointed, entire, flat, many-ribbed, rough, somewhat glaucous leaves, and jagged bearded stipules. The flowers are in a solitary, terminal, dense, smooth spike, two or three inches long. The calyx is four-flowered, tumid, imbricated, abrupt, with a short compressed point. In the upper part of the spike it is more elongated; and in this situation the corolla is more or less awned. The grain is imbricated in four rows.

The native country of wheat is unknown; but its cultivation is supposed to have spread from Sicily over Europe. It is now an object of culture in almost all countries having a temperate climate. Sown in the autumn, it stands the winter, and ripens its seeds in the following summer. Numerous varieties have been produced by cultivation, some of which are usually described as distinct species. Among these may perhaps be ranked *T. æstivum*, or spring wheat, distinguished by its long beards, and *T. compositum*, or Egyptian wheat, by its compound spikes. The seeds are too well known to need description. They are prepared for use by grinding and sifting, by which the interior farinaceous part is separated from the husk. The former is divided according to its fineness into different portions, but so far as regards its medical relations may be considered under one head, that of *farina* or *flour.* The latter is called *bran*, and constitutes from 25 to 33 per cent.

Flour is white, inodorous, and nearly insipid. Its chief constituents are starch, gluten, albumen, saccharine matter, and gum, the proportions of which are not constant. Clifford Richardson (*Bulletin* No. 9, *U. S. Department of Agriculture*, 1886) gives as the average of 27 analyses of wheat the following composition: moisture, 9·25; ash, 1·84; oil, 2·30; sugar, 3·50; dextrine and soluble starch, 2·30; starch, 67·88; albuminoids soluble in 80 per cent. alcohol, 3·58; albuminoids insoluble in 80 per cent. alcohol, 7.45; fibre, 1·90: total, 100.* The gummy substance found in wheat flour is not precisely identical with ordinary gum; as it contains nitrogen, and does not yield mucic acid by the action of nitric acid. The starch, which is by far the most abundant ingredient, is much employed in a separate state. (See *Amylum.*) The gluten, however, is not less important; as it is to the large proportion of this principle in wheat flour that it owes its superiority over that from other grains for the preparation of bread. The gluten here alluded to is the substance first noticed as a distinct principle by Beccaria. It is the soft, viscid, fibrous mass which remains, when wheat flour, enclosed in a linen bag, is exposed to the action of a stream of water, and at the same time pressed with the fingers till the liquor comes away colorless. But this has been ascertained to consist, in fact, of two different substances. When boiled in alcohol, one portion of it is dissolved, while another remains unaffected. Einhof ascertained that the part of the glutinous mass left behind by alcohol is identical with *vegetable albumen*, while the dissolved portion only is strictly entitled to the name of *gluten*, which had been previously applied to the whole mass. As these two principles are contained in numerous vegetable products, and as they are frequently referred to in this work,

* A very elaborate investigation into the phosphates in wheat grain, as to their bases, the relative proportion of the soluble and insoluble phosphates, the relative quantity in which they exist in different parts of the grains, and other interesting points, has been made by F. Crace Calvert, and published in the *Chemical News* (Sept. 10, 1869, p. 121), to which the reader is referred. We have space for a very few only of the facts developed. One of the facts, which had been previously shown by Fresenius, is that almost the whole of the ashes of wheat consists of phosphates. Of these, nearly two-thirds are soluble in water, and are mainly phosphates of potassium and magnesium; the insoluble salts being phosphates of calcium and iron, with a little of the insoluble magnesian phosphate $Mg_3(PO_4)_2$. Another highly important fact is that by far the larger proportion of the phosphates exists in the parts separated in the sifting of the flour; and our fine white bread is, therefore, greatly deficient in one of the most essential elements of nutrition. Besides this reason for preferring brown or bran-bread to the whitest, another exists: there is a peculiar ferment, discovered by M. Mège-Mouries, in the inner cortical part of the wheat, which is rejected in the fine white flour, which rapidly changes starch into sugar, and thus greatly promotes the panary fermentation.

it is proper that they should be briefly noticed. They both contain nitrogen, and both, when left to themselves in a moist state, undergo putrefaction. From these circumstances, and from close resemblance to certain proximate animal principles in chemical habitudes and relations, they are sometimes called, in old works on chemistry, *vegeto-animal substances*. They are separated from each other by boiling the gluten of Beccaria, above referred to, with successive portions of alcohol, till the liquid, filtered while yet hot, ceases to become turbid on cooling. The proper gluten dissolves, and may be obtained by adding water to the solution, and distilling off the alcohol. Large cohering flakes float in the liquor, which, when removed, form a viscid elastic mass, consisting of the substance in question with slight impurity. The part left behind by the alcohol is coagulated albumen.

Pure *gluten*, sometimes called *vegetable fibrin*, is a pale yellow, adhesive, elastic substance, which, by drying, becomes more deeply yellow and translucent. It is almost insoluble in water, and quite insoluble in ether, and in the oils both fixed and volatile. Hot alcohol dissolves it much more readily than cold; and from its solution in boiling alcohol it separates unchanged when the liquor cools. It is soluble in the dilute acids, and in caustic alkaline solutions, in consequence of forming soluble compounds with the acids and alkalies. With the earths and metallic oxides it forms nearly insoluble compounds, which are precipitated when earthy or metallic salts are added to the solution of gluten in liquor potassæ. Corrosive sublimate precipitates it from its acid as well as alkaline solutions, and, added in solution to moist gluten, forms a compound with it, which, when dry, is hard, opaque, and incorruptible. Gluten is precipitated by infusion of galls. Its name originated in its adhesive property. It exists in most farinaceous grains, and in the seeds of some leguminous plants.

Vegetable albumen is destitute of adhesiveness, and, when dried, is opaque, and of a white, gray, or brown color. Before coagulation, it is soluble in water, but insoluble in alcohol. By heat it coagulates and becomes insoluble in water. It is dissolved by solutions of the caustic alkalies. Most of the acids, if added to its solution in excess, precipitate compounds of the acids respectively with the albumen, which, though soluble in pure water, are insoluble in that liquid when acidulated. It is not, however, precipitated by an excess of phosphoric or acetic acid. Its relations to the earthy and metallic salts are similar to those of gluten. Corrosive sublimate precipitates it from its solutions, except from those in phosphoric and acetic acids, and, when added in a state of solution to moist albumen, forms with it a hard, opaque compound. It is also precipitated by infusion of galls. This principle derived its name from its very close resemblance to animal albumen. It is associated with gluten in most of the farinaceous grains, is a constituent of all the seeds which form a milky emulsion with water, and exists in all the vegetable juices which coagulate by heat.

The mixture of vegetable fibrin and albumen which constitutes the gluten of Beccaria, exercises an important influence over starch, which, with the presence of water, and the aid of a moderate heat, it converts partly into gum and partly into sugar. The production of saccharine matter in the germination of seeds and in malting, which is an example of germination, is thus explained. The gluten becomes acid in the process, and loses the property of reacting on starch.

It is thought by many chemists that *vegetable albumen* is identical in all respects with *animal albumen*, and the *gluten* of vegetables with animal *fibrin*; and that both these principles, as well as another named *casein*, found also both in the animal and vegetable kingdoms, belong to a class of compounds termed *proteids*. *Proteids* consist of nitrogen, carbon, hydrogen, oxygen, and sulphur, and their average composition may be expressed by the empirical formula $C_{72}H_{112}N_{18}O_{22}S$.

A poisonous alkaloid has been detected by Mr. Ballaud in flour which had been kept in sacks for twelve or eighteen months. (See *P. J. Tr.*, 1885, p. 368.)

It is scarcely necessary to state that bread is formed by making flour into a paste with water, with the addition of yeast, setting it aside to ferment, and then exposing it to the heat of an oven. The fermentation excited by the yeast is accompanied with the extrication of carbonic acid gas, which, being retained by the tenacity of the gluten, forms innumerable little cells throughout the mass, and thus renders the bread light.* Alcohol is also generated during the fermentation, most of which is driven off from the bread in baking; but a small portion remains, averaging, according to Mr. Thos. Polas, 0·314 per cent. (*Chem. News*, May 30, 1873, p. 271.)

Medical Properties and Uses. Wheat flour in its unaltered state is seldom used in medicine. It is sometimes sprinkled on the skin in erysipelatous inflammation, and various itching or burning eruptions, particularly the nettlerash; though rye flour is generally preferred for this purpose.

Bread is more employed. An infusion of toasted bread in water is a nutritive drink, well adapted to febrile complaints. Within our experience, no drink has been found more grateful in such cases than this infusion, sweetened with a little sugar, and flavored by lemon-juice. Boiled with milk, bread forms a good emollient poultice, which may be improved by the addition of a little perfectly fresh lard. Slices of it steeped in lead-water, and the crumb mixed with the fluid and confined within gauze, afford convenient modes of applying this preparation to local inflammations. The crumb (*mica panis*) is, moreover, frequently used to give bulk to minute doses of very active medicines, administered in the form of pill. It should be recollected that it always contains common salt, which is incompatible with certain substances, as, for example, nitrate of silver.

Bran is sometimes used in decoction, as a demulcent in catarrhal affections and complaints of the bowels. When taken in substance, it is laxative, and may be used with advantage to prevent costiveness. Bran bread, made from the unsifted flour, is an excellent laxative article of diet in some dyspeptic cases. The action of the bran is probably mechanical, consisting in the irritation produced upon the mucous membrane of the bowels by its coarse particles. Bran also forms an excellent demulcent bath.

Off. Prep. Br. Cataplasma Fermenti.

FEL BOVIS. *U. S.* *Ox Gall.*

(FĔL BŌ'VIS.)

"The fresh gall of Bos Taurus. Linné. (*Class*, Mammalia. *Order*, Ruminantia.)" *U. S.*

Recent researches of a very thorough character have thrown more light on the subject of the constituents of gall. The most characteristic constituents of all galls of whatever origin are, first, the sodium or potassium salts of certain resinous acids known collectively as the "gall-acids," and, secondly, certain coloring matters known as "gall-pigments." The gall-acids thus far made known are *glycocholic acid*, $C_{26}H_{43}NO_6$; *taurocholic acid*, $C_{26}H_{45}NSO_7$; *hyoglycocholic acid*, $C_{27}H_{43}NO_5$; *hyotaurocholic acid*, $C_{27}H_{45}NSO_6$; and *chenotaurocholic acid*, $C_{29}H_{49}NSO_6$. Of these, the first two occur in ox gall as sodium salts, although sometimes (in green galls) the first one is absent. The bilicholic acid and bilifellinic acid of Berzelius, as well as fellic and fellinic acids, appear to have been mixtures. The solutions of these

* Clifford Richardson gives the following result of the analysis of ordinary family loaf bread: water, 37·30 per cent.; soluble albuminoids, 1·19; insoluble albuminoids, 0·35; fat, 0·60; sugar, 2·16; dextrine, 2·85; starch, 47·03; fibre, 0·85; ash, 1·17: total, 100.

Adulteration of bread. Among the adulterations of bread practised by the bakers, alum, employed to cause whiteness, and thus cover defects in the flour, is perhaps the one which has most attracted notice, and which, being sometimes noxious, it is most important to be able to test. One of the means of detection recommended, is that of incineration, by which the bread is consumed, while the alum, if there be any, is left behind. But this method is somewhat tedious; and logwood has been recommended as being at once most convenient, and, according to Mr. John Horsley, "*perfectly reliable*," if applied as he directs. The following is Mr. Horsley's method, by which in the county of Gloucester, England, alone, in the course of two surveys, he succeeded in obtaining 200 convictions out of some thousands of cases examined by him. He first makes a tincture of logwood by digesting, for 8 hours, two drachms of freshly cut chips in 5 oz. of methylated spirit and filtering; next makes a saturated solution of carbonate of ammonium in distilled water; then mixes a teaspoonful of each solution with a wineglass of water in a white-ware dish, thus forming a pink-colored liquid; and lastly immerses a portion of the suspected bread, "for five minutes or so," in the mixed fluids. If alum be present, the bread, placed on a plate to drain, will in the course of an hour or two assume a blue color; if not present, the pink color fades away. The appearance of a greenish color on drying will indicate the presence of copper. (*Chem. News*, May 17, 1872, p. 1872.) For some modifications of this method by Herz, see *Archiv d. Pharm.*, 1886, p. 676.)

gall-acids, as well as their alkaline salts, give on addition of sugar and a drop of sulphuric acid a clear and strong purplish red color (Pettenkofer's gall test). Drechsel modifies Pettenkofer's test as follows. Add to the concentrated alkaline solution of the biliary salts syrupy phosphoric acid. Next add a little cane sugar, and heat the test-tube by setting it in the neck of a flask containing boiling water. After a short heating a characteristic red or reddish violet color will make its appearance, even if only traces of biliary acids are present. (*N. R.*, 1882, p. 120.) They are also decomposed by the action of baryta water into non-nitrogenous acids and amide-compounds, as will be seen in the following reactions:

$$\underset{\text{Glycocholic acid.}}{C_{26}H_{43}NO_6} + H_2O = \underset{\text{Cholic acid.}}{C_{24}H_{40}O_5} + \underset{\text{Glycine.}}{C_2H_5NO_2}$$

$$\underset{\text{Taurocholic acid.}}{C_{26}H_{45}NO_7S} + H_2O = \underset{\text{Cholic acid.}}{C_{24}H_{40}O_5} + \underset{\text{Taurine.}}{C_2H_7NO_3S}.$$

The gall-pigments are very unstable organic coloring matters, so that their individuality cannot be said to be very thoroughly established. The recent researches of Staedeler (*Verhand. d. Naturf. Ges. in Zürich*, 8) and R. Maly (*Ann. Ch. und Pharm.*, 132, p. 129) have, however, given us a better knowledge of them. They are *bilirubin*, $C_{32}H_{36}N_4O_6$; *biliverdin*, $C_{32}H_{36}N_4O_8$; *bilifuscin*, $C_{16}H_{20}N_2O_4$ (?); and *biliprasin*, $C_{16}H_{22}N_2O_6$ (?). Of these, the first two seem to exist originally in the gall, and the others are probably derived from them. Hoppe-Seyler (*Deut. Chem. Ges. Ber.*, 7, p. 1065) has shown that the hæmoglobin and hæmatin of the blood can be changed into hydrobilirubin, a derivative of bilirubin, so that the origin of these gall-pigments seems to be clearly shown.

Ox gall contains in addition *cholesterine*, *choline*, *urea*, fats, which are the *glycerides of acetic and propionic acids*, mucus, and some inorganic salts, such as sodium and potassium chlorides, sodium, potassium, calcium, and magnesium phosphates.

The *sodium glycocholate* and *taurocholate* may be separated in the following manner. Dry ox-bile is treated with absolute alcohol, and the tincture precipitated by ether in excess. Both salts are deposited, and the glycocholate crystallizes upon standing, the taurocholate remaining in an amorphous form, resembling oily or resinous matter. They may be separated more completely by taking advantage of their different relations to the acetate and subacetate of lead. Both the acids are precipitated by the subacetate, the glycocholate only by the acetate. If the deposit above referred to be dissolved in water, solution of acetate of lead will throw down a glycocholate of lead, while the addition of the subacetate of lead to the remainder will precipitate the taurocholate. The acids may be separated from the salts of lead by sulphuric acid, and then recombined with soda.

Properties. "A brownish green or dark green, somewhat viscid liquid, having a peculiar odor, a disagreeable, bitter taste, and a neutral or faintly alkaline reaction. Sp. gr. 1·018–1·028. A mixture of 2 drops of Ox Gall and 10 C.c. of Water, when treated, first with a drop of freshly prepared solution of 1 part of sugar in 4 parts of water, and afterward with sulphuric acid, cautiously added, until the precipitate first formed is redissolved, gradually acquires a cherry-red color, changing successively to carmine, purple, and violet." *U. S.*

Off. Prep. Fel Bovis Inspissatum; Fel Bovis Purificatum.

FEL BOVIS INSPISSATUM. *U. S.* *Inspissated Ox Gall.*

(FĔL BŎ'VĬS ĬN-SPĬS-SĀ'TŬM.)

"Fresh Ox Gall, *one hundred parts* [or twenty ounces av.], To make *fifteen parts* [or three ounces av.]. Heat the Ox Gall to a temperature not exceeding 80° C. (176° F.), strain it through muslin, and evaporate the strained liquid, on a water-bath, in a porcelain capsule, to *fifteen parts* [or three ounces av.]." *U. S.*

FEL BOVIS PURIFICATUM. *U. S., Br.* *Purified Ox Gall.*

(FĔL BŎ'VĬS PŪ-RĬ-FĬ-CĀ'TŬM.)

Fel Bovinum Purificatum, *Br.;* **Fel Tauri Depuratum,** *P.G.;* **Extractum Fellis Bovini; Fiel de Bœuf purifiée,** *Fr.;* **Gereinigte Ochsengalle (Rindsgalle),** *G.*

"The purified gall of the Ox; Bos Taurus." *Br.*

"Fresh Ox Gall, *three parts* [or sixteen ounces av.]; Alcohol, *one part* [or six fluidounces]. Evaporate the Ox Gall in a porcelain capsule, on a water-bath, to *one part* [or five and a half ounces av.], then add to it the Alcohol, agitate the mixture thoroughly, and let it stand, well covered, for twenty-four hours. Decant the clear solution, filter the remainder, and, having mixed the liquids and distilled off the Alcohol, evaporate to a pilular consistence." *U. S.*

"Fresh Ox Bile *one pint* [Imp. meas.]; Rectified Spirit *a sufficiency*. Evaporate the bile to five fluidounces [Imp. meas.], and mix it with half a pint [Imp. meas.] of the spirit by agitation in a bottle, setting the mixture aside for twelve hours or until the sediment subsides. Decant the clear solution, and filter the remainder, washing the filter and contents with a little more of the spirit. Distil off most of the spirit from the mixed liquids, and evaporate the residue in a porcelain dish by the heat of a water-bath until it acquires a suitable consistence for forming pills." *Br.*

The object of this preparation is to furnish purified concentrated Ox Gall in a condition fitted for internal administration. The addition of Alcohol to the concentrated liquid is for the purpose of separating mucilaginous matter.

Properties. The U. S. Pharmacopœia describes Purified Ox Gall, and requires it to respond to the following tests. "A yellowish green, soft solid, having a peculiar odor, and a partly sweet and partly bitter taste. It is very soluble in water and in alcohol. A solution of 1 part of Purified Ox Gall in about 100 parts of water, behaves towards sugar and sulphuric acid as the solution mentioned under Ox Gall. (See *Fel Bovis.*) The aqueous solution of Purified Ox Gall should yield no precipitate on the addition of alcohol." *U. S.*

Medical Properties and Uses. Bile was formerly highly valued as a remedy in numerous complaints, and was considered peculiarly applicable to cases attended with deficient biliary secretion. It is supposed to be tonic and laxative. The dose of purified Ox Gall is from five to ten grains (0·33 to 0·65 Gm.). Dr. Bonorden has found the most extraordinary effects, in the resolution of hypertrophies, from bile applied directly to the parts affected. Hypertrophy of the mammæ and that of the tonsils are particularly mentioned as yielding with surprising facility to this application; but good may be expected from it in all cases of the affection in which the part can be reached. He employs a mixture of 3 parts of inspissated bile, 1 part of extract of conium, 2 of soda soap, and 8 of olive oil, to be rubbed on the part four times a day. He has also found advantage in similar affections of the eye, as opacity of the cornea, pannus, and staphyloma, from bile dropped into the eye, or applied by a hair pencil, several times a day. (*Med. Times and Gaz.*, Oct. 1858, p. 353.)

Refined ox gall, much used by limners and painters, is prepared, according to Gray, in the following manner. Take of "fresh ox gall, one pint; boil, skim, add one ounce of alum, and keep it on the fire for some time; to another pint, add one ounce of common salt in the same manner; keep them bottled up for three months; then decant off the clear; mix them in an equal proportion; a thick yellow coagulum is immediately formed, leaving the refined gall clear and colorless."

FERRI ARSENIAS. *Br.* *Arseniate of Iron.*

(FĚR'RĪ ĂR-SĒ'NĬ-ĂS.)

Ferrous Arseniate; Arséniate de Fer, *Fr.;* Arsensaures Eisen, *G.*

"Take of Sulphate of Iron *twenty and three-quarter ounces* [avoir.]; Arseniate of Sodium, dried at 300° F. (148°·9 C.), *fifteen and three-quarter ounces* [avoir.]; Bicarbonate of Sodium *four and a half ounces* [avoir.]; Boiling Distilled Water *a sufficiency*. Dissolve the Arseniate of Sodium in about five pints [Imp. meas.], and the Sulphate of Iron in about six pints [Imp. meas.] of the water, mix the two solutions, adding the Bicarbonate of Sodium dissolved in a little distilled water. Stir thoroughly. Collect the white precipitate which has formed on a calico filter, and wash until the washings cease to be affected by a diluted solution of chloride of barium. Squeeze the washed precipitate between folds of strong linen in a screw press, and dry it on porous bricks in a warm-air chamber the temperature of which shall not exceed 100° F. (37°·8 C.)." *Br.*

This is an officinal of the first British Pharmacopœia, which as yet is the only one that has adopted it. The washed precipitate described in the process is ferrous arseniate ($Fe_3As_2O_8$). A portion of ferrous arseniate remains dissolved in the solution. This is precipitated by the sodium bicarbonate, with the evolution of carbonic acid gas.

Arseniate of iron is white when first formed, but quickly turns green on exposure to the air during the process of washing and drying, and finally becomes a ferroso-ferric arseniate, of the probable composition, $3Fe(FeO)AsO_4.16H_2O$. It is an amorphous powder, without smell or taste, insoluble in water, but readily dissolved by hydrochloric acid. The British Pharmacopœia gives the following characters of the salt. Its solution in hydrochloric acid causes a copious light blue precipitate with ferrocyanide of potassium, and a still more abundant one, of a deeper color, with ferricyanide of potassium. A small quantity, boiled with an excess of caustic soda, and filtered, gives, when exactly neutralized by nitric acid, a brick-red precipitate on the addition of solution of nitrate of silver. The former test proves the presence both of the ferrous and ferric oxides, the latter, of arsenic acid. The solution in hydrochloric acid, when diluted, gives no precipitate with chloride of barium, showing the absence of any sulphate. "One hundred grains dissolved in an excess of sulphuric acid diluted with water continues to give a blue precipitate with ferricyanide of potassium, until at least 225 grain-measures of the volumetric solution of bichromate of potassium have been added." *Br.* This test proves that there is a due proportion of ferrous oxide present; for the bichromate of potassium oxidizes the ferrous oxide, and until this is wholly converted into ferric oxide, a blue precipitate continues to be produced, ceasing, however, when the conversion is complete.

Medical Properties. The arseniate of iron is said to unite the virtues of the two metals which enter into its composition; but the quantity of iron in any permissible dose is so small as to be nearly or quite insignificant; and the activity of the medicine is in fact due to the arsenic alone. The complaints in which it has been found efficient are those in which arsenic in other forms has proved to be a most valuable remedy; and, judging from our own observation, there is no one of them in which the common solution of arsenite of potassium will not produce all the effects that can be obtained from the arsenical preparations, with which this ought undoubtedly to be ranked rather than with the chalybeates. Should the coexistence of an anæmic state of the system with any disease requiring the use of arsenic, indicate the joint use of iron, it would be unsafe to depend on the arseniate of iron, alone. This remedy is peculiarly useful in chronic affections of the skin, especially those of a scaly character, as lepra, psoriasis, and the advanced stage of eczema and impetigo. It is useful also in lupus, and, mixed with twelve times its weight of simple cerate, may be employed externally in cancerous ulcers, though much caution is requisite. The dose is from the eighth to the tenth of a grain (0·008–0·006 Gm.), of which about one-half only is ferrous oxide; given in pill, three times a day. (See *Syrupus Ferri Arseniatis*, Part II., National Formulary.)

FERRI CARBONAS SACCHARATUS. *U.S.* *Saccharated Carbonate of Iron.* [*Saccharated Ferrous Carbonate.*]

(FĔR'RĪ CĂR-BŌ'NĂS SĂC-CHA-RĀ'TŬS.)

Ferri Carbonas Saccharata, *Br.;* Ferrum Carbonicum Saccharatum, *P.G.;* Carbonas Ferrosus Saccharatus; Saccharure de Carbonate ferreux, *Fr.;* Zuckerhaltiges Kohlensaures Eisen, *G.*

"Sulphate of Iron, *ten parts* [or five ounces av.]; Bicarbonate of Sodium, *seven parts* [or three and a half ounces av.]; Sugar, in fine powder, *sixteen parts* [or eight ounces av.]; Distilled Water, *a sufficient quantity.* Dissolve the Sulphate of Iron in *forty parts* [or twenty fluidounces] of hot Distilled Water, and the Bicarbonate of Sodium in *one hundred parts* [or three pints] of warm Distilled Water, and filter the solutions separately, and allow them to cool. Add the solution of Sulphate of Iron gradually to the solution of Bicarbonate of Sodium contained in a capacious flask, and mix thoroughly by shaking. Fill up the flask with boiling Distilled Water, and set the mixture aside for two hours. Draw off the supernatant liquid from the precipitate by means of a siphon, and then fill the flask again with hot

Distilled Water and shake it. Pour off the clear liquid and repeat the operation until the decanted liquid gives but a slight turbidity with test-solution of chloride of barium. Transfer the drained precipitate to a porcelain capsule containing the Sugar, and mix intimately; evaporate the mixture to dryness, by means of a water-bath, and reduce the product to powder. Keep the powder in small, well-stopped vials." *U. S.*

"Take of Sulphate of Iron *two ounces* [avoirdupois]; Carbonate of Ammonium *one ounce and a quarter* [avoird.]; Boiling Distilled Water *two gallons* [Imperial measure]; Refined Sugar *one ounce* [avoird.]. Dissolve the Sulphate of Iron and the Carbonate of Ammonium each in half a gallon [Imp. meas.] of the Water, and mix the two solutions with brisk stirring in a deep cylindrical vessel, which is then to be covered as accurately as possible. Set the mixture by for twenty-four hours, and from the precipitate which has subsided separate the supernatant solution by a siphon. Pour on the remainder of the Water, stir well, and, after subsidence, again remove the clear solution. Collect the resulting carbonate on a calico filter, and, having first subjected it to expression, rub it with the Sugar in a porcelain mortar. Finally dry the mixture at a temperature not exceeding 212° F. (100° C.)." *Br.*

This is a new U. S. officinal preparation; the process is identical with that of the former German Pharmacopœia. It is to be regretted that the author of the formula did not adopt the expedient of adding sugar or syrup to the solutions of the two salts, to protect the precipitate as soon as it was formed, as was recommended by Vallet. When solutions of ferrous sulphate and sodium carbonate are mixed together, there are formed, by double decomposition, sodium sulphate which remains in solution, and ferrous carbonate which falls as a pale blue precipitate. This precipitate begins immediately to alter in nature by the absorption of oxygen, and, if washed and dried in the ordinary way, becomes ferric oxide, associated with a small quantity of the ferrous carbonate, which has escaped change. As the preparations of iron containing ferrous oxide are the most esteemed, the change which this precipitate undergoes has always been a matter of regret, and various attempts have been made to prevent it. Saccharine matter has been ascertained to possess the required preservative properties; and, in the preparation under consideration, it is used to prevent the ferrous carbonate as first precipitated from passing into the ferric hydrate.

Dr. Becker, a German physician, was the first to suggest the use of saccharine matter as a means of protection against the absorption of oxygen; and the idea was carried out by Klauer, a German chemist, who first made the saccharated carbonate of iron. The use of boiling distilled water in the process is to avoid the action of the air contained in unboiled water. The washed precipitate is pressed so as to free it from water as far as possible, and then incorporated with the sugar in fine powder. The mode of treating the precipitate unnecessarily exposes it to the action of the air; and the late London method of incorporating it with the sugar immediately after washing, was on this account preferable. The final drying heat should not exceed 54·5° C. (130° F.) (See *Archiv d. Pharm.*, Jan. 1878; *N. R.*, 1878, p. 116; 1881, pp. 69, 285.)

Properties. "A greenish gray powder, gradually oxidised by contact with air, odorless, having at first a sweetish, afterward a slightly ferruginous taste, and a neutral reaction. It is only partially soluble in water; but completely soluble, with copious evolution of carbonic acid gas, in diluted hydrochloric acid, forming a clear, yellow liquid. This solution affords a blue precipitate with test-solution either of ferrocyanide or of ferricyanide of potassium, but should not be rendered more than slightly turbid by test-solution of chloride of barium (limit of sulphate). If 8 Gm. of the Saccharated Carbonate of Iron be dissolved in water with an excess of hydrochloric acid, and the solution mixed with 33 C.c. of the volumetric solution of bichromate of potassium, the mixture should still afford a blue color or precipitate with test-solution of ferricyanide of potassium (presence of at least 15 per cent. of ferrous carbonate)."* *U. S.*

* *Saccharated Oxide of Iron. Saccharum Ferrugineum.* This is a combination of sugar and ferric oxide. It is soluble and of a pure sweet taste. According to the method of Siebert, to prepare it dissolve two parts of iron in twenty-four parts of nitric acid, sp. gr. 1·2; evaporate the

Saccharated carbonate of iron is in small coherent lumps, usually of a grayish brown color, permanent in the air, having a sweet, styptic taste, and wholly and readily soluble in warm hydrochloric acid, diluted with half its volume of water, with effervescence. According to the British Pharmacopœia, it is a "carbonate of iron ($FeCO_3$, + H_2O), mixed with peroxide of iron and sugar, the carbonate (if reckoned as anhydrous) forming about one-third of the mixture." The presence of sesquioxide of iron is a defect, which is avoided in Vallet's ferruginous mass.

Its solution in dilute hydrochloric acid is but slightly affected by ferrocyanide of potassium, showing the presence of the ferric salt in only small proportion, but yields a copious blue precipitate with the ferricyanide, proving the abundance of the ferrous compound. The same solution should give but a very slight precipitate with chloride of barium, evincing that very little sulphate either of iron or of soda has escaped the washing process. "Thirty grains dissolved in excess of phosphoric acid, and diluted with water, continue to give a blue precipitate with ferricyanide of potassium until at least 287·5 grain-measures of the volumetric solution of bichromate of potassium have been added." *Br.* This test, like the present officinal one, determines the quantity of ferrous salt present, requiring the stated amount of the bichromate to convert it into the ferric chloride.

Medical Properties. This preparation is an excellent chalybeate, possessing the advantages of having nearly all the iron in it in the ferrous state, and of being readily soluble in acids. Originally introduced into the officinal list by the Edinburgh College, it appeared for the first time in the Dublin and London Pharmacopœias of 1850 and 1851. It is undoubtedly more active than the subcarbonate of iron, and must be used in a smaller dose. It is, however, inferior to Vallet's ferruginous mass, in the preparation of which the anti-oxidizing influence of saccharine matter is more fully applied. The dose of the saccharated carbonate of iron is from five to thirty grains (0·33–1·95 Gm.), given in the form of pill.

Off. Prep. Br. Pilula Ferri Carbonatis.

FERRI CHLORIDUM. *U.S.* *Chloride of Iron.* [*Ferric Chloride.*]

Fe_2Cl_6. $12H_2O$; 540·2. (FĔR'RĪ CHLŌ'RĮ-DŬM.) Fe_2Cl_3. 12HO; 270·1.

Ferrum Sesquichloratum, *P.G.;* Ferrum Muriaticum Oxydatum, Chloridum vel Chloruretum Ferricum, Ferri Perchloridum; Ferric Chloride; Perchlorure de Fer, Chlorure ferrique, *Fr.;* Eisenchlorid, *G.*

"Iron, in the form of fine wire and cut into small pieces, *fifteen parts* [or two ounces av.]; Hydrochloric Acid, *eighty-six parts* [or nine and a half fluidounces]; Nitric Acid, Distilled Water, each, *a sufficient quantity.* Put the Iron Wire into a flask capable of holding double the volume of the intended product, pour upon it *fifty-four parts* [or six fluidounces] of Hydrochloric Acid previously diluted with *twenty-five parts* [or three fluidounces] of Water, and let the mixture stand until effervescence ceases; then heat it to the boiling point, filter through paper, and, having rinsed the flask and Iron Wire with a little boiling Distilled Water, pass the rinsings through the filter. To the filtered liquid add *twenty-seven parts* [or three fluidounces] of Hydrochloric Acid, and pour the mixture slowly and gradually, in a stream, into *eight parts* [or six fluidrachms] of Nitric Acid, contained in a capacious porcelain vessel. After effervescence ceases, apply heat, by means of a sand-bath, until the liquid is free from nitrous odor; then test a small portion with freshly-prepared test-solution of ferricyanide of potassium. Should this reagent produce a blue color, add a little more Nitric Acid and evaporate off the excess. Then add the remaining *five parts* [or half a fluidounce] of Hydrochloric Acid, and enough Distilled Water to make the whole weigh *sixty parts* [or eight ounces av.], and set this aside, covered with glass, until it forms a solid, crystalline mass. Lastly, break it into pieces, and keep the fragments in a glass-stoppered bottle, protected from light." *U. S.*

filtrate to fifteen parts; when *quite cool* dissolve twelve parts of sugar in the filtrate, and add an excess of a solution of twelve parts of sugar in twelve parts of 20 per cent. water of ammonia. After setting aside for twenty-four hours, precipitate this with four or five times its volume of strong alcohol; collect the precipitate, partially dry with bibulous paper, intimately mix the moist mass with its own weight of powdered sugar, dry by a moderate heat. It is a good antidote for arsenic. (*A. J. P.*, xl. 324, 326. See also *Neues Repertor. für Pharm.*, xviii. 86.)

This formula of the U. S. Pharmacopœia has been adopted with but little alteration from that of Wittstein. (*Pract. Pharm. Chem., Darby's Transl.*, p. 265.) When iron is heated with hydrochloric acid, water is decomposed, the hydrogen escapes with effervescence, and the oxygen uniting with the iron forms ferrous oxide, which reacts with the hydrochloric acid to form water and ferrous chloride.* The next step of the process is to convert the ferrous chloride into the ferric salt. This is effected by treating it with hydrochloric and nitric acids, and heating till red fumes no longer escape. The following reaction explains this: $6FeCl_2 + 2HNO_3 + 6HCl = 3Fe_2Cl_6 + 2NO + 4H_2O$. The solution is then evaporated, and, on cooling, concretes into a crystalline mass. The relative proportions of iron and the two acids are adjusted very nearly to the production of these results. There are two crystallized hydrates, one, $Fe_2Cl_6 + 6H_2O$, which is very deliquescent, the other, $Fe_2Cl_6 + 12H_2O$, which is less so, but which, when stood over sulphuric acid, liquefies and slowly deposits crystals of the first hydrate, $Fe_2Cl_6 + 6H_2O$, losing half of its water of hydration.

Properties. It is in fragments of a crystalline structure, an orange-yellow color, inodorous, and of a strong chalybeate and styptic taste and an acid reaction. It is deliquescent, very soluble in water, and soluble also in alcohol and ether. "On ignition the salt suffers partial decomposition. The dilute aqueous solution yields a brown-red precipitate with water of ammonia, a blue one with test-solution of ferrocyanide of potassium, and a white one, insoluble in nitric acid, with test-solution of nitrate of silver. If the iron be completely precipitated from a solution of the salt by an excess of water of ammonia, the filtrate should not yield either a white or a dark colored precipitate with hydrosulphuric acid (zinc, copper), nor should it leave a fixed residue on evaporation and gentle ignition (fixed alkalies). On adding a clear crystal of ferrous sulphate to a cooled mixture of equal volumes of concentrated sulphuric acid and a moderately dilute solution of the salt, the crystal should not become colored brown, nor should there be a brownish black zone developed around it (abs. of nitric acid). A few drops of a solution of the salt, added to freshly prepared test-solution of ferricyanide of potassium, should impart to the latter a pure greenish brown color without a trace of blue (abs. of ferrous salt). A one per cent. solution of the salt in Distilled Water, when boiled in a test-tube, should remain clear (abs. of oxychloride)." *U. S.* It contains a variable proportion of water according to the crystalline forms it is made to assume, having about 40 per cent. or twelve mols. when in fine acicular crystals, and only 22 per cent. or five mols. when in the form of larger tables. (*Brande and Taylor.*) Its solution in water gives with ammonia a brown precipitate of ferric oxide, and does not yield a blue one with ferricyanide of potassium, proving the absence of ferrous chloride.†

The sesquichloride of iron is used almost exclusively in the form of tincture or liquor; and in reference to its effect and application we refer to the *Tinctura Ferri Chloridi* and *Liquor Ferri Chloridi*. As a solid, it keeps indefinitely without change. When used, it may be dissolved in water in such proportions as may be required. Six, three, two, and one and a half drachms to a fluidounce of water have been recommended; the stronger solutions being used in the treatment of varices, the weaker for injection into aneurisms, and for application to bleeding surfaces, etc. Mr. J. Z. Lawrence, of England, has used it as a styptic in a semi-deliquesced state and found it extremely efficient. He keeps it in a bottle, in which it gradually deliquesces; and, while it is in this condition, he applies the thick liquid portion, by means of a brush of spun-glass, to the bleeding surface.

* The Paris Pharmaceutical Society have adopted the following preparations of ferrous chloride, made by dissolving iron in hydrochloric acid, and evaporating the filtered solution rapidly to dryness.

Syrup of Ferrous Chloride. Dissolve 5 grammes of dry ferrous chloride in 20 grammes of orange-flower water, and add 800 grammes syrup of gum and 175 grammes syrup of orange-flower. (See, also, *Syrupus Ferri Protochloridi*, Part II., National Formulary.

Pills of Ferrous Chloride. Dry ferrous chloride, powdered marshmallow-root, each 10 grammes, mucilage sufficient. Make into 100 pills, which are to be silvered.

† *Incompatibles with Ferric Chloride.* The following list is given (*L'Union Pharmaceutique*, 1872) by M. Bouilhon. Salts of silver; mercurous salts; alkalies, their carbonates and bicarbonates; the arsenites and arseniates; borate of sodium; tannin and vegetable astringents; gums; vegetable extracts and vegetable infusions; albumen; casein.

FERRI CITRAS. *U.S.* *Citrate of Iron.* [*Ferric Citrate.*]

(FĔR'RĪ CĬ'TRĂS.)

$Fe_2(C_6H_5O_7)_2.6H_2O$; 597·8. $Fe_2O_3, C_{12}H_5O_{11}.6HO$; 298·9.

Ferrum Citricum Oxydatum, *P.G.;* Citras Ferricus; Ferric Citrate, *E.;* Citrate de Sesquioxyde de Fer, Citrate ferrique, *Fr.;* Citronensaures Eisenoxyd, Eisencitrat, *G.*

"Solution of Citrate of Iron, *a convenient quantity.* Evaporate the Solution, at a temperature not exceeding 60° C. (140° F.), to the consistence of syrup, and spread it on plates of glass, so that, when dry, the salt may be obtained in scales." *U. S.*

Properties. Citrate of iron is in "transparent, garnet-red scales, permanent in the air, odorless, having a very faint, ferruginous taste, and an acid reaction. Slowly but completely soluble in cold water, and readily so in boiling water; insoluble in alcohol. When strongly heated, the salt emits fumes having the odor of burnt sugar, and finally leaves a residue amounting to 26 per cent. of the original weight, which should not have an alkaline reaction (abs. of fixed alkalies). The aqueous solution of the salt is not precipitated, but is rendered darker by water of ammonia. If heated with solution of potassa, it affords a brown-red precipitate, without evolving any vapor of ammonia. On adding test-solution of ferrocyanide of potassium to an aqueous solution of the salt, a bluish green color or precipitate is produced, which is increased and rendered dark blue by the subsequent addition of hydrochloric acid (difference from citrate of iron and ammonium). If a solution of the salt be deprived of its iron by boiling with an excess of solution of potassa, the concentrated and cooled filtrate precipitated with test-solution of chloride of calcium, and the new filtrate heated to boiling, a white, granular precipitate will be produced." *U. S.*

Medical Properties. Citrate of iron was introduced to the notice of the profession, in 1831, by M. Béral, of Paris. It is a pleasant chalybeate, and is best given in solution. Prof. Procter found that a solution of this salt in distilled water, containing 240 grains in a fluidounce, keeps perfectly, and is very convenient for dispensing. It may be given in the dose of ten minims (0·6 C.c.), containing five grains (0·33 Gm.) of the salt, several times a day. (See *Liquor Ferri Citratis.*)

Off. Prep. Ferri et Quininæ Citras.

FERRI ET AMMONII CITRAS. *U.S., Br.* *Citrate of Iron and Ammonium.* [*Ammonio-Ferric Citrate.*]

(FĔR'RĪ ĔT AM-MŌ'NI-Ī CĬ'TRĂS.)

Ferri et Ammoniæ Citras, *Br.;* Ferrum Citricum Ammoniatum, *P.G.;* Ferri Ammonio-Citras, Ferro-Ammonium Citricum; Ammonio-Citrate of Iron, Soluble Citrate of Iron, *E.;* Citrate de Fer et d'Ammoniaque (de Fer ammoniacal), Citrate ferrique ammoniacal, *Fr.;* Citronensaures Eisenoxyd-Ammonium (Ammoniak), *G.*

"Solution of Citrate of Iron, *three parts* [or one pint]; Water of Ammonia, *one part* [or seven fluidounces]. Mix the Solution of Citrate of Iron with the Water of Ammonia, evaporate the mixture, at a temperature not exceeding 60° C. (140° F.), to the consistence of syrup, and spread it on plates of glass, so that, when dry, the salt may be obtained in scales. Keep the product in well-stopped bottles in a dark place." *U. S.*

"Take of Solution of Persulphate of Iron *ten fluidounces, or a sufficiency;* Solution of Ammonia *twenty-three fluidounces, or a sufficiency;* Citric Acid *four ounces* [avoir.]; Distilled Water *a sufficiency.* Mix sixteen fluidounces [Imp. meas.] of the Solution of Ammonia with two pints [Imp. meas.] of Distilled Water, and to this add gradually the Solution of Persulphate of Iron, previously diluted with two pints [Imp. meas.] of distilled water, stirring them constantly and briskly, and taking care that ammonia is, even finally, in slight excess as indicated by the odor. Let the mixture stand for two hours, stirring it occasionally, then put it on a calico filter, and, when the liquor has drained away, wash the precipitated ferric hydrate with distilled water until that which passes through the filter ceases to give a precipitate with chloride of barium. Dissolve the Citric Acid in four fluidounces [Imp. meas.] of Distilled Water, and having applied the heat of a water-bath, add the ferric hydrate, previously well drained, and stir them together until nearly the whole of the hydrate has dissolved, or until the citric acid is saturated with ferric hydrate (prepared, if necessary, from more of the solution of persulphate of iron). Let the solution cool, then add five and a half fluidounces [Imp. meas.] of solution of ammonia. Filter through flannel, adding some distilled water if necessary; evaporate to the consistence of syrup, the presence of a very slight excess of ammonia being maintained, and dry in thin layers on flat porcelain or glass plates at a temperature not exceeding 100° F. (37°·8 C.). Remove the dry salt in flakes, and keep it in a stoppered bottle." *Br.**

In the U. S. Pharmacopœia, the process consists simply in evaporating a mixture of solution of citrate of iron and water of ammonia. In the British, ferric hydrate is first precipitated from a solution of the ferric sulphate, then digested at a moderate heat with a solution of citric acid, and lastly neutralized by ammonia. It has, however, been found by Dr. Squibb that a heat above 82·1° C. (180° F.) acts injuriously in the preparation of the citrate of iron; and the boiling heat directed in the British Pharmacopœia of 1864 was, therefore, improper. (*A. J. P.*, xxvii. 297.) This error has been corrected in the present Br. Pharmacopœia, which directs that the salt should be dried at a heat not above 38° C. (100° F.). In the U. S. formula the citrate of iron is used already prepared, in the British it is prepared in the process. The direction as to the evaporation, at the close of the original British process, was not sufficiently explicit. The solution should be concentrated to a syrupy consistence, as ordered in the U. S. and existing British formulas, before being poured out on porcelain or glass to dry; and it is important that the heat employed in the concentration should not exceed that indicated.

Prof. J. U. Lloyd (*N. R.*, 1879, p. 323) states that it is usually difficult to adjust accurately the quantity of the ammonia in this process, and proposes to use a definite quantity of a fixed salt, like citrate of ammonium, instead. His process will be found in the foot-note.† R. Rother recommends the following method: Dissolve 272 parts of ferric citrate in three or four times its weight of water with heat, add 79 parts of ammonium carbonate, evaporate, and scale in the usual manner. (*A. J. P.*, 1887, p. 166.)

Off. Prep. Ferri et Strychninæ Citras; Liquor Ferri et Quininæ Citratis; Vinum Ferri Citratis.

Off. Prep. Br. Vinum Ferri Citratis.

Properties. Ammonio-citrate of iron is more soluble than the citrate. It is in "transparent, garnet-red scales, deliquescent on exposure to damp air, odorless, having a saline, mildly ferruginous taste, and a neutral reaction. Readily and wholly soluble in water; insoluble in alcohol. When strongly heated, the salt emits fumes having the odor of burnt sugar, and finally leaves a residue amounting to about 25 per cent. of the original weight, which should not have an alkaline reaction (abs. of fixed alkalies). The aqueous solution of the salt is not precipitated, but is rendered darker by water of ammonia. If heated with solution of potassa, it affords a brown-red precipitate, and vapor of ammonia is evolved. On adding test-solution of ferrocyanide of potassium to an aqueous solution of the salt, no blue color or precipitate is produced unless the solution is acidulated with hydrochloric acid (difference from citrate of iron). If a solution of the salt be deprived of its iron by boiling with an excess of solution of potassa, the concentrated and cooled filtrate precipitated with test-solution of chloride of calcium, and the new filtrate heated to boiling, a white, granular precipitate will be produced." *U. S.* It is almost insoluble in alcohol. It is neutral to test-paper ("feebly reddens litmus paper," *Br.*); an alkaline

* For a formula for *citrate of iron and bismuth*, see *P. J. Tr.*, 3d ser., v. 832.

† Prepare a solution of citrate of ammonium from citric acid 8 oz. av., and ammonia water q. s. Add the ammonia water to the citric acid until in slight excess, then evaporate the solution until it measures sixteen fluidounces.

Then take of solution of tersulphate of iron 16 fluidounces; citric acid 4 ounces avoir.; distilled water and ammonia water, each, a sufficient quantity; solution of citrate of ammonium 5 fluidounces. Prepare hydrated oxide of iron from the solution of tersulphate of iron. Having drained it, place in an evaporating dish and add the citric acid, warm upon a steam or water-bath, and stir until the citric acid is dissolved, then add the solution of citrate of ammonium and stir until the hydrated oxide is dissolved, filter and evaporate to the consistence of thick syrup, and spread upon glass with a brush, and dry. The yield will be 4234 grains.

solution from which the iron has been thrown down, if acidulated with hydrochloric acid in slight excess, does not yield a crystalline deposit, showing that the acid is not the tartaric. When incinerated in the air, it leaves about thirty per cent. of peroxide of iron, *Br.* Its precise chemical constitution is not determined; but Méhn (*Jahresb.*, 1873, p. 570), on evaporating a solution of ferrous citrate in ammonia to dryness, obtained a salt of the formula $Fe_2(NH_4)_7.C_6H_5O_7)_3 + 3H_2O$. This salt is a pleasant chalybeate, in doses of five grains (0·33 Gm.). According to Dr. Paris, it may be mixed with the carbonated alkalies without decomposition, and given in a state of effervescence with citric acid. It should be prescribed when the citrate of iron is desired in solution, as it is not suited for administration in the form of pills, owing to the presence of ammonia, which renders it too soluble, and causes the pills to flatten after they have been made, and frequently to cohere in one solid mass. The officinal citrate of iron should always be used for pills, as it is more slowly dissolved.

FERRI ET AMMONII SULPHAS. *U. S.* *Sulphate of Iron and Ammonium.* [*Ammonio-Ferric Sulphate. Ammonio-Ferric Alum.*]

(FĔR'RĪ ĔT ĄM-MŌ'NĮ-Ī SŬL'PHĂS.)

$Fe_2(NH_4)_2(SO_4)_4.24H_2O$; 963·8. $Fe_2O_3, 3SO_3. NH_4O, SO_3. 24HO$; 481·9.

Ferrum Sulfuricum Oxydatum Ammoniatum, *P.G.;* Ferrum Ammonio-Sulphuricum, Ferri Ammonio-Sulphas, Sulphas Ammonico-Ferricus; Sulfate de Fer et d'Ammoniaque, Sulfate de Fer (ferrique) ammoniacal, Alun de Fer ammoniacal, *Fr.;* Schwefelsaures Eisenoxyd-Ammonium, Ammoniakalischer Eisenalaun, *G.*

"Sulphate of Iron and Ammonium should be kept in well-stopped bottles." *U. S.*

The present Pharmacopœia does not give a process for preparing this salt; that of U. S. P. 1870 will be found below.*

This is an ammonia iron-alum, in which the place of the aluminium oxide (alumina) is occupied by the ferric oxide. It is prepared by heating the solution of tersulphate of iron with sulphate of ammonium until the latter salt is dissolved, and then allowing the solution to cool. The two salts unite to form the sulphate of iron and ammonium, which, being insoluble in the amount of liquid employed, crystallizes when it cools. The process is based on that of Wm. Hodgson (*A. J. P.*, 1856, p. 305).

"Ammonio-ferric alum is in octohedral crystals, of a pale violet color, and sour astringent taste, slowly efflorescent on exposure, and having a slightly acid reaction. Soluble in three parts of water at 15° C. (59° F.), and in 0·8 part of boiling water; insoluble in alcohol. When strongly heated, the crystals fuse, lose their water of crystallization, swell up, and finally leave a pale brown residue. The aqueous solution of the salt yields a blue precipitate with test-solution of ferrocyanide of potassium. With solution of potassa it affords a brown-red precipitate, and if the mixture be heated, vapor of ammonia is evolved. With test-solution of chloride of barium it produces a white precipitate insoluble in hydrochloric acid. If all the iron be precipitated from a solution of the salt by heating with an excess of solution of potassa, the resulting filtrate, when mixed and heated with test-solution of chloride of ammonium in excess, should not yield a white, gelatinous precipitate (abs. of aluminium)." *U. S.* According to H. Rose, the pure salt is white, and gives a colored solution with water, in consequence of the formation of a basic ferruginous salt. This decomposition is prevented by dissolving it in dilute sulphuric acid, when the solution is colorless.

Instead of sulphate of ammonium, sulphate of potassium may be employed with the solution of tersulphate of iron, in which case a potassa iron-alum is produced, called *potassio-ferric alum*, which has all the properties, physical and remedial, of the ammonio-ferric salt; and the two appear to have been indiscriminately used.

The iron-alums were brought to the notice of the Pharmaceutical Society of

* *Ferri et Ammonii Sulphas.* "Take of Solution of Tersulphate of Iron *two pints*; Sulphate of Ammonium *four troyounces and a half*. Heat the Solution of Tersulphate of Iron to the boiling point, add the Sulphate of Ammonium, stirring until it is dissolved, and set the liquid aside to crystallize. Wash the crystals quickly with very cold water, wrap them in bibulous paper, and dry them in the open air." *U. S.* 1870.

London, in Dec. 1853, by Mr. Lindsley Blyth, as a new remedy, prescribed in St. Mary's Hospital. Dr. Tyler Smith found them to be more astringent than common alum, and devoid of the stimulating effects of the other salts of iron. Ferric alum is certainly useful in passive leucorrhoeas, and its saturated solution has been strongly recommended as a styptic. The dose is from five to ten grains (0·33–0·65 Gm.), to be repeated twice or three times a day.

FERRI ET AMMONII TARTRAS. *U. S.* *Tartrate of Iron and Ammonium.* [*Ammonio-Ferric Tartrate.*]

(FĔR'RĪ ĔT AM-MŌ'NĮ-Ī TÄR'TRĀS.)

Ferri Ammonio-Tartras; Ammonio-Tartrate of Iron; Tartrate de Fer et d'Ammoniaque, Tartrate ferrique ammoniacal, *Fr.;* Weinsaures Eisenoxyd-Ammonium, *G.*

"Solution of Tersulphate of Iron, *ninety parts* [or thirteen fluidounces]; Tartaric Acid, *sixty parts* [or twelve ounces av.]; Water of Ammonia, *seventy-two parts* [or fourteen and a half fluidounces]; Carbonate of Ammonium, Distilled Water, Water, each, *a sufficient quantity.* To the Water of Ammonia, previously diluted with *one hundred and eighty parts* [or two and a quarter pints] of cold Water, add, constantly stirring, the Solution of Tersulphate of Iron, previously diluted with *nine hundred parts* [or ten pints] of cold Water. Pour the whole on a wet muslin strainer, allow the precipitate to drain, then return it to the vessel and mix it intimately with *one thousand parts* [or twelve pints] of cold Water. Again drain it on the strainer and repeat the operation once, or oftener, until the washings cause but a slight cloudiness with test-solution of chloride of barium. Then allow the precipitate to drain completely. Dissolve one half of the Tartaric Acid in *one hundred and thirty parts* [or one and a half pints] of Distilled Water, neutralize the solution exactly with Carbonate of Ammonium, then add the other half of the Tartaric Acid and dissolve by the application of a gentle heat. Then, while continuing the heat, which should not exceed 60° C. (140° F.), add the magma of hydrated oxide of iron, in small portions at a time, until it is no longer dissolved. Filter the solution, evaporate it, at the before-mentioned temperature, to the consistence of syrup, and spread it on plates of glass, so that, when dry, the salt may be obtained in scales. Keep the product in well-stopped bottles, in a dark place." *U. S.*

This process does not differ essentially from that of Prof. Procter. (*A. J. P.*, 1841, p. 276.) Tartrate of ammonium is prepared, which is converted into bitartrate by the addition of tartaric acid; and the excess of acid is then combined with hydrated oxide of iron freshly prepared from the officinal solution of the tersulphate. A double salt of tartrate of ammonium and iron is thus made in solution, which is obtained by filtering and concentrating the solution. The salt, theoretically, must be considered as consisting of one mol. of tartaric acid and two mol. of base, one consisting of ammonia and the other of ferric oxide, $2(FeO)NH_4C_4H_4O_6.3H_2O$. It is hardly probable that the salt has exactly this chemical composition, as the scaled salts cannot be said to be definite compounds. C. N. Lake believes that the officinal proportion of tartaric acid is excessive, and that the sixty parts should be reduced to fifty-eight parts. (*Proc. N. Y. State Pharm. Assoc.*, 1886, p. 167.)

This salt is in "transparent scales varying in color from garnet-red to yellowish brown, only slightly deliquescent, without odor, having a sweetish and slightly ferruginous taste, and a neutral reaction. Very soluble in water, but insoluble in alcohol. When strongly heated, the salt emits fumes having the odor of burnt sugar, and finally leaves a residue amounting to about 25 per cent. of the original weight, which should not have an alkaline reaction (abs. of fixed alkalies). The aqueous solution of the salt is not precipitated, but is rendered darker by water of ammonia. If heated with solution of potassa, it yields a brown-red precipitate, and vapor of ammonia is evolved. On adding test-solution of ferrocyanide of potassium to an aqueous solution of the salt, no blue color or precipitate is produced unless the solution is acidulated with hydrochloric acid. If a solution of the salt be deprived of iron, by boiling with an excess of solution of soda, the concentrated and cooled filtrate, when supersaturated with acetic acid, affords a white, crystalline precipitate." *U. S.*

It is a mild chalybeate, and may be given in a dose of from ten to thirty grains (0·65–1·95 Gm.).

FERRI ET POTASSII TARTRAS. *U. S., Br.* *Tartrate of Iron and Potassium.* [*Potassio-Ferric Tartrate.*]

(FĔR′RĪ ĔT PO-TĂS′SI-Ī TĂR′TRĂS.)

Ferrum Tartaratum, *Br.;* Tartarated Iron; Tartarus Ferratus, *P. G.;* Ferri Potassio-Tartras, Ferrum Tartarisatum, Tartras Ferrico-Potassicus, s. Potassico-Ferricus, s. Ferrico-Kalicus; Ferro-Tartrate of Potassium; Tartrate de Fer et de Potasse, Tartrate ferrico-potassique, Tartare chalybé, Tartre martial, *Fr.;* Weinsaures Eisenoxyd-Kali, Eisenweinstein, *G.*

"Solution of Tersulphate of Iron, *twelve parts* [or thirteen fluidounces]; Bitartrate of Potassium, *four parts* [or six ounces av.]; Distilled Water, *thirty-two parts* [or three pints]; Water of Ammonia, Water, each, *a sufficient quantity.* To *ten parts* [or fifteen fluidounces] of Water of Ammonia, diluted with *twenty parts* [or two pints] of cold Water, add, constantly stirring, the Solution of Tersulphate of Iron, previously diluted with *one hundred parts* [or nine pints] of cold Water. Pour the whole on a wet muslin strainer, allow the precipitate to drain, then return it to the vessel and mix it intimately with *one hundred and twenty parts* [or eleven pints] of cold Water. Again drain it on the strainer, and repeat the operation once, or oftener, until the washings produce but a slight cloudiness with test-solution of chloride of barium. Put the drained precipitate into a stone-ware or porcelain vessel, add to it *thirty-two parts* [or three pints] of Distilled Water, heat the mixture, on a water-bath, to a temperature not exceeding 60° C. (140° F.), add the Bitartrate of Potassium, and stir until the hydrated oxide of iron is dissolved. Filter while hot, and let the filtrate stand in a cool, dark place for twenty-four hours; then stir it well with a porcelain or glass spatula, so that the precipitate which has formed in it may be thoroughly incorporated with the liquid. Now add, very cautiously, just enough Water of Ammonia to dissolve the precipitate, evaporate the solution, in a porcelain vessel, to the consistence of thick syrup, and spread it on plates of glass, so that, when dry, the salt may be obtained in scales. Keep the product in well-stopped bottles, in a dark place." *U. S.*

"Take of Solution of Persulphate of Iron *six fluidounces* [Imperial measure]; Solution of Ammonia *eleven fluidounces* [Imp. meas.]; Acid Tartrate of Potassium, in powder, *two ounces* [avoirdupois]; Distilled Water *a sufficiency.* Mix the Solution of Ammonia with *three pints* [Imp. meas.] of Distilled Water, and to this add gradually the Solution of Persulphate of Iron previously diluted with two pints [Imp. meas.] of Distilled Water, stirring constantly and briskly. Let the mixture stand for two hours, stirring it occasionally, then put it on a calico filter, and, when the liquid has drained away, wash the precipitate with Distilled Water until that which passes through the filter ceases to give a precipitate with chloride of barium. Mix the washed and drained precipitate intimately with the Acid Tartrate of Potassium in a porcelain dish, and let the mixture stand for twenty-four hours; then, having applied heat, not exceeding 140° F. (60° C.), add gradually a pint [Imp. meas.] of Distilled Water, and stir constantly until nothing more will dissolve. Filter; evaporate at a temperature not exceeding 140° F. (60° C.) to the consistence of syrup, and dry it in thin layers on flat porcelain or glass plates in a drying closet at not much above 100° F. (37°·8 C.). Remove the dry salt in flakes and keep it in stoppered bottles." *Br.*

The object of these processes is to combine the excess of acid in the bitartrate of potassium with oxide of iron. In both, the plan of Soubeiran in the main is adopted; namely, that of dissolving the moist hydrated oxide to saturation in a mixture of the bitartrate and water, aided by a moderate heat. The oxide is obtained from the solution of tersulphate of iron, which is precipitated by ammonia. Potassa, which was used in the former British process, is not a good precipitant; because the alkali adheres obstinately to the precipitated oxide, and cannot be completely separated even by repeated washings. The oxide should be gradually added to the bitartrate and water, heated to 60° C. (140° F.), as recommended by Soubeiran, at which temperature the oxide dissolves more readily and in larger quantity than when a higher temperature is employed. Besides, in the latter case, a portion of the ferric oxide is converted into ferrous oxide. (*Gmelin's Handbook*, x. 315.) In the U. S. process the addition of water of ammonia to the cooled filtrate dissolves the precipitated insoluble ferric tartrate, and is in accordance with the recommendation of Prof. J. U. Lloyd (*N. R.*, 1879, p. 324), who asserts that this modification renders the salt more soluble without interfering with its stability. G. H. Chas. Klie suggested this improvement in *A. J. P.*, 1876, p. 170. (See also *N. R.*, 1878, p. 21.) In both formulas, the liquid is poured out on a plane surface, so as to dry in scales. When duly carried into effect, they yield a product at all times identical, and having all the required qualities of the salt.*

The late Dr. Ure proposed the *tartrate of iron* for medical use. He made it by acting on clean iron filings, or bits of iron wire, with a solution of tartaric acid. It is a pulverulent salt, insoluble in water, and possessing a mild chalybeate taste.

Properties. Tartrate of iron and potassium, as obtained by the above formulas, is in "transparent, garnet-red scales, only slightly deliquescent, without odor, having a sweetish, slightly ferruginous taste, and a neutral reaction. Very soluble in water, but insoluble in alcohol ["sparingly soluble in spirit," *Br.*]. When strongly heated, the salt emits fumes having the odor of burnt sugar, and finally leaves a dark brown residue, having a strongly alkaline reaction and effervescing with acids. The aqueous solution of the salt is not precipitated, but is rendered darker by water of ammonia. If heated with solution of potassa, it affords a brown-red precipitate, and a slight odor of ammonia is evolved. On adding test-solution of ferrocyanide of potassium to an aqueous solution of the salt, no blue color or precipitate is produced, unless the solution is acidulated with hydrochloric acid. If a solution of the salt be deprived of its iron by boiling with an excess of solution of soda, the concentrated and cooled filtrate, when supersaturated with acetic acid, will afford a white, crystalline precipitate." *U. S.* It has a sweetish slightly chalybeate taste. Its solution does not change the color of litmus, and at common temperatures is not precipitated by potassa, soda, or ammonia. In boiling solution, soda precipitates oxide of iron, without evolution of ammonia; and the filtered solution, acidulated with hydrochloric acid, deposits a crystalline substance when it cools; the latter test showing the presence of tartrate of potassium, the former that of the sesquioxide of iron without ammonia, and both together the character of the salt. According to the view of its nature taken in the U. S. Pharmacopœia, it is a double salt, consisting of one mol. of tartrate of iron and one of tartrate of potassium ($Fe_2(C_4H_4O_6)_3 + K_2C_4H_4O_6 + H_2O$). Flückiger (*Pharmaceutische Chemie*, 2d ed., p. 573, 1888), on the

* *Another method of preparing this salt.* M. Roger, having found the tartrate of iron and potassium, as existing in the shops of Paris, a very variable salt, seldom presenting perfect identity of composition in any two specimens, and ascribing this result to the imperfection of the prevalent mode of preparing it, which requires a large amount of water, and consequently a prolonged evaporation, resulting in the reduction of the oxide, and the production of a yellowish insoluble ferrous salt, and which is attended besides with various other inconveniences, proposes the following method, which he conceives to be free from these objections, and to present in all instances an identical product. The newly-proposed method consists in causing, as a first step, strongly hydrated oxide of iron to be dissolved in tartaric acid to complete saturation, for which purpose the water of hydration of the oxide is sufficient at a temperature of 38° C. to 49° C. (100° to 120° F.). The solution takes place completely and quickly; and the point of saturation is known when the liquid, at first clear, becomes turbid, thickens, and at last concretes in the form of a jelly. No more of the oxide, which is in slight excess, is now to be added. Upon this jelly is to be poured, little by little, a very concentrated solution of *pure* carbonate of potassium, of which the quantity to be used should be the proper molecular weight to correspond with that of the tartaric acid employed. But this precision as to the quantity of the carbonate is not absolutely necessary; as the cessation of effervescence is a sufficient criterion of saturation. Should, however, the solution, upon testing it, be found slightly acid, the solution of carbonate of potassium should be cautiously added till the liquid becomes slightly alkaline. The vessel is then to be removed from the water-bath, and the whole allowed to cool. Twelve hours afterwards, the liquid is decanted, filtered, and evaporated by means of a water-bath, with constant agitation, to a syrupy consistence. It is then to be spread by means of a brush, in thin layers, on plates of glass, which are to be placed in the drying room. The salt is thus obtained in beautiful spangles, of a deep garnet-red. Or it may be dried in moulds of tinned iron with a large surface: but in this case, instead of scales, it forms little black masses not unlike jet. Thus prepared, it always presents the same composition, dissolves in water without residue, and, besides, is little disposed to deliquescence, so that it may be readily employed in pills. The solution, however, is slow in forming, as the salt at first agglomerates at the bottom of the vessel; but in half an hour it is complete, and may be kept long unchanged. (*Journ. de Pharm.*, Juin, 1861, p. 401.)

other hand, considers the salt formed to be one in which (Fe_2O_2) is present as a bivalent group, and gives it the formula $C_4H_4O_6K_2 + C_4H_4O_6(Fe_2O_2) + 4H_2O$. "By incinerating 50 grains at a red heat, washing what is left with distilled water, and again incinerating, a residue of peroxide is obtained, weighing 15 grains." (*Br.*) The salt is incompatible with astringent vegetable infusions, which give rise to a dark-colored precipitate.

Medical Properties. Tartrate of iron and potassium is an agreeable chalybeate, and is preferred by M. Mialhe, who conceives that it is more readily absorbed than any other ferruginous preparation. It is also well borne by the stomach, whether taken fasting, or with the food. From its slight taste and ready solubility, it is one of the best ferruginous preparations for children. The dose for an adult is from ten grains to half a drachm (0·65–1·95 Gm.), given preferably in solution.

FERRI ET QUININÆ CITRAS. *U.S., Br.* *Citrate of Iron and Quinine.*

(FĔR'RĪ ĔT QUĬ-NĪ'NÆ CĪ'TRĂS—kwẹ-nī'nē.)

Ferri et Quiniæ Citras, *Br.*, 1867, *U.S.* 1870; Citrate of Iron and Quinia; Citrate de Fer et de Quinine, *Fr.*; Chininum Ferro-Citricum, *P.G.*; Citronensaures Eisen-Chinin, *G.*

"Citrate of Iron, *eighty-eight parts* [or twenty-two ounces av.]; Quinine, dried at 100° C. (212° F.), until it ceases to lose weight, *twelve parts* [or three ounces av.]; Distilled Water, *a sufficient quantity*, To make *one hundred parts* [or about twenty-five ounces av.]. Dissolve the Citrate of Iron in *one hundred and sixty parts* [or thirty-eight fluidounces] of Distilled Water, by heating on a water-bath, at a temperature not exceeding 60° C. (140° F.). To this solution add the Quinine and stir constantly until it is dissolved. Lastly, evaporate the solution, at a temperature not exceeding 60° C. (140° F.), to the consistence of syrup, and spread it on plates of glass, so that, when dry, the salt may be obtained in scales. Keep the product in well-stopped bottles, in a dark place." *U.S.*

"Take of Solution of Persulphate of Iron *four and a half fluidounces*; Sulphate of Quinine *one ounce* [avoirdupois]; Diluted Sulphuric Acid *twelve fluidrachms* [Imperial measure]; Citric Acid *three ounces and thirty grains* [avoird.]; Solution of Ammonia, Distilled Water, of each, *a sufficiency*. Mix eight fluidounces [Imp. meas.] of the Solution of Ammonia with two pints [Imp. meas.] of Distilled Water, and to this add the solution of Persulphate of Iron previously diluted with two pints of Distilled Water, stirring them constantly and briskly. Let the mixture stand for two hours, stirring it occasionally, then put it on a calico filter, and, when the liquid has drained away, wash the precipitated ferric hydrate with Distilled Water until that which passes through the filter ceases to give a precipitate with chloride of barium.

"Mix the Sulphate of Quinine with eight [fluid]ounces of Distilled Water, add the Diluted Sulphuric Acid, and when the salt is dissolved precipitate the quinine with a slight excess of Solution of Ammonia. Collect the precipitate on a filter, and wash it with a pint and a half of Distilled Water.

"Dissolve the Citric Acid in five [fluid]ounces of Distilled Water, and, having applied the heat of a water-bath, add the ferric hydrate previously well drained; stir them together, and, when the hydrate has dissolved, add the precipitated quinine, continuing the agitation until this also has dissolved. Let the solution cool, then add in small quantities at a time twelve fluidrachms of Solution of Ammonia diluted with two fluidounces of Distilled Water, stirring the solution briskly, and allowing the quinine which separates with each addition of ammonia to dissolve before the next addition is made. Filter the solution, evaporate it to the consistence of a thin syrup, then dry it in thin layers on flat porcelain or glass plates at a temperature of 100° F. (37°·8 C.). Remove the dry salt in flakes, and keep it in a stoppered bottle." *Br.*

The present process differs in several particulars from that formerly officinal; the solution of citrate of iron has been replaced by a definite weight of citrate of iron, and, instead of using freshly precipitated quinine, the moisture is driven off entirely, and the perfectly dry alkaloid is used. There has been very little gain in saving time by the change, because of the slow solubility both of the citrate of iron and quinine, and this is particularly so if the temperature is strictly adhered to. The *officinal* citrate of iron and quinine has never been very largely used, because of its slow solubility, the manufacturers supplying a salt which is readily soluble, due to the presence of ammonia. By the introduction of a solution of citrate of iron and quinine (see *Liquor Ferri et Quininæ Citratis*) the salt is now furnished in a very convenient liquid form for use in solutions, whilst the above comparatively insoluble salt is retained for use in pills, for which it is much better adapted than the soluble salt of the manufacturers.

The use of sulphate of iron by the former Br. process is abandoned, and the solution of the persulphate retained. From this the freshly precipitated hydrate of iron is obtained by precipitation with ammonia. The next step is to separate quinine from the sulphate, by simply dissolving the salt in water with the aid of sulphuric acid, and then precipitating by ammonia. Thirdly, the hydrate and quinine are dissolved successively, aided by the heat of a water-bath, in solution of citric acid, whereby a citrate of iron and of quinine is obtained. The ammonia is added in order to render the citrate of iron and quinine more soluble by the agency of a portion of citrate of ammonium. It is important that the ammonia should not be added in excess; on the contrary, the solution should retain a slight acid reaction. (*Fleurot.*) After evaporation, the salt is dried, as in the other process, on glass or porcelain, so as to be obtained in thin scales.

The U. S. and Br. preparations are essentially different; both consist of citric acid, ferric oxide, and quinine; the British, however, containing the important addition of citrate of ammonium. No analysis of either salt has been made that determines precisely its chemical composition. Both are undoubtedly mere mixtures of the citrates of iron and quinine, the British containing citrate of ammonium.

The characters of the U. S. salt, as given in the Pharmacopœia, are the following. "Transparent, thin scales, varying in color from reddish brown to yellowish brown, slowly deliquescent on exposure to air, odorless, having a bitter and mildly ferruginous taste, and a slightly acid reaction. Slowly but wholly soluble in cold water, more readily so in hot water, and but slightly soluble in alcohol. When strongly heated, the salt emits fumes having the odor of burnt sugar, and finally leaves a residue which should not have an alkaline reaction (abs. of fixed alkalies). On supersaturating the aqueous solution of the salt with a slight excess of water of ammonia, the color of the liquid is deepened and a white, curdy precipitate is thrown down, which is soluble in ether and answers to the reactions of quinine. (See *Quinina.*) A small portion of the filtrate, when mixed with test-solution of ferrocyanide of potassium, does not produce a blue color or precipitate unless it is acidulated with hydrochloric acid. If another portion of the filtrate be deprived of its iron by boiling with an excess of potassa, the concentrated and cooled filtrate precipitated by test-solution of chloride of calcium, and the new filtrate heated to boiling, a white, granular precipitate will be produced. On heating the solution of the salt with potassa, no vapor of ammonia should be evolved. The salt contains 12 per cent. of dry quinine. It may be assayed as follows: Dissolve 4 Gm. of the scales in 30 C.c. of water, in a capsule, with the aid of heat. Cool, and transfer the solution to a glass separator, rinsing the capsule; add an aqueous solution of 0·5 Gm. of tartaric acid, and then solution of soda in decided excess. Extract the alkaloid by agitating the mixture with four successive portions of chloroform, each of 15 C.c. Separate the chloroformic layers, mix them, evaporate them in a weighed capsule, on a water-bath, and dry the residue at a temperature of 100° C. (212° F.). It should weigh 0·48 Gm." *U. S.*

Amorphous quinine or chinoidine is sometimes substituted for the crystallizable alkaloid. Dr. de Vrij proposes a method of detecting this fraud, which depends upon the fact that oxalic acid forms with crystallizable quinine, in a chloroformic solution, white crystals of oxalate of quinine without discoloration. (See *N. R.*, 1881, p. 10.)

The British citrate is described as in thin scales of a greenish golden-yellow color, of a bitter and chalybeate taste, somewhat deliquescent (which does not seem to be the case with our officinal salt), and entirely soluble in cold water. "The solution is very slightly acid, and is precipitated reddish brown by solution of soda, white by solution of ammonia, blue by ferrocyanide and ferricyanide of potassium, and grayish black by tannic acid. When burned with exposure to air, it leaves a residue which when moistened with water is not alkaline to test paper [oxide of iron]. Fifty grains, dissolved in a fluidounce of water, and treated with a slight excess of ammonia, give a white precipitate [quinine] which, when dissolved out by successive treatments of the fluid with ether or chloroform and the latter evaporated, and the residue dried until it ceases to lose weight, weighs seven and a half grains. The precipitate is almost entirely soluble in pure ether [showing the absence of cinchonine and quinidine] and when burned leaves but a minute residue." *Br.* Mr. Umney states (*P. J. Tr.*, 3d ser., iv.) that the salt prepared according to the British formula will not stand this test, and that fifty grains of it will not yield more than 7·1 grains of quinine. When dissolved by the aid of an acid, it forms a solution which, decolorised by a little purified animal charcoal, turns the plane of polarization strongly to the left; a character of quinine; cinchonine turning it to the right. (*Squire.*) The salt is said to be sometimes adulterated by cinchonine, which would be at once detected by the test of solubility in ether and the effect on polarized light, above given. Oscar Zinn (*A. J. P.*, 1877, p. 550) examined six commercial samples, two of which contained no quinine, but cinchonine. H. G. Drueding found three out of six samples deficient in quinine. As it occurs in the British market, it is of exceedingly variable composition, containing, according to Mr. J. C. Braithwaite, who examined 35 different specimens, a proportion of quinine varying from 1·5 to 17 per cent. (*P. J. Tr.*, 1868, p. 157.) The proportion of alkaloid appears to be usually below the standard. (A. W. Gerrard, *Ibid.*, March, 1873, p. 763.) According to Mr. C. H. Wood (*Ibid.*, 2d ser., x. 644), this salt undergoes a rapid change of composition when exposed to the direct rays of the sun.

The new officinal process of assay will doubtless bring to light all shortcomings.* (See results of examination of commercial citrate of iron and quinine by E. C. Federer, *Proc. Mich. Pharm. Assoc.*, 1887, or *Pharm. Era*, 1887, p. 357.)

Citrate of iron and quinine combines the virtues of its two bases, and may be given in all cases in which they are jointly indicated, preferably in pill form. The dose, as a tonic, is five or six grains (0·33–0·4 Gm.), containing about a grain (0·065 Gm.) of quinine, three or four times a day. This dose may be increased, if deemed advisable. (See *Liquor Ferri et Quininæ Citratis.*)

FERRI ET STRYCHNINÆ CITRAS. *U. S.* *Citrate of Iron and Strychnine.*

(FĔR'RĪ ĔT STRȲCH-NĪ'NÆ CĪ'TRĂS.)

Ferri et Strychninæ Citras, *U. S.* 1870; Citrate de Fer et de Strychnine, *Fr.*; Citronensaures Eisen-Strychnin, *G.*

"Citrate of Iron and Ammonium, *ninety-eight parts* [or four hundred and ninety grains]; Strychnine, *one part* [or five grains]; Citric Acid, *one part* [or five grains]; Distilled Water, *one hundred and twenty parts* [or eleven fluidrachms], To make *one hundred parts.* Dissolve the Citrate of Iron and Ammonium in *one hundred parts* [or nine fluidrachms] of Distilled Water, and the Strychnine, together with the Citric Acid, in *twenty parts* [or two fluidrachms] of Distilled Water. Mix the two solutions, evaporate the mixture, by means of a water-bath, at a temperature not exceeding 60° C. (140° F.), to the consistence of syrup, and spread it on plates

* R. Rother, on the plea of more uniform composition, uses anhydrous quinine, and proposes the following formula for citrate of iron and quinine. Ferric citrate, 8·16 grammes; citric acid, 2·16 grammes; sodium bicarbonate, 1·68 grammes; quinine trihydrite, 3·78 grammes; or quinine anhydrite, 3·24 grammes; water sufficient. Place the ferric citrate, sodium bicarbonate, and 20 C.c. of water in a porcelain capsule of convenient size and apply heat, constantly stirring the mixture until perfect solution has resulted. Now place the quinine, citric acid, and 20 C.c. of water in a similar capsule, and apply heat whilst stirring the mixture, until the combination is completed. Pour the solution into this magma, apply heat, and when all has dissolved, evaporate the solution at a moderate temperature, to a syrupy consistence, and spread it on glass plates to dry in the warm open air, so that the salt may form in scales. (*A. J. P.*, 1885, pp. 121–126.)

of glass, so that, when dry, the salt may be obtained in scales. Keep the product in well-stopped bottles, in a dark place." *U. S.*

Citrate of iron and strychnine, although long used in medicine, was first recognized in 1870. The present formula does not differ essentially from that of 1870.

This salt is well adapted for administration in pilular form, but should never be prescribed in solution. Dr. Squibb has shown that a whitish deposit will begin to settle from the solution within two or three hours after it is made, and continue to increase for several days; the deposit was found to contain fifty per cent. of strychnine. When water of ammonia or citrate of ammonium was added, the precipitate was redissolved, but the solution could not be made permanent by the addition, as the precipitate reappeared. There might be dangerous or alarming symptoms if this solution were dispensed without shaking. (*Ephemeris*, June, 1888, p. 1128.)

Properties. "Transparent, garnet-red scales, deliquescent on exposure to air, odorless, having a bitter and slightly ferruginous taste, and a slightly acid reaction. Readily and wholly soluble in water, and but slightly soluble in alcohol. When strongly heated, the salt emits fumes having the odor of burnt sugar, and finally leaves a residue which should not have an alkaline reaction (fixed alkalies). On heating the aqueous solution of the salt with solution of potassa, a brown-red precipitate is produced and vapor of ammonia is evolved. If 1 Gm. of the salt be dissolved in 4 C.c. of water, in a small test-tube, then 1 C.c. of solution of potassa added, and the mixture shaken with 2 C.c. of chloroform, the residue left on evaporating the chloroform will answer to the reactions of strychnine. (See *Strychnina.*) On adding test-solution of ferrocyanide of potassium to a dilute aqueous solution of the salt, no blue color or precipitate is produced unless the solution is acidulated with hydrochloric acid. If a solution of the salt be deprived of its iron by boiling with an excess of solution of potassa, the concentrated and cooled filtrate precipitated with test-solution of chloride of calcium, and the new filtrate heated to boiling, a white, granular precipitate will be produced." *U. S.*

Medical Properties. It is an efficient tonic, but has no advantages over the two active substances it contains when given conjointly in an uncombined state, and has the great disadvantage that the dose of one principle cannot be varied independently of that of the other. It occurs in beautiful red scales, of an intensely bitter, scarcely ferruginous taste, and is very soluble in water. It contains one per cent. of strychnine, there being in five grains one-twentieth of a grain of the alkaloid. The dose is three to five grains (0·20–0·33 Gm.) in pill or solution.

FERRI HYPOPHOSPHIS. *U. S.* *Hypophosphite of Iron.* [*Ferric Hypophosphite.*]

$Fe_2(H_2PO_2)_6$; 501·8. (FĔR'RĪ HȲ-PO-PHŎS'PHIS.) $Fe_2O_3(2HO, PO)_3$; 250·9.

Ferrum Hypophosphorosum, Hypophosphis Ferricus; Hypophosphite de Fer, *Fr.;* Unterphosphorigsaures Eisenoxyd, *G.*

This is among the hypophosphites brought into notice in consequence of their recommendation by Dr. Churchill in the treatment of phthisis, in which they were thought to be useful by the introduction of phosphorus into the system. This particular salt may be considered preferable to others, when a marked condition of anæmia indicates a deficiency of iron in the tissues. It may be made by the action of hypophosphorous acid on carbonate of iron formed by precipitation from the sulphate; but as some difficulty has been found in obtaining this acid perfectly pure, Mr. C. H. Wood, of London, prefers the plan of double decomposition. He proposes that sulphate of iron and hypophosphite of calcium be made to react on each other in molecular proportions, represented by 480 grains of crystallized sulphate of iron and 326 grains of commercial hypophosphite; in the latter an allowance of 10 per cent. being made for impurities ordinarily found in that salt. These quantities will yield 320 grains of the hypophosphite of iron; and the reaction will be represented by the following formula: $Ca(H_2PO_2)_2 + FeSO_4 = CaSO_4 + Fe(H_2PO_2)_2$. Sulphate of calcium is precipitated, and ferrous hypophosphite is held in solution. (*P. J. Tr.*, 1868, p. 342.) In this condition the salt is a ferrous compound; but on evaporation the ferrous salt becomes ferric, and acquires the properties as detailed in the Pharmacopœia. Of this the following description is given in the late edition of that work.

Properties. "A white or grayish white powder, permanent in the air, odorless and nearly tasteless, only slightly soluble in water, more readily so in presence of hypophosphorous acid, freely soluble in hydrochloric acid or in solution of citrate of sodium, forming with the latter a green solution. When strongly heated in a dry test-tube, the salt evolves a spontaneously inflammable gas (phosphoretted hydrogen), and, on ignition, leaves behind ferric pyrophosphate. The salt is readily oxidized by nitric acid or other oxidizing agents. It should be completely soluble in acetic acid (abs. of ferric phosphate). This solution, when mixed with test-solution of oxalate of ammonium, should not afford a white precipitate soluble in hydrochloric acid (abs. of calcium)." *U. S.*

Syrup of hypophosphite of iron may be prepared by simply adding syrup to the solution of the hypophosphite, remaining after the separation of the sulphate of calcium, in the process of Mr. Wood above given. If two and a half ounces of water are used in the process, and the paste resulting from the precipitation of the sulphate of calcium be pressed out, the remaining liquid, after filtration, will form with seven times its volume of syrup a liquid containing two grains of the hypophosphite in a fluidrachm. (*P. J. Tr.*, April, 1868.) But in this form, if the syrup be not thoroughly enclosed, it quickly absorbs oxygen, and in a few hours begins to exhibit the formation of a precipitate, rendering it in a short time unfit for use. A little phosphoric or citric acid added to the syrup will obviate this result; but it is better perhaps at once to form a syrup from materials which will not be liable to this objection. Mr. Wood employs the following process. "Take of granulated sulphate of iron 480 grs., hypophosphite of lime 326 grs., diluted phosphoric acid f℥i, water f℥iss, syrup q. s. Dissolve, without heat, the sulphate of iron in the phosphoric acid, previously mixed with the water. Rub the hypophosphite to fine powder, and pour on it the solution of the sulphate. Triturate together for two or three minutes, then pour the mixture on a piece of damp calico, and squeeze out the liquid with the hands. Filter this solution, and add to it seven times its volume of strong syrup. The resulting syrup will contain two grains of the hypophosphite of iron in each fluidrachm." The dose may be from 2 to 6 fluidrachms (7·5–22·50 C.c.).

Prof. C. L. Diehl prepares the syrup from a freshly precipitated magma, produced by precipitating a solution of calcium hypophosphite with solution of chloride of iron and dissolving the magma by the aid of potassium citrate. (*Proc. A. P. A.*, 1882, p. 71; see, also, National Formulary, Part II.) This salt may be given in states of system where deficient powers of the cerebral centres are attended with an anæmic state of the blood. The phosphorus is supposed to serve as a nutrient to the brain, and the iron supplies red corpuscles to the circulation. It may be given in pill or powder in the dose of from five to ten grains; but a more eligible form, and one generally preferred, is that of syrup.

FERRI IODIDUM SACCHARATUM. *U. S.* *Saccharated Iodide of Iron.* [*Saccharated Ferrous Iodide.*]

(FĔR'RĪ I-ŎD'I-DŬM SĂC-CHA-RĀ'TŬM.)

Ferrum Iodatum Saccharatum, *P.G.;* Zuckerhaltiges Jodeisen, *G.*

"Iron, in the form of fine wire, and cut into small pieces, *six parts* [or thirty grains]; Iodine, *seventeen parts* [or eighty-five grains]; Distilled Water, *twenty parts* [or one and a half fluidrachms]; Sugar of Milk, *eighty parts* [or four hundred grains]. Mix the Iron, Iodine, and Distilled Water in a flask of thin glass, shake the mixture occasionally until the reaction ceases, and the solution has acquired a green color and lost the smell of Iodine; then filter it through a wetted filter into a porcelain capsule containing *forty parts* [or two hundred grains] of Sugar of Milk. Rinse the flask and Iron Wire with a little Distilled Water, pass the rinsings through the filter into the capsule, and evaporate, on a water-bath, constantly stirring, until a dry mass remains. Transfer the mass quickly to a heated iron mortar containing the remainder of the Sugar of Milk, and reduce the whole to powder. Transfer the powder at once to small, well-dried bottles, which must be securely stopped, and kept in a cool and dark place." *U. S.*

This is a new officinal preparation; it is identical with the Saccharated Iodide of

Iron of the German Pharmacopœia, and consists of ferrous iodide preserved by contact with sugar of milk. It is a more stable form of administering ferrous iodide than the salt in its pure state. (See *Ferri Iodidum.*)*

Properties. The Pharmacopœia gives the following description. "A yellowish white or grayish powder, very hygroscopic, odorless, having a sweetish, ferruginous taste, and a slightly acid reaction. Soluble in 7 parts of water at 15° C. (59° F.), forming an almost clear solution; only partially soluble in alcohol. When strongly heated, the compound swells up, chars, evolves the odor of iodine and of burnt sugar, and, on ignition, leaves a residue which should yield nothing soluble to water (abs. of salts of alkalies). The aqueous solution yields a blue precipitate with test-solution of ferricyanide of potassium. If mixed with some gelatinized starch and afterward with a little chlorine water, the solution assumes a deep blue color. This color should not be developed in the aqueous solution by gelatinized starch alone (abs. of free iodine). On mixing an aqueous solution of 5 Gm. of Saccharated Iodide of Iron with a solution of 1 Gm. of nitrate of silver, and filtering, the filtrate should still produce a precipitate or cloudiness with test-solution of nitrate of silver (presence of at least 20 per cent. of ferrous iodide)." *U. S.*

Medical Properties. The medical properties of this preparation are identical with those of the iodide of iron. The dose is two to five grains (0·13 to 0.33 Gm.).

FERRI LACTAS. *U. S.* *Lactate of Iron.* [*Ferrous Lactate.*]

(FĔR'RĪ LĂC'TĂS.)

$Fe(C_3H_5O_3)_2 . 3H_2O$; 287·9. $FeO, C_6H_5O_5 . 3HO$; 143·95.

Ferrum Lacticum, *P.G.;* Lactas Ferrosus; Lactate de Fer, *Fr.;* Milchsäures Eisenoxydul, Eisenlactat, *G.*

A formula for this salt was omitted in the late U. S. P. revision. In the process of U. S. P. 1870,† the lactic acid unites with the iron, forming lactate of iron, a part of which crystallizes when the solution cools, and the remainder is obtained by evaporation and crystallization. It may be more cheaply prepared, on the large scale, by digesting the impure acid first obtained in M. Louradour's process, with iron filings, or by reaction between sulphate of iron and the lactate of calcium or lactate of zinc prepared as a step in obtaining lactic acid. The following is M. Gobley's process for making lactate of calcium, preparatory to its conversion into lactate of iron. Add to 2 pints of skim-milk, diluted with twice its bulk of water, and con-

* *Tasteless Salts of Iron.* A class of preparations of iron have been introduced by Mr. J. L. A. Creuse, of Brooklyn, N. Y. (*A. J. P.*, xiv. 214). It has long been known that the citrate of ammonium has the property of rendering soluble many ordinarily insoluble preparations of iron. Mr. Creuse believes that all the salts of ferric oxide form chemical combinations with all the alkaline (ammonium, sodium, potassium, lithium) citrates, which combinations are all greenish, soluble in water, nearly insoluble in alcohol, free from ferruginous taste, perfectly stable, and so resisting decomposition as to form no precipitate with Peruvian bark; indeed, chemical reagents do not reveal the iron in them unless strong acids or sulphuretted hydrogen be used. None of these salts coagulate the blood; they cannot be used as styptics.

Tasteless Iodide of Iron is prepared in the following manner: 126·3 grains of iodine are combined with iron in the usual way to obtain the solution of ferrous iodide; this is filtered and 63 grains of iodine dissolved in it; a solution of 201 grains of citric acid is exactly saturated with potassa and then added gradually to the first solution. When the apple-green color has been developed the solution is evaporated, with gentle stirring, to dryness, when cauliflower-like masses of acicular crystals will be obtained. These are stable except in direct sunlight. (See *Syrupus Ferri Citro-Iodidi*, National Formulary, Part II.)

Tasteless Chloride of Iron is made by adding an alkaline citrate in solution to a solution of sesquichloride of iron, in such proportion that there shall be two molecules of the former to three molecules of chlorine. Usually from 120 to 140 grains of citric acid saturated with soda, potassa, or ammonia are required for the preparation of an ounce of a tincture of corresponding strength to the officinal tincture. The addition should be made to the liquor, and the final solution must not contain more than 40 per cent. of alcohol. R. Rother affirms that these so-called salts are mere mixtures of citrate of iron and iodide or chloride of the alkali used. (*A. J. P.*, 1876, p. 171; see, also, *Syrupus Ferri Protochloridi*, National Formulary, Part II.)

† "Take of Lactic Acid *a fluidounce;* Iron, in the form of filings, *half a troyounce;* Distilled Water *a sufficient quantity.* Mix the Acid with a pint of Distilled Water in an iron vessel, add the Iron, and digest the mixture on a water-bath, supplying Distilled Water, from time to time, to preserve the measure. When the action has ceased, filter the solution, while hot, into a porcelain capsule, and set it aside to crystallize. At the end of forty-eight hours, decant the liquid, wash the crystals with a little alcohol, and dry them on bibulous paper. By evaporating the mother-water in an iron vessel to one-half, filtering while hot, and setting the liquid aside, more crystals may be obtained." *U. S.* 1870.

tained in an earthen pan, 64 drachms of powdered lactose, and 51 drachms of powdered chalk. Allow the whole to ferment for eleven or twelve days, at a temperature of from 26·6° C. to 32·2° C. (80° to 90° F.), supplying water as it evaporates. Transfer the liquor to a capsule, heat it gradually to boiling, and stir it constantly. Boil for a quarter of an hour to coagulate casein, allow the insoluble matters to subside, and strain the liquid through flannel. The clear liquid is a solution of lactate of calcium. In this process the casein of the milk, acting as a ferment, converts not only the lactose of the milk, but the lactose added, into lactic acid; a result which would not take place were it not for the presence of the chalk, which saturates the lactic acid as it is formed, and prevents it from uniting with the casein, whereby the power of the latter as a ferment would be destroyed. (*Journ. de Pharm.*, 3e sér., vi. 54.) (See also other methods under *Acidum Lacticum*, p. 79.) Lactate of calcium may be expeditiously converted into lactate of iron by the following process of M. Lepage. Dissolve 100 parts of lactate of calcium, obtained by M. Gobley's process, in 500 parts of boiling water; dissolve also 68 parts of pure crystallised sulphate of iron in 500 parts of cold distilled water. Mix the filtered solutions in a matrass, acidulate slightly with lactic acid, and heat in a water-bath, stirring frequently until the double decomposition is completed. Then filter to separate the sulphate of calcium, and evaporate rapidly to one-half, either in an iron vessel, or in a porcelain capsule containing a few turnings of iron. Filter again, and set aside to crystallize; and, having washed the crystals in a funnel with a little alcohol, dry them on bibulous paper. (*Journ. de Pharm.*, 3e sér., ix. 272.) In relation to the precautions to be observed in preparing this lactate, so as to prevent the partial oxidation of the iron, see *A. J. P.*, 1853, p. 556.*

Lactate of iron is in "pale, greenish white, crystalline crusts or grains, permanent in the air, odorless, having a mild, sweetish, ferruginous taste, and a slightly acid reaction. Soluble in 40 parts of water at 15° C. (59° F.), and in 12 parts of boiling water; almost insoluble in alcohol, but freely soluble in solution of citrate of sodium, yielding a green solution. When heated on platinum foil, the salt froths up, gives out thick, white acrid fumes, and chars, a brown-red residue being finally left. The aqueous solution yields a blue precipitate with test-solution of ferricyanide of potassium. If the salt be boiled for fifteen minutes with nitric acid of the sp. gr. 1·200, white, granular mucic acid will be deposited on cooling the liquid. An aqueous solution of the salt should not be rendered more than faintly opalescent by test-solution of acetate of lead (limit of sulphate, citrate, tartrate, etc.)." *U. S.* It has an acid reaction, and possesses a mild, sweetish, ferruginous taste. The aqueous solution quickly becomes yellow, in consequence of the iron passing to a higher state of oxidation. M. Louradour has seen several samples of this lactate, variously adulterated; as with effloresced sulphate of iron, starch, and lactin; the sophistication being concealed by the sale of the salt in powder. These impurities may be detected by appropriate reagents; but M. Louradour recommends, as a simpler way of avoiding them, the rejection of the salt when not in crystalline crusts.

Medical Properties. Lactate of iron has the general medical properties of the ferruginous preparations, and has been especially used in chlorosis by Andral, Fouquier, Bouillaud, and other Parisian doctors. As much as 12 or even 20 grains (0·80–1·3 Gm.) may be given in the course of a day. It may be administered in lozenge, pill, or syrup. The *lozenge* may be made of one grain (0·065 Gm.) of the lactate to twelve (0·80 Gm.) of sugar; and the *pill*, of one grain (0·065 Gm.) of the salt, with an equal weight of some inert powder free from astringent matter, and sufficient honey. The following is the formula for a *syrup* proposed by M. Cap. Take of lactate of iron *a drachm;* white sugar *twelve ounces and a half;*

* *Ferric Lactate.* Instead of the officinal ferrous lactate, Louis P. Carbonell recommends the ferric lactate, which he succeeded in obtaining in light brown transparent scales by following the process for the other scale preparations of iron, taking particular care fully to saturate the acid and to avoid high temperature during the whole operation. If the first precaution be overlooked, a more or less pasty mass will be the result, and if the temperature rise too high, a pulverulent salt will be obtained. The scaled salt is freely soluble in water and alcohol.

Lactate of iron and quinine and *lactate of iron and strychnine* may also be obtained in brown scales, have a bitter ferruginous taste, and are soluble in alcohol and water. (*A. J. P.*, 1876, p. 459.)

boiling distilled water *six fluidounces and a half.* Rub the salt to powder with half an ounce of the sugar; and dissolve the mixture quickly in the boiling water. Pour the solution into a matrass placed on a sand-bath, and add to it the rest of the sugar in small pieces. When the sugar is dissolved, filter the syrup, and, as soon as it is cold, transfer it to bottles which must be well stopped. This syrup has a very light amber color, and contains about four grains of the salt to the fluidounce. The dose is from two to four fluidrachms (7·5–15 C.c.). Bread, called *chalybeate bread*, containing lactate of iron in the proportion of about a grain (0·065 Gm.) to the ounce (31·1 Gm.), has been used with advantage by chlorotic patients in one of the hospitals of Paris. The bread is not injured in taste or quality.

Off. Prep. Syrupus Hypophosphitum cum Ferro.

FERRI OXALAS. *U. S.* *Oxalate of Iron.* [*Ferrous Oxalate.*]

$FeC_2O_4.H_2O$; 161·9. (FĔR'RĪ ŎX'A-LĂS.) $FeO, C_2O_3.HO$; 80·95.

Ferrum Oxalicum, Oxalas Ferrosus; Oxalate de Fer, *Fr.;* Oxalsaures Eisenoxydul, *G.*

No process for this salt is given in the present Pharmacopœia; that of U. S. of 1870 will be found in the foot-note.*

Oxalate of iron was officinal for the first time in 1870. It is "a pale yellow, or lemon-yellow, crystalline powder, permanent in the air, odorless and nearly tasteless, very slightly soluble in cold or hot water, but soluble in cold, concentrated hydrochloric acid, and in hot diluted sulphuric acid. When heated in contact with air, it decomposes with a faint combustion, and, on ignition, leaves a residue, amounting to not less than 49·3 per cent. of the original weight. On heating the salt with excess of test-solution of carbonate of sodium, it is decomposed, yielding a precipitate, which, when dissolved in diluted hydrochloric acid, affords a blue precipitate with test-solution of ferricyanide of potassium, and a filtrate which, when supersaturated with acetic acid, yields, with test-solution of chloride of calcium, a white precipitate soluble in hydrochloric acid." *U. S.*

It is no doubt capable of acting as a feeble chalybeate, but possesses no advantages over other iron preparations. The dose is two to three grains (0·13–0·20 Gm.).

FERRI OXIDUM HYDRATUM. *U.S.* *Hydrated Oxide of Iron.* [*Ferric Hydrate.*]

$Fe_2(HO)_6$; 213·8. (FĔR'RĪ ŎX'I-DŬM HȲ-DRĀ'TŬM.) $Fe_2O_3.3HO$; 106·9.

Ferri Peroxidum Hydratum, *Br.;* Ferri Sesquioxidum; Ferri Oxidum Rubrum; Hydrous Peroxide of Iron; Ferric Oxyhydrate; Ferrugo; Hydrated Peroxide of Iron, Hydrated Sesquioxide of Iron, Moist Peroxide of Iron; Hydras Ferricus; Sesquioxide (Peroxyde) de Fer hydraté humide, Hydrate de Peroxyde de Fer gélatineux, *Fr.;* Feuchtes Eisenoxydhydrat, Gegengift der Arsenigensäure, *G.*

"Solution of Tersulphate of Iron, *ten parts* [or three fluidounces]; Water of Ammonia, *eight parts* [or three and a quarter fluidounces]; Water, *a sufficient quantity.* To the Water of Ammonia, previously diluted with *twenty parts* [or eight fluidounces] of cold Water, add, constantly stirring, the Solution of Tersulphate of Iron, previously diluted with *one hundred parts* [or two and a half pints] of cold Water. Pour the whole on a wet muslin strainer, and allow the precipitate to drain; then return it to the vessel and mix it intimately with *one hundred and twenty parts* [or three pints] of cold Water. Again drain it on the strainer and repeat the operation. Lastly, mix the precipitate with enough cold Water to make the mixture weigh *twenty parts* [or eight ounces av.]. When Hydrated Oxide of Iron is to be made in haste for use as an antidote, the washing may be performed more quickly, though less perfectly, by pressing the strainer forcibly with the hands until no more liquid passes, and then adding enough Water to make the whole weigh about *twenty parts* [or eight ounces av.].

"*Note.* The ingredients for preparing Hydrated Oxide of Iron, as an antidote,

* "Take of Sulphate of Iron *two troyounces;* Oxalic Acid *four hundred and thirty-six grains;* Distilled Water *a sufficient quantity.* Dissolve the Sulphate of Iron in thirty fluidounces, and the Oxalic Acid in fifteen fluidounces of Distilled Water. Filter the solutions, and, having mixed them with agitation, set aside the mixture until the precipitate is deposited. Decant the clear liquid, wash the precipitate until the washings cease to redden litmus, and dry it with a gentle heat." *U. S.*

should always be kept on hand, in bottles holding, respectively, about *ten troy ounces* or *three hundred grammes* of Solution of Tersulphate of Iron, and about *eight troy ounces* or *two hundred and forty grammes* of Water of Ammonia." *U. S.*

"Take of Solution of Persulphate of Iron *four fluidounces*; Solution of Soda *thirty-three fluidounces*; Distilled Water *a sufficiency*. Mix the Solution of Persulphate of Iron with a pint [Imperial measure] of the Distilled Water, and add this gradually to the Solution of Soda, stirring them constantly and briskly. Let the mixture stand two hours, stirring it occasionally, then put it on a calico filter, and, when the liquid has drained away, wash the precipitate with Distilled Water, until what passes through the filter ceases to give a precipitate with chloride of barium. Dry it at a temperature not exceeding 212° F. (100° C.) until it ceases to lose weight, then reduce it to fine powder." *Br.*

This preparation was introduced into the U. S. Pharmacopœia on account of its importance as an antidote to arsenious acid. It is frequently used in the officinal processes as the source of iron, when it is desired to produce a ferric compound, but the directions for making it always accompany the preparation in which it is used, because of the difficulty of preserving the ferric hydrate. In the former processes the first step was to convert the sulphate of iron into the tersulphate; but in the present the officinal solution of tersulphate of iron (persulphate, *Br.*) is taken already containing the iron in the proper state of oxidation. This is simply treated with water of ammonia (*U. S.*), or diluted solution of soda (*Br.*), which throws down the oxide combined with water, constituting the hydrated oxide required.

It is the duty of the apothecary to be always prepared to make this antidote, by keeping the necessary solutions for its precipitation. Magnesia is probably a better precipitant than either of those officinal. (See next article.) In most cases of arsenical poisoning minutes are of immense importance, and time must be lost in washing the precipitated iron if the officinal process is adhered to. Magnesia is not only not irritant, but is itself antidotal to arsenic; so that the precipitated mass may be given at once to the patient. The oxide should not be kept in stock, but when ordered as an antidote should be made fresh.

The British preparation differs from the officinal one in the important particular that it is in fine powder and contains but 10 per cent. of moisture, the *moist peroxide of iron* having been abandoned at the last revision as a separate preparation on account of its instability and both processes merged into one.

Properties. Hydrated oxide of iron, as directed to be kept by the U. S. formula, "is a brown-red magma, wholly soluble in hydrochloric acid, without effervescence." The hydrated oxide ($Fe_2O_3,2H_2O$) loses, by the British process, one-half of its combined water, and is converted into the monohydrated sesquioxide (Fe_2O_3,H_2O), which is the present officinal preparation. As prepared by the Dublin process, in which it was heated to redness, it lost the second molecule of water, and became the anhydrous sesquioxide (Fe_2O_3), identical with the *colcothar* of commerce.

The monohydrated sesquioxide is a reddish brown, tasteless, insoluble powder, differing from colcothar in containing a molecule of water. Hence, "heated to dull redness in a test-tube it gives off moisture." *Br.* It should not be deliquescent, and should dissolve entirely in hydrochloric acid without effervescence. Its solution in diluted hydrochloric acid yields a copious blue precipitate with the ferrocyanide of potassium, but none with the ferricyanide; showing that it contains ferric oxide but no ferrous oxide. If it contain copper, its hydrochloric solution will deposit this metal on a bright piece of iron. M. Dawies states that, if the hydrated oxide recently prepared be kept for four or five days in boiling water, it loses a large proportion of its water, containing at the end of that time only 5·77 per cent. The larger portion of the oxide has, therefore, become dehydrated; and the same thing happens at a lower temperature, 41·1° C. (106° F.), in two or three months. It becomes of a brick-red color, and is but slightly soluble in nitric acid. (*Journ. de Pharm.*, 4e sér., iv. 400.) This oxide is not used as a medicine. It is employed in making iron plaster and reduced iron, for which purposes other forms of oxidised iron would answer as well. The former Dublin *rubigo ferri* or *rust of iron*, formed by exposing moistened iron wire to the air till converted into rust, is essentially the sesquioxide, containing a little carbonate of iron, and does not differ very essentially from the subcarbonate of iron formerly officinal.*

If exposed to a red heat it loses the combined water, and becomes the anhydrous sesquioxide, less easily soluble in acids, improper for medicinal use, and altogether without effect as an antidote. Kept for some time in the pulpy state, it loses half its combined water, and becomes less soluble in acids, and less efficient as an antidote. Dr. Hirsch has given some useful details in making precipitated oxide of iron upon a comparatively large scale in *Amer. Drug.*, 1884, p. 66.

Medical Properties and Uses. The hydrated oxide of iron is not an eligible ferruginous preparation for medical use. Its antidotal powers in poisoning by arsenic, the manner in which it acts, the circumstances which impair its efficiency, and the mode of using it, are fully explained under *Acidum Arseniosum*. Its power of rendering arsenious acid insoluble is readily shown by agitating a solution of the acid with a considerable excess of the moist oxide, filtering, and then testing the filtered solution for the acid; not a trace of the metal can be detected, even by sulphuretted hydrogen. It is stated, however, to be inferior as an antidote to the saccharated oxide of iron. The hydrated oxide, as obtained by the U. S. formula, contains a little ammonia, which is thought by some to assist its antidotal powers. At least it has been ascertained that the sesquioxide, when precipitated by potassa as formerly directed by the Dublin College, is less efficient than when precipitated by ammonia, and must be employed in quantities three or four times as large to produce the same effect. The dry hydrate, rubbed up with water, is in the same proportion weaker than the pulpy hydrate. Subcarbonate of iron (formerly officinal) possesses antidotal powers to arsenic, though in an inferior degree; but this statement will not apply to it, after it has been exposed to a red heat, to which it is improperly subjected by some manufacturing chemists. By ignition it becomes anhydrous, and altogether inefficient as an antidote.

Off. Prep. Emplastrum Ferri; Trochisci Ferri.

Off. Prep. Br. Emplastrum Ferri.

FERRI OXIDUM HYDRATUM CUM MAGNESIA. *U.S.*

Hydrated Oxide of Iron with Magnesia.

(FĔR'RĪ ŎX'Į-DŬM HȲ-DRĀ'TŬM CŬM MĂG-NĒ'ȘĮ-Ą.)

Antidotum Arsenici, *P.G.;* Antidote to Arsenious Acid; Gegengift der Arsenigensäure, *G.*

"Solution of Tersulphate of Iron, *one thousand grains* (65·00 Gm.); Magnesia,

* *Ferri Subcarbonas.* U. S. 1870; *Subcarbonate of Iron; Sesquioxide of Iron; Red Oxide of Iron; Precipitated Carbonate of Iron; Aperitive Saffron of Mars.* "Take of Sulphate of Iron *eight troyounces;* Carbonate of Sodium *nine troyounces;* Water *eight pints.* Dissolve the salts separately, each in four pints of the Water; then mix the solutions thoroughly, and set aside the mixture until the precipitate has subsided. Then pour off the supernatant liquid, wash the precipitate with water until the washings pass nearly tasteless, and dry it on bibulous paper without heat." *U. S.* 1870.

When the solutions of carbonate of sodium and sulphate of iron are mixed together, a hydrated ferrous carbonate, of a pale blue color, is thrown down, and sulphate of sodium remains in solution. The precipitate, during the washing and drying, absorbs oxygen, and loses nearly all its carbonic acid, whereby it is converted almost entirely into ferric oxide. The direction to dry the precipitate without heat is important: as even a moderate elevation of temperature has been shown, by the experiments of Mr. J. A. Rex, to modify the resulting product unfavorably, diminishing its solubility in hydrochloric acid in proportion to the heat employed. (*A. J. P.*, May, 1862, p. 193.)

Properties. Subcarbonate of iron is a reddish brown powder, of a disagreeable, slightly styptic taste; insoluble in water, and not readily dissolved by any acid except hydrochloric, with which it effervesces slightly. When of a bright red color it should be rejected, as this color shows that it has been injured by exposure to heat. After precipitation from its hydrochloric solution by ammonia or potassa, either of which throws down the sesquioxide of iron, the supernatant liquor should give no indications of containing any metal in solution by the test of sulphuretted hydrogen or ferrocyanide of potassium. It is incompatible with acids and acidulous salts. In composition it is a hydrated ferric oxide, containing a little ferrous carbonate. By exposure to a red heat, it absorbs oxygen, and loses water and carbonic acid, being converted into the *astringent saffron of Mars* of the French Codex. After ignition it is no longer a subcarbonate, but is converted into the pure sesquioxide, which is less soluble in acids, and less efficient as a medicine than the preparation in its original state. Hence it is wrong to expose the subcarbonate to a red heat, as some manufacturing chemists are in the habit of doing, in order to give it a bright red color.

Medical Properties and Uses. Subcarbonate of iron is a rather feeble ferruginous tonic, nearly free from astringency, and causing, even in the largest doses, no obvious effects save only a very slight gastric disturbance. It has been especially commended in neuralgia in doses of a teaspoonful (3·75 C.c.). The ordinary chalybeate dose is five grains (0·33 Gm.).

one hundred and fifty grains (10 Gm.); Water, *a sufficient quantity*. Mix the Solution of Tersulphate of Iron with twice its weight of Water, and keep the mixture in a well-stopped bottle. Rub the Magnesia with Water to a smooth and thin mixture, transfer this to a bottle capable of holding *thirty-two fluidounces* or about *one liter*, and fill it up with Water. When the preparation is wanted for use, mix the two liquids by adding the Magnesia mixture, gradually, to the Iron solution, and shake them together until a homogeneous mass results.

"*Note.* The diluted Solution of Tersulphate of Iron and the mixture of Magnesia with Water, should always be kept on hand, ready for immediate use." *U. S.*

This is a new officinal preparation. It has been introduced for the purpose of furnishing a ready and efficient antidote against Arsenious Acid. It is almost identical with the *Antidotum Arsenici* of the German Pharmacopœia, and experience has shown its effectiveness. Ferric hydrate is produced when the mixture of magnesia is added to the diluted solution of tersulphate of iron, and as the magnesia is in excess and acidity thus prevented, no harm can result from not separating the by-products of the reaction. When mixed as officinally directed, and ready for use, it contains ferric hydrate with magnesium sulphate and hydrate. It has been shown that no soluble compound with arsenic is formed when it is used as an antidote, and the presence of the magnesium salts, from a therapeutical point of view, is not at all objectionable. (See *Acidum Arseniosum*, p. 36.)

FERRI PHOSPHAS, *U. S., Br.* *Phosphate of Iron.* [*Ferric Phosphate.*]

(FĔR'RĪ PHŎS'PHĂS.)

Ferrum Phosphoricum, *P.G.;* Phosphas Ferroso-Ferricus; Ferroso-Ferric Phosphate; Phosphate de Fer, Phosphate ferroso-ferrique. *Fr.;* Phosphorsaures Eisenoxydul (Eisenoxydul-Oxyd), *G.*

"Ferrous phosphate, $Fe_3(PO_4)_2 8H_2O$, at least 47 per cent.; with ferric phosphate and some oxide." *Br.*

"Citrate of Iron, *five parts* [or ten ounces av.]; Phosphate of Sodium, *six parts** [or twelve ounces av.]; Distilled Water, *ten parts* [or nineteen fluidounces]. Dissolve the Citrate of Iron in the Distilled Water by heating on a water-bath. To this solution add the Phosphate of Sodium and stir constantly, until it is dissolved. Evaporate the solution at a temperature not exceeding 60° C. (140° F.), to the consistence of thick syrup, and spread it on plates of glass, so that, when dry, the salt may be obtained in scales. Keep the product in well-stopped bottles, in a dark place." *U. S.*

"Take of Sulphate of Iron *three ounces* [avoirdupois]; Phosphate of Sodium *two and three-quarter ounces* [avoird.]; Bicarbonate of Sodium *three-quarters of an ounce* [avoird.]; Boiling Distilled Water *a sufficiency*. Dissolve the Sulphate of Iron in *thirty fluidounces* [Imp. meas.] of the Water, and the Phosphate of Sodium in a similar quantity of water. When each solution has cooled to between 100° and 130° F. (37°·8 and 54°·4 C.) add the latter to the former, pouring in also a solution of the Bicarbonate of Sodium in a little Distilled Water. Mix thoroughly. Transfer the precipitate to a calico filter, and wash it with hot distilled water, till the filtrate ceases to give a precipitate with chloride of barium. Finally dry the precipitate at a temperature not exceeding 120° (48°·9 C.)." *Br.*

It is to be regretted that another title was not chosen for this preparation by the Committee of Revision; for the phosphate of iron made by the U. S. Pharm. 1880 is altogether different from the salt formerly officinal, not only in appearance and solubility, but in chemical composition. As obtained by the present process, it is not a definite chemical compound, but a mixture, which should probably be called sodio-ferric citro-phosphate, and bears a resemblance to the pyrophosphate, which is now directed to be made by a similar process. (See *Ferri Pyrophosphas.*)

The British phosphate of iron is a very different salt. By double decomposition ferrous phosphate and sodium sulphate are produced, the former precipitating as a

* C. N. Lake recommends 4½ parts of phosphate of sodium instead of 6 parts. (See *Proc. New York State Pharm. Assoc.*, 1886, p. 170.)

white bulky powder, which soon changes on exposure to a greenish blue, and ultimately to a slate color; a portion of sulphuric acid is liberated from the ferrous sulphate during the reaction, and this retaining in solution some of the ferrous phosphate, requires the addition of the solution of sodium bicarbonate to decompose it and set free the remainder of the ferrous phosphate. This salt, when first formed, is represented by the formula $Fe_3(PO_4)_2$; but the strong affinity of its ferrous oxide for oxygen causes the gradual production of sesquisalt, which, therefore, to a certain extent always exists in the preparation; hence the British authority requires it to contain at least 47 per cent. of ferrous phosphate, $Fe_3(PO_4)_2 8H_2O$.

Phosphate of iron, as made by the U. S. Pharmacopœia, is in "thin, bright green, transparent scales, permanent in dry air when excluded from light, odorless, having an acidulous, slightly saline taste, and a slightly acid reaction. Freely and completely soluble in water, but insoluble in alcohol. The aqueous solution of the salt is rendered blue by test-solution of ferrocyanide of potassium, but does not yield a blue precipitate with this reagent, unless it has been acidulated with hydrochloric acid. When heated with solution of potassa in excess, a brown-red precipitate is thrown down, and the filtrate, after being supersaturated with acetic acid, yields a light yellow precipitate with test-solution of nitrate of silver (difference from pyrophosphate). 100 parts of the salt represent about 13·5 parts of metallic iron." *U. S.* When made by the British process, it is in the form of a powder of a bright slate color, insoluble in water, but soluble in acids. The solution in dilute hydrochloric acid gives a blue precipitate with both ferricyanide and ferrocyanide of potassium, but much the more copiously with the former, proving the presence both of ferrous and ferric oxide, but a great preponderance of ferrous oxide. When treated with tartaric acid and an excess of ammonia, and subsequently with the *solution of ammonio-sulphate of magnesium* (see *Tests*, Part III.), it lets fall a crystalline precipitate. If the preparation contain arsenic, it will be detected by producing a dark precipitate on the surface of a slip of pure copper introduced into the solution. "Thirty grains dissolved in hydrochloric acid, continue to give a blue precipitate with ferricyanide of potassium until at least two hundred and seventy-nine grain-measures of the *volumetric solution of bichromate of potassium* have been added." *Br.* This shows the presence of 47 per cent. of ferrous phosphate.

Phosphate of iron, dissolved to saturation in a boiling solution of metaphosphoric acid (HPO_3), under the name of *superphosphate of iron*, was proposed as a new remedy, in Jan. 1851, by Dr. Routh, of London. Mr. Thomas Greenish, of the same city, states that the solution of the salt, on cooling, hardens into a mass of pilular consistence, soluble in water in all proportions, and free from any disagreeable or inky taste.

Medical Properties. Phosphate of iron possesses the general properties of the ferruginous preparations, and has been given with advantage in amenorrhœa and dyspepsia. The dose is from five to ten grains (0·33–0·65 Gm.).*

Off. Prep. Syrupus Ferri Quininæ et Strychninæ Phosphatum.

Off. Prep. Br. Syrupus Ferri Phosphatis.

* *Compound Syrup of Phosphate of Iron. Chemical Food.* For a formula for a compound syrup of phosphate of iron by Mr. Wiegand, made by introducing into it the phosphates of calcium, potassium, and sodium, and for remarks on the pharmacy of the phosphates by Prof. Procter, see *A. J. P.*, 1854 (pp. 111 and 112). A formula similar to Mr. Wiegand's, communicated by Mr. Edward Parrish, as probably representing the process for a secret preparation considerably used in this city, may be found in *A. J. P.*, 1857 (p. 573). These formulas are too complicated to have any therapeutic value. Nevertheless, as the preparations have had much vogue, under the name of *chemical food*, we give the formula of Mr. Parrish from the journal referred to. "Take of Sulphate of Iron ʒx; Phosphate of Soda ʒxii; Phosphate of Lime ʒxii; Glacial Phosphoric Acid ℥xx; Carbonate of Soda ℈ij; Carbonate of Potassa ʒi; Hydrochloric Acid, Water of Ammonia, each, q. s.; Powdered Cochineal ʒij; Water q. s. to make f℥xx; Sugar ℔iij (troy); Oil of Orange ♏x. Dissolve the Sulphate of Iron in f℥ij, and the Phosphate of Soda in f℥iv of boiling Water. Mix the solutions, and wash the precipitated phosphate of iron till the washings are tasteless. Dissolve the Phosphate of Lime in f℥iv of boiling Water with sufficient Hydrochloric Acid to make a clear solution, precipitate it with Water of Ammonia, and wash the precipitate. To the freshly precipitated phosphates add the Phosphoric Acid previously dissolved in Water. When clear, add the Carbonates of Soda and Potassa, and afterwards sufficient Hydrochloric Acid to dissolve the precipitate. Now add Cochineal mixed with the Sugar, apply heat, and, when the syrup is formed, strain and flavor it. Each teaspoonful contains about one grain of phosphate of iron and two and

FERRI PYROPHOSPHAS. *U. S.* *Pyrophosphate of Iron.* [*Ferric Pyrophosphate.*]

(FĔR'RĪ PȲ-RQ-PHŎS'PHĂS.)

Ferrum Pyrophosphoricum cum Ammonio Citrico, *P.G.;* Pyrophosphas Ferricus cum Citrate Ammonico; Pyrophosphate of Iron with Ammonium Citrate; Pyrophosphate de Fer citro-ammoniacal, *Fr.;* Pyrophosphorsaures Eisenoxyd mit Citronensauren Ammonium, *G.*

"Citrate of Iron, *nine parts* [or nine ounces av.]; Pyrophosphate of Sodium, *ten parts** [or ten ounces av.]; Distilled Water, *eighteen parts* [or seventeen fluidounces]. Dissolve the Citrate of Iron in the Distilled Water by heating, on a water-bath. To this solution add the Pyrophosphate of Sodium and stir constantly until it is dissolved. Evaporate the solution, at a temperature not exceeding 60° C. (140° F.), to the consistence of thick syrup, and spread it on plates of glass, so that, when dry, the salt may be obtained in scales. Keep the product in well-stopped bottles, in a dark place." *U. S.*

The process now officinal differs very materially from that of the U. S. Pharmacopœia, 1870. In the latter, phosphate of sodium was converted into the pyrophosphate by moderately igniting it; this was dissolved in water, and the solution mixed with a diluted solution of tersulphate of iron, when ferric pyrophosphate was precipitated; this was washed with cold water and dissolved in a solution of citrate of ammonium. The process was completed by evaporating the solution sufficiently, and then spreading it out to dry on glass or porcelain, so that the salt was obtained in scales.† This formula was based upon a method, proposed by M. E. Robiquet to the Academy of Medicine at Paris, in Feb. 1857, of preparing pyrophosphate of iron for use, by dissolving a gelatinous precipitate of the salt in a solution of citrate of ammonium, and forming a syrup with the solution.

The view which obtained when this process was first made officinal was, that a double salt was formed, consisting of ferric pyrophosphate and ammonium citrate, which might be called ammonio-ferric citro-ortho phosphate. According to R. Rother (*A. J. P.*, 1876, p. 174), there was an excess of ferric citrate in the pyrophosphate of iron of the U. S. P. 1870, and it was believed to be a complex mixture of the colloid salts, ammonio-ferric pyrophosphate, ammonio-ferric citrate, and free ferric citrate, as shown in the reaction $2(Fe_4 3P_2O_7) + 6(NH_4)_3C_6H_5O_7 = Fe_4 3P_2O_7 \cdot 3(NH_4)_4P_2O_7 + 2(FeC_6H_5O_7 \cdot (NH_4)_3C_6H_5O_7) + 2(FeC_6H_5O_7)$. By mixing two molecules of ferric citrate and one of ammonium pyrophosphate a compound analogous to the officinal preparation was obtained, containing the same proportion of ammonio-ferric pyrophosphate, but mixed with twice as much ammonio-ferric citrate and free ferric citrate. Rother's views have been adopted by the Committee of Revision, as well as the salt which he recommended, in which ammonia was replaced by soda, because of the greater stability of the latter. Pyrophosphate of Iron, U. S. P. 1880, consists probably of sodio-ferric pyrophosphate, sodio-ferric citrate, and free ferric citrate.

The sodio-ferric pyrophosphate, dried at 100° C., is considered by Flückiger (*Pharm. Chem.*, 2d ed., p. 607, 1888) to have the following composition: $Fe_4(P_2O_7)_3 + 3Na_4P_2O_7 + 14H_2O$.

a half grains of phosphate of lime, with smaller quantities of the alkaline phosphates, all in perfect solution." The objection to such preparations as this is not that each of the ingredients may not be useful, but that they are so numerous that a morbid state of system must be extremely rare in which they can all be indicated, and every medicine is more or less noxious if given when it is not needed. The probability is that the therapeutic value of the preparation depends mainly on its ferruginous ingredient, and that, as a general rule, its therapeutic effects may be equally well if not better obtained from a simple syrup of phosphate of iron.

Simple Syrup of Phosphate of Iron. Subsequently, Mr. Wiegand gave a formula for a simple syrup of phosphate of iron, made by dissolving the recently precipitated salt in hydrochloric acid, and adding the requisite quantity of sugar. By a misprint the phosphate of sodium taken is double what it should be. The same writer has proposed to make a syrup of the phosphates of iron and calcium, by dissolving in the above a definite quantity of recently precipitated phosphate of calcium, made by double decomposition between solutions of chloride of calcium and phosphate of sodium. See his formulas in *A. J. P.*, 1855 (p. 104).

* C. N. Lake asserts that a better salt may be made by diminishing the proportion of pyrophosphate of sodium to eight parts. (*Proc. N. Y. State Pharm. Assoc.*, 1886, p. 170.)

† For these processes in detail and Soubeiran's *Syrup of Pyrophosphate of Iron*, see U. S. D., 15th edition, page 682.

Properties. "Thin, apple-green, transparent scales, permanent in dry air when excluded from light, but turning dark on exposure to light, odorless, having an acidulous, slightly saline taste, and a slightly acid reaction. Freely and completely soluble in water, but insoluble in alcohol. The aqueous solution of the salt is rendered blue by test-solution of ferrocyanide of potassium, but does not yield a blue precipitate with this reagent, unless it has been acidulated with hydrochloric acid. When heated with solution of potassa in excess, a brown-red precipitate is thrown down, and the filtrate, after being supersaturated with acetic acid, yields a white precipitate with test-solution of nitrate of silver (difference from phosphate). 100 parts of the salt represent about 11·5 parts of metallic iron." *U. S.*

Medical Properties. It is a very good chalybeate, mild yet efficient in its action on the system, without disagreeable taste, and, from its solubility, readily administered in any form that may be desirable, whether that of pill, simple solution in water,* or syrup. The dose is from two to five grains (0·13–0·33 Gm.). A syrup may be readily prepared by dissolving it in water, and adding simple syrup.

FERRI SULPHAS. *U. S., Br.* *Sulphate of Iron.* [*Ferrous Sulphate.*]

$FeSO_4.7H_2O$; 277·9. (FĔR'RĪ SŬL'PHĂS.) $FeO, SO_3.7HO$; 138·95.

Green Vitriol; Ferrum Sulfuricum Purum, *P.G.;* Sulfas Ferrosus, Ferrum Vitriolatum Purum, Vitriolum Martis Purum; Ferrous Sulphate; Sulfate (Protosulfate) de Fer, Sulfate ferreux, *Fr.;* Schwefelsaures Eisenoxydul, *G.*

"Take of Iron Wire *four ounces* [avoirdupois]; Sulphuric Acid *four fluidounces* [Imperial measure]; Distilled Water *one pint and a half* [Imp meas.]. Pour the Water on the Iron placed in a porcelain dish, add the Sulphuric Acid, and, when the disengagement of gas has nearly ceased, boil for ten minutes. Filter now through paper, and, after the lapse of twenty-four hours, separate the crystals which have been deposited from the solution. Let these be dried on filtering paper placed on porous bricks, and preserved in a stoppered bottle." *Br.*

The object of this process is to make a pure sulphate of iron by direct combination. Sulphuric acid, in a concentrated state, acts but imperfectly on iron; but when diluted, a vigorous action takes place, the oxygen of the water converts the metal into an oxide, with which the sulphuric acid unites, and hydrogen is evolved. The theoretical quantities for mutual reaction are 56 of iron to 98 of acid. This proportion is one part of iron to one and three-quarters of acid. The *British Council* uses an excess of acid, the weight of acid taken being 7·38 avoirdupois ounces, instead of 7. An excess of iron, however, is desirable, as it tends to secure the production of a perfect ferrous sulphate. A process for this salt was given in the U. S. P. 1870, which was based upon the method of Bonsdorff. This chemist found that, when a perfect sulphate of iron was formed in solution by heating dilute sulphuric acid with an excess of iron, it might be crystallized free from sesquioxide, provided a little excess of sulphuric acid were added to the liquid before filtration, in order to prevent the formation of any sesquioxide during the process; at the same time avoiding, as much as possible, the contact of the air. Hence the directions in the former U. S. formula to acidulate with sulphuric acid, to cause the funnel to touch the bottom of the receiving vessel, which avoids the dropping of the liquid through the air, and to cover the vessel containing the concentrated liquid, when it is set aside to crystallize.

Properties. Sulphate of iron is in the form of "large, pale, bluish green, monoclinic prisms, efflorescent and absorbing oxygen on exposure to air, without odor, having a saline, styptic taste, and an acid reaction. Soluble in 1·8 parts of water at 15° C. (59° F.), and in 0·3 part of boiling water; insoluble in alcohol. When quickly heated, the crystals fuse. When slowly heated to 115° C. (239° F.), they fall to powder and lose 38·86 per cent. of their weight (water of crystallization). "42·1 grains dissolved in water acidulated with sulphuric acid continue to give a blue precipitate with ferricyanide of potassium until about 500 grain-measures of

* *Liquor Ferri Pyrophosphatis.* A permanent solution may be made by Rother's process by dissolving 120 grains of pyrophosphate of iron in five fluidrachms of water with the aid of heat, filtering whilst hot, mixing the filtrate with two fluidrachms of glycerin, and adding enough water through the filter to make one fluidounce. (*Drug. Circ.*, 1886, p. 99.)

the *volumetric solution of bichromate of potassium* have been added." *Br.* The aqueous solution of the salt affords a blue precipitate with test-solution of ferricyanide of potassium, and a white precipitate, insoluble in hydrochloric acid, with test-solution of chloride of barium. When acidulated with sulphuric acid, the solution should yield no colored precipitate (copper), and not more than a faint white turbidity with hydrosulphuric acid (limit of ferric salt). If 4·167 Gm. of Sulphate of Iron are dissolved in water acidified with diluted sulphuric acid, and the solution treated with volumetric solution of bichromate of potassium, until a drop no longer gives a blue color with test-solution of ferricyanide of potassium, the required number of C.c. of the volumetric solution multiplied by *two* (2), equals the percentage of unoxidized ferrous sulphate in crystals." *U. S.* As prepared by Bonsdorff's method, ferrous sulphate is blue verging to green. When it becomes more green than blue, or entirely green, an indication is afforded that it contains some sesquioxide. By exposure to the air the crystals absorb oxygen, and become first green, and ultimately covered with a yellow efflorescence of subsulphate, insoluble in water. Sometimes the crystals are quite permanent when made by Bonsdorff's method, owing to the slight excess of acid which they contain. The aqueous solution is bluish green; but by standing it attracts oxygen, and becomes first green and then reddish, depositing, in the mean time, a portion of sesquisulphate, having the composition $Fe_2(SO_4)_3 + Fe_2O_3 + 8H_2O$. (Wittstein, *Chem. Gaz.*, May 15, 1849; from *Buchner's Repert.*) At a red heat it loses its acid, and is converted into the anhydrous sesquioxide of iron called *colcothar*. It is incompatible with the alkalies and their carbonates, soaps, lime-water, the chlorides of calcium and barium, the borate and phosphate of sodium, nitrate of silver, and the acetate and subacetate of lead. It is decomposed also by astringent vegetable infusions, the tannic and gallic acids of which form, if any sesquioxide be present, a black compound of the nature of ink. The extent to which this change lessens the activity of the salt is not well ascertained. Sulphate of iron, as kept in the shops, is often the impure commercial sulphate, which is not fit for medicinal use.* The perfectly pure salt is precipitated white by ferrocyanide of potassium; but that of ordinary purity gives a greenish precipitate, more or less deep, with this test, owing to the presence of some sesquioxide of iron. Copper may be detected by immersing in the solution a bright piece of iron, on which a cupreous film will be deposited. Both copper and zinc may be discovered by sesquioxidizing the iron by boiling the solution of the salt with nitric acid, and then precipitating the iron by an excess of ammonia. If the filtered solution is blue, copper is present; and if it contains zinc, this will be separated in flakes of white oxide, on expelling the excess of ammonia by ebullition.

It is often desirable to protect the sulphate of iron against the oxidation to which it is liable on exposure. Sugar acts as a preservative in the case of this salt, as in that of protiodide of iron. It may be added to the solution, or incorporated with the sulphate in substance. M. E. Latour has given a formula for crystallizing the salt with sugar. Mr. Geo. Welborn has found a small lump of camphor, wrapped in tissue paper, and placed in the bottle with the sulphate, to prevent its oxidation. (*P. J. Tr.*, May, 1868, p. 537.) M. Pavesi, of Mortara, effects the same object by incorporating it with an equal weight of gum arabic, by evaporating a joint solution of the two substances with a gentle heat. (*Journ. de Pharm.*, 4e sér., iii. 49.)

Medical Properties and Uses. Sulphate of iron is a very astringent chalybeate.

* *Commercial Sulphate of Iron. Copperas.* This was formerly officinal in the London Pharmacopœia, in which it was employed for preparing the pure sulphate. It is manufactured on a large scale for the purposes of the arts, from the native sulphide of iron, or iron pyrites, by roasting, oxidation by exposure to air and moisture, and lixiviation. The constituents of the mineral become sulphuric acid and ferrous oxide, which, by their union, form the salt. Sulphate of iron is also obtained in many chemical processes as a collateral product, as in the manufacture of alum, in the precipitation of copper from solutions of sulphate of copper by scraps of iron, etc.

Commercial sulphate of iron is far from being pure. Besides containing some sesquioxide of iron, it is generally contaminated with metallic and earthy salts; such as those of copper, zinc, alumina, and magnesia. Two principal kinds occur in the market; one in large grass-green crystals, the surface of which is studded with ochreous spots; the other, of a bluish green color, and ordinarily mixed with the powder of the effloresced salt. The commercial sulphate should never be dispensed by the pharmacist until it has undergone purification by recrystallization from a slightly acid solution.

In overdoses it produces nausea, vomiting, griping, and purging, and other evidences of gastro-enteric irritation or inflammation. Its astringency fits it especially for use when anæmia is conjoined with marked relaxation, or a tendency to immoderate discharges; such as passive hemorrhages, colliquative sweats, diabetes, chronic mucous catarrh, leucorrhœa, gleet, etc. Externally, the solution is used in chronic ophthalmia, leucorrhœa, and gleet, made of various strengths, from one or two to eight or ten grains of the salt to the fluidounce of water. M. Velpeau has found it an excellent remedy in erysipelas, applied topically in the form of solution or ointment. In forty cases in which it was tried, it cut short the disease in from 24 to 48 hours. The solution was made of three and a half drachms of the salt to a pint of water, and applied by compresses, kept constantly wet. In a few cases convenience required the application of the ointment, made of eight parts of the salt to thirty of lard. An ointment, made of one or two parts of the sulphate to sixty of lard, was found by M. Devergie to be particularly efficacious in certain skin diseases, especially in the different forms of eczema. In scaly affections it had no effect. The dose is one or two grains (0·065–0·13 Gm.), in the form of pill, which should be made from the dry sulphate. (See *Ferri Sulphas Exsiccata.*)

The sulphate of iron, usually in the form of the impure salt or commercial copperas, is a powerful disinfectant, although, according to experiments, its germicidal power is very feeble. When thrown into a mass of decomposing organic matter, a portion of it is at once precipitated as a sulphide or as an oxide by the sulphuretted hydrogen and ammonia present. It is asserted that ferric sulphate is capable of uniting with organic substances to form definite stable compounds, and that animal substances kept in a 3 per cent. solution of neutral ferric sulphate for a length of time and afterwards removed from it mummify without decomposition. (*New Remedies*, Dec. 1883, 685.)

Off. Prep. Ferri Sulphas Exsiccatus; Ferri Sulphas Præcipitatus; Ferri Carbonas Saccharatus; Liquor Ferri Subsulphatis; Liquor Ferri Tersulphatis; Mistura Ferri Composita; Pilula Aloes et Ferri; Massa Ferri Carbonatis; Pilulæ Ferri Compositæ.

Off. Prep. Br. Ferri Sulphas Exsiccata; Pilula Aloes et Ferri.

FERRI SULPHAS EXSICCATUS. *U.S.* *Dried Sulphate of Iron.* [*Dried Ferrous Sulphate.*]

$Fe SO_4. H_2 O$; 169·9. (FĔR'RĪ SŬL'PHĂS ĔX-SĬC-CĀ'TŬS.) $FeO, SO_3. HO$; 84·95.

Ferri Sulphas Exsiccata, *Br.;* Ferrum Sulfuricum Siccum, *P.G.;* Sulfate de Fer desséché, *Fr.;* Entwässertes Schwefelsaures Eisenoxydul, *G.*

"Sulphate of Iron, in coarse powder, *a convenient quantity*. Expose the Sulphate of Iron, in an unglazed earthen vessel, to a moderate heat, occasionally stirring, until it has effloresced. Then increase the heat to 149° C. (300° F.), and maintain it at that temperature until the salt ceases to lose weight. Lastly, reduce the residue to fine powder, and keep it in well-stopped bottles." *U. S.*

"Take of Sulphate of Iron *four ounces*. Expose it in a porcelain or iron dish to a temperature of 212° F. (100° C.) until aqueous vapor ceases to be given off. Reduce the residue, which should weigh rather less than two and a half ounces [avoird.], to a fine powder, and preserve it in a stoppered bottle." *Br.*

Properties. "A grayish white powder, soluble in water with the exception of a small residue, and answering to the reactions and tests of sulphate of iron. (See *Ferri Sulphas.*) 100 parts of crystallized sulphate of iron yield about 61 per cent. of the dried salt." *U. S.* "Ten grains dissolved in distilled water acidulated with sulphuric acid continue to give a blue precipitate with ferricyanide of potassium until at least 191 grain-measures of the *volumetric solution of bichromate of potassium* have been added, corresponding to at least 97½ per cent. of pure dried sulphate of iron." *Br.*

In these processes six mols. out of seven of the water of crystallization of the salt are driven off. The heat should not exceed 149° C. (300° F.), otherwise the salt itself would suffer decomposition. Dried sulphate of iron is used for making pills, the crystallized sulphate not being adapted to that purpose. In prescribing the dried sulphate it is necessary to recollect that three grains are equivalent to five of the crystallized salt.

Off. Prep. Pilulæ Aloes et Ferri.

FERRI SULPHAS PRÆCIPITATUS. *U.S.* *Precipitated Sulphate of Iron.* [*Precipitated Ferrous Sulphate.*]

(FĔR'RĪ SŬL'PHĂS PRÆ-CĬP-Ĭ-TĀ'TŬS.)

$Fe\,SO_4.\,7H_2\,O$; 277·9. $FeO,\,SO_3.\,7HO$; 138·95.

Ferri Sulphas Granulata, *Br.;* Granulated Sulphate of Iron.

"Sulphate of Iron, *one hundred parts* [or sixteen ounces av.]; Distilled Water, *one hundred and seventy parts* [or twenty-six fluidounces]; Sulphuric Acid, *four parts* [or two and a half fluidrachms]; Alcohol, *a sufficient quantity.* Dissolve the Sulphate of Iron in the Distilled Water, previously mixed with the Sulphuric Acid, and filter the solution. Allow the filtrate to become cold, pour it gradually, with constant stirring, into an equal volume of Alcohol [or two pints], and set the mixture aside for one day in a well-covered vessel. Drain the crystalline powder, which has settled in a funnel, wash it with Alcohol, until the washings cease to redden blue litmus paper, fold it in a piece of muslin and press it gently. Finally, spread the powder on bibulous paper and dry it quickly in the sunlight, or in a dry-room, at the ordinary temperature, and keep it in well-stopped bottles." *U. S.*

"Take of Iron Wire *four ounces* [avoirdupois]; Sulphuric Acid *four fluidounces* [Imperial measure]; Distilled Water *one pint and a half* [Imp. meas.]; Rectified Spirit *eight fluidounces* [Imp. meas.]. Pour the Water on the Iron placed in a porcelain capsule, add the Sulphuric Acid, and, when the disengagement of gas has nearly ceased, boil for ten minutes, and then filter the solution into a jar containing the Spirit, stirring the mixture so that the salt shall separate in minute granular crystals. Let these, deprived by decantation of adhering liquid, be transferred on filtering paper to porous tiles, and dried by exposure to the atmosphere. They should be preserved in a stoppered bottle." *Br.*

This preparation is officinal for the first time. The product is identical with the granulated sulphate of iron of the British Pharmacopœia. The process of the U. S. Pharmacopœia has the advantage of being more manageable and convenient, sulphate of iron being used directly instead of being made by the action of sulphuric acid on the metal. The directions given in the first part of the British process are precisely the same as those laid down by the British Council for making Sulphate of Iron; but the hot solution of the iron in the sulphuric acid, instead of being allowed to filter into an empty vessel, is made to drop into a portion of rectified spirit, the mixture being stirred while it cools. The acid directed is in excess; and the filtrate is consequently an acid solution of ferrous sulphate mixed with spirit. The stirring as the mixture cools, finely granulates the salt, which separates perfectly pure; the spirit holding in solution any tersulphate of iron which may have been formed, and the excess of acid dissolving any free sesquioxide. This process, in its main features, is that of M. Berthemot. (See 8th ed. U. S. D.)

Properties. Precipitated sulphate of iron is a "very pale bluish green, crystalline powder, efflorescent in dry air, but, when in contact with moisture, becoming gradually oxidized, without odor, having a saline and styptic taste, and an acid reaction. Soluble in 1·8 parts of water at 15° C. (59° F.) and in 0·3 part of boiling water; insoluble in alcohol. It should respond to the same reactions and tests as Sulphate of Iron." (See *Ferri Sulphas.*) Barckhauser, Salzer, and others have stated that ferrous sulphate precipitated by alcohol did not always contain 7 molecules of water, and it could not be relied upon for making volumetric solutions because of this lack of uniformity in composition. Caro (*Annalen*, clxv. 29) and Schlickum (*Pharm. Zeitung*, No. 49), on the other hand, maintain that precipitated ferrous sulphate is constant in composition, and Schlickum proved that if the precipitation took place in the cold it always contained 7 molecules of water, but *boiling* with strong alcohol diminished the proportion of water of crystallization.

"If 4·167 Gm. of precipitated sulphate of iron are dissolved in water acidified with diluted sulphuric acid, and the solution treated with volumetric solution of bichromate of potassium, until a drop no longer gives a blue color with test-solution of ferricyanide of potassium, the required number of C.c. of the volumetric solution, multiplied by *two* (2), equals the percentage of unoxidised ferrous sulphate in crystals." *U.S.* "41·7 grains dissolved in distilled water acidulated with sulphuric acid continue to give a blue precipitate with ferricyanide of potassium until 500 grain-measures of the *volumetric solution of bichromate of potassium* have been added." *Br.* When carefully dried it undergoes no change by keeping. It appears to have been introduced into the catalogue of the Dublin Pharmacopœia of 1850, as the best form of the sulphate for conversion into the officinal dried salt; and its peculiar state of aggregation would seem to fit it for that purpose; yet this intention, if it existed, seems to have been overlooked in the revision of the British Pharmacopœia, in which the granulated salt is not directed in the formula for the dried sulphate. The reason for its retention was probably that it is less liable to oxidation on exposure than the sulphate in its ordinary form, and experience has shown that it is admirably adapted for dispensing.

Off. Prep. Br. Syrupus Ferri Phosphatis.

FERRI VALERIANAS. *U.S.* *Valerianate of Iron.* [*Ferric Valerianate.*]

(FĔR'RĪ VA-LĒ-RI-Ā'NĂS.)

$Fe_2(C_5H_9O_2)_6$; 717·8. $Fe_2O_3.3C_{10}H_9O_3$; 358·9.

"Valerianate of Iron should be preserved in small, well-stopped vials, in a cool and dark place." *U. S.*

This preparation, which was officinal in the old Dublin Pharmacopœia, has been introduced into the new United States Pharmacopœia. It is rarely used, because of its insolubility. It may be made by precipitating a diluted solution of tersulphate of iron with a solution of sodium valerianate, collecting and washing the precipitate.

Properties. It is officinally described as "a dark tile-red, amorphous powder, permanent in dry air, having a faint odor of valerianic acid, and a mildly styptic taste. Insoluble in cold water, but readily soluble in alcohol. Boiling water decomposes it, setting free the valerianic acid and leaving ferric hydrate. When slowly heated, the salt parts with its acid without fusing, but when rapidly heated, it fuses and gives off inflammable vapors having the odor of butyric acid. On ignition, ferric oxide remains. Mineral acids decompose the Valerianate, forming the respective ferric salts and liberating valerianic acid." *U. S.*

FERRUM. *U.S.*, *Br.* *Iron.*

Fe; 55·9. (FĔR'RŬM.) Fe; 27·95.

"Metallic Iron, in the form of fine, bright, and non-elastic wire." *U. S.* "Annealed iron wire having a diameter of 0·005 of an inch, or wrought iron nails; free from oxide." *Br.*

Fer, *Fr.*; Eisen, *G.*; Ferro, *It.*; Hierro, *Sp.*; Mars, *Fr.*

In the U. S. Pharmacopœia, this metal is employed in different preparations, in the form of wire; it was officinal in 1850 as *Ferri Ramenta*, Iron Filings.

Iron is the most abundant and useful of the metals, and so interwoven with the wants of mankind that the extent of its consumption by a nation may be taken as an index of progress in civilisation. It is universally diffused in nature, not only in the mineral but also in the vegetable and animal kingdoms. There are very few minerals in which traces of it are not to be found, and it is an essential constituent in many parts of animals, but particularly in the blood. It is one of the few metals which are not deleterious to the animal economy.

Iron occurs, 1, native (almost exclusively, however, of meteoric origin); 2, sulphuretted in the minerals, pyrites (simple ferric sulphide), pyrrotine or magnetic pyrites, and arsenopyrite or mispickel (a sulph-arsenide of iron); 3, oxidised, embracing the magnetic, specular, red, brown, and argillaceous oxides of iron, together with chromite (mixed oxides of iron, chromium, and magnesium), and franklinite (mixed oxides of iron, manganese, and zinc); 4, in saline combination, forming carbonate, sulphate, phosphate, and arseniate of iron. Those minerals of iron which admit of being worked to advantage are called iron ores. These include the different native oxides, and the carbonate (spathic iron). The best iron is obtained from varieties of the native oxide, usually called magnetic iron ore and specular iron ore. These occur abundantly in Sweden, and furnish the superior iron of that country. The upper peninsula of Michigan now yields similar ores. As a general rule, those ores yield the best iron which occur in primitive formations.

Extraction. The mode of extracting iron from its ores varies somewhat with the nature of the ore; but the general principles of the operation are the same for all. The ore, previously broken into small pieces and roasted, is exposed to the action of an intense heat, urged by an air-blast, in contact with carbonaceous matter, such as charcoal, coke, or anthracite, and in connection with some flux, capable of fusing with the impurities of the ore. The flux varies with the nature of the ore, and is generally limestone. Fluorspar is occasionally used, but is not often found in sufficiently large deposits to be available. The flux, whatever it may be, enters into fusion with the impurities, and forms what is called the slag, which is a fusible silicate of lime chiefly; while the carbonaceous matter, acting on the oxide of iron, reduces it to the metallic state.

The reduced metal, from its density, occupies the lower part of the furnace, and is protected from the action of the air by the melted slag which floats on its surface. When the reduction is completed, the slag is allowed to run out by a hole in the side of the furnace, and the melted metal by an aperture at the bottom, the latter being received into long triangular moulds, where it solidifies in masses, known in commerce by the name of *pig* or *cast iron.* In this state the metal is brittle and far from being pure; as it contains from 3 to 6 per cent. of carbon, with silicon, phosphorus, sulphur, and manganese. It is purified, and brought to the state of *malleable iron*, by being fused and subjected, while stirred, to the action of a current of air on its surface. By these means the carbon is nearly burnt out, and the other impurities are oxidized and made to rise to the surface as a slag. Instead of this process, called "refining," usage in this country and England substitutes what is termed "pig-boiling," that is, the pig iron is at once submitted to the operation of puddling without previous refining. The "puddling" process consists in heating the charge of pig iron on the hearth of a reverberatory furnace in contact with ferric oxide and in a reducing flame. The silicon is first burnt out, and then the carbon gradually disappears; the phosphorus goes into the "tap cinder" as phosphide and phosphate; the sulphur also in part does so as sulphur dioxide and in part remains in the cinder as ferrous sulphide. As the metal approaches to purity, it becomes tough and less liquid, and its particles agglutinate so as to form semi-fused lumps, though the temperature of the furnace continues the same. These lumps are then taken out of the furnace, and their particles, by means of ponderous hammers moved by steam or water power, or by great pressure, are forced together so as to form one tenacious mass. The metal is finally rolled out into bars of a convenient size, when it constitutes the malleable iron of commerce.

The third form of commercial iron, known as "steel," is made either by the *cementation* process, or by the *Bessemer* process. In the former case, wrought iron is packed with charcoal and heated until combination takes place, and the resulting steel is cast into ingots. In the latter case, cast-iron is melted in large vessels called converters, when a blast of air is blown through the mass, burning out the requisite amount of carbon, and then, after addition of a small amount of *spiegeleisen*, or of manganiferous cast-iron, the finished product is run into moulds. Steel contains from one-half to one per cent. of carbon.

Iron mines occur in most countries, but more particularly in northern ones. In Spain, the principal mines furnish spathic iron and the red oxide. The chief iron ores of France are the spathic iron, and the specular, brown, and argillaceous oxides; of Germany, the spathic iron and brown oxide. The island of Elba is celebrated for its rich and abundant specular iron ore.

In the United States iron is abundant. The principal ores that are worked are the magnetic, red, and brown oxides. The magnetic oxide is found in large beds in Essex Co., N. Y., on the borders of Lake Champlain, and in the Lake Superior district; the red oxide in New York, New Jersey, Pennsylvania, and especially in a very pure state in Missouri, at Iron Mountain and Pilot Knob; the brown oxide in Eastern Pennsylvania.

Properties. Iron is a hard, malleable, ductile, and tenacious metal, of a grayish white color and fibrous texture, a slightly styptic taste, and a sensible odor when rubbed. In tenacity it yields only to nickel and cobalt. (*Deville.*) Its sp. gr. is about 7·7 (7·8, *U. S.*), and its fusing point very high. It possesses the magnetic and welding properties. It is combustible, and, when heated to whiteness, burns in atmospheric air, and with brilliant scintillations in oxygen gas. At a red heat, its surface is converted into black oxide, and at common temperatures, by the combined agency of air and moisture, it becomes covered with a reddish matter, called *rust*, which is the hydrated sesquioxide. It combines with all the non-metallic elements, except hydrogen and nitrogen, and with most of the metals. It forms three compounds with oxygen, a monoxide and sesquioxide, which, by their union, form the native magnetic oxide, and a trioxide, which forms an acid called ferric acid. The *monoxide*, or ferrous oxide, is of a dark blue color, attracted by the magnet, and spontaneously combustible in the air, being converted into sesquioxide. It is the base of green vitriol, and of the green salts of iron generally. It is very prone to absorb oxygen; and hence the salts which contain it are soon partially converted, when in solution, into salts of the sesquioxide. Its formula is FeO, consisting of one atom of iron, Fe, and one of oxygen, O, making its mol. wt. $56 + 16 = 72$. The *sesquioxide*, or ferric oxide, is readily obtained by dissolving iron in hydrochloric acid, precipitating by ammonia, and igniting the precipitate. It is of a red color, not attracted by the magnet, and forms salts, which for the most part have a reddish color. Its formula is Fe_2O_3, consisting of two atoms of iron, Fe, and three atoms of oxygen, O, making its mol. wt. $112 + 48 = 160$. An allotropic variety of the sesquioxide, soluble in water, and not responding to the ordinary tests of iron, has been discovered by M. Pean de Saint-Gilles. The *native black oxide*, the magnetic oxide of mineralogists, consists of one molecule of FeO, and one molecule of Fe_2O_3, making its mol. wt. $72 + 160 = 232$. Under the name of *Ferri Oxidum Magneticum*, the British Pharmacopœia has a preparation consisting of this oxide with three mols. of water. *Ferric acid*, discovered by Frémy, may be obtained, in union with potassa, by passing chlorine through a very concentrated solution of the alkali, holding the hydrated sesquioxide in suspension, or by fusing iron filings with nitre. This acid consists of one atom of iron 56, and three of oxygen $48 = 104$. Iron forms a number of important salts.

Iron is readily detected, even in minute quantities, by bringing it to the state of sesquisalt in solution, and adding ferrocyanide of potassium or tincture of galls; the former of which will strike a deep blue, the latter a black color. Bringing it to the state of sesquisalt is readily effected by boiling the solution containing it with a little nitric acid.

General Therapeutic Effects of Iron. The preparations of iron are pre-eminently tonic, and peculiarly well fitted to improve the quality of the blood, when impoverished from any cause. Hence they are useful in diseases characterized by debility, especially when the consequence of inordinate discharges. The diseases in which they are usually employed are chronic anæmia or chlorosis, hysteria, fluor albus, scrofula, rickets, passive hemorrhages, dyspepsia when dependent on deficient energy of the digestive function, and neuralgia. They are contraindicated in all inflammatory diseases, producing, when injudiciously employed, heat, thirst, headache, difficulty of breathing, and other symptoms of an excited circulation. In order to understand their effect in improving the blood, it must be borne in mind that this fluid always contains iron, as an essential constituent of the red corpuscles. The amount in ten thousand parts of blood, according to different authorities, is 2·3 parts (Le Canu), 2·4 (Denis), 5·5 (Becquerel and Rodier), 8·7 (Poggiale), mean 4·7. In anæmia the blood is deficient in iron, not because the red corpuscles contain less of the metal, for they, individually considered, always contain the normal quantity; but because there are fewer of them. (*Becquerel and Rodier.*) The question here arises, which are the preparations of iron best adapted to promote the formation of the red constituent of the blood, and what are the conditions of their administration most favorable to their efficient action? According to M. Bouchardat, the preparations most easily assimilated are metallic iron and the ferrous oxide; and, when the latter is in saline combination, it should be united either with carbonic acid, or with some organic acid. He holds that, when the iron is combined with a mineral acid, such as the sulphuric or phosphoric, the preparation acts solely as an astringent. Quevenne did not go so far as this, but believed that the mineral acid salts were not well adapted for assimilation, and that they were less so in proportion to their astringent power.

Quevenne laid it down as a rule, that, when the iron preparations are given with the view of improving the blood, they should be taken with the meals, and not on an empty stomach. Doses, thus given, are well borne, which often cause uneasiness and pain, when taken fasting. The gastric juice of the empty stomach is usually alkaline; and Quevenne proved that reduced iron, introduced, through a fistulous opening, into the stomach of fasting dogs, was not acted on, and was without effect in exciting the secretion. The juice, during digestion, is acid, and has been shown by the experiments of Quevenne to be in a favorable state for dissolving iron. The ferruginous preparations, it is true, were found to be unequally soluble; for, while iron filings were freely soluble, the subcarbonate of iron was but slightly attacked. It was observed that the acidity of the gastric juice was but little diminished by the solution of the iron; which fact can be explained only by supposing that the presence of the metal caused a nearly proportional increase of the acid secretion. Assuming these observations to be accurate, it is easy to perceive why the ferruginous preparations should be taken with the food, selecting of course those most soluble in the gastric juice. The digested iron, being intimately blended with the digested food, is in a favorable state for secondary assimilation. In the use of ferruginous preparations, it is necessary to persevere for several months, in order to reap the fullest benefit. Even after the cure appears to be accomplished, it is safest to continue them, in diminishing doses, for a considerable time.

IRON WIRE. *Ferri Filum. U. S.* 1850.

Fil de Fer, *Fr.;* Eisendraht, *G.;* Fil di Ferro, *It.;* Hilo de Hierro, *Sp.*

IRON FILINGS. *Ferri Ramenta. U. S.* 1850. *Limatura Ferri.*

Limailles de Fer, *Fr.;* Eisenfeilicht, *G.;* Limatura di Ferro, *It.;* Limatura de Hierro, *Sp.*

Iron, when employed in pharmaceutical operations, should be of the purest kind; and hence the Pharmacopœias generally direct it, when wanted in small masses, to be in the form of *iron wire*, which is necessarily made from the purest, because the softest and most ductile, iron, and is readily cut into pieces. The wire is very flexible and without elasticity.

Iron filings are usually obtained from the workshops of the blacksmith; but, as furnished from this source, they are generally very impure, and unfit for medicinal use. M. Gobley, upon examining thirty-six samples of iron filings, found but three exempt from copper. The rest, besides wood, sand, and oxide of iron, contained as high as 2 per cent. of this metal. Iron filings cannot be completely purified by the magnet; as they often have adhering to them bits of foreign matter, which are carried up with them. The only way to obtain them pure, is to file a piece of pure iron with a clean file. The French Codex directs iron in an *impalpable powder*, prepared by porphyrizing bright and clean iron filings without water. A dull black powder is formed, which must be carefully preserved from moisture. An impalpable powder of the metal, *Ferrum Reductum*, is officinal.

FERRUM REDUCTUM. *U.S.* *Reduced Iron.*

(FĔR'RŬM RE-DŬC'TŬM.)

Ferrum Redactum, *Br., P.G.,* U. S. P. 1870; Ferri Pulvis, *U. S.* 1850; Powder of Iron; Ferrum Hydrogenio Reductum, Ferrum Ope Hydrogenii Paratum; Iron reduced by Hydrogen, Iron by Hydrogen; Fer réduit par l'Hydrogène, *Fr.;* Reducirtes Eisen, *G.*

A process for this form of iron is no longer officinal; that of U. S. P. 1870 will be found in the foot-note.*

* *Ferrum Redactum.* "Take of Subcarbonate of Iron *thirty troyounces.* Wash the Subcarbonate thoroughly with water until no traces of sulphate of sodium are indicated by the appropriate tests,

"Take of Strong Solution of Perchloride of Iron, Solution of Ammonia, Zinc granulated, Sulphuric Acid, Chloride of Calcium, Distilled Water, of each, *a sufficiency*. Dilute the strong solution of Perchloride of Iron with five volumes of water; pour the mixture into such a quantity of Solution of Ammonia, diluted with five volumes of water, that the whole after thorough stirring has a distinct odor of ammonia. Wash the precipitated ferric hydrate until the washings are no longer rendered cloudy by solution of nitrate of silver. Dry the precipitate.

"Introduce the resulting ferric oxyhydrate into an iron tube, confining it to the middle part of the tube by plugs of asbestos. Pass the tube through a furnace, and when it has been raised to a strong but not bright red heat, cause it to be traversed by a stream of hydrogen gas developed by the action on the zinc of some of the sulphuric acid diluted with eight times its volume of water. The gas before entering the tube must be rendered quite dry by being made to pass first through the remainder of the sulphuric acid, and then through a tube eighteen inches long packed with small fragments of the chloride of calcium. The farther end of the iron tube is to be connected by a cork with a bent tube dipping under water; and when the hydrogen is observed to pass through the water at about the rate that it bubbles through the sulphuric acid, the furnace is to be allowed to cool down to the temperature of the atmosphere, a slow current of hydrogen being still continued. The reduced iron is then to be withdrawn, and enclosed in a dry well-stoppered bottle." *Br.*

This preparation was introduced into the United States and Dublin Pharmacopœias of 1850, and is retained in the present edition of our own, although the process for it has been abandoned. It consists of metallic iron in fine powder, obtained by reducing the sesquioxide by hydrogen at a dull red heat. The subcarbonate of the U. S. Pharm. 1870, which is essentially the sesquioxide of iron, is deprived of water by calcination, and then subjected to the reducing influence of a stream of hydrogen, purified from sulphuretted hydrogen and other acid by passing successively through a solution of subacetate of lead and milk of lime. The hydrogen unites with the oxygen of the sesquioxide to form water, and leaves the iron in the metallic state. The subcarbonate should be perfectly free from sulphate of sodium, which it is apt to contain when imperfectly washed. If this salt be present, it will be reduced by the hydrogen to the state of sulphide of sodium, which will contaminate and spoil the metallic iron formed, and cause the preparation, when taken, to give rise to unpleasant eructations. The heat should be carefully regulated; for if it fall below dull redness, part of the oxide will escape reduction; and, if it exceed that point considerably, the particles of reduced iron will agglutinate, and the preparation will be heavy and not readily pulverizable. The British process is not so well fitted for practical purposes as that of the U. S. Pharm. 1870. In the last revision of the British Pharmacopœia, instead of directing a certain quantity of hydrated peroxide of iron, a process is given in the formula for making the ferric oxyh .rate by precipitating a solution of ferric chloride. The direction to dry the hydrogen is unnecessary. On the subject of powder of iron, manufacturing chemists will find it useful to consult the paper of MM. Soubeiran and Dublanc, in which

and calcine it in a shallow vessel until free from moisture. Then spread it upon a tray, made by bending an oblong piece of sheet-iron in the form of an incomplete cylinder, and introduce this into a wrought-iron reduction-tube, of about four inches in diameter. Place the reduction-tube in a charcoal furnace; and, by means of a self-regulating generator of hydrogen, pass through it a stream of that gas, previously purified by bubbling successively through solution of subacetate of lead, diluted with three times its volume of water, and through milk of lime, severally contained in four-pint bottles, about one-third filled. Connect with the further extremity of the reduction-tube a lead tube bent so as to dip into water. Make all the junctions air-tight by appropriate lutes; and, when the hydrogen has passed long enough to fill the whole of the apparatus to the exclusion of atmospheric air, light the fire, and bring that part of the reduction-tube, occupied by the Subcarbonate, to a dull-red heat, which must be kept up so long as the bubbles of hydrogen, breaking from the water covering the orifice of the lead tube, are accompanied by visible aqueous vapor. When the reduction is completed, remove the fire, and allow the whole to cool to the ordinary temperature, keeping up, during the refrigeration, a moderate current of hydrogen through the apparatus. Withdraw the product from the reduction-tube, and, should any portion of it be black instead of iron-gray, separate such portion for use in a subsequent operation. Lastly, having powdered the Reduced Iron, keep it in a well-stopped bottle. When thirty troyounces of Subcarbonate of Iron are operated on, the process occupies from five to eight hours." *U. S.* 1870.

full directions are given for purifying the hydrogen, constructing the furnace, regulating the heat, and avoiding explosions. (*A. J. P.*, xviii., p. 303. For improvements by Prof. Procter, see *A. J. P.*, xix., p. 11.)

Since the tenth edition of this work was published, several processes have been proposed for obtaining powder of iron. Mr. Arthur Morgan, of Dublin, recommended the use of dried ferrocyanide of potassium, thoroughly mixed with anhydrous red oxide of iron, and calcined with pure carbonate of potassium at a low red heat. The product contains all the iron in a reduced state, mixed with soluble matters, which are carefully washed away. (See *A. J. P.*, 1854, p. 450.) A similar process to the above has been proposed by a German chemist, named Zängerle; the oxalate of iron being substituted for the red oxide. (See *P. J. Tr.*, 1857, p. 565.) Prof. Wöhler recommended the use of the same oxalate, not in connection with ferrocyanide of potassium, but as a suitable compound of iron for reduction by hydrogen. W. Müller found that oxide of iron obtained by heating the metal in the air is reduced when moist at 293° C. (559·4° F.); when quite dry, at 305° to 339° C. (581° to 642·2° F.); the oxalate moist, at 278° C. (532·4° F.). Another eligible compound for reduction is the crystalline powder of oxide of iron, prepared by fusing, in a clay crucible, pure dried sulphate of iron with three times its weight of chloride of sodium, and then washing the melted mass when cold, until everything soluble is removed. (*Wöhler.*) M. Crolas prepares a pure oxide of iron by adding chloride of barium to the solution of the chloride of iron to precipitate the contaminating sulphate, getting rid of the chloride of barium by crystallization and precipitating by solution of ammonia. The chloride of ammonium is driven off by heat. (*Journ. de Pharm.*, 4e sér., xx. 30.) The process of M. Eugène Fegueux consists in reducing the oxide of iron by carbonic oxide, formed by passing a stream of carbonic acid over red-hot charcoal in the reduction-tube, before it reaches the oxide of iron. The carbonic acid, thus reduced to carbonic oxide, is formed again by the deoxidizing of the ferruginous oxide.

Under the name of "*alcoholized iron*," a powder of iron has been introduced into this country, said to be prepared, in the eastern parts of Germany, by attrition of iron filings with honey, by some cheap method, as by attachment to a saw-mill or steam machinery. It has the appearance of powdered plumbago, but under the magnifying glass is seen to contain particles with the metallic lustre, and rounded as if by friction. It is soluble in diluted sulphuric acid, with the escape of hydrogen free or nearly so from sulphur; but a small quantity of a black powder remains undissolved. (*A. J. P.*, 1867, p. 11.) The relation of the epithet "alcoholized" to this powder is not very obvious, as this name was given originally to iron obtained by passing alcohol vapor over oxide of iron. It is not much inferior to reduced iron, and is better than some preparations sold by that name.

Properties. Powder of iron, called by the French *fer reduit*, is a light, tasteless powder, soft to the touch, of an iron-gray color, and without metallic lustre. If black, the preparation is to be rejected as not being fully deoxidized. When thrown into a dilute acid, it causes a lively effervescence of hydrogen without odor. A small portion of it, struck on an anvil with a smooth hammer, forms a scale having a brilliant metallic lustre. It takes fire upon the application of a burning body. On account of its great liability to oxidation, it should be kept in a dry bottle, well stopped. A black powder, having a composition corresponding with that of the magnetic oxide of iron, has been sold in London and Edinburgh under the name of Quevenne's iron. The spurious powder may be known by its having a black instead of an iron-gray color, and by its effervescing but slightly with acids. In the process for making reduced iron, part of the sesquioxide almost always escapes full deoxidation, and comes out of the tube a black color. This part should be rejected, instead of being sold as reduced iron, as appears to have been done by some manufacturing chemists. If the preparation has been very badly made, its solution in dilute sulphuric acid will produce an intensely red color with sulphocyanide of potassium. It is officinally described as "a very fine, grayish black, lustreless powder, permanent in dry air, without odor or taste, and insoluble in water or alcohol. When ignited in contact with air, it is converted into ferric oxide.

When treated with diluted sulphuric acid, it causes the evolution of nearly odorless hydrogen gas, and, on being warmed, it is dissolved without leaving a residue." *U. S.*

Tests of Purity. The Pharmacopœia gives a quantitative test, which is based on Carles's method* and that of the British Pharmacopœia. "If 1 Gm. of Reduced Iron be digested with 3·5 Gm. of iodine, 2·5 Gm. of iodide of potassium, and 50 C.c. of distilled water for two hours, the resulting filtrate should have a green color, and should not be rendered blue by gelatinized starch (presence of at least 80 per cent. of metallic iron)." *U. S.* "Ten grains added to an aqueous solution of fifty grains of iodine and fifty grains of iodide of potassium, and digested in a small flask and gently heated, leaves not more than five grains undissolved, which should be entirely soluble in hydrochloric acid." *Br.* Schacht (*Pharm. Zeitung; N. R.*, 1877, p. 207) proposes the following tests of purity. "It should be completely soluble in warm, diluted, pure hydrochloric acid, and the evolved gas (hydrogen) must be entirely indifferent against paper impregnated with lead acetate. When treated for half an hour with 25 parts of a solution of ferric chloride of spec. grav. 1·300, in a glass-stoppered vial, under repeated shaking, it is entirely dissolved."

J. Creuse communicated a valuable paper to the Amer. Pharm. Association in 1874, in which he showed the deficiencies of many brands of commercial iron by hydrogen, and recommended a test based on an estimation of the amount of hydrogen liberated from a definite weight of the reduced iron. O. Wilner (*Farmaceutisk Tiddskrift*, Aug. 1880; *A. J. P.*, 1881, p. 15) states that, 1. The amount of metallic iron in reduced iron can be accurately determined by treatment with mercuric chloride and titration with potassium permanganate. 2. If metallic iron is treated by the aid of a gentle heat with an excess of a concentrated solution of mercuric chloride, mercurous chloride and metallic mercury are separated, and the metallic iron passes as ferrous chloride into solution; the ferrous and ferric oxides which may be present remain undissolved, and therefore do not prevent the estimation of the amount of metallic iron in the reduced iron. 3. The amount of ferrous oxide in the preparation may be estimated by treating the same portion with hydrochloric acid, digesting the mixture in a closed vessel until the finely divided ferrous oxide becomes dissolved, and titrating with potassium permanganate. 4. The ferric chloride which is thus formed at the same time has no appreciable action upon the precipitated metallic mercury and mercurous chloride.

Medical Properties. Powder of iron, reduced from the oxide by hydrogen, was first prepared for medicinal purposes by Quevenne and Miquelard, of Paris. It is one of the best of chalybeate tonics, nearly free from astringency, and, according to Quevenne and M. Costes, of Bordeaux, yields the largest proportion of iron into the gastric juice. The chief objection to it is the difficulty of obtaining it well prepared. Much of the powder of iron found in the shops is not to be depended on, in consequence of imperfect reduction. Observations to determine its therapeutic value, compared with that of the other ferruginous preparations, were made by M. Costes, for nearly four years, at the Saint-André hospital, of Bordeaux, and with results highly favorable to it. The dose is from three to six grains (0·20–0·40 Gm.) several times a day, given in powder or pill. It is sometimes prepared with chocolate in the form of lozenges.

Off. Prep. Pilulæ Ferri Iodidi.

FICUS. *U. S., Br.* *Fig.*

(FĪ′CŬS.)

"The fleshy receptacle of Ficus Carica, Linné (*Nat. Ord.* Urticaceæ, Artocarpeæ), bearing fruit upon its inner surface." *U. S.* "The dried fruit of Ficus Carica." *Br.*

* P. Carles estimates the proportion of iron by the use of a titrated solution of iodine, containing 4·53 grammes of iodine and 5 grammes of iodide of potassium in a hundred cubic centimetres; one cubic centimetre of this solution is equivalent to ·01 gramme of iron. 0·1 gramme of the iron to be tested should be put in 5 grammes of water in a matrass and heated. Then the solution should be added from a burette. Sometimes a little continuance of the heat is necessary for the perfection of the reaction, which changes the color of the liquid persistent yellow. Before accepting the readings of the burette the residue should be tested with hydrochloric acid. Any effervescence shows that the iron has not fully combined with the iodine. (*Journ. de Pharm.*, 4e sér., xx. 178.)

Caricæ, *P.G.*; Ficus Passa, Fici, Fructus Caricæ; Figues, *Fr.*; Feigen, *G.*; Fichi, *It.*; Higos, *Sp.*

Gen. Ch. Common receptacle turbinate, fleshy, converging, concealing the florets in the same or distinct individuals. MALE. *Calyx* three-parted. *Corolla* none. *Stamens* three. FEMALE. *Calyx* five-parted. *Corolla* none. *Pistil* one. *Seed* one, covered with the closed, persistent, somewhat fleshy calyx. *Willd.*

Ficus Carica. Willd. *Sp. Plant.* iv. 1131; Woodv. *Med. Bot.* p. 714, t. 244. The fig-tree, though often not more than twelve feet high, sometimes rises in warm climates twenty-five or even thirty feet. Its trunk, which seldom exceeds seven inches in diameter, is divided into numerous spreading branches, covered with a brown or ash-colored bark. Its large, palmate leaves, usually divided into five obtuse lobes, are deep green and shining above, pale green and downy beneath, and stand alternately on strong, round footstalks. The flowers are situated within a common receptacle, placed upon a short peduncle in the axils of the upper leaves. This receptacle, the walls of which become thick and fleshy, constitutes what is commonly called the fruit; though this term is, strictly speaking, applicable to the small seed-like bodies found in great numbers on the internal surface of the receptacle, to which they are attached by fleshy pedicels. Cultivation has produced in the fig, as in the apple and peach, a great diversity in shape, size, color, and taste. It is usually, however, turbinate, or top-shaped, umbilicate at the large extremity, of the size of a small pear, of a whitish, yellowish, or reddish color, and of a mild, mucilaginous, saccharine taste. The dried figs can be partially restored to their original shape by soaking.

The fig-tree is supposed to have come originally from the Levant. It was introduced at a very early period into various parts of the south of Europe, and is now very common throughout the whole basin of the Mediterranean, particularly in Italy and France. To hasten the ripening of the fruit, it is customary to puncture it with a sharp-pointed instrument covered with olive oil. The ancient process of *caprification* is still practised in the Levant. It consists in attaching branches of the wild fig-tree to the cultivated plant. The fruit of the former contains great numbers of the eggs of an insect of the genus Cynips, the larvæ of which, as soon as they are hatched, spread themselves over the cultivated fruit, and, by conveying the pollen of the male organs over which they pass to the female florets, hasten the impregnation of the latter, and cause the fig to come quickly to perfection, which might otherwise ripen very slowly, or wither and drop off before maturity. Some authors attribute the effect to the piercing of the fruit by the young insects. According to Landerer, the unripe fig contains an irritant juice, which inflames the skin, and may even disorganize it. (See *A. J. P.*, xxxiii. 215.)

The figs, when perfectly ripe, are dried by the heat of the sun, or in ovens. Those imported into this country come chiefly from Smyrna, packed in drums or boxes. They are more or less compressed, and are usually covered in cold weather with a whitish saccharine efflorescence, which melts in the middle of summer, and renders them moist. The best are yellowish or brownish, somewhat translucent when held to the light, and filled with a sweet viscid pulp, in which are lodged numerous small yellow seeds. They are much more saccharine than the fresh fruit. Their chief constituents are grape sugar, which is present in the dried fruit to the amount of 60–70 per cent., and gum or mucilage.

Medical Properties and Uses. Figs are nutritious, laxative, and demulcent. In the fresh state they are considered, in the countries where they grow, a wholesome and agreeable aliment, and have been employed from time immemorial. They are apt, however, when eaten freely, to produce flatulence, pain in the bowels, and diarrhœa. Their chief medical use is as a laxative article of diet in constipation. They occasionally enter into demulcent decoctions; and, when roasted or boiled, and split open, are sometimes applied as a cataplasm to the gums.

Off. Prep. Confectio Sennæ.

FŒNICULUM. *U.S.* *Fennel.*

(FŒ-NĬCŬ-LŬM—fe-nĭk'yū-lŭm.)

"The fruit of Fœniculum vulgare. Gaertner. (*Nat. Ord.* Umbelliferæ, Orthospermæ.)" *U.S.* "The dried fruit of cultivated plants of Fœniculum capillaceum, *Gilib.* (Fœniculum vulgare, *Gaert.*)." *Br.*

Fœniculi Fructus, *Br.;* Fructus Fœniculi, *P. G.;* Fennel Fruit (Seed), Sweet Fennel Fruit; Fenouil, Fruits (Semences) de Fenouil, *Fr.;* Fenchel, Fenchelsamen, *G.;* Finnocchio, *It.;* Hinojo, *Sp.*

The plant producing fennel-seed was attached by Linnæus to the genus *Anethum*, but was separated from it by De Candolle, and placed, with three or four others, in a new genus styled *Fœniculum*, which has been generally adopted by botanists. The *Anethum Fœniculum* of Linnæus embraced two varieties, the *common* or *wild fennel*, and the *sweet fennel;* the latter being the plant usually cultivated in the gardens of Europe. These are considered by De Candolle as distinct species, and named respectively *Fœniculum vulgare* and *Fœniculum dulce*, but the correctness of the opinion of the great Swedish botanist is now generally admitted.

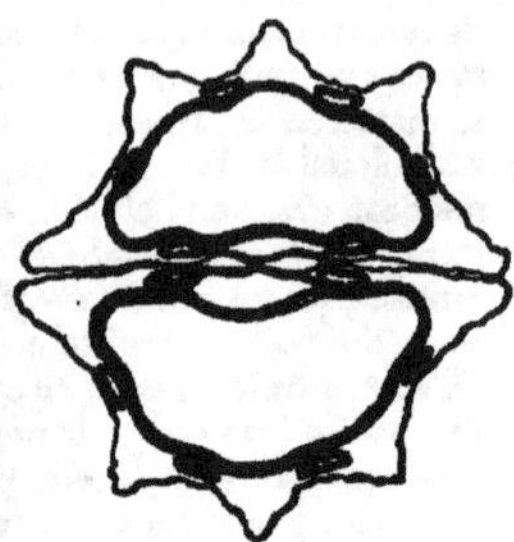

Transverse section of Fennel, magnified to show the oil-tubes.

Gen. Ch. *Calyx* a tumid obsolete rim. *Petals* roundish, entire, involute, with a squarish blunt lobe. *Fruit* nearly taper. *Half-fruits* with five prominent bluntly keeled ridges, of which the lateral are on the edge, and rather broadest. *Vittæ* single in the channels, 2 on the commissure. *Involucre* none. *Lindley.*

Fœniculum vulgare. De Cand. *Prodrom.* iv. 142.—*Anethum Fœniculum.* Linn.; Woodv. *Med. Bot.* p. 127, t. 49. *Common Fennel* has a biennial or perennial tapering root, and an annual, erect, round, striated, smooth, green, and copiously branching stem, which usually rises three or four feet in height. The leaves, which stand alternately at the joints of the stem, upon membranous striated sheaths, are many times pinnate, with long, linear, pointed, smooth, deep green leaflets. The flowers are in large, flat, terminal umbels, with from thirteen to twenty rays, and destitute both of general and partial involucres. The corolla consists of five petals, which, as well as the stamens, are golden-yellow. The fruit is ovate, rather less than two lines in length by about a line in breadth, and of a dark color, especially in the channels. The plant is a native of Europe, growing wild upon sandy and chalky ground throughout the continent, and is also abundant in Asia, possibly extending as far as China. The variety *F. officinale* of Merat and De Lens is chiefly characterized by its fruit being twice as long as that of the ordinary plant, and also a little curved, of a less dark color, with prominent ridges, and a persistent peduncle. It is sweeter and more aromatic than common fennel-seed.

F. dulce. De Cand. *Prodrom.* iv. 142. *Sweet Fennel* bears a general resemblance to *F. vulgare*, but differs in having its stem somewhat compressed at the base, its radical leaves somewhat distichous, and the number of rays in the umbel only from 6 to 8. It is also a much smaller plant, being only about a foot high; its flowers appear earlier; and its young shoots or turiones are sweeter and edible. In Italy it is cultivated as a garden vegetable, the shoots being eaten boiled or as a salad.

The roots of fennel were formerly employed in medicine, but are generally inferior in virtues to the fruit, which is now the only officinal portion. It is stated that manufacturers of the oil usually distil the whole plant. Commerce is partly supplied from the product of our own gardens; but much the larger portion of the medicine is imported from Europe, and chiefly, as we have been informed, from Germany. During the winter of 1879 much of the seed in the German market was adulterated with fennel-seed partially deprived of its oil. The fennel-seed cultivated here is sweeter and more aromatic than that from abroad, probably in consequence of its greater freshness.

Fennel-seeds (half-fruits) are oblong oval, from one to three or four lines in length, flat on one side, convex on the other, not unfrequently connected by their flat surfaces, straight or slightly curved, brownish or of a dark grayish green color, with fine prominent, obtuse, yellowish ridges on the convex surface. On section the vittæ or oil-tubes are seen to be very well developed, and to be situated one between each pair of ridges and two upon the flat face of each mericarp. There are two varieties of fennel seed; one which is probably the product of the wild fennel growing in the south of France, is from one to two lines long, dark-colored, rather flat, almost always separate, and without footstalks: the other is from three to five lines in length, lighter-colored, with much more prominent ridges, often conjoined by their flat surface, and very frequently provided with a footstalk. They do not differ essentially in aromatic properties. The odor of fennel-seed is fragrant, its taste warm, sweet, and agreeably aromatic. It yields its virtues to hot water, but more freely to alcohol. The essential oil may be separated by distillation with water. (See *Oleum Fœniculi.*) From 960 parts of the seed, Neumann obtained 20 parts of volatile and 120 of fixed oil.

Medical Properties and Uses. Fennel-seed was used by the ancients. It is one of our most grateful aromatics, and in this country is much employed as a carminative, and as a corrigent of other less pleasant medicines, particularly senna and rhubarb. It is recommended for these purposes by the absence of any highly excitant property. An infusion may be prepared by introducing two or three drachms of the seeds into a pint of boiling water. The dose of the bruised or powdered seeds is from a scruple to half a drachm (1·3–1·95 Gm.). In infants the infusion is frequently employed as an enema for the expulsion of flatus.

Off. Prep. Pulvis Glycyrrhizæ Compositus.

Off. Prep. Br. Aqua Fœniculi; Pulvis Glycyrrhizæ Compositus.

FRANGULA. *U.S.* *Frangula.* [*Buckthorn.*]

(FRĂN'GŪ-LA.)

"The bark of Rhamnus Frangula, Linné (*Nat. Ord.* Rhamnaceæ), collected at least one year before being used." *U. S.* "The dried bark of Rhamnus Frangula, *Linn.* Collected from the young trunk and moderate-sized branches, and kept at least one year before being used." *Br.*

Rhamni Frangulæ Cortex, *Br.;* Frangula Bark; Alder Buckthorn; Cortex Frangulæ, *P.G.;* Bourdaine, Bourgène, *Fr.;* Faulbaumrinde, *G.*

Gen. Ch. *Calyx* four- to five-cleft, the tube campanulate lined with the disk. *Petals* small, short-clawed, notched at the end, wrapped around the short stamens, or sometimes none. *Ovary* from two- to four-celled. *Drupe* berry-like, containing two to four separated seed-like nutlets. *Gray's Manual.*

R. frangula. Linn. *B. & T.* 65.—*Frangula vulgaris.* Reichert. The *Alder Buckthorn* is an erect glabrous shrub ten to fifteen feet high, without thorns, with broadly ovate obtuse leaves, with the margins entire or slightly sinuate, the under side sometimes slightly downy, and the rather numerous lateral veins diverging equally almost from the whole length of the midrib. Flowers all hermaphrodite, two or three together in each axil, with the calyx, teeth, petals, and stamens in fives. Fruit dark purple, the size of a pea. This plant grows in hedges and bushy places throughout Europe and Russian Asia, except in the far north.

It is probable that most of the species of the genus Rhamnus have cathartic properties. An article upon *R. Purshiana,* D. C., will be found on page 1286, as it is officinal in the Br. Pharmacopœia. The *R. catharticus,* Linn., or common buckthorn, grows in Europe along with the officinal species, and has become naturalized in this country. Its bark is probably often sold for the officinal article. It is distinguished by its more spreading, thorny habit, and its diœcious flowers, which are thickly clustered in the axils and have their parts in fours. The leaves also are more acute, have their margins finely serrate and their lateral veins mostly proceeding from the proximal half of the midrib. The fruit is black.*

* The berries, which are ripened in September, are of the size of a pea, round, somewhat flattened at top, black, smooth, shining, with four seeds in a green, juicy parenchyma. Their odor is unpleasant, their taste bitterish, acrid, and nauseous. Their blackish, expressed juice was formerly recognized in the Br. Ph. under the name of *Rhamni Succus.* It has the color, odor, and taste of the parenchyma, is reddened by the acids, and from deep green is rendered light green by the alkalies. Upon standing it soon begins to ferment, and becomes red in consequence of the formation of acetic acid. Evaporated to dryness, with the addition of lime or an alkali, it forms the color called by painters *sap-green.* The dried fruit of another species, *R. infectorius,* yields a rich yellow color, and is employed in the arts under the name of *French berries.* M. Fleury obtained a peculiar crystallizable principle, *rhamnin;* but he did not ascertain whether it possessed cathartic properties. (See *Journ. de Pharm.,* xxvii. 666.) Winckler obtained from the ripe fruit a principle which he called *cathartin,*

Properties. This bark is officinally described as "quilled, about one twenty-fifth of an inch (1 mm.) thick; outer surface gray brown, or blackish brown, with numerous small, whitish, transversely-elongated, suberous warts; inner surface smooth, pale brownish yellow; fracture in the outer layer short, of a purplish tint; in the inner layer fibrous and pale yellow; nearly inodorous; taste sweetish and bitter." *U. S.*

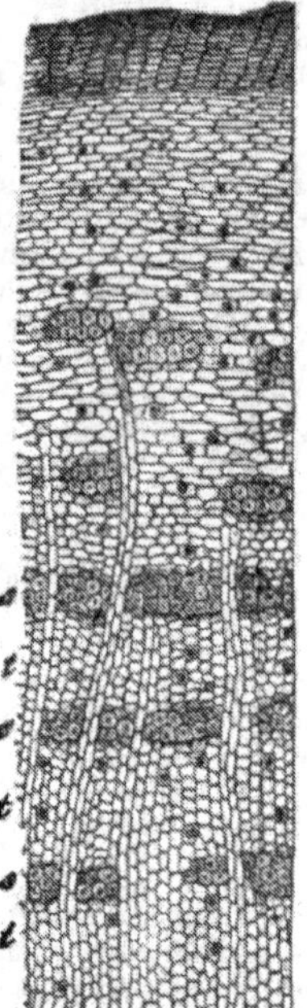

Frangula bark. *t*, bast-parenchyma; *s*, bundles of bast-cells. (After Berg.)

According to Prof. Schrenk (*Amer. Drug.*, April, 1887), the bark of *Rhamnus frangula* can be distinguished from that of *R. Purshiana* (*Cascara sagrada*) by the absence of the irregular angular sclerenchymatous cells, which in *R. Purshiana* are wedged together in large compact groups, increasing in size and number towards the surface, and causing the short fracture of the outer bark.

It is not certainly known which of the several bodies isolated from frangula bark is the purgative principle. The most important body, *frangulin*, the *rhamnoxanthin* ($C_{20}H_{20}O_{10}$) of Buchner and Binswanger, may be obtained by Phipson's process by macerating the bark for three or four days in carbon disulphide, then permitting the liquid to evaporate, exhausting the residue with alcohol, which leaves the fatty matter behind, evaporating the alcoholic liquid to dryness, and recrystallizing from ether. As thus obtained it is in fine yellow crystals, melting at about 249° C. (480·2° F.), and subliming in golden-yellow needles. It is insoluble in water, soluble in 160 parts of warm 80 per cent. alcohol, nearly insoluble in cold alcohol, soluble in hot fixed oils, benzin, and oil of turpentine. It communicates its color to cotton, silk, and wool. Faust (*Archiv d. Pharm.*, 187, 8) first proved the glucoside character of frangulin by boiling it in alcoholic solution with hydrochloric acid, obtaining glucose and *frangulinic acid*, $C_{14}H_{10}O_5$. This forms fine microscopic needles of reddish color, fusing at 248°–250° C. Liebermann and Waldheim (*Ber. d. Chem. Ges.*, 9, p. 1775) obtained in this decomposition instead of frangulinic acid *emodin*, $C_{15}H_{10}O_5$, which they consider to be trioxymethylanthraquinone. Frangulinic acid, on the other hand, would be a dioxyanthraquinone and an isomer of alizarine.

Medical Properties. In its fresh state this drug is very irritant to the gastro-intestinal mucous membrane, producing, when taken in sufficient quantity, violent catharsis, accompanied by vomiting, and much pain. During drying it is said to lose much of its irritant powers, and the dried bark is affirmed to resemble rhubarb in its action: hence the directions of the British Pharmacopœia that the bark should be at least one year old. A *decoction* (half ounce to the half pint) may be used in tablespoonful doses, or a dessertspoonful of an *elixir*, four fluidounces of

and believes that the rhamnin of Fleury, which was obtained from the unripe berries, is converted into that principle and grape sugar as the fruit matures. (*Chem. Gaz.*, viii. 282.) Lefort (*Journ. de Pharm.*, 1866, p. 420) studied Fleury's rhamnin, and describes it as forming pale yellow, translucent tables. It is scarcely soluble in cold water, soluble in hot alcohol, insoluble in ether or bisulphide of carbon. It is very soluble in caustic alkalies, from which it is precipitated by mineral acids. He gives it the formula $C_{12}H_{12}O_5 + 2H_2O$. Lefort also found a principle, *rhamnegin*, soluble in cold water, but otherwise agreeing in properties with rhamnin. Schützenberger (1868) decomposed rhamnegin, proving it to be a glucoside, having the formula $C_{24}H_{32}O_{14}$, and yielding *rhamnetin*, $C_{12}H_{10}O_5$, and a sugar isomeric with mannit. Schützenberger also finds a body isomeric with rhamnegin, and distinguishes the two as α *rhamnegin* and β *rhamnegin*, which, with Lefort's rhamnin, are present in buckthorn juice.

Liebermann and Hörmann (*Ber. Chem. Ges.*, xi. (1878), pp. 952, 1618) confirm Schützenberger's results, and give the name of *xanthorhamnin* to his α rhamnegin. They find his formula $C_{12}H_{10}O_5$ for rhamnetin to be correct, but get results that give for xanthorhamnin rather the formula $C_{48}H_{66}O_{29}$. Both the berries and their expressed juice are active hydragogue cathartics, apt to cause nausea and severe griping, and at one time much used in dropsy and also in rheumatism and gout. The dose of the recent berry is said to be about a scruple (1·3 Gm.), of the dried a drachm (3·9 Gm.), of the expressed juice a fluidounce (30 C.c.).

the fluid extract to twelve of elixir of orange, or the officinal fluid extract in doses of fifteen to thirty minims (0·9 to 1·9 C.c.).

Off. Prep. Extractum Frangulæ Fluidum.

Off. Prep. Br. Extractum Rhamni Frangulæ; Extractum Rhamni Frangulæ Liquidum.

GALBANUM. *U.S., Br.* *Galbanum.*

(GĂL'BA-NŬM.)

"A gum-resin obtained from Ferula galbaniflua, Boissier et Buhse, and probably from other allied plants. (*Nat. Ord.* Umbelliferæ, Orthospermæ.)" *U.S.* "A gum-resin obtained from Ferula galbaniflua, *Boiss. and Bohse;* Ferula rubricaulis, *Boiss.;* and probably other species." *Br.*

Gummi-Resina Galbanum; Galban, Mutterharz, *G.;* Galbano, *It., Sp.*

It is uncertain from what plant galbanum is derived. At one time it was supposed to be the product of *Bubon Galbanum*, an umbelliferous plant of the eastern coast of Africa. It has also been referred to the *Ferula Ferulago* of Linnæus, the *Ferula galbanifera* of Lobel, which inhabits the coast of the Mediterranean, and is found also in Transylvania and the Caucasus. But no part of either of these plants has the odor of galbanum; and it is, therefore, scarcely probable that they yield the drug. Mr. Don, having found the seeds taken from a parcel of galbanum to belong to an undescribed genus of umbelliferous plants, and concluding that they came from the same source as the gum-resin itself, gave the title of Galbanum to the new genus, and named the species *Galbanum officinale.* This was rather hastily adopted by the London College; as it is by no means certain that the same plant produced the seeds and the gum-resin. Specimens of a plant were received in England from Persia having a concrete juice adhering to them, which was taken by Dr. Lindley for galbanum: and that botanist, finding that the plant belonged to an undescribed genus, named it *Opoïdia*, with the specific name *galbanifera.* Dr. Pereira, however, found the substance not to be galbanum; and this supposed origin of the drug, therefore, must be considered as more than doubtful. A German traveller, F. A. Buhse, who has resided in Persia, states that, in 1848, he met with the *galbanum* plant on the declivities of the Demavend, near the southern coast of the Caspian. He saw the gum-resin exuding spontaneously from the plant, and was informed by the natives that the drug was collected from it. The plant is a Ferula, and has received the name of *F. galbaniflua*, Boissier and Buhse. Buhse also states that the Persian galbanum is yielded by a second plant, which is doubtfully distinct from *F. galbaniflua;* this is the *F. rubricaulis*, Boissier (*F. erubescens*, Berg). Galbanum is said to be obtained by making incisions into the stem, or cutting it off a short distance above the root. A cream-colored juice exudes, which concretes upon exposure to the air. A portion of juice also exudes spontaneously from the joints, and hardens in the shape of tears. The drug is brought from India and the Levant.

Properties. Galbanum usually appears in the form of masses composed of whitish, reddish, or yellowish tears, from the size of a pin's head to that of a pea, and larger, irregularly agglutinated by a darker colored yellowish brown or greenish substance, more or less translucent, and generally mixed with pieces of stalk, seeds, or other foreign matters. It is also found, though rarely in our markets, in the state of distinct roundish tears, about as large as a pea, of a yellowish white or pale brownish yellow color, shining externally as if varnished, translucent, and often adhering together. Galbanum has in cool weather the consistence of firm wax, but softens in summer, and by the heat of the hand is rendered ductile and adhesive. At 100° C. (212° F.) it is sufficiently liquid to admit of straining; and it generally requires to be strained before it can be used. A dark brown or blackish color, a consistence always soft, the absence of whitish grains, a deficiency in the characteristic odor and taste, and the intermixture of earthy impurities, are signs of inferiority.

The odor of galbanum is peculiar and disagreeable; its taste bitterish, warm, and acrid; its sp. gr. 1·212. Triturated with water, it forms an imperfect milky solution, which on standing deposits the greater portion of what was taken up. Wine and vinegar act upon it in a similar manner. Alcohol dissolves a considerable proportion, forming a yellow tincture, which has the smell and taste of galbanum, and becomes milky with water, but affords no precipitate. In dilute alcohol it is wholly soluble, with the exception of impurities. Ether dissolves the greater portion. "When moistened with alcohol, galbanum acquires a purple color on the addition of a little hydrochloric acid." *U. S.* It contains volatile oil, resin, and mucilage. The oil, amounting to 7 per cent., is a slightly yellowish liquid, partly consisting of a hydrocarbon, $C_{10}H_{16}$, boiling at from 170° to 180° C. The greater part of oil of galbanum, however, consists of hydrocarbons of a much higher boiling point. The crude oil is dextrogyrate. The resin, constituting about 60 per cent., is very soft, and dissolves in ether or in alkaline liquids, even in milk of lime, but only partially in bisulphide of carbon. When heated with hydrochloric acid for some time, it yields *umbelliferone*, $C_9H_6O_3$, which may be dissolved from the acid liquid by means of ether or chloroform, and obtained on evaporation in colorless acicular crystals. The aqueous solution of umbelliferone exhibits, especially on addition of an alkali, a brilliant blue fluorescence, which is destroyed by an acid. If a small fragment of galbanum is immersed in water, a fluorescence is produced by a drop of ammonia. Asafœtida shows the same, but ammoniacum does not.

Galbanum submitted to dry distillation yields a thick oil of brilliant blue color. This oil on rectification yields a greenish portion, and then a superb blue oil. Kachler (*Ber. Ch. Ges.*, 1871, p. 36) found a colorless oil, $C_{10}H_{16}$, and a blue oil, $C_{10}H_{14}O$, boiling at 289° C. The blue oil, according to Kachler, after purification, agrees with the blue oil of the flowers of *Matricaria Chamomilla.*

By fusing galbanum resin with potash, Hlasiwetz and Barth (*Ann. Ch. Pharm.*, 130, p. 354) obtained *resorcin*, together with acetic and volatile fatty acids.

According to Ludewig, a gum-resin, designated as *Persian galbanum*, is received in Russia by the way of Astracan or Orenburg, and is the kind used in that country. It comes enclosed in skins, and is in masses of a reddish brown color with whitish streaks, of a disagreeable odor, somewhat like that of asafœtida, and of an unpleasant, bitter, resinous taste. It is so soft as to melt with a slight elevation of temperature. It differs from common galbanum in its odor, in its color, which is never greenish, and in the absence of tears, and is probably derived from a different plant. It abounds in impurities. This variety of galbanum is probably the same as that obtained by Dr. Aitchison in Afghanistan, which on chemical examination yielded volatile oil, 3·108; resin (ether extractive 61·2, alcohol extractive 7·576), 68·776; water extractive (gum), 17·028; insoluble matter, 10·56 per cent. (*P. J. Tr.*, Dec. 11, 1886.)

Medical Properties and Uses. Galbanum was known to the ancients. It is stimulant, expectorant, and antispasmodic, and is considered as intermediate in power between ammoniac and asafœtida. It has chiefly been used in chronic affections of the bronchial mucous membrane, amenorrhœa, and chronic rheumatism. It is occasionally applied externally as a plaster to indolent swellings, with the view of promoting resolution or suppuration. The dose is from ten to twenty grains (0·65–1·3 Gm.), and may be given in pill, or triturated with gum arabic, sugar, and water, so as to form an emulsion.

Off. Prep. Emplastrum Asafœtidæ; Emplastrum Galbani; Pilulæ Galbani Compositæ.

Off. Prep. Br. Emplastrum Galbani; Pilula Asafœtidæ Composita.

GALLA. *U.S., Br.* *Nutgall.* [*Galls.*]

(GAL'LA.)

"Excrescences on Quercus lusitanica, Webb, *var.* infectoria, De Candolle (*Nat. Ord.* Cupuliferæ), caused by the punctures and deposited ova of Cynips Gallæ tinctoriæ. Olivier. (*Class*, Insecta. *Order*, Hymenoptera.)" *U. S.* "Excrescences on Quercus lusitanica, *Webb*, *var.* infectoria (Quercus infectoria, *Oliv.*), caused by the puncture and deposit of an egg or eggs of Cynips Gallæ tinctoriæ." *Br.*

Gallæ, *P.G.;* Gale Halepense, vel Heroica, vel Levantica, vel Tinctoria, vel Quercina; Galle de Chêne, Noix de Galle, *Fr.;* Galläpfel, *G.;* Galla, *It.;* Agallas de Levante, *Sp.*

Many plants, when pierced by certain insects, particularly those of the genus *Cynips*, are affected at the points of puncture with a morbid action, resulting in excrescences, which, as they are derived from the juices of the plant, partake more or less of its chemical character. Most of the oaks are occasionally thus affected; and the resulting excrescences, having in a high degree the astringency of the plant, have been employed for various practical purposes. They are known by the name of *galls*, a term which, as well as their use in medicine, has been handed down from the ancients. *Quercus infectoria*, *Q. Ægilops*, *Q. excelsa*, *Q. Ilex*, *Q. Cerris*, and *Q. Robur* have been particularized as affording this product; but it is now generally admitted, on the authority of Olivier, that the officinal galls are derived chiefly, if not exclusively, from *Q. infectoria*.*

QUERCUS. See *Quercus Alba.*

Quercus infectoria. Willd. *Sp. Plant.* iv. 436; Olivier, *Voy. Orient.* t. 14 *et* 15; Carson, *Illust. of Med. Bot.* ii. 40, pl. 85. The *dyer's oak* is a small tree or shrub, with a crooked stem, seldom exceeding six feet in height. The leaves are obtusely toothed, smooth, of a bright green color on both sides, and stand on short footstalks. The acorn is elongated, smooth, two or three times longer than the cup, which is sessile, somewhat downy, and scaly. This species of Quercus grows, according to Olivier, throughout Asia Minor, from the Archipelago to the confines of Persia. Captain M. Kinnier found it also in Armenia and Kurdistan; General Hardwicke observed it growing in the neighborhood of Adwanie; and it probably pervades the middle latitudes of Asia.

The gall originates from the puncture of the *Cynips quercûsfolii* of Linnæus, the *Diplolepis gallæ tinctoriæ* of Geoffroy, a hymenopterous insect or fly, with a fawn-colored body, dark antennæ, and the upper part of its abdomen shining brown. The insect pierces the shoots and young boughs, and deposits its egg in the wound. This irritates the part, and a small tumor quickly rises, which is the result of a morbid growth, exhibiting various cells under the microscope, but no proper vegetable fibre. The egg grows with the gall, and is soon converted into a larva, which feeds upon the vegetable matter around it, and thus forms a cavity in the centre of the excrescence. The insect at length becomes a fly, and escapes by eating its way out. The galls are in perfection when fully developed, before the egg has been hatched, or the fly has escaped. Collected at this period, they are called, from their dark color, *blue*, *green*, or *black galls*, and are most highly esteemed. Those which are gathered later and have been injured by the insect are *white galls*. They are usually larger, less heavy and compact, and of a lighter color than the former.

The galls collected in Syria and Asia Minor are brought to this country chiefly from the ports of Smyrna and Trieste, or from London. As they are produced abundantly near Aleppo, it has been customary to designate them by the name of

* Under the name of *Chinese galls*, a product has been brought from China, supposed to be caused by an insect allied to the Aphis, as such an insect has been found in the interior of them. They are irregularly spindle-shaped, often more or less bent, with obtusely pointed protuberances, about two inches long by an inch in diameter at the central thickest part, of an ash color and a soft velvety feel, very light, hollow, with translucent walls about a line in thickness, of a slight odor recalling that of ipecacuanha, and a bitter astringent taste. From an examination of fragments of leaves and petioles found among these galls, Dr. Schenck concluded that the tree on which they are found is a species of Rhus; but, according to M. Decaisne, professor at the Museum of Natural History in Paris, their true source is probably the *Distylium racemosum* of Zuccarini (*Flor. Japon.*, i. p. 178, t. 94), a large tree of Japan, the leaves of which produce a velvety gall, resembling the one in question. (Guibourt, *Hist. Nat. des Drogues*, 1850, iii. 703.) More recently, however, it has been asserted by Mr. Daniel Hanbury that this opinion of Decaisne is erroneous (*P. J. Tr.*, Feb. 1862, p. 421); as, in his examination of the packages imported from China and Japan, he has found remains of different parts of a species of Rhus, but never any of a Distylium. Besides, the form of the galls of the Distylium, as figured by Siebold and Zuccarini, is entirely different. The species of Rhus which yields the commercial Chinese galls is the *R. semi-alata.* (Murray.) The Chinese make great use of this product both in dyeing and as a medicine. L. A. Buchner, Jr., has found it to contain 65 per cent. of tannic acid identical with that of the officinal galls. (*Pharm. Centralblatt*, July, 1851, p. 526.) It is recommended by Stenhouse for the manufacture of gallic acid, being preferable for this purpose to the officinal galls, in consequence of its less amount of coloring matter. (*P. J. Tr.*, Dec. 1862.) An inferior kind of galls is produced in great quantities in England, by the attack of the *Cynips Kollari* of Hartig, upon the common English oak; but they have been ascertained to contain little tannic acid, and are of little value.

that town; though the designation, however correct it may formerly have been, is now wholly inapplicable, as they are obtained from many other places, and the produce of different parts of Asiatic Turkey is not capable of being discriminated, at least in our markets. Great quantities of galls, very closely resembling those from the Mediterranean, have been brought to the United States from Calcutta. Dr. Royle states that they are taken to Bombay from Bussorah through the Persian Gulf. We are, nevertheless, informed that galls are among the products of Moultan. Those of France and other southern countries of Europe have a smooth, shining reddish surface, are little esteemed, on account of their small yield of tannin, and are seldom brought to the United States.

Properties. Galls are nearly round, from the size of a pea to that of a very large cherry, with a surface usually studded with small tuberosities, in the intervals of which it is smooth. The best are externally of a dark bluish or lead color, sometimes with a greenish tinge, internally whitish or brownish, hard, solid, brittle, with a flinty fracture, a striated texture, and a small spot or cavity in the centre, indicating the presence of the undeveloped or decayed insect. Their powder is of a light yellowish gray. Those of inferior quality are of a lighter color, sometimes reddish or nearly white, of a loose texture, with a large cavity in the centre, communicating externally by a small hole through which the fly has escaped. The U. S. P. directs that "light, spongy and whitish-colored Nutgalls should be rejected," but allows "in the centre a cavity containing either the partly developed insect, or pulverulent remains left by it," and therefore permits white galls of good quality. Galls have a bitter, very astringent taste, and when whole are inodorous or nearly so, but bruised or in powder they have a decided and peculiar though not very strong smell. The tannin of galls, usually known as *gallo-tannic acid*, appears to exist in the galls, in part at least, as a glucoside, but one very easily broken up by ferments like pectase into glucose and *di-gallic acid*, $C_{14}H_{10}O_9$, which is the material, therefore, extracted from the galls. This di-gallic acid may be considered as the anhydride of *gallic acid*, $C_7H_6O_5$, formed from two molecules of this latter by the elimination of one molecule of water. Commercial tannin yields from 0 to 22 per cent. of glucose, showing the presence of varying amounts of the unaltered glucoside. Galls yield on an average from 65 to 77 per cent. of tannin. (See *Acidum Tannicum* and *Acidum Gallicum*, pages 114 and 60.) All the soluble matter of galls is taken up by forty times their weight of boiling water, and the residue is tasteless. Alcohol dissolves seven parts in ten, ether five parts. (*Thompson's Dispensatory.*) A saturated decoction deposits upon cooling a copious pale yellow precipitate. The infusion or tincture affords precipitates with sulphuric and hydrochloric acids, lime-water, and the carbonates of ammonium and potassium; with solutions of acetate and subacetate of lead, the sulphates of copper and iron, the nitrates of silver and mercury, and tartrate of antimony and potassium; with solution of gelatin; and with the infusions of Peruvian bark, columbo, opium, and many other vegetables, especially those containing alkaloids, with most of which tannic acid forms insoluble compounds. The infusion of galls reddens litmus paper, is rendered orange by nitric acid, milky by the corrosive chloride of mercury, and has its color deepened by ammonia; but yields no precipitate with either of these reagents. Sulphate of zinc was said by Dr. A. T. Thomson to occasion a slow precipitate, but this result was not obtained by Dr. Duncan. Infusion of galls is rendered more permanent by the addition of 10 per cent. of glycerin.

A variety of galls was imported into Germany, which was said to be derived from Central Asia, especially from the provinces of Khokan, Khiva, and Bucharia, where they are used in dyeing. They are of various forms, some being long, others round, cylindrical, or angular; and sometimes they are grouped upon a single stalk, and covered with little elevations. They differ from all other galls by their color, being on one side yellow, and on the other of a fine red. Most of them present a little opening; and in the interior are eggs and larvæ of a peculiar species of Aphis. They have yielded, on analysis, 43·10 per cent. of tannin, 3·03 of a green wax, 16 of cellulose, and an undetermined quantity of fecula and volatile oil. (R. Palne, *Journ. de Pharm.*, Avril, 1873, p. 336.)

Medical Properties and Uses. Galls are powerfully astringent, but are no longer used internally.*

Off. Prep. Tinctura Gallæ; Unguentum Gallæ.

Off. Prep. Br. Acidum Gallicum; Acidum Tannicum; Tinctura Gallæ; Unguentum Gallæ; Unguentum Gallæ cum Opio.

GAULTHERIA. *U.S.* *Gaultheria.* [*Wintergreen.*]

(GÂUL-THĒ'RI-Ą—gâwl-thē'rĭ-ą.)

Boxberry, Checkerberry; Feuilles de Gaulthérie (de Paloninier), Thé du Canada, Thé de Terreneuve, *Fr.*; Canadischer Thee, Bergthee, *G.*

"The leaves of Gaultheria procumbens. Linné. (*Nat. Ord.* Ericaceæ.)" *U. S.*

Gen. Ch. *Calyx* five-cleft, bibracteate at the base. *Corolla* ovate. *Capsule* five-celled, invested with the berried calyx. *Pursh.*

Gaultheria procumbens. Willd. *Sp. Plant.* ii. 616; Bigelow, *Am. Med. Bot.* iii. 27; Barton, *Med. Bot.* i. 171. This is a small, indigenous, shrubby, evergreen plant, with a long, creeping, horizontal root, which sends up at intervals one or two erect, slender, round, reddish stems. These are naked below, leafy at top, and usually less than a span in height. The *leaves* are short-petiolate, obovate or roundish-oval, about an inch and a half (4 centimeters) long, and three-quarters of an inch (2 centimeters) or more broad, acute, revolute at the edges with a few mucronate serratures, coriaceous, shining, bright green above, paler beneath, of unequal size, and supported irregularly on short red petioles. The flowers, of which not more than from three to five are usually on each stem, stand upon curved, drooping, axillary peduncles. The calyx is white, five-toothed, and furnished at its base with two concave cordate bracts, described by some as an outer calyx. The corolla is white, ovate, or urceolate, contracted at the mouth, and divided at the border into five small acute segments. The stamens have curved, plumose filaments, and oblong orange-colored anthers opening on the outside. The germ, which rests upon a ring having ten teeth alternating with the ten stamens, is roundish, depressed, and surmounted by an erect filiform style, ending in an obtuse stigma. The fruit is a small, five-celled, many-seeded capsule, with a fleshy covering, formed by the enlarged calyx, and presenting the appearance of a bright scarlet berry.

The plant extends from Canada to Georgia, growing in large beds in mountainous tracts, or in dry barrens and sandy plains, beneath the shade of shrubs and trees, particularly of other evergreens, as the Kalmiæ and Rhododendra. It is abundant in the pine-barrens of New Jersey. In different parts of the country, it is variously called *partridge-berry*, *deer-berry*, *tea-berry*, *wintergreen*, and *mountain-tea*. The flowers appear from May to September, and the fruit ripens at corresponding periods. Though the leaves only are officinal, all parts of the plant are endowed with the peculiar flavor for which these are employed, and which is found in several other plants, particularly in the bark of *Betula lenta*, or sweet birch. The fruit possesses it in a high degree, and, being at the same time sweetish, is much relished by some persons, and forms a favorite article of food with partridges, and other wild animals. To the very peculiar aromatic odor and taste which belong to the whole plant, the leaves add a marked astringency. The aromatic and medicinal properties of wintergreen reside exclusively in a volatile oil which is officinal and which alone is used in internal medicine. (See *Oleum Gaultheriæ.*)

Off. Prep. Syrupus Sarsaparillæ Compositus.

GELSEMIUM. *U.S., Br.* *Gelsemium.* [*Yellow Jasmine.*]

(ĢEL-SĒM'Ĭ-ŬM.)

"The rhizome and rootlets of Gelsemium sempervirens. Aiton. (*Nat. Ord.*

* *Aromatic Syrup of Galls.* The following old formula based upon one of Dr. Physick's is still sometimes employed. Macerate for twenty-four hours half an ounce of powdered galls, two drachms of bruised cinnamon, and two drachms of bruised nutmeg, in half a pint of brandy; then percolate, and, when the liquor has ceased to pass, add enough diluted alcohol to yield half a pint of filtered liquor. Put this into a shallow capsule, suspend over it two ounces of sugar on a slip of wire-gauze, and set the tincture on fire. The sugar melts with the flame, and falls into the liquid beneath. When the combustion ceases, agitate and filter. A highly astringent aromatic syrup is obtained, a fluidrachm of which may be given in diarrhœa. (*A. J. P.*, xxvii. 416.)

Loganiaceæ.)" *U.S.* "The dried rhizome and rootlets of Gelsemium nitidum, *Michaux* (Gelsemium sempervirens, *Aiton*)." *Br.*

Gen. Ch. *Calyx* five-parted. *Corolla* funnel-form, with a spreading border, five-lobed, nearly equal. *Anthers* oblong, sagittate. *Style* long and slender. *Stigmas* two, two-parted. *Capsule* elliptical, flat, two-valved, two-celled. *Seeds* flat, attached to the margin of the valves.

Gelsemium sempervirens. Gray, *Man. of Bot.*—*Gelseminum nitidum.* Michaux.—*Bignonia sempervirens.* Willd. *Sp. Plant.* iii. 291. Figured in *A. J. P.*, xxvii. 197. The *yellow* or *Carolina jasmine* is one of the most beautiful climbing plants of our Southern States, ascending lofty trees, and forming festoons from one tree to another, and in its flowering season, in the early spring, scenting the atmosphere with its

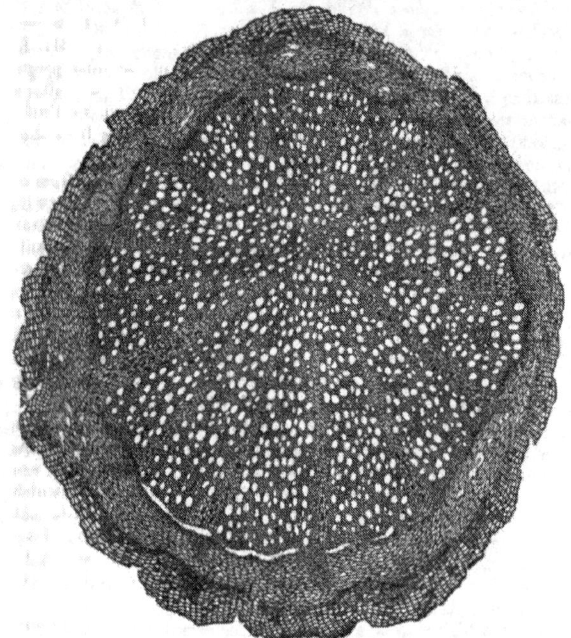

Gelsemium, transverse section.

delicious odor. The stem is twining, smooth, and shining; the leaves perennial, opposite, shortly petiolate, lanceolate, entire, dark green above, and paler beneath; the flowers in axillary clusters, large, of a deep yellow color, and fragrant, with a very small, five-leaved calyx, and a funnel-shaped corolla, having a spreading, five-lobed, nearly equal border. The fruit is a flat, compressed capsule, divisible into two parts, two-celled, and furnished with flat seeds, which adhere to the margins of the valves. The plant grows in rich, moist soils along the sea-coast from Virginia to the south of Florida. The flowers are said to be poisonous.

Properties. As we have seen it in commerce, the rhizome is sliced into pieces, about an inch in length, cylindrical or split, very light and fibrous, of a dirty yellowish white color, but darker where the epidermis remains, of a slight feebly narcotic odor, and a bitterish, not unpleasant taste. It is officinally described as "cylindrical, long, or cut in sections, occasionally an inch and a quarter (3 cm.) thick, the roots much thinner; externally light brown-yellow with purplish brown, longitudinal lines; tough; fracture splintery; bark thin, with silky bast-fibres, closely adhering to the pale yellowish, porous wood, having fine, medullary rays, and in the rhizome a thin pith." The figure (page 721) shows in transverse section the widening of the medullary rays from within outwards; another microscopic character, said by Prof. Rothrock to be diagnostic, is the more or less complete division of the pith into four parts by plates of large, thin-walled cells. (*A. J. P.*, 1884, 130.) Gelsemium yields its virtues to water, and readily to diluted alcohol. Analyzed by Mr. Henry Kollock, it was found to contain gum, starch, pectic acid, albumen, gallic acid, fixed oil, a fatty resin, a dry acrid resin, yellow coloring matter, volatile oil, extractive, lignin, a peculiar alkaloid called *gelsemine*, salts of potassa, lime, and magnesia, iron and silica. The alkaloid, however, was not obtained sufficiently pure to admit of a full investigation of its properties. (*A. J. P.*, xxvii. 203.) After Mr. Kollock's experiments, the alkaloid was obtained in a crystalline form, but still impure, by Prof. Maisch, from a tincture of the root, by a process of which a very brief abstract is given in *A. J. P.*, 1869, p. 36, by Mr. C. L. Eberle, who, in the same paper, publishes the results of his own investigation. Mr. Eberle not only extracted gelsemine, but satisfactorily established its alkaline properties, and proved that it was not contained in the wood of the root. Soon afterwards, the chemistry of Yellow Jasmine was more thoroughly investigated by Prof. Theo. G. Wormley. (*A. J. P.*, 1870, p. 1.) He obtained pure gelsemine from the root, and a peculiar acid, which he called *gelseminic* (gelsemic) acid.

Gelsemic or *Gelseminic Acid.* Prof. Wormley obtains the acid from a fluid extract of the root, which is actually a concentrated tincture, by evaporating it on a water-bath to about one-eighth of its volume, adding to the residue several times its bulk of pure water, allowing the mixture to stand until the supernatant liquid is nearly or quite clear, then transferring to a filter, washing the solids well with water, and reducing the filtrate thus obtained, together with the washings, on a water-bath, to about the volume of the concentrated fluid extract. To this, filtered if necessary, hydrochloric acid is added in the proportion of a drop of the pure acid to each fluidounce of the original fluid extract; the acidulated liquid is then agitated with twice its volume of ether; and, after the liquids have separated, the ethereal portion is decanted, the aqueous liquid again agitated with a similar quantity of ether, which is in its turn decanted, and the watery part finally washed with about its volume of ether. On mixing the ethereal liquids thus obtained, and allowing them to evaporate spontaneously, the gelsemic acid is left, chiefly in the form of nearly colorless groups of crystals, together with more or less yellowish or brownish resinous matter. From this the crystals are separated by washing with a little cold absolute alcohol, which dissolves the resin, with but a little of the crystals. To purify the crystals further, they are mixed with a little hot water, and extracted from the mixture when cool by chloroform, which, on spontaneous evaporation, yields them nearly if not quite colorless.

The acid, when pure, is colorless, inodorous, almost tasteless, and readily crystallizable, usually in groups or tufts of fine needles. It has strong neutralizing powers; combining with bases to form completely neutral salts, of which those formed with alkalies are freely soluble, while the others are at best but sparingly soluble in water. The acid itself is freely soluble in chloroform and ether, but slightly so in cold water, which takes up only about one-thousandth of its weight of the acid. Hot water dissolves it more freely, but on cooling deposits it in long, slender needles. The action of concentrated nitric acid may be considered as a test. If a drop of this acid be added to gelsemic acid or any of its salts, it forms a yellow, reddish, or red solution, which, if treated with ammonia in excess, becomes of a deep blood-red color, lasting for hours. The $\frac{1}{1000}$ of a grain will exhibit these changes. Caustic potassa, soda, or ammonia, added to the acid, causes it to become intensely yellow, and forms with it highly fluorescent solutions. The acid is fusible, and, at a high heat, volatilizable without change.

Robbins (*Deut. Chem. Ges.*, 1876, p. 1182), who has also investigated gelsemic acid, states that it is identical with *æsculin* (the glucoside of the horse-chestnut), and gives it the formula $C_{15}H_{16}O_9 + 1\frac{1}{2}H_2O$. Dragendorff (*Jahresb. für Pharmacog., Pharm. und Toxicol.*, 1878, p. 640) reinvestigated the constituents of Gelsemium sempervirens, and found æsculin and gelsemine, extracting the former out of an acid solution by chloroform and the latter from an alkaline solution by benzin and chloroform. Schwartz (*Inaugural Dissertation*, Dorpat, 1882) also found æsculin, the identity of which he established by a series of reactions, and some *æsculetin*, presumably from the decomposition of portions of the æsculin. The subject has since (*A. J. P.*, July, 1882) been re-examined by Prof. Wormley, who finds that gelsemic acid differs from æsculin in the following well-marked particulars: 1, in crystallization, the gelsemic acid crystallizes much more readily; 2, its insolubility in water and ether, the gelsemic acid is more soluble in ether and less soluble in water than æsculin; 3, gelsemic acid is not soluble in hydrochloric acid, while æsculin is; 4, corrosive sublimate gives a copious yellow precipitate with gelsemic acid, while it gives no result with æsculin; 5, sulphate of copper and acetate of lead yield precipitates with gelsemic acid differing from those of the same reagents with æsculin. Wormley, therefore, concludes that they are "very different substances."

Gelsemine, Gelsemia. This may be obtained, according to Wormley, from the concentrated extract from which gelsemic acid has been separated by ether, by rendering it slightly alkaline with potassa (Schwartz (*loc. cit.*) prefers soda solution on account of the too great energy of the caustic potassa), then agitating repeatedly with chloroform, which dissolves the alkaloid with some impurities, and yields it, when evaporated at a very moderate heat, in the form of a hard, gum-like, yellowish, or brownish yellow solid. If this be treated with a little water, and acidulated with hydrochloric acid, it yields the alkaloid with some impurities to the liquid, which, if now filtered, evaporated to about one-sixteenth by volume of the original fluid extract employed, and then treated with a slight excess of caustic potassa, will give up the alkaloid in the form of a more or less white precipitate. This, upon being separated, and allowed to dry, shrinks greatly, and becomes dark. To purify it, the dry mass is powdered, and dissolved, with the aid of a few drops of hydrochloric acid, in a little water, from which the alkaloid is precipitated by a slight excess of caustic potassa, and then taken up by ether, which leaves it, on spontaneous evaporation, in the state of a very hard, brittle, and transparent mass, strongly adhering to the surface of the vessel employed. If now detached and pulverized, it forms a powder nearly or quite colorless. If still colored, it may be again treated with ether.

Gelsemine was obtained in a much purer state than had been previously made by A. W. Gerrard. (*A. J. P.*, 1883, p. 258.) It is a brittle, transparent solid, crystallizing with difficulty from alcohol. Boiling water sparingly dissolves it. It softens at 38° C., and fuses at 45° C. The pure base gives no color reaction with strong nitric acid, and the mixture is scarcely changed in color by heating. Strong sulphuric acid has no apparent action upon it; but if to the mixture a little manganic oxide be added and rubbed with a glass rod a deep crimson-red is obtained, passing to green. This reaction is so delicate that it can be demonstrated with a solution of 1 in 100,000. If this reaction is performed upon the pure alkaloid, the color is sufficiently intense to cause it to be mistaken for strychnine; but if a parallel experiment be carried on with strychnine, the two alkaloids cannot be mistaken, for the strychnine gives an intense purple, passing to red. Gerrard analyzed the alkaloid with care, and gives the formula $C_{12}H_{14}NO_2$ as its correct composition. F. A. Thompson (*Pharm. Era*, 1887, p. 3) announced the presence of a second alkaloid, which he called *gelseminine*. After obtaining a solution of the alkaloids as sulphates he agitates it with an alkali and ether; the ethereal solution is shaken with water acidulated with hydrochloric acid, and the alkaloids are converted into hydrochlorates; hydrochlorate of gelseminine being easily soluble, and hydrochlorate of gelsemine less soluble, the latter is deposited on standing, and may be obtained pure by repeated crystallizations. He asserts that gelseminine differs greatly in physical and chemical properties from gelsemine; but, as he had not succeeded in obtaining it absolutely pure, does not give the differences.

Medical Properties.* Gelsemium produces in the healthy adult agreeable sensa-

* Gelsemium is said to have been long popularly employed as a vermifuge in the Southern and Southwestern States; but its more valuable properties have been known but for a few years. Their discovery was accidental. A planter of Mississippi, laboring under an obstinate bilious fever, directed his servant to get a particular root from the garden, and prepare a tea from it. The tea was

tions of languor, with muscular relaxation, so that the subject finds some difficulty in moving the eyelids, and keeping the jaws closed. More largely taken, it occasions dizziness, dimness of vision, dilated pupil, general muscular debility, and universal prostration; reducing the frequency and force of the pulse, and the frequency of respiration. After very pronounced poisonous doses the symptoms which have just been enumerated are intensified,—double or impaired vision, ptosis, dilated insensible pupils, falling of the lower jaw, loss of power of enunciation, and excessive muscular relaxation are associated with slow, labored breathing, which in some cases is interrupted by violent spells of dyspnœa; consciousness is long unimpaired, but is apt to be lost before death, and in rare cases unconsciousness has been present even although recovery followed. Of the various symptoms of gelsemium poisoning the most characteristic are the dropping of the jaw and the ocular manifestations, combined with general muscular relaxation. The effects usually begin in half an hour, but sometimes almost at once. According to Prof. Wormley, death has occurred at periods which vary from one to seven and a half hours. Twelve minims of the fluid extract are said to have proved fatal to a boy three years old, and thirty-five drops of a tincture of the bark have caused death in one hour and a half. In several instances a drachm of the fluid extract has under treatment been recovered from. Dr. M. P. Hatfield has recorded a case in which fifteen grains of a resinoid extract of gelsemium caused death in a woman in one hour.

The treatment of poisoning by gelsemium should consist in evacuating the stomach, maintaining absolute rest in the horizontal position, keeping up the bodily temperature, if required, by external warmth, and administering spinal and arterial stimulants. We have very little experimental data as to the physiological antidotes to gelsemium. Our general knowledge indicates that morphine, atropine, strychnine, and digitalis given hypodermically should be of service in the treatment of the poisoning, and Dr. Courtright (quoted by Wormley) narrates a case in which the hypodermic injection of three grains of morphine, in divided doses, within a few moments was followed by marked improvement and recovery, although the patient had taken between one and two teaspoonfuls of the tincture of gelsemium. The combined injection of atropine and morphine probably affords the best available treatment.

Recent physiological studies, whilst by no means complete, have thrown much light upon the action of gelsemium. The muscular weakness which it causes is always associated with a depression of reflex activity, and is the result of a direct paralyzing influence upon the spinal cord, as probably is also the diminution of sensibility; the nerves and muscles not being sensibly affected by the poison. The action upon the circulation is less marked than upon the nervous system, the heart and arterial pressure not being much affected by therapeutic doses. After toxic amounts there is great depression of the circulation, which has been shown by Dr. I. Ott to be at least in part due to a direct action upon the heart. The dilatation of the pupil which is present in poisoning with the drug, and which is also produced by its local application to the eye, is probably due to a paralysis of the oculo-motor nerve; to which also may be ascribed the palsy of accommodation and of the external rectus muscle. The diseases in which the medicine has been prescribed are intermittent, remittent, typhoid, and yellow fevers, the irritative fevers of childhood, inflammation of the lungs and pleura, dysentery, rheumatism and other inflammatory affections, neuralgia, dysmenorrhœa, morbid wakefulness, delirium tremens, trismus nascentium, chorea, hysteria, and epilepsy. The drug is, however, not applicable to the treatment of low fevers, and is not sufficiently powerful as a cardiac depressant to be relied upon in very sthenic inflammations; its use should be chiefly restricted to spasmodic and neuralgic affections. In supraorbital neuralgia and in odontalgia it has been especially commended.

prepared accordingly, and drunk by the invalid, who was soon afterwards affected with great prostration, and especially muscular debility, so that he could not raise a limb, but without stupor. These effects gradually passed off, and with them the fever. The servant had made a mistake in the root, and dug that of the Gelsemium instead of the one intended. The planter, having made this discovery, employed the root afterwards with success upon his own plantation and in the neighborhood. The remedy passed into the hands of irregular practitioners, and was used by the "eclectic physicians" before its virtues came to the knowledge of the profession.

There is much testimony as to its antiperiodic properties; and it may be used as an adjuvant to quinine in the treatment of remittent fever. Dr. James D. McGarghey praises it especially in cases of intermittent, when the attacks are disposed to return obstinately and irregularly. (*Phila. Med. Times*, March 7, 1874.) It has also been employed with a measure of success in controlling cardiac palpitations.

Gelsemium should be administered in the form either of the tincture or of the fluid extract; the dose of the tincture being ten minims (0·6 C.c.), that of the fluid extract two minims (0·12 C.c.); to be repeated, if necessary, every 2, 4, or 6 hours, and be gradually increased till the object is obtained, or some obvious effect is produced on the system.

The alkaloid gelsemine is exceedingly powerful. Prof. Wormley injected one-eighth of a grain into a strong cat, with the result of death in one and a half hours. He also found, as the average result of several experiments, that eight fluidounces of the fluid extract yield 3·20 grains of the pure alkaloid. On the basis of this result, the dose of gelsemine may be estimated at the 200th or 300th of a grain, supposing all the virtue of the root to reside in the alkaloid. But this estimate probably exceeds its strength; and the proper dose can be determined only by a series of carefully conducted trials.

Off. Prep. Extractum Gelsemii Fluidum; Tinctura Gelsemii.

Off. Prep. Br. Extractum Gelsemii Alcoholicum; Tinctura Gelsemii.

GENTIANA. *U.S.* *Gentian.*

(GĔN-TI-Ā'NA—jĕn-she-ā'na.)

"The root of Gentiana lutea. Linné. (*Nat. Ord.* Gentianaceæ.)" *U.S.* "The dried root of Gentiana lutea." *Br.*

Gentianæ Radix, *Br.;* Gentian Root; Radix Gentianæ, *P.G.;* Radix Gentianæ Rubræ (vel Luteæ vel Majoris); Racine de Gentiane (de Gentiane jaune), Gentiane jaune, *Fr.;* Enzian, Enzianwurzel, Bitterwurzel, Rother Enzian, *G.;* Genziana, *It.;* Genciana, *Sp.*

Gen. Ch. Corolla one-petalled. *Capsule* two-valved, one-celled, with two longitudinal receptacles. *Willd.*

Gentiana lutea. Willd. *Sp. Plant.* i. 1331; Woodv. *Med. Bot.* p. 273, t. 95; Carson, *Illust. of Med. Bot.* ii. 12, pl. 60. *Yellow Gentian* is among the most remarkable of the species which compose this genus, both for its beauty and great comparative size. From its thick, long, branching, perennial root, an erect, round stem rises to the height of three or four feet, bearing opposite, sessile, ovate, acute, five-nerved leaves of a bright green color, and somewhat glaucous. The lower leaves, which spring from the root, are narrowed at their base into the form of a petiole. The flowers are large and beautiful, of a yellow color, peduncled, and placed in whorls at the axils of the upper leaves. The calyx is monophyllous, membranous, yellowish, and semi-transparent, splitting when the flower opens, and reflected when it is fully expanded; the corolla is rotate, and deeply divided into five or six lanceolate, acute segments; the stamens are five or six, and shorter than the corolla. This plant grows among the Apennines, the Alps, the Pyrenees, and in other mountainous or elevated regions of Europe. The root is the only part employed.

Several other species possess analogous virtues, and are used for similar purposes. The roots of *G. purpurea* and *G. punctata*, inhabiting the same regions as *G. lutea*, and of *G. Pannonica*, growing in Austria, are said to be often mingled with the officinal, from which they are scarcely distinguishable. The *G. macrophylla* of Pallas is used in Siberia; one indigenous species, *G. Catesbæi*,* growing in the

* *Gentiana Catesbæi.* The blue gentian has a perennial, branching, somewhat fleshy root, and a simple, erect, rough stem, rising eight or ten inches in height, and bearing opposite leaves, which are ovate-lanceolate, acute, and rough on their margin. The flowers are of a palish blue color, crowded, nearly sessile, and axillary or terminal. The divisions of the calyx are linear-lanceolate, and longer than the tube. The corolla is large, ventricose, plaited, and divided at its border into ten segments, of which the five outer are more or less acute, the five inner bifid and fringed. The number of stamens is five, and the two stigmas are seated on the germ. The capsule is oblong, acuminate, with two valves, and a single cell. *G. Catesbæi* grows in the grassy swamps of North and South Carolina, where it flowers from September to December. It was named by Walter and Elliot in honor of Catesby, by whom it was delineated nearly a century ago. The dried root is said to have at first a mucilaginous and sweetish taste, which is soon succeeded by an intense bit-

Southern States, formerly had a place in the secondary catalogue of the U. S. Pharmacopœia, and is reputed to be but little inferior to the officinal species. *G. quinqueflora*, growing throughout the Northern and Northwestern States, is said to be much used in domestic practice.

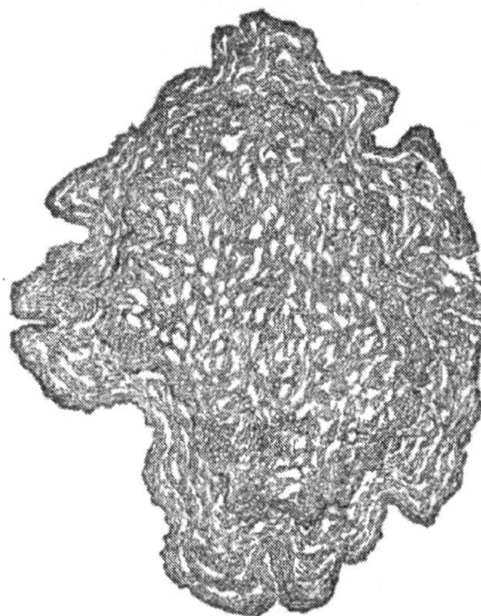

Gentian, transverse section.

Properties. As found in the shops, gentian is in pieces of various dimensions and shape, usually of considerable length, consisting sometimes of longitudinal slices, sometimes of the root cut transversely, twisted, wrinkled externally, sometimes marked with close transverse rings of a grayish brown color on the outside, yellowish or reddish within, and of a soft, spongy texture. It is officinally described as occurring "in nearly cylindrical pieces or longitudinal slices, about one inch (25 mm.) thick, the upper portion closely annulate, the lower portion longitudinally wrinkled; externally deep yellowish brown; internally lighter; somewhat flexible and tough when damp; rather brittle when dry; fracture uneven; the bark rather thick, separated from the somewhat spongy meditullium by a black cambium line; odor peculiar, faint, more prominent when moistened; taste sweetish and persistently bitter." *U. S.*

There is no distinct pith, no distinct liber-cells, starch granules, or raphides. (For further details, see *P. J. Tr.*, July, 1872, p. 42.) The odor is feeble, but decided and peculiar. The taste is slightly sweetish and intensely bitter, without being nauseous. The powder is yellowish. Water and alcohol extract the taste and virtues of the root.

Kromayer, in 1862, first obtained the bitter principle of gentian in a state of purity, and gave it the name of *gentio-picrin*, and the formula $C_{20}H_{30}O_{12}$. It is a neutral body, crystallizing in colorless needles, which readily dissolve in water. It is soluble in spirit of wine, but in absolute alcohol only when aided by heat; it does not dissolve in ether. A solution of caustic soda forms with it a yellow solution. Under the influence of dilute acids, gentio-picrin is resolved into glucose and an amorphous yellowish brown neutral substance named *gentiogenin*. Fresh gentian roots yield about $\frac{1}{10}$ per cent. of gentio-picrin. Another constituent is *gentianin* or *gentisin*, $C_{14}H_{10}O_5$. It forms tasteless, yellowish prisms, subliming with partial decomposition at a temperature over 300° C., sparingly soluble in alcohol, and, with alkalies, yields intensely yellow, crystallizable compounds, easily decomposed by carbonic acid. Hlasiwetz and Habermann showed, in 1875, that when *gentianin* was melted with caustic potash, it yielded *phloroglucin*, $C_6H_3(OH)_3$, and *oxysalicylic acid*, $C_6H_3.(OH_2)COOH$. The latter was at first called *gentianic* or *gentisinic acid*.

Prof. Maisch believes that tannin is absent from gentian root, and states that the dark, olive green coloration observed when ferric chloride is added to its preparations is due to gentisic acid (*A. J. P.*, 1876, p. 117). Ville (*A. J. P.*, 1877, p. 429) and Davies (*P. J. Tr.*, 1879, p. 220) maintain that there is a small quantity of

terness, approaching nearly to that of the officinal gentian. Alcohol and boiling water extract its virtues, and the tincture and decoction are even more bitter than the root in substance. It may be given in powder in the dose of from fifteen to thirty grains, or in the form of extract, infusion, wine, or tincture, which may be prepared in the manner directed for the similar preparations of foreign gentian.

tannin in gentian root. Prof. Patch (*A. J. P.*, 1876, p. 188) found that an alcoholic solution of an ethereal extract of gentian yielded a dark green coloration with ferric salts, but if the alcoholic solution were diluted with water it yielded no precipitate with gelatin. Subsequently (*Proc. A. P. A.*, 1881) he showed there was a principle associated with the resinous matter in gentian (but which was not isolated in a state of purity), that produced the reactions of a tannin, viz., a greenish black color with ferric chloride, and precipitates with tartar emetic, cinchonidine sulphate, and gelatin.

M. Louis Magnes found in the root, when perfectly dried at 100° C. (212° F.), 15 per cent. of glucose, and 12 per cent. in the root in its ordinary state. (*A. J. P.*, pp. 333–4.) When gentian is macerated in cold water, it undergoes the vinous fermentation, in consequence of the presence of this saccharine principle. From the fermented infusion a spirituous liquor is obtained by distillation, which, though bitter and unpleasant to the smell, is said to be relished by the Swiss and Tyrolese. A. Meyer (*Pharm. Centralb.*, 1882, May) obtained a sweet principle which he called *gentianose*, $C_{16}H_{66}O_{31}$, by precipitating the filtered juice with alcohol, treatment with ether, and crystallization from alcohol. It does not reduce Fehling's solution. Infusion of gentian is precipitated by tannic acid and the soluble salts of lead, but is compatible with the salts of iron.

Medical Properties and Uses. Gentian possesses, in a high degree, the tonic powers which characterise the simple bitters. It excites the appetite, invigorates digestion, moderately increases the temperature of the body and the force of the circulation, and operates in fact as a general corroborant. In very large doses, however, it is apt to load and oppress the stomach, to irritate the bowels, and even to occasion nausea and vomiting. It has been known as a medicine from the highest antiquity, and is said to have derived its name from Gentius, a king of Illyria. Many of the complex preparations handed down from the Greeks and Arabians contain it among their ingredients; and it enters into most of the stomachic combinations employed in modern practice. It may be used in all cases of pure debility of the digestive organs, or where a general tonic impression is required. Dyspepsia, atonic gout, amenorrhœa, hysteria, scrofula, intermittent fever, diarrhœa, and worms are among the many affections in which it has proved useful; but it is the condition of the stomach and of the system generally, not the name of the disease, which must be taken into consideration in prescribing it; and there is scarcely a complaint in which it can be advantageously given under all circumstances. Its powder has been applied externally to malignant and sloughing ulcers. It should be administered only in the form of preparation. A syrup may be prepared by forming a saccharated infusion by means of percolation, and incorporating this at a boiling heat with simple syrup; or, perhaps more eligibly, by dissolving two drachms of the extract of gentian, and afterwards fifteen ounces of sugar, in half a pint of water. The porous property of the root causes it to expand with moisture, and it has been employed, as a substitute for sponge tent, in the enlargement of strictured passages.

Off. Prep. Extractum Gentianæ; Extractum Gentianæ Fluidum; Tinctura Gentianæ Composita.

Off. Prep. Br. Extractum Gentianæ; Infusum Gentianæ Compositum; Tinctura Gentianæ Composita.

GERANIUM. *U. S.* *Geranium.* [*Cranesbill.*]

(GE-RĀ'NI-ŬM.)

"The rhizome of Geranium maculatum. Linné. (*Nat. Ord.* Geraniaceæ)." *U. S.*

Cranesbill Root; Racine de Bec-de-Grue tacheté, Racine de Pied-de-Corneille, *Fr.*; Fleckstorchschnabel-Wurzel, *G.*

Gen. Ch. Calyx five-leaved. *Corolla* five-petalled, regular. *Nectary* five melliferous glands, united to the base of the longer filaments. *Arilli* five, one-seeded, awned, at the base of a beaked receptacle; awns simple, naked, neither spiral nor bearded. *Willd.*

Geranium maculatum. Willd. *Sp. Plant.* iii. 705; Bigelow, *Am. Med. Bot.* i. 84; Barton, *Med. Bot.* i. 149. This plant has a perennial, horizontal, fleshy root, which is furnished with short fibres, and sends up annually an herbaceous stem, with several radical leaves. The stem is erect, round, dichotomously branched, from one to two feet high, of a grayish green color, and thickly covered, in common with the petioles and peduncles, with reflexed hairs. The leaves are deeply divided into three, five, or seven lobes, which are variously incised at their extremities, hairy, and of a pale green color, mottled with still paler spots. Those which rise from the root are supported on footstalks eight or ten inches long; those of the stem are opposite, the lower petiolate, the upper nearly sessile, with lanceolate or linear stipules. The flowers are large, and usually of a purple color. The peduncles spring from the forks of the stem, and severally support two flowers upon short pedicels. The calyx is composed of five oblong, ribbed, cuspidate leaves; the petals are five, obovate, and entire; the stamens ten, with oblong, deciduous anthers, the five alternate filaments being longer than the others, and having glands at their base; the germ is ovate, supporting a straight style as long as the stamens, and surmounted by five stigmas. The fruit consists of five aggregate, one-seeded capsules, attached by a beak to the persistent style, curling up and scattering the seeds when ripe.

The cranesbill is indigenous, growing throughout the United States, in moist woods, thickets, and hedges, and generally in low grounds. It flowers from May to July. The root should be collected in autumn.

Properties. Geranium occurs in pieces from one to three inches long, from a quarter to half an inch in thickness, somewhat flattened, contorted, wrinkled, tuberculated, and beset with slender fibres. It is externally of an umber-brown color, internally reddish gray, compact, inodorous, and of an astringent taste, without bitterness or other unpleasant flavor. "The bark is thin; the wood-wedges yellowish, small, forming a circle near the cambium line; the medullary rays broad; the central pith large, and the rootlets thin and fragile." Water and alcohol extract the virtues of geranium. According to Dr. Edward Staples, it contains tannic and gallic acids, mucilage, red coloring matter, resin, and a crystallizable vegetable principle. (*A. J. P.*, 1829, p. 171.) The Messrs. Tilden found, besides tannic and gallic acids, gum, pectin, sugar, starch, albumen, resin soluble in alcohol, oleoresin soluble in ether only, coloring matter, chlorophyll, lignin, and various salts. (*P. J. Tr.*, 1863, p. 22.) Tannic and gallic acids are probably the sole active ingredients.

Medical Properties and Uses. Geranium is one of our best indigenous astringents, and may be employed for all the purposes to which these medicines are applicable. The absence of unpleasant taste, and of other offensive qualities, renders it peculiarly serviceable in the case of infants, and persons of very delicate stomach. Diarrhœa, chronic dysentery, cholera infantum in the latter stages, and the various hemorrhages are the forms of disease in which it is most commonly used, and with greatest advantage; but care should be taken, before it is administered, that the condition of the system and of the part affected is such as not to contraindicate the use of astringents. As an application to indolent ulcers, an injection in gleet and leucorrhœa, and a gargle in relaxation of the uvula and aphthous ulcerations of the throat, it answers the same purpose as kino, catechu, and other medicines of the same class. It is a popular domestic remedy in various parts of the United States, and is said to be employed by the Indians. It may be given in substance, decoction, tincture, or extract. The dose of the powder is twenty or thirty grains (1·3–1·95 Gm.); that of a decoction, made by boiling an ounce of the root in a pint and a half of water to a pint, from one to two fluidounces (30–60 C.c.); that of the fluid extract, twenty to thirty minims (1·25 to 1·9 C.c.). The medicine is sometimes given to children, boiled in milk.

Off. Prep. Extractum Geranii Fluidum.

GLYCERINUM. *U.S.*, *Br.* *Glycerin.*

(GLỸÇ-Ē-RĪ′NŬM.)

Glycerina, *U. S.* 1870; Glycerine; Glycerinum, *P.G.;* Glycérine, *Fr.;* Oelsüss, *G.*

"A liquid obtained by the decomposition of fats and fixed oils, and containing not less than 95 per cent. of absolute Glycerin [$C_3H_5(HO)_3$; **92.** — $C_6H_5O_3.3HO$; 92.]" *U.S.* "A sweet principle, $C_3H_5(HO)_3$, obtained by reaction of fats and fixed oils with aqueous fluids, and containing a small percentage of water." *Br.*

In the process for making lead plaster, litharge, olive oil, and water are boiled together, when the olein of the oil is decomposed by the lead oxide, according to the following reaction: $2(C_3H_5(OC_{18}H_{33}O)_3) + (PbO)_3 + (H_2O)_3 = 2(C_3H_5(OH)_3) + 3(Pb(OC_{18}H_{33}O)_2)$, when we obtain lead oleate or plaster and free glycerin. (See *Emplastrum Plumbi.*) It follows, therefore, that the plaster, while still hot and in the liquid state, contained glycerin diffused through it. It was this process that was used for preparing glycerin in the formula of U. S. P. 1850. In accordance with this, when the liquid plaster is mixed with an equal measure of boiling water, and the mixture stirred briskly, a solution of glycerin is obtained; which, after having been decanted, and evaporated to a limited extent, is freed from lead by sulphuretted hydrogen. The liquid is then filtered to separate sulphide of lead, heated to free it from sulphuretted hydrogen, and finally evaporated to expel the water, which is known to be all removed when the mass ceases to lose weight.

Glycerin was discovered in 1789 by Scheele, by whom it was called the *sweet principle of oils.* It is produced not only during the saponification of the fats and oils by oxide of lead in forming lead plaster, but also during the same process when effected by potassa and soda in the manufacture of soap; the alkalies uniting with the oily acids, and setting the glycerin free. Soap-makers' waste is an abundant source of glycerin; but when thus obtained, it is apt to have more or less odor, which even percolation through animal charcoal does not always remove. The two methods of saponification by which glycerin has been obtained on a large scale are the process of Wilson and Payne, of decomposing the fats by superheated steam and after distillation, and the lime autoclave process of Milly. A new process, lately patented by Michaud Frères, of Paris, and operated by the Continental Glycerine Co., of New York, decomposes the fats by high-pressure steam in the presence of a small quantity of zinc oxide. The glycerin is obtained pure, and the fat acids can be saponified afterwards. The process of Mr. Richard A. Tilghman, of this city (the patent for which was obtained in 1854, and, after years of litigation, is at last sustained, 1888), consists in subjecting fatty bodies to the action of water at a high temperature under pressure, whereby the fats, which are *glycerides* or ethers of the fatty acids, are broken up into free glycerin and free fatty acids, the water supplying the elements of hydrogen and oxygen necessary for that change. The reaction is as follows for the case of a fat like stearin: $C_3H_5(OC_{18}H_{35}O)_3 + (H.OH)_3 = C_3H_5(OH)_3 + 3(C_{18}H_{35}O.OH)$. (*A. J. P.*, March, 1855, p. 121.) Through a distillatory apparatus containing palm oil, heated steam between 550° and 600° is passed. The oil is decomposed into free acids and glycerin, which, together with water, distil over, and, condensing in the receiver, separate into two layers, the lower of which is glycerin. If this, as first procured, contain too much water, it must be concentrated; if discolored, it must be redistilled with vapor. (*P. J. Tr.*, 1861, p. 350.) Ordinary impure glycerin may be purified by distillation with steam under pressure. Though, when distilled alone, it is partially decomposed, giving off pungent vapors of *acrolein*, yet in a current of superheated steam it passes over unchanged at temperatures between 204·4° C. and 260° C. (400° F. and 500° F.). (*Brande & Taylor.*) Very pure glycerin is now produced in the United States in immense quantities. The census of 1880 reported 7,117,825 lbs. as produced that year, of which one-half was used for nitroglycerin manufacture. The European production, according to the best authorities, is at present about 9000 tons yearly. The importation into the United States for 1887 was 12,765,072 lbs. For interesting statistics of its manufacture in Cincinnati, see *Pharm. Era*, 1887, p. 70. (See *Nitroglycerin*, Part II.)

Properties. Glycerin is, "a clear, colorless liquid, of syrupy consistence, oily to the touch, hygroscopic, without odor, very sweet and slightly warm to the taste, and neutral in reaction. It is soluble, in all proportions, in water and in alcohol, also in a mixture of 3 parts of alcohol and 1 part of ether, but insoluble in ether, chloroform, benzol, or fixed oils. Its sp. gr. should not be less than 1·250, corresponding to the presence of at least 95 per cent. of absolute Glycerin. In solution with water it is slowly vaporized, with steam, at 100° C. (212° F.); exposed alone to higher temperature, it yields acrid decomposition vapors of a characteristic odor, with a little Glycerin vapor, and at 290° C. (554° F.) it boils, and is decomposed.

If a fused bead of borax, on a loop of platinum wire, be moistened with Glycerin previously made slightly alkaline with diluted solution of soda, and after a few minutes held in a colorless flame, the latter will be tinted deep green." *U. S.* This last officinal test is that of Senier and Lowe. (*Jour. Chem. Society*, Sept. 1878.) In properties, glycerin is intermediate between water and the oils. When exposed to the air it gradually absorbs moisture. As already stated, though decomposed by a high heat in its unmixed state, yet with water under pressure it is volatilizable unchanged at a temperature between 204·4° C. and 260° C. (400° F. and 500° F.). Cooled down rapidly, it only becomes more viscid, without congealing, even when a temperature of —40° C. is attained; but, if kept for some time at a temperature of about 0° C. (32° F.), it gradually forms hard but deliquescent crystals, which melt only at about 22° C. (71·6° F.).* This fact is now utilized as a means of concentrating and purifying glycerin. According to Mr. G. F. Wilson, glycerin, when of the density 1·24, contains 94 per cent. of anhydrous glycerin; when of the density 1·26, 98 per cent. A table by Dr. Wilhelm Lenz (*Zeitsch. f. Anal. Chem.*, 1880, p. 297), showing the percentage of absolute glycerin in mixtures of glycerin and water, which was obtained by a quantitative determination of the carbon in the various dilutions by ultimate analysis, will be found in U. S. D., 15th ed., p. 712. The following table by Prof. W. W. J. Nicol, of England, has been constructed after careful determinations, aided by Dr. A. B. Lyons's data on expansion of glycerin solutions. (*Pharm. Era*, 1888, p. 55.)

Per cent. Glycerin.	Sp. Gr. at 15° C. —59° F.	Per cent. Glycerin.	Sp. Gr. at 15° C. —59° F.	Per cent. Glycerin.	Sp. Gr. at 15° C. —59° F.	Per cent. Glycerin.	Sp. Gr. at 15° C. —59° F.
1	1·00236	26	1·06500	51	1·13265	76	1·20131
2	1·00473	27	1·06765	52	1·13539	77	1·20404
3	1.00711	28	1·07031	53	1·13814	78	1·20677
4	1·00949	29	1·07297	54	1·14088	79	1·20949
5	1·01189	30	1·07564	55	1·14362	80	1·21221
6	1·01430	31	1·07832	56	1·14637	81	1·21493
7	1·01673	32	1·08100	57	1·14912	82	1·21766
8	1·01917	33	1·08370	58	1·15187	83	1·22038
9	1·02163	34	1·08639	59	1·15462	84	1·22310
10	1·02409	35	1·08908	60	1·15737	85	1·22583
11	1·02655	36	1·09176	61	1·16011	86	1·22855
12	1·02910	37	1·09445	62	1·16286	87	1·23128
13	1·03177	38	1·09713	63	1·16561	88	1·23400
14	1·03410	39	1·09983	64	1·16837	89	1·23673
15	1·03652	40	1·10253	65	1·17113	90	1·23945
16	1·03905	41	1·10525	66	1·17387	91	1·24217
17	1·04160	42	1·10798	67	1·17662	92	1·24487
18	1·04416	43	1·11071	68	1·17937	93	1·24756
19	1·04672	44	1·11345	69	1·18212	94	1·25021
20	1·04930	45	1·11618	70	1·18487	95	1·25285
21	1·05189	46	1·11893	71	1·18761	96	1·25547
22	1·05449	47	1·12167	72	1·19035	97	1·25809
23	1·05712	48	1·12441	73	1·19309	98	1·26072
24	1·05973	49	1·12716	74	1·19583	99	1·26335
25	1·06236	50	1·12990	75	1·19857	100	1·26598

Glycerin possesses extensive powers as a solvent, and is an excellent excipient for many medicinal substances. It dissolves bromine and iodine, the iodide of sulphur,

* Mr. Wm. Crookes gives an account, in the *Chem. News* of Jan. 18, 1867, of 5 tons of glycerin imported into London from Germany in casks of 8 cwt. each, which, though when it left the continent it was in its ordinary state of a viscid liquid, was found, on reaching London, to have become solidified into a mass of very hard, brilliant crystals. The same result has been noticed in Vienna, in a mass of glycerin which had been in an iron tank more than a year. (*Chem. News*, April 5, 1867, p. 174.) The crystalline mass noticed by Mr. Crookes yielded pure glycerin when melted. Frozen glycerin has been examined by Mr. Wallace Procter and Prof. Henry Trimble (*A. J. P.*, 1885, p. 273); the crystals had the sp. gr. 1·2618, and the portion which had not been solidified had the sp. gr. 1·235.

the chlorides of potassium and sodium, the fixed alkalies, some of the alkaline earths, lime, for example, for which it increases the solvent powers of water (*Journ. de Pharm.*, Juin, 1874), and a large number of neutral salts. It also dissolves the vegetable acids, particularly tannic acid. It is a good solvent of pepsin, and is used for the extraction of this principle from the mucus of the stomach. Two parts and a half of glycerin dissolve one of sugar, and three and a half parts, one of gum. When starch-paste and glycerin are heated together, a turbid liquid is formed, which deposits on cooling; the supernatant liquid holding starch in solution. (*Journ. de Pharm.*, Nov. 1868, pp. 361–2.) Prof. J. S. Blockley, of London, has ascertained that certain neutral vegetable substances are far more soluble in glycerin than in water. Thus salicin dissolves in eight parts of cold glycerin, and santonin in eighteen parts when boiling. The latter solution, when of half this strength, forms on cooling an almost solid mass. It is not always a good solvent for alkaloids or their salts, and will *sometimes precipitate the latter from their watery solutions.* Glycerin, next to alcohol, is the best solvent of iodine. Iodine and iodide of potassium, when dissolved in it, form *iodized glycerin*, the medical applications of which are given under iodine. (See *Iodinium.*)* It combines with potassa and baryta, and also with sulphuric acid. Glycerin is not susceptible of becoming rancid, or of fermenting spontaneously; but will generate a portion of alcohol under the combined influence of chalk, and of a ferment formed of cheese or animal tissue. During this change there is no intermediate formation of glucose, provided carbonate of calcium is present. (*Berthelot.*) Glycerin does not evaporate when exposed to the air; nor can it be distilled without decomposition, unless in the presence of water or steam. When decomposed by heat, it emits extremely irritating vapors. At a full red heat it takes fire, and burns with a blue flame. In consequence of the high temperature required for its volatilization, it has been proposed to use it for an evaporating bath, in which a heat beyond that of boiling water is required. Glycerin is antiseptic, and has been recommended by Mr. Warington and M. Demarquay to preserve alimentary substances and objects of natural history, and to inject bodies for dissection. According to Dr. W. Fraser, it does not answer to keep pathological preparations; as they are completely softened by its action. M. Berthelot, of Paris, has succeeded in combining glycerin with a number of acids, both mineral and organic, forming three distinct series of neutral compounds. Among others he has united it with the fatty acids, producing, by synthesis, the organic fatty substances, stearin, palmitin, olein, etc. Glycerin has been formed artificially from tribromallyl, by Wurtz, and from trichlorhydrin, by Friedel and Silva. Neither synthesis is practical on a large scale, nor could they compete with its preparation from natural fats. By Pasteur it has been ascertained to be one of the products of the vinous fermentation. Glycerin is a triatomic alcohol, being a compound of the triad radical (C_3H_5) with 3(OH) groups. In the natural fats, the three H atoms of these OH groups are replaced by fatty acid radicals like stearyl, $C_{18}H_{35}O$, palmityl, $C_{16}H_{31}O$, and oleyl, $C_{18}H_{33}O$. The natural fats are, therefore, compounds of an alcohol radical with an organic acid, and are true ethers, to which the special names of *glycerides* have been given.

The solvent and preservative properties as well as agreeable taste and permanent consistence of glycerin render it very useful as a menstruum in pharmacy; and a

* The following table, by Klever, gives a general view of the solvent powers of glycerin. 100 parts of glycerin dissolving the annexed quantities of substances:

	PARTS.		PARTS.		PARTS.		PARTS.
Acidum arseniosum..	20	Brucine..................	2·25	Morphine................	0·45	Sodii bicarbonas......	8
" arsenicum....	20	Calcii sulphid.........	5	Morphinæ acetas.....	20	" boras..............	60
" benzoicum...	10	Cinchonine.............	0·30	" murias...	20	" carbonas..........	98
" boracicum...	10	Cinch. sulphas........	6·70	Phosphorus............	0·20	" chloras...........	20
" oxalicum....	15	Cupri acetas..........	10	Plumbi acetas.........	20	Sulphur..................	0·10
" tannicum....	50	" sulphas..........	30	Potassii arsenias......	50	Strychnine..............	0·25
Alumen.................	40	Ferr. et potas. tart...	8	" chloras.......	3·50	Strychninæ nitras...	4
Ammonii carbonas..	20	" lactas.............	16	" bromidum...	25	" sulphas.	22·50
" murias....	20	" sulphas..........	25	" cyanidum...	32	Urea.......................	50
Antimon. et pot. tart.	5·50	Hydrarg. chlorid. corrosiv.	7·50	" iodidum......	40	Veratrine................	1
Atropine................	3			Quinine..................	0·50	Zinci chloridum.......	50
Atropinæ sulphas....	33	" cyanidum.	27	Quininæ tannas......	0·25	" iodidum.........	40
Barii chloridum......	10	Iodinium.................	1·90	Sodii arsenias.........	50	" sulphas..........	35

(*Neues Jahrb. für Pharm.*, 1869, Mai u. Juni, 315.)

class of preparations consisting of medicinal substances dissolved in it has come into extensive use. The British Pharmacopœia has adopted such a class, under the name of *Glycerina* or *glycerines*. This title is not now available because these terminations are reserved for alkaloids, whilst the term *glyceroles*, adopted from the French, is objectionable, as the termination has been used as designative of certain proximate principles. But the U. S. title, *Glycerita* or *glycerites*, is satisfactory.

Impurities and Tests. Glycerin is occasionally deficient in density and consistency. According to M. Dalpiaz, it is sometimes perfectly colorless from being bleached by chlorine, when it is apt to contain chloride of calcium, as well as free chlorine. The latter may be detected by rendering the suspected sample slightly blue by a few drops of sulphate of indigo, and then adding a little sulphuric acid, when, if free chlorine be present, the blue color will disappear. The Pharmacopœia furnishes the following tests. "Glycerin should be neutral to litmus paper. Upon warming a portion of 5 or 6 Gm. with half its weight of diluted sulphuric acid, no butyric or other acidulous odor should be developed. A portion of 2 or 3 Gm., gently warmed with an equal volume of sulphuric acid in a test-tube, should not become dark colored (abs. of cane sugar). A portion of about 2 Gm., heated in a small, open porcelain or platinum capsule, upon a sand-bath, until it boils, and then ignited, should burn and vaporize so as to leave not more than a dark stain (abs. of sugars and dextrin, which leave a porous coal). A portion heated to about 85° C. (185° F.), with test-solution of potassio-cupric tartrate, should not give a decided yellowish brown precipitate, and the same result should be obtained, if, before applying this test, another portion be boiled with a little diluted hydrochloric acid for half an hour (abs. of sugars). After full combustion no residue should be left (metallic salts). Diluted with 10 times its volume of distilled water, portions should give no precipitates or colors, when treated with test-solution of nitrate of silver, chloride of barium, chloride of calcium, sulphide of ammonium, or oxalate of ammonium (acrylic, hydrochloric, sulphuric, or oxalic acids, iron or calcium salts)." *U. S.* Lime may be detected by oxalate of ammonium; lead, by hydrosulphate of ammonium; and sulphuric acid, by a soluble salt of baryta. Diluted, and boiled with a solution of potassa, it is not altered in color, showing the absence of glucose. Trommer's test is probably still more effectual. Chloroform was proposed as a test of sugar, in consequence of the complete insolubility of sugar in it, while glycerin was said to be very soluble; but subsequently chloroform has been shown to be incapable of dissolving glycerin, though readily forming an even mixture, which separates into its two constituents, on standing. (*Chem. News*, Feb. 25, 1870, p. 87.) The absence of sugar is shown, if, upon the addition of two drops of concentrated sulphuric acid, and the application of heat, no brown discoloration is observed. (*Journ. de Pharm.*, Nov. 1863, p. 405.) The late Prof. Procter believed that the most satisfactory method of detecting cane sugar is to dilute a little glycerin with three parts of water, then add a few grains of tartaric acid, and boil for a short time. Cane sugar, if present, is thus converted into glucose, which may be detected by adding first a solution of sulphate of copper, and then the solution of potassa to the heated liquid, when the formation of the reddish suboxide of copper will afford the requisite proof. (*A. J. P.*, 1867, p. 110.) According to M. Hager, sugar or dextrine may be detected in the following manner. Dilute the glycerin with water, add molybdate of ammonium and some drops of nitric acid, and boil. If these impurities are present, a blue color is produced; if not, it remains colorless. (*Ibid.*, May, 1869, p. 206.)*

Among the most injurious impurities of glycerin are thought to be oxalic and formic acids, the latter of which is especially irritating to the skin, so as to unfit

* As impure glycerin is often irritant to the skin, and thus unfitted for some of the most important uses of this principle, it is very important to have a test by which this kind of impurity may be detected. According to M. Hager, if equal volumes of the irritating glycerin and pure sulphuric acid be mixed in a glass tube, there will be an immediate disengagement of gas; and, after the escape of gas has ceased, and the mixture allowed to rest, a renewed agitation will cause a new development of gas; and this phenomenon may be repeated several times; whereas, if the glycerin be pure and unirritant, there is a rise of temperature, and there may be a slight discoloration, but no effervescence, and only the production of a few bubbles of air on agitation. (*Journ. de Pharm. et de Chim.*, Nov. 1867, p. 360.)

glycerin for some of the purposes for which it is most employed. The oxalic acid is said to result from the action of sulphuric acid employed in purifying glycerin; the formic, from the reaction between glycerin and oxalic acid. They may be detected by the U. S. P. tests. Mr. Henry Bower, of Philadelphia, who manufactures very pure glycerin, says that nitrate of silver is the most reliable test. Glycerin which shows no reaction with this salt, he considers suitable for all uses. (*A. J. P.*, 1868, p. 265.) For a method of extracting glycerin from mixtures containing sugar and glucose, see a paper by Prof. Prescott. (*N. R.*, 1878, p. 354.) For methods of determining glycerin in mixtures or its detection in wines, etc., see *Chem. News*, 1882, p. 36; *A. J. P.*, 1882, p. 284; *Schweiz. Wochensch. f. Pharm.*, 1881, p. 307; *Chem. News*, 1886, p. 15; *Amer. Drug.*, 1886, p. 85.

Medical Properties. The uses of glycerin as a vehicle of other medicines have been already given. When given internally, it is laxative, and it has also been suggested as a substitute for cod-liver oil in phthisis, etc. Dr. R. P. Cotton, however, has tried it in the Consumption Hospital at Brompton, and shown that it has generally but little influence, and that as a remedial agent it will bear no comparison with cod-liver oil. When injected directly into the blood, glycerin produces in the lower animals violent nervous symptoms and death, but this action is probably due to the mechanical alteration of the viscidity of the vital fluid. All our physiological evidence goes to show that glycerin has, unless in very immoderate quantities, no distinct physiological or therapeutic properties other than those of a feeble laxative. Although at various times much lauded in tuberculous diseases and in diabetes, it has entirely failed to gain the confidence of the profession, and is now very rarely employed.

Glycerin has come into extensive use as an *external* remedy. Its emollient virtues and undrying property adapt it to the treatment of skin diseases in which a softening and soothing application is required. It appears to have been first employed externally, in 1846, by Mr. Thomas De la Rue, of London, whose observation of its utility led Mr. Startin to try it in the Hospital for Skin Diseases, where it came into extensive use. The principal cutaneous diseases in which it has been found beneficial are pityriasis, lepra, herpes, eczema, psoriasis, prurigo, and lichen. It is a useful addition to lotions in the incrusted form of lupus, and in various syphilitic and strumous eruptions. It is also useful in chapped skin and excoriated surfaces. Added to poultices, in a proportion varying from one-fourth to one-sixteenth, it has the effect of keeping them soft for a long time. To collodion it gives a plasticity which renders it often better suited to skin affections. Incorporated in very small proportion with extracts and pills, it keeps them soft and free from mouldiness. M. Devergie, in giving the results of his trials of glycerin in skin diseases, thinks its virtues have been exaggerated, and that it is not superior to pure lard and similar fatty substances; though it has the advantages of liquidity and freedom from odor. In cases of deafness, from deficiency, accumulation, or hardness of the cerumen, and attended with dryness of the meatus, glycerin is an excellent remedy, introduced into the canal by means of raw cotton saturated with it. Glycerin may be used in the form of an ointment.*

Glycerin has been recommended by M. Vogel as a substitute for the common water-bath. A temperature of 100° C. (212° F.) can be applied by means of it, without the diffusion of unpleasant odors, as from fixed oils or paraffine used in the same way. (*Journ. de Pharm.*, Oct. 1868, p. 315.)

Off. Prep. Extracta; Extracta Fluida; Glycerita; Tincturæ, etc.

Off. Prep. Br. Extractum Cinchonæ Liquidum; Glycerinum Acidi Carbolici; Glycerinum Acidi Gallici; Glycerinum Acidi Tannici; Glycerinum Aluminis; Glycerinum Amyli; Glycerinum Boracis; Glycerinum Plumbi Subacetatis; Glycerinum Tragacanthæ; Lamellæ; Linimentum Iodi; Linimentum Potassii Iodidi cum

* Mr. Ecky's *glycerin ointment* is made as follows. Take of spermaceti *half an ounce*; white wax *a drachm*; oil of almonds *two fluidounces*; glycerin *a fluidounce*. Melt the spermaceti and wax with the oil of almonds by a moderate heat. Then, having poured the melted liquid into a Wedgwood mortar, add the glycerin, and rub until the ingredients are thoroughly mixed and cool. This ointment may be used with advantage in chaps and excoriations.

Sapone; Mel Boracis; Pilula Aloes et Myrrhæ; Pilula Rhei Composita; Pilula Saponis Composita; Tinctura Kino; Unguentum Iodi.

GLYCERITA. *Glycerites.*

(GLY̆Ç-E-RĪ'TA.)

Glycerina, *Br.;* Glycerines.

These are solutions of medicinal substances in glycerin. In the thirteenth edition of the Dispensatory various reasons were adduced for preferring the name glycerates for these preparations, but, as the revisers of the U. S. Pharmacopœia have since adopted that of glycerites, these reasons are omitted. The U. S. name is certainly much better than the English. (See p. 713.)

Glycerin has valuable properties as a solvent and vehicle of medicinal substances. Such are its not unpleasant taste and bland character; its wide range of solvent power, which adapts it sometimes as a menstruum where neither water nor alcohol could be advantageously used, and enables it to retain in solution insoluble substances so frequently deposited from infusions and decoctions; and its preservative influence, which often protects against oxidation, and, by a destructive agency upon all of the lowest forms of vegetable and animal life, prevents the various fermentative processes so destructive of organic bodies. Another important property, as a vehicle for external remedies, is the permanence of its liquid character, so that it does not, like water and alcohol, dry up when applied to the skin; resembling in this respect, as well as in its demulcent quality, the fixed oils, without their tendency to rancidity. Hence it has of late come into extensive use in the preparation of medicinal solutions, which under the name of *Glycérés* found admission into the French Codex of 1866, and are now recognized by both the United States and British Pharmacopœias.* In the last revision of the U. S. Pharmacopœia *all* of the formerly officinal glycerites were dropped, including two of the most valuable and frequently used, glycerite of tannic and carbolic acids. Two new glycerites were introduced, Glyceritum Amyli and Glyceritum Vitelli.

GLYCERINUM ACIDI CARBOLICI. *Br.* *Glycerine of Carbolic Acid.*

(GLY̆Ç-E-RĪ'NŬM ĂÇ'I-DĪ CĂR-BŎL'I-CĪ.)

Glycérole d'Acide phénique, Glycérine phénique, *Fr.;* Phenol-Glycerit, *G.*

"Take of Carbolic Acid *one ounce* [avoirdupois]; Glycerine *four fluidounces* [Imperial measure]. Rub them together in a mortar until the acid is dissolved; or the mixture may be warmed." *Br.*

For the uses of this preparation, see *Acidum Carbolicum* (p. 47). It is nearly identical in strength with the *Glyceritum Acidi Carbolici* of U. S. P. 1870, which was made by mixing *one troyounce* of carbolic acid with *four fluidounces* of glycerin. It may be used internally or locally, and for both purposes should in general be diluted with water at the time of application. Four and a half minims represent about a grain of the acid. The dose is from five to ten minims (0·3–0·6 C.c.).

GLYCERINUM ACIDI GALLICI. *Br.* *Glycerine of Gallic Acid.*

(GLY̆Ç-E-RĪ'NŬM ĂÇ'I-DĪ GĂL'LI-CĪ.)

Glycérole d'Acide gallique, *Fr.;* Gallussäure-Glycerit, *G.*

"Take of Gallic Acid *one ounce* [avoirdupois]; Glycerine *four fluidounces* [Im-

* *Glyceritum Picis Liquidæ.* U. S. 1870. *Glycerite of Tar.* "Take of Tar *a troyounce;* Carbonate of Magnesium, in powder, *two troyounces;* Glycerin *four fluidounces;* Alcohol *two fluidounces;* Water *ten fluidounces.* Having mixed the Glycerin, Alcohol, and Water, rub the Tar in a mortar, first with the Carbonate of Magnesium, and then with six fluidounces of the mixed liquids gradually added, and strain with expression. Rub the residue in like manner with half the remaining liquid, and strain as before. Repeat the process again with the remaining liquid. Put the residue into a percolator, add gradually the expressed liquids previously mixed, and afterwards a sufficient quantity of water to make the liquid which passes measure a pint." *U. S.*

This is a very excellent preparation of tar, which may be used either externally or internally. The formula is essentially the same as that proposed by Mr. J. B. Moore, although employing one-third less of the magnesium salt (*A. J. P.,* 1869, p. 115). As first made it is of a reddish brown color; after a time it is apt to deposit pitchy matter, which should be separated by filtration. An ounce of it represents half a fluidrachm of tar. The dose is a drachm to a half ounce (3·75–15 C.c.).

perial measure]. Stir them together in a porcelain dish, and apply a temperature not exceeding that of a water-bath until complete solution is effected." *Br.*

This preparation was dropped at the last revision of the U. S. Pharmacopœia. The strength of the *Glyceritum Acidi Gallici* of U. S. P. 1870 was *one troyounce* of gallic acid to *four fluidounces* of glycerin the manipulation being the same as in the British.

Prof. T. E. Thorpe cautions against the use of a temperature higher than 100° C. (212° F.), because of the conversion of the gallic acid into poisonous pyrogallic acid. (*Year-Book of Pharmacy*, 1882, p. 469.)

Glycerin is peculiarly fitted for a vehicle of gallic acid, which it readily dissolves, while the acid is but sparingly soluble in water. For the uses of this glycerite, see *Acidum Gallicum* (p. 62). The solution contains one grain of gallic acid in about four and a half minims of glycerin, and the dose is from twenty to sixty minims (1·25–3·75 C.c.).

GLYCERINUM ACIDI TANNICI. *Br.* *Glycerine of Tannic Acid.*

(GLȲÇ-Ḙ-RĪ'NŬM ĂÇ'Ị-DĪ TĂN'NỊ-ÇĪ.)

Glycérole de Tannin, Glycérine tannique, *Fr.;* Tannin-Glycerol, *G.*

"Take of Tannic Acid *one ounce* [avoirdupois]; Glycerine *four fluidounces* [Imperial measure]. Stir them together in a porcelain dish, and apply a temperature not exceeding that of a water-bath until complete solution is effected." *Br.*

This, the most valuable of all glycerites, was unfortunately dropped at the last revision of the U. S. Pharmacopœia: the strength of the British preparation very closely corresponds with that of the *Glyceritum Acidi Tannici*, U. S. P. 1870, which was *one troyounce* of tannic acid to *four fluidounces* of glycerin.

This preparation may be used, both internally and externally, for most of the purposes to which tannic acid is applied. (See *Acidum Tannicum*, p. 117.) Dr. S. Ringer esteems it highly as a remedy in ozæna and other sanious or purulent discharges from the nostrils and ears, being omitted if the symptoms present an acute form. He has found it also very serviceable in the early stages of eczema, and in impetigo; the scabs being removed before it is applied; and considers it extremely useful in chronic inflammation and superficial ulceration of the fauces, with a relaxed, moist, and granular appearance of the pharyngeal mucous membrane. (*Am. Journ. of Med. Sci.*, Jan. 1869, p. 241.) The solution contains one grain of tannic acid in between four and five minims; and the dose is from ten to forty minims (0·6–2·5 C.c.).

On the whole, it is a most useful preparation of tannic acid for external use; as circumstances require it the officinal strength may be altered by directions of the physician; a very concentrated solution, two parts of glycerin to one of tannin, may be made by the aid of a moderate heat. This applied daily to nipples, during the later months of pregnancy, will usually prevent the occurrence of "sore nipples" during suckling.

GLYCERINUM ALUMINIS. *Glycerine of Alum.*

(GLȲÇ-Ḙ-RĪ'NŬM Ạ-LŪ'MỊ-NĬS.)

"Take of Alum, in powder, *one ounce* [avoir.]; Glycerine *five fluidounces* [Imp. meas.]. Stir them together in a porcelain dish, gently applying heat until solution is effected. Set aside; and pour off the clear fluid from any deposited matter." *Br.*

This is a new and valuable addition to the British Pharmacopœia. It has the astringency of the glyceride of tannin without the tendency to soil the linen or blacken in contact with iron. It was proposed by Dr. R. W. Parker. Its medical properties are those of alum. (*A. J. P.*, 1886, p. 296.)

GLYCERITUM AMYLI. *U.S.* *Glycerite of Starch.*

(GLȲÇ-Ḙ-RĪ'TŬM Ạ-MȲ'LĪ.)

Glycerinum Amyli, *Br.;* Glycerine of Starch; Unguentum Glycerini, *P. G.;* Glycamyl, Plasma Glycéré d'Amidon, Glycérat simple (d'Amidon), *Fr.;* Stärke-Glycerit, *G.*

"Starch, *ten parts* [or one ounce av.]; Glycerin, *ninety parts* [or seven fluidounces], To make *one hundred parts.* Rub them together in a mortar until they are intimately mixed. Then transfer the mixture to a porcelain capsule, and apply a heat gradually raised to 140° C. (284° F.), and not exceeding 144° C. (291° F.), stirring constantly, until the starch-granules are completely dissolved and a translucent jelly is formed." *U. S.*

"Take of Starch *one ounce* [avoir.]; Glycerine *five fluidounces* [Imp. meas.]; Distilled Water *three fluidounces* [Imp. meas.]. Stir them together in a porcelain dish, and apply heat, stirring constantly, until the starch particles are completely broken and a translucent jelly is formed." *Br.*

Of these preparations it is only necessary to say that, with the exception of an inconsiderable difference in the proportions, they are the same as that brought into notice in 1858 by Mr. G. F. Schacht under the name of *plasma*, as a substitute for ointments, the emollient and demulcent properties of which they possess, without their inconvenience, whether used simply, or as a vehicle for other substances to be employed locally. Mr. Schacht prepares plasma by mixing 70 grains of starch in powder, and a fluidounce of glycerin, heating to 240° F. until the union is effected, and stirring constantly. The stirring should be continued moderately, during the cooling, to secure a proper consistence. As the plasma is liable to absorb moisture, it should be kept in well-closed vessels. (*P. J. Tr.*, Oct. 1866, p. 210.)

Pharm. Uses. Br. Suppositoria Acidi Carbolici cum Sapone; Suppositoria Acidi Tannici; Suppositoria Morphinæ cum Sapone.

GLYCERINUM BORACIS. *Br. Glycerine of Borax.*

(GLĬÇ-Ę-RĪ′NŬM BO̧-RĀ′CĬS.)

Glycérole de Borax, *Fr.*; Borax-Glycerol, *G.*

"Take of Borax, in powder, *one ounce* [avoir.]; Glycerine *four fluidounces* [Imp. meas.]; Distilled Water *two fluidounces* [Imp. meas.]. Rub them together in a mortar until the borax is dissolved; or heat gently until solution is effected." *Br.*

The *Glyceritum Sodii Boratis* of U. S. 1870 was of the strength of *one troy-ounce* to *four fluidounces.* Otherwise it did not differ from the British preparation.

The demulcent properties and sweet taste of this preparation render it a useful and convenient method of applying borax to the infantile thrush, and other forms of sore mouth in children. It has been very highly commended in facial erysipelas by Prof. D. M. Salazar, of Madrid. The part should be freely painted with it and then covered with raw cotton. (*N. Y. Med. Record*, viii. 311.)

GLYCERINUM PLUMBI SUBACETATIS. *Br. Glycerine of Subacetate of Lead.*

(GLĬÇ-Ę-RĪ′NŬM PLŬM′BĪ SŬB-ĂÇ-Ę-TĀ′TĬS.)

"Take of Acetate of Lead *five ounces* [avoir.]; Oxide of Lead, in powder, *three and a half ounces* [avoir.]; Glycerine *one pint* [Imp. meas.]; Distilled Water *twelve fluidounces* [Imp. meas.]. Mix together and boil for a quarter of an hour; then filter and evaporate until the water is dissipated." *Br.*

This glycerite originated with Dr. Balmanno Squire, of London, but the process made officinal is that recommended by Dr. R. W. Parker. (See *A. J. P.*, 1886, p. 296.) It is a powerful sedative astringent, and may be employed as a local application in various external inflammations.

GLYCERINUM TRAGACANTHÆ. *Br. Glycerine of Tragacanth.*

(GLĬÇ-Ę-RĪ′NŬM TRĂG-Ą-CĂN′THÆ.)

"Take of Tragacanth, in powder, *one hundred and ten grains;* Glycerine *one fluidounce* [Imp. meas.]; Distilled Water *seventy-four fluidgrains.* Mix the tragacanth with the glycerine in a mortar, add the water, and rub until a translucent homogeneous jelly is produced." *Br.*

This new officinal has been introduced into the British Pharmacopœia mainly to serve as an excipient for pills.

GLYCERITUM VITELLI. *U.S.* *Glycerite of Yolk of Egg.* [*Glyconin.*]

(GLÏÇ-Ȩ-RĪ'TŬM VĮ-TĔL'LĪ.)

"Fresh Yolk of Egg, *forty-five parts* [or thirteen ounces av.]; Glycerin, *fifty-five parts* [or sixteen ounces av.], To make *one hundred parts*. Rub the Yolk of Egg with the Glycerin gradually added, until they are thoroughly mixed." *U. S.*

Under the name of *Glyconin* there has been employed in France for many years, both for medical purposes and for those of the toilet, an emulsion made of glycerin and the yolk of eggs. When these two substances are rubbed together, they unite to form a very intimate mixture, which does not separate. It has the consistence of honey, and forms an opaque emulsion with water. It may be preserved almost indefinitely. The usual proportions of the ingredients are four parts of the yolk of eggs and five parts of pure glycerin. Attention was called to its usefulness as a vehicle for the administration of cod-liver oil by Mr. Geo. C. Close, of Brooklyn, N. Y., in 1874,* and it has since been repeatedly recommended for this purpose, and as a basis emulsion for general purposes. See, also, papers by Mr. Close in *Proc. A. P. A.*, 1884 and 1886. It is itself not medicinal, but is used as a protective local application in burns, erysipelas, fissure of the nipples, and various cutaneous affections.

GLYCYRRHIZA. *U.S.* *Glycyrrhiza.* [*Liquorice Root.*]

(GLÏÇ-ŸR-RHĪ'ZĄ—glis-ir-rī'zą.)

Glycyrrhizæ Radix, *Br.;* Radix Liquiritiæ Glabræ, *P. G.;* Radix Glycyrrhizæ Hispanicæ; Spanish Licorice Root; Réglisse, Bois doux, Racine douce; Bois de Réglisse, *Fr.;* Spanisches Süssholz, Spanische Süssholzwurzel, Süssholzwurzel, *G.;* Liquirizia, *It.;* Regaliza, *Sp.*

"The root of Glycyrrhiza glabra. Linné. (*Nat. Ord.* Leguminosæ, Papilionaceæ.)" *U. S.* "The root and subterranean stems or stolons, fresh and dried, of Glycyrrhiza glabra, *Linn.*" *Br.*

Gen. Ch. Calyx bilabiate; upper lip three-cleft, lower undivided. *Legume* ovate compressed. *Willd.*

Glycyrrhiza glabra. Willd. *Sp. Plant.* iii. 1144; Woodv. *Med. Bot.* p. 420, t. 152; Carson, *Illust. of Med. Bot.* i. 38, pl. 32. The liquorice plant has a perennial root, which is round, succulent, tough, and pliable, furnished with sparse fibres, rapid in its growth, and in a sandy soil penetrates deeply into the ground. The stems are herbaceous, erect, and usually four or five feet in height, have few branches, and are garnished with alternate, pinnate leaves, consisting of several pairs of ovate, blunt, petiolate leaflets, with a single leaflet at the end, of a pale green color, and clammy on their under surface. The flowers are violet or purple, formed like those of the pea, and arranged in axillary spikes supported on long peduncles. The calyx is tubular and persistent. The fruit is a compressed, smooth, acute, one-celled legume, containing from one to six small kidney-shaped seeds. There are two very distinct varieties of the plant, yielding the root; the typical form, which is smooth throughout, and the variety, *G. glandulifera*, W. K., in which the stem, leaves, and pods are more or less roughly glandular or pubescent.

The plant is a native of the south of Europe, Barbary, Syria, and Persia; and is cultivated in England,† the north of France, and Germany. Much of the root imported into this country comes from Messina and Palermo in Sicily. It is also largely produced in the north of Spain, where it is an important article of commerce. It is probable that a portion of the root from Italy and Sicily is the product

* *Glyconin Emulsion of Cod-Liver Oil.* The formula proposed by Mr. Close, and at one time largely used by Drs. Andrews, Beard, and others, is as follows. Cod-Liver Oil 4 fluidounces, Glyconin 9 fluidrachms, Aromatic Spirit of Ammonia 1 fluidrachm, Sherry Wine 2 fluidounces, Diluted Phosphoric Acid 4 fluidrachms, Essence of Bitter Almond (made by dissolving 1 fluidrachm of the volatile oil in half a pint of alcohol) 2 fluidrachms. The cod-liver oil is to be added *very slowly* to the glyconin with brisk stirring, and the other ingredients added in the order named.

† Most of the liquorice root of commerce appears to be the product of wild plants, but it has been successfully cultivated in England (*A. J. P.*, 1874, 473) and in Syria (*P. J. Tr.* xvi. 647). Although the attempts to produce it in the United States have hitherto met with no great success, we can see no reason why in some of the lowlands of the South-eastern States it should not flourish. An interesting report upon the production of liquorice root in Spain was made by Mr. H. C. Marsten, United States consul, and may be found abstracted in *New Remedies*, Jan. 1882.

of *G. echinata*, which grows wild in Apulia. This species is also abundant in the south of Russia, where, according to Hayne, sufficient extract is prepared from it to supply the whole Russian empire. Large quantities of liquorice root are now imported for the purpose of making the Extract, the imports for 1887 being 79,603,835 pounds, valued at $1,670,041.

A species of Glycyrrhiza, *G. lepidota*, grows abundantly about St. Louis, in the State of Missouri, and flourishes along the banks of the Missouri River to its source. It is probably the same as the liquorice plant mentioned by Mackenzie as growing on the northern coast of this continent. Mr. Nuttall states that its root possesses in no inconsiderable degree the taste of liquorice.

Properties. The liquorice root of the shops is in long pieces, varying in thickness from a few lines to two inches, fibrous when not peeled, externally grayish brown and longitudinally wrinkled by desiccation, internally yellowish, pliable, tough, without smell, and of a sweet mucilaginous taste, mingled with a slight degree of acrimony. "Fracture coarsely fibrous; bark rather thick; wood porous, but dense, in narrow wedges; medullary rays linear; taste sweet, somewhat acrid. The underground stem, which is often present, has the same appearance, but contains a thin pith." *U. S.* There are two chief varieties of it, the Spanish and the Russian. The roots of the latter form are much larger than the Spanish, and their taste has more or less bitterness mixed with its sweetness. Mr. Henry N. Rittenhouse informs us that commercially the roots are preferred in the following order: 1, Italian; 2, Spanish; 3, Syrian; 4, Turkish; 5, Russian,—the Italian being the sweetest and the Russian the most bitter. Liquorice root is often worm-eaten and more or less decayed. The best pieces are those which have the brightest yellow color internally, and of which the layers are distinct. The bark is chiefly liber, consisting of parenchymatous tissue with bast-cells, which are stained yellow by iodine, and are arranged so as to make ordinary liber bundles, and also a sort of net-work. A character said by Prof. Rothrock (*A. J. P.*, 1884, 129) to be diagnostic is the occurrence in the wood and parenchyma of bundles composed of numerous bast-cells, surrounded by a sheath of large cells containing crystals of oxalate of calcium. In the Russian root the prosenchymatous wood-cells are larger than in the Spanish. The powder is of a grayish yellow color, when the root is pulverized without being deprived of its epidermis; of a pale sulphur-yellow, when the epidermis has been removed. Robiquet found the following ingredients in liquorice root: 1, a peculiar transparent yellow substance, called *glycyrrhizin*, of a sweet taste, scarcely soluble in cold water, very soluble in boiling water, with which it gelatinizes on cooling, thrown down from its aqueous solution by acids, readily soluble in cold alcohol, insusceptible of the vinous fermentation, yielding no oxalic acid by the action of the nitric, and therefore wholly distinct from sugar; 2, a crystallizable principle named *agedoïte* by Robiquet, but subsequently proved to be identical with *asparagin*; 3, starch; 4, albumen; 5, a brown acrid resin; 6, a brown nitrogenous extractive matter; 7, lignin; 8, salts of lime and magnesia, with phosphoric, sulphuric, and malic acids. The chief constituent, *glycyrrhizin*, Gorup-Besanez (*Ann. Ch. und Pharm.*, 118, p. 236) considered to be a glucoside, having the composition $C_{24}H_{36}O_9$. On boiling with dilute acids it breaks up into glycyrretin and an uncrystallizable sugar capable of fermentation. Roussin (*Journ. de Pharm. et de Chim.*, July, 1875, p. 6) found that the sweet taste of the root was not owing to the free glucoside, but to its compound with ammonia. Habermann (*Ann. Ch. und Pharm.*, 197, p. 105) found that glycyrrhizin-ammonia was the acid ammonium salt of glycyrrhizic acid, a nitrogenous acid, and gave the formula $C_{44}H_{63}NO_{18}.NH_4$ for it. (See *Glycyrrhizinum Ammoniatum.*) He succeeded in extracting from the commercial "ammoniacal glycyrrhizin" *glycyrrhizic acid*, which may be considered to be the active constituent of liquorice. It was obtained by dissolving the crude glycyrrhizin in glacial acetic acid at a boiling temperature, rapidly filtering, again treating the crystalline parts of the filtrate in the same manner, and finally purifying by repeated crystallizations from 90 per cent. alcohol. Its properties are peculiar, and account to a great extent for the singular behavior of liquid liquorice preparations. With water, in which the substance is but little soluble at ordinary temperature, it forms a transparent, faintly yellow jelly. On mixing 1 Gm. of the body with 100 C.c. of water, the mixture after a few hours becomes so jelly-like that the open vessel may be inverted without losing any substance. It is insoluble in ether, but slightly soluble in absolute alcohol (even boiling), more so in alcohol of 90 per cent., and especially so when hot. Its solubility increases with the decrease of the percentage of alcohol. The apparent glucosidal character of glycyrrhizic acid Habermann explains by the fact that it breaks up on boiling with dilute sulphuric acid into *glycyrrhetin* and *parasaccharic acid*, according to the reaction $C_{44}H_{63}NO_{18} + 2H_2O = C_{32}H_{47}NO_4 + 2C_6H_{10}O_8$. (*Ann. d. Chem.*, 197, 105; *N. R.*, Sept. 1879.) By fusing glycyrrhizin with caustic potash, Weselsky and Benedikt (*Deutsch. Chem. Ges.*, 1876, p. 1158) obtained *paraoxybenzoic acid*.

Medical Properties and Uses. Liquorice root is an excellent demulcent, well adapted to catarrhal affections, and to irritations of the mucous membrane of the bowels and urinary passages. It is best given in the form of decoction, either alone, or combined with other demulcents. It is frequently employed as an addition to the decoctions of acrid or irritating vegetable substances, such, for example, as seneka and mezereon, the acrimony of which it covers, while it renders them more acceptable to the stomach. Before being used, it should be deprived of its cortical part, which is somewhat acrid, without possessing the peculiar virtues of the root. The decoction may be prepared by boiling an ounce of the bruised root, for a few minutes, in a pint of water. By long boiling, the acrid resinous principle is extracted. Perhaps, however, to this principle may in part be ascribed the therapeutical virtues of liquorice root in chronic bronchial diseases. The powder is used in the preparation of pills, either to give due consistence, or to cover their surface and prevent them from cohering.

For formulas for Aromatic Elixir and Syrup of Liquorice, see Part II., *National Formulary*.

Off. Prep. Extractum Glycyrrhizæ Fluidum; Extractum Glycyrrhizæ Purum; Glycyrrhizinum Ammoniatum; Pulvis Glycyrrhizæ Compositus; Decoctum Sarsaparillæ Compositum; Extractum Sarsaparillæ Fluidum Compositum; Massa Hydrargyri; Pilula Ferri Iodidi; Pulvis Morphinæ Compositus; Syrupus Sarsaparillæ Compositus; Tinctura Rhei Dulcis.

Off. Prep. Br. Confectio Terebinthinæ; Decoctum Sarsæ Compositum; Extractum Glycyrrhizæ; Extractum Glycyrrhizæ Liquidum; Infusum Lini; Pilula Ferri Iodidi; Pilula Hydrargyri; Pulvis Glycyrrhizæ Compositus.

GLYCYRRHIZINUM AMMONIATUM. *U.S.* *Ammoniated Glycyrrhizin.*

(GLȲÇ-ȲR-RHĮ-ZĪ′NŬM ĄM-MŌ-NĮ-Ā′TŬM—glĭs-ĭr-rĭ-zī′nŭm.)

"Glycyrrhiza, in No. 20 powder, *one hundred parts* [or sixteen ounces av.]; Water, Water of Ammonia, Sulphuric Acid, each, *a sufficient quantity*. Mix *ninety-five parts* [or six pints] of Water with *five parts* [or five fluidounces] of Water of Ammonia, and, having moistened the powder with the mixture, macerate for twenty-four hours. Then pack it moderately in a cylindrical percolator and gradually pour water upon it until *five hundred parts* [or five pints] of percolate are obtained. Add to the percolate, slowly and while stirring, a sufficient quantity of Sulphuric Acid, so long as a precipitate is produced. Collect this on a strainer, wash it with cold Water, redissolve it in Water with the aid of Water of Ammonia, filter, if necessary, and again add Sulphuric Acid so long as a precipitate is produced. Collect this, wash it, dissolve it in a sufficient quantity of Water of Ammonia previously diluted with an equal volume of Water, and spread the clear solution upon plates of glass, so that, on drying, the product may be obtained in scales." *U.S.*

This is a new officinal preparation; its introduction is a result of the very important researches of Z. Roussin, communicated to the Société de Pharmacie of Paris, June 2, 1875. This investigator noticed that *glycyrrhizin*, the sweet principle of liquorice root, was insipid when compared with the root itself, and suspected that it existed in a modified form in the root. Experiment showed that alkalies developed the sweet taste, and he ultimately proved that the alkali with which it was combined in the root was ammonia, and that glycyrrhizin played the part of an acid. He named the compound *glycyrrhizate of ammonium*, and called attention to the fact that liquorice root which had lost a portion of its sweetness through fermentation and the development of acetic acid and precipitation of insoluble glycyrrhizin could be restored to its former sweetness if allowed to remain a sufficient length of time in an ammoniacal atmosphere. The officinal process for ammoniated glycyrrhizin is closely modelled after Roussin's, with the exception of the substitution of percolation by a slightly ammoniated menstruum for maceration and expression with cold water. Roussin purified his product by redissolving it in alcohol and precipitating with ether; this is deemed unnecessary for a preparation which is intended to be useful without being expensive. (See *Proc. A. P. A.*, 1876, p. 544.) Connerade has proposed some modification of Roussin's method; his process is as follows. "Macerate ground liquorice root with one and a half parts by weight of water, strain, wash the residue with a very small quantity of water, heat the mixed liquids to boiling to coagulate albumen, strain again, and then add diluted sulphuric acid (1 in 10), as long as a precipitate is produced. Let this settle, decant the liquid, and dissolve the precipitate in solution of ammonia, diluted with nine parts of water. Filter the latter and evaporate it to dryness. The compound then remains as a brown, friable varnish, unaltered by air, of a pure, sweet taste, easily soluble in cold water, and imparting to the latter, even when diluted to 1 in 1000 parts, an amber color. The yield is about 10 per cent. of the weight of the root." (*N. R.*, March, 1881.)

Properties. The following is the description given in the U. S. Pharmacopœia. "Dark brown or brownish red scales, inodorous, of a very sweet taste, and soluble in water and in alcohol. The aqueous solution, when heated with potassa or soda, evolves vapor of ammonia. On supersaturating the aqueous solution with an acid, a substance (Glycyrrhizin) is precipitated, which, when dissolved in hot water, forms a jelly on cooling. This substance, when washed with diluted alcohol and dried, appears as an amorphous, yellow powder, of a strong, bitter-sweet taste, and an acid reaction." *U. S.*

Medical Properties and Uses. This substance appears to possess the medical properties of liquorice, and may be used as an elegant substitute for it in mixtures which are neither acid nor alkaline. The dose of it is from five to fifteen grains.

GOSSYPII RADICIS CORTEX. *U. S.* *Cotton Root Bark.*

(GOS-SȲP'Ĭ-Ī RA-DĪ'CĬS CÔR'TĔX.)

"The bark of the root of Gossypium herbaceum, Linné, and of other species of Gossypium. (*Nat. Ord.* Malvaceæ.)" *U. S.*

Cottonroot Bark; Écorce de la Racine de Cotonnier, *Fr.*; Baumwollen-Wurzelrinde, *G.*

Gen. Ch. *Calyx* cup-shaped, obtusely five-toothed, surrounded by a three-parted involucel, with dentate-incised, cordate leaflets, cohering at the base. *Stigmas* three to five. *Capsule* three to five-celled, many-seeded. *Seeds* surrounded by a tomentose wool. *De Cand.*

In consequence of changes produced in the plants of this genus by cultivation, botanists have found great difficulty in determining which are distinct species, and which are merely varieties. De Candolle describes thirteen species in his Prodromus, and mentions six others, but considers them all uncertain. Royle describes eight and admits others. Schwartz thinks they may all be referred to one original species. The plants inhabit different parts of tropical Asia and Africa, and many of them are cultivated for their cotton in climates adapted to their growth. The species from which most of the cotton of commerce has been thought to be obtained, is the one specially indicated by the U. S. Pharmacopœia. According to Dr. Royle, it is the India cotton which is produced by *G. herbaceum*, while *G. Barbadense* furnishes all the cotton of North America, and *G. Peruvianum* that produced in Brazil, Peru, and other parts of South America. (See *A. J. P.*, 1858, p. 339.) Dr. A. W. Chapman, however, in his *Flora of the Southern United States* (N. Y., 1860, p. 58), states that the numerous varieties of the cotton-plant are now referred to two species, the *long-staple*, or *sea-island*, to *G. album* (Haw.), and the *short-staple*, or *upland*, to *G. nigrum* (Haw.).

Gossypium herbaceum. Linn. *Sp. Plant.* 975; De Cand. *Prodrom.* i. 456. This is a biennial or triennial plant, with a branching stem from two to six feet high, and palmate hoary leaves, the lobes of which are somewhat lanceolate and acute. The flowers are pretty, with yellow petals, having a purple spot near the claw. The leaves of the involucel or outer calyx are serrate. The capsule opens when ripe, and displays a loose white tuft of long slender filaments, which surround the seeds and adhere firmly to the outer coating. The plant is a native of Asia, but is cultivated in most tropical countries. It requires a certain duration of warm weather to perfect its seeds, and, in the United States, does not mature north of Virginia.

The herbaceous part of the plant contains much mucilage, and has been used as a demulcent. The seeds yield by expression a fixed oil of the drying kind, which is employed for making soap and other purposes. (See *Oleum Gossypii.*) The bark of the root has been supposed to possess medical virtues, and is now recognized by the U. S. Pharmacopœia. Another officinal portion, and that for which the plant is cultivated, is the filamentous substance surrounding the seeds. This when separated constitutes the cotton of commerce.

Cotton seeds have been employed in our Southern States with great asserted success in the treatment of intermittents. In a communication from Prof. H. R. Frost to the *Charleston Medical Journal* for May, 1850, it is stated, on the authority of Dr. W. K. Davis, of Monticello, that this application of the cotton seed originated with a planter in Newberry District, South Carolina, who had often used the remedy in intermittents, and never failed to effect a cure. A pint of the seeds is boiled in a quart of water to a pint, and a teacupful of the decoction is given to the patient in bed, an hour or two before the expected return of the chill.

Properties. Cotton Root Bark is officinally described as "in thin, flexible bands or quilled pieces; outer surface brownish-yellow, with slight, longitudinal ridges or meshes, small, black circular dots, or short, transverse lines, and dull, brownish orange patches, from the abrasion of the thin cork; inner surface whitish, of a silky lustre, finely striate; bast fibres long, tough, and separable into papery layers; inodorous; taste very slightly acrid and faintly astringent." *U. S.* Prof. E. S. Wayne, of Cincinnati, found in it a peculiar acid resin, colorless and soluble in water, when pure, but absorbing oxygen on exposure, and then becoming red and insoluble in water. It is deposited by the fluid extract on standing. He suggests that this may be the active principle of the root; but the fact has not been determined. (*A. J. P.*, 1872, p. 289.)

William C. Staehle (*A. J. P.*, 1875, p. 457) made an examination of this resin, and obtained results somewhat different from those of Prof. Wayne. Staehle's percolate was of a dark, reddish brown color, whilst Wayne's was pale amber. This is accounted for, however, by the presence of a principle which is colorless in the fresh bark, but of a dark red in bark which has been exposed to air and light. W. A. Taylor noticed that the change in color from pale amber to dark red took place in an alcoholic tincture. (*A. J. P.*, 1876, p. 403.) Staehle found the resin soluble in 14 parts of alcohol, 15 parts of chloroform, 23 parts of ether, and 122 parts of benzol.

Medical Properties. It has been employed by Dr. Bouchelle, of Mississippi, who believes it to be an excellent emmenagogue, and not inferior to ergot in promoting uterine contraction. He states that it is habitually and effectually resorted to by the slaves of the South for producing abortion, and thinks that it acts in this way without injury to the general health. To assist labor, he employs a decoction made by boiling four ounces of the inner bark of the root in a quart of water to a pint, and gives a wineglassful (60 C.c.) every twenty or thirty minutes. (*West. Journ. of Med. and Surg.*, Aug. 1840.) These opinions of Dr. Bouchelle have been confirmed by various Southern medical practitioners, and Dr. H. I. Garrigues asserts that the cotton-root has great powers in arresting hemorrhage and ameliorating the other symptoms of uterine fibroids, but, for some reason, the drug has not yet come into general use. Dr. Bellany, of Columbus, Georgia, says that the root should be gathered as late as possible in the fall before frost. The officinal fluid extract may be used in doses of half a fluidrachm to one fluidrachm (1·9 to 3·75 C.c.), repeated at short intervals if necessary.

Off. Prep. Extractum Gossypii Radicis Fluidum.

GOSSYPIUM. *U.S., Br.* *Cotton.* [*Purified Cotton. Absorbent Cotton.*]

(GOS-SYP'I-ŬM.)

"The hairs of the seed of Gossypium herbaceum, Linné, and of other species of Gossypium (*Nat. Ord.* Malvaceæ), freed from adhering impurities and deprived of fatty matter." *U. S.* "The hairs of the seed of Gossypium barbadense, *Linn.*; and of other species of Gossypium, from which fatty matter and all foreign impurities have been removed." *Br.*

Bonelyax, Lana (Lanugo, s. Pili) Gossypii; Coton, *Fr.;* Baumwolle, *G.;* Cotone, *It.;* Algodon, *Sp.*

Cotton consists of "white, soft, fine filaments, under the microscope appearing as flattened, hollow and twisted bands, spirally striate and slightly thickened at the edges; inodorous, tasteless, insoluble in water, alcohol, or ether; soluble in an ammoniacal solution of sulphate of copper." It is without smell or taste, soluble in strong alkaline solutions, and decomposed by the concentrated mineral acids. In chemical character it is identical with lignin. By nitric acid it is converted into that remarkable explosive substance denominated gun cotton, for an account of which, see *Pyroxylinum* and *Collodium.* Officinal cotton is made by boiling the raw cotton in a diluted alkaline solution. A soap is formed through the union of the fatty matter with the alkali, and this is subsequently dissolved out by repeated washings. Mr. F. L. Slocum published in 1881 a process for preparing it. For details see the foot-note.* The U. S. P. tests are as follows. "Cotton should be perfectly free from all perceptible impurities, and, on combustion, should not leave more than 0·8 per cent. of ash. When thrown upon water, it should immediately absorb the latter and sink, and the water should not acquire either an acid or an alkaline reaction." *U. S.* The latter test proves the absence of fatty matter, for if even a small quantity be present the cotton will float in water. Repeated experiments have proven that cotton will take fire and burn spontaneously, if impregnated with olive oil, linseed oil, or almost any other fixed oil, and allowed to stand. (*P. J. Tr.*, 1872, p. 225.) Cotton, analyzed by M. Schunck, was found, independently of cellulose, ($C_6H_{10}O_5$), of which it chiefly consists, to contain vegetable wax, a fatty acid, coloring matter, pectic acid, and a little of an albuminoid substance. (*Journ. de Pharm.*, Sept. 1868, p. 233.) For medical use it should be carded into thin sheets.† It is said that air passed through cotton loses the property of inducing fermentation, on account of the microscopic organisms being strained out of it; and this fact has been utilized in preserving infusions by placing them in bottles, containing corks armed with tubes, loosely filled with cotton, and drawing the infusion from a stopcock near the bottom.

Medical Properties. Cotton has been used from time immemorial for the fabrication of cloth; but it is only of late that it has entered the catalogue of medicines. The use of cotton as a filtering medium and in the preparation of medicated waters has already been alluded to. It is chiefly employed in recent burns and scalds; an application of it adopted from popular practice. It is said to relieve the pain, dimin-

* Take of the best quality of carded cotton batting, any desired quantity, and boil it with a 5 per cent. solution of caustic potassa or soda for one-half hour, or until the cotton is entirely saturated with the solution, and the alkali has saponified all oily matter. Then wash thoroughly, to remove all soap, and nearly all alkali; press out the excess of water, and immerse in a 5 per cent. solution of chlorinated lime for 15 or 20 minutes; again wash, first with a little water, then dip in water acidulated with hydrochloric acid, and thoroughly wash with water; press out the excess of water, and again boil for 15 or 20 minutes in a 5 per cent. solution of caustic potassa or soda; now wash well, dipping in the acidulated water and washing thoroughly with pure water. Afterwards press out and dry quickly.

The amount of loss by this process is practically 10 per cent. A sample of 360 grs. lost, on boiling with alkali and bleaching, 15 grs., or 4·17 per cent., and 270 grs. of this bleached sample lost, on again boiling with an alkali, 14 grs., or 5·18 per cent., a total loss of 9·35 per cent. (*A. J. P.*, 1881, p. 53.)

† *Wood Wool.* Under this name Prof. Bruns has introduced finely grained, purified wood-fibre, such as is used in making paper. It may be medicated like cotton. (*N. R.*, 1883, p. 361.)

ish the inflammation, prevent vesication, and very much to hasten the cure. Whatever advantages result from it are probably ascribable to the absorption of effused liquids, and the protection of the part affected from the air. It is applied in thin and successive layers; and benefit is said to result from the application of a bandage when the skin is not too much inflamed. We have, however, seen cotton do much harm in burns, by becoming consolidated over a vesicated surface and acting as a mechanical irritant. Such a result may be prevented by first dressing the burn with a piece of fine linen spread with simple ointment. Cotton is also recommended in erysipelas, and as a dressing for blisters; and we have found it useful, applied in a large bunch over parts affected with rheumatism, especially in lumbago.* It has also been used as a dressing for wounds, including amputation and other operations by the surgeons; being largely applied to injured surfaces, and confined in its place by bandages, which are allowed to remain undisturbed, in order to prevent the injurious influence of the impure hospital air, and the access to the wounds of organic germs, which dispose to suppuration and septic disease. (See *Bost. Med. & Surg. Journ.*, May, 1872, p. 325; Aug. 1874, p. 197; *Arch. Gén.*, Dec. 1871; *Journ. de Pharm.*, Jan. 1872.)

Off. Prep. Pyroxylinum. *Off. Prep. Br.* Pyroxylin.

GRANATUM. *U.S.* *Pomegranate.*

(GRĄ-NĀ'TŬM.)

"The bark of the root of Punica Granatum. Linné. (*Nat. Ord.* Granataceæ.)" *U.S.* "The dried bark of the root." *Br.*

Granati Radicis Cortex, *Br.;* Cortex Radicis Granati, *P.G.;* Écorce de la Racine de Grenadier (de Balaustier), Écorce de Granade, *Fr.;* Granatwurzelrinde, Granatäpfelschale, *G.;* Malicorio, Scorza del Melogranati, *It.;* Corteza de Granada, *Sp.*

Gen. Ch. *Calyx* five-cleft, superior. *Petals* five. *Pome* many-celled, many-seeded. *Willd.*

Punica Granatum. Willd. *Sp. Plant.* ii. 981; Woodv. *Med. Bot.* p. 531, t. 190; Carson, *Illust. of Med. Bot.* i. 45, pl. 38. The pomegranate is a small shrubby tree, attaining in favorable situations the height of twenty feet, with a very unequal trunk, and numerous branches which sometimes bear thorns. The leaves are opposite, entire, oblong or lance-shaped, pointed at each end, smooth, shining, of a bright green color, and placed on short footstalks. The flowers are large, of a rich scarlet color, and stand at the end of the young branches. The petals are roundish and wrinkled, and are inserted into the upper part of the tube of the calyx, which is red, thick, and fleshy. The fruit is a globular berry, about the size of an orange, crowned with the calyx, covered with a reddish yellow, thick, coriaceous rind, and divided internally into many cells, which contain an acidulous pulp, and numerous oblong, angular seeds.

This tree grows wild upon both shores of the Mediterranean, in Arabia, Persia, Bengal, China, and Japan, has been introduced into the East and West Indies, and is cultivated in all civilized countries where the climate is sufficiently warm to allow the fruit to ripen. In higher latitudes, where it does not bear fruit, it is raised in gardens and hot-houses for the beauty of its flowers, which become double and acquire increased splendor of coloring by cultivation. Doubts have been entertained as to its original country. The name of *Punicum malum*, applied by the ancients to its fruit, implies that it was abundant at an early age in the vicinity of Carthage.

* Absorbent cotton has been medicated in various ways and come largely into use. (See *Iodinized Cotton*, under *Iodinum.*) *Picric Cotton* is prepared by dissolving 0·25 Gm. of picric acid in 25 Gm. of ether, or of 94 per cent. alcohol, and immersing in the solution 10 Gm. of clean cotton, and drying. *Salicylic Cotton* (5 per cent.) may be prepared by Prof. Brun's process, by saturating 1 kilogramme of cotton with 4 litres of a solution of 50 Gm. of salicylic acid, 20 Gm. of castor oil in 3·930 litres of alcohol. *Benzoic Cotton* is made in the same way, substituting benzoic for salicylic acid. (*A. J. P.*, Dec. 1878.) *Chlorinated Cotton.* Prof. Pavesi subjects cotton moistened with glycerin, and suspended at the top of a large wide-mouthed bottle, to the action of chlorine vapor, generated by adding sulphuric acid to chlorinated lime. (*N. R.*, July, 1880.)
generated by adding sulphuric acid to chlorinated lime. (*N. R.*, July, 1880.) Mr. Joseph W. England communicates in *A. J. P.*, 1887, p. 173, practical formulas for preparing the following medicated cottons and gauzes: *Borated Cotton, Benzoated Cotton, Salicylated Cotton, Naphthalinated Cotton, Iodoformized Cotton, Carbolized Cotton, Sublimated Cotton, Carbolized Gauze, Sublimated Gauze, Absorbent Canton Flannel.*

The fruit, for which the plant is cultivated, varies much in size and flavor. It is said to attain greater perfection in the West Indies than in its native country. The edible pulp is red, succulent, pleasantly acid, and sweetish. The flowers were recognized by the Dublin College, and the seeds are officinal in France.

Rind of the Fruit. This is presented in commerce under the form of irregular fragments, hard, dry, brittle, of a yellowish or reddish brown color externally, paler within, without smell, and of an astringent, slightly bitter taste. It contains a large proportion of tannin, and, in countries where the tree abounds, has been employed for tanning leather.

Flowers. The flowers, sometimes called *balaustines*, are inodorous, have a bitterish, astringent taste, and impart a violet-red color to the saliva. They contain tannic and gallic acids, and were used by the ancients in dyeing.

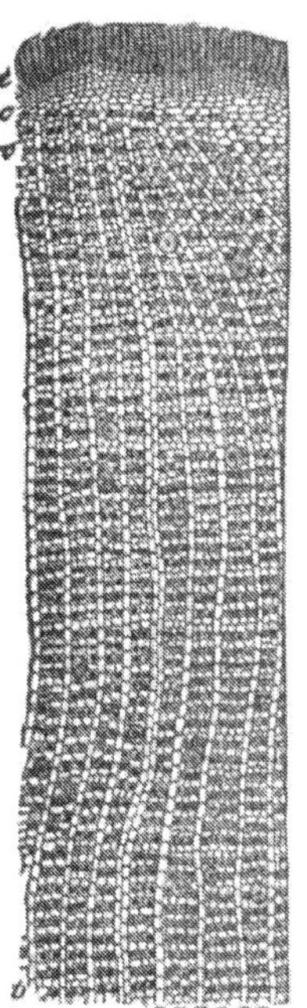
Pomegranate bark. *e*, cork layer; *o*, middle bark; *s*, inner bark; *r*, medullary rays; *g*, bast-tissue. (After Berg.)

Bark of the Root. The roots of the pomegranate are hard, heavy, knotty, ligneous, and covered with a bark which is yellowish gray or ash-gray on the outer surface, and yellow on the inner. As officinally described, the bark is "in thin quills or fragments, from two to four inches (5 to 10 cm.) long, little over one twenty-fifth of an inch (1 mm.) thick; outer surface yellowish gray, free from lichens; somewhat warty, or longitudinally and reticulately ridged; inner surface smooth, finely striate, grayish yellow; fracture short, granular, greenish yellow, indistinctly radiate." *U. S.* It has little or no smell, colors the saliva yellow when chewed, and leaves in the mouth an astringent taste without disagreeable bitterness. The infusion of the bark yields a deep blue precipitate with salts of iron, and a yellowish white precipitate with solution of gelatin. The inner surface of the bark, steeped in water and then rubbed on paper, produces a yellow stain, which, by the contact of sulphate of iron, is rendered blue, and by that of nitric acid acquires a slight rose tint, which soon vanishes. (*Ibid.*, xvii. 438.) These properties serve to distinguish this bark from those of the box root and barberry, with which it is said to be sometimes adulterated. When used, it should be separated from the ligneous portion of the root, as the latter is inert.*

The bark contains more than 22 per cent. of tannic acid, which Rembold (*Ann. der Ch. und Pharm.*, 143, p. 285) found to consist for the most part of a peculiar variety called *punico-tannic acid*, $C_{20}H_{16}O_{13}$; when boiled with dilute sulphuric acid, it is resolved into *ellagic acid*, $C_{14}H_8O_9$, and sugar. Punico-tannic acid is accompanied by common tannic acid, yielding by means of sulphuric acid gallic acid, which appears sometimes to pre-exist in the bark.

Pomegranate bark also yields a considerable quantity of *mannit*, which was formerly described under the names of *punicin* or *granatin*. The active power of the root, however, is due, according to Tanret (*Comp.-Rend.*, 86, p. 1270, and 87, p. 358), to an alkaloid *pelletierine*, $C_8H_{13}NO$, a dextrogyrate liquid boiling at 195° C. The alkaloid is easily soluble in water, alcohol, and ether, and specially so in chloroform. It has strong basic properties, and precipitates many metallic salts. 1000 parts of dry bark yielded 4 parts of the alkaloid.

* Dr. C. Harz stated in 1870 that the commercial bark, sold as the bark of the root of the pomegranate, consisted really, in great measure, of that of the stem; a little of the proper root-bark being occasionally intermingled with it. The root-bark, the author observes, "has large cells; and at a distance from the cambium, the cells of the medullary rays are not elongated but quadratic. The trunk-bark, as well as that of the root, has anthelmintic properties." (*A. J. P.*, 1870, p. 226.) A minute description of the microscopic character of the root-bark, by which it may be distinguished, is contained in *P. J. Tr.* (1873, p. 703).

In a later communication (*Comp.-Rend.*, 88, p. 716), Tanret announces that he has found three additional volatile bases in the bark, a liquid left-rotating one, a liquid optically inactive one, and a crystallizable inactive one, which latter has the formula $C_9H_{15}NO + 2H_2O$, fuses at 46° C., and boils at 246° C. His process for obtaining these alkaloids is as follows. "A mixture of the salts of the alkaloids is prepared by mixing the powdered bark with a milk of lime, exhausting with water, shaking the resulting liquor with chloroform and neutralizing the latter with dilute acid. A solution of the mixed alkaloids is thus obtained in which one or other of them predominates, according to the source of the bark. Two of the four alkaloids are displaced from their salts by bicarbonate of sodium, and two are not. This solution is therefore treated with an excess of bicarbonate of sodium and shaken with chloroform, and this in its turn is agitated with dilute sulphuric acid. The resulting solution contains the sulphates of two alkaloids, to which the names of "*methylpelletierine*," $C_9H_{17}NO$, and "*pseudopelletierine*," $C_9H_{15}NO$, have been given. Caustic potash is then added to the first liquor, and upon repeating the treatment with chloroform and acid there is obtained a solution of the sulphates of "pelletierine" and "*isopelletierine*." (*P. J. Tr.*, 1880, p. 829.) Carl J. Bender (*Pharm. Centralh.*, 1885, p. 6) found three bases in pomegranate bark, one crystallizable and two amorphous. He objects to the name pelletierine, and substitutes "*punicine*." Wm. F. Junkuns analysed pomegranate bark, and believes that the alkaloïd exists in the bark as a tannate. (*A. J. P.*, 1884, p. 137.)

Medical Properties and Uses. The rind of the pomegranate fruit was formerly recognized by the U. S. Pharmacopœia. It is astringent, and in the form of decoction is sometimes employed in diarrhœa and colliquative sweats, and, more frequently, as an injection in leucorrhœa, and as a gargle in sore throat in the earlier stages, or after the inflammatory action has in some measure subsided. The powdered rind has also been recommended in intermittent fever. The flowers have the same medical properties, and are used for the same purposes. The bark of the root was used by the ancients as a vermifuge, and is recommended in the writings of Avicenna, but was unknown in modern practice till brought into notice by Dr. F. Buchanan, who learned its powers in India. The Mahometan physicians of Hindostan consider it a specific against tænia. One of these practitioners, having relieved an English gentleman in 1804, was induced to disclose his secret, which was then made public. The French writers prefer the product of the wild pomegranate, growing on the borders of the Mediterranean, to that of the plant cultivated in gardens for ornamental purposes. The bark may be administered in powder or decoction; but the latter form is usually preferred. The decoction is prepared by macerating two ounces of the bruised bark in two pints of water for twenty-four hours, and then boiling to a pint. Of this a wineglassful may be given every half-hour, hour, or two hours, until the whole is taken. It often nauseates and vomits, and usually purges. Portions of the worm often come away soon after the last dose. It is recommended to give a dose of castor oil and to diet the patient strictly on the day preceding the administration of the remedy; and, if it should not operate on the bowels, to follow it by castor oil, or an enema. If not successful on the first trial, it should be repeated daily for three or four days, until the worm is discharged. It appears to have been used by the negroes of St. Domingo before its introduction into Europe.

The efficacy of pelletierine as a tænicide has been abundantly confirmed, and it appears to be established that the tannate is the most effective and the least dangerous form of the remedy; probably because its insolubility prevents its rapid absorption and enables it to come in prolonged contact with the worm. The experiments of Dr. Dujardin-Beaumetz have shown that the pelletierine alkaloids act upon the higher animals like curare, causing paralysis of the motor nerves, without affecting sensation or muscular contractility. The same authority asserts that hypodermic injections of six grains produce in man severe vertigo, muscular weakness, and great retinal congestion. Double vision has also been noted, and Galezowski has been led by it to prescribe pelletierine in paralysis of the third and sixth pairs of nerves; he affirms that he has succeeded in bringing relief after the failure of iodide of potassium and blisters. The proper dose of the tannate of pelletierine is variously given by authorities. It has been stated to be one-half to three-quarters of a grain (0·03 to 0·05 Gm.) (*Bull. Thérap.*, xcvi., xcvii.), but others place it as high as eight grains (0·52 Gm.). Commercially, it occurs almost exclusively as a syrupy solution, put up, we believe, under the supervision of its discoverer, each bottle containing a single dose, it is stated, of about five grains. We have seen pronounced temporary general palsy produced in a female adult by this dose. The dose of pomegranate rind and flowers in powder is from twenty to thirty grains (1·3–1·95 Gm.). A decoction may be prepared in the proportion of an ounce of the medicine to a pint of water, and given in the dose of a fluidounce (30 C.c.). The remedy should always be given after a twelve hours' fast, and be followed in two hours by a brisk cathartic. The seeds are demulcent.

Off. Prep. of the Bark of the Root. Br. Decoctum Granati Radicis.

GRINDELIA. *U.S.* *Grindelia.*

(GRĬN-DĒ'LĮ-Ą.)

"The leaves and flowering tops of Grindelia robusta. Nuttall. (*Nat. Ord.* Compositæ.)" *U. S.*

Gen. Ch. *Heads* solitary, terminating leafy branches, or occasionally more or less corymbose, heterogamous with the rays fertile, or in one species homogamous (rayless), many-flowered. *Involucre* hemispherical or globular, commonly coated with resin or balsam; its scales very numerous, imbricated, narrow, with coriaceous, appressed, bare, and slender, more or less spreading or squarrose, green tips. *Receptacle* flat or convex, foveolate. *Rays* numerous, narrow. *Branches* of the style tipped with a lanceolate or linear appendage. *Akenes* compressed or turgid, or the outermost somewhat triangular, glabrous, truncate. *Pappus* of two to eight caducous awns or stout corneous bristles. Biennial or perennial, and mostly coarse herbs, with sessile or partly clasping leaves, often viscid or resinous, and middle-sized or rather large heads of yellow flowers. *Torrey & Gray.*

This genus inhabits the western side of both North and South America. Most if not all of the species produce a resinous exudation, especially from the flower-heads, and it is probable that medical properties are common to the genus.

G. robusta, Nuttall, is an herbaceous plant, from one to three feet high, very glabrous, with leaves varying from broadly spatulate or oblong to lanceolate, or the upper cordate and clasping, commonly obtuse, sharply more or less serrate; the scales of the involucre are produced into long circinate, squarrose, awn-like tips; the pappus of two to three, rarely five, nearly smooth, flattish awns; akenes mostly one- to three-toothed at the apex.

Grindelia squarrosa, Dunal, is in general a less leafy and bushy plant than *G. robusta*, but so closely resembles some varieties of the latter, that after a careful study of various published descriptions and of the specimens in the herbarium of the Academy of Natural Sciences, we are not satisfied of this specific distinctness. The character pointed out by Torrey and Gray, that in *robusta* the leaves are broader at the base than above, does not hold; for in a specimen in the herbarium of the Philadelphia Academy of Natural Sciences labelled in Nuttall's handwriting, and, therefore, probably the type of *G. robusta*, the leaves are not broader at the base; whilst in various specimens of *G. squarrosa* they are not narrowed at the base. The most constant distinctive characters in the specimens at hand are that *G. robusta* has a more leafy involucre and its leaves usually are more coarsely serrate; but Watson describes a variety of *G. robusta* in which the upper leaves are entire. There is no constant difference in the scales of the involucre.

Properties. The officinal description of grindelia is as follows. "Leaves about two inches (5 cm.) or less long, varying from broadly spatulate or oblong to lanceolate, sessile or clasping, obtuse, more or less sharply serrate, pale green, smooth, finely dotted, brittle; heads many-flowered; the involucre hemispherical, about half an inch (12 mm.) broad, composed of numerous, imbricated, squarrosely tipped scales; ray-florets yellow, ligulate, pistillate; disk-florets yellow, tubular, perfect; pappus consisting of about three awns of the length of the disk-florets." *U. S.*

As it occurs in commerce, grindelia is in the form of the whole dried herb; the stems are about eighteen inches in length, light brownish, very frequently stripped of their leaves, but with some of the floral heads adherent. The brittle leaves are much broken, and with separated floral heads are mixed with the stem. The taste is warmish, peculiar, and very persistent. The specimens we have examined seemed to contain numerous floral heads, some according with those of the typical *G. robusta*, others without trace of involucral leaves. Some of the latter may have been removed, it is true, by accidents of carriage; but if *G. squarrosa* and *robusta* be distinct species, it would appear that they are indiscriminately collected. The activity of the drug probably resides in the resinous exudation. Dr. C. J. Rademaker obtained from it an oil, the odor of which closely resembled that of oil of turpentine, resin, and a crystalline body, having an alkaline reaction: the constituents deserve further chemical investigation. (*N. R.*, 1876, p. 205.)

Medical Properties and Uses. According to Dr. Buffington, when given to the lower animals in very large doses grindelia produces narcosis, with dilated pupils, slowing of the action of the heart from stimulation of the inhibitory nerves, and elevation of the blood-pressure from stimulation of the vaso-motor centre. Dobroklowsky has found that on the isolated frog's heart it acts in small doses as a stimulant and in large doses as a paralyzant. Grindelia is not, however, used in practical medicine for its influence upon the circulation, but as an antispasmodic, especially in asthma. Dobroklowsky found that it acts upon the motor nerves and muscles, but Buffington states that it paralyzes first the sensory nerve-trunks, then the sensory side of the spinal cord, and afterwards involves the motor nerve-trunks and cord. In practical medicine it has been found especially valuable in asthma, and in bronchitis when there is a distinct tendency to dyspnœa and bronchial spasm. It seems probable that it not only exerts an antispasmodic influence, but also stimulates the bronchial mucous membrane, and it may be confidently exhibited in chronic bronchitis, especially of the aged. It has been employed with asserted success in hooping-cough. Its active principles appear to be excreted from the kidneys; hence after large doses there are sometimes evidences of renal irritation; and in chronic catarrh of the bladder good has been effected by its stimulant influence upon the mucous membrane of the viscus. As a local application, grindelia has been employed with asserted advantage in burns, vaginitis, genito-urinary catarrh, etc., applied either in the form of a poultice or in solution.

Off. Prep. Extractum Grindeliæ Fluidum.

GUAIACI LIGNUM. *U. S., Br.* *Guaiacum Wood.*

(GUĀ'IĀ-CĪ LĬG'NŬM—gwī'yą-sī.)

"The heart-wood of Guaiacum officinale, Linné, and of Guaiacum sanctum, Linné. (*Nat. Ord.* Zygophyllaceæ.)" *U. S.* "The heart-wood of Guaiacum officinale, *Linn.*, or of Guaiacum sanctum, *Linn.* For use in pharmacy the wood, as usually imported, should be deprived of its sap-wood, and the heart-wood reduced to the form of chips, raspings, or shavings." *Br.*

Lignum Guajaci, *P.G.;* Lignum Sanctum (vel Benedictum, vel Vitæ); Lignum Vitæ; Bois de Gayac, *Fr.;* Guajakholz, Franzosenholz, Pockenholz, *G.;* Legno Guaiaco, *It.;* Guayaco, *Sp.*

Gen. Ch. *Calyx* five-cleft, unequal. *Petals* five, inserted into the calyx. *Capsule* angular, three- or five-celled. *Willd.*

Guaiacum officinale. Willd. *Sp. Plant.* ii. 538; Woodv. *Med. Bot.* p. 557, t. 200; Carson, *Illust. of Med. Bot.* i. 25, pl. 17. This is a large tree, of very slow growth. When of full size it is from forty to sixty feet high, with a trunk four or five feet in circumference. The branches are knotted, and covered with an ash-colored striated bark. That of the stem is of a dark gray color, variegated with greenish or purplish spots. The leaves are opposite, and abruptly pinnate, consisting of two, three, and sometimes four pairs of leaflets, which are obovate, veined, smooth, shining, dark green, from an inch to an inch and a half long, and almost sessile. The flowers are of a rich blue color, stand on long peduncles, and grow to the number of eight or ten at the axils of the upper leaves. The seeds are solitary, hard, and of an oblong shape.

G. sanctum, L., is distinguished from *G. officinale* by its five-celled fruit and its oblong or obliquely obovate, or sometimes rhomboid-ovate leaflets, six to eight to each leaf. It grows in Cuba and some other of the West India Islands, and in the Bahama Islands. Its wood is smaller than that of *G. officinale*, and is said by Fée to be paler and less dense.

G. officinale grows in the West Indies, particularly in Hayti and Jamaica, and is found also in the warmer parts of the neighboring continent. All parts of the tree are possessed of medicinal properties; but the wood and the concrete juice only are officinal. The bark, though much more efficacious than the wood, is not kept in the shops. It is said that other species of Guaiacum contribute to the supplies brought into the market. *G. sanctum* of Linnæus, and *G. arboreum* of De Candolle, are particularly specified.

Guaiacum wood is imported from Hayti and other West India islands, in the shape of logs or billets, covered with a thick gray bark, which presents on its inner surface, and upon its edges when broken, numerous shining crystalline points. These were supposed by Guibourt to be benzoic acid, by others a resinous exudation from the vessels of the plant; but Dr. Otto Berg has determined that they are crystals of sulphate of calcium. The billets are used by the turners for the fabrication of various instruments and utensils, for which the wood is well adapted by its extreme hardness and density. It is kept by the druggists and apothecaries in the state of shavings or raspings, which they obtain from the turners. It is commonly called *lignum vitæ*, a name which obviously originated from the supposition that the wood was possessed of extraordinary remedial powers.

Properties. Guaiacum wood is hard and heavy. The color of the sap-wood is yellow, that of the older and central layers greenish brown, that of the shavings a mixture of the two. It is said that, when the wood is brought into a state of minute division, its color is rendered green by exposure to the air, and bluish green by the action of nitric acid fumes; and the latter change may be considered as a test of its genuineness. (*Duncan.*) An easier test is a solution of corrosive sublimate, which, added to the shavings and slightly heated, causes a bluish green color in the genuine wood. (*Chem. Gaz.*, No. 80, Feb. 1846.) Guaiacum wood is almost without smell unless rubbed or heated, when it becomes odorous. When burnt it emits an agreeable odor. It is bitterish and slightly pungent, but requires to be chewed for some time before the taste is developed. It contains, according to Trommsdorf, 26 per cent. of resin, and 0·8 of a bitter pungent extractive, upon both of which, probably, though chiefly on the former, its medicinal virtues depend. (See *Guaiaci Resina.*) It yields its virtues but partially to water. One pound of the wood afforded to Geiger two ounces of extract.

Medical Properties and Uses. Guaiacum wood ranks among the stimulant diaphoretics. It is said to have been introduced to the notice of European practitioners by the natives of Hispaniola, soon after the discovery of America. It was used in Europe so early as 1508, and attained great celebrity as a remedy for lues venerea; but more extended experience has proved it to be wholly inadequate to the cure of that disease; and it is now employed simply to palliate the secondary symptoms, or to assist the operation of other and more efficient remedies. It is thought to be useful also in chronic rheumatism and gout, scrofula, certain cutaneous eruptions, ozæna, and other protracted diseases dependent on a depraved or vitiated condition of the system. It is usually exhibited in decoction, and in combination with other medicines, as in the compound decoction of sarsaparilla. As but a small portion of the guaiac contained in it is soluble in water, the probability is that its virtues have been greatly overrated, and that the good which has followed its employment resulted rather from the more active medicines with which it is associated, or from the attendant regimen, than from the wood itself. The simple decoction may be prepared by boiling an ounce in a pint and a half of water down to a pint, the whole of which may be administered in divided doses during the twenty-four hours. An aqueous extract is directed by the French Codex.

Off. Prep. Decoctum Sarsaparillæ Compositum; Syrupus Sarsaparillæ Compositus.
Off. Prep. Br. Decoctum Sarsæ Compositum.

GUAIACI RESINA. *U. S., Br.* *Guaiac.*

(GUĂĪ'Ą-CĪ RĘ-ȘĪ'NĄ—gwā'yą-sī.)

"The resin of the wood of Guaiacum officinale. Linné. (*Nat. Ord.* Zygophyllaceæ.)" *U. S.* "The resin obtained from the stem of Guaiacum officinale, *Linn.*, or of Guaiacum sanctum, *Linn.*, by natural exudation, by incision, or by heat." *Br.*

Resina Guajaci, *P.G.;* Guaiacum; Guaiacum Resin; Résine de Gayac, *Fr.;* Guajak, Guajakharz, *G.;* Resina de Guajaco, *It.;* Resina de Guayaco, *Sp.*

For a description of *Guaiacum officinale*, see *Guaiaci Lignum*, p. 727.

Guaiac is the concrete juice of this tree. It is obtained in several different modes. The most simple is by spontaneous exudation, or by incisions made into the trunk. Another method is by sawing the wood into billets about three feet long, boring them longitudinally with an auger, then placing one end of the billet on the fire, and receiving in a calabash the melted guaiac, which flows out through the hole at the opposite extremity. But the plan most frequently pursued is probably to boil the wood, in the state of chips or sawdust, in a solution of common salt, and skim off the matter which rises to the surface. Guaiac is brought to this market from the West Indies. It is usually in large irregular pieces of various size, in which small fragments of bark, sand, and other impurities are mixed with the genuine guaiac, so as to give to the mass a diversified appearance. Sometimes we find it in small roundish homogeneous portions, separate or agglutinated; sometimes in homogeneous masses, prepared by melting and straining the drug in its impure state. It is probable that the guaiac, obtained from the billets in the manner above described, is of uniform consistence.*

Properties. The masses are irregular or somewhat globular, of a glassy lustre and resinous fracture. They are of a deep greenish brown or dark olive color on their external surface, and internally wherever the air can penetrate. The predominant hue of those parts not exposed to the air is reddish brown or hyacinthine, diversified, however, with shades of various colors. The odor is feeble but fragrant, and is rendered stronger by heat. The taste, which is at first scarcely perceptible, becomes acrid after a short period; and a permanent sense of heat and pungency is left in the mouth and fauces. Guaiac is brittle, and when broken presents a shining glass-like surface, conchoidal or splintery, with the smaller fragments more or less translucent. It is readily pulverized; and the powder, at first of a light gray color, becomes green on exposure to the light. Its sp. gr. varies from 1·2 to 1·23. It softens in the mouth, and melts with a moderate heat. Water dissolves a small proportion of guaiac, not exceeding nine parts in 100, forming an infusion of a greenish brown color and sweetish taste, which, upon evaporation, yields a brown substance soluble in hot water and alcohol, but scarcely so in ether. Alcohol takes up the whole, with the exception of impurities. The tincture is of a deep brown color, is decomposed by water, and affords blue, green, and brown precipitates, with the mineral acids. It is colored blue by nitric acid, by chlorine, and by tincture of the chloride of iron, and usually by spirit of nitrous ether; and is similarly changed when treated successively by dilute hydrocyanic acid, and solution of sulphate of copper. Either in substance or tincture, guaiac gives a blue color to gluten and substances containing it, to mucilage of gum arabic, to milk, and to various freshly cut roots, as the potato, carrot, and horseradish. It is soluble also in ether, alkaline solutions, and sulphuric acid. The solution in sulphuric acid is of a rich claret color, deposits, when diluted with water, a lilac precipitate, and, when heated, evolves charcoal. Exposed to air and light, guaiac absorbs oxygen and becomes green, and the change takes place rapidly in the sunshine. Tincture of guaiac has been used for the detection of blood-stains, which it does by the blue color produced by it, when in contact with the red coloring matter of blood, in connection with some ozonized substance, especially peroxide of hydrogen. (*Guy's Hosp. Reports*, 3d ser., xiii. 432.)

It may be used also to distinguish the blood of man and other mammals, in which

* Under the name of *Resina Guaiaci Peruviana Aromatica* there is a substance circulating in European commerce, which probably has no relation to guaiac. For a summary of our knowledge concerning it, see *A. J. P.*, 1877, p. 18.

the corpuscles are non-nucleated, from that of other classes, as birds, fishes, and reptiles, which have nucleated corpuscles. The following method of applying the test, made known by Dr. R. M. Bertolet, microscopist of the Philadelphia Hospital, has the advantage that it will present the evidence to the spectator, and thus be made to give conviction in jury trials. A microscopic preparation, duly mounted, is carefully irrigated with a simple tincture of guaiac resin, and then, under glass, exposed to the action of a very small quantity of an ethereal solution of peroxide of hydrogen. The mammalian corpuscles will exhibit a uniform blue coloration throughout, of different shades in the different corpuscles, while, if the blood corpuscle is nucleated, the nucleus is seen as a well-defined and deep blue body, with a delicate violet-colored medium around it. (*Am. Journ. of Med. Sci.*, Jan. 1874, p. 129.)

The composition of guaiacum resin was ascertained by Hadelich (*Journ. für pr. Chem.*, 87, p. 335) to be as follows. Guaiaconic acid 70·3 per cent., guaiaretic acid 10·5 per cent., guaiac beta-resin 9·8 per cent., gum 3·7 per cent., ash constituents 0·8 per cent., guaiacic acid, coloring matter (guaiac yellow), and impurities 4·9 per cent. Of these constituents, *guaiaretic acid*, $C_{20}H_{26}O_4$, was discovered by Hlasiwetz in 1859. It may be extracted from the crude resin by alcoholic potash or by quicklime, forming a crystalline salt with the former and an amorphous compound with the latter. The free acid is obtained by decomposing one of these salts with hydrochloric acid and crystallising from alcohol. The crystals, which are soluble in ether, alcohol, benzol, chloroform, carbon disulphide, or acetic acid, but not in ammonia or in water, melt below 80° C., and may be volatilized without decomposition. They are not colored blue by oxidizing agents. If the mother-liquor from the potassium salt of the guaiaretic acid be decomposed with hydrochloric acid and the precipitate washed with water, ether will extract *guaiaconic acid*, $C_{19}H_{20}O_5$. This compound, discovered by Hadelich in 1862, is a light brown amorphous substance, fusing at 100° C. It is without acid reaction, but decomposes alkaline carbonates, forming salts easily soluble in water and alcohol. It is insoluble in water, benzol, or bisulphide of carbon, but dissolves in ether, chloroform, acetic acid, or alcohol. With oxidizing agents it assumes a transient blue tint. After the extraction of the guaiaconic acid, there remains a substance insoluble in ether, to which the name of *Guaiac Beta-resin* has been applied. Its composition does not appear to differ greatly from that of guaiaconic acid.

Guaiacic acid, $C_{12}H_{16}O_6$, obtained in 1841 by Thierry, from guaiacum wood, or from the resin, crystallizes in colorless needles. Hadelich states that not more than one part in 20,000 can be obtained from the resin.

Guaiac yellow, the coloring matter of guaiacum resin, was first observed by Pelletier. It crystallizes in pale yellow quadratic octahedra, having a bitter taste, but is not a glucoside.

Guaiac resin also yields interesting products on dry distillation. First, according to Hlasiwetz, is obtained *guaiacene*, C_5H_8O, at 118° C., next, *guaiacol*, $C_6H_4\left\{\begin{matrix}OCH_3\\OH\end{matrix}\right.$, being the methyl ether of pyrocatechin, at 205°–210° C., and with it *kreosol*, $C_6H_3(CH_3)_2OH$, and finally, *pyroguaiacin*, $C_{38}H_{44}O_6$ (according to Wiesner, $C_{18}H_{18}O_3$), in pearly scales, melting at 180° C.

According to Lieben and Zeisel (*Ber. d. Chem. Ges.*, xiv. p. 932), guaiacene is the aldehyd of tiglic acid, $C_5H_8O_2$, and can be made synthetically from a mixture of acetaldehyd and propionaldehyd.

It will be inferred, from what has been said, that the mineral acids are incompatible with the solutions of guaiac.

Adulterations. This drug is sometimes adulterated with the resin of the pine. The fraud may be detected by the terebinthinate odor exhaled when the sophisticated guaiac is thrown upon burning coals, as well as by its partial solubility in hot oil of turpentine. This liquid dissolves resin, but leaves pure guaiac untouched. Amber is said to be another adulteration. Nitric acid affords an excellent test of guaiac. If paper moistened with the tincture be exposed to the fumes of this acid, it speedily becomes blue. Purgotti proposed guaiac resin as a test for copper. (See *A. J. P.*, June, 1880.)

Medical Properties and Uses. Guaiac is stimulant and alterative, producing, when swallowed, a sense of warmth in the stomach, with dryness of the mouth and thirst, and promoting various secretions. If given to a patient when covered warm in bed, especially if accompanied with opium and ipecacuanha, or the antimonials, and assisted by warm drinks, it often excites profuse perspiration; and hence it has been usually ranked among the diaphoretics. If the patient be kept cool during its administration, it is sometimes directed to the kidneys, the action of which it promotes. In large doses it purges; and it is thought by some practitioners to be possessed of emmenagogue powers. It has been given with asserted advantage in chronic rheumatism, gouty affections, secondary syphilis, scrofulous diseases, and cutaneous eruptions. It was much relied upon by the late Dr. Dewees in the cure of amenorrhœa and dysmenorrhœa. Dr. James Jackson, of Boston, recommends it occasionally as a laxative, in the dose of a drachm.

The medicine is given in substance or tincture. The dose of the powder is from ten to thirty grains (0·65–1·95 Gm.), which may be exhibited in pill or bolus, in the shape of an emulsion formed with gum arabic, sugar, and water, or as a syrup.* An objection to the form of powder is that it quickly aggregates. Guaiac is sometimes administered in combination with alkalies, with which it readily unites. Several European Pharmacopœias direct a *soap of guaiac*, under the name of *sapo guaiacinus*, to be prepared by diluting the liquor potassæ with twice its weight of water, boiling lightly, then adding guaiac gradually, with continued agitation, so long as it continues to be dissolved, and finally filtering, and evaporating to the pilular consistence. One scruple (1·3 Gm.) may be taken daily in divided doses.

Off. Prep. Pilulæ Antimonii Compositæ; Tinctura Guaiaci; Tinctura Guaiaci Ammoniata.

Off. Prep. Br. Mistura Guaiaci; Pilula Hydrargyri Subchloridi Composita; Tinctura Guaiaci Ammoniata.

GUARANA. *U.S.* *Guarana.*†

(GUA-RÄ'NA.)

"A dried paste prepared from the crushed or ground seeds of Paullinia Sorbilis. Martius. (*Nat. Ord.* Sapindaceæ.)" *U.S.*

Paullinia, Brazilian Cocoa, Guarana Bread; Paò de Guarana, *Indian*; Pasta Guarana, *P.G.*; Guarana, *Fr.*, *G.*

Gen. Ch. *Capsule* pyriform, septicidal. *Stem* climbing. *Leaves* compound. *Bentham and Hooker.*

There are described of the genus Paullinia 80 species, all of them confined in their geographical range to Eastern South America, except one, which has strayed to Western Africa. The name of the genus was given in honor of Christ. Fred. Paullini, a German medico-botanical writer, who died in 1712.

P. Sorbilis. Martius, *Reise in Brasil*, vol. iii. p. 1098; *B. & T.* 67.—*Guarana uva.* This woody climber grows in the northern and western provinces of Brazil, ripening its seeds in October and November. The leaves are alternate, on long stalks, impari-pinnate, with five oblong oval, coarsely irregularly sinuate-dentate leaflets, five to six inches long by two to three broad, contracted into a shortly attenuated blunt point. The flowers are arranged in axillary, spicate panicles, four inches or more in length. The fruit is about the size of a grape, ovoid or pyriform, on a short peduncle, with a short strong beak, glabrous, with six longitudinal ribs. The three-valved pericarp is thin, tough, and strongly hairy within. Another species, the *P.*

* *Syrup of Guaiac.* Dr. T. C. Craig. (*A. J. P.*, July, 1880.) Powd. Guaiac Resin, 640 grains; Caustic-Potassa, 58 grains; White Sugar, ℔j (avoird.); Water, q. s. Dissolve the Potassa in 8 fluidounces of water; moisten the Guaiac with this solution; pack it in a percolator and gradually pour on the remainder of the solution; when this ceases dropping, add sufficient water to make the percolate measure eight fluidounces; add the sugar and dissolve.

† It is said to have been by mistake that *Paullinia* and *guarana* have been considered identical; the former term being applicable exclusively to the product of the two species of Paullinia above referred to, while the latter belongs properly to a preparation made by the aborigines, belonging to the tribe Guaranas, whence its name. This second substance contains the seeds of the Paullinia, but is a mixture of various substances, among them chocolate and farina, the precise composition of which is most carefully kept secret by the natives. (*Ann. de Thérap.*, 1858, p. 76.)

Cupana, growing on the banks of the Orinoco River, is said also to be used in making guarana. (*Ann. de Thérap.*, 1858, p. 70.)

Preparation and Properties. The seeds, which look like small horse-chestnuts, are contained in a three-celled, three-valved, coriaceous capsule, are lenticular and almost thorny, and invested with a flesh-colored arillus, which is easily separable when dry. Guarana is made exclusively by the Guaranis, a tribe of South America Indians, and probably varies in the details of its preparation, as it certainly does i appearance and quality. The general method of manufacture is said to be by powdering the seed in a mortar, or upon a chocolate-stone previously heated, mixing the powder with a little water, exposing it for some time to the dew, then kneading it into a paste, mixing with this some of the seeds, either whole or merely bruised, and finally forming, probably with the addition of various foreign matters, a mixture which is shaped into cylindrical or globular masses. After having been dried and hardened in the sun, or by the smoke of a fire, these masses are of a reddish brown color, rugose on the surface, very hard, with an irregular fracture, and of a marbled appearance when broken, due to the fragments of the seeds and their black testa imbedded in the mass. Paullinia is of a somewhat astringent and bitterish taste, and, in this as well as in its odor, bears some resemblance to chocolate, though not oleaginous. It swells up and softens in water, which partially dissolves it. Martius found in it a crystallizable principle, which he named *guaranine*, but which has been proved by MM. Berthemot and Dechastelus to be identical with *caffeine*. Alexander Bennett, in an elaborate series of physiological experiments, has confirmed this identity.* The discovery of caffeine in plants belonging to distinct natural families, namely, the coffee and tea plants, the Paraguay tea, and the Paullinia, is a highly interesting result of recent chemical investigations. It is said to be more abundant in the Paullinia than in either of the other vegetables; 5·07 per cent. having been found by Dr. Stenhouse in Paullinia, while he got only 2·13 from good black tea, 1·00 per cent. from coffee, and 1·2 from Paraguay tea. (*P. J. Tr.*, xvi. 213.) According to Berthemot and Dechastelus, it exists in the seeds united with tannic acid, with which it appears to form two compounds, one crystallizable and soluble in water, the other of a resinoid appearance and insoluble. Besides these ingredients, the seeds contain free tannic acid, gum, albumen, starch, and a greenish fixed oil. (*Journ. de Pharm.*, xxvi. 514.) For a method of preparing guaranine, see *Journ. de Pharm.*, 4e sér., xviii. 224. Rochefontaine and Gusset prepare guaranine by mixing one part of calcined magnesia with five parts of powdered guarana, moistening with water, and after standing 24 hours, exhausting the mass with boiling chloroform, evaporating the chloroform, treating the residue with boiling water, filtering, and evaporating over sulphuric acid. (*A. J. P.*, 1886, p. 248.) Dr. F. V. Greene, U. S. N., prefers a process for obtaining caffeine from guarana similar to one proposed by Prof. Wayne for its extraction from tea and coffee. The details of the method are as follows. The powdered guarana is intimately mixed with three times its weight of finely divided litharge, and the mixture boiled in distilled water, until, on allowing the temperature to fall below the boiling point, the insoluble portion is found to subside rapidly, leaving the supernatant liquid clear, and without color. When cool, the clear liquid is filtered, and the precipitate is transferred to the filter and washed with boiling water, the washing to be continued as long as yellowish precipitates are produced with either phosphomolybdic acid solution, auric or platinic chloride. A stream of sulphuretted hydrogen gas is now passed through the filtrate, and the sulphide of lead thus formed separated by filtration. The solution is evaporated on a water-bath to expel the excess of sulphuretted hydrogen, filtered to remove a trace of sulphur, finally evaporated to the crystallizing point, and the caffeine, which crystallizes out on cooling, removed from the mother-liquor and pressed between folds of bibulous paper. After being thus treated, the crystals will be found to be perfectly white. Dr. F V. Greene has shown that the tannic acid from guarana has different properties from that found in other plants, and proposes to call it *paullinitannic acid*. (*A. J. P.*, 1877, p. 390.) M. Fournier has found in paullinia, besides tannate of caffeine, the following principles: gum, starch, an acrid green fixed oil, a concrete volatile

* This identity has recently been denied by Dr. T. J. Mays. (See H. C. Wood's *Therapeutics*.)

oil, an aromatic liquid volatile oil soluble in water with a little alcohol, another liquid volatile oil scarcely soluble in water, a peculiar principle not precisely determined, and tannic acid. (*Ibid.*, Avril, 1861, p. 291.) Dr. E. R. Squibb examined commercial guarana, and obtained 4·38 per cent. of alkaloid in good specimens. On account of the uncertainty of the composition of guarana, he recommends fluid extract of green coffee as a substitute. (See Part II., *National Formulary;* also, *Ephemeris*, 1884, p. 612.)

Medical Properties and Uses. The effects of guarana upon the system are chiefly those of its alkaloid, although it contains enough tannin to have an appreciable influence. It is habitually employed by the Indians, either mixed with articles of diet, as with cassava or chocolate, or in the form of drink, prepared by scraping it, and suspending the powder in sweetened water, precisely as other nations use teas, coffees, etc. It is also considered by the Indians useful in the prevention and cure of bowel complaints. Dr. Gavrelle, who was formerly physician to Dom Pedro, in Brazil, and there became acquainted with the virtues of this medicine, called the attention of the profession to it some years since in France. He had found it advantageous in the diarrhœa of phthisis, sick headache, paralysis, tedious convalescence, and generally as a tonic. It has since been employed in various affections, but is now chiefly used in migraine or nervous sick headaches, administered when the attack is developing. It may be given in substance, in the quantity of one or two drachms (3·9–7·8 Gm.), rubbed into powder and mixed with sweetened water; but the fluid extract may be substituted in equivalent doses.

Off. Prep. Extractum Guaranæ Fluidum.

GUTTA-PERCHA. *U. S., Br.* *Gutta-Percha.*

(GŬT'TA PĔR'CHA.)

"The concrete exudation of Isonandra Gutta. Hooker. (*Nat. Ord.* Sapotaceæ.)" *U. S.* "The concrete juice of Dichopsis Gutta (Isonandra Gutta, *Hook.*), and of several other trees of the natural order Sapotaceæ." *Br.*

Gutta-Percha Depurata, *P.G.;* Gutta-Taban; Gutta-Percha, *Fr.*, *G.*

This valuable product of the East Indies was first brought into notice by Dr. Wm. Montgomerie, a British army surgeon, who became acquainted with its singular properties in the year 1842, at Singapore, and in the following year sent specimens of it to Europe. It is the product of a large tree growing in the southern extremity of the Malayan Peninsula, the islands of Singapore and Borneo, and probably many other islands in the neighborhood. *Isonandra gutta* is of considerable magnitude, with a trunk commonly three feet and sometimes as much as six feet in diameter, having numerous ascending branches, which are crowded with leaves at their extremities. The flowers are small and white; the leaves petiolate, oblong, four or five inches long by two in breadth, bright green above and brownish beneath.*

Dr. Montgomerie states that the natives procure the gutta-percha by the very wasteful mode of cutting down the tree, stripping off the bark, and then collecting the milky juice, which is put into convenient recipients, and coagulates on exposure to the air. Twenty or thirty pounds are thus collected from each tree; but the probability is that the product would be much greater if obtained by tapping the tree, and thus preserving it for future use. In consequence of the abundance in which it is collected, and the wasteful methods pursued, fears are entertained that the tree will before long be extirpated. The exportations from Singapore (which port furnishes the bulk of all the gutta-percha of commerce) now amount to four and a

* *Bulata.* Under the name of *bulata*, the product of *Sapota Mulleri*, a tree growing in great abundance in Dutch Guiana in South America, has recently attracted considerable attention, having been imported into England from Demerara. It is said to have properties which will render it, in some instances, a useful substitute for gutta-percha, which it resembles in elasticity and exceeds in ductility, while requiring a much higher heat to soften. Its solubilities in various menstrua do not seem to have been determined; but they are probably analogous to those of gutta-percha and caoutchouc. It is the concrete juice of the *Sapota Mulleri*, or *bullet tree.* The idea is entertained that it may serve as a good insulating material for submarine telegraphic wires. Another possible substitute for gutta-percha has been found in the concrete juice of an *Apocynea* growing in Ceylon, named *Alstonia scholaris.* (*P. J. Tr.*, 2d ser., vi. 490. See also *Caoutchouc*, Part II.)

half million kilogrammes annually, valued at three and a quarter million dollars. As found in commerce gutta-percha is generally impure, containing fragments of vegetable matter and earth. From these it may be freed by kneading it in hot water, or by melting it with oil of turpentine, straining, and evaporating. It may also be purified by means of chloroform. One part of gutta-percha cut into small pieces, put into a flask with 20 parts of chloroform, and frequently shaken, will be fully dissolved in two or three days. To this solution, which cannot be readily filtered, add one-fourth of a part of water, shaking the mixture, and then allowing it to rest for two weeks. The impurities rise or sink, and the clear intervening liquid yields pure gutta-percha by the distillation of the chloroform. (*Chem. Centralbl.*, Feb. 1857, p. 108.) A more satisfactory method is probably by dissolving one part of gutta-percha in twenty of boiling benzol, shaking the solution frequently with sulphate of calcium, which upon standing two or three days carries down with it the coloring matter, then decanting the clear liquid, and adding it, in small portions at a time, to alcohol, agitating continually. During this process the gutta-percha is deposited perfectly white. Thorough desiccation requires an exposure of several weeks, but it may be hastened by rubbing in a mortar. (*Journ. de Pharm.*, Août, 1863, p. 138.)*

Properties. Gutta-percha is of a dull white or whitish color, often with reddish brown streaks, of a feeble odor, tasteless, at ordinary temperatures hard and almost horny, somewhat flexible in thin pieces, having an unctuous feel under the fingers, and very tenacious. Its sp. gr. is 0·9791. (*Soubeiran.*) At about 49° C. (120° F.), it becomes softer and more flexible, but is still elastic, resisting, and tenacious. At 66° C. to 71° C. (150° F. to 160° F.), it is soft, very plastic, and capable of being welded and moulded into any form; "plastic above 120° F. (48°·8 C.)" *Br.* It can be softened, either by means of hot water or by dry heat. On cooling it reassumes its former state, and retains any form which may have been given to it. In the softened state it is readily cut with a knife, though with some difficulty when cold. Exposed to a heat of 166° C. (330° F.), it loses a portion of water, and on hardening becomes translucent and gray; but it recovers its original characters if immersed in water. Subjected to igneous distillation, it yields volatile products, resembling closely the volatile oil obtained from caoutchouc by the same process. Heated in an open vessel, it melts, foams up, and takes fire, burning with a brilliant flame and smoke. A portion thus melted retains the state of a viscid fluid on cooling. Gutta-percha is a non-conductor of electricity. It is insoluble in water, alcohol, alkaline solutions, and the weak acids. Ether and the volatile oils soften it in the cold, and imperfectly dissolve it with the aid of heat. Oil of turpentine dissolves it perfectly, forming a clear colorless solution, which yields it unchanged by evaporation. It is also dissolved by bisulphide of carbon, chloroform, and benzol and benzin. According to Soubeiran, it contains, besides pure gutta-percha, small portions of a vegetable acid, casein, and two resins one soluble in ether and oil of turpentine, the other in alcohol. (*Journ. de Pharm.*, 3e sér., xi. 22.) Freed from these impurities, it has an ultimate composition closely analogous to if not identical with that of caoutchouc. For a particular account of the distinctive properties of pure gutta-percha, and the two resins mixed with it, the reader is referred to an article by M. Payen, in the *Journ. de Pharm.* (3e sér., xxii. 183), also in the *Chem. Gaz.* (x. 353). According to Baumhauer, pure gutta-percha, as it issues from the tree, is a hydrocarbon, with the formula $C_{10}H_{16}$, which

* *Pure white gutta-percha.* For dental purposes, as for filling carious hollows, it is desirable that gutta-percha should be purified, and rendered perfectly white. But what is sold as such in the market is said to consist largely of the white oxide of zinc, and is on this account badly adapted to the purpose intended. Mr. F. Baden Benger recommends the following method of purification for dentists' use. He states that good crude gutta-percha will yield at least 75 per cent. of the purified. Four ounces of the gutta-percha, in small pieces, are to be digested for a few days with five pounds of methylated chloroform; and the solution thus formed should be filtered in such a way as to permit little or no loss of chloroform. To the liquid thus filtered, which should be nearly colorless, an equal bulk of alcohol should be added, or a sufficiency to precipitate the gutta-percha, which will separate as a white mass. This is to be washed with alcohol, pressed in a cloth, and dried by exposure to the air. In this state, the gutta-percha is perfectly white, but too porous for use. To give it the proper consistence, it should be boiled for half an hour in a porcelain capsule, and rolled into cylinders while hot. The dentist can prepare this himself with sufficient economy, if he guard against the loss of chloroform. This may be separated from alcohol by washing with water, and the alcohol from the water by distillation. (*P. J. Tr.*, Sept. 1868, p. 160.)

he calls *gutta*, and by the oxidation of which, in various degrees, the different bodies constituting gutta-percha are produced. This hydrocarbon can be separated by treating gutta-percha with dilute hydrochloric acid, and boiling the residue with ether, which deposits the gutta on cooling; but the ethereal treatment must be frequently repeated to obtain it quite pure. (*Journ. für prakt. Chem.*, lxxviii. 279.) M. Arppe considers gutta-percha as a mixture of six different resins, which may have been formed from a hydrocarbon, $C_{10}H_{16}$. (See *Chem. Gaz.*, ix. 471.) Oudemans (*Jahresber.*, 1859, p. 517) finds two resinous products in gutta-percha: *fluavil*, fusing at 42° C., with the formula $C_{20}H_{32}O$, and soluble in cold alcohol, and *albane*, fusing at 140° C., with the formula $C_{10}H_{16}O$, and soluble in chloroform, bisulphide of carbon, and ether, from which last it crystallizes out on cooling. Gutta-percha resists putrefaction strongly; but in certain situations, as when employed to protect underground telegraph wires passing near the roots of the oak, it has been observed to undergo speedy decomposition, in consequence, as is supposed, of the action of fungi. (*P. J. Tr.*, xvii. 193.)

Gutta-percha has been applied to many useful and ornamental purposes. Its plasticity when moderately heated, great firmness and tenacity at ordinary temperatures, and insolubility in water and alcohol are the properties to which it chiefly owes its value. By immersing it in hot water, it is made susceptible of being formed into any desirable shape; so that utensils of various kinds, ornamental impressions, casts, sheets, bands, cords, sticks, tubes, etc., applicable to numerous purposes in the arts, may be made from it with great facility. To give it greater pliability, it is sometimes mixed with the tar resulting from the igneous decomposition of caoutchouc, or with its own tar and lampblack. It may be vulcanized in the same manner as caoutchouc, and undergoes a similar change of properties. (See *Caoutchouc.*) In the dissolved state it may be employed as a varnish, impervious to moisture.

Medical Uses. Gutta-percha has been introduced into surgery, in order to preserve limbs and joints in fixed positions, and has been used beneficially in club-foot, fractures, and diseases of the joints. It is employed for these purposes in the shape of bands, two or three inches broad and about a line thick, which, being softened in water, are applied in this state, and, when they harden, form a firm case for the limb. Holes should be made through the bands, for the escape of the vapor from the surface. It may in some cases be applied by moulding it, in its soft state, upon the part to be kept at rest, as to the hip and adjacent parts of the body and thigh, in cases of hip-joint disease, for which, when dried, it will form a support equal to the most accurately carved wooden splint. It is also used for the formation of catheters and other tubes, splints, stethoscopes, bougies, specula, pessaries, and various other instruments useful in surgery. In fractures it is much used as a splint; sometimes, after softening by immersion in warm water at the time, it is applied as a bandage without difficulty, and, hardening afterwards, acts as a splint to the injured limb. The officinal Liquor Gutta-Perchæ affords a liquid which, when applied by means of a camel's-hair pencil, forms, on the evaporation of the solvent, a thin, elastic covering, which completely excludes the air, and acts like an artificial cuticle to the part. Another application of gutta-percha is to serve as a vehicle of certain caustic substances, particularly chloride of zinc, and caustic potassa. The preparation is made by reducing the caustic substance to fine powder, and then thoroughly mixing it with its weight of gutta-percha, melted at the lowest possible temperature. (See *Potassa*, and *Zinci Chloridum.*) A great advantage of the preparation is that it may be made into any desirable form, and will retain that form when applied for a considerable length of time.

Off. Prep. Liquor Gutta-Perchæ.

HÆMATOXYLON. *U.S.* *Hæmatoxylon.* [*Logwood.*]

(HÆ-MA-TŎX'Y-LŎN.)

"The heart-wood of Hæmatoxylon Campechianum. Linné. (*Nat. Ord.* Leguminosæ, Papilionaceæ.)" *U.S.* "The sliced heart-wood of Hæmatoxylum Campechianum." *Br.*

Hæmatoxyli Lignum, *Br.;* Lignum Campechianum, *P.G.;* Lignum Cœruleum; Bois d'Inde, Bois de Sang, Bois de Campêche, *Fr.;* Blauholz, Campecheholz, Blutholz, Kampeschenholz, *G.;* Legno di Campeggio, *It.;* Palo de Campeche, *Sp.*

Gen. Ch. Calyx five-parted. *Petals* five. *Capsule* lanceolate, one-celled, two-valved, with the valves boat-form. *Willd.*

Hæmatoxylon Campechianum. Willd. *Sp. Plant.* ii. 547; Woodv. *Med. Bot.* p. 455, t. 163; Carson, *Illust. of Med. Bot.* i. 33, pl. 25. This is a tree of middle size, usually not more than twenty-four feet high, though, under favorable circumstances, it sometimes rises forty or fifty feet. The trunk, seldom exceeding twenty inches in diameter, is often very crooked, and is covered with a dark rough bark. The

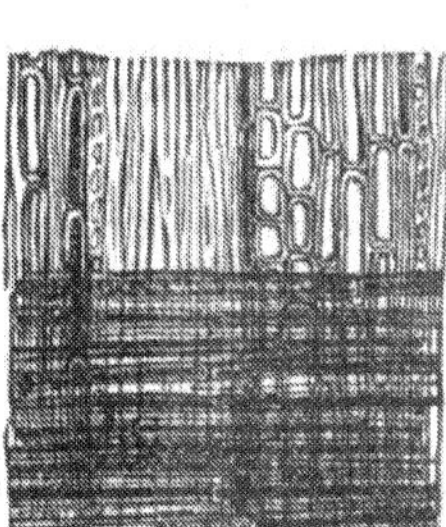

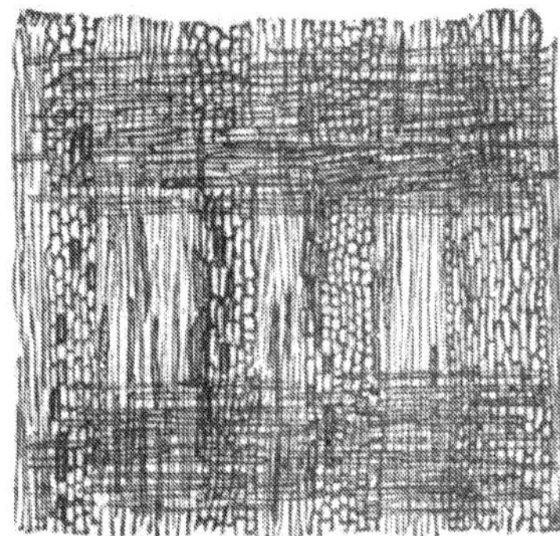

Hæmatoxylon, longitudinal section, as seen under high and low powers.

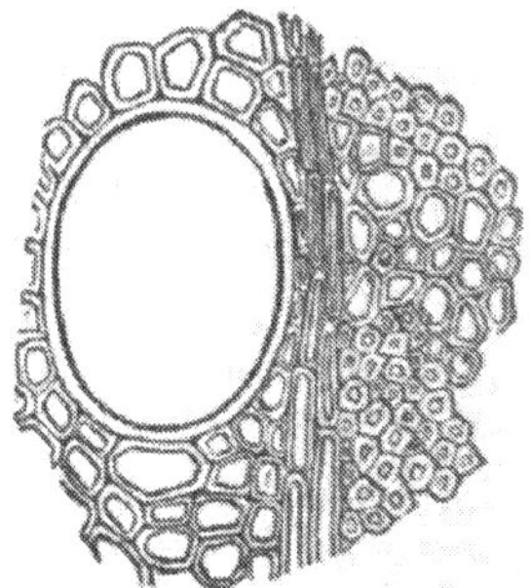

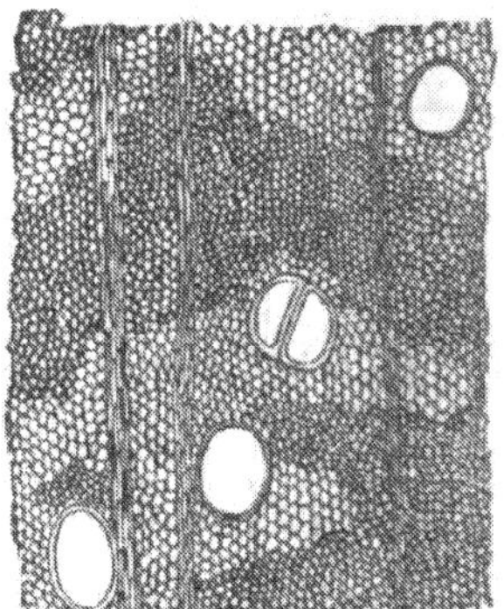

Hæmatoxylon, transverse section, as seen under high and low powers.

branches are also crooked, with numerous smaller ramifications, which are beset with sharp spines. The sap-wood is yellowish, but the interior layers are of a deep red color. The leaves are alternate, abruptly pinnate, and composed of three or four pairs of sessile, nearly obcordate, obliquely nerved leaflets. The flowers, which are in axillary spikes or racemes near the ends of the branches, have a brownish purple calyx and lemon-yellow petals. They exhale an agreeable odor, said to resemble that of the jonquil.

The tree is a native of Campeachy, the shores of Honduras Bay, and other parts of tropical America, and has become naturalized in Jamaica. The wood, which is the part used in medicine, is a valuable article of commerce, and largely employed in dyeing. It comes to us in logs deprived of the sap-wood, and having a blackish brown color externally. For medical use it is cut into chips, or rasped into coarse powder, and in these states it is kept in the shops.

Properties. Logwood is hard, compact, heavy, of a deep red color, becoming purplish black by exposure, internally brown-red, and marked with irregular, concentric circles, splitting irregularly, of a slight peculiar odor, and a sweet, somewhat astringent taste. Logwood is generally kept in the shops in small chips or coarse powder of a dark brown-red color, often with a greenish lustre. When chewed it colors the saliva dark pink. It imparts its color to water and to alcohol. The infusion made with cold water, though red, is less so than that with boiling water. It affords precipitates with sulphuric, nitric, hydrochloric, and acetic acids, alum, sulphate of copper, acetate of lead, and sulphate of iron, striking a bluish black color with the last-mentioned salt. (*Thompson's Dispensatory.*) Precipitates are also produced with it by lime-water and gelatin. Chevreul found in logwood a volatile oil, an oleaginous or resinous matter, a brown substance the solution of which is precipitated by gelatin (*tannin*), another brown substance soluble in alcohol but insoluble in water or ether, a nitrogenous substance resembling gluten, free acetic acid, various salts, and a peculiar principle, called *hæmatoxylin* or *hématin*, on which the coloring properties of the wood depend. This is obtained by digesting the aqueous extract in alcohol, evaporating the tincture till it thickens, then adding a little water, and submitting the liquid to a new but gentle evaporation. Upon allowing it to rest, hæmatoxylin is deposited in crystals, which may be purified by washing with alcohol and drying. Thus procured, the crystals are shining, of a yellowish rose color, bitterish, acrid, and slightly astringent to the taste, readily soluble in boiling water, forming an orange-red solution which becomes yellow on cooling, and soluble also in alcohol and ether. According to Erdmann, who obtained hæmatoxylin by the process of Chevreul, substituting ether for alcohol, its crystals, when quite pure, are colorless, without a tinge of redness; its taste is sweet, like that of liquorice, without bitterness or astringency; and it is not of itself a coloring substance, but affords beautiful red, blue, and purple colors, by the joint action of an alkaline base and the oxygen of the air. He obtained from logwood 9 to 12 per cent. of crystallized hæmatoxylin, to which he gave the formula $C_{16}H_{14}O_6$. It crystallizes with 1 or with 3 molecules of water, and is readily soluble in hot water or alcohol, but sparingly in cold water or in ether. (*Journ. für pr. Chem.*, 36, p. 205.)

By the combined action of ammonia and oxygen dark violet crystalline scales of *hæmatëin*, $C_{16}H_{12}O_6 + 3H_2O$, are produced. They show a fine green hue, which is also very commonly observable on the surface of the logwood chips of commerce. Hæmatein may again be transformed into hæmatoxylin by means of hydrogen or of sulphurous acid. Commercial extract of logwood extracted from the wood by boiling water contains both hæmatoxylin and hæmatein.

Medical Properties and Uses. Logwood is a mild astringent, devoid of irritating properties, and well adapted to the treatment of that relaxed condition of bowels which is apt to succeed cholera infantum. It is also occasionally used with advantage in ordinary chronic diarrhœa and chronic dysentery. The only officinal preparation is the extract. Dose, ten to twenty grains (0 65–1·3 Gm.).

Off. Prep. Extractum Hæmatoxyli.

HAMAMELIS. *U. S.* *Hamamelis.* [*Witchhazel.*]

(HĂM-A-MĒ'LĬS.)

"The fresh leaves of Hamamelis virginica, Linné (*Nat. Ord.* Hamamelaceæ), collected in autumn." *U. S.*

Gen. Ch. Flowers in little axillary clusters or heads, usually surrounded by a scale-like three-leaved involucre. *Calyx* four-parted, and with two or three bractlets at its base. *Petals* four, strap-shaped, long and narrow, spirally involute in the bud. *Stamens* eight, very short; the four alternate with the petals anther-bearing, the others imperfect and scale-like. *Styles* two, short. *Pod* opening loculicidally from the top. *Gray's Manual.*

H. Virginica. L. *Witch-hazel* is an indigenous shrub, from five to fifteen feet high, growing in almost all sections of the United States, usually on hills or in stony places, and often on the banks of streams. It is the only species of the genus found in Eastern North America, and is specifically characterized by its leaves being obovate or oval, wavy-toothed, and somewhat downy when young. The seeds are black and shining externally, white, oily, and farinaceous within, and edible like the hazelnut. It is remarkable for the late appearance of its yellow flowers, which expand in September or October, and continue till the weather becomes very cold in winter. The fruit, which is a nut-like capsule not unlike the hazelnut, ripens in the following autumn, and is often mingled on the same plant with the new blossoms.

Properties. The leaves of the witchhazel are officinally described as "short-petiolate, about four inches (10 cm.) long, obovate or oval, slightly heart-shaped and oblique at the base, sinuate-toothed, nearly smooth; inodorous; taste astringent and bitter." *U. S.* The bark, which is sometimes used, has a bitter, astringent, somewhat sweetish, and pungent taste.

Walter B. Cheney examined witchhazel bark, and found tannin, resin, extractive, but no indication of an alkaloid or other crystalline principle. (*A. J. P.*, 1886, p. 418.) It contains a trace of volatile oil, however. Dr. John Marshall, of the University of Pennsylvania, also found that hamamelis root contains tannic acid and a trace of volatile oil, but no other active substance. (*Therap. Gaz.*, ii. 295.)

Medical Properties. The bark of the witchhazel is said to have first attracted attention on account of its use by the North American Indians as a sedative application to external inflammations. It was many years ago strongly recommended by Dr. James Fountain and Dr. N. S. Davis (*N. Y. Jour. Med.*, x. 208; *Trans. Amer. Med. Assoc.*, i. 350) in hemorrhage of the lungs and stomach. Dr. Fountain also used with alleged great advantage an ointment prepared from lard and the decoction of equal parts of hamamelis, white-oak bark, and apple-tree bark. Of late years the professional attention has been very strongly directed to the remedy on account of the enormous sale of a much vaunted proprietary remedy said to be made by distilling the bark with very dilute alcohol (six per cent. solution), and used externally for sprains and bruises, and internally for most of the diseases to which flesh is heir. The pecuniary success of this remedy probably has depended in very small part upon the virtues of the witchhazel, which seems to possess no active physiological properties. At least we have injected a very concentrated distillate in large quantities into frogs and into mammals without perceiving any more effects than would be produced by the injection of similar quantities of distilled water, and Dr. Guy, in Paris, has reached similar conclusions. The fluid extract of the drug has been used as a remedy in various forms of venous dilatation and engorgement. It was very strongly commended by Dr. Jno. H. Musser in varicose veins (*Phila. Med. Times*, vol. xiii. 499), and has been used by some practitioners with good results in cases of hemorrhoids, but has failed to yield in other hands corresponding advantage. (See *Boston Med. and Surg. Journ.*, April 16, May, 1885; also *Bull. Gén. de Thérap.*, vol. cvi. p. 94.) The dose of the fluid extract given by Dr. Musser was a teaspoonful four times a day. It may, however, be given in double the quantity with impunity, and probably in such doses is advantageous through the gallic acid which it contains.

Off. Prep. Extractum Hamamelidis Fluidum.

HEDEOMA. *U.S.* *Hedeoma.* [*Pennyroyal.*]

(HĔD-Ē-Ō'MA.)

"The leaves and tops of Hedeoma pulegioides. Persoon. (*Nat. Ord.* Labiatæ.)" *U. S.*

Herbe de Pouliot américaine, *Fr.;* Amerikanischer Poley, *G.*

This herb, first attached to the genus *Melissa*, and afterwards to *Cunila*, is at present universally considered by botanists as belonging to the *Hedeoma* of Persoon. It has been confounded by some with *Mentha Pulegium*, or European pennyroyal.

Gen. Ch. *Calyx* bilabiate, gibbous at the base, upper lip three-toothed, lower two; dentures all subulate. *Corolla* ringent. *Stamens* two, sterile; the two fertile stamens about the length of the corolla. *Nuttall.*

Hedeoma pulegioides. Barton, *Med. Bot.* ii. 165.—*Cunila pulegioides.* Willd. *Sp. Plant.* i. 122. This is an indigenous annual plant, from nine to fifteen inches high, with a small, branching, fibrous, yellowish root, and a pubescent, quadrangular stem, which sends off numerous slender erect branches. The leaves are opposite, having short petioles, about half an inch long, oblong-lanceolate or oval, nearly acute, attenuated at the base, remotely serrate, rough or pubescent, and prominently veined and glandular on the under surface. The flowers are very small, pale blue, supported on short peduncles, and arranged in axillary whorls along the whole length of the branches. They have a tubular-ovoid, two-lipped and five-toothed calyx, and a pale blue, spotted, two-lipped corolla, containing two sterile and two fertile exserted stamens. The plant is common in all parts of the United States, preferring dry grounds, and, where abundant, scenting the air for a considerable distance with its grateful odor. Both in the recent and dried state it has a pleasant aromatic smell, and a warm, pungent, mint-like taste. It readily imparts its virtues to boiling water. The volatile oil upon which they depend may be separated by distillation, and employed instead of the herb itself. For the chemical nature of the oil, see *Oleum Hedeomæ*.

Medical Properties and Uses. Pennyroyal is a gently stimulant aromatic, and may be given in flatulent colic and sick stomach, or to qualify the action of other medicines. Like most of the aromatic herbs, it possesses the property, when administered in warm infusion, of promoting perspiration, and of exciting the menstrual flux when the system is predisposed to the effort. A large draught of the warm tea is in popular practice often given at bedtime, in recent cases of suppression of the menses, the feet having been previously bathed in warm water.

HEMIDESMI RADIX. *Br. Hemidesmus Root.* [*Indian Sarsaparilla.*]

(HĔM-Ĭ-DĔS'MĪ RĀ'DĬX.)

"The dried root of Hemidesmus indicus, *R.*" *Br.* (*Nat. Ord.* Asclepiadaceæ.)

Nunnari, *E.*; Racine de Hemidesmus, *Fr.*; Hemidesmus-Wurzel, *G.*

Gen. Ch. Corolla rotate. *Filaments* connate at the base, not united above, inserted into the tube of the corolla. *Anthers* cohering separate from the stigma, with twenty pollen-masses. *Stigma* flattish, pointless.

Hemidesmus Indicus. R. Brown, *Hort. Kew.* ii. 75; Lindley, *Flor. Med.* p. 543.—*Periploca Indica.* Willd. *Sp. Plant.* i. 1251. This is a climbing plant, with twining, woody, slender stems, and opposite petiolate leaves, which are entire, smooth, shining, and of a firm consistence. The leaves vary much in size and shape, some being linear and acute, others broad-lanceolate, and others again oval or ovate. The flowers are small, green on the outside, purple within, and disposed in axillary racemes. The calyx is five-parted, with acute divisions; the corolla flat, with oblong, pointed divisions. The fruit consists of two long, slender, spreading follicles.

This plant is common over the whole peninsula of Hindostan. The officinal portion is the root, which has long been used in India as a substitute for sarsaparilla. It is long, slender, tortuous, cylindrical, and little branched, consisting of a ligneous centre, and a brownish, corky bark, marked with longitudinal furrows and transverse fissures. The microscopic characters of this root are curious and of much interest to the structural botanist. (See *P. J. Tr.*, 1872, p. 62.) It has an aromatic odor and bitter taste. Mr. Garden obtained from it a peculiar volatilizable acid principle, which he named *smilasperic acid*, under the erroneous impression that the root was derived from *Smilax aspera.* Pereira proposed to call it *hemidesmic acid.* Scott (*Chem. Gazette*, 1843, p. 378) also obtained a stearopten by distillation with water, presumably the same material. It has not been further investigated.

Medical Properties and Uses. Indian sarsaparilla is said to be tonic, diuretic, and alterative. It was introduced into Great Britain from India, and was employed for some time under the name of *smilax aspera.* It is used for the same purposes as sarsaparilla. In some instances it is said to have proved successful in syphilis when that medicine had failed; but it cannot be relied on. The native practitioners in India are said to employ it in nephritic complaints, and in the sore mouth of children. It is used in the form of infusion or decoction, made in the proportion of two ounces of the root to a pint of water. A pint may be given in wineglassful doses, in the course of the day. A syrup is directed in the British Pharmacopœia. (See *Syrupus Hemidesmi.*)

Off. Prep. Br. Syrupus Hemidesmi.

HIRUDO. *Br.* *The Leech.*

(HI-RŪ'DŌ.)

"Sanguisuga medicinalis (*Savigny*), the *Speckled Leech*; and S. officinalis (*Sav.*), the *Green Leech*." *Br.*

Hirudinea, *P.G.;* Sangsue, *Fr.;* Blutegel, *G.;* Mignátta, *It.;* Sanguijuela, *Sp.*

HIRUDO. *Class* 1, Annelides. *Order* 3, Abranchiatæ. *Family* 2, Asetigeræ. *Cuvier.*

The leech belongs to that class of invertebrated articulated animals called *Annelides.* This class contains the worms with red blood, having soft retractile bodies composed of numerous segments or rings, breathing generally by means of branchiæ, with a nervous system consisting in a double knotted cord, destitute of feet, and supplying their place by the contractile power of their segments or rings. The third order of this class—*Abranchiatæ*—comprehends those worms which have no apparent external organ of respiration. This order is again divided into two families, to the second of which—the *Asetigeræ*, or those not having setæ to enable them to crawl—the leech belongs.

It is an aquatic worm with a flattened body, tapering towards each end, and terminating in circular flattened disks, the hinder one being the larger of the two. It swims with a vertical undulating motion, and moves when out of the water by means of these disks or suckers, fastening itself first by one and then by the other, and alternately stretching out and contracting its body. The mouth is placed in the centre of the anterior disk, and is furnished with three cartilaginous lens-shaped jaws at the entrance of the alimentary canal. These jaws are lined at their edges with fine sharp teeth, and meet so as to make a triangular incision in the flesh. The head is furnished with small raised points, supposed by some to be eyes. Respiration is carried on through small apertures ranged along the inferior surface. The nervous system consists of a cord extending the whole length, furnished with numerous ganglions. The intestinal canal is straight, and terminates in the anus, near the posterior disk. Although hermaphrodite, leeches mutually impregnate each other. They are oviparous; and the eggs, varying from six to fifteen, are contained in a sort of spongy, slimy cocoon, from half an inch to an inch in diameter. These are deposited near the edge of the water, and hatched by the heat of the sun. The leech is torpid during the winter, and casts off from time to time a thick slimy coating from its skin. It can live a considerable time in sphagnous moss, or in moistened earth, and is frequently transported in this manner to great distances.

Savigny has divided the genus Hirudo of Linnæus into several genera. The true leech is the Sanguisuga of this author, and is characterised by its three lenticular jaws, each armed with two rows of teeth, and by having ten ocular points. Several species are used for medical purposes, of which the most common are the gray and the green leech of Europe, both of which are varieties of the *Hirudo medicinalis* of Linnæus; and the *Hirudo decora* of this country.

1. *Hirudo medicinalis.* Linn. *Ed. Gmel.* i. 3095.—*Sanguisuga officinalis.* Savigny, *Mon. Hir.* p. 112, t. 5, f. 1. *The green leech.* — *Sanguisuga medicinalis.* Savigny, *Mon. Hir.* p. 114, t. 5, f. 2. *The gray leech.* Many of the best zoologists regard the *Sanguisuga officinalis* and *S. medicinalis* of Savigny as mere varieties. They are both marked with six longitudinal dorsal ferruginous stripes, the four lateral ones being interrupted or tessellated with black spots. The color of the black varies from a blackish to a grayish green. The belly in the first variety is of a yellowish green color, free from spots, and bordered with longitudinal black stripes. In the second it is of a green color, bordered and maculated with black. This leech varies from two to four inches in length. It inhabits marshes and running streams, and is abundant throughout Europe.*

* A variety of the leech has come into use in Europe, called in commerce *African leeches.* They are of a beautiful light green color, varying to a deep green, and often inclining to red, with black points on the back, and broad streaks of a bright orange yellow, which are black towards the abdomen. They correspond perfectly with the *Sanguisuga interrupta* of Moquin-Tandon. These leeches draw very well. (*P. J. Tr.*, x. 38.) The leeches from Algiers, called in French commerce *dragons* (*Sanguisuga troctena* of Moquin-Tandon), of which considerable numbers have been taken

The great use made of leeches in the modern practice of medicine has occasioned them to become a considerable article of commerce. They are collected in Spain, France, Italy, Germany, and Sweden, and carried in large numbers to London and Paris. They are also frequently brought to this country; as the practitioners in some of our large cities use only the foreign leech, although our own waters furnish an inexhaustible supply of this useful worm.*

2. *Hirudo decora.* Say, *Colonel Long's Second Expedition*, ii. 268. The medicinal leech of America has been described by Say under the name of *Hirudo decora*, in the Appendix to the Second Expedition of Colonel Long. Its back is of a deep pistachio-green color, with three longitudinal rows of square spots. These spots are placed on every fifth ring, and are twenty-two in number. The lateral rows of spots are black, and the middle range, of a light brownish orange color. The belly is of the latter color, variously and irregularly spotted with black. The American leech sometimes attains the length of four or five inches, although its usual length is from two to three. It does not make so large and deep an incision as the European leech, and draws less blood.

The indigenous leech is much used in the city of Philadelphia. The practitioners of New York and Boston are supplied chiefly from abroad. The leeches employed in Philadelphia are generally brought from Bucks and Berks Counties, in Pennsylvania, and occasionally from other parts of the State.

The proper preservation of leeches is an object of importance to the practitioner, as they are liable to a great and sudden mortality. They are usually kept in jars, in clear, soft water, which should be changed twice a week in winter, and every other day in summer. The jar must be covered with a linen cloth, and placed in a situation not liable to sudden changes of temperature. They will live a long time and continue active and healthy, without any other attention than that of frequently changing the water in which they are kept. M. Derheims has proposed the following excellent method of preserving them. In the bottom of a large basin or trough of marble he places a bed, six or seven inches deep, of a mixture of moss, turf, and fragments of wood. He strews pebbles above, so as to retain them in their place without compressing them too much, or preventing the water from freely penetrating them. At one end of the trough, and about midway of its height, is placed a thin slab of marble or earthenware, pierced with numerous holes, and covered with a bed of moss, which is compressed by a thick layer of pebbles. The reservoir being thus disposed is half filled with water, so that the moss and pebbles on the shelf shall be kept constantly moist. The basin is protected from the light by a linen cover stretched over it. By this arrangement the natural habits of the leech are not counteracted. One of these habits, essential to its health, is that of drawing itself through the moss and roots to clear its body from the slimy coat which forms on its skin and is a principal cause of its disease and death. Mr. James Baues recommends that, when kept in jars, they should be cleansed by means of a whisk of very fine broom

to France, are said by M. A. de Quatrefages, contrary to former opinion, to be quite equal to the European. (*Journ. de Pharm.*, 3e sér., xxxiii. 105.) It is stated (*P. J. Tr.*, June, 1867, p. 735) that great numbers of leeches are collected in Australia, and sent to Melbourne, whence a large proportion are exported to Europe and America, chiefly to London and Paris in the former continent, and San Francisco, Panama, and New York in the latter. It is estimated that two or three millions annually pass through the hands of the Murray River Fishing Company. The leech is said (*Ibid.*, March, 1865, p. 461) to abound in almost every river and lagoon in Australia, and to differ from the ordinary English leech only, that the olive streaks are much lighter in the former. They are collected by throwing into the water a fresh sheep-skin, to which they attach themselves. They bear transportation wonderfully well. In Hindostan and the island of Ceylon, where the varieties of leeches are said to be more numerous than in any other part of the world, it is stated by Mr. P. L. Simmonds, that the propagation of the kind used in medicine is carefully kept secret. (*P. J. Tr.*, Dec. 1870, p. 522.)

* Attempts have been made, in France, on a large scale, to propagate leeches for sale. This is done by means of natural meadows, in which numerous small ponds are made, where the leeches, with certain cautions as to nourishment and preservation, multiply and grow so rapidly as to become a source of profit. In order that they may propagate, it is necessary that they should be fed on blood, which is given them either by causing animals, as horses, cows, etc., to be driven into the meadows, or by obtaining blood from slaughter-houses, and, after depriving it of fibrin by agitation, immersing the animals for a time in it while yet warm. (See *Journ. de Pharm.*, Jan. 1854, p. 5, and Mai, 1854, p. 336.)

or willow, when the water is changed. M. Lahache, an apothecary at Bruyères, strongly recommends the carrageen or Irish moss (*Chondrus crispus*), as admirably adapted to the habits and wants of the leech, furnishing the animal, as he supposes, with nutriment, as it does not die of inanition when thus kept. The water should be renewed in the jars daily. (*Journ. de Pharm. et de Chim.*, 4e sér., iii. 128.) Mr. Alfred Allchin keeps them in aquaria with growing water-plants and snails, which keep the water pure.* (*A. J. P.*, xxviii. 222.)

Medical Uses. Leeches afford the least painful and in many instances the most effectual means for the local abstraction of blood. They are often applicable to parts which, either from their situation or their great tenderness when inflamed, do not admit of the use of cups; and, in the cases of infants, are under all circumstances preferable to that instrument. They are indeed a powerful therapeutic agent, and give to the physician, in many instances, a control over disease which he could obtain in no other way. Their use is in great measure restricted to the treatment of local inflammation; and, as a general rule, they should not be resorted to until the force of the circulation has been diminished by bleeding from the arm, or in the natural progress of the complaint.

In applying leeches to the skin, care should be taken to shave off the hair, if there be any, and to have the part well cleansed with soap and water, and afterwards with pure water. If the leech do not bite readily, the skin should be moistened with a little blood, or milk and water. It is said to bite more freely if the skin is previously reddened by a sinapism, and then washed perfectly clean. Sometimes the leech is put into a large quill open at both ends, and applied with the head to the skin until it fastens itself, when the quill is withdrawn. If it be desirable that the leech shall bite in a particular spot, this end may be attained by cutting a small hole in a piece of blotting-paper, and then applying this moistened to the skin, so that the hole shall be immediately over the spot from which the blood is to be taken. Leeches continue to draw blood until they are gorged, when they drop off.† The quantity of blood which they draw varies with the part to which they are applied, and the degree of inflammation existing in it. From the loose and vascular textures they will abstract more than from those which are firm and compact, and more from an inflamed than from a healthy part. As a general rule, our leechers apply six for every fluidounce of blood. A single European leech will draw from half an ounce to an ounce. The quantity may often be much increased by bathing the wound with warm water. Leeches will continue to suck after their tails are cut off, which is sometimes done, although it is a barbarous practice.‡ It is said that they will draw better if put into cold beer, or diluted wine, and allowed to remain until they become very lively. They may be separated from the skin at any time by sprinkling a little salt upon them. After they drop off, the same application will make them disgorge the blood they have swallowed. Some leechers draw the leeches from the tail to the head through their fingers, and thus squeeze out the blood, after which all that is necessary is to put them in clean water, and change it frequently.§ Leeches which are

* For other methods of keeping leeches, also for raising them, see *U. S. D.*, 14th ed., p. 472.

† As a very efficient mode of applying leeches, it is recommended, after having moistened the skin with pure warm water, to put the leeches into a tumbler half full of cold water, and by an adroit movement invert it upon the part. The leeches are said to attach themselves so rapidly that it seems to the patient as though they made but a single bite. When they are all attached, the glass is to be carefully removed, the water being absorbed, as it runs off on one side, by a sponge or linen cloths.

‡ Under the name of *bdellatomy*, a practice has been introduced into Germany, of making a small incision in the side of the leech while drawing. The blood escapes through the wound, and the animal will continue to suck for a long time, so that one will perform the office of many in the quantity of blood taken.

§ MM. Soubeiran and Bouchardat, after numerous experiments upon the different modes of fitting the gorged leeches for use again, came to the conclusion that a carefully managed pressure is the best. Two conditions, however, are necessary to success; one that they should be disposed to disgorge the blood, and the other that they should be immersed in warm water previously to the stripping. The first object is effected by common salt. The following plan is recommended. The leeches are to be thrown into a solution of 16 parts of common salt in 100 of water, from which they are to be taken out one by one, and, being held by the tail, are to be dipped into water which feels hot to the hand, but yet can be borne by it, and then passed lightly between the fingers. Thus treated, they easily give up the blood. After being stripped, they should be placed in ves-

gorged with blood should be kept in a vessel by themselves; as they are more subject to disease, and often occasion a great mortality among the others. They should not be again used until they have recovered their activity. In cases where the bleeding from leech-bites continues longer than is desirable, it may be stopped by continued pressure, with the application of lint, by the use of collodium, or by touching the wounds with lunar caustic. A little cotton, impregnated with a saturated solution of alum in boiling-hot water, and, after it has become sufficiently cool, but before the alum has begun to crystallize, pressed upon the wound, will often prove effectual. Another mode of repressing the hemorrhage is to press upon the bite a piece of thin caoutchouc, previously softened upon one side by heat, so as to become adhesive. If lunar caustic be applied, the stick must first be brought to a fine point, which is to be inserted in the wound. Some have even recommended the use of a fine wire made red hot. When the part wounded is without a bony basis, pressure may be made by pinching the wound between the fingers. It may sometimes be necessary, in the case of a deep bite, to sew the wound, which is readily done with a single stitch of the needle, that need not penetrate deeper than the cutis.*

HORDEUM DECORTICATUM. *Br.* *Pearl Barley.*

(HÖR'DE-ŬM DE-CŎR-TI-CĀ'TŬM.)

"The dried seed of Hordeum distichon, *Linn.*, divested of its integuments. From plants cultivated in Britain." *Br.* (*Nat. Ord.* Graminaceæ.)

Hordeum, *U. S.* 1870; Hordeum Perlatum; Orge perlé, Orge, *Fr.;* Perlgerste, Perlgraupen, Gerstengraupen, *G.;* Orzo, *It.;* Cebada, *Sp.*

Gen. Ch. *Calyx* lateral, two-valved, one-flowered, three-fold. *Willd.*

Several species of Hordeum are cultivated in different parts of the world. The most common are *H. vulgare* and *H. distichon*, both of which have been introduced into the United States.

1. *Hordeum vulgare.* Willd. *Sp. Plant.* i. 472; Loudon's *Encyc. of Plants*, p. 73. The culm or stalk of common barley is from two to four feet in height, fistular, and furnished with alternate, sheathing, lanceolate, roughish, and pointed leaves. The flowers are all perfect, and arranged in a close terminal spike, the axis of which is dentate, and on each tooth supports three sessile flowers. The calyx or outer chaff has two valves. The corolla or inner chaff is also composed of two valves, of which the interior is larger than the other, and terminates in a long, rough, serrated awn or beard. The seeds are arranged in four rows.

2. *H. distichon.* Willd. *Sp. Plant.* i. 473; Loudon's *Encyc. of Plants*, p. 73. This species is distinguished by its flat spike or ear, which on each flat side has a double row of imperfect or male florets without beards, and on each edge, a single

sels containing fresh water, which should be renewed once a day. At the end of eight or ten days, they are fit for reapplication. (*Journ. de Pharm.*, 3e sér., xi. 343 and 350.) It is said that, in the French military hospitals, a mixture of one part of vinegar with eight parts of water is preferred to salt water for promoting disgorgement. (*Lond. Med. Times and Gaz.*, Oct. 1856, p. 375.) It has been stated that, if the leeches, after being stripped, be put into water sweetened with a little white sugar, and the solution be renewed several times, at intervals of six or twelve hours, they will speedily recover their activity, and may be reapplied two or three times in the course of a few days. Immersion in camphor-water, for a few moments, is said by Mr. Boyce to cause them to vomit the blood. They should afterwards be put into clean water, to be changed in half an hour. Dr. Frodsham, of England, has found camphor-water preferable either to salt water or diluted vinegar, for disposing the gorged leech to part with blood. M. Grannat, a French military pharmaceutist, has found the natural process of disgorging preferable to all others. He placed some gorged leeches in wooden tubs, containing at bottom a little clay and water, and renewed the water every forty-eight hours. After eight days, the leeches, now in good health, were transferred to a pond prepared for the purpose, where they propagated. He put 1000 leeches in the pond, and at the end of a year had taken out 850 fit for service, without interfering with the reproduction. (*Journ. de Pharm.*, 3e sér., xx. 186.) M. Vayson's plan of preserving leeches has been highly recommended. It consists simply in putting them, after stripping, if they have been used, in an earthenware vessel of the shape of an inverted truncated cone, with holes in the bottom so small as to prevent the escape of the leech, and filled with turfy earth. After the introduction of the leech, the opening is to be closed with a coarse cloth. The vessel is then placed in a tub containing water four inches deep. If to be sent to a distance, the earth in the vessel should be moistened throughout.

* An instrument has been invented called the *mechanical leech*, by which the attempt has been made to imitate the action of the leech in drawing blood. It consists essentially of two parts, one for making the puncture, and the other for abstracting blood through the agency of atmospheric pressure. In other words, it is a minute cupping instrument. (*Am. Journ. Med. Sci.*, xvi. 207.)

row of bearded perfect or hermaphrodite florets. The seeds, therefore, are in two rows, as indicated by the specific name of the plant.

The original country of the cultivated barley is unknown. The plant has been found growing wild in Sicily, and various parts of the interior of Asia. *H. vulgare* is said by Pursh to grow in some parts of the United States, apparently in a wild state. The seeds are used in various forms.

1. In their natural state they are oval, oblong, pointed at one end, obtuse at the other, marked with a longitudinal furrow, of a yellowish color externally, white within, having a faint odor when in mass, and a mild sweetish taste. Careful analyses of barley have been made, which agree in the main, though differing in some details, especially as to whether any sugar exists in the barley before malting.

Pillits found (*Zeit. für Anal. Chem.*, 1872, p. 62) in the dry barley 14·3 per cent. of insoluble albuminates, 2·1 per cent. of soluble albuminates, 62·6 per cent. of starch, 1·9 per cent. of dextrin, 2·7 per cent. of sugar, 1·7 per cent. of extractive material, 3·1 per cent. of fat, 1·4 per cent. of soluble ash, 1·2 per cent. of insoluble ash, and 8·9 per cent. of lignin. The presence of sugar seems to have been shown by Kühnemann (*Deutsch. Chem. Ges.*, 1875, p. 387, and 1876, p. 1385), who found a crystallized dextrogyrate sugar which did not reduce alkaline copper solution, and an amorphous lævogyrate mucilaginous substance called *sinistrin*. According to Kühnemann, barley does not contain dextrin.

Clifford Richardson (*Bulletin Department of Agriculture*, No. 9, 1886, p. 77) gives the following as the average composition of American barley: water, 6·47 per cent.; ash, 2·87; oil, 2·67; sugar, etc., 7·02; dextrine and soluble starch, 3·55; starch, 62·09; albumenoids soluble in 80 per cent. alcohol, 3·66; albumenoids insoluble in 80 per cent. alcohol, 7·86; fibre, 3·81: total, 100·00. He finds, moreover, that on an average the grain makes up 84·78 per cent. and the hull 15·22 per cent. of the barley.

2. *Malt* consists of the seeds made to germinate by warmth and moisture, and then baked so as to deprive them of vitality. It is in the form of malt that barley is so largely consumed in the manufacture of malt liquors. (See *Maltum.*)

An interesting substance, called *diastase*, was discovered by MM. Payen and Persoz in the seeds of barley, oats, and wheat, and in the potato. It is found, however, only after germination, in which process the production of it appears to be the first step. Germinated barley seldom contains it in larger proportion than two parts in a thousand. It is obtained by bruising freshly germinated barley, adding about half its weight of water, expressing strongly, treating the viscid liquid thus obtained with sufficient alcohol to destroy its viscidity, then separating the coagulated albumen, and adding a fresh portion of alcohol, which precipitates the diastase in an impure state. To render it pure, it must be redissolved as often as three times in water, and precipitated by alcohol. For an account of the mode of preparing diastase from malt, recommended by M. Perrot, see the *Journal de Pharmacie*, Juillet, 1874, p. 43. It is solid, white, tasteless, soluble in water and weak alcohol, but insoluble in the latter fluid when concentrated. Though without action upon gum and sugar, it has the extraordinary property, when mixed, in the proportion of only one part to 2000, with starch suspended in water, and maintained at a temperature of about 71·1° C. (160° F.), of converting that principle into dextrin and *maltose*. This latter is a variety of sugar produced only by this action of malt. It was first recognized by Dubrunfaut, but has been more thoroughly studied by O'Sullivan and by Schulze. Its formula is $C_{12}H_{22}O_{11} + H_2O$, which molecule of water of crystallization it loses at 100°–110° C. (or, as Richter proposes, it may have the formula $C_{18}H_{34}O_{17}$). O'Sullivan explains the action of diastase upon starch by the following reactions:

At 63° C. — $C_{18}H_{30}O_{15} + H_2O = C_{12}H_{22}O_{11} + C_6H_{10}O_5$.

" 64°–70° C. — $2(C_{18}H_{30}O_{15}) + H_2O = C_{12}H_{22}O_{11} + 4(C_6H_{10}O_5)$.

" 70° C. — $4(C_{18}H_{30}O_{15}) + H_2O = C_{12}H_{22}O_{11} + 10(C_6H_{10}O_5)$. (*Chem. Soc. Journ.*, 10, p. 597.)

The crystals of maltose, $C_{12}H_{22}O_{11} + H_2O$, are soluble in water and alcohol, they reduce Fehling's solution, and, according to O'Sullivan, are equal to 63·9–65·5 per cent. of dextrose, but, according to Schulze, they are equal to 66–67 per cent. dextrose, and show a specific rotatory power of $[\alpha] = 150°$ to the right.

The whole of the starch undergoes this change, except the teguments of the granules, amounting to about 4 parts in 1000. The change which barley undergoes during germination, and in malting, is of a similar character. The purity of diastase may be tested by mixing 0·05 parts of it with 200 parts of paste containing 10 parts of starch; after standing, the resulting liquid should filter rapidly, and decolorize five times its volume of Fehling's solution. The name of *maltine* has been given to the diastase of malt; and this principle has been found identical with the salivary ferment in its action on alimentary substances. Indeed, according to M. Coutara, the two ferments, vegetable and animal, appear to be identical, not only in the action referred to, but in their chemical and physical properties; and consequently there is but one diastase, whether vegetable or animal. (*Arch. Gén.*, Avril, 1870, p. 501.)

3. *Hulled barley* is merely the grain deprived of its husk, which, according to Einhoff, amounts to 18·75 parts in the hundred.*

4. *Barley meal* is formed by grinding the seeds, previously deprived of their husk. It has a grayish white color, and contains, according to Fourcroy and Vauquelin, an oleaginous substance, sugar, starch, nitrogenous matter, acetic acid, phosphates of calcium and magnesium, silica, and iron. It may be made into a coarse, heavy, hard bread, which in some countries is much used for food.

5. *Pearl barley* (*hordeum perlatum*) is the seed deprived of all its investments, and afterwards rounded and polished in a mill. It is in small round or oval grains, having the remains of the longitudinal furrow of the seeds, and of a pearly whiteness. It is wholly destitute of hordein, and abounds in starch, with some gluten, sugar, and gum. This is the proper form of barley for medicinal use.

Medical Properties. Barley is one of the mildest and least irritating of farinaceous substances, and, though not medically used in its solid state, forms, by decoction with water, a drink admirably adapted to febrile and inflammatory complaints, and much employed from the time of Hippocrates to the present. Pearl barley is the form usually preferred for the preparation of the decoction, made by pouring four pints of boiling water on two troyounces of pearl barley and boiling away to two pints, and straining. Malt affords a liquor more demulcent and nutritious, and the decoction of malt may be prepared by boiling from two to four ounces in a quart of water and straining. When hops are added, the decoction takes the name of wort, and acquires tonic properties, which render it useful in debility, especially when attended with suppuration.

Off. Prep. Br. Decoctum Hordei.

HUMULUS. *U.S.* *Hops.*

(HŪ'MŬ-LŬS.)

"The strobiles of Humulus Lupulus. Linné. (*Nat. Ord.* Urticaceæ, Cannabineæ.)" *U.S.* "The dried strobiles of Humulus Lupulus, *Linn.*. from plants cultivated in England." *Br.*

Lupulus, *Br.;* Hop; Strobili Humuli, s. Lupuli; Hop; Houblon, *Fr.;* Hopfen, *G.;* Luppolo, *It.,* Lupolo Hombrecillo, *Sp.*

Gen. Ch. MALE. *Calyx* five-leaved. *Corolla* none. FEMALE. *Calyx* one-leafed, obliquely spreading, entire. *Corolla* none. *Styles* two. *Seed* one, within a leafy calyx. *Willd.*

Humulus Lupulus. Willd. *Sp. Plant.* iv. 769; Bigelow, *Am. Med. Bot.* iii. 163. The root of the hop is perennial, and sends up numerous annual, angular, rough, flexible stems, which twine around neighboring objects in a spiral direction, from

* M. Lemoine, a French pharmaceutist, proposes a chemical method of decorticating barley and other seeds. Putting 100 parts of the seeds into a wooden vessel, he pours upon them 15 parts of sulphuric acid, stirs the mixture for 15 or 20 minutes, applying in the case of barley a gentle heat, then adds 50 parts of water, which he decants after a very few moments of constant agitation. After sufficient washing, and the neutralization of the last remains of acid by solution of carbonate of sodium or potassium, he puts the grain upon a piece of cloth with large meshes stretched upon a frame, where he allows it to drain for about an hour, then transfers it to a similar cloth, and exposes it to a current of air for several days to dry. (*Journ. de Pharm.*, Mars, 1863, p. 223.)

left to right, and climb to a great height. The leaves are opposite, and stand upon long footstalks. The smaller are sometimes cordate; the larger have three or five lobes; all are serrate, of a deep green color on the upper surface, and, together with the petioles, extremely rough, with minute prickles. At the base of the footstalks are two or four smooth, ovate, reflexed stipules. The flowers are numerous, axillary, and furnished with bracts. The male flowers are a yellowish white, and arranged in panicles; the female, which grow on a separate plant, are pale green, and disposed in solitary, peduncled aments, composed of membranous scales, ovate, acute, and tubular at the base. Each scale bears near its base, on its inner surface, two flowers, consisting of a roundish compressed germ, and two styles, with long filiform stigmas. The aments are converted into ovate membranous cones or strobiles, the scales of which contain, each, at its base, two small seeds, surrounded by a yellow, granular powder.

The hop is a native of North America and Europe. It is occasionally found growing wild in the Eastern States, and, according to Mr. Nuttall, is abundant on the banks of the Mississippi and the Missouri. In parts of New England, New York, and Michigan, it is extensively cultivated, and most of the hops consumed in the United States are supplied by those districts. The part of the plant used is the fruit or strobiles. These when fully ripe are picked, dried by artificial heat, packed in bales, and sent into the market under the name of hops.

Hops consist of numerous thin, translucent, veined, leaf-like scales, which are of a pale greenish yellow color, and contain near the base two small, round, black seeds. They are officinally described as "ovate, about an inch and a quarter (3 cm.) long, consisting of a thin, hairy, undulated axis and many obliquely ovate, membranous, greenish scales, in the upper part reticulately veined, and toward the base parallel-veined, glandular and surrounding a sub-globular achene." *U. S.* Though brittle when quite dry, they are pulverized with great difficulty. Their odor is strong, peculiar, somewhat narcotic, and fragrant; their taste very bitter, aromatic, and slightly astringent. Their aroma, bitterness, and astringency are imparted to water by decoction; but the first-mentioned property is dissipated by long boiling. The most active part of hops is a substance formed on the surface of the scales, and, in the dried fruit, existing in the state of very small granules. This substance was called *lupulin* by the late Dr. A. W. Ives, of New York, by whom its properties were first investigated and made generally known; though it was previously noticed by Sir J. E. Smith, of England, and M. Planche, of France. The scales themselves, however, are not destitute of virtues, and contain, as shown by MM. Payen and Chevallier, the same active principles as the lupulin, though in less proportion.*

* Hops are often subjected in Germany to the fumes of burning sulphur, from the supposition that they keep better when thus treated. Besides, by being partially bleached by the process, old hops, which have suffered from time, having become darker, generally spotted, and weaker, assume a brighter appearance, as if fresher, and generally command a better price in the market. To detect the consequent presence of sulphurous acid, the brewers put a silver spoon in a mixture of hops and water, under the impression that it will produce a black stain upon the silver. But this test will answer only when applied within a fortnight after the use of the sulphur. A more delicate method is that of Dr. Heidenreich, who puts 20 or 30 cones of the hops in a flask with zinc and hydrochloric acid, and passes the hydrogen evolved through solution of acetate of lead. If sulphurous acid be present, sulphuretted hydrogen will be produced, which will occasion a dark precipitate with the solution. But even this plan often fails when the hops have been kept more than three or four weeks. A modification of this test has been proposed by Dr. R. Wagner. For the solution of acetate of lead used in Heidenreich's method, there is to be substituted a solution of nitro-prusside of sodium, so weak as to have a very light brown color, to which have been added a few drops of solution of potassa. If the gas evolved contain the minutest proportion of sulphur, a violet color will be produced when the first bubble passes into the solution; and this will by a continuance of the process become a magnificent purple. The least trace of sulphurous acid may thus be found; but, a few months after the sulphuring of hops, none at all can be detected. (*Chem. Gaz.*, April 1, 1856; from *Comptes-Rendus.*)

Hops are said to be sometimes threshed in order to separate the lupulin, which is sold separately. Their efficiency is thus, no doubt, greatly impaired. Hops thus treated have the scales more or less broken; and any parcel presenting this appearance may be suspected. Hops often contain a variable quantity of lupulin, in consequence of the granules of this substance separating, especially on agitation, and seeking the lower portion of the mass, which thus becomes richer, while the upper is poorer. They should always be examined in reference to the lupulin they contain, and, if nearly or quite destitute of it, should be deemed of inferior value, and not to be used medicinally, though not worthless.

LUPULINA. *U. S. Lupulin.* This is obtained separate by rubbing or threshing and sifting the strobiles, of which it constitutes from one-sixth to one-tenth by weight. It is in the state of a yellowish powder, mixed with minute particles of the scales, from which it cannot be entirely freed when procured by a mechanical process. It has the peculiar flavor of hops, and appeared to MM. Lebaillif and Raspail, when examined by the microscope, to consist of globules filled with a yellow matter, resembling in this respect the pollen of vegetables; but, from the investigations of M. Personne, it would seem to be of the nature of a gland, commencing in a cell formed among those of the epidermis, and, when fully developed, secreting a resinous matter. (*Journ. de Pharm.*, 3e sér., xxvi. 242.) It is inflammable, and when moderately heated becomes somewhat adhesive. The odor of lupulinic grains resides in the essential oil. This is obtained to the extent of 0·9 per cent. by distilling hops with water. Personne stated that it contained *valerol*, $C_6H_{10}O$, which passes into valerianic acid; the latter in fact occurs in the glands, yet, according to Mehn, only to the extent of 0·1 to 0·17 per cent. When distilled from the fresh strobiles the oil has a greenish color, but a reddish brown when old hops have been employed. It is devoid of rotatory power, neutral to litmus paper, and gives no remarkable coloration with concentrated sulphuric acid. The bitter principle formerly called *lupulin* or *lupulite* was first isolated by Lermer (*Journ. für pr. Chem.*, 101, p. 137), who called it the *bitter acid of hops* (*Hopfenbittersaüre*). It crystallizes in large brittle rhombic prisms, and possesses the peculiar bitter taste of beer. Its composition is $C_{32}H_{50}O_7$. The main contents of the hop gland consists of wax (*myricyl palmitate* according to Lermer) and resins, one of which is crystalline and unites with bases. Besides the constituents of the glands, hops contain, according to Etti, *humulo-tannic acid* and *phlobaphene.* The former is a whitish, amorphous mass, soluble in alcohol, hot water, or acetic ether, not in ether. By heating the humulo-tannic acid to 130° C., or by boiling its aqueous or alcoholic solution, it gives off water and is transformed into phlobaphene, a dark red amorphous substance, $(C_{25}H_{24}O_{13})^2 - H_2O = C_{50}H_{46}O_{25}$. The latter substance, on boiling it with dilute mineral acids, again loses water, and furnishes glucose. From raw phlobaphene, ether removes the bitter principles of hops, a colorless crystallizable and a brown amorphous resin, besides chlorophyll and essential oil. (*Pharmacographia*, 2d ed., pp. 553 and 555.)

The existence of a peculiar alkaloid in hops, suggested by Lermer in 1863, has been determined by Griessmayer. A concentrated decoction of hops was distilled with potassa or magnesia, the distillate neutralized with hydrochloric acid, evaporated to dryness, and treated with cold absolute alcohol to remove ammonium chloride; the alcoholic liquid was heated to boiling and cooled, when much trimethylamine chloride crystallized. The residuary liquid was filtered, the filtrate evaporated, first by a water-bath and then spontaneously, the residue was redissolved in water in a narrow cylinder, agitated with potassa and ether, and the ethereal liquid allowed to evaporate spontaneously. The remaining alkaline liquid had a peculiar odor recalling that of conine, and a cooling but not bitter taste. It soon exhibited small crystals, and finally solidified completely. The author supposed that these crystals were impurities, and that the pure alkaloid is liquid or gaseous. He proposes for it the name of *lupuline.* (*A. J. P.*, 1874, p. 360.)

Lastly, Etti found arabic (pectic) acid, phosphates, nitrates, malates, citrates, and also sulphates, chiefly of potassium, to occur in hops. The amount of ash afforded by hops dried at 100° C. would appear to be on an average about 6–7 per cent.

Dr. H. Bungener has isolated from hops a bitter crystalline substance, $C_{25}H_{35}O_4$, which is insoluble in water, but soluble in alcohol and alkaline solutions. He believes it to be identical with Lermer's hop-bitter acid, to be feebly acid, and possessing the character of an aldehyd. (*P. J. Tr.*, 1884, p. 1008.)

Medical Properties and Uses. Hops are tonic and slightly narcotic, and have been highly recommended in diseases of general or local debility, associated with morbid vigilance, or other nervous derangement. Diuretic properties have also been ascribed to them. The complaints in which they have been used are dyspepsia, and the nervous tremors, wakefulness, and delirium of drunkards.

An *infusion*, prepared with half an ounce of hops and a pint of boiling water, may be given in the dose of two fluidounces (60 C.c.) three or four times a day. The tincture is now the only officinal preparation of hops, but the alcohol probably acts more decidedly upon the system than the hops. (See *Tinctura Humuli.*) A pillow of hops has proved useful in allaying restlessness and producing sleep in nervous disorders. They should be moistened with water containing a trace of glycerin previously to being placed under the head of the patient, in order to prevent rustling. Fomentations with hops, and cataplasms made by mixing them with some emollient substance, are often beneficial in local pains and tumefactions.

The effects of hops may be obtained most conveniently by the use of *lupulin*, though Dr. Fronmüller, having after two trials with it obtained no soporific effect, denies it a place among the narcotics with hypnotic properties. (*B. and F. Med.-Chir. Rev.*, April, 1867, pp. 526–7.) Dr. Wm. Byrd Page, of Philadelphia, has found this substance very effectual as an antaphrodisiac, in the treatment of gonorrhœa, spermatorrhœa, and other irritated conditions of the genito-urinary apparatus; and the same result has been obtained by other practitioners. We have found it apparently effectual in irritable bladder, when other narcotics had failed. The dose of lupulin in substance is from six to twelve grains (0·4–0·8 Gm.), given in the form of pills, which may be made by simply rubbing the powder in a warm mortar till it acquires the consistence of a ductile mass, and then moulding it into the proper shape.* Lupulin may be incorporated with poultices, or formed into an ointment with lard, and used externally for the same purposes as hops.

Off. Prep. Tinctura Humuli.

Off. Prep. of Hops. Br. Extractum Lupuli; Infusum Lupuli; Tinctura Lupuli.

Off. Prep. of Lupulin. Extractum Lupulinæ Fluidum; Oleoresina Lupulinæ.

HYDRARGYRI CHLORIDUM CORROSIVUM. *U.S. Corrosive Chloride of Mercury.* [*Corrosive Sublimate. Mercuric Chloride.*]

$HgCl_2$; 270·5. (HȲ-DRĂR′ǤY̧-RĪ ǤHLŌ′RĮ-DŬM CŎR-RǪ-SĪ′VŬM.) $HgCl$; 135·25.

Hydrargyri Perchloridum, *Br.;* Hydrargyrum Bichloratum Corrosivum, *P.G.;* Sublimatus Corrosivus, Chloruretum (Chloretum) Hydrargyricum, Hydrargyrum Corrosivum Sublimatum, Hydrargyri Bichloridum; Corrosive Chloride of Mercury, Perchloride of Mercury, Bichloride of Mercury; Deuto-chlorure de Mercure, Sublimé corrosif, Chlorure mercurique, *Fr.;* Ætzendes Quecksilberchlorid, Ætzender Quecksilbersublimat, *G.*

A formula for this salt has been very properly omitted from the U. S. Pharmacopœia. The process of 1870 will be found in the foot-note.†

"Take of Persulphate of Mercury *twenty ounces* [avoirdupois]; Chloride of Sodium, dried, *sixteen ounces* [avoird.]; Black Oxide of Manganese, in fine powder, *one ounce* [avoird.]. Reduce the Persulphate of Mercury and the Chloride of Sodium each to fine powder, and, having mixed them and the Oxide of Manganese thoroughly by trituration in a mortar, put the mixture in an apparatus adapted for sublimation, and apply sufficient heat to cause vapors of perchloride of mercury to rise into the less heated part of the apparatus which has been arranged for their condensation." *Br.*

In order to understand the above process and that of the U. S. P. 1870, which is the same in principle, it is necessary to premise that corrosive sublimate is mercuric chloride, consisting of two atoms of chlorine and one of mercury. By boiling sulphuric acid in excess with mercury to dryness, a white salt (mercuric sulphate) is formed, according to the reaction, $2H_2SO_4 + Hg = HgSO_4 + SO_2 + 2H_2O$. (See *Hydrargyri Sulphas.*) When this is mixed with chloride of sodium (common salt),

* Dr. Dyce Duckworth, of St. Bartholomew's Hospital, London, recommends, as the result of his own observation, the aromatic spirit of ammonia as a better solvent of lupulin than any other yet proposed. He offers the following formula. "Lupulin ℥ij, Aromatic Spirit of Ammonia Oj. Macerate for seven days, with occasional agitation, then filter, and add sufficient of the menstruum to make up a pint. The dose of this *Tinctura Lupulinæ Ammoniata* is from ♏xx to f℥j." (*P. J. Tr.*, Oct. 1868.)

† "Take of Mercury *twenty-four troyounces;* Sulphuric Acid *thirty-six troyounces;* Chloride of Sodium *eighteen troyounces.* Boil the Mercury with the Sulphuric Acid, by means of a sand-bath, until a dry white mass is left. Rub this, when cold, with the Chloride of Sodium in an earthenware mortar; then sublime with a gradually increasing heat." *U.S.*

and the mixture exposed to a subliming heat, a mutual decomposition takes place, according to the reaction: $HgSO_4 + (NaCl)_2 = Na_2SO_4 + HgCl_2$. The mercuric chloride thus formed sublimes and the sodium sulphate remains behind. The quantities for mutual decomposition are two mols. of chloride of sodium and one mol. of mercuric sulphate. The British formula differs from that of the U. S. P. 1870 in ordering sulphate of mercury ready formed, instead of preparing it as the first step of the process, and in the use of a small proportion of black oxide of manganese, intended to convert into mercuric any mercurous salt that may be in the sulphate, and thus prevent the formation of mercurous chloride. (See *Hydrargyri Sulphas.*)

The names given in the two Pharmacopœias to this important chloride do not exactly correspond. It is called the corrosive chloride of mercury in the U. S. Pharmacopœia, and perchloride in the British. We prefer the former, as indicating, beyond any possibility of mistake, the article intended, as well as its corrosive property. Perchloride and subchloride are hardly sufficiently distinctive, when a mistake may be so serious as that of confounding corrosive sublimate and calomel. In the first British Pharmacopœia corrosive sublimate was recognized as the officinal title, which was a sufficient guarantee of security; but, unfortunately, it was deemed proper, immediately after the officinal title, and in close connection with it, to define the salt as chloride of mercury, in conformity with the view, adopted in that work, of the atomic weight of mercury. With many persons calomel is still the chloride of mercury, so that there is some chance that, should calomel be prescribed by this title, corrosive sublimate may be dispensed for it, with dangerous if not fatal effects to the patient. Indeed, death has, at least in one recorded instance, occurred in consequence of this confusion of nomenclature; and our officinal guides should take especial care to guard against such mistakes, instead of contributing to them.

Preparation and Properties. The first step in making corrosive sublimate is to form mercuric sulphate, by heating sulphuric acid and the metal together in an iron pot, so arranged as to carry off the unwholesome fumes of sulphurous oxide, which are copiously generated. The dry salt obtained is then mixed with the common salt, and the mixture sublimed in an iron pot lined with clay, and covered by an inverted earthen pan. The late Dr. A. T. Thomson, of London, took out a patent for forming corrosive sublimate, on the large scale, by the direct combination, by combustion, of gaseous chlorine with heated mercury. The product is stated to be perfectly pure, and to be afforded at a lower price than the sublimate made in the usual way. In order that the combination may take place, the mercury need not be heated to its boiling point, but only to a temperature between 149° C. and 204° C. (300° and 400° F.). According to Dr. Maclagan, corrosive sublimate, made by this process, is liable to the objection that a proportion of calomel is always formed, occasionally amounting to 10 per cent.

It may sometimes be useful to know how to make a small quantity of corrosive sublimate on an emergency. This may be done by dissolving mercuric oxide (red precipitate) in hydrochloric acid, evaporating the solution to dryness, dissolving the dry mass in water, and crystallising. Here a double decomposition takes place, resulting in the formation of water and the bichloride.

"Heavy, colorless, rhombic crystals or crystalline masses, permanent in the air, odorless, having an acrid and persistent, metallic taste, and an acid reaction. Soluble in 16 parts of water and in 3 parts of alcohol at 15° C. (59° F.); in 2 parts of boiling water, in 1·2 parts of boiling alcohol, and in 4 parts of ether. When heated to about 265° C. (509° F.), the salt fuses; at a higher temperature it sublimes unchanged, and without residue. The aqueous solution of the salt yields a reddish or yellowish precipitate on the addition of lime-water, and, on the addition of test-solution of nitrate of silver, a white precipitate insoluble in nitric acid, but soluble in ammonia. If 1 Gm. of the salt be dissolved in boiling water, then mixed with 5 C.c. of strong solution of soda (sp. gr. about 1·260) in a long test-tube, and about 0·5 Gm. of fine aluminium wire, cut into small pieces, be added (a loose plug of cotton being pushed a short distance down the tube), the generated gas should not impart any tint to paper wet with test-solution of nitrate of silver, and kept over the mouth of the test-tube for half an hour (abs. of arsenic)." *U. S.*

Ether is capable of removing corrosive sublimate, to a considerable extent, from its aqueous solution, when agitated with it. According to M. Mialhe, ether will not dissolve it when accompanied by a considerable quantity of mercuric oxide, and a chloride of an alkalifiable metal. Sulphuric, nitric, and hydrochloric acids dissolve it without alteration. When heated it melts, and readily sublimes in dense, white, acrid vapors, which condense, on cool surfaces, in white, shining needles. Its aqueous solution renders green the syrup of violets, and is precipitated brick-red, becoming yellow, by the fixed alkalies and alkaline earths, and white by ammonia. (See *Hydrargyrum Ammoniatum.*) The former precipitate is mercuric oxide, which has the property of evolving oxygen, and of being reduced to metallic globules when exposed to heat. This oxide is formed in the process for preparing *aqua phagedænica*, called also *lotio flava* or *yellow wash*, which is obtained by mixing half a drachm of corrosive sublimate with a pint of lime-water. Corrosive sublimate forms, with chloride of ammonium and chloride of sodium, compounds which are more soluble than the uncombined mercurial salt. It is on this account that aqueous solutions of sal ammoniac, or of common salt, dissolve much more corrosive sublimate than simple water. The combination of corrosive sublimate with chloride of ammonium was formerly called *sal alembroth*, or *salt of wisdom*. According to F. Hinterberger, corrosive sublimate is capable of combining with quinine and cinchonine. (*Chem. Gaz.*, ix. 211.) By dissolving one part of corrosive sublimate and a hundred parts of common salt in distilled water and evaporating to dryness, a soluble preparation is obtained which does not coagulate albumen. (*A. J. P.*, xliv. 11.)

Corrosive sublimate has the property of retarding putrefaction. Animal matters immersed in its solution shrink, acquire firmness, assume a white color, and become imputrescible. On account of this property it is usefully employed for preserving anatomical preparations.

Test of Purity and Incompatibles. Pure corrosive chloride of mercury sublimes, when heated, without residue, and its powder is entirely and readily soluble in ether. Consequently, if a portion of any sample should not wholly dissolve in ether, or if it should not evaporate entirely, the presence of some impurity is proved. If calomel be present, and it frequently is, it will not be wholly soluble in water.* Arsenic is reported to be a frequent impurity in corrosive sublimate. (See paper by J. Granville Smith, *A. J. P.*, 1877, p. 397.) It can be readily detected by the test of U. S. P. 1880. (See p. 748.) Corrosive sublimate is incompatible with many of the metals, the alkalies and their carbonates, soap, lime-water, tartar emetic, nitrate of silver, the acetates of lead, the sulphides of potassium and sodium, the soluble iodides, and all the sulphydrates. It is decomposed by many vegetable and some animal substances. According to Dr. A. T. Thomson, it produces precipitates in infusions or decoctions of chamomile, horseradish, columbo, catechu, cinchona, rhubarb, senna, simaruba, and oak-bark. MM. Mialhe and Lepage have shown that corrosive sublimate is slowly converted into calomel by syrup of sarsaparilla and syrup of honey, but is not changed by contact with pure syrup.

Medical Properties and Uses. Corrosive sublimate is a very powerful preparation, operating quickly, and, if not properly regulated, producing violent effects. It is less apt to salivate than most other mercurials. In minute doses, suitably repeated, it may exert its peculiar influence without any obvious alteration of the vital functions, except, perhaps, a slight increase in the frequency of the pulse, and in the secretions from the skin and kidneys. Sometimes, however, it purges; but this effect may be obviated by combining it with a little opium. In larger doses it occasions nausea, vomiting, griping pain in the bowels, diarrhœa, and other symptoms of gastric and intestinal irritation, and in still larger quantities produces all the effects of a violent corrosive poison. It has long been used as a remedy in syphilis, in all stages of which it has been highly recommended. It is said to remove the symptoms more speedily than other mercurials; whilst its action is less unpleasant, as the

* M. Bullot, having noticed in some corrosive sublimate an insoluble portion consisting of minute yellowish granules, found on examination that it was an aniline product. He surmised that the drug had been thrown into commerce after having been used in the preparation of aniline dyes. (*Journ. de Pharm.*, 4e sér., xviii. 414.)

mouth is less liable to be made sore. It is especially useful in the advanced stages of the disorder, when there is no cachexia. When a very rapid impression is desired it is not as useful as calomel. It is also used advantageously in some chronic cutaneous affections, and in obstinate chronic rheumatism. It is usually associated with alterative or diaphoretic medicines, such as the antimonials, and the compound decoction or syrup of sarsaparilla; and, in order to obviate the irritation it is apt to produce, it may often be advantageously united with opium. There is no doubt that many of the substances, in connection with which it is employed, alter its chemical condition; but it does not follow that, even in its altered state, it may not be very useful as a remedy.

Externally employed, corrosive sublimate is stimulant and escharotic. A solution in water, containing from an eighth to half a grain in the fluidounce, is employed as an injection in gleet, and as a collyrium in chronic venereal ophthalmia. A stronger solution, containing one or two grains in the fluidounce, is an efficacious wash in lepra, and other scaly eruptions. Dissolved in water, in the proportion of five to ten grains to the fluidounce, it may be used with much benefit in venereal ulcers of the throat, to which it should be applied by means of a camel's-hair pencil. With lime-water it forms the *aqua phagedænica* of the older writers, employed as a wash for ill-conditioned ulcers. The powdered chloride has been used as an escharotic, but is, in general, inferior to nitrate of silver or caustic potassa. In *onychia maligna*, however, it is employed with great advantage, mixed with an equal weight of sulphate of zinc, and sprinkled thickly upon the surface of the ulcer, which is then to be covered with a pledget of lint saturated with tincture of myrrh. The whole diseased surface is thus removed, and the ulcer heals.* This practice originated, we believe, with the late Dr. Perkins, of Philadelphia, and was highly recommended by Dr. Physick. Dr. Geo. B. Wood often employed it with success. A solution of corrosive sublimate in collodion (four parts to thirty) has been used as a caustic, for the destruction of nævi materni, and for other purposes. It can be very accurately applied, but its use requires care, as fatal poisoning has followed a single application of the alcoholic solution of corrosive sublimate to a moderate surface of ringworm. (*London Lancet*, 1871, ii. 413.) It is applied by means of a camel's-hair pencil.

The dose of corrosive sublimate is from the twelfth to the eighth of a grain (0·005 to 0·007 Gm.) preferably given after meals, in pill, or solution. The pill is usually prepared with crumb of bread; and care should be taken that the medicine be equally diffused through the pilular mass, before it is divided.

Toxicological Properties. Swallowed in poisonous doses, it produces burning heat in the throat, excruciating pain in the stomach and bowels, excessive thirst, anxiety, nausea and frequent retching with vomiting of bloody mucus, diarrhœa and sometimes bloody stools, small and frequent pulse, cold sweats, general debility, difficult respiration, cramps in the extremities, faintings, insensibility, convulsions, and death. The mucous membrane of the stomach exhibits, on dissection, signs of the operation of a violent corrosive poison. These symptoms are sometimes followed or conjoined with others indicating an excessive mercurial action upon the system, such as inflammation of the mouth and salivary glands, profuse salivation,

* *Antiseptic Dressings.* The following directions are given in *Pharm. Rundschau*, Prague, for antiseptic dressings to be used in the German army.

Corrosive Sublimate Gauze. Dissolve 50 Gm. mercuric chloride in 5000 Gm. alcohol, and add 7500 Gm. distilled water, 2500 Gm. glycerin, and 0·5 Gm. fuchsin, the latter being added for the purpose of readily distinguishing the corrosive sublimate gauze from others. Four hundred metres of gauze are well kneaded in this solution and allowed to soak for fifteen minutes; the gauze is then strongly pressed and well dried on wash-lines, being protected from light and dust.

Corrosive Sublimate Cotton. Absorbent cotton is soaked in the above solution and dried in loose layers.

Corrosive Sublimate Catgut. A 5 per cent. aqueous solution of corrosive sublimate is prepared, in which thin catgut is soaked for about eight hours, and the thicker kinds for ten or twelve hours. The catgut is subsequently kept in vials with alcohol.

Corrosive Sublimate Silk is prepared by soaking well-washed ligature silk in a solution of 5 parts of corrosive sublimate in 100 parts of water and 20 parts of glycerin. After drying it is wrapped in oiled silk or other water-proof material; and before using, it is dipped into a 3 per cent. phenol solution, or a 1 per cent. solution of corrosive sublimate.

fetid breath, etc. The only symptom of corrosive sublimate poisoning which distinguishes it from poisoning by antimony, arsenic, or other corrosive metallic irritant is the fact that the stools are very frequent, smallish, and composed chiefly of mucus and blood. A case is on record of death, in an infant, from the constitutional effects of corrosive sublimate sprinkled upon an excoriated surface; and, in two instances of children, the one seven, and the other nine years old, death, with all the symptoms of internal poisoning, followed the application to the scalp of an ointment, said to consist of one part of the corrosive chloride to four parts of tallow. (*Dub. Quarterly*, Aug. 1854, p. 70.) In the inferior animals, in whatever mode introduced into the system, it produces symptoms and lesions similar to those which it causes in man. In the treatment of poisoning by corrosive sublimate, Orfila recommends the free use of the white of eggs beaten up with water. The albumen forms an insoluble and comparatively innocent compound with the corrosive sublimate; and the liquid by its bulk dilutes the poison, and distends the stomach so as to produce vomiting. It is, however, asserted by M. Lassaigne that this compound of albumen and corrosive sublimate, when recently precipitated, is soluble in acid and alkaline liquids, and in solutions of the chlorides of potassium, sodium, and calcium. (See *Journ. de Pharm.*, xxiii. 510.) It is also soluble in an excess of albumen, whether introduced into the stomach, or previously existing there. It is, therefore, important, at the same time that the antidote is used, to evacuate the stomach before the newly formed compound can be dissolved. If eggs cannot be procured, wheat flour may be substituted; gluten having, according to M. Taddei, the same effect as albumen. Milk also has been recommended, in consequence of the insoluble compound which casein forms with the poison. Besides the antidotes mentioned, Peruvian bark, meconic acid, ferrous sulphide, and iron filings have been proposed, all of which have the property of decomposing corrosive sublimate. The ferrous sulphide was found quite successful by M. Mialhe in experiments upon dogs, if given immediately after the poison was swallowed, but failed when delayed for ten minutes. Dr. T. H. Buckler, of Baltimore, made some successful experiments on lower animals upon the antidotal properties of a mixture of gold dust and iron filings (*Med. and Surg. Journ.*, 1843); and a case of poisoning by corrosive sublimate has been recorded by Dr. C. Johnston, of the same city, in which this antidote was employed with the apparent effect of saving life, after albumen had been used without effect. Dr. Johnston, however, employed the reduced iron of the Pharmacopœia, and gold leaf, arranging them in alternate layers, so as to make boluses of convenient size. (*Am. Journ. of Med. Sci.*, April, 1863, p. 340.) The method of operating of this antidote will be understood when the action of gold and iron as a test for corrosive sublimate is explained in the succeeding paragraph. It is of the utmost importance that whatever antidote is used should be given without delay, and in this respect the one nearest at hand may be considered the best. Under all circumstances the stomach should be rapidly and thoroughly washed out by abundance of mucilaginous fluids, the stomach-pump being used if necessary. The after-effects should be treated like other forms of toxic gastro-enteritis, *i.e.*, by local bloodletting or counter-irritation, demulcent drinks, opiates, etc.

Tests for Corrosive Sublimate. On account of the extreme virulence of this chloride as a poison, the reagents by which it may be detected form a subject of study of the utmost importance, as connected with medico-legal investigations. The best tests for determining its mercurial nature, mentioned in the order of their delicacy, are ferrocyanide of potassium, lime-water, carbonate of potassium, iodide of potassium, ammonia, sulphuretted hydrogen, and stannous chloride. *Ferrocyanide of potassium* gives rise to a white precipitate (ferrocyanide of mercury), becoming slowly yellowish, and at length pale blue. *Lime-water* throws down a yellow precipitate of hydrated mercuric oxide. *Carbonate of potassium* causes a brick-red precipitate of mercuric carbonate. *Iodide of potassium* produces a very characteristic pale scarlet precipitate of mercuric iodide. This precipitate frequently appears at first yellow, especially if the corrosive sublimate be present in minute proportion. *Ammonia* gives rise to a white, flocculent precipitate, the officinal ammoniated mercury, or white precipitate. *Sulphuretted hydrogen* occasions a black precipitate of mercuric sulphide; and the same precipitate is thrown down by ammonium sulphydrate. Finally, *protochloride of tin* (stannous chloride) causes a grayish black precipitate (mercury in a finely divided state). Taking the results of Devergie, the relative delicacy of these tests may be expressed numerically as follows: Ferrocyanide of potassium 1½; lime-water 4; carbonate of potassium 7; iodide of potassium 8; ammonia 36; sulphuretted hydrogen or ammonium sulphydrate 60; and stannous chloride 80. Wormley (*Micro-Chemistry of Poisons*, 2d ed., p. 348) states that the reaction of stannous chloride is interfered with or entirely prevented by the presence of alkaline chlorates, and also of free nitric acid. He especially commends, however, the copper test, which is as follows: *A bright plate of copper*, immersed in a solution containing corrosive sublimate, is instantly tarnished, and, after the lapse of half an hour, becomes covered with a grayish white powder. *A polished piece of gold*, moistened with the *clear* mercurial solution, and touched through the liquid with a piece of iron, contracts a white stain. This test, which was proposed by Mr. Sylvester and simplified by Dr. Paris, is conveniently applied by moistening, with the suspected solution, a gold coin or ring, and touching it through the moistened spot with the point of a penknife. The object of the iron is to form with the gold a simple galvanic circle, which enables the latter metal to precipitate the mercury on its surface. Nearly all the above tests merely prove the presence of mercury. To determine whether the metal is united with chlorine, the mercurial liquid may be precipitated by lime-water, and the filtered solution, acidulated with nitric acid, then tested with nitrate of silver. If the mercury is in the state of chloride, the filtered solution will be one of chloride of calcium, which, with nitrate of silver, will yield a heavy, white precipitate (chloride of silver), insoluble in nitric acid, but soluble in ammonia. The nitrate of silver may be added directly to the mercurial liquid; and, if it contain corrosive sublimate, chloride of silver will fall, but probably mixed with calomel.

By the combined indications of the foregoing tests, corrosive sublimate may be infallibly detected, unless it exists in very minute quantity, associated with organic substances, by which its presence is often greatly obscured. When it exists in organic mixtures, made by boiling the contents or substance of the stomach in distilled water, Dr. Christison recommends that a preliminary trial be made with the protochloride of tin, on a small portion filtered for the purpose. If this causes a grayish black color, he shakes the mixture, as recommended by Orfila, with a fourth of its bulk of cold ether, which dissolves the corrosive sublimate, and rises to the surface. The ethereal solution is then evaporated to dryness, and the dry salt obtained is dissolved in hot water, whereby a pure solution is procured, in which the poison may be readily detected by the ordinary tests. In using ether, however, it must be borne in mind that, as ascertained by M. Mialhe, the presence of a considerable quantity of mercuric oxide, and of a chloride of an alkalifiable metal, prevents the solvent power of ether. If the trial test should produce a light gray color, the corrosive sublimate is indicated in still less quantity, and Dr. Christison recommends to proceed in the following manner. Treat the unfiltered mixture with protochloride of tin, as long as any precipitate is formed, which will have a slate-gray color. Collect, wash, and drain it on a filter, and, having removed it without being dried, boil it, in a glass flask, with a moderately strong solution of caustic potassa, until all the lumps disappear. The alkali will dissolve all animal and vegetable matter; and, on allowing the solution to remain at rest, a heavy grayish black powder will subside, which consists chiefly of metallic mercury, and in which small globules of the metal may sometimes be seen with the naked eye, or by the aid of a magnifier. Wormley (*loc. cit.*) suggests boiling the organic mixture with water acidulated with hydrochloric acid, and testing the filtered solution with a strip of copper foil. Probably advantage might be derived from the process of dialysis, in separating corrosive sublimate, among other crystallizable substances, from the colloidal matters contained in organic mixtures. (See *Dialysis.*)

Off. Prep. Hydrargyri Iodidum Rubrum; Hydrargyri Oxidum Flavum; Hydrargyrum Ammoniatum.

Off. Prep. Br. Hydrargyri Iodidum Rubrum; Hydrargyri Oxidum Flavum; Hydrargyrum Ammoniatum; Liquor Hydrargyri Perchloridi; Lotio Hydrargyri Flava.

HYDRARGYRI CHLORIDUM MITE. *U.S.* *Mild Chloride of Mercury.* [*Calomel. Mercurous Chloride.*]

Hg_2Cl_2; 470·2. (HY-DRÄR'GY-RĪ CHLŌ'RĮ-DŬM MĪ'TĒ.) Hg_2Cl; 235·1.

Hydrargyri Subchloridum, *Br.;* Hydrargyrum Chloratum Mite, *P.G.;* Hydrargyri Chloridum, Hydrargyrum Chloratum (Muriaticum), Mercurius Dulcis, Chloruretum Hydrargyrosum; Submuriate of Mercury, Protochloride of Mercury; Calomelas; Subchloride of Mercury; Protochlorure ou Sous-muriate de Mercure, Calomèle, *Fr.;* Quecksilberchlorür, *G.*

Very properly, a process for this compound has been omitted from the present Pharmacopœia, as it cannot be made by the pharmacist conveniently. For process of U. S. P. 1870, see foot-note.*

"Take of Persulphate of Mercury *ten ounces* [avoirdupois]; Mercury *seven ounces* [avoird.]; Chloride of Sodium, dried, *five ounces* [avoird.]; Boiling Distilled Water *a sufficiency*. Moisten the Persulphate of Mercury with some of the Water, and rub it and the Mercury together until globules are no longer visible; add the Chloride of Sodium, and thoroughly mix the whole by continued trituration. Sublime by a suitable apparatus into a chamber of such size that the Calomel, instead of adhering to its sides as a crystalline crust, shall fall as a fine powder on its floor. Wash this powder with boiling Distilled Water, until the washings cease to be darkened by a drop of sulphydrate of ammonium. Finally, dry at a temperature not exceeding 212° F. (100° C.)." *Br.*

The object of the above process is to obtain the mercurous chloride. This chloride, according to the view generally received by chemists, consists of two atoms of mercury combined with two of chlorine (some chemists consider it to contain only one atom of each), so that it has relatively only half as much chlorine as corrosive sublimate. In the U. S. process, as in the case of corrosive sublimate, mercuric sulphate is first formed; but instead of being immediately sublimed with the chloride of sodium, it undergoes a preparatory trituration with a quantity of mercury equal to that employed in forming it. This trituration may be conceived to take place between one mol. of mercuric sulphate and one atom of metallic mercury, which are thus converted into one mol. of mercurous sulphate, according to the reaction: $HgSO_4 + Hg = Hg_2SO_4$. The one mol. of mercurous sulphate thus formed, being heated with two of common salt, the two atoms of chlorine in the latter sublime in union with the two of mercury in the former, and generate one mol. of mercurous chloride, Hg_2Cl_2; while one molecule of sodium sulphate, Na_2SO_4, remains as a residue. It is hence apparent that the residue of this process and of that for corrosive sublimate is the same.

The calomel, as sublimed, is liable to contain a little corrosive sublimate; and hence the direction of the U. S. Pharmacopœia of 1870 to wash it with boiling distilled water until ammonia produces no precipitate with the washings. Ammonia occasions a white precipitate (ammoniated mercury) so long as the washings contain corrosive sublimate; and, when it ceases to produce this effect, the operator may rest satisfied that the whole of the poisonous salt has been removed. According to M. Berthé, calomel, in contact with hot water, is converted, to a small extent, into corrosive sublimate; and hence he recommends that the portion of water to be tested should be cold when passed through the calomel.

The British process is a modification of that of the old Dublin Pharmacopœia, including, like that, no directions for making the mercuric sulphate; because this salt is made by a separate formula, being designated as *sulphate of mercury*. It omits, however, as unnecessary, a partial preliminary sublimation, to test the production of corrosive sublimate, and, immediately after a thorough mixture of the materials, proceeds to the final sublimation. An improvement was to cause the va-

* "Take of Mercury *forty-eight troyounces*; Sulphuric Acid *thirty-six troyounces*; Chloride of Sodium *eighteen troyounces*; Distilled Water *a sufficient quantity*. Boil, by means of a sand-bath, twenty-four troyounces of the Mercury with the Sulphuric Acid, until a dry white mass is left. Rub this, when cold, with the remainder of the Mercury, in an earthenware mortar, until they are thoroughly mixed. Then add the Chloride of Sodium, and, having rubbed it with the other ingredients until globules of Mercury cease to be visible, sublime the mixture into a large chamber so that the sublimate may fall in powder. Wash the sublimed matter with boiling Distilled Water, until the washings afford no precipitate with water of ammonia, and dry it." *U. S.*

pors to enter for condensation a chamber of considerable size, so that they might fall in powder, instead of condensing on the sides of the receiver in a crystalline mass. The necessity of pulverizing the calomel is thus avoided. The Br. Pharmacopœia directs the powder to be washed; but, instead of using ammonia as a test of the absence of corrosive sublimate in the washings, directs for the purpose sulphide of ammonium, which throws down a black precipitate if corrosive sublimate is present.

Preparation on the Large Scale. The process for making calomel, by means of mercuric sulphate, was originally practised at Apothecaries' Hall, London. The proportions taken and the mode of proceeding in that establishment are, according to Mr. Brande, as follows: 50 lbs. of mercury are boiled to dryness with 70 lbs of sulphuric acid, in a cast-iron vessel; and 62 lbs. of the dry salt formed are triturated with 40½ lbs. of mercury till the globules disappear, and the whole is mixed with 34 lbs. of common salt. The mixture is sublimed from an earthenware retort into an earthenware receiver, and the product is from 95 to 100 lbs. of calomel in mass. This is then ground to an impalpable powder, and washed with a large quantity of distilled water.

The object of bringing calomel into a state of minute division is more perfectly accomplished by the method of Mr. Joseph Jewell, of London, improved by M. Ossian Henry. It consists in causing the calomel in vapor to come in contact with steam in a large receiver, whereby it is condensed into an impalpable powder, and perfectly washed from corrosive sublimate in the same operation. Calomel made by this process, sometimes called Jewell's or Howard's *hydrosublimate of mercury*, is free from all suspicion of containing corrosive sublimate, is much finer than when obtained by levigation and elutriation, and possesses more activity as a medicine. This kind of calomel is included in the French Codex under a distinct name (*mercure doux à la vapeur*). M. Soubeiran, of Paris, has perfected a process for obtaining calomel as an impalpable powder, by substituting the agency of cold air for that of steam for the purpose of condensing it; a process which he believes to be precisely the same as that pursued by the English manufacturers, and which produces a calomel equal to the best English. A description of his apparatus may be found in the *Journal de Pharmacie* (3e sér., ii. 507), and of the English apparatus, as described by F. C. Calvert, in the same journal (3e sér.. iii. 121). Both these papers are copied into the *A. J. P.* (xv. 89 and 93). Calomel may also be prepared in the dry way by taking four parts of corrosive sublimate and rubbing it up in a mortar with three parts of mercury, after moistening the mass with alcohol. The powder is then dried and sublimed in glass flasks. The powder should be dried sharply before sublimation, so as to drive off any trace of uncombined mercury. A comparative examination of English and American calomel was undertaken separately in 1885 by Profs. Bedford and Patch. (See *Proc. A. P. A.*, 1885, pp. 476, 477.) Whilst there was no reason for preferring English calomel, none of the samples exhibited more than traces of mercuric chloride.

Prof. Wöhler has proposed to obtain calomel, in the humid way, by precipitating a solution of corrosive sublimate by a stream of sulphurous acid, taking advantage of a reaction first observed by Vogel. Calomel obtained in the humid way, called *precipitated calomel*, was formerly officinal with the Dublin College, and was adopted in the French Codex. This form of calomel is of doubtful utility; and, when obtained by Prof. Wöhler's process, it is a crystalline powder, which is unfit for use unless after elaborate levigation and elutriation.

Properties. When in mass its form and appearance depend on the shape and temperature of the subliming vessel. In this state it is generally in the form of a white, fibrous, crystalline cake, the interior surface of which is often studded with shining transparent crystals, having the shape of quadrangular prisms, and a texture somewhat horny and elastic. When the mass is scratched it yields a yellow streak, which is very characteristic. Its sp. gr. is 7·2. Prof. Patch found in his examination (*Proc. A. P. A.*, 1885, p. 477) the specific gravity of calomel to vary from 6·94 to 7·93, the standard being water at 39° F. The officinal form of this chloride is that of powder, in which state it is always kept in the shops. The powder has a light buff or ivory color, if obtained by the levigation of sublimed masses; but if condensed at once in the form of an impalpable powder, as is the case with Jewell's calomel and in the officinal processes, it is perfectly white. To protect it from the action of the light, it should be kept in a dark place, or in bottles painted black, or covered with black paper. By the action of the fixed alkalies or alkaline earths it immediately becomes black, in consequence of the formation of mercurous oxide, reducible by heat to the metallic state. The preparation employed under the name of *lotio nigra* or *black wash*, as a local application to syphilitic ulcers, etc., is made by adding *a drachm* of calomel to *a pint* of lime-water. By double decomposition between the calomel and lime, the black suboxide precipitates, and chloride of calcium remains in solution, indicated by yielding a copious white precipitate with nitrate of silver. The oxide, however, is not pure, but associated with undecomposed calomel. Before being applied, the wash should be well shaken.

"A white, impalpable powder, permanent in the air, odorless and tasteless, and insoluble in water, alcohol, or ether. When strongly heated, it is wholly volatilized, without melting. The salt is blackened by water of ammonia. A portion heated in a dry glass tube with dried carbonate of sodium, yields metallic mercury. Distilled water or alcohol, after having been agitated with a portion of the salt, and filtered, should not be affected by hydrosulphuric acid nor by test-solution of nitrate of silver (abs. of mercuric chloride), nor should the aqueous or alcoholic filtrate leave any residue on evaporation (fixed soluble impurities). On heating the salt with solution of potassa, no odor of ammonia should be evolved; and acetic acid, agitated with the salt and filtered, should remain unaffected by hydrosulphuric acid or by test-solution of nitrate of silver (abs. of and difference from ammoniated mercury)." *U. S.*

Tests of Purity and Incompatibles. Calomel, when pure, completely sublimes on the application of heat, a property which detects all fixed impurities, such as carbonate, sulphate, and phosphate of calcium, sulphate of barium, and carbonate of lead. Under the influence of an elevated temperature, especially in the presence of alcohol or water, it gives rise to a small quantity of corrosive sublimate. (*M. Berthé.*) Calomel strikes a black color, free from reddish tinge, by the action of the fixed alkalies; and the black oxide thus produced is brought by heat to the metallic state. The buff color indicates the absence of corrosive sublimate; but whiteness by no means shows the presence of this impurity. Its freedom from the corrosive chloride may be determined by washing a portion of it in warm distilled water, and then testing the water with ammonia, which will cause a white precipitate (ammoniated mercury), should the water have taken up any of the poisonous chloride. (See also the *U. S. P.* 1880, *Tests*, p. 754.) An easy method of detecting corrosive sublimate, proposed by M. Bonnewyn, is to put some of the suspected powder upon a well-polished surface of iron, and then moisten it with a drop of alcohol or ether. If the calomel be pure the surface will remain quite unaffected, while it will be blackened by corrosive sublimate if present only in the proportion of one to 50,000. (*Journ. de Pharm. et de Chim.*, 4e sér., ii. 79.) The presence of any soluble chloride whatever in the calomel would be detected by the production of a precipitate with the washing by nitrate of silver. Soluble salts of mercury may be detected by rubbing the suspected calomel with ether on a bright surface of copper, when the metal will become amalgamated, and exhibit a white stain. When this test shows impurity, the soluble salt present is probably corrosive sublimate. Calomel, containing corrosive sublimate, acts violently on the bowels; and, when the impurity has been present in considerable amount, has been known to cause death. Besides being incompatible with the alkalies and alkaline earths, calomel is also decomposed by the alkaline carbonates, soaps, sulphydrates, and, according to some authorities, by iron, lead, and copper. By boiling with the alkaline formiates it is decomposed, and metallic mercury liberated. (H. Rose, *Annal. der Physik und Chem.*, cvi. 500.) According to M. Lebeaux, calomel should not be prescribed with iodine; unless the prescriber intends to give mercuric iodide (red iodide), when the dose must be reduced accordingly. (*Annuaire de Thérap.*, 1857, p. 180.) It should not be given at the same time with nitrohydrochloric acid, for fear of generating corrosive sublimate. One of the authors has been informed of a case in which death, with symptoms of violent gastro-intestinal irritation, followed their joint use. Agreeably to the experiments of M. Deschamps, calomel is decomposed by bitter almonds and by hydrocyanic acid. In the former case corrosive sublimate, mercuric cyanide, and chloride of ammonium are formed; in the latter, corrosive sublimate and mercuric cyanide only. Hence this writer considers it very dangerous to associate calomel with bitter almonds or hydrocyanic acid in prescription. This conclusion has been confirmed by M. Mialhe and M. Prenleloup; and, more recently, it has been shown by Dr. E. Riegel that cherry laurel water has the power of converting calomel into corrosive sublimate. According to M. Mialhe, calomel is in part converted into corrosive sublimate and metallic mercury by chloride of ammonium, and by the chlorides of sodium and potassium, even at the temperature of the body; and hence he believes that the conversion may take place in the primæ viæ. Popular belief coincides with M. Mialhe's views in regard to the power of common salt to increase the activity of calomel. More recently M. Mialhe has extended his observations, and now believes that all the preparations of mercury yield a certain amount of corrosive sublimate by reacting with solutions of the chlorides of potassium, sodium, and ammonium. The mercuric oxide and similarly constituted compounds are most prone to undergo this change. Even metallic mercury digested with the chlorides named, is partly converted, under the influence of the air, into corrosive sublimate. Dr. Gardner denies the assertion of M. Mialhe, that calomel is converted into corrosive sublimate by chlorides of the alkali metals, maintaining that it is merely rendered soluble by their solutions. The results, however, of M. Mialhe have been confirmed experimentally by Dr. A. Fleming, of Pittsburg, Pa. (*A. J. P.*, Sept. 1857.) M. Bauwens, of Ghent, recognizing the conversion of calomel into corrosive sublimate in the body by these chlorides, explains by this fact the relatively less powerful action of large than of small doses of calomel. He also states that physicians near the sea, where the water is brackish, seldom prescribe calomel, and that naval surgeons have been obliged to abstain from giving it to sailors who eat salt meat. Dr. H. Peake, of Arkadelphia, Arkansas, has known many instances in which salivation has been induced by the joint use of calomel and vegetable acids, in the forms of sour fruit, vinegar, buttermilk, etc., where the mercurial alone would not have induced it. (*N. O. Med. and Surg. Journ.*, Nov. 1858, p. 724.)

Medical Properties and Uses. Calomel unites to the general properties of the mercurials those of a purgative and anthelmintic. It is the most valuable of the mercurial preparations. Whether the object is to bring the system under the general influence of mercury, or to produce its alterative action upon the hepatic or other secretory function, calomel, on account both of its certainty and its mildness, is preferred to all other preparations, with the single exception of the blue pill, which, though less certain, is still milder, and is sometimes preferably employed. When used with the above objects, the tendency to purge which it sometimes evinces, even in very small doses, must be restrained by combining it with opium.

As a purgative, calomel owes its chief value to its tendency to act on the liver, the secretory function of which it stimulates. It is usually slow and somewhat uncertain in its cathartic effect, and, though itself but slightly irritating, sometimes occasions severe griping pain with bilious vomiting, attributable to the acrid character of the bile which it causes the liver to secrete. It is peculiarly useful in the commencement of bilious fevers, in hepatitis, jaundice, bilious and painter's colic, dysentery, especially that of tropical climates, and all other affections attended with congestion of the portal system, or torpidity of the hepatic function. The difficulty with which it is thrown from the stomach renders it highly useful in some cases of obstinate vomiting, when other remedies are rejected. In the cases of children it is peculiarly valuable from the facility of its administration. In the treatment of worms, it is often useful as an aid to other remedies, acting probably not only as a purgative, but also as an irritant to the worms, either by its immediate influence, or that of the acrid bile which it causes to flow. The slowness and uncertainty of its action, and its liability to salivate if too long retained in the bowels, render it proper either to follow or combine it with other cathartics, in order to insure its purgative effect. When given alone, it should be followed, if it do not operate in six or seven hours, by a dose of castor oil or sulphate of magnesium. The cathartics with which it is most frequently combined are jalap, rhubarb, aloes, scammony, colocynth, and gamboge. It is often added in small quantities to purgative combinations, with a view to its influence on the liver.

In very large doses, calomel is supposed by some to act directly as a sedative, and with this view has been given in yellow and malignant bilious fevers, violent dysentery, malignant cholera, etc. The quantities which have been administered in such affections, with asserted impunity and even advantage, are almost incredible. A common dose is one or two scruples, repeated every half hour, or hour, or less frequently, according to the circumstances of the case. We have had no experience in this mode of administering calomel. It is, however, unquestionable that the effects obtained from calomel are not at all proportionate to the size of the dose. This is evidently due to the peculiarities of its absorption. It seems to be established that it is not, as was at one time supposed, converted in the stomach into corrosive sublimate, but is precipitated by the alkaline juices of the intestine in the form of black oxide, which black oxide is itself soluble in alkaline liquors and also in fatty matters. A small quantity of calomel coming into the intestines is, therefore, at once converted into black oxide and fully exhausts all the solvent power of the alkaline juices, which may therefore be unable to take up any more rapidly a large than a small amount of the drug. It is further probable that in some cases in which minute doses of calomel are given in powdered form, the excessive action of the drug is due to the conversion of some of the calomel into corrosive sublimate.*

Externally applied, calomel is often used as an efficient alterative and desiccant in venereal and other ulcers, herpetic eruptions, etc.

In syphilis, calomel vapor-baths once or twice a week are often of service. They may be extemporized by pouring an ounce and a half of water into a dish, putting a scruple of calomel in it, and heating by means of a spirit lamp, the patient being seated on a chair over the dish, and surrounded by blankets closely wrapped around the neck, spread out below.

The dose as an alterative, in functional derangement of the liver, is from half a grain to a grain (0·03 to 0·065 Gm.) every night, or every other night, followed in the morning, if the bowels are not opened, by a gentle saline laxative. When the stomach or bowels are very irritable, as in cholera and diarrhœa, from an eighth to a quarter of a grain (0·008 to 0·016 Gm.) may be given every hour or two, so as to amount to one or two grains (0·065 to 0·13 Gm.) in the course of the day. With a view to salivation, the dose is from half a grain to a grain (0·03 to 0·065 Gm.) three or four times a day, to be increased considerably in urgent cases. Sometimes, very minute doses, as the twelfth of a grain (0·005 Gm.) or less, given very frequently, so as to amount to the ordinary quantity in twenty-four hours, will operate more effectually as a sialagogue than larger doses. When large doses are given with this view, it is often necessary to combine them with opium. As a purgative, from five to fifteen grains (0·33 to 1 Gm.) or more may be exhibited. The cathartic action is not increased in proportion to the dose, and enormous quantities have been given with impunity. On the other hand, the most effective method of influencing the liver and other intestinal glands is the exhibition of one-quarter to one-half grain

* G. Vulpius has investigated the conditions which favor the formation of corrosive sublimate in calomel mixtures, and reaches the following conclusions:

1. No sublimate forms in the course of twenty-four hours in mixtures of calomel with white sugar, milk sugar, magnesia, carbonate of magnesium, and sodium bicarbonate.

2. No such formation takes place in three months in mixtures of calomel with magnesia, magnesium carbonate, and sugar.

3. Minute traces of corrosive sublimate are found at the expiration of the same time in a mixture of calomel, bicarbonate of sodium, and sugar of milk.

4. A large quantity of corrosive sublimate forms in the same time in a mixture of calomel, bicarbonate of sodium, and cane sugar.

5. Calomel powders, containing magnesia or sodium bicarbonate alone, will contain corrosive sublimate, if digested with water.

6. The formation of corrosive sublimate in mixtures of calomel and alkalies digested in water for a short time is not favored, but on the contrary prevented, by the presence of hydrochloric acid in the water, the acid neutralizing, to a certain extent, the alkalies which cause the formation. (*A. J. P.*, July, 1879.)

doses every hour until the effect is produced or five or six grains have been taken. Even in very small single doses of not more than one, two, or three grains (0·065, 0·13, or 0·20 Gm.), calomel purges some individuals briskly. In these persons, large doses, though they do not proportionably increase the evacuation, often occasion spasmodic pain in the stomach and bowels. For children larger doses are generally required in proportion than for adults. Not less than two or three grains (0·13–0·20 Gm.) should be given as a purge to a child two or three years old; and this quantity often fails to act, unless assisted by castor oil or some other cathartic. Calomel may be given in pill made with gum arabic and syrup, or in powder mixed with syrup or molasses.

Off. Prep. Pilulæ Antimonii Compositæ; Pilulæ Catharticæ Compositæ.

Off. Prep. Br. Lotio Hydrargyri Nigra; Pilula Hydrargyri Subchloridi Composita; Unguentum Hydrargyri Subchloridi.

HYDRARGYRI CYANIDUM. *U.S.* *Cyanide of Mercury.* [*Mercuric Cyanide.*]

$Hg(CN)_2$; 251·7. (HȲ-DRĂR'ǤY̆-RĪ CȲ-ĂN'I-DŬM.) $Hg\,C_2\,N$; 125·85.

Hydrargyri Cyanuretum, *U. S.* 1850; Hydrargyrum Cyanatum (Borussicum), Cyanuretum Hydrargyricum, Mercurius Cyanatus vel Borussicus; Cyanuret of Mercury, Bicyanide of Mercury, Prussiate of Mercury; Prussiate ou Cyanure ou Bicyanure de Mercure, *Fr.;* Cyanquecksilber, Quecksilber-Cyanid, *G.*

A process for this preparation is no longer officinal; that of U. S. P. 1870 is appended.*

The formula of U. S. P. 1870 is based upon that of Winckler. Hydrocyanic acid is generated by the action of sulphuric acid on the ferrocyanide of potassium, and, being received in a vessel containing water and a portion of red oxide of mercury, reacts with the oxide, according to the reaction: $(HCN)_2 + HgO = Hg(CN)_2 + H_2O$, generating, by double decomposition, water, and mercuric cyanide which is held in solution. Sufficient red oxide of mercury is not used at first to saturate the whole of the hydrocyanic acid generated, because, should there happen to be any excess of the red oxide, there would be produced on evaporation, instead of the substance wanted, a peculiar salt composed of cyanide and red oxide of mercury, which would crystallize in small acicular crystals. Hence, a portion of the water still containing uncombined hydrocyanic acid is set aside, to be added to the liquid in which the acid had been completely saturated by the addition of red oxide, and thus at least neutralize any oxide of mercury that might be present in it in excess. A surplus of hydrocyanic acid would be of no disservice, except the loss of material incurred, as it is evaporated in the subsequent concentration. "Cyanide of Mercury should be kept in well-stopped bottles, protected from light." *U. S.*

Properties, etc. "Colorless or white, prismatic crystals, becoming dark-colored on exposure to light, odorless, having a bitter, metallic taste, and a neutral reaction. Soluble in 12·8 parts of water and in 15 parts of alcohol at 15° C. (59° F.); in 3 parts of boiling water and in 6 parts of boiling alcohol. When slowly heated, the salt decomposes into metallic mercury and cyanogen gas, which is inflammable, burning with a purplish flame. On further heating, the blackish residue, containing globules of metallic mercury, is wholly dissipated. On adding hydrochloric acid to the aqueous solution, hydrocyanic acid vapor is evolved. A five per cent. aqueous solution of the salt, when mixed with a dilute aqueous solution of iodide of potassium, should not yield a red or reddish precipitate soluble in excess of either liquid (abs. of mercuric chloride)." *U. S.*

* "Take of Ferrocyanide of Potassium *five troyounces;* Sulphuric Acid *four troyounces and one hundred and twenty grains;* Red Oxide of Mercury, in fine powder, Water, each, *a sufficient quantity.* Dissolve the Ferrocyanide of Potassium in twenty fluidounces of Water, and add the solution to the Sulphuric Acid, previously diluted with ten fluidounces of Water, and contained in a glass retort. Distil the mixture nearly to dryness into a receiver, containing ten fluidounces of Water and three troyounces of Red Oxide of Mercury. Set aside two fluidounces of the distilled liquid, and to the remainder add, with agitation, sufficient Red Oxide to destroy the odor of hydrocyanic acid. Then filter the solution, and, having added the reserved liquid, evaporate the whole in a dark place, in order that crystals may form. Lastly, dry the crystals, and keep them in a well-stopped bottle, protected from the light." *U. S.* 1870.

In composition, it is a normal cyanide of mercury, consisting of one atom of the metal 199·7, and two of cyanogen 52 = 251·7; its formula being $HgCy_2$, or $Hg(CN)_2$.

Cyanide of mercury acts on the animal economy as a potent poison. In medicinal doses it sometimes causes ptyalism, but does not produce epigastric pain like corrosive sublimate. It has been occasionally used as a remedy in syphilis. M. Desmartis praises it highly in syphilis, particularly when there are long-continued obscure pains. Prochorow gives from 25 to 30 drops of a one per cent. solution hypodermically without causing local irritation, and with great asserted benefit, in chronic syphilis. Dose, internally, from one-sixteenth to one-eighth of a grain (0·004–0·008 Gm.).

HYDRARGYRI IODIDUM RUBRUM. *U.S., Br.* *Red Iodide of Mercury.* [*Biniodide of Mercury. Mercuric Iodide.*]

$Hg\,I_2$; 452·9. (HȲ-DRÄR′ǴY̧-RĪ Ī-ŎD′Į-DŬM RŬ′BRŬM.) $Hg\,I$; 226·45.

Hydrargyrum Biiodatum Rubrum, *P.G.;* Mercurius Iodatus Ruber, Deutoioduretum Hydrargyri, Ioduretum Hydrargyricum; Deuto-iodure (Bi-iodure) de Mercure, Iodure mercurique, *Fr.;* Quecksilberjodid, Rothes Jodquecksilber, *G.*

"Corrosive Chloride of Mercury, *nine parts* [or one ounce av.]; Iodide of Potassium, *eleven parts* [or five hundred and thirty-five grains]; Distilled Water, *a sufficient quantity.* Dissolve the Corrosive Chloride of Mercury in *one hundred and fifty parts* [or one pint] of warm Distilled Water, and the Iodide of Potassium in *thirty parts* [or three fluidounces] of Distilled Water, and filter the solutions separately. Add the solution of Corrosive Chloride of Mercury, when cold, to the solution of Iodide of Potassium, constantly stirring. Collect the precipitate on a filter, wash it with Distilled Water until the washings cease to give a precipitate with test-solution of nitrate of silver, and dry it, between sheets of bibulous paper, at a temperature not exceeding 40° C. (104° F.). Keep the product in well-stopped bottles." *U. S.*

"Take of Perchloride of Mercury *four ounces* [avoirdupois]; Iodide of Potassium *five ounces* [avoird.]; Boiling Distilled Water *four pints* [Imperial measure]. Dissolve the Perchloride of Mercury in three pints [Imp. meas.], and the Iodide of Potassium in the remainder of the Water, and mix the two solutions. When the temperature of the mixture has fallen to that of the atmosphere, decant the supernatant liquor from the precipitate, and, having collected the latter on a filter, wash it twice with cold distilled water, and dry it at a temperature not exceeding 212° F. (100° C.)." *Br.*

In the above processes for forming mercuric iodide, which may be considered as identical, a double decomposition takes place between corrosive sublimate and iodide of potassium, resulting in the formation of chloride of potassium which remains in solution, and mercuric iodide which precipitates. The precipitate is soluble in the reacting salts, and hence a loss of part of it is incurred by an excess of either. It is best, however, to have a slight excess of the iodide of potassium, which is furnished by the proportion taken in the formulas; as then the decomposition of the whole of the corrosive sublimate is insured, and any contamination of the mercuric iodide by it prevented. The late process of the Edinburgh College consisted in a combination of the ingredients by trituration in due proportion with the aid of alcohol; but, after the red powder was obtained, it was treated with a boiling solution of common salt, which dissolved the mercuric iodide to the exclusion of any contaminating mercurous iodide; and the solution, thus obtained, on cooling, deposited the pure mercuric salt in crystals. Mr. F. R. Williams states that in the manufacture of the red iodide on a large scale the amount of water required by the officinal processes is very troublesome. He remedies it by using chloride of ammonium, so as to get a very concentrated solution of corrosive sublimate, which he adds to a concentrated solution of the iodide. The addition of the chloride of ammonium does not interfere with the reaction, but is of material service in assisting in the solution of the corrosive sublimate. (*P. J. Tr.*, June, 1873.)

Dr. Chas. L. Mitchell has improved upon the process of Williams, and we give his process in the foot-note.*

Properties. As obtained by the late Edinburgh process, it is in splendid crimson acicular crystals. Köhler has found, however, that it crystallizes better from boiling hydrochloric acid. (*Ber. der Deutsch. Chem. Ges.*, 1879, p. 608.) It also crystallizes well from hot saturated solutions in acetone, glacial acetic acid, absolute alcohol, amyl alcohol, and nitric acid of 1·2 sp. gr. When heated the mass becomes yellow at about 150° C. (302° F.), melting at 254° C. (489·2° F.) to a blood-red liquid, and sublimes at 349° C. in yellow rhombic scales, which become red on cooling. "It is entirely volatilized by a heat under redness." *Br.*

Mercuric iodide is a dimorphous substance, having a different crystalline form in its red and yellow states. According to Schiff, it is only in its yellow form that it is soluble in alcohol; and hence it is that, when separated by water from its alcoholic solution, it falls in this condition. (*Ann. der Chem. und Pharm.*, cix. 371.) It forms definite compounds with the iodides of the alkali metals. The compound formed with iodide of potassium has been used as a medicine. (See *Iodohydrargyrate of Potassium*, in Part II.) "When digested with solution of soda it assumes a reddish brown color, and the fluid, cleared by filtration and mixed with solution of starch, gives a blue precipitate on being acidulated with nitric acid," showing that it is an iodide. Mercuric iodide consists of one atom of mercury 199·7, and two of iodine 253·2 = 452·9, and its formula is HgI_2. It combines with mercurous iodide, so as to form a yellow *sesqui iodide*, represented by the formula $HgI + HgI_2$ or Hg_2I_3.

"A scarlet red, crystalline powder, permanent in the air, odorless and tasteless, almost insoluble in water, soluble in 130 parts of alcohol at 15° C. (59° F.), and in 15 parts of boiling alcohol; also soluble in solution of iodide of potassium, or of mercuric chloride.† When heated, the salt turns yellow, but reassumes its red color on cooling. On ignition it is wholly dissipated. On heating the salt with solution of soda and adding a little sugar of milk, metallic mercury is precipitated. If the salt be heated with sulphuric acid and some black oxide of manganese, vapor of iodine will be given off. Water agitated with the salt, and filtered, should remain unaffected by test-solution of nitrate of silver (abs. of soluble iodide, chloride)." *U. S.*

Medical Properties and Uses. Mercuric iodide is a powerful irritant poison. It has been used in similar diseases with the mercurous iodide, namely, in scrofula and syphilis, but is much more active. It is especially valuable in old, obstinate cases of syphilis, as in syphilitic rheumatic pains and diseases of the bones, thickening of the dura mater, etc. There seems to be in these cases no practical difference between its action and that of corrosive sublimate, although sometimes it is better borne by the stomach than is the latter preparation. The dose is the sixteenth of a grain (0·004 Gm.) gradually increased to the fourth (0·016 Gm.), given in pill. It is sometimes administered in water with iodide of potassium so as to make a solution of potassio-mercuric iodide.‡

M. Cazenave considers mercuric iodide as the best topical application in lupus. He applies it in thin layers, every six or eight days, to small portions of the ulcerated

* *Hydrargyri Iodidum Rubrum, Mitchell's Process.* Mercury, 1000 grs.; Nitric Acid, 1700 grs. Iodide Potassium, 1662 grs. or q. s.; Distilled Water, q. s. (Instead of the mercury and nitric acid ℥v ʒi ℈ii of Liq. Hydrarg. Nit. can be used.) Dissolve the mercury in the nitric acid by the aid of a little heat (in large quantities this is not necessary, as the reaction between the acid and mercury generates sufficient heat), and dilute with an equal bulk of water. Then add the iodide potassium, dissolved in 8 fluidounces of water, until no farther precipitation ensues, being careful towards the last to add the solution very gradually, so as to avoid dissolving the mercuric iodide in an excess of the liquid. Collect the precipitate on a filter, wash well with distilled water, drain and dry. (*A. J. P.*, 1876, p. 116.)

† Bourgoin has given solubilities different from these. (See *Amer. Drug.*, 1885, p. 97.) For paper on solubility in fatty bodies, by C. Méhu, see *P. J. Tr.*, 1885, p. 327.

‡ A syrup has been largely used in the French hospitals and in this country which has received the name of *Sirop Gibert*. It is made by dissolving *three* grains of *red iodide of mercury* and *one hundred and two grains* of *iodide of potassium* in *three fluidrachms* of water, filtering, and adding sufficient simple syrup to make *ten fluidounces*. Each tablespoonful contains about one-seventh of a grain of red iodide of mercury and five grains of iodide of potassium.

surface at a time, in the form of a caustic ointment, made of equal parts of the iodide, oil, and lard. The application produces severe pain, and gives rise to a sharp inflammation, which soon terminates, leaving the ulcer in an improved condition, with a tendency to cicatrize smoothly, and on a level with the surrounding skin. (*Ann. de Thérap.*, 1852, p. 175.)

Off. Prep. Liquor Arsenii et Hydrargyri Iodidi.

Off. Prep. Br. Liquor Arsenii et Hydrargyri Iodidi; Unguentum Hydrargyri Iodidi Rubri.

HYDRARGYRI IODIDUM VIRIDE. *U.S.* *Green Iodide of Mercury.* [*Protiodide of Mercury. Mercurous Iodide.*]

Hg_2I_2; 652·6. (HȲ-DRÄR'GY-RĪ Ī-ŎD'Ĭ-DŬM VĬR'Ĭ-DĒ.) Hg_2I; 326·3.

Hydrargyri Iodidum, *U.S.* 1850; Iodide of Mercury; Hydrargyrum Iodatum Flavum, *P.G.*; Hydrargyrum Iodatum, Hydrargyri Iodidum, Iodaretum Hydrargyrosum; Yellow Iodide of Mercury; Protiodure de Mercure, Iodure mercureux, *Fr.*; Quecksilberjodür, Gelbes Jodquecksilber, *G.*

"Mercury, *eight parts* [or one ounce av.]; Iodine, *five parts* [or two hundred and seventy-four grains]; Alcohol, *a sufficient quantity*. Pour about *three parts* [or half a fluidounce] of Alcohol into a mortar containing the Mercury, add the Iodine in several, successive portions, and triturate the mixture, adding sufficient Alcohol from time to time to keep the mass constantly moist, and taking care that it shall neither become too hot, nor be exposed to light during the various steps of the process. Continue the trituration until all globules of Mercury have disappeared, and the mixture has become nearly dry and has acquired a greenish yellow color. Then add sufficient Alcohol to reduce the whole to a thin paste, pour this into a bottle, let it stand for several days, and then wash the Iodide twice with about *fifty parts* [or half a pint] of Alcohol each time, and decant the washings. Transfer the Iodide to a filter and continue washing with Alcohol until the washings are no longer affected by hydrosulphuric acid. Lastly, dry the product in a dark place, between sheets of bibulous paper, at a temperature not exceeding 40° C. (104° F.). Keep the product in well-stopped bottles, protected from light." *U. S.*

The present process for this preparation is an improvement over that of U. S. P. 1870, in directing the gradual addition of the iodine to the mixture of alcohol and mercury; this prevents volatilization. The Br. Pharmacopœia dropped this salt at its last revision, and the omission has been rather severely criticised.

This process for forming the mercurous iodide is a case of simple combination, the alcohol facilitating the union by dissolving the iodine. The drug may be prepared by precipitation, by adding a solution of iodide of potassium to one of mercurous nitrate; but, as it is difficult to prepare mercurous nitrate, without being mixed with some mercuric nitrate, the green iodide, when thus obtained, is apt to be contaminated with red iodide. M. Roland Seeger suggests double decomposition between mercurous acetate and iodide of potassium. (*A. J. P.*, 1859, p. 204.) M. Boutigny proposes to decompose calomel by iodide of potassium, and gives the following formula. Twenty-nine drachms of calomel are mixed with twenty of pulverized iodide of potassium in a glass mortar, and twelve ounces of boiling distilled water poured upon the mixture. After cooling the liquid is decanted, and the precipitate washed on a filter with distilled water, and dried in the shade. (See *A. J. P.*, viii. 326.) This process did not succeed with Mr. Charles Bullock, of this city, when he used the reacting ingredients in quantities six times those recommended by M. Boutigny. Mr. John Canavan, of New York, ascribes the failure to insufficient trituration, which, to insure complete reaction, must be long continued. If the reaction be imperfect, the water washes away not only chloride of potassium, but also iodide of potassium, holding in solution a part of the mercurous iodide formed, which is ultimately decomposed into mercuric iodide and metallic mercury. The experiments of Prof. J. M. Maisch, of this city, tend to confirm this view. He further found that a boiling temperature enables chloride of potassium to decompose the mercurous iodide perceptibly, and infers that the use of cold water would give a purer product. He therefore concludes that the process of Boutigny cannot be depended upon for giving a pure mercurous iodide, and that we must fall back on the Pharmacopœia process. As prepared by the U. S. formula of 1850, it was liable to contain a little red iodide; but this is obviated in the present edition by the direction to wash it, near the close of the operation, with alcohol. It is known to be free from the red iodide when the alcoholic washings produce no permanent cloudiness with a large quantity of water. According to Mr. F. R. Williams, a boiling solution of common salt is much more efficacious as well as much more economical than alcohol as a solvent for washing out the red from the green iodide. (*P. J. Tr.*, June, 1873, p. 1016.) Even when purified, however, it generally contains a little metallic mercury, and, according to Dr. Squibb, a considerable portion of the yellow iodide; but these are of little consequence compared with the red iodide, which should always be carefully sought for, and separated if found. (*A. J. P.*, Jan. 1857.) M. P. Yrou has prepared the green iodide by subliming iodine with an excess of mercury, and subsequently washing it with dilute nitric acid. (*Journ. de Pharm.*, 4e sér., xviii. p. 167.) Mr. George A. Haffa precipitates a solution of mercurous nitrate with potassium iodide, and obtains mercurous iodide of a yellow or green color according to the density of the solution. The solution of mercurous nitrate is prepared by acting upon 15,000 grs. of mercury with a cold mixture of nitric acid (6000 grs.) and water (4000 grs.), placing the vessel in cold water and stirring the contents constantly until the reaction has entirely ceased; the white crystalline mass, without being separated from the excess of metallic mercury, is then dissolved in water acidulated with nitric acid (1 oz. to the gallon) until the solution measures four pints. For preparing *green mercurous iodide*, six ounces of a solution of mercurous nitrate are mixed with six pints of water, and there is added in a continuous stream, and with constant stirring, a solution of potassium iodide (3 oz. in 54 oz. of water); the precipitate is washed with water and dried without the aid of heat. *Yellow mercurous iodide* is prepared in the same manner, except that two ounces of solution of mercurous nitrate diluted with water (8 pints) are used with a solution of potassium iodide (1 oz. in 4 pints of water). This salt darkens much more quickly when exposed to the light than that made by the pharmacopœial process. (*A. J. P.*, 1886, p. 12.) Stoman practically confirms these results. (*Ber. d. Deutsch. Chem. Ges.*, 1887, p. 2818; see, also, *Pharm. Era*, 1888, p. 97.)

From experiments by Mr. C. H. Wood, it appears that the green iodide is a mixture of red iodide and metallic mercury. By continuing the trituration, the powders become more and more yellow, and at length have only a tinge of green. He infers that the pure mercurous iodide is yellow, and that the green color is owing to an admixture of the blue of the mercury with the yellow of the mercurous iodide.* (*P. J. Tr.*, 1868, 503.) Flückiger (*Pharmaceutische Chemie*, 2d ed., 1888, p. 472) agrees with this view, and says that by slow sublimation, at a very gentle heat, the true mercurous iodide can be gotten in small transparent yellow crystals of the quadratic system which are related to the forms of calomel.

Properties. "A dull green to greenish yellow powder, becoming more yellow by exposure to air, and darker by exposure to light, odorless and tasteless, almost insoluble in water, and wholly insoluble in alcohol or ether. When strongly heated, the salt is volatilized without residue. When added to a solution of iodide of potassium, the salt is decomposed into metallic mercury which precipitates and mercuric iodide which dissolves. If 10 C.c. of alcohol are shaken with 1 Gm. of the salt and filtered, the filtrate should not produce more than a very faint, transient opalescence, when dropped into water; and when 5 C.c. of the filtrate are evaporated from a white porcelain surface, not more than a very faint red stain should remain behind (abs. of more than traces of mercuric iodide)." *U. S.* Its sp. gr. is

* Patrouillard recommends Dublanc's process, which consists in triturating together a mixture of mercuric (red) iodide and of metallic mercury, in the following proportions: Mercuric iodide 227 parts; mercury 100 parts. The red iodide may easily be obtained of absolute purity, and in a state of perfect dryness; besides, during the trituration, there is no risk of loss by volatization. The mixture should merely be moistened with alcohol of eighty per cent., so as to form a thin paste, and well triturated; the reaction takes place in a very short time, and the product is of a dark greenish yellow color. By way of precaution, it should be washed with boiling alcohol. (*Rép. de Pharm.*, 1877, 549; *N. R.*, Nov. 1877.)

7·75. If quickly and cautiously heated, it sublimes in red crystals, which afterwards become yellow. "Gradually heated in a test-tube, it yields a yellow sublimate, which, upon friction, or after cooling, becomes red, while globules of metallic mercury are left in the bottom of the tube." *Br.* 1867. It is generally considered to be composed of two atoms of mercury united with two atoms of iodine, Hg_2I_2, $399·4 + 253·2 = 652·6$, although some chemists make its formula HgI, consisting of one atom of mercury 199·7, and one of iodine $126·6 = 326·3$.

Medical Properties and Uses. Green iodide of mercury is used in advanced syphilis. The dose is half a grain (0·033 Gm.) daily, gradually increased to two grains (0·13 Gm.). It should never be given at the same time with iodide of potassium, which converts it immediately into red iodide and metallic mercury. (Mialhe, *Journ. de Pharm.*, 3e sér., ix. 36.)

HYDRARGYRI OXIDUM FLAVUM. *U.S., Br.* *Yellow Oxide of Mercury.* [*Yellow Mercuric Oxide.*]

Hg O; 215·7. (HȲ-DRĂR'ǤȲ-RĪ ŎX'Ĭ-DŬM FLĀ'VŬM.) Hg O; 107·85.

Hydrargyrum Oxydatum Via Humida Paratum, *P.G.*; Hydrargyrum Oxidatum Flavum vel Præcipitatum; Precipitated Oxide of Mercury; Oxide de Mercure jaune ou précipité, *Fr.*; Praecipitirtes (Gelbes) Quecksilberoxid, *G.*

"Corrosive Chloride of Mercury, *one part* [or one ounce av.]; Solution of Potassa, *nine parts* [or eight and a half fluidounces]; Distilled Water, *a sufficient quantity*. Dissolve the Corrosive Chloride of Mercury in *one hundred parts* [or about six pints] of warm Distilled Water and filter the solution. Pour the filtrate into the Solution of Potassa, previously diluted with *one hundred parts* [or six pints] of Distilled Water, stirring constantly, and set the liquid containing the precipitate aside for twenty-four hours. Then decant the supernatant, clear liquid from the precipitate, and wash the latter repeatedly by the affusion and decantation of Distilled Water, using about *one hundred parts* [or six pints] of Water each time. Continue the washing on a strainer until the washings cease to be affected by test-solution of nitrate of silver. Let the precipitate drain, and dry it, between sheets of bibulous paper, in a dark place, at a temperature not exceeding 40° C. (104° F.). Keep the product in well-stopped bottles, protected from light." *U. S.*

"Take of Perchloride of Mercury *four ounces* [avoir.]; Solution of Soda *two pints* [Imp. meas.]; Distilled Water *a sufficiency*. Dissolve the Perchloride of Mercury in four pints [Imp. meas.] of Distilled Water, aiding the solution by the application of heat, and add this to the Solution of Soda. Stir them together; allow the yellow precipitate to subside; remove the supernatant liquor by decantation; thoroughly wash the precipitated oxide on a calico filter with Distilled Water, and finally dry it by the heat of a water-bath." *Br.*

The process adopted for this preparation is that of Dr. Hoffmann. Both the Pharmacopœias direct the alkaline solution in excess, and the addition of the corrosive sublimate to the alkali. Both these points are important, for if the corrosive sublimate be in excess, brown oxychloride will be formed towards the last of the decomposition; and when the alkali is added to the solution of corrosive sublimate, the same compound will be formed from the first, and is with difficulty decomposed by an excess of alkali. The solution of potassa should be as free as possible from carbonate, to prevent the formation of brown carbonate of mercury. The mercuric chloride is precipitated by the alkalies, chloride of potassium or of sodium being left in solution. The object of the subsequent washing is to remove the chloride of potassium and the excess of the alkali.*

Properties. The officinal yellow oxide is of a yellow color similar to that of the yolk of eggs, and is a completely amorphous powder, exhibiting no evidence of crys-

* Dr. Charles L. Mitchell proposes an improvement on the officinal process, which avoids the use of large vessels when it is made on a large scale. He takes solution of mercuric nitrate (prepared by dissolving mercury in an excess of nitric acid), any convenient quantity; solution of soda, U. S. P., a sufficient quantity. The solution of mercuric nitrate is diluted with an equal bulk of water, and solution of soda added until in slight excess. The yellow precipitate is collected, washed well, and dried.

talline particles even under the microscope. Yellow oxide of mercury differs only from the red, by being amorphous and in a much more minute state of division; the red oxide, by trituration, acquiring an orange and finally a yellow color. In consequence of its different state of aggregation, it presents some peculiarities in its chemical relations, and is much more quickly acted on by reagents than is the red oxide. Thus, oxalic acid, which acts on the red oxide only with the aid of heat, immediately combines with the yellow oxide at ordinary temperatures, producing the white oxalate; and while the latter oxide, in contact with chlorine, gives up oxygen to that element, forming hypochlorous acid and corrosive sublimate, the former exercises scarcely any influence on the gas at common temperatures. It is described in the U. S. Pharmacopœia as

"A light orange-yellow, heavy, impalpable powder, permanent in the air, and turning darker on exposure to light, odorless and tasteless, insoluble in water or alcohol, but wholly soluble in nitric or hydrochloric acid. When strongly heated it assumes a red color; at a higher temperature it is decomposed, giving off oxygen and separating metallic mercury, and is finally volatilized without leaving a residue. When digested, on a water-bath, for fifteen minutes, with a strong solution of oxalic acid, it forms mercuric oxalate of a white color (diff. from red mercuric oxide)." *U. S.* I. Comere explains in a paper in *Rép. de Pharm.*, 1881, p. 199, the various conditions and modifications in the process necessary to make the oxide vary in color. (*N. R.*, 1882, p. 149.)

Medical Properties. The attention which has been recently paid to the yellow oxide, is owing to its peculiar applicability to the local treatment of diseases of the eye, in consequence of its amorphous character. Mr. B. Squire, of England, was the first to notice publicly this use of the oxide (*P. J. Tr.*, 2d ser., vi. 512). At present the yellow oxide is very largely used by oculists throughout the world. The red oxide, however carefully it may be triturated, even though in a perfectly impalpable state, still shows under the microscope crystalline particles, which, in contact with the conjunctiva, cause more or less irritation; and it can, therefore, be readily understood that, in the ordinary mode of preparing it for use as an ointment, it may sometimes be productive of serious annoyance. From this objection the yellow oxide is entirely exempt.

Off. Prep. Oleatum Hydrargyri; Unguentum Hydrargyri Oxidi Flavi.

Off. Prep. Br. Oleatum Hydrargyri.

HYDRARGYRI OXIDUM RUBRUM. *U. S., Br.* *Red Oxide of Mercury.* [*Red Precipitate. Red Mercuric Oxide.*]

Hg O; 215·7. (HȲ-DRĂR'GY̧-RĪ ŎX'Į-DŬM RŪ'BRŬM.) Hg O; 107·85.

Hydrargyri Nitrico-oxidum; Hydrargyrum Oxydatum Rubrum, *P.G.;* Hydrargyri Nitrico-oxydum, Mercurius Corrosivus Ruber vel Precipitatus, Oxidum Hydrargyricum; Deut-oxide ou Peroxide de Mercure, Oxide mercurique, Précipité rouge, Poudre de Jean de Vigo, *Fr.;* Rother Praecipitat, Quecksilber Praecipitat, Rothes Quecksilberoxid, *G.*

A process for this oxide has been omitted from the present Pharmacopœia; that of U. S. P. 1870 is appended.*

"Take of Mercury, by weight, *eight ounces* [avoirdupois]; Nitric Acid *four fluidounces and a half* [Imperial measure]; Water *two fluidounces* [Imp. meas.]. Dissolve half the Mercury in the Nitric Acid diluted with the Water, evaporate the solution to dryness, and with the dry salt thus obtained, triturate the remainder of the Mercury until the two are uniformly blended together. Heat the mixture in a porcelain dish, with repeated stirring, until acid vapors cease to be evolved." *Br.*

In this process the mercury is dissolved by the nitric acid, forming either mercuric nitrate, or a mixture of this with mercurous nitrate. The resulting mass when exposed to a strong heat is decomposed, giving out red nitrous fumes, and assuming successively a yellow, orange, and brilliant purple-red color, which becomes orange-red on cooling. These changes are owing to the gradual separation and decompo-

* "Take of Mercury *thirty-six troyounces;* Nitric Acid *twenty-four troyounces;* Water *two pints.* Dissolve the Mercury, with the aid of a gentle heat, in the Acid and Water previously mixed, and evaporate to dryness. Rub the dry mass into powder, and heat it in a very shallow vessel until red vapors cease to rise." *U. S.* 1870.

sition of the nitric acid, by the oxygen of which the mercurous oxide, if any be present, is converted into mercuric oxide, while nitrogen dioxide gas escapes, and becomes nitrogen tetroxide on contact with the air. The mercuric oxide is left behind; but in general not quite free from the nitrate, which cannot be wholly decomposed by heat, without endangering the decomposition of the oxide itself, and the volatilization of the metal. The preparation is commonly called *red precipitate.*

The name of *red oxide of mercury*, by which it is now designated in most of the Pharmacopœias, is appropriate, as nitrate of mercury exists in it merely as an accidental impurity; and there is no occasion to distinguish the preparation from the oxide obtained by calcining mercury, the latter not being officinal, and perhaps never employed.

In the preparation of this mercurial, various circumstances influence the nature of the product, and must be attended to, if we desire to procure the oxide with that fine bright orange-red color, and shining scaly appearance, usually considered desirable. Among these circumstances is the condition of the nitrate of mercury submitted to calcination. According to Gay-Lussac, it should be employed in the form of small crystalline grains. If previously pulverized, as directed in the officinal processes, it will yield an orange-yellow powder; if it be in the state of large and dense crystals, the oxide will have a deep orange color. Care must also be taken that the mercury and acid be free from impurities. It is highly important that sufficient nitric acid be employed fully to saturate the mercury. M. Payssé, who paid great attention to the manufacture of red precipitate, recommended 70 parts of nitric acid from 34° to 38° Baumé, to 50 parts of mercury. This, however, is an excess of acid. We have been told by a skilful practical chemist of Philadelphia that he has found, by repeated experiment, 7 parts of nitric acid of 35° Baumé, to be sufficient fully to saturate 6 parts of mercury. Less will not answer, and more will be useless. It is not necessary that the salt should be removed from the vessel in which it is formed; and it is even asserted that the product is always more beautiful when the calcination is performed in the same vessel. A matrass may be used with a large flat bottom, so that an extended surface may be exposed, and all parts heated equally. The metal and acid having been introduced, the matrass should be placed in a sand-bath, and covered with sand up to the neck. The solution of the mercury should be favored by a gentle heat, which should afterwards be gradually increased till red vapors appear, then maintained as equably as possible till these vapors cease, and at last slightly elevated till oxygen gas begins to escape. This may be known by the increased brilliancy with which a taper will burn if placed in the mouth of the matrass, or by its rekindling if partially extinguished. Too high a temperature must be carefully avoided, as it decomposes the oxide, and volatilizes the mercury. At the close of the operation, the mouth of the vessel should be stopped, and the heat gradually diminished, the matrass being still allowed to remain in the sand-bath. These last precautions are said to be essential to the fine red color of the preparation. It is best to operate upon a large quantity of materials, as the heat may be thus more uniformly maintained. The direction in the British, to rub a portion of mercury with the nitrate before decomposing it, renders the process more economical; as the nitric acid, which would otherwise be dissipated, is thus employed in oxidizing an additional quantity of the metal.

As the process is ordinarily conducted in laboratories, the nitrate of mercury is decomposed in shallow earthen vessels, several of which are placed upon a bed of sand, in the chamber of an oven or furnace, provided with a flue for the escape of the vapors. Each vessel may conveniently contain ten pounds of the nitrate. There is always loss in the operation thus conducted.*

* Under the name of *Hydrargyri Oxydum Rubrum*, the Dublin College formerly directed a preparation, called by the elder chemists *hydrargyrum præcipitatum per se*, or *precipitate per se*, and sometimes *calcined mercury*, made by exposing the metal to a heat near its boiling point, or about 315·5°C (600° F.), in a matrass with a broad bottom and narrow mouth. The vapors rising were condensed in the upper part of the vessel; and a circulation was thus kept up within it, during which the mercury slowly combined with oxygen, being converted first into a black and then into a red powder. But the process was very slow, requiring several weeks for the complete oxidation of the metal; and, as the product, which was pure mercuric oxide, had no peculiar virtues to recom-

Properties, etc. Red precipitate, well prepared, has a brilliant red color, with a shade of orange, a shining scaly appearance, and an acrid taste. It is very slightly soluble in water, of which Dr. Barker found 1000 parts to take up 0·62 of the oxide. Dr. Christison found 1 part of the oxide to be dissolved by about 7000 parts of boiling water, and the solution to give a black precipitate with sulphuretted hydrogen. Tannic acid precipitates metallic mercury from an aqueous solution of the oxide, especially when heated. (Bullock, *Proc. A. P. A.*, 1858, p. 306.) It is insoluble in cold alcohol and ether. (*Ibid.*) Nitric and hydrochloric acids dissolve it without effervescence. "Heavy, orange-red, crystalline scales, or a crystalline powder, becoming more yellow the finer it is divided, permanent in the air, odorless and tasteless, insoluble in water or alcohol, but wholly soluble in nitric or hydrochloric acid. When strongly heated it turns darker, without emitting reddish fumes (abs. of nitrate); at a higher temperature it is decomposed, giving off oxygen and separating metallic mercury, and is finally volatilised without residue. When digested, on a water-bath with a strong solution of oxalic acid, it does not change color within two hours (difference from yellow mercuric oxide)." *U. S.* It is essentially mercuric oxide, consisting of one atom of the metal 199·7, and one of oxygen 16 = 215·7, or, according to the Br. Pharmacopœia, consisting of one atom of mercury 100, and one of oxygen 8 = 108; but, in its ordinary state, it always contains a minute proportion of nitric acid, probably in the state of subnitrate. According to Brande, when rubbed and washed with a solution of potassa, edulcorated with distilled water, and carefully dried, it may be regarded as nearly pure mercuric oxide. It is said to be sometimes adulterated with brickdust, red lead, etc.; but these may be readily detected, as the oxide of mercury is wholly dissipated if thrown upon red-hot iron. The disengagement of red vapors, when it is heated, indicates the presence of nitrate of mercury. The same or some other saline impurity would be indicated, should water, in which the oxide has been boiled, afford a precipitate with lime-water.

Medical Properties and Uses. This preparation is too harsh and irregular in its operation for internal use; but is still employed externally as a stimulant and escharotic either in the state of powder or of ointment, although to a great extent supplanted by the yellow oxide. In the former state it is sprinkled on the surface of chancres, and indolent, flabby, or fungous ulcers. The powder should be finely levigated.*

Off. Prep. Liquor Hydrargyri Nitratis; Unguentum Hydrargyri Oxidi Rubri.
Off. Prep. Br. Unguentum Hydrargyri Oxidi Rubri.

HYDRARGYRI PERSULPHAS. *Br. Persulphate of Mercury.*

Hg, SO₄; 295·4. (HȲ-DRÄR′ǤY̆-RĪ PĔR-SŬL′PHĂS.) **Hg O SO₃; 148.**

Hydrargyri Sulphas. *Br.*, 1867; Sulphate of Mercury; Mercurius Vitriolatus, Hydrargyrum Sulphuricum, Sulphas Mercurius; Mercuric Sulphate, Persulfate ou Deuto-sulfate de Mercure, Sulfate mercurique, *Fr.*; Schwefelsaures Quecksilberoxid, *G.*

"Take of Mercury, by weight, *twenty ounces* [avoirdupois]; Sulphuric Acid *twelve fluidounces* [Imperial measure] Heat the Mercury with the Sulphuric Acid in a porcelain vessel, stirring constantly, until the metal disappears, then continue the heat until a dry white salt remains." *Br.*

Mercury is not acted on by cold sulphuric acid; but, when boiled with an excess of this acid to dryness, it is changed to mercuric sulphate at the expense of part of the acid, sulphurous acid being copiously evolved. Persulphate of mercury, as obtained by a separate formula, is peculiar to the British Pharmacopœia; it was formed as the first step of the processes of the U. S. P. 1870 for corrosive sublimate, calomel, and turpeth mineral. The adoption of a separate formula and distinct officinal name for this salt is certainly a convenience; as it obviates the necessity of repeating the directions for obtaining the same substance in several formulas. On

mend it over the oxide procured in the ordinary mode, it was properly discarded by the College. The oxide made in this way is in minute, sparkling, crystalline scales, of a deep red color, becoming still deeper by heat.

* *Black Oxide of Mercury. Oxidum Hydrargyri Nigrum.* U. S. 1850. This preparation has been dropped from both Pharmacopœias, and is now very rarely used. For a full account of its preparation, uses, and properties, see U. S. Dispensatory, 14th edition, p. 1256.

account of its various uses, it requires to be made on a large scale by the manufacturing chemist; and the process is generally performed in a cast-iron vessel, which should be conveniently arranged for the escape and decomposition of the sulphurous acid fumes, which otherwise become a serious nuisance to the neighborhood. The best way to effect this purpose is to allow them to pass off through a very lofty chimney filled with coke, over which a stream of water is made to trickle.

Properties, etc. Mercuric sulphate is in the form of a white crystalline powder, becoming yellow by the affusion of water, and entirely volatilizable by heat. It consists of one atom of mercury 199·6, and one group, SO_4, characteristic of sulphates 96, or $HgSO_4 = 295·4$. It has no medical uses.

Off. Prep. Br. Hydrargyri Perchloridum; Hydrargyri Subchloridum.

HYDRARGYRI SUBSULPHAS FLAVUS. *U.S.* *Yellow Subsulphate of Mercury.* [*Basic Mercuric Sulphate.* *Turpeth Mineral.*]

(HȲ-DRÄR'ǤȲ-RI SŬB-SŬL'PHĂS FLĀ'VŬS.)

Hg (HgO)₂ SO₄; 727·1. 3HgO, SO₃; 363·55.

Hydrargyri Sulphas Flava, *U. S.* 1870; Hydrargyri Subsulphas, Mercurius Emeticus Flavus, Sulphas Hydrargyricus Flavus, Hydrargyrum Sulphuricum Flavum, Turpethum Minerale; Sulfate jaune de Mercure, Turbith minéral, Sulfate trimercurique, *Fr.*; Basischwefelsaures Quecksilberoxyd, Mineralischer Turpeth, *G.*

"Mercury, *ten parts* [or four ounces av.]; Sulphuric Acid, *five parts* [or two ounces av.]; Nitric Acid, *four parts* [or nine fluidrachms]; Distilled Water, *a sufficient quantity.* Upon the Mercury, contained in a capacious flask, pour the Sulphuric Acid, then gradually add the Nitric Acid, previously mixed with *three parts* [or one fluidounce] of Distilled Water, and digest at a gentle heat until reddish fumes are no longer given off. Transfer the mixture to a porcelain capsule, and heat it on a sand-bath, frequently stirring, until a dry, white mass remains. Reduce this to a fine powder and throw it, in small portions at a time, and constantly stirring, into *two hundred parts* [or five pints] of boiling Distilled Water. When all has been added, continue the boiling for ten minutes, then allow the mixture to settle, decant the supernatant liquid, transfer the precipitate to a strainer, wash it with warm Distilled Water until the washings no longer have an acid reaction, and dry it in a moderately warm place." *U. S.*

By referring to the articles on corrosive sublimate and calomel, it will be found that the peculiar salt which is generated by boiling sulphuric acid with mercury to dryness, is directed to be made as the first step for obtaining these chlorides; and here the same salt is again directed to be formed in preparing turpeth mineral. The nitric acid assists in the process by hastening the formation of the sulphate. We have already stated that this salt is normal mercuric sulphate. When thrown into boiling or even warm water it is instantly decomposed, and an insoluble salt is precipitated, which is the turpeth mineral. Its composition is Hg_3SO_6, or, more clearly expressed, $HgSO_4 + 2HgO$; that is, a compound of one mol. of mercuric sulphate and two mols. of mercuric oxide.

Properties, etc. Yellow sulphate of mercury is a lemon-yellow powder, of a somewhat acrid taste. It dissolves in 2000 parts of cold, and about 600 of boiling water. "A heavy, lemon-yellow powder, permanent in the air, odorless, and almost tasteless, insoluble in water or alcohol, but soluble in nitric or hydrochloric acid. When heated, the salt turns red, becoming yellow again on cooling. At a red heat it is volatilized without residue, evolving vapors of mercury and of sulphurous acid. The salt should be soluble in 20 parts of hydrochloric acid without residue (abs. of mercurous salt)." *U. S.* It was originally called *turpeth mineral*, from its resemblance in color to the root of *Ipomæa Turpethum.*

Medical Properties and Uses. Turpeth mineral is alterative, and powerfully emetic and errhine. As an alterative, it has been given in leprous disorders and glandular obstructions. It has been usefully employed as an emetic, repeated every few days, in chronic enlargement of the testicle. It operates with great promptness, and sometimes excites ptyalism. Dr. Hubbard, of Maine, recommends it highly as an emetic in croup, on the ground of its promptness and certainty, and of its not producing catharsis, or the prostration caused by antimony. This practice has been followed with alleged extraordinarily good results by Dr. Fordyce Barker, of New York, and other practitioners, but is not without danger, since Dr. A. McPhedran reports (*Med. News*, vol. xliii. 1883) a case in which a child five months old was killed by two powders given as emetics at intervals of fifteen minutes. No vomiting ensued, but vio'ent purging came on in the course of a short time, with intense abdominal pain and other symptoms of poisoning, resembling those caused by corrosive sublimate. A second similar case occurred in the practice of Dr. Cameron, of Toronto, Canada. The dose for a child two years old is two or three grains (0·13 or 0·20 Gm.), repeated in fifteen minutes, if it should not operate. As an errhine, it has been used with benefit in chronic ophthalmia; but it sometimes produces salivation when thus employed. The dose as an alterative is from a quarter to half a grain (0·016 to 0·03 Gm.); as an emetic from two to five grains (0·13 to 0·33 Gm.). When employed as an errhine, one grain (0·065 Gm.) may be mixed with five (0·33 Gm.) of starch or powdered liquorice root.

Turpeth mineral, in an overdose, acts as a poison. One drachm (3·9 Gm.) of it is said to have killed a boy 16 years old. (*Lond. Med. Gaz.*, March, 1847.)

HYDRARGYRI SULPHIDUM RUBRUM. *U.S.* *Red Sulphide of Mercury.* [*Red Mercuric Sulphide. Cinnabar.*]

Hg S; 231·7. (HȲ-DRĂR'GY̆-RĪ SŬL'PHI-DŬM RŪ'BRŬM.) Hg S; 115·85.

Hydrargyri Sulphuretum Rubrum, *U.S.* 1870; Cinnabaris; Hydrargyrum Sulfuratum Rubrum, *P.G.;* Sulfuretum Hydrargyricum; Sulfure rouge de Mercure, *Fr.;* Rothes Schwefelquecksilber, Zinnober, *G.*

"Take of Mercury, *forty troyounces;* Sulphur, *eight troyounces.* To the Sulphur, previously melted, gradually add the Mercury, with constant stirring, and continue the heat until the mass begins to swell. Then remove the vessel from the fire, and cover it closely to prevent the contents from inflaming. When the mass is cold, rub it into powder, and sublime." *U. S.* 1870.

This preparation has been discarded, we think somewhat prematurely, by the British Council.

Mercury and sulphur, when heated together, unite with great energy, and a product is obtained, which by sublimation becomes the red or mercuric sulphide. In order to render the combination more prompt, the sulphur is first melted; and the addition of the mercury should be made gradually, while the mixture is constantly stirred. Dr. Barker recommends the addition of the metal by straining it upon the melted sulphur through a linen cloth, whereby it falls in a minutely divided state. When the temperature has arrived at a certain point, the combination takes place suddenly with a slight explosion, attended with the inflammation of the sulphur, which must be extinguished by covering the vessel. A black mass will thus be formed, containing generally an excess of sulphur, which, before the sublimation is performed, should be got rid of by gently heating the matter, reduced to powder, on a sand-bath. The sublimation is best performed, on a small scale, in a closely stopped glass matrass, which should be placed in a crucible containing sand, and, thus arranged, exposed to a red heat. The equivalent quantities for forming this sulphide are 32 of sulphur and 199·7 of mercury.

Preparation on the Large Scale. Cinnabar is seldom prepared on a small scale, being made in large quantities for the purposes of the arts. Until within a few years it was nearly all manufactured in Europe, but it is now made to an enormous extent in this country. In Holland, where it is largely manufactured, the sulphur is melted in a cast-iron vessel, and the mercury is added in a divided state, by causing it to pass through chamois leather. As soon as the combination has taken place, the iron vessel is surmounted by another, into which the cinnabar is sublimed. The larger the quantity of the materials employed in one operation, the finer will be the tint of the product. It is also important in the manufacture to use the materials pure, and to drive off any uncombined sulphur which may exist in the mass, before submitting it to sublimation. In the United States, Martin's method, consisting of the agitation together of quicksilver, sulphur, and an alkaline sulphide, appears to have the preference. Another process for its manufacture in the wet way very largely employed is Brunner's. (*Wagner's Chem. Tech.*, 12th ed., 1886, p. 149.)

Properties, etc. "Brilliant, dark red, crystalline masses, or a fine, bright, scarlet powder, permanent in the air, odorless, and tasteless, insoluble in water, alcohol, nitric or hydrochloric acid, or in dilute solutions of alkalies. It is dissolved by nitro-hydrochloric acid with separation of sulphur. When heated, the salt becomes brown and then black, but, on cooling, it reassumes its red color. At a higher temperature it takes fire, burns with a bluish flame, emitting the odor of burning sulphur, and is finally volatilised without residue. On dissolving the salt in nitro-hydrochloric acid and adding an excess of stannous chloride, metallic mercury is precipitated. If the salt be treated with warm solution of potassa, the filtrate, after being acidulated with hydrochloric acid, should not yield a yellow or orange-colored precipitate (arsenic, antimony), nor should it produce a colored precipitate with acetate of lead (chromates, iodides, or other sulphides). If the salt be digested with diluted nitric acid for five minutes, the filtrate, after being much diluted, should not be darkened by hydrosulphuric acid (abs of red oxide of mercury or of lead)." *U. S.* In close vessels at a red heat it sublimes without decomposition, and condenses in a mass, composed of a multitude of small needles. When duly levigated, it furnishes a brilliant red powder, which is the paint called *vermilion.* The same compound occurs native, being the sole ore from which mercury is extracted. The preparation, if purchased in powder, should be carefully examined; as, in that state, it is sometimes adulterated with red lead, dragon's blood, or chalk. If red lead be present, acetic acid, digested with it, will yield a yellow precipitate (iodide of lead) with iodide of potassium. Dragon's blood may be detected by alcohol, which will take up the coloring matter of that substance, if present; and, if chalk be mixed with it, effervescence will be excited on the addition of an acid. This sulphide consists of one atom of mercury 199·7, and one of sulphur 32=231·7.

Medical Properties and Uses. Cinnabar is at present only employed by fumigation, as a rapid sialagogue, in syphilitic affections, when it is desired to obtain an immediate mercurial impression. Half a drachm may be thrown on a red-hot iron, in a close apartment, the fumes inhaled as they arise. These consist of sulphurous acid gas and mercurial vapor, the former of which must prove highly irritating to the patient's lungs. A better substance for mercurial fumigation is the black oxide of mercury.*

HYDRARGYRUM. *U. S., Br.* *Mercury.* [*Quicksilver.*]

Hg; 199·7. (HȲ-DRÄR'GY-RŬM.) **Hg; 99·85.**

Quicksilver; Mercurius, Argentum Vivum; Mercure, Vif Argent, *Fr.*; Quecksilber, *G.*; Mercurio, *It.*; Azógue, *Sp.* and *Port.*

Mercury is found pure, forming an amalgam with silver, in the form of protochloride (native calomel), but most abundantly as the sulphide or native cinnabar. Mines of this metal are found at Almaden in Spain, at Idria in Carniola, in the duchy of Deux-ponts, in Belluno a province of Venetia,† in Corsica, in the Philippine Islands and China, near Huancavelica in Peru, near Azogue in New Granada, at Durango in Mexico, and at New Almaden, New Idria, and other localities in Santa Clara County, California, about sixty-six miles from San Francisco. The most ancient mine is that of Almaden in Spain, which was worked before the Christian era. This mine, and the mines of California, are the most productive at the present day; the Spanish mine yielding about three millions of pounds, and the California more than this amount annually. The ore in all the mines mentioned is cinnabar.

* *Black Sulphide of Mercury. Æthiops Mineral. Hydrargyri Sulphuretum Nigrum.* Though very properly discarded from the Pharmacopœias, this has too long occupied a place in the catalogue of the Materia Medica to be passed over without some notice. The following was the formula of the U. S. Pharmacopœia of 1850, for its preparation. "Take of Mercury, Sulphur, each, a pound. Rub them together till all the globules disappear." *U. S.* It is now very rarely used. For an account of its properties, see U. S. Dispensatory, 14th edition, p. 1259.

† For an account of these Italian mines and the mode of working them, see *P. J. Tr.*, March, 1878.

The cinnabar from old Almaden is of a dull red color in mass, of a dull brick-red color when in fine powder, and of the sp. gr. 3·6. That from New Almaden is of a bright red color, slightly inclining to purple, not so hard as the Spanish ore, of a brilliant vermilion color in powder, and having the sp. gr. 4·4. The California cinnabar is richer in mercury, because purer, than the Spanish; the former yielding about 70, the latter about 38 per cent. of mercury, according to the analysis of Mr. Adam Bealey. The California mine had been long known to the Indians, but its commercial value was first made known about 1843, by a Mexican, named Castillero, who became its first owner. At present it is in the hands of Americans. (See *P. J. Tr.*, Feb. 1855; also a paper by Dr. Ruschenberger, U.S.N., in *A. J. P.*, March, 1856.) Dr. Ruschenberger has detected selenium in California cinnabar. A quicksilver ore has been found in Macon County, Tennessee, where it is said to exist in vast quantities. According to Mr. E. S. Wayne, it is a talcose rock, and contains mercury in the metallic state, yielding 7·5 per cent. of the metal. (*A. J. P.*, 1868, p. 76.) Mercury has also been found in the island of Borneo, district of Sarawak. (*Chem. News*, Nov. 5, 1869, p. 224.)

Extraction, etc. Mercury is obtained almost exclusively from the sulphide or native cinnabar. It is extracted by two principal processes. According to one process, the mineral is picked, pounded, and mixed with lime. The mixture is then introduced into cast-iron retorts, which are placed in rows, one above the other, in an oblong furnace, and connected with earthenware receivers, one-third full of water. Heat being applied, the lime combines with the sulphur, so as to form sulphide and sulphate of calcium; while the mercury distils over, and is condensed in the receivers. The other process is practised at Almaden in Spain. Here a square furnace is employed, the floor of which is pierced with many holes, for the passage of the flame from the fireplace beneath. In the upper and lateral part of the furnace, holes are made, communicating with several rows of *aludels*, formed of adapters passing into one another, which terminate in a small chamber that serves both as condenser and receiver. The mineral, having been picked by hand and pulverized, is kneaded with clay, and formed into small masses, which are placed on the floor of the furnace. Heat being applied, the sulphur burns, and the volatilized mercury passes through the aludels to be condensed in the chamber. The process pursued at New Almaden is described by Dr. Ruschenberger. (See *A. J. P.*, March, 1856.)

Mercury, as found in commerce, is contained in cylindrical wrought-iron bottles, called flasks, each containing 76½ pounds. Since the regular working of the California mine of New Almaden, the importation of the metal from Spain and Austria has gradually diminished, and at present the domestic production is sufficient not only to supply the home consumption, but to give an excess for exportation. The different mines of California were, in the year 1862, said to be yielding mercury at the rate of four millions of pounds per annum (*A. J. P.*, Sept. 1862, p. 410), and in 1877 the yield had increased to over six million pounds, but in 1881 it had decreased to four and a half million pounds, and in 1886 to 2,293,547 pounds. The exports are made principally to China, Mexico, Chili, and Peru. The chief uses of the metal are in mining silver and gold, in preparing vermilion, in making thermometers and barometers, in silvering looking-glasses, and in forming various pharmaceutical compounds.

Properties. Mercury is "a shining, silver-white metal, liquid at temperatures above —40° C. (—40° F.), odorless and tasteless, and insoluble in ordinary solvents, but soluble in nitric acid without residue. Sp. gr. 13·5. At the common temperature it volatilizes very slowly, more rapidly as the temperature increases, and at 350° C. (662° F.) it boils, being finally volatilized without residue. When globules of Mercury are dropped upon white paper, they should roll about freely, retaining their globular form, and leaving no streaks or traces. It should be perfectly dry and present a bright surface. On boiling 5 Gm. of distilled water with 5 Gm. of Mercury, and 4·5 Gm. of hyposulphite of sodium, in a test-tube, for about one minute, the Mercury should not lose its lustre and should not acquire more than a slightly yellowish shade (abs. of more than slight traces of foreign metals)." *U. S.* When perfectly pure it undergoes no alteration by the action of air or water, but in its ordinary state suffers a slight tarnish. When heated to near the boiling point, it gradually combines with oxygen, and is converted into mercuric oxide; but at the temperature of ebullition it parts with the oxygen with which it had combined, and is reduced again to the metallic state. Its sp. gr. is 13·5, and its atomic weight 199·7. It boils at 357·25° C. (669° F.), yielding a colorless vapor, and congeals at —39·4° C. (—39° F.), forming a malleable solid of tin-white color. It is a good conductor of heat, and its specific heat is small. It is not attacked by hydrochloric acid, nor by cold sulphuric acid; but boiling sulphuric acid or cold nitric acid dissolves it, producing mercurous sulphate and mercurous nitrate respectively; with the extrication, in the former case, of sulphurous acid; in the latter, of nitrogen dioxide becoming hyponitric acid fumes. Its combinations are numerous, and several of them constitute important medicines. It forms two series of compounds, the *mercurous* compounds containing the group $(Hg_2)^{II}$, and the *mercuric* compounds containing the single atom Hg^{II}.

Mercury, as it occurs in commerce, is in general sufficiently pure for pharmaceutical purposes. Occasionally it contains foreign metals, as lead, tin, zinc, and bismuth. Mr. Brande informs us that, in examining large quantities of this metal in the London market, he found it only in one instance intentionally adulterated. When impure, the metal has a dull appearance, leaves a trace on white paper, is deficient in due fluidity and mobility, as shown by its not forming perfect globules, is not totally dissipated by heat, and, when shaken in a glass bottle, coats its sides with a pellicle, or, if very impure, deposits a black powder. If agitated with strong sulphuric acid, the adulterating metals become oxidized and dissolved, and thus the mercury may to a limited extent be purified. Lead is detected by shaking the suspected metal with equal parts of acetic acid and water, and then testing the acid by sulphate of sodium, or iodide of potassium. The former will produce a white, the latter a yellow precipitate, if lead be present. Bismuth is discovered by dropping a nitric solution of the mercury, prepared without heat, into distilled water, when subnitrate of bismuth will be precipitated. The complete solubility of the metal in nitric acid shows that tin is not present; and, if sulphuretted hydrogen does not act upon hydrochloric acid previously boiled upon the metal, the absence of contaminating metals is shown.

Mercury may be purified by digesting it with a small portion of weak nitric acid, or with a solution of mercuric chloride (corrosive sublimate); whereby all the ordinary contaminating metals will be removed. The purification by nitric acid is, according to L. Meyer (*Zeit. Anal. Chem.*, ii. 241), best effected as follows. The metal is allowed to flow in a very thin stream from a small opening in a glass funnel into a wide glass tube 1·25 m. high and 5 cm. in diameter, which contains a mixture of water and 100 C.c. of nitric acid. A narrow tube is fastened to the bottom of this, from which the pure metal flows; it has then only to be washed with water and dried. The above operation may have to be repeated several times, and the metal if pure must leave no residue when dissolved in pure nitric acid, evaporated to dryness and ignited. Mercury, however, is usually purified by distillation. To separate mechanical impurities, moisture, small quantities of oxide, mercury may be filtered by collecting it in a sound piece of chamois leather and gathering the corners together, forcibly squeezing the particles through the pores of the leather.

The British Pharmacopœia of 1864 gave the following process for the purification of mercury, using for this purpose an impure form of the metal, under the name of *Commercial Mercury* or *Quicksilver*.

"Take of Mercury of Commerce *three pounds* [avoirdupois]; Hydrochloric Acid *three fluidrachms;* Distilled Water *a sufficiency*. Place the Commercial Mercury in a glass retort or iron bottle, and applying heat cause two pounds and a half of the metal to distil over into a flask employed as a receiver. Boil on this for five minutes the Hydrochloric Acid diluted with nine fluidrachms of Distilled Water, and having, by repeated affusions of Distilled Water and decantations, removed every trace of acid, let the mercury be transferred to a porcelain capsule, and dried first by filtering paper, and finally on a water-bath." *Br.*

Mercury, being much more volatile than the contaminating metals, rises first in distillation, while they are left behind. But it is necessary to avoid pushing the distillation too far; for in that event, some of the foreign metals are apt to be carried over. The British Council, on account of this danger, directed only five-sixths of the mercury to be distilled. The distilled product is boiled for a few minutes with diluted hydrochloric acid, which, while it does not attack the mercury, dissolves any contaminating metals which may have passed over. The distillation is directed to be performed from a glass retort or iron bottle; but it is more conveniently conducted from the latter, over a common fire, into water contained in a receiver. In small operations a wash hand basin will answer for a receiver. Millon has ascertained the curious fact, that the presence of so small a quantity as one ten-thousandth of lead or zinc in mercury raises its boiling point. M. Violette has made known a method of distilling mercury, or amalgamated silver, which presents many advantages. It consists in subjecting the metal, in iron vessels, to a current of high-pressure steam, which serves the double purpose of imparting the necessary heat, and carrying over the mercurial vapor by a mechanical agency. (*Philos. Mag.*, Dec. 1850.) As it is difficult and troublesome to purify mercury by distillation, it is better to purchase pure samples of the metal, which may always be found in the market.

Mercury is detected with great delicacy by Smithson's process, which consists in the use of a plate of tin, lined with one of gold, in the form of a spiral. When immersed in a mercurial solution, this galvanic combination causes the precipitation of the mercury on the gold, which consequently contracts a white stain. In order to be sure that the stain is caused by mercury, the metal must be volatilized in a small tube, so as to obtain a characteristic globule. MM. Danger and Flandin have improved on Smithson's process. (See *Chem. Gaz.*, No. 61, p. 191.) A minute portion of any of the preparations of mercury, either in the solid state or in concentrated solution, being placed on a bright plate of copper, and a drop of a strong solution of iodide of potassium added, a silvery characteristic stain will immediately appear on the copper.

Medical Properties. Mercury in its uncombined state is inert; but, in combination, acts as a peculiar and universal stimulant. When exhibited in minute division, as it exists in several preparations, it produces its peculiar effects; but this does not prove that the uncombined metal is active, but only that the condition of minute division is favorable to chemical combination, and consequently to its solution in the stomach. Its compounds exhibit certain general medical properties and effects which belong to the whole as a class; while each individual preparation is characterized by some peculiarity in its operation. In this place we shall consider the physiological action of mercury, and the principles by which its administration should be regulated; while its effects as modified in its different combinations will be noticed under the head of the several preparations. Of the modus operandi of mercury we know nothing, except that it possesses a peculiar alterative power over the vital functions. This alterative power is sometimes exerted, without being attended with any other vital phenomenon than the removal of disease; while at other times it is accompanied with certain obvious effects, such as a quickened circulation, a frequent jerking pulse, and increased activity of all the secretory functions, particularly those of the salivary glands and the liver.

When mercury acts slowly as an alterative, there is not the least apparent disturbance of the circulation. When it operates decidedly and obviously, it is very prone to cause an immoderate flow of saliva, and produce the condition denominated ptyalism or salivation. Mercury has been detected in most of the solids and fluids of the body, including the blood. When in the blood it cannot be detected by the ordinary tests, on account of its intimate union with the organic matter of that liquid. To discover it, the blood must be subjected to destructive distillation. The liver is the organ which retains mercury the longest. It has been detected in that viscus, though absent in the lungs, heart, bile, and spinal marrow.*

Mercury has been used in almost every disease, but too often with evil results. In functional derangement of the digestive organs, mercurials in minute doses often exert a salutary operation, subverting the morbid action, and that, too, by their slow, alterative effect, without affecting the mouth. In these cases no decided disturb-

* For a method of detecting mercury in the urine, see *P. J. Tr.*, Aug. 1873, p. 145.

ance of the vital functions takes place; but the alvine discharges, if clay-colored, are generally restored to their natural hue: whether the liver be torpid and obstructed as in jaundice, or pouring out a redundancy of morbid bile as in melæna, the judicious use of mercury seems equally efficacious in unloading the viscus, or restoring its secretion to a healthy state. In chronic inflammation of the mucous and serous membranes, the alterative effects of mercury are sometimes attended with much benefit. In many of these cases effusion has taken place; and, under these circumstances, the mercury often proves useful, as well by promoting absorption as by removing the chronic inflammation on which the effusion depends. Hence, it is often given with advantage in chronic forms of meningitis, bronchitis, pleuritis, pneumonia, dysentery, rheumatism, etc., and in hydrocephalus, hydrothorax, ascites, and general dropsy.

Mercury may also be advantageously resorted to in certain states of febrile disease. In some forms of remittent and typhoid fever, a particular stage is marked by a parched tongue, torpor of the bowels, scanty urine, and dryness of the surface. Here the very cautious employment of mercury is sometimes serviceable. It acts in such cases by increasing the secretions.

In syphilitic affections, mercury, until of late years, was held to be indispensable. Of its mode of action in these affections we know nothing. Without entering into the question of the necessity of mercury in venereal complaints, we are free to admit that the discussion which has grown out of it has shown that this remedy has frequently been unnecessarily resorted to in syphilis.

For inducing the specific effects of mercury on the constitution, blue pill or calomel is generally resorted to. In order to procure what we have called the slow alterative effects of the metal, from half a grain to a grain (0·03 to 0·067 Gm.) of blue pill may be given in the twenty-four hours, or from a sixth to a fourth of a grain (0·01 to 0·016 Gm.) of calomel; or, if a gentle ptyalism be our object, two or three grains (0·13 or 0·20 Gm.) of the former, or a grain of the latter (0·067 Gm.) two or three times a day. Where the bowels are peculiarly irritable, it is often necessary to introduce the metal by means of friction with mercurial ointment; and where a speedy effect is desired, the internal and external use of the remedy may be simultaneously resorted to.

The first observable effects of mercury in inducing ptyalism are a coppery taste in the mouth, a slight soreness of the gums, and an unpleasant sensation in the sockets of the teeth, when the jaws are firmly closed. Shortly afterwards the gums begin to swell, a line of whitish matter is seen along their edges, and the breath is infected with a peculiar and very disagreeable smell, called the mercurial fetor. The saliva at the same time begins to flow; and, if the affection proceed, the gums, tongue, throat, and face become much swollen; ulcerations attack the lining membrane of the mouth and fauces; the jaws become excessively painful; the tongue is coated with a thick whitish fur; and the saliva flows in streams from the mouth. It occasionally happens that the affection of the mouth proceeds to a dangerous extent, inducing extensive ulceration, gangrene, and even hemorrhage. The best remedies are astringent and detergent gargles, used weak at first, as the parts are extremely tender. In cases attended with swelling and protrusion of the tongue, the wash is best applied by injection, by means of a large syringe. We have found lead-water among the best applications in these cases; and dilute solutions of chlorinated soda or of chlorinated lime, while they correct the fetor, will be found to exert a curative influence on the ulcerated surfaces. A wash of nitrate of silver, made by dissolving eight grains (0·52 Gm.) in a fluidounce (30 C.c.) of water, has also been used with benefit. As excessive ptyalism and its frequent attendants of severe inflammation and ulceration of the mouth and fauces are not at all essential to the remedial constitutional effects of mercury, it becomes desirable if possible to moderate or prevent them; and for this purpose it is believed that the simultaneous use of chlorate of potassium is very effective. (See *N. R.*, Jan. 1873, p. 217.)

While the system is under the action of mercury, the blood is more watery than in health, less charged with albumen, fibrin, and red globules, and loaded with a fetid fatty matter. (*Dr. S. Wright*, quoted by *Christison.*) When drawn from a vein, it exhibits the same appearance as in inflammation.

In the foregoing observations, we have described the ordinary effects of mercury, but occasionally, in peculiar constitutions, its operation is quite different, being productive of a dangerous disturbance of the vital functions. The late Mr. Pearson gave a detailed account of this occasional peculiarity in the operation of mercury, in his work on the venereal disease. The symptoms which characterize it are a small and frequent pulse, anxiety about the præcordia, pale and contracted countenance, great nervous agitation, and alarming debility. Their appearance is the signal for discontinuing the mercury; as a further perseverance with it might be attended with fatal consequences. Mercury also produces a peculiar eruption of the skin, which is described by writers under the various names of *hydrargyria*, *eczema mercuriale*, and *lepra mercurialis*.

Those who work in mercury, and are, therefore, exposed to its vapor, such as water-gilders, looking-glass silverers, and quicksilver miners, are injured seriously in their health, and not unfrequently affected with shaking palsy, attended with vertigo and other cerebral disorders. The miners are often salivated.

Many plants, exposed to the influence of the vapor spontaneously rising from mercury in confined air, perish in a few days; while, if sulphur be placed by the side of the metal, no effect of the kind is experienced. (Boussingault, *Journ. de Pharm. et de Chim.*, Sept. 1867, p. 176.) A probable inference from this fact is, that workmen, necessarily exposed to the vapor of mercury, might be protected by the presence of sulphur in sufficient quantity.

Mercury is sometimes given in the metallic state, in the quantity of a pound or two, in obstruction of the bowels, to act by its weight; but the practice is of doubtful advantage.

HYDRARGYRUM AMMONIATUM. *U. S., Br.* *Ammoniated Mercury.* [*White Precipitate. Mercurammonium Chloride.*]

NH_2HgCl; 251·1. (HȲ-DRÄR′ǤY̨-RŬM ĄM-MŌ-NĮ-Ā′TŬM.) NH_2Hg_2Cl; 251·1.

Hydrargyri Precipitatum Album; Hydrargyri Ammonio-Chloridum.

"Corrosive Chloride of Mercury, *ten parts* [or one ounce av.]; Water of Ammonia, Distilled Water, each, *a sufficient quantity*. Dissolve the Corrosive Chloride of Mercury in *two hundred parts* [or twenty fluidounces] of warm Distilled Water; filter the solution and allow it to cool. Pour the filtrate gradually, and constantly stirring, into *fifteen parts* [or one and a half fluidounces] of Water of Ammonia, taking care that the latter shall remain in slight excess. Collect the precipitate upon a filter, and when the liquid has drained from it as much as possible, wash it twice with a mixture of *twenty parts* [or two fluidounces] of Distilled Water and *one part* [or fifty minims] of Water of Ammonia. Finally, dry the precipitate, between sheets of bibulous paper, in a dark place, at a temperature not exceeding 30° C. (86° F.)." *U. S.*

"Take of Perchloride of Mercury *three ounces* [avoirdupois]; Solution of Ammonia *four fluidounces*; Distilled Water *a sufficiency*. Dissolve the Perchloride of Mercury in three pints of the Distilled Water with the aid of heat; pour the Solution into the Ammonia, diluted with one pint of water, constantly stirring; collect the precipitate on a filter, and wash it well with cold Distilled Water until the liquid which passes through ceases to give a precipitate when dropped into a solution of nitrate of silver acidulated with nitric acid. Lastly, dry the product at a temperature not exceeding 212° F. (100° C.)." *Br.*

The Pharmacopœias now agree in obtaining white precipitate by precipitating a solution of corrosive sublimate by ammonia. When ammonia, in slight excess, is added to a cold solution of corrosive sublimate, chloride of ammonium is formed in solution, and the white precipitate of the Pharmacopœias is thrown down. The precipitate is washed twice, according to the U. S. formula, according to the British, with greater precision, until they cease to give evidence of the presence of a chloride by producing a precipitate with nitrate of silver acidulated with nitric acid. The matter washed away is chloride of ammonium and the excess of ammonia employed; and hence the washings, agreeably to the directions of the British formula, are tested with an acid solution of nitrate of silver. The white precipitate forms according to the following reaction: $HgCl_2 + 2NH_3 = NH_4Cl + NH_2HgCl$. In other words, one molecule of corrosive sublimate reacts with two of ammonia, and yields one molecule of ammonium chloride and one of *mercur-ammonium chloride*, or white precipitate. As the molecular weight of corrosive sublimate is 270·5, and of the ammonium needed 34, if water of ammonia be taken containing 10 per cent. of ammonia gas, the proportions would be 270·5 to 340. The Pharmacopœia directs 10 parts of sublimate to 15 of water of ammonia. A method of making white precipitate, said to be employed by large manufacturers, substitutes chloride of ammonium and carbonate of sodium for ammonia. As the product contains less mercury than the officinal preparation, and is in commerce, it is important to be able to distinguish the two. According to Prof. Redwood, this can be done by heating, the officinal preparation volatilizing without fusing, the unauthorised, fusing before volatilizing; Prof. Attfield has, however, shown that fusibility does not necessarily indicate that the specimen contains only 65 per cent. of mercury, or infusibility demonstrate that it contains the officinal proportion of 79½ per cent. The commercial variety differs somewhat from the present officinal preparation in composition, its formula being $N_2H_6HgCl_2$ (or *mercur-diammonium chloride*). See paper by F. X. Moerck, *A. J. P.*, 1888, p. 80.

Properties. "White, pulverulent pieces, or a white powder, permanent in the air, odorless and tasteless, and insoluble in water or alcohol. At a temperature below a red heat the salt is decomposed without fusion, and at a red heat it is wholly volatilized. When heated with solution of potassa, the salt becomes yellow and evolves vapor of ammonia. It is completely soluble in a cold solution of hyposulphite of sodium, with evolution of ammonia; on heating this solution for a short time, it separates red mercuric sulphide, which, on protracted boiling, turns black. The salt should be soluble in hydrochloric acid without residue (mercurous salt), and without effervescence (carbonate). Its solution in acetic acid should not be rendered turbid by diluted sulphuric acid (lead)." *U. S.*

Adulteration with white lead, chalk, or sulphate of calcium may be detected by exposing a sample to a strong red heat, when these impurities will remain. Should starch be mixed with it, a charred residue will be obtained on the application of heat. Lead or starch may be found by digesting it with acetic acid, and testing the acetic solution with the compound solution of iodine, which will give a yellow precipitate if lead, and a blue one if starch be present. The absence of mercurous oxide is shown by its not being blackened when rubbed with lime-water. Ammoniated mercury is used only as an external application.

Mercur-diammonium chloride is said to produce an ointment more translucent and less beautifully white than the genuine, and more apt to become yellow on being kept. (Mr. J. Borland, *P. J. Tr.*, Dec. 1867, p. 262.)

Ammoniated mercury has been swallowed by mistake. It is highly poisonous, producing gastric pain, nausea, and purging. For an account of a recovery, after half a drachm was swallowed, see *London Lancet*, July 4, 1857. The remedies employed were an emetic of sulphate of zinc, and milk to allay the gastro-intestinal irritation.

Off. Prep. Unguentum Hydrargyri Ammoniati.
Off. Prep. Br. Unguentum Hydrargyri Ammoniati.

HYDRARGYRUM CUM CRETA. *U.S., Br.* *Mercury with Chalk.*

(HȲ-DRĂR'ǤY-RŬM CŬM CRĒ'TA.)

Mercure avec la Craie, Poudre de Mercure crayeux, *Fr.;* Quecksilber mit Kreide, *G.*

"Mercury, *thirty-eight parts;* Sugar of Milk, in fine powder, *twelve parts;* Prepared Chalk, *fifty parts;* Ether, Alcohol, each, *a sufficient quantity*, To make *one hundred parts.* Mix the Mercury, Sugar of Milk, and *twelve parts* of the Chalk in a suitable mortar; moisten the mass with a mixture of *equal parts* of Ether and Alcohol, and triturate it briskly. Gradually add the remainder of the Chalk, dampen the powder occasionally with a mixture of Ether and Alcohol made in the same proportions as before, and continue the trituration until globules of Mercury are no longer visible under a magnifying power of ten diameters, and the powder is of a uniform, gray color, and dry." *U. S.*

"Take of Mercury, by weight, 1 ounce [avoir.]; Prepared Chalk 2 ounces [avoir.]. Rub the mercury and chalk in a porcelain mortar until metallic globules cease to be visible to the naked eye, and the mixture acquires a uniform gray color." *Br.*

When mercury is triturated with certain dry and pulverulent substances, such as chalk or magnesia, it gradually loses its fluidity and metallic lustre, and becomes a blackish or dark gray powder. A similar change takes place when it is rubbed with viscid or greasy substances, such as honey or lard. The globules disappear, so as in some instances not to be visible even through a good lens; and the mercury is said to be extinguished. It was formerly thought that the metal was oxidized in the process. At present, the change is generally ascribed to the mechanical division of the metal, which in this state is supposed to be capable of acting on the system. There is good reason, however, to believe that in this, as in all the analogous preparations of mercury, in which the metal is extinguished by trituration, a very small portion is converted into mercurous oxide, while by far the greater part remains in the metallic state.

Robert B. Matter suggests an improved process whereby labor and time are saved; it is as follows; Mix twelve parts of finely powdered gum arabic with twelve parts of prepared chalk, triturate it with sufficient water to form a rather thin paste, add thirty-eight parts of mercury, and continue the trituration until the globules of mercury have disappeared. Now add thirty-eight parts of finely powdered prepared chalk and sufficient water to form a thin paste, triturate, and when all the globules of mercury have disappeared, place the mortar in a hot water-bath. The mixture distributed around the sides of the mortar will dry rapidly, when it can be easily scraped out, powdered in a clean mortar, passed through bolting cloth, or a fine sieve, and finally rubbed lightly in a clean dry mortar; 8 ounces may be made by this process in an hour. (*A. J. P.*, 1886, p. 119.)

Mercury with chalk is a smooth grayish powder, insoluble in water. Globules of mercury can generally be seen in it with the aid of a microscope; as the metal can scarcely be completely extinguished with chalk alone by any length of trituration. Mr. Jacob Bell found that, by powerfully pressing it, a considerable quantity of metal was separated in the form of globules. Mr. Phillips states that the extinguishment of the mercury is greatly accelerated by the addition of a little water. Dr. Stewart, of Baltimore, proposed the following process, by which he stated that the preparation might be completed in a short time, so that no globules should be visible with a powerful lens. Three ounces of mercury and six ounces of resin are to be rubbed together for three hours; five ounces of chalk are to be added, and the trituration continued for an hour; the mixture is then to be heated with alcohol so as to dissolve the resin; and the remaining powder is to be dried on bibulous paper, and well rubbed in a mortar. (*A. J. P.*, xv. 162.) But Professor Procter showed that the preparation thus made contains mercuric oxide, and is, therefore, injuriously harsh in its operation. (*Ibid.*, xxii. 113.) It is said that the precipitated black oxide is sometimes added with a view to save time in the trituration; but this must be considered as an adulteration, until it can be shown that the same oxide exists, in the same proportion, in the preparation made according to the officinal directions. Dr. Ed. Jenner Coxe, of New Orleans, found that the extinguishment of the mercury may be effected much more speedily than in the ordinary manner, by putting the ingredients into a quart bottle, to be well corked, and kept in constant agitation till the object is attained. A portion of the chalk may be thus shaken with the metal until no globules can be seen, and the process completed by trituration with the remainder of the chalk in a mortar. This mode of proceeding was suggested to Dr. Coxe by Mr. W. Hewson, of Augusta, Ga. (*Ibid.*, xxii. 317.) Dr. Squibb, having ascertained that the preparation cannot be satisfactorily made in this way on a large scale (*Proc. A. P. A.*, 1858, p. 424), has invented a machine for accomplishing the same object, by which the requisite motion is imparted to the materials contained in two large bottles, and which is said to answer the purpose well. By means of this apparatus, Dr. Squibb prepares mercury with chalk on a large scale, mixing the materials in the officinal proportions, but aiding the extinguishment of the metal by adding about one-seventh of its weight of honey, and adding this to the chalk made into a paste with water and afterwards drying. (*Ibid.*, 1859, p. 359.) It has been shown that the preparation thus made resists oxidation most effectually; owing probably to the presence of saccharine matter. (J. P. Remington, *A. J. P.*, Jan. 1869.) W. E. Bibby (*A. J. P.*, 1876, p. 269) recommends the rubbing of 3 troyounces of mercury, 4 troyounces of prepared chalk, and 1 troyounce of sugar of milk together in a mortar into an impalpable powder and passing through a fine sieve. As found in commerce, mercury with chalk, instead of being the mild preparation intended, sometimes acts very harshly, causing vomiting, gastric pains, etc. This has been ascribed to the presence of antimony or arsenic, which, however, must be rare; and the ordinary cause of the harshness is no doubt mercuric oxide, produced in minute proportion either during the trituration, or by the spontaneous change which occurs with time; mercurous oxide becoming mercuric oxide by the influence of light. The only sure method to guard against such results is to test the preparation carefully before dispensing it. (See *A. J. P.*, 1878, p. 325.) If the mercury contained in it be volatilized by heat, and the remaining chalk be dissolved by dilute acetic acid, the solution should not be colored by sulphuretted hydrogen. The presence of any probable metallic impurity may be detected in this way. To detect mercuric oxide, a portion of the powder may be treated with diluted hydrochloric acid with a moderate heat, and the solution tested by stannous chloride, which, if there be any mercuric oxide present, will cause a precipitation of metallic mercury as a black powder.

Medical Properties and Uses. Mercury with chalk is a very mild mercurial, similar in its properties to the blue mass, but much weaker. It is sometimes used as an alterative, particularly in the complaints of children attended with deficient biliary secretion, indicated by white or clay-colored stools. The chalk is antacid, and, though in small quantity, may sometimes be a useful accompaniment of the mercury in diarrhœa. Eight grains of the U. S. preparation contain about three grains of mercury. The dose is from five grains to half a drachm (0·33–1 95 Gm.) twice a day. Two or three grains (0·13–0·20 Gm.) is the dose for a child. It should not be given in pill with substances which become hard on keeping; as the contraction of the mass presses together the particles of mercury, which, in time, appear in globules in the interior of the pill.

HYDRASTIS. *U. S.* *Hydrastis.* [*Golden Seal.*]

(HȲ-DRĂS'TIS.)

"The rhizome and rootlets of Hydrastis Canadensis. Linné. (*Nat. Ord.* Ranunculaceæ.)" *U. S.*

Rhizoma Hydrastis; Golden Seal, Yellow Root, Yellow Puccoon, Orange Root, Indian Dye, Indian Turmeric; Racine d'Hydrastis de Canada, *Fr.;* Canadische Gelbwurzel, *G.*

Gen. Ch. *Calyx* of three petalloid sepals, falling when the flower opens. *Ovaries* in a roundish ovoid head. *Stigmas* subsessile, dilated, flat, rounded at the apex. *Carpels* fleshy, one or two-seeded, cohering in a compound berry.

Hydrastis Canadensis. Gray, *Manual of Bot.* p. 14; figured in Griffith's *Med. Bot.* p. 82.—*Yellow-root, Orange-root, Yellow Puccoon.* This is a small, herbaceous, perennial plant, with a thick, fleshy, yellow rhizome, from which numerous long radical fibres proceed, and an erect, simple, pubescent stem, from six inches to a foot in height. There are usually but two leaves, which are unequal, one sessile at the top of the stem, the other attached to it a short distance below by a thick roundish footstalk, causing the stem to appear as if bifurcate near the summit. The leaves are pubescent, roundish-cordate, with from three to seven, but generally five lobes, which are pointed and unequally serrate. A solitary flower stands upon a peduncle rising from the basis of the upper leaf. It is whitish, rose-colored, or purplish, without corolla, but with a colored calyx, the sepals of which closely resemble petals, and are very caducous, falling very soon after the flower has expanded. The fruit is a globose, compound, red or purple berry, half an inch or more in diameter, composed of many minute granules, each containing one, or more rarely two seeds. The plant grows in moist, rich woodlands, in most parts of the United States, but abundantly in the North and West. The fruit bears a close resemblance to the raspberry, but is not edible. The root is the part used. The Indians employed it for staining and dyeing yellow, and it is said to impart a rich and permanent yellow, and with indigo a fine green to wool, silk, and cotton.

Properties. The fresh root is juicy and loses much of its weight in drying. The dried caudex is officinally described as "about an inch and a half (4 cm.) long and a quarter of an inch (6 mm.) thick; oblique, with short branches, somewhat annulate and longitudinally wrinkled; externally yellowish gray; fracture short, waxy, bright reddish yellow, with a thickish bark, about ten narrow wood-wedges, broad medullary rays, and large pith. Rootlets thin, brittle, with a thick, yellow bark and subquadrangular, woody centre." *U. S.* Many of the detached rootlets are mixed with the rhizomes in mass. The color of the rhizome, though yellow in the recent root, becomes of a dark yellowish brown by age; that of the rootlets and the interior of the root is yellow, and of the powder still more so. The odor is strong, sweetish, and somewhat narcotic, the taste bitter and peculiar. The medicine imparts its virtues and coloring matters to water and alcohol. Examined by Mr. Alfred A. B. Durand, of Philadelphia, it was found to contain albumen, starch, fatty matter, resin, yellow coloring matter, sugar, lignin, and various salts. He also discovered a peculiar nitrogenous, crystallizable substance, for which he proposed the provisional name of *hydrastin*, until it should be determined whether it was, as he suspected, an alkaloid. (*A. J. P.*, 1851, p. 112.) Since that time it has been ascertained that the claims of this principle to be considered as an alkaloid were just, and it has definitely taken the name of *hydrastine*, of which *hydrastin* and *hydrastia* are merely synonymes. It has also been determined that the root contains another alkaloid, to which it owes its yellow color, and which is probably identical with the yellow coloring matter of Mr. Durand. Mr. F. Mahla first ascertained that this new alkaloid of hydrastis is *berberine** (*Am. Journ. of Sci. and Arts*, Jan. 1862, p. 43). It exists

* *Berberine.* This alkaloid appears to have been first discovered, in 1826, in a species of Xanthoxylum, by Chevallier and Pelletan, who, from its color and taste, named it *xanthopicrite*. Buchner and Herberger, in 1835, found it in *Berberis vulgaris*, and named it berberine; but none of these chemists were aware of its alkaline properties. Indeed, the substance obtained by them, at least the berberine of Buchner, must have been a native salt of the proper alkaloid, which was not, therefore, procured in a pure state. Subsequently Fleitmann demonstrated its basic character, and published an account of several of its salts. It is not confined to the barberry, but has been found, by various chemists, in several other plants, particularly those combining bitterness and a yellow color, as in various products of *Cocculus palmatus*, *Hydrastis Canadensis*, *Xanthorrisa apiifolia*, *Coptis Teeta*, *Xanthoxylum Clava Herculis*, *Coscinium fenestratum*, and others belonging to the natural families of Berberaceæ, Menispermaceæ, and Ranunculaceæ. Indeed, few if any of the known alkaloids are so widely diffused as this appears to be in the vegetable kingdom. A list of all the plants from which it has been obtained is contained in *A. J. P.* (Sept. 1863, p. 456).

Berberine may be obtained most readily from its sulphate. Prof. Procter has given the following process for preparing it, based upon a suggestion of Mr. Merrill, of Cincinnati. The coarsely powdered root is to be exhausted by repeated decoction with boiling water, and the mixed liquids, after filtration, are to be evaporated to a soft extract. This is to be digested several times with stronger alcohol, in the proportion of a pint to half a pound of the root, until exhausted, one-fourth of its bulk of water is to be added to the tincture, and five-sixths of the alcohol to be distilled off. To the residue, while still hot, sulphuric acid is to be added in excess, and the liquid allowed to cool. The sulphate of berberine is deposited in crystals, and, having been purified by recrystallization, is to be decomposed by the addition, in excess, to its solution in boiling water, of freshly precipitated protoxide of lead, the solution being kept hot until the decomposition is completed. This may be known by the absence of a precipitate when acetate of lead is added to a drop of the clear liquid. The liquid is then to be filtered, and set aside to crystallise. Thus obtained, berberine is in the form of a yellow powder, which, under the microscope, appears to consist of groups of minute, acicular crystals. It has a bitter taste, is soluble in about 100 parts of cold water, still less soluble in cold alcohol, freely soluble in both these liquids when hot, and insoluble in ether. It forms salts of difficult solubility with hydrochloric and sulphuric acids, and is distinguished by being copiously precipitated by the former acid from its cold watery solution in the form of crystals of the hydrochlorate. It is freely dissolved by acetic acid, which forms with it a readily soluble salt. (*A. J. P.*, Jan. 1864, p. 10.) Its formula is, according to Fleitmann, $C_{42}H_{40}N_2O_{11}$, but, on the more recent authority of Perrins, $C_{20}H_{17}NO_4$. (*P. J. Tr.*, April, 1863, p. 464.) Hlasiwetz (*Ann. Ch. Pharm.*, 115, p. 45) also confirms this formula, which may therefore be assumed as correct. The *hydrochlorate of berberine*, which is the salt that has attracted most notice, may be readily obtained by using hydrochloric instead of sulphuric acid in the above process, and purifying the precipitate by

in large proportion in hydrastis, constituting, according to Perrins, nearly 4 per cent. There can be no doubt that this medicine owes much of its virtues to berberine. For a valuable paper by Prof. J. U. Lloyd on the preparation of Salts of Berberine, see *A. J. P.*, 1879, p. 11. A substance, obtained by the precipitation of an infusion of the root by hydrochloric acid, has been for some time known and used by the "Eclectics," under the name of hydrastin; it consists of variable proportions of hydrastine, berberine, and resin (*A. J. P.*, 1876, p. 386), and the reader must be cautious not to confound this substance with the alkaloid to which the name properly belongs.

Hydrastine, which is the characteristic alkaloid, may be obtained by exhausting the powdered root as far as possible with water by percolation, adding hydrochloric acid to the infusion so as to precipitate the berberine in the form of hydrochlorate, and treating the mother-liquor with solution of ammonia in slight excess. The hydrastine is precipitated, in an impure state, and may be purified by repeated solution in boiling alcohol, which deposits it in crystals on cooling. A little animal charcoal may be used towards the close of the process, in order to completely deprive the crystals of color. To Mr. Mahla, of Chicago, and Mr. Perrins, of London, is due the credit of having fully investigated the properties of this alkaloid.* Hydrastine crystallizes in brilliant, four-sided prisms, which are white or colorless when pure, inodorous, and almost tasteless in consequence of their insolubility in the saliva, but become bitter and somewhat acrid in saline combination. It melts at 135° C. (275° F.), is decomposed at a higher temperature, and is inflammable. It is nearly insoluble in water, but is readily dissolved by alcohol, ether, chloroform, and benzol. It has an alkaline reaction, and with the acids forms salts, most of which are readily soluble in water, and, according to Mr. Merrill, of Cincinnati, either uncrystallizable, or crystallizable with difficulty. The alkalies and tannic acid precipitate it from its saline solutions. With sulphuric acid and bichromate of potassium or red oxide of lead, it assumes a red color; but it differs from strychnine in exhibiting no tint of blue or violet. Its composition is $C_{22}H_{23}NO_6$ (*Mahla*). Mr. Perrins obtained 1·5 per cent. of it from the root, and, having given five grains of it to a rabbit, without any other effect than a slight uneasiness which soon ceased, concluded justly that it was not poisonous.

It is highly probable, from the odor of hydrastis, that, besides the two alkaloids here mentioned, it contains also an active volatile principle; but this has not yet been isolated. Mr. A. K. Hale, of Ann Arbor, Michigan, has ascertained that there is another alkaloid in hydrastis, somewhat resembling berberine, but quite distinct. To the neutral mother-liquor of hydrastine, he added water of ammonia in great excess, say 10 per cent., which caused a yellow precipitate, darker than berberine, and more soluble in water than this latter. Its alcoholic solution shows a neutral reaction; it dissolves in cold nitric acid less readily than berberine; the solution becomes red on heating. It dissolves in hot sulphuric acid with reddish brown color; is more easily soluble in cold potash solution than berberine, and gives with double potassium quicksilver iodide a slighter yellow precipitate. Mr. Hale did not name it, or determine its ultimate composition. (*A. J. P.*, 1873, p. 248.) Mr. Hale's results have since been confirmed by J. C. Burt (*A. J. P.*, 1875, p. 481),

solution in hot alcohol, and subsequent refrigeration. It is in fine acicular crystals, of a bright yellow color, and intensely bitter taste, very slightly soluble in cold water, to which, however, it imparts a deep yellow color, slightly soluble also in cold alcohol, but dissolved in large proportion by both liquids when hot. By concentrated nitric acid both this salt and its base are decomposed, with the production of a dark red color, and the escape of nitrous fumes. A process for *Hypophosphite of Berberine*, by Prof. J. U. Lloyd, may be found in *A. J. P.*, July, 1877. Parsons (*N. R.*, 1879, p. 109) analysed *Phosphate of Berberine*, and believes the formula to be $C_{20}H_{17}NO_4.2H_3PO_4$.

According to the studies of Falck and Guenste, berberine causes in dogs and rabbits restlessness, convulsive tremblings, hurried respiration, and diarrhœa, followed, if the dose has been large enough, by decrease of the breathing-rate, wide-spread paralysis, dyspnœa, convulsions, and death. In man as yet no serious symptoms have been recorded as produced by it. Buchner is stated to have taken nearly twenty grains without causing anything more serious than a loose stool. It has been employed in internal medicine as a simple bitter, in doses of two to five grains (0·13 to 0·33 Gm.).

* For a paper by Mr. Mahla, see *Amer. Journ. of Sci. and Arts*, July, 1863, p. 57, and for another by Mr. J. Dyson Perrins, of London, *P. J. Tr.*, 1862, p. 546.

who states that the yield of the third alkaloid is less than that of hydrastine or berberine, and by H. Lerchen (*A. J. P.*, 1878, p. 470), who proposes the name of *xanthopuccine* for it.

Prof. F. B. Power believes that hydrastine and berberine are the sole alkaloids in hydrastis, and that the fluorescence of solutions is due to hydrastine alone. (*Proc. A. P. A.*, 1886, p. 429.)

Medical Properties and Uses. Very diversified powers have been claimed for hydrastis. Thus, while all admit its tonic properties, it is considered by different practitioners as aperient, alterative in its influence on the mucous membranes, cholagogue, deobstruent in reference to the glands generally, diuretic, antiseptic, etc. It has been employed in dyspepsia and other affections requiring tonic treatment, in jaundice and other functional disorders of the liver, as a laxative in constipation and piles, and as an alterative in various diseases of the mucous membranes, as catarrh, chronic enteritis, cystirrhœa, leucorrhœa, gonorrhœa, etc., being used in the latter complaints both internally and locally. By some it is used as one of the best substitutes for quinine in intermittents.

The physiological action of hydrastine has been studied by Dr. Roberts Bartholow (*Lloyd's Drugs and Medicines of North America*), Dr. Mays (*Therapeutic Gazette*, 1886), Dr. Fellner (*Centralbl. Med. Wissen.*, Nov. 1884), and others. It produces in both cold- and warm-blooded animals violent tetanic convulsions, rapidly ending in death from cramp asphyxia. These convulsions appear to be spinal, and are accompanied by great heightening of the reflex activity. According to the experiments of Bartholow and Mays, the drug exhausts the excitability of the motor nerves, but this action seems to be very feeble. The experiments of Dr. Mays show that when the alkaloid is applied locally to a sensory nerve it lessens very distinctly its irritability. When given internally, it is asserted by Dr. Mays to cause an anæsthesia which is principally centric. According to the experiments of Fellner, small doses of the alkaloid produce rise of the arterial pressure, preceded by a slight fall, whilst large doses produce depression of the arterial pressure. After the division of the spinal cord the drug was powerless to cause rise of the arterial pressure, and it would appear, therefore, that it acts chiefly upon the vaso-motor centre. The fall of the arterial pressure appears to be in part due to a direct action upon the heart, as Dr. Bartholow has shown that the alkaloid, when placed upon the exposed heart of the frog, induces diastolic arrest with loss of electric excitability. Slavatinski (*London Lancet*, May, 1886) states that, finally, in poisoning with the drug the vaso-motor centre is paralyzed. Both Fellner and Slavatinski affirm that hydrastine has a distinct ecbolic action, producing uterine contractions in the non-pregnant uterus, and abortion in pregnant rabbits. Dr. Slavatinski reports a case of premature labor caused by hypodermic injections of two to three grammes,

Under the name *hydrastin* there is sold commercially a substance consisting of berberine, hydrastine, and probably some resin. Employing this, Professor Rutherford (*Brit. Med. Journ.*, 1879, vols. i. and ii.) found in his experiments upon the lower animals marked increase in the biliary excretion. When locally applied the preparations of hydrastis have a very remarkable effect upon mucous membrane. They have been used with asserted excellent results in chronic gastro-intestinal catarrhs, and especially in those due to alcohol. In the second stages of gonorrhœa, after the acute inflammation has been subdued, hydrastin, or the fluid extract suspended in mucilage, is of very great service. Five grains of the commercial impure hydrastin, or ten to twenty minims of the fluid extract, may be used to the ounce of injection. It is probable that in otorrhœa, nasal, vaginal, and other mucous catarrhs, equally good results might be obtained. Hydrastin has also been employed as an antiperiodic, and probably has the action of a simple bitter upon the stomach.

The proper internal dose of pure hydrastin cannot be considered as settled; the commercial drug is usually impure, and may often be administered in doses of five to ten grains (0·33 Gm. to 0·66 Gm.). The dose of the pure alkaloid is given by Dr. Mays as one-fourth of a grain (0·016 Gm.). The fluid extract of hydrastis is an excellent preparation.* In regard to other forms of preparation, the root may be treated like columbo or gentian.

Off. Prep. Extractum Hydrastis Fluidum; Tinctura Hydrastis.

HYOSCYAMINÆ SULPHAS. *U. S.* *Sulphate of Hyoscyamine.*

(HȲ-OS-CȲ-A-MĪ'NÆ SŬL'PHĂS.)

$(C_{17}H_{23}NO_3)_2.H_2SO_4$; 676. $C_{34}H_{23}NO_6.HO, SO_3$; 338.

"The neutral sulphate of an alkaloid prepared from Hyoscyamus." *U. S.*

Sulfate d'Hyoscyamine, *Fr.;* Hyoscyaminum Sulfuricum, Schwefelsaures Hyoscyamin, *G.*

Although Brandes announced the existence of an alkaloid in the seeds of Hyoscyamus niger, the process which he used to obtain it was not successful in other hands. The credit of first isolating the alkaloid *hyoscyamine* or *hyoscyamia* from the plant must be given to Geiger and Hesse, who obtained it as long ago as 1833. Höhn and Reichardt's process, in which the seed is used as the source, is as follows. They treat hyoscyamus seed, first with ether to separate fatty matter, then with alcohol acidulated with a few drops of sulphuric acid, and afterwards distil the alcoholic solution. The watery residue is to be neutralized by soda, and the liquid precipitated by a solution of tannin. The precipitate having been placed on a porcelain plate to dry, is mixed while yet moist with an excess of lime, and then exhausted by strong alcohol. The alcoholic solution is treated with sulphuric acid, then with soda, and finally with ether, which dissolves the liberated hyoscyamine. By distilling off the ether a colorless oleaginous liquid is left, which at length concretes. (*Journ. de Pharm.*, Mai, 1872, p. 385.)

These investigators gave to hyoscyamine the formula $C_{15}H_{23}NO_3$, but Ladenburg has shown by a study of its decomposition products that it is isomeric with atropine, $C_{17}H_{23}NO_3$. Ladenburg has made within the last few years what is the most complete study of atropine and hyoscyamine that we have, and has established their relations to each other in a clearer light. According to him (*Ber. der Chem. Ges.*, xiii., pp. 251, 909, and 1549), *Hyoscyamus* contains two alkaloids, a crystalline one, to which the name of *hyoscyamine* is given, and which is the one hitherto studied under that name, and an amorphous one, which remains in the mother-liquor after the removal of the crystallizable alkaloid, and comes into commerce as a brown thickish syrup. It can be extracted by the formation of the gold salt, which is less soluble than hyoscyamine gold chloride. This alkaloid, for which he proposes the name *hyoscine*, and which has the same formula ($C_{17}H_{23}NO_3$) as *hyoscyamine*, yields different decomposition products upon decomposition by baryta water. Hyoscyamine treated with boiling baryta water assimilates a molecule of water and splits up into what were called *hyoscinic acid*, $C_9H_{10}O_3$, and *hyoscine*, $C_8H_{15}NO$, but which Ladenburg shows to be simply identical with the decomposition products of atropine, *tropic acid* and *tropine*. Hyoscine, on the other hand, yields *tropic acid*, $C_9H_{10}O_3$, and *pseudotropine*, $C_8H_{15}NO$. Inasmuch as Ladenburg (*Ber. der Chem. Ges.*, xii., p. 941) has succeeded in effecting the synthesis of *atropine* by the combination of tropic acid and tropine (the two decomposition products which are common to the two alkaloids *atropine* and *hyoscyamine*), we must look for the differences between these two, to physical and molecular sources rather than chemical.

Hyoscyamine crystallizes in colorless, transparent, silky needles, fusing at 108·5° C., is inodorous, of an acrid, disagreeable taste, slightly soluble in water, very soluble in alcohol and ether, and volatilizable with little change if carefully distilled. It is quickly altered by contact with water and an alkali, and when heated with potassa or soda is completely decomposed, with the disengagement of ammonia. It neutralizes

* *Liquor Hydrastinæ.* Under the names of *Liquid Hydrastis, Fluid Hydrastis, Colorless Hydrastis*, etc., preparations of the alkaloids of hydrastis have been largely used. In some cases these solutions have been made directly from the drug by depriving a fluid extract of coloring matter, in others the alkaloid has been dissolved in a suitable liquid. Gust. Steinmann (*A. J. P.*, 1887, p. 296) examined several samples and found hydrastine in each, combined with either sulphuric or hydrochloric acid, besides aluminium, potassium, boric acid, etc., in small proportion; by dissolving 20 grains of hydrastine sulphate or chloride in a pint of a solution of glycerin and water (sp. gr. 1·15), a liquid is produced from which the asserted good results can be obtained.

the acids, forming crystallizable salts,* and is precipitated by infusion of galls. The alkaloid and its salts are very poisonous; and the smallest quantity, introduced into the eye, produces dilatation of the pupil, which continues long.

Hyoscine has been known in commerce as *amorphous hyoscyamine.* The best salts, according to Prof. Edlefsen, to prepare and dispense are the *hydrobromate* and *hydriodate.*

Hydriodate of hyoscine crystallizes from water, in which it is only moderately soluble, in small, hemihedral prisms, which mostly have a slight yellowish color. Dried at 100° C. (212° F.), the salt had the composition: $C_{17}H_{23}NO_3.HI.\frac{1}{2}H_2O$.

Hydrobromate of hyoscine is very easily soluble in water. It forms large colorless, transparent, and sharply defined crystals, sometimes of 1 to 2 cm. in length. They are rhombic, sphenoid, hemihedral prisms, which, when exposed in the desiccator over sulphuric acid, lose three molecules (12·27 per cent.) of water. Afterwards dried at 100° C. (212° F.) in vacuo, they yield nothing more. The composition is $C_{17}H_{23}NO_3.HBr.\frac{1}{2}H_2O$, when dry; when crystallised, the water amounts to $3\frac{1}{2}H_2O$. (*Ber. der Chem. Ges.*, 1881, p. 1870; *N. R.*, 1882, p. 51.)

The double gold chloride, $C_{17}H_{23}NO_3HCl + AuCl_3$, is less soluble than the corresponding gold salt of hyoscyamine, and so serves to separate them when together.

Properties. The Pharmacopœia describes the sulphate of hyoscyamine as "small golden yellow, or yellowish white scales or crystals, or a yellowish white, amorphous powder, deliquescent on exposure to air, odorless, having a bitter and acrid taste, and a neutral reaction. Very soluble in water and in alcohol. When heated on platinum foil, the salt chars and is finally completely dissipated. An aqueous solution of the salt is not precipitated by test-solution of platinic chloride. With chloride of gold it yields a precipitate, which, when recrystallized from boiling water acidulated with hydrochloric acid, is deposited, on cooling (without rendering the liquid turbid) in brilliant, lustrous, golden yellow scales (difference from atropine). The aqueous solution yields, with test-solution of chloride of barium, a white precipitate insoluble in hydrochloric acid." *U. S.* The sulphate of hyoscyamine has been selected as the most suitable salt for use, on account of its being more soluble than the alkaloid.

Medical Properties. Owing to the facts that until very recently commercial hyoscyamine has usually been contaminated with hyoscine, and that few careful studies of a chemically pure hyoscyamine have been made, its exact influence upon the human system is not positively determined. The studies of Dr. J. C. Shaw appear, however, to prove that hyoscyamine acts upon the nervous system and the circulation, including the heart and the vaso-motor system, precisely as does atropine, except as regards respiration, which appears in most cases to have been slowed rather than increased in rapidity, an indication that hyoscyamine, unlike atropine, is not a respiratory stimulant. Dr. Shaw also found that hyoscyamine is less powerful as a mydriatic and more powerful as a soporific than is atropine. On the other hand, in studies upon normal men, Dr. Richter could not perceive that hyoscyamine had a tendency to produce sleep. Prof. Sydney Ringer, in a careful comparative study of hyoscyamine and atropine in acute mania, was unable to detect any important differences in the action of the two substances. The dose of commercial hyoscyamine varies greatly according to its purity, but one-fortieth of a grain of the pure alkaloid has produced violent poisoning, with symptoms similar to those caused by atropine.

Hyoscine. Various observers have noted that the impure amorphous hyoscyamine is more powerful than is the crystallized alkaloid. These observations, with the chemical fact that amorphous hyoscyamine is chiefly hyoscine, in 1884 led Dr. H. C. Wood to make a careful physiological study of that alkaloid upon the lower animals and to apply it to clinical medicine. It was found that the pure hyoscine produced in the frog, motor reflex paralysis, due to a depression of the spinal cord; and that in mammals it caused disturbance of respiration, loss of muscular power, pronounced tendency to stupor, and, finally, death by asphyxia. It exerted very little influence upon the circulation even when in toxic doses. It became evident

* Ladenburg states that the simple salts of hyoscyamine do not crystallise, although the double salts do.

that the drug was a depressant of the principal cerebral centres, of the respiratory centres, and also of the lower motor centres of the spinal cord. In man, the ingestion of hyoscine in decided doses is followed in a very short time by dryness of the mouth, flushings of the face, great sleepiness, associated in some cases with delirious mutterings, and giddiness akin to that of alcoholic intoxication. The respirations are usually lessened in frequency, and the pulse-rate is also somewhat diminished. Dilatation of the pupils is usually, but not invariably, produced. After toxic doses these symptoms are intensified; whilst the frequent loss or impairment of the power of swallowing, and a peculiar hoarseness of the voice, with, in some cases, laryngeal dyspnœa, indicate that the muscles of the larynx, as well as those of the pharnyx, have a special tendency to be paralyzed by the alkaloid; the respiration becomes not only slow and full, but sometimes takes on a distinctly Cheyne-Stokes character; the skin is not dry, as in atropine-poisoning, but is frequently covered with sweat. No cases of fatal poisoning are on record. One-fourth of a grain of very impure hyoscine produced in the case of Dr. Hutchinson profound muscular relaxation, with quiet coma, lasting for eleven hours. In applying hyoscine to the treatment of disease, Dr. H. C. Wood found that it is a valuable soporific, especially useful in those cases in which the wakefulness is complicated with or due to cerebral excitement. In insomnia produced by overwork, when the brain seems to lose the capability of ceasing its action, hyoscine is of service; but it is especially valuable in active delirious conditions, such as occur in acute mania or in exacerbations in the course of chronic mania. In those cases in which morphine increases the cerebral excitement hyoscine usually acts most happily. According to the statements of Drs. Bruce and Tirard, it is an entirely safe remedy in cases of severe kidney disease when morphine is contraindicated. Dr. H. C. Wood has found that it is an efficient remedy in the treatment of sexual excitement, such as nymphomania, spermatorrhœa, and allied affections, and that it will almost invariably control excessive seminal emissions. Hyoscine rarely, if ever, produces much more serious after-effects than a little dryness of the throat and headache, and does not disturb the alimentary canal. The reports of later clinicians indicate that excessive susceptibility to its influence is a not infrequent idiosyncrasy, and it is even affirmed that $\frac{1}{1200}$ of a grain has caused alarming symptoms. It is probable, however, that much larger doses were taken in these cases than is alleged. On account of its tendency to produce pharyngeal and laryngeal paralysis, it should not be employed in such diseases as scarlet fever or diphtheria when there is a tendency to throat difficulties. Being practically tasteless, hyoscine is readily given in food or drink without the knowledge of the patient. It acts well when taken by the mouth, but is especially efficient and prompt when administered hypodermically, and never produces local irritation. The effects of a hypodermic dose are usually manifested inside of ten minutes, and persist for six or eight hours. The dose by the mouth is from $\frac{1}{120}$ to $\frac{1}{30}$ of a grain; for hypodermic injections $\frac{1}{150}$ to $\frac{1}{100}$ of a grain. On account of the susceptibility of some persons to it, the commencing dose by the mouth should not be over $\frac{1}{120}$ of a grain, by injection $\frac{1}{150}$ of a grain: after cautious trial, doses larger than the maximum just given may be employed.

HYOSCYAMUS. *U. S.*, *Br.* *Hyoscyamus.* [*Henbane.*]

(HŸ-OS-CӮ'Ą-MŬS.)

Hyoscyami Folia, *Br.*

"The leaves of Hyoscyamus niger, Linné (*Nat. Ord.* Solanaceæ), collected from plants of the second year's growth." *U. S.* "The fresh leaves and flowers, with the branches to which they are attached, of Hyoscyamus niger, *Linn.*; also the leaves separated from the branches and flowering tops, carefully dried; collected from biennial plants, growing wild or cultivated in Britain, when about two-thirds of the flowers are expanded." *Br.*

Hyoscyami Folia, *Br.*, *U. S.* 1870; Herba Hyoscyami; Feuilles de Jusquiame noir, *Fr.*; Bilsenkraut, *G.*

Gen. Ch. *Corolla* funnel-form, obtuse. *Stamens* inclined. *Capsules* covered with a lid, two-celled. *Willd.*

Hyoscyamus niger. Willd. *Sp. Plant.* i. 1010; Woodv. *Med. Bot.* p. 204, t. 76; Carson, *Illust. of Med. Bot.* ii. 19, pl. 66. Henbane is usually a biennial plant, with a long, tapering, whitish, fleshy, somewhat branching root, not unlike that of parsley, for which it has been eaten by mistake, with poisonous effects. The stem, which rises in the second year, is erect, round, branching, from one to four feet high, and thickly furnished with leaves. These are large, oblong-ovate, deeply sinuated with pointed segments, undulated, soft to the touch, and at their base embrace the stem. The upper leaves are generally entire. Both the stem and leaves are hairy, viscid, and of a sea-green color. The flowers form long, one-sided, leafy spikes, which terminate the branches, and hang downwards. They are composed of a calyx with five pointed divisions, a funnel-shaped corolla, with five unequal, obtuse segments at the border, five stamens inserted into the tube of the corolla, and a pistil with a blunt, round stigma. Their color is an obscure yellow, beautifully variegated with purple veins. The fruit is a globular two-celled capsule, covered with a lid, invested with the persistent calyx, and containing numerous small seeds, which are discharged by the horizontal separation of the lid. The whole plant has a rank offensive smell.

H. niger is susceptible of considerable diversity of character, causing varieties which have by some been considered as distinct species. Thus, the plant is sometimes annual, the stem simple, smaller, and less downy than in the biennial plant, the leaves shorter and less hairy and viscid, and the flowers often yellow without the purple streaks. It has been ascertained that much difference of medical properties is connected with these diversities of character; and the British Pharmacopœia directs the biennial variety as the most efficient.

The plant is found in the northern and eastern sections of the United States, occupying waste grounds in the older settlements, particularly graveyards, old gardens, and the foundations of ruined houses. It grows in great abundance about Detroit, in Michigan. It is not, however, a native of this country, having been introduced from Europe. In Great Britain, and on the continent of Europe, it grows abundantly along the roads, around villages, amidst rubbish, and in uncultivated places. Both varieties were formerly cultivated in England, but at present the biennial is solely or chiefly grown. The annual plant flowers in July or August, the biennial in May or June. For an account of the cultivation of the biennial variety of *H. niger* at Hitchen, Herts, England, see *P. J. Tr.*, Feb. 1860.

H. albus, so named from the whiteness of its flowers, is used in France indiscriminately with the former species, with which it appears to be identical in medicinal properties.

All parts of *Hyoscyamus niger* are active. The leaves are officinally described as "ovate, or ovate-oblong, sometimes ten inches (25 cm.) long and four inches (10 cm.) broad; sinuate-toothed, the teeth large, oblong or triangular; grayish green, glandular, hairy; midrib prominent; odor heavy, narcotic; taste bitter and somewhat acrid." *U. S.* Much of the efficacy of henbane depends upon the time at which it is gathered. The leaves should be collected soon after the plant has flowered. In the biennial plant, those of the second year are preferred to those of the first. The latter, according to Dr. Houlton, are less clammy and fetid, yield less extractive, and are medicinally much less efficient. It is said that the plant is sometimes destroyed by severe winters in England, and that no leaves of the second year's growth are obtainable. This is, perhaps, one of the causes of the great uncertainty of the medicine as found in commerce. The root also is said to be much more poisonous in the second year than in the first.*

* The several products of the henbane plants are placed by Mr. R. Usher (*P. J. Tr.*, Aug. 1867) in the following order, as to efficiency: 1, the leaves of the biennial plant of the second year's growth; 2, the biennial plant of the first year; 3, the British annual henbane; 4, the German annual henbane. The last two, though most extensively used, are really nearly valueless, and should always be rejected. The British annual so nearly resembles the biennial of the second year, having flowers, that the two may be easily mistaken for one another; but a sufficient distinction is that the annual plant "possesses no flavor or aroma." Besides, the leaves are much shorter; and occasionally there is a pure primrose blossom, which never happens with the biennial, which is beautifully streaked. The biennial plant is so liable to the attacks of worms, that at one time little of the second year's growth was collected, and the market was consequently supplied with a very inferior article.

Properties. The recent leaves have, when bruised, a strong, disagreeable, narcotic odor, somewhat like that of tobacco. Their taste is mucilaginous and very slightly acrid. When dried, they have little smell or taste. Thrown upon the fire, they burn with a crackling noise, as if they contained a nitrate, and at the same time emit a strong odor. Their virtues are completely extracted by diluted alcohol. The watery infusion is of a pale yellow color, insipid, with the narcotic odor of the plant. The leaves were analysed by Lindbergsen, who obtained from them a narcotic principle. They contain a large proportion of nitrate of potassium; Mr. F. Mahla having obtained, as nearly as he could estimate from his experiments, 2 per cent. of that salt. (*A. J. P.*, 1859, p. 402.) The seeds are very small, roundish, compressed, somewhat kidney-shaped, a little wrinkled, of a gray or yellowish gray color, of the odor of the plant, and an oleaginous, bitterish taste. Geiger and Hesse (1833) were the first to demonstrate the existence of an alkaloid in hyoscyamus. Ladenburg has shown (1880) that there are two alkaloids in the plant—one crystallizable, *hyoscyamine*, and the other amorphous, *hyoscine*. (See *Hyoscyaminæ Sulphas*, p. 802.)

Höhn (*Ann. Chem. Pharm.*, 157, 98) obtained from the seeds a bitter principle which proved to be a glucoside. He calls it *hyoscypicrin*, and gives it the formula $C_{27}H_{52}O_{14}$.

From experiments made by Mr. Hirtz upon the relative medicinal power of extracts from the seeds and from the leaves, he inferred that the former had ten times the strength of the latter.

Henbane leaves yield, by destructive distillation, a very poisonous empyreumatic oil.

Medical Properties and Uses. Hyoscyamus was known to the ancients, and was employed by some of the earlier modern practitioners, but had fallen into disuse, and was almost forgotten, when Baron Störck again introduced it into notice. By this physician and some of his successors it was prescribed in numerous diseases, and, if we may credit their testimony, with the happiest effects; but subsequent experience of its operation has been such as very much to narrow the extent of its application. It is at present used almost exclusively to relieve pain, procure sleep, or quiet irregular nervous action; and is not supposed to exercise any specific curative influence over particular diseases. It is similar in its physiological action to belladonna, and in poisonous doses produces similar symptoms, but it is more of a hypnotic and much feebler. It is chiefly employed to allay nervous irritation, in hysteria, and in various pectoral diseases with cough; also to prevent griping by the vegetable cathartics. In Europe, where the fresh leaves are readily obtained, it is often applied externally in the shape of lotion, cataplasm, or fomentation, to allay pain and irritation, in scrofulous or cancerous ulcers, scirrhous, hemorrhoidal, or other painful tumors, gouty and rheumatic swellings, and nervous headache. The diagnosis between hyoscyamus and belladonna-poisoning can scarcely be made with certainty without a history. The treatment of the two poisonings is identical. (See *Belladonna*.)

Henbane may be given in fluid or solid extract or in tincture. The dose of the leaves is from five to ten grains (0·33–0·65 Gm.), of the seeds somewhat smaller. The common extract, or inspissated juice of the fresh leaves (*Extractum Hyoscyami, Br.*), is exceedingly variable in its operation, being sometimes active, sometimes almost inert. The usual dose is two or three grains (0·13–0·20 Gm.), repeated and gradually increased till its effects are obtained. The alcoholic extract, prepared from the recently dried leaves (*Extractum Hyoscyami Alcoholicum, U. S.*), is said to be more certain. The dose of this to begin with is one or two grains (0·065–0·13 Gm.), which may be increased gradually to twenty or thirty grains (1·3–1·95 Gm.). An extract from the seeds would, no doubt, be much more efficacious. The dose of the tincture is one or two fluidrachms (3·75–7·5 C.c.).

Off. Prep. Abstractum Hyoscyami; Extractum Hyoscyami Alcoholicum; Extractum Hyoscyami Fluidum; Tinctura Hyoscyami.

inferior article. For an account of an interesting investigation on the physical distinctions between annual and biennial plants, see *Amer. Drug.*, 1884, p. 142, or *Proc. A. P. A.*, 1885, p. 123.

Off. Prep. Br. Extractum Hyoscyami; Succus Hyoscyami; Tinctura Hyoscyami.

ICHTHYOCOLLA. *U. S.* *Isinglass.*

(ĬCH-THY̆-Ō-CŎL′LĄ.)

"The swimming-bladder of Acipenser Huso, Linné, and of other species of Acipenser (*Class*, Pisces; *Order*, Sturiones)." *U. S.*

Colla Piscium, *P.G.;* Fish-glue; Ichthyocolle, Colle de Poisson, *Fr.;* Hausenblase, Fischleim, *G.;* Colla di Pesce, *It.;* Cola de Pescado, *Sp.*

Isinglass is a gelatinous substance, prepared chiefly from the sounds or swimming bladders of fishes, especially those of different species of sturgeon. Though not retained in the British Pharmacopœia, it still has a place in that of the United States, and is universally kept in the shops. In most fishes there is a membranous bag, placed in the anterior part of the abdomen, communicating frequently, though not always, by means of a duct, with the œsophagus or stomach, and containing usually a mixture of oxygen and nitrogen gases in various proportions. From the supposition that it was intended by its expansion or contraction to enable the fish to rise or sink in the water, it has been denominated *swimming bladder*. It is of different shape in different fishes, and consists of three coats, of which the two interior are thin and delicate, the outer tough and of a silvery whiteness.

The *Acipenser Huso*, or *beluga* of the Russians, is particularly designated by the Pharmacopœia as the species of sturgeon from which isinglass is procured; but three others, the *A. Ruthenus*, or sterlet, *A. sturio*, or common sturgeon, and *A. stellatus*, or starred sturgeon, also furnish large quantities to commerce. All these fish inhabit the interior waters of Russia, especially the Volga and other streams which empty into the Caspian Sea. Immense numbers are annually taken, and consumed as food by the Russians. The air-bags are removed from the fish, and, having been split open and washed in water in order to separate the blood, fat, and adhering extraneous membranes, are spread out, and when sufficiently stiffened are formed into cylindrical rolls, the ends of which are brought together and secured by pegs. The shape given to the roll is that of a staple, or more accurately that of a lyre, which it firmly retains when dried. Thus prepared it is known in commerce by the name of *staple isinglass*, and is distinguished into the *long* and *short staple*. Sometimes the membranes are dried in a flat state, or simply folded, and then receive the name of *leaf* or *book isinglass*. The scraps or fragments of these varieties, with various other parts of the fish, are boiled in water, which dissolves the gelatin, and upon evaporation leaves it in a solid state. This is called *cake isinglass*, from the shape which it is made to assume. It is sometimes, however, in globular masses. Of these varieties, the *long staple* is said to be the best; but the finest *book isinglass* is not surpassed by any brought to this country. It is remarkable for its beautiful iridescence by transmitted light. One hundred grains of this isinglass dissolve in ten ounces of water, forming a tremulous jelly when cold, and yield but two grains of insoluble residuum. That in *cakes* is brownish, of an unpleasant odor, and employed only in the arts. Inferior kinds, with the same commercial titles, are said to be prepared from the peritoneum and intestines of the fish. An inferior Russian product, known in English commerce by the name of *Samovy isinglass*, is procured, according to Pereira, from the *Silurus Glanis*. It comes, like the better kind, in the shape of *leaf*, *book*, and *short staple*.

Isinglass, little inferior to the Russian, is made in Iceland from the sounds of the cod and ling. It is said also to be prepared by the fishermen of Newfoundland. We receive from Brasil the air-bladders of a large fish, prepared by drying them in their distended state. They are oblong, tapering, and pointed at one end, bifid with the remains of their pneumatic duct at the other, and of a firm consistence. The Brazilian isinglass is inferior to the Russian. Considerable quantities have been manufactured in New England, as formerly supposed, from the intestines of the cod, and of other allied fishes. This sort is in the form of thin ribbons several feet in length, and from an inch and a half to two inches in width. One hundred grains dissolve almost entirely in water, leaving but two grains of insoluble membrane, and form a tremulous jelly when cold with eight ounces of water. It is, therefore, as pure and nearly as strong a gelatin as the Russian isinglass; but it retains a fishy taste and odor, which render it unfit for culinary or medicinal purposes. Isinglass of good quality has also been made in New York from the sounds of the weak-fish —*Otolithus regalis* of Cuvier (Storer, *Rep. on Fishes of Mass.*, p. 33)—and perhaps of other fishes caught in the neighborhood. The sounds are dried whole, or merely split open, and vary much in size and texture, weighing from a drachm to an ounce. An article called "*refined or transparent isinglass*" is made by dissolving the New England isinglass in hot water, and spreading the solution to dry on oiled muslin. It is in very thin transparent plates, and is an excellent glue, but retains a strong fishy odor. A variety of Ichthyocolla, called India or China Isinglass, has been consumed largely in China from time immemorial, and became known to the Europeans of India about 1839. It is now found in the markets of London, where it is chiefly employed in clarifying beer. (*Journ. de Pharm.*, Fév. 1870, p. 153.) It is the swimming bladder derived from two species of *Polynemus*, and from several other species of fish in the Indian waters. (*Ibid.*, Janv. 1873, p. 77.) Preparations such as *Nelson's* and *Coxe's gelatin* are largely used now as substitutes for isinglass in making jellies. They are made from selected bones, and the gelatin is concentrated in vacuo and filtered clear, and often bleached with sulphurous acid. (See *Glue*, Part II.)

Mr. C. T. Carney states that the New England isinglass is prepared, not as supposed from the intestines of fish, but from the sounds of the hake (*Gadus merlucius*), by the following process. Having been taken from the fish, split open, cleansed, and dried, they are soaked in water till sufficiently soft, then passed through rollers so as to form a large, homogeneous, dough-like sheet, which is cut into strips, and then again passed through rollers till reduced to a ribbon-like form. The pieces thus prepared are thoroughly dried, and folded into bundles. (*Proc. A. P. A.*, 1857.)

According to Dr. V. Griessmayer, the skin of the ray (*Raja*, a tribe of deep-sea fishes, with flat body and naked and often leather-like skin) has been much used recently, particularly in France, in place of isinglass, as clarifying agent in brewing. The skin of the thornback or rough ray (*Raja clavata*) is, according to Jericka, the best for this purpose. The clarifying mixture prepared from this is without color, odor, or taste, and clears any turbid liquid within 12 hours, or at least within 3 days if the liquid is kept in a very cold place. This new clarifier is said to be much superior to either Russian or American isinglass. (*Dingler's Pol. Journ.*, vol. 230, 335; *N. R.*, Feb. 1879.)

Isinglass is sometimes kept in the shops cut into fine shreds, and is thus more easily acted on by boiling water.

Properties. In its purest form it is "in separate sheets, sometimes rolled, of a horny or pearly appearance; whitish or yellowish, semi-transparent, iridescent, inodorous, insipid; almost entirely soluble in boiling water and in boiling diluted alcohol. The solution in 24 parts of boiling water forms, on cooling, a transparent jelly." *U. S.* The inferior kinds are yellowish and more opaque. In cold water it softens, swells up, and becomes opalescent. Boiling water entirely dissolves it, with the exception of a minute proportion of impurities, amounting, according to Mr. Hatchet, to less than 2 per cent. The solution on cooling assumes the form of a jelly, which consists of pure gelatin and water. Isinglass is in fact the purest form of *gelatin* with which we are acquainted, and may be used whenever this principle is required as a test. It is insoluble in alcohol, but is dissolved readily by most of the diluted acids, and by alkaline solutions. It has a strong affinity for tannin, with which it forms an insoluble compound. Boiled with sulphuric acid, it is converted into a peculiar substance, called *glycocoll* or *sugar of gelatin*, which is in reality *amido-acetic acid* $C_2H_3(NH_2)O_2$. Its aqueous solution speedily putrefies. (See *Glue*, Part II.)

An ingenious adulteration of isinglass has been practised in London, apparently by rolling a layer of gelatin between two layers of the genuine substance. This may be detected by the disagreeable odor and taste of the adulterated drug, and the effects of water upon it. Genuine isinglass, cut into shreds and treated with water, becomes opalescent and more opaque than before; while the shreds, though they soften and swell, remain unbroken, and, when examined by the microscope, are seen to be decidedly fibrous. Gelatin, on the contrary, when similarly treated, becomes more transparent than before; the shreds are disintegrated, and the structure appears amorphous under the microscope. In the adulterated article, both these characters are presented in layers more or less distinct. (*P. J. Tr.*, ix. 505.)

A *false isinglass* has been imported into England from Para, in Brazil, consisting of the dried ovary of a large fish. It has somewhat the form of a bunch of grapes, consisting of ovoid or roundish masses, attached by a footstalk to a central axis. It is not gelatinous, and is unfit for the purposes to which isinglass is applied. (See *A. J. P.*, xxv. 144.)*

F. Prolius has made an examination of various kinds of European isinglass to determine their comparative value; his results are arranged in tabular form in *P. J. Tr.*, 1884, p. 900.

Medical Properties and Uses. Isinglass has no peculiar medical properties. It may be given internally, in the form of jelly, as a slightly nutritious article of diet; but it has no advantage over the jelly made from calves-feet. Three drachms impart sufficient consistency to a pint of water. It is employed for clarifying liquors, and imparting lustre to various woven fabrics. Added in small quantities to vegetable jellies, it gives them a tremulous appearance, which they want when unmixed. As a test of tannin it is used in solution, in the proportion of a drachm to ten fluidounces of distilled water. It forms the basis of the *English court-plaster.*

Off. Prep. Emplastrum Ichthyocollæ.

IGNATIA. *U. S.* *Ignatia.* [*Bean of Saint Ignatius.*]

(IG-NĀ'TI-Ą—ĭg-nā'she-ą.)

"The seed of Strychnos Ignatii. Bergius. (*Nat. Ord.* Loganiaceæ.)" *U. S.*

Semen Ignatiæ, Faba Ignatii, Faba Sancti Ignatii, *Lat.;* Fève igasurique, Fève de Saint Ignace, *Fr.;* Ignatiusbohne, Bittere Fiebernuss, Ignasbohnen, *G.;* Fava di Santo Ignasio, *It.;* Haba de Santo Ignacio, *Sp.*

STRYCHNOS. See *Nux Vomica.*

Strychnos Ignatia. Lindley, *Flor. Med.* 530.—*Ignatia amara.* Linn. *Suppl.* This species of Strychnos is a tree of middling size, with numerous long, cylindrical, glabrous, vine-like branches, which bear opposite, nearly sessile, oval, pointed, entire, and very smooth leaves. The flowers are long, nodding, white, tubular, fragrant, and arranged in short, axillary racemes. The fruit is of the size and shape of a pear, with a smooth, whitish, ligneous rind, enclosing about twenty seeds, imbedded in a dry medullary matter, and lying one upon the other. The seeds are the part used. The tree is a native of the Philippine Islands, where the seeds were highly esteemed as a medicine, and, having attracted the attention of the Jesuits, were honored with the name of their founder.

Prof. Flückiger and Arthur Meyer have made a microscopical examination of the fruit of *Strychnos Ignatii;* they show that there exists between the seed of this fruit and that of *S. Nux Vomica* a very close structural analogy. (*P. J. Tr.*, 1881, p. 1.)

Properties. The seeds are about an inch long, rather less in breadth, still less in thickness, convex on one side, obscurely angular, with two, three, or four faces on the other, and marked at one end with a small depression indicating their point

* *Japanese Isinglass.* Two forms of this substance are described by Mr. Hanbury, one in irregularly four-sided sticks, about eleven inches long, very light and porous, the other in long shrivelled strips about one-eighth of an inch thick. It is translucent, yellowish white, without smell or taste, insoluble in cold water, but swelling up and softening under its influence, and dissolved in great measure by boiling water, with which it gelatinises on cooling. The peculiarities of this substance are owing to a principle denominated *gelose* by Payen, which resembles gelatin in its gelatinising property, but differs in its chemical relations, and is probably peculiar. It resembles the carrageenin of Irish moss, but has a greater gelatinizing power. The jelly formed by dissolving it in boiling water, and allowing the solution to cool, requires a higher temperature to liquefy it than gelatin jelly, and does not melt in the mouth. Gelose differs from gelatin in not being precipitated by tannic acid, and from rice jelly in not being rendered blue by iodine. Japan isinglass is used for the same purposes as that of animal origin. It is derived, according to Mr. Hanbury, from different species of various genera of sea-weed, and especially *Gelidium corneum.* (See *A. J. P.*, 1860, p. 354.) The term *Agar Agar*, in the East Indies, is applied to several sea-weeds prepared for food. (See Part II.; also, *Proc. A. P. A.*, xxvi. 173; *P. J. Tr.*, xi. 137.)

of attachment. They are externally of a pale brown color, apparently smooth, but covered in fact with a short down or efflorescence, which may be removed by scraping them with a knife. They are somewhat translucent, and their substance is very hard and horny. They have no smell, but an excessively bitter taste. They are officinally described as "about an inch and a fifth (3 cm.) long, oblong or ovate, irregularly angular, dull brownish or blackish, very hard, horny; fracture granular, irregular; the albumen somewhat translucent, enclosing an irregular cavity with an oblong embryo; inodorous; very bitter." *U. S.* To Pelletier and Caventou they yielded the same constituents as nux vomica, and, among them, 1·2 per cent. of strychnine, and 0·5 per cent. of brucine. Analyzed by Mr. J. M. Caldwell, they were found to contain the two alkaloids, strychnine and brucine, combined with igasuric acid, and, besides these, a volatile principle, extractive, gum, resin, coloring matter, fixed oil, and bassorin, but no starch or albumen. (*A. J. P.*, 1857, p. 298.) Flückiger, on the other hand, found 1·78 per cent. of nitrogen, corresponding to about 10 per cent. of albuminoid matter. (*Pharmacographia*, p. 433.) In consequence of the relatively larger proportion of strychnine which they yield, they have been used instead of nux vomica, in the preparation of that alkaloid, when their cost would permit of the substitution, but the nux vomica bean has been imported in such large quantities, and is now so low in price, that the ignatia bean is rarely used for this purpose.

Medical Properties and Uses. MM. Magendie and Delile proved that ignatia acts on the human system in the same manner as nux vomica, and modern research has confirmed this, only showing that the preparations of ignatia are stronger than those of nux vomica. The two medicines are used for precisely similar purposes. (See *Nux Vomica.*) The dose of the officinal abstract is from a half grain to a grain (0·03–0·065 Gm.) in pill three times a day. The officinal tincture is a good preparation.

Off. Prep. Abstractum Ignatiæ; Tinctura Ignatiæ.

ILLICIUM. *U.S.* *Illicium.* [*Star Anise.*]

(ĬL-LĬ'CI-ŬM—ĭl-lĭsh'e-ŭm.)

Anisi Stellati Fructus, *Br.;* Star-Anise Fruit.

"The fruit of Illicium anisatum. Loureiro. (*Nat. Ord.* Magnoliaceæ.)" *U. S.*
"The dried fruit of Illicium anisatum, *Linn.* From plants cultivated in China." *Br.*

Gen. Ch. *Flowers* hermaphrodite or rarely polygamously diœcious. *Sepals* two to three imbricate. *Carpels* in a verticillate simple series or single, compressed, dehiscent by their superior margin.

This genus inhabits Asia and America. Many of its species are possessed of aromatic properties. *I. Floridanum*, a small evergreen tree or shrub with oblong-lanceolate, acuminate leaves, which grows westward from Florida along the coast bounding the Gulf of Mexico, has its bark, leaves, and probably also seed-vessels, endowed with a spicy odor and taste, analogous to those of anise. Another species, *I. parviflorum*, a shrub found by Michaux in the hilly regions of Georgia and Carolina, has a flavor closely resembling that of sassafras root. The *Illicium anisatum* is a small tree, twenty-five or thirty feet high, bearing small yellow and white flowers, and when cultivated yielding fruit only once in two years, and at the commencement but sparingly.

Illicium anisatum was examined by C. E. Schlegel (*A. J. P.*, 1885, p. 426), who found *saponin* in the aqueous extract; in the alcoholic extract a crystalline principle of a strong musk-like odor, which did not show alkaloidal or glucoside reactions; and oil of star-anise. *I. Floridanum* was examined by Henry C. C. Maisch (*A. J. P.*, 1885, p. 278), who obtained from the leaves, besides essential oil, crystals of a glucoside to which probably the bitter taste of the leaves is due. The root-bark and the capsules both yielded a neutral crystalline principle insoluble in alcohol and ether, but soluble in chloroform, melting at 110° C. (230° F.), which was not further examined.

The *I. religiosum*, or *Shikimi*, of India, is very poisonous, causing vomiting, epileptiform convulsions, with dilated pupil and exceedingly cyanosed countenance: * in it has been found by Mr. J. F. Eykman (*P. J. Tr.* xi. 1046) a crystalline, excessively poisonous principle, for which the name of *Shikimin* has been proposed. The accompanying cuts portray the differences in the capsules of several species.

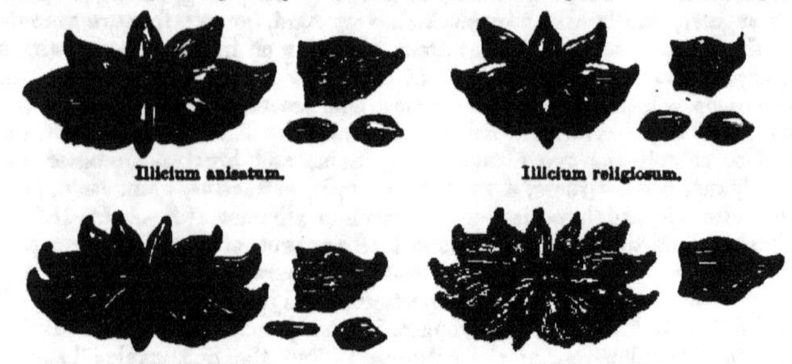

Illicium anisatum. Illicium religiosum.

Illicium Griffithii. Illicium magus.

Properties. "The fruit is pedunculate, and consists of eight stellately arranged carpels, which are boat-shaped, about half an inch (12 mm.) long, rather woody, wrinkled, straight-beaked, brown, dehiscent on the upper suture, internally red-brown, glossy, and with a single, flattish, oval, glossy, brown-yellow seed; odor anise-like; taste of the carpels sweet and aromatic, and of the seeds oily. Star-anise should not be confounded with the very similar but poisonous fruit of *Illicium religiosum*, Siebold, the carpels of which are more woody, shrivelled, and have a thin, mostly curved beak, a faint clove-like odor, and an unpleasant taste." *U. S.*

Star-anise is used principally as a source of oil of anise, which is prepared by distillation not only in Southwestern China, but also in enormous quantities in Annam,

* The following table gives the distinctive characters which, according to Mr. J. F. Eykman, distinguish the oil of *Illicium religiosum* from allied oils. (*P. J. Tr.*, xi. 1048.)

	Ol. Anisi Vulgaris.	Oleum Foeniculi.	Ol. Illicii Anisati.	Ol. Illicii Religiosi.
Constituents......	Chiefly solid and liquid anethol.	Small quantity of terpene boiling at 190° C., and liquid and solid anethol.	Chiefly solid and liquid anethol.	Rather much of a terpene boiling at 173° to 176° C.; liquid anethol boiling at 232° to 233° C.
Melting Point ...	+6° to 18° C.	—2° to +18° C.	About 0° C.	Not solid when cooled 20° C.
Specific Gravity..	About 0·908.	0·94 to 0·998.	0·978.	1·006.
Molecular Rotation.	0° to +0·5°.	+13° to +19·6°	0° to —0·4.°	—8·6°.
Alcoholic Hydrochloric Acid.	Colorless, afterwards reddish, then pale red.	Colorless.	Colorless.	Colorless, afterwards blue.
Chloral Reagent	Colorless, afterwards yellow and brownish.	Colorless, then beautiful red.	Colorless, then beautiful red.	Colorless, afterwards dirty brown yellow.
Ammoniacal Silver Solution.	In 24 hours no reduction.	Like ol. anisi vulgaris.	Like ol. anisi vulgaris.	Reduction in a few hours.
Hager's Reaction	In alcohol, a portion of the sulphuric acid and oil mixture remains undissolved as a thick mass adhering to the sides of the tube.	Mixture of oil, sulphuric acid and alcohol is perfectly clear.	Like ol. anisi vulgaris.	Mixture is nearly clear; separation of a little reddish white deposit.
10 drops of oil, with 60 drops of ether and about 0·150 gramme of sodium.	Colorless; after 4 hours the mixture nearly colorless; deposit yellowish white.	....	Colorless; after 4 hours liquid and deposit yellow.	Colorless; quickly bluish; after 4 hours liquid pale yellow, deposit yellow.

Eykman (*Pharm. Jour.*, 1885, p. 985) has since shown that in the essential oil of the fruit of *Illicium religiosum*, *safrol*, $C_{10}H_{10}O_2$, is found, accompanied by *eugenol*, $C_{10}H_{12}O_2$. On the other hand, the chief constituent of the oil of *Illicium anisatum*, as stated before, is anethol, $C_{10}H_{12}O$.

a province of Cochin China, where it is enclosed in tinned vessels and sent into commerce through China.

INFUSA. *U. S.* *Infusions.*

(IN-FŪ'SA.)

Tisanes, Infusions, *Fr.;* Infusionen, Aufgüsse, *G.*

These are aqueous solutions obtained by treating with water, without the aid of ebullition, vegetable products only partially soluble in that liquid. The water employed may be hot or cold, according to the objects to be accomplished. Infusions are generally prepared by pouring boiling water upon the vegetable substance, and macerating in a tightly closed vessel till the liquid cools. The soluble principles are thus extracted more rapidly, and, as a general rule, in a larger proportion than at a lower temperature. Some substances, moreover, are dissolved in this manner, which are nearly or quite insoluble in cold water. A prolonged application of heat is in some instances desirable; and this may be effected by placing the vessel near the fire. Cold water is preferred when the active principle is highly volatile, when it is injured by heat, or when any substance of difficult solubility at a low temperature exists in the vegetable, which it is desirable to avoid in the infusion. A longer continuance of the maceration is necessary in this case; and, in warm weather, there is sometimes danger that spontaneous decomposition may commence before the process is completed. When a strong infusion is required, the *process of percolation* may be advantageously resorted to. The water employed should be free from saline impurities, which frequently produce precipitates and render the infusion turbid. Fresh river, rain, or distilled water is usually preferable to that of pumps or springs, except when the latter are known to produce water which will not react with any of the constituents of the infusion.

The substance to be acted on should be sliced or bruised, or in the state of powder; but, unless when percolation is employed, this last condition is seldom requisite, and is always inconvenient, as it requires that the infusion should be filtered through paper in order completely to separate the undissolved portion. In other cases, it is sufficient to strain through fine linen or muslin. When percolation is resorted to, the substance should be more or less finely powdered. The United States Pharmacopœia furnishes a general formula for infusions, which is to be used when the proportions are not specified, and is as follows:

General Formula for Infusions, U. S. P.

"An ordinary infusion, the strength of which is not directed by the physician, nor specified by the Pharmacopœia, shall be prepared by the following formula.

"Take of

The Substance, coarsely comminuted, *ten parts* [or one ounce av.];
Boiling Water, *one hundred parts* [or ten fluidounces];
Water, *a sufficient quantity*,

To make *one hundred parts* [or ten fluidounces].

"Put the substance into a suitable vessel, provided with a cover, pour upon it the Boiling Water, cover the vessel tightly, and let it stand two hours. Then strain, and pass enough Water through the strainer to make the Infusion weigh *one hundred parts* [or measure ten fluidounces].

"*Caution.* The strength of infusions of energetic or powerful substances should be specially prescribed by the physician." *U. S.*

Infusions are usually prepared in glazed earthenware or porcelain vessels fitted with covers. Mr. Brande suggests the use of clean metallic vessels, which, when finely polished, retain the heat for a longer time; but they are also more liable to chemical alteration, and may sometimes injuriously affect the preparation. Vessels of block-tin are generally well adapted for the purpose.*

As infusions do not keep well, especially in warm weather, they should be made extemporaneously and in small quantities. In this country they are usually prepared in families, and the propriety of their introduction into the Pharmacopœia has been doubted; but it is desirable to have certain fixed standards for the regulation of the medical practitioner; and it is sometimes convenient to direct infusions from the apothecary, for whose guidance officinal formulas are necessary. Physicians would, indeed, find an advantage in more frequently directing them to be prepared by the pharmacist, instead of leaving their preparation to the carelessness or want of skill of attendants upon the sick. Infusions may be kept during hot weather, and for many months, by straining them *while hot*, and pouring them at once into bottles provided with accurately ground stoppers. The bottle must be full, the stopper being made to displace its bulk of the fluid. A common bottle with a cork stopper may be used, if the softened corks be forced into the full bottle, tied down and at once dipped into hot sealing wax. The hotter the liquid and freer from air, the better will the infusion keep. Prof. Almén (Upsala, Sweden) has proposed a very efficient method of preserving infusions. (*A. J. P.*, April, 1875.) It is as follows. The infusion or decoction is heated for some time in a water-bath at 100° C. (212° F.), and the bottle then fitted with a tight cork, through which a glass tube passes, lightly filled with cotton wool. The cork has a second opening, through which a glass tube passes nearly to the bottom of the bottle; this tube is bent at a

* *Alsop's Infusion Jar.* This presents a very neat and effectual method of making the hot infusions. It consists of an earthenware mug, represented in the marginal figure, with a spout (*d*) proceeding from the bottom, and placed closely to the side of the vessel to prevent fracture; a perforated plate or diaphragm (*b*), supported on a ledge (*c*), at about one-quarter or one-third of the height of the vessel from the top; and a lid (*a*), which may be fastened on by a string through holes (*ff*). The material to be submitted to infusion is placed on the perforated plate, and the hot water poured in so as to cover it, the vessel having been previously warmed so as not to chill the liquid. As the water becomes impregnated, it acquires an increased specific gravity, and sinks to the bottom, its place being supplied by the unsaturated portion; and this circulation goes on until the whole of the soluble matter is extracted. In order to maintain a due warmth, the vessel may be placed upon a stove or an iron plate near the fire. The advantage of the process is that the material is subjected to the solvent power of the least impregnated portion of the menstruum. Such jars may now be had in Philadelphia. In order that the vessel may be adapted for the preparation of different quantities of infusions, it would be an advantage to have ledges arranged within, at different heights, so that the diaphragm may be supported at any desirable point. The surface of the liquid (*e*) should of course always be above the medicinal substance placed upon the diaphragm. (See *A. J. P.*, viii. 89.)

Squire's Infusion Mug. Mr. Squire, of London, has modified this jar by adding a colander of queensware, which is closely covered with a lid, and descends into the jar so as to form a diaphragm for the support of the substance to be infused. It has the advantage that the material, after having been exhausted, may be lifted out without disturbing the infusion. In the margin is a figure of the mug. It is made of queensware, of the capacity of two pints, into which a thimble-shaped colander descends to somewhat less than half its depth, supported on the rim of the mug by a projecting ledge, with a carefully fitted cover, which closes the whole. The substance to be submitted to infusion is introduced into the colander either before or after it has been fitted to the mug; the water, hot or cold, as the case may be, is then poured in so as to fill the lower vessel, and cover the materials in the upper; and, the cover having been applied, the vessel is set aside for the length of time required. The colander is then to be lifted out, and the infusion is ready for use. For preparing small quantities of infusion, a half pint for example, the mug must be made of a smaller size.

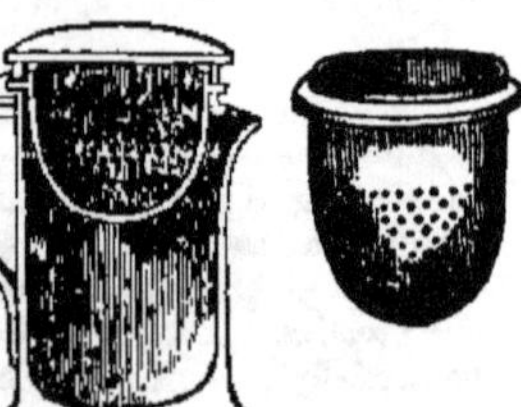

sharp angle and has fitted to it a piece of india-rubber tubing, to which a pinch-cock is attached, by means of which the contents may be drawn, as wanted. By making very concentrated infusions, as suggested by Mr. Donovan, with a mixture of three parts of water and one of alcohol, they may be long kept, and when used can be diluted with water to the proper strength. Thus, if made four times as strong as the officinal infusion, they may be diluted with three measures of water. The proportion of alcohol would thus be very small; but it might still be medically injurious; and infusions should not be prepared in this way unless with the cognisance of the prescriber.

Mr. Battley, of London, has introduced a set of preparations, which he calls *inspissated infusions*, the advantages of which are that the virtues are extracted by cold water, are not injured by heat used in the evaporation, are in a concentrated state, and are not impaired by time. To prepare them he macerates the material, coarsely powdered, bruised, or finely sliced, in twice its weight of cold distilled water, pressing the solid matter into the liquid repeatedly by a rammer or the hand; then allows the liquid to drain out, or expresses it in the case of highly absorbent substances; and repeats the process, with an amount of water equal to that which has been separated, until the strength is exhausted. Four or six hours of maceration are usually sufficient. The infusion is then to be concentrated by evaporation at a temperature not exceeding 71·1° C. (160° F.) to the sp. gr. 1·200, and as much alcohol is to be added as will make its sp. gr. 1·100. These preparations are very analogous to the *fluid extracts* already treated of. As a general rule, it would probably be preferable to prepare the infusion by the process of percolation. The inspissated infusions must be diluted when administered. The presence of alcohol, though in small quantity, would sometimes be a serious objection. (*P. J. Tr.*, x. 129.)

As we have already treated of the chemical relations and medical properties of the substances used in infusion, it would be useless repetition to enlarge upon these points in the following details. We shall touch upon them only in cases of peculiar interest, or where changes requiring particular notice may grow out of the nature of the process.

The former officinal preparations of this class, omitted in the present U. S. Pharmacopœia, are the infusions of Angustura, Chamomile, Buchu, Columbo, Capsicum, Cloves, Cascarilla, Catechu, Red Cinchona, Thoroughwort, Compound Gentian, Hops, Juniper, Rhatany, Compound Flaxseed, Pareira Brava, Tar, Quassia, Rhubarb, Compound Rose, Sage, Senna, Serpentaria, Spigelia, Tobacco, Dandelion, Valerian, Ginger.

INFUSUM ANTHEMIDIS. *Br. Infusion of Chamomile.*

(IN-FŪ'SŬM ĂN-THĔM'I-DĬS.)

Infusum Chamomillæ Romanæ; Tisane de Chamomille romaine, *Fr.;* Römisch-Kamillenthee, *G.*

"Take of Chamomile Flowers *half an ounce* [avoirdupois]; Boiling Distilled Water *ten fluidounces* [Imp. meas.]. Infuse in a covered vessel, for fifteen minutes, and strain." *Br.*

As this preparation has been dismissed from the U. S. Pharmacopœia, it must now be made according to the general formula (see page 788), unless otherwise directed; if so made, it will be three times the strength of that of the Pharm. 1870. Under these circumstances the British preparation is to be preferred; even this is sufficiently concentrated to be quite unpalatable to most patients.

The infusion of chamomile has the odor and taste of the flowers. It affords precipitates with gelatin, yellow Cinchona bark, sulphate of iron, tincture of chloride of iron, nitrate of silver, corrosive chloride of mercury, and the acetates of lead. As a tonic it is given cold, in the dose of one or two fluidounces (30–60 C.c.) several times a day. To assist the operation of emetic medicines it should be administered in the tepid state, and in large draughts. The infusion prepared by maceration in cold water is more grateful to the palate and stomach than that made with boiling water, but is less efficient as an emetic.

INFUSUM AURANTII. *Br.* *Infusion of Orange Peel.*

(IN-FŪ'ṢŬM ÂU-RĂN'TI-Ī—âw-răn'she-ī.)

Tisane d'Écorce d'Orange, *Fr.;* Pomeranzenschalen-Aufguss, *G.*

"Take of Bitter Orange Peel, cut small, *half an ounce* [avoirdupois]; Boiling Distilled Water *ten fluidounces* [Imp. meas.]. Infuse in a covered vessel, for fifteen minutes, and strain." *Br.*

This infusion is given as a grateful stomachic, in the dose of one or two fluidounces (30 or 60 C.c.).

INFUSUM AURANTII COMPOSITUM. *Br.* *Compound Infusion of Orange Peel.*

(IN-FŪ'ṢŬM ÂU-RĂN'TI-Ī CQM-PŎṢ'I-TŬM.)

Tisane d'Ecorce d'Orange composée, *Fr.;* Pomeranzen- und Citronenschalen-Aufguss, *G.*

"Take of Bitter Orange Peel, cut small, *one quarter of an ounce* [avoirdupois]; Fresh Lemon Peel, cut small, *fifty-six grains;* Cloves, bruised, *twenty-eight grains;* Boiling Distilled Water *ten fluidounces* [Imperial measure]. Infuse in a covered vessel, for a quarter of an hour, and strain." *Br.* A grateful stomachic in the dose of one or two fluidounces (30 or 60 C.c.).

INFUSUM BRAYERÆ. *U.S.* *Infusion of Brayera.*

(IN-FŪ'ṢŬM BRĀY-Ĕ'RÆ.)

Infusum Cusso, *Br.;* Infusion of Kousso; Tisane de Cousso, *Fr.;* Kossotrank, *G.*

"Brayera, in No. 20 powder, *six parts* [or one ounce av.]; Boiling Water, *one hundred parts* [or one pint]. Pour the Boiling Water upon the Brayera, and let it macerate in a covered vessel until cool. This Infusion should be dispensed without straining." *U.S.*

"Take of Kousso, in coarse powder, *one half of an ounce* [avoirdupois]; Boiling Distilled Water *eight fluidounces* [Imp. meas.]. Infuse in a covered vessel, for fifteen minutes. Not to be strained." *Br.* The whole may be taken for a dose.

This is a new officinal infusion, which has been introduced with a view of affording an efficient method of administering kousso. It is of the same strength as the British infusion. The unusual direction to dispense an infusion without straining argues little faith in the ability of the menstruum to exhaust the drug. The dose would be half a pint (236 C.c.).

INFUSUM BUCHU. *Br.* *Infusion of Buchu.*

(IN-FŪ'ṢŬM BŪ'ÇHŪ—bū'kū.)

Infusum Diosmæ s. Barosmæ; Tisane de Bucco, *Fr.;* Buchuaufguss, *G.*

"Take of Buchu Leaves, bruised, *half an ounce* [avoirdupois]; Boiling Distilled Water *ten fluidounces* [Imp. meas.]. Infuse in a covered vessel, for half an hour, and strain." *Br.*

This infusion was dropped at the last revision. If made by the general formula (see page 812), it will be one and a half times the strength of the preparation of U. S. P. 1870. It has the odor, taste, and medical virtues of the leaves, and affords a convenient method of administering the medicine. The dose of the British preparation is one or two fluidounces (30 or 60 C.c.).

INFUSUM CALUMBÆ. *Br.* *Infusion of Calumba.*

(IN-FŪ'ṢŬM CA-LŬM'BÆ.)

Tisane de Colombo, *Fr.;* Kolombo-Infusion, *G.*

"Take of Calumba Root, cut small, *half an ounce* [avoirdupois]; Cold Distilled Water *ten fluidounces* [Imp. meas.]. Macerate in a covered vessel, for half an hour, and strain." *Br.*

This preparation was not retained in the present Pharmacopœia. When made by the general formula (see page 812) it will be three times as strong as the infusion of U. S. P. 1870.

The infusion of Columbo is apt to spoil very quickly, especially in warm weather. It has been generally supposed that the cold infusion would keep better than the hot, because it contains no starch. Mr. Thomas Greenish, however, upon comparing specimens of the two infusions, found that the spontaneous change began sooner in the cold than in the hot, though the former was clearer. Columbo contains starch and albumen. Cold water extracts the latter without the former; hot water the former with comparatively little of the latter, which is partially coagulated by the heat. Both starch and albumen are liable to spontaneous change; but the former is much the more permanent of the two. Hence it is, according to Mr. Greenish, that the hot infusion keeps best. Indeed, he ascribes the change which takes place in the starch of the hot infusion chiefly to the agency of a little albumen, which has escaped coagulation. According to these views, the best plan of preparing infusion of columbo is to exhaust the root with cold water, by which the starch is left behind, and then to heat the infusion to the boiling point in order to coagulate the albumen. (*A. J. P.*, xviii. 141; from *P. J. Tr.*) Upon comparing specimens of the cold and hot infusion, we have not found the results of Mr. Greenish fully confirmed. The cold infusion appeared to keep better than the hot. Nevertheless, the plan of preparing the infusion above proposed is probably the best. The infusion of columbo is not disturbed by salts of iron, and may be conveniently administered in connection with them. The dose of the British infusion is two fluidounces (60 C.c.) three or four times a day.

INFUSUM CARYOPHYLLI. *Br.* *Infusion of Cloves.*

(ĮN-FŪ′ṢŬM CĂR-Y̧-Ǫ-PHY̆L′LĪ.)

Tisane de Girofle, *Fr.;* Gewürznelken-Infusion, *G.*

"Take of Cloves, bruised, *a quarter of an ounce* [avoirdupois]; Boiling Distilled Water *ten fluidounces* [Imp. meas.]. Infuse in a covered vessel, for half an hour, and strain." *Br.*

It is fortunate that this infusion is rarely used, for it was dropped at the last revision of the U. S. Pharmacopœia. If made by the general formula (page 788), it will be at least six times the strength of the preparation of U. S. P. 1870.

The infusion of cloves affords precipitates with lime-water, and with the soluble salts of iron, zinc, lead, silver, and antimony. (*Phillips.*) The dose of the British infusion is about two fluidounces (60 C.c.).

INFUSUM CASCARILLÆ. *Br.* *Infusion of Cascarilla.*

(ĮN-FŪ′ṢŬM CĂS-CA̧-RĬL′LÆ.)

Tisane de Cascarilla, *Fr.;* Kaskarilla-Aufguss, *G.*

"Take of Cascarilla Bark, in No. 20 powder, *one ounce* [avoirdupois]; Boiling Distilled Water *ten fluidounces* [Imp. meas.]. Infuse in a covered vessel, for half an hour, and strain." *Br.*

This infusion was also dropped at the last revision of the U. S. Pharmacopœia; a preparation made by the general formula (see page 812) will be one and a half times the strength of the infusion of cascarilla of U. S. P. 1870.

This infusion affords precipitates with lime-water, infusion of galls, nitrate of silver, acetate and subacetate of lead, sulphate of zinc, and sulphate of iron. The dose of the British infusion is two fluidounces (60 C.c.).

INFUSUM CATECHU. *Br.* *Infusion of Catechu.*

(ĮN-FŪ′ṢŬM CĂT′Ę-CHŪ—kat′ę-kū.)

Infusum Catechu Compositum, *U. S.* 1870; Infusion of Catechu, *E.;* Tisane de Cachou Composée, *Fr.;* Catechuaufguss mit Zimmt, *G.*

"Take of Catechu, in coarse powder, *one hundred and sixty grains;* Cinnamon Bark, bruised, *thirty grains;* Boiling Distilled Water *ten fluidounces* [Imperial measure]. Infuse in a covered vessel, for half an hour, and strain." *Br.*

This is an elegant mode of administering catechu. The dose is from one to three fluidounces (30 to 90 C.c.), repeated three or four times a day, or more frequently.

INFUSUM CHIRATÆ. *Br.* *Infusion of Chiretta.*

(IN-FŪ'SŬM CHI-RĀ'TÆ—ki-rā'tē.)

Tisane de Chiretta, *Fr.;* Chiretta-Thee, *G.*

"Take of Chiretta, cut small, *a quarter of an ounce* [avoirdupois]; Distilled Water, at 120° F. (48°·9 C.), ten *fluidounces* [Imp. meas.]. Infuse in a covered vessel, for half an hour, and strain." *Br.*

The dose of this simple bitter is from one to three fluidounces (30 to 90 C.c.).

INFUSUM CINCHONÆ. *U.S.* *Infusion of Cinchona.*

(IN-FŪ'SŬM CĬN-CHŌ'NÆ—sin-kō'nē.)

Infusum Cinchonæ Acidum, *Br.;* Infusion of Yellow Bark; Infusion of Calisaya Bark; Tisan de Quinquina jaune, *Fr.;* Kalisaya-Rindenaufguss, *G.*

"Cinchona, in No. 40 powder, *six parts* [one ounce av.]; Aromatic Sulphuric Acid, *one part* [eighty minims]; Water, *a sufficient quantity*, To make *one hundred parts* [or one pint]. Mix the Acid with *fifty parts* [or half a pint] of Water, and moisten the powder with *three parts* [or half a fluidounce] of the mixture; pack it firmly in a conical glass percolator, and gradually pour upon it, first, the remainder of the mixture, and afterward, Water, until the Infusion weighs *one hundred parts* [or measures one pint]. When no variety of Cinchona is specified by the physician directing this Infusion, use Yellow Cinchona." *U. S.*

"Take of Red Cinchona Bark, in No. 40 powder, *half an ounce* [avoir.]; Aromatic Sulphuric Acid *one fluidrachm* [Imp. meas.]; Boiling Distilled Water *ten fluidounces* [Imp. meas.]. Infuse in a covered vessel for one hour, and strain." *Br.*

Though the infusion with boiling water is more quickly prepared than the cold infusion, and therefore better adapted to cases of emergency, yet the former is a more elegant preparation, not turbid like the latter, and at least equally efficient. We, therefore, prefer the process of the U. S. Pharmacopœia, provided it be skilfully conducted.

The U. S. infusion is an efficient preparation. Water extracts from bark the kinates of quinine and cinchonine, but leaves behind the compounds which these principles form with the cinchotannic acid. The simple infusion, therefore, is rather feeble. But the addition of the acid insures the solution of all or nearly all the active matter. Dr. Geo. B. Wood placed much reliance in this infusion. It would be best to macerate the bark with the acidulated water some time before it is introduced into the percolator.

The infusion of cinchona, made without acid, affords precipitates with the alkalies, alkaline carbonates, and alkaline earths; the soluble salts of iron, zinc, and silver; corrosive chloride of mercury, arsenious acid, and tartar emetic; gelatinous solutions; and various vegetable infusions and decoctions, as those of galls, chamomile, columbo, cascarilla, horseradish, cloves, catechu, orange-peel, foxglove, senna, rhubarb, valerian, and simaruba. In some instances the precipitate occurs immediately, in others not for several hours. Few, however, of these substances diminish the efficacy of the infusion, as they do not affect the active principles. The alkalies, alkaline earths, and vegetable astringents are really incompatible. As gallic, tartaric, and oxalic acids form salts with quinine of somewhat difficult solubility, the neutral and soluble gallates, tartrates, and oxalates produce in the infusion slight precipitates of corresponding salts of the alkaloids; but these are redissolved by an excess of the acid. Tartrate of antimony and potassium does not precipitate the alkaloids. Solutions of iodine are incompatible, forming with the alkaloids insoluble compounds. For an account of the chemical reactions of the infusions of different varieties of Cinchona bark, see *A. J. P.* (ix. 128).

The simple infusion of cinchona may be advantageously administered in cases which require tonic treatment, but do not call for the full powers of the bark. The acid infusion has all the powers of cinchona itself. The medium dose is two fluidounces (60 C.c.), equivalent to a drachm of the bark.

INFUSUM CUSPARIÆ. *Br.* *Infusion of Cusparia.*

(IN-FŪ'SŬM CŬS-PĀ'RI-Æ.)

Tisane d'Angustura, *Fr.;* Angustura-Aufguss, *G.*

"Take of Cusparia Bark, in No. 40 powder, *half an ounce* [avoirdupois]; Distilled Water, at 120° F. (48°·9 C.), *ten fluidounces* [Imp. meas.]. Infuse in a covered vessel, for one hour, and strain." *Br.*

Under the name of *Infusum Angusturæ* this preparation was officinal in the U.S. Pharm. 1870, made in the proportion of half a troyounce of angustura bark in a pint of water. Made according to the general formula, page 812, it would be three times the strength of the infusion formerly officinal. The dose of the British infusion is two fluidounces (60 C.c.), repeated every two, three, or four hours.

INFUSUM DIGITALIS. *U. S., Br.* *Infusion of Digitalis.*

(IN-FŪ'SŬM DIǤ-I-TĀ'LĬS.)

Tisane de Digitale, *Fr.;* Fingerhutaufguss, *G.*

"Digitalis, in No. 20 powder, *three parts* [or fifty-five grains]; Cinnamon, in No. 20 powder, *three parts* [or fifty-five grains]; Boiling Water, *one hundred and eighty-five parts* [or seven and a half fluidounces]; Alcohol, *fifteen parts* [or six fluidrachms]; Water, *a sufficient quantity,* To make *two hundred parts* [or half a pint]. Pour the Boiling Water upon the mixed powders, and macerate for two hours in a covered vessel. Then strain, add the Alcohol, and pass enough Water through the strainer to make the infusion weigh *two hundred parts* [or measure half a pint]." *U. S.*

"Take of Foxglove leaves, dried, *twenty-eight grains;* Boiling Distilled Water *ten fluidounces* [Imp. meas.]. Infuse in a covered vessel, for fifteen minutes, and strain." *Br.*

The U. S. P. infusion does not differ essentially from that formerly officinal. Mr. D. E. Prall (*A. J. P.*, 1878, p. 423) proved that the abundant precipitate in the old infusion was caused by the tincture of cinnamon, and recommended a simple infusion without any aromatic. The present process affords a preparation which keeps moderately well, but it is not entirely free from precipitation, which may be prevented by replacing one fluidounce of water in a pint of the infusion with one fluidounce of glycerin, as proposed by M. F. E. Valentine. (*A. J. P.*, 1884, p. 504.)

The U. S. infusion is essentially the same as that employed by Withering. It affords precipitates with sulphate of iron, acetate of lead, tannic acid, and infusion of cinchona. The dose has usually been stated at half a fluidounce (15 C.c.), repeated twice a day under ordinary circumstances, every eight hours in urgent cases, until the system is affected. The proportion of digitalis is scarcely half as great in the British preparation, and the dose is proportionably larger. It will not escape the close observer, that the stated dose of digitalis in infusion is much larger than in substance, for which there does not appear to be a good reason, but which accounts for the fact that many physicians assert that they get better results from the infusion than from the digitalis itself. The British Pharmacopœia, though its infusion has only about half the strength of ours, gives its dose as from two to four fluidrachms (7·5 to 15 C.c.).

INFUSUM ERGOTÆ. *Br.* *Infusion of Ergot.*

(IN-FŪ'SŬM ĔR'GO-TÆ.)

Tisane de Seigle ergoté, *Fr.;* Mutterkornaufguss, *G.*

"Take of Ergot, crushed, *a quarter of an ounce* [avoirdupois]; Boiling Distilled Water *ten fluidounces* [Imp. meas.]. Infuse in a covered vessel, for half an hour, and strain." *Br.*

The dose of this infusion is two fluidounces (60 C.c.).*

* *Infusum Eupatorii.* U.S. 1870. *Infusion of Thoroughwort.* "Take of Thoroughwort or Boneset [the dried herb] *a troyounce;* Boiling Water *a pint.* Macerate for two hours in a covered vessel, and strain." *U. S.* 1870. As a tonic, this infusion should be taken cold in the dose of one or two fluidounces (30 or 60 C.c.) three or four times a day, or more frequently; as an emetic and diaphoretic, in large tepid draughts. It is popularly called *boneset tea.*

INFUSUM GENTIANÆ COMPOSITUM. *Br.* *Compound Infusion of Gentian.*

(IN-FŪ'ṢŬM ĢĔN-TI-Ā'NÆ COM-PŎṢ'I-TŬM—jĕn-she-ā'nē.)

Tisane de Gentiane composée, *Fr.;* Enzianaufguss, *G.*

"Take of Gentian Root, sliced, Bitter-Orange Peel, cut small, of each, *fifty-five grains;* Fresh Lemon Peel, cut small, *one quarter of an ounce* [avoir.]; Boiling Distilled Water *ten fluidounces* [Imp. meas.]. Infuse in a covered vessel, for half an hour, and strain." *Br.*

"Take of Gentian, in moderately coarse powder, *half a troyounce;* Bitter Orange Peel, in moderately coarse powder, Coriander, in moderately coarse powder, each, *sixty grains;* Alcohol *two fluidounces;* Water *a sufficient quantity.* Mix the Alcohol with fourteen fluidounces of Water, and, having moistened the mixed powders with three fluidrachms of the menstruum, pack them firmly in a conical percolator, and gradually pour upon them first the remainder of the menstruum, and afterwards Water, until the filtered liquid measures a pint." *U. S.* 1870.

It is, in our opinion, unfortunate that this, the most esteemed of all infusions, should have been dropped by the Committee of Revision of the Pharm. 1880. We have inserted the formula of the U. S. P. 1870, as it will doubtless continue to be largely prescribed. It should be designated, however, as U. S. P. 1870. It has been the custom with some physicians to prescribe a concentrated infusion made with one-fourth the quantity of menstruum directed by the formula of U. S. P. 1870. This permits the use of a valuable tonic with the presence of but a trifling amount of alcohol. This concentrated preparation keeps well, and it may be diluted with the right quantity of the proper menstruum by the pharmacist to make the infusion of U. S. P. 1870.

The use of the alcohol is to assist in dissolving the bitter principle, and at the same time to contribute towards the preservation of the infusion, which, without this addition, is very apt to spoil. It has, however, been abandoned by the British Pharmacopœia, and lemon peel substituted; this is a very doubtful improvement. The dose is a fluidounce (30 C.c.) repeated three or four times a day.

INFUSUM JABORANDI. *Br.* *Infusion of Jaborandi.*

(IN-FŪ'ṢŬM JĂB Q-RĂN'DĪ.)

"Take of Jaborandi, cut small, *half an ounce* [avoir.]; Boiling Distilled Water *ten fluidounces* [Imp. meas.]. Infuse in a covered vessel, for half an hour, and strain." *Br.*

This is a good preparation of jaborandi, and is useful in those cases where the effects of the drug are increased by large dilution with water, as in promoting diaphoresis. (See *Pilocarpus.*) The dose of the infusion is from one to two fluidounces (30 or 60 C.c.).

INFUSUM KRAMERIÆ. *Br.* *Infusion of Rhatany.*

(IN-FŪ'ṢŬM KRA-MĒ'RI-Æ.)

Tisane de Ratanhia, *Fr.;* Ratanha-Aufguss, *G.*

"Take of Rhatany Root, in coarse powder, *half an ounce* [avoirdupois]; Boiling Distilled Water *ten fluidounces* [Imp. meas.]. Infuse in a covered vessel, for half an hour, and strain." *Br.*

The infusion of rhatany is undoubtedly most efficient when prepared by the mode of percolation, with cold water, from the root in a state of moderately coarse powder, as directed in the U. S. process of 1870. The dose of the infusion is one or two fluidounces (30 or 60 C.c.).

INFUSUM LINI. *Br.* *Infusion of Linseed.*

(IN-FŪ'ṢŬM LĪ'NĪ.)

Tisane de Lin, *Fr.;* Leinsamen-Aufguss, *G.*

"Take of Linseed *one hundred and fifty grains;* Dried Liquorice Root, in No. 20 powder, *fifty grains;* Boiling Distilled Water *ten fluidounces.* Infuse in a covered vessel, for two hours, and strain." *Br.*

This is nearly identical with the *Compound Infusion of Flaxseed* of the U. S. P. 1870.* It is a useful demulcent drink in inflammatory affections of the mucous membrane of the lungs and urinary passages. It may be taken *ad libitum.*

INFUSUM LUPULI. *Br.* *Infusion of Hop.*

(ĬN-FŪ'ṢŬM LŪ'PŪ-LĪ.)

Infusum Humuli, *U. S.* 1870; Tisane de Houblon, *Fr.;* Hopfenaufguss, *G.*

"Take of Hop *half an ounce* [avoirdupois]; Boiling Distilled Water *ten fluidounces* [Imp. meas.]. Infuse in a covered vessel, for one hour, and strain." *Br.*

The infusion of hops U. S. P. 1870 was made exactly like the above, except that the strength was half a troyounce to a pint. As it was dropped at the last revision, it must now be made by the general formula, page 812 (unless otherwise directed), which will make it three times the strength of the former infusion.

The dose of the British infusion is one or two fluidounces (30 or 60 C.c.).†

INFUSUM MATICÆ. *Br.* *Infusion of Matico.*

(ĬN-FŪ'ṢŬM MĂT'Ĭ-ÇÆ.)

Tisane de Matico, *Fr.;* Matico-Aufguss, *G.*

"Take of Matico Leaves, cut small, *half an ounce* [avoirdupois]; Boiling Distilled Water *ten fluidounces* [Imp. meas.]. Infuse in a covered vessel, for half an hour, and strain." *Br.*

The dose of this infusion is two fluidounces (60 C.c.).‡

INFUSUM PRUNI VIRGINIANÆ. *U. S.* *Infusion of Wild-cherry.*

(ĬN-FŪ'ṢŬM PRŪ'NĪ VĬR-ǴĬN-Ĭ-Ā'NÆ.)

Tisane d'Écorce de Cerisier sauvage, *Fr.;* Wildkirschen-Thee, *G.*

"Wild-cherry, in No. 40 powder, *four parts* [or half an ounce av.]; Water, *a sufficient quantity,* To make *one hundred parts* [or twelve fluidounces]. Moisten the powder with *six parts* [or six fluidrachms] of Water, and macerate for one hour; then pack it firmly in a conical glass percolator, and gradually pour Water upon it until the Infusion weighs *one hundred parts* [or measures twelve fluidounces]." *U. S.*

This is a peculiarly suitable object for officinal direction, as, in consequence of the volatile nature of one of its active ingredients, and for another reason (see *Prunus Virginiana*), it is better prepared with cold water than in the ordinary mode. The infusion of wild-cherry bark is one of the preparations to which the process of percolation or displacement is well adapted. In this way the virtues of the bark can be more rapidly and thoroughly exhausted than by maceration alone. In order to allow time for the reaction necessary to the production of the hydrocyanic acid, an hour's preliminary maceration is directed, which might perhaps be advantageously

* "Take of Flaxseed *half a troyounce;* Liquorice Root, bruised, *one hundred and twenty grains;* Boiling water *a pint.* Macerate for two hours in a covered vessel, and strain." *U. S.* 1870.

† *Infusum Juniperi,* U. S. 1870. *Infusion of Juniper.* "Take of Juniper, bruised, *a troyounce;* Boiling water *a pint.* Macerate for an hour in a covered vessel, and strain." *U. S.* 1870. The whole quantity may be taken in twenty-four hours, in doses of two or three fluidounces (60 or 90 C.c.).

‡ *Infusum Pareiræ.* U. S. 1870. *Infusion of Pareira Brava.* "Take of Pareira Brava, bruised, *a troyounce;* Boiling Water *a pint.* Macerate for two hours in a covered vessel, and strain." *U. S.* 1870. The infusion of pareira brava is highly esteemed by some English practitioners as a remedy in irritation and chronic inflammation of the urinary passages, and has been found useful in catarrh of the bladder. The dose is one or two fluidounces (30 or 60 C.c.). Brodie employed a *decoction* of the root, which he prepared by boiling half an ounce in three pints of water down to a pint, and gave in the quantity of from eight to twelve fluidounces daily. The Br. Pharmacopœia has substituted the decoction for the infusion.

Infusum Picis Liquidæ, U. S. 1870; *Infusion of Tar. Tar Water.* "Take of Tar *a pint;* Water *four pints.* Mix them, and shake the mixture frequently during twenty-four hours. Then pour off the infusion, and filter through paper." *U.S.* Water takes from tar a small portion of acetic acid, empyreumatic oil including creasote, and resinous matter, acquiring a sharp empyreumatic taste, the odor of tar, and the color of Madeira wine. Thus impregnated it is stimulant and diuretic, and may be taken in the quantity of one or two pints daily. It is also used as a wash in chronic cutaneous affections, and is said to have proved beneficial, by injection into the bladder, in some cases of chronic cystitis.

somewhat lengthened. If kept in a warm place this preparation undergoes a rapid alteration, and even under the best of circumstances is unstable. According to the experiments of Mr. J. B. Moore (*A. J. P.*, 1873, p. 242) two fluidounces of glycerin to the pint of menstruum is of great advantage in delaying the change. When properly made, infusion of wild-cherry bark is beautifully transparent, has the color of Madeira wine, and the agreeable bitterness and peculiar flavor of the bark. The dose is two or three fluidounces (60 or 90 C.c.) three or four times a day, or more frequently when a strong impression is required.

INFUSUM QUASSIÆ. *Br.* *Infusion of Quassia.*

(ĮN-FŪ'ȘŬM QUAS'SĮ-Æ—kwŏsh'ę-ē.)

Tisane de Quassie, *Fr.*; Quassia-Aufguss, *G.*

"Take of Quassia Wood, in chips, *fifty-five grains*; Cold Distilled Water *ten fluidounces* [Imp. meas.]. Macerate in a covered vessel, for half an hour, and strain." *Br.*

The dropping of this infusion at the last revision of the U. S. Pharm., and the substitution of the general formula in its place (p. 812), will result in making a preparation six times the strength of that of the U. S. P. 1870. Boiling water may be employed when it is desirable to obtain the preparation quickly; but cold water affords a clearer infusion. The half-hour maceration directed in the British Pharmacopœia, considering that cold water is used, appears to us to be too short for the exhaustion of the wood. The dose is two fluidounces (60 C.c.) three or four times a day.

INFUSUM RHEI. *Br.* *Infusion of Rhubarb.*

(ĮN-FŪ'ȘŬM RHĒ'Ī.)

Tisane de Rhubarbe, *Fr.*; Rhabarber-Aufguss, *G.*

"Take of Rhubarb Root, in thin slices, *a quarter of an ounce* [avoirdupois]; Boiling Distilled Water *ten fluidounces* [Imp. meas.]. Infuse in a covered vessel, for half an hour, and strain." *Br.*

In order that the rhubarb may be exhausted, it should be digested with the water near the fire, at a temperature somewhat less than that of boiling water. It is customary to add some aromatic, such as cardamom, fennel-seed, or nutmeg, which improves the taste of the infusion, and renders it more acceptable to the stomach. One drachm of either of these spices may be digested in connection with the rhubarb.

This infusion may be given as a gentle laxative, in the dose of one or two fluidounces (30 or 60 C.c.), every three or four hours till it operates. It is occasionally used as a vehicle for tonic, antacid, or more active cathartic medicines. The stronger acids and most metallic solutions are incompatible with it.

As infusion of rhubarb was not retained in the present Pharmacopœia, the general formula, page 812, must be used (unless otherwise directed), which will make a preparation six times the strength of that of the U. S. P. 1870.

INFUSUM ROSÆ ACIDUM. *Br.* *Acid Infusion of Roses.*

(ĮN-FŪ'ȘŬM RŌ'ȘÆ AÇ'Į-DŬM.)

Infusum Rosæ Compositum, *U. S.* 1870; Compound Infusion of Rose; Acid Infusion of Rose, Tisane de Rose composée, *Fr.*; Saurer Rosenaufguss, *G.*

"Take of Dried Red-rose Petals, broken up, *a quarter of an ounce* [avoirdupois]; Diluted Sulphuric Acid *one fluidrachm*; Boiling Distilled Water *ten fluidounces* [Imp. meas.]. Add the Acid to the Water, infuse the Petals in the mixture in a covered vessel, for half an hour, and strain." *Br.*

The formula of the U. S. P. 1870 is preferable to that of the British Pharm. on account of the presence of sugar. It is unfortunate, in our opinion, that this elegant infusion was dropped at the last revision of the U. S. Pharmacopœia. We append the formula of the U. S. P. 1870. "Take of Red Rose [dried petals] *half a troyounce*; Diluted Sulphuric Acid *three fluidrachms*; Sugar [refined], in coarse powder, *a troyounce and a half*; Boiling Water *two pints and a half*. Pour the Water upon the Rose in a covered glass or porcelain vessel; add the Acid, and macerate for half an hour. Lastly, dissolve the Sugar in the liquid, and strain." *U. S.*

The red roses serve little other purpose than to impart a fine red color and a slight astringent flavor to the preparation, which owes its medicinal virtues almost exclusively to the sulphuric acid. According to Mr. J. B. Barnes, one part of glycerin added to eight or nine parts of infusion of rose increases greatly its brightness and transparency. It is refrigerant and astringent, and affords a useful and not unpleasant drink in hemorrhages and colliquative sweats. It is much used by British practitioners as a vehicle for saline medicines, particularly sulphate of magnesium, the taste of which it serves to cover. It is also employed as a gargle, usually in connection with acids, nitre, alum, or tincture of Cayenne pepper. The dose is from two to four fluidounces (30 to 118 C.c.).*

INFUSUM SENEGÆ. *Br.* *Infusion of Senega.*

(ĮN-FŪ'ṢŬM SĔN'Ę-GÆ—sĕn'ę-jē.)

Tisane de Polygale de Virginie, *Fr.;* Senega-Aufguss, *G.*

"Take of Senega Root, in No. 20 powder, *half an ounce* [avoirdupois]; Boiling Distilled Water *ten fluidounces* [Imp. meas.]. Infuse in a covered vessel, for half an hour, and strain." *Br.*

The dose of the preparation is from one to three fluidounces (30 to 90 C.c.).

INFUSUM SENNÆ. *Br.* *Infusion of Senna.*

(ĮN-FŪ'ṢŬM SĔN'NÆ.)

Tisane de Séné, *Fr.;* Senna-Aufguss, *G.*

"Take of Senna *one ounce* [avoirdupois]; Ginger, sliced, *twenty-eight grains;* Boiling Distilled Water *ten fluidounces* [Imp. meas.]. Infuse in a covered vessel, for half an hour, and strain." *Br.*

"Take of Senna *a troyounce;* Coriander, bruised, *sixty grains;* Boiling Water *a pint.* Macerate for an hour in a covered vessel, and strain." *U. S.* 1870.

We prefer the coriander of the U. S. Pharmacopœia, 1870, to the ginger of the British. The strength of the British preparation has been doubled in the present edition of the Pharmacopœia, and is now nearly twice as great as that of the U. S. infusion of 1870. The infusion deposits, on exposure to the air, a yellowish precipitate, which is said to aggravate its griping tendency; it should, therefore, not be made in large quantities. It is customary to connect with it manna and some one of the saline cathartics, which increase its efficacy, and render it less painful in its operation. (See *Infusum Sennæ Compositum.*) The dose of the infusion is about four fluidounces (118 C.c.). The cold infusion, especially if made by percolation from the coarsely powdered leaves, while probably not inferior in strength to that prepared with boiling water, is said to be less unpleasant to the taste.

Off. Prep. Br. Mistura Sennæ Composita.

INFUSUM SENNÆ COMPOSITUM. *U. S.* *Compound Infusion of Senna.* [*Black Draught.*]

(ĮN-FŪ'ṢŬM SĔN'NÆ CQM-PŎS'Į-TŬM.)

Tisane de Séné composée, *Fr.;* Senna-Aufguss, *G.*

"Senna, *six parts* [or half an ounce av.]; Manna, *twelve parts* [or one ounce av.]; Sulphate of Magnesium, *twelve parts* [or one ounce av.]; Fennel, bruised, *two parts* [or seventy-three grains]; Boiling Water, *one hundred parts* [or half a pint]; Water, *a sufficient quantity,* To make *one hundred parts* [or half a pint]. Pour the Boiling Water upon the solid ingredients and macerate in a covered vessel until cool. Then strain, and add enough Water through the strainer to make the Infusion weigh *one hundred parts* [or measure half a pint]." *U. S.*

* *Infusum Salviæ.* U. S. 1870. *Infusion of Sage.* "Take of Sage *half a troyounce; Boiling* Water *a pint.* Macerate for half an hour in a covered vessel, and strain." *U. S. P.* 1870. This preparation is less used internally than as a gargle, or as a vehicle for other substances, such as alum, employed in this way.

This preparation is the Black Draught of European Pharmacy, and it is an excellent form of administering these cathartics in a liquid condition. The simple infusion of senna was dropped in the last revision of the British Pharmacopœia; and the above, which more closely corresponds with *senna tea*, used as a popular purgative draught, substituted. The dose is about four fluidounces (118 C.c.).

INFUSUM SERPENTARIÆ. *Br.* *Infusion of Serpentary.*

(IN-FŪ'SŬM SĔR-PĔN-TĀ'RI-Æ.)

Tisane de Serpentaire, *Fr.;* Schlangenwurzel-Aufguss, *G.*

"Take of Serpentary Rhizome, in No. 20 powder, *quarter of an ounce* [avoirdupois]; Boiling Distilled Water *ten fluidounces* [Imp. meas.]. Infuse in a covered vessel, for half an hour, and strain." *Br.*

The infusion of serpentaria having been dropped at the last revision of the U. S. Pharmacopœia, the general formula, page 812, must be used (unless otherwise specified), which will make an infusion three times the strength of the U. S. 1870 preparation. The dose of the British preparation is one or two fluidounces (30 or 60 C.c.), every two hours in low forms of fever, but less frequently in chronic affections.*

INFUSUM UVÆ URSI. *Br.* *Infusion of Bearberry.*

(IN-FŪ'SŬM Ū'VÆ ŬR'SĪ.)

Tisane d'Uva Ursi, *Fr.;* Bärentraubenblätter-Aufguss, *G.*

"Take of Bearberry Leaves, bruised, *half an ounce* [avoirdupois]; Boiling Distilled Water *ten fluidounces* [Imp. meas.]. Infuse in a covered vessel, for one hour, and strain." *Br.* The dose is one or two fluidounces (30 or 60 C.c.) three or four times a day.

INFUSUM VALERIANÆ. *Br.* *Infusion of Valerian.*

(IN-FŪ'SŬM VA-LĒ-RI-Ā'NÆ.)

Tisane de Valériane, *Fr.;* Baldrian-Aufguss, *G.*

"Take of Valerian Rhizome, bruised, *quarter of an ounce* [avoir.]; Boiling Distilled Water *ten fluidounces* [Imp. meas.]. Infuse in a covered vessel, for one hour, and strain." *Br.*

This is another of the infusions dropped at the last revision of the U. S. Pharmacopœia. It must now be made by the general formula, page 812 (unless otherwise specified), and it will therefore be six times the strength of that of the U. S. P. 1870.

The dose of the British infusion is two fluidounces (60 C.c.), repeated three or four times a day, or more frequently.†

INJECTIONES HYPODERMICÆ. *Hypodermic Injections.*

(IN-JĔC-TI-Ō'NĒS HȲ-PO-DĔR'MI-CÆ—in-jĕk-shŏ'ō-nĕz.)

Under this head are classed preparations which are recognised in the British Pharmacopœia for hypodermic application. Camphor water is selected as the vehicle for two of them on account of its antiseptic properties, but it is very doubtful if their introduction will prove of practical value, on account of the great likelihood of their being dispensed in a partially decomposed condition. Hypodermic injections should never be prepared in advance of actual requirements.

* *Infusum Spigeliæ.* U. S. 1870. *Infusion of Spigelia.* "Take of Spigelia *half a troyounce;* Boiling Water *a pint.* Macerate for two hours in a covered vessel, and strain." U. S. 1870. The dose of this infusion, for a child two or three years old, is from four fluidrachms to a fluidounce (15 to 30 C.c.); for an adult, from four to eight fluidounces (118 to 236 C.c.), repeated morning and evening. A quantity of senna equal to that of the spigelia is usually added, in order to insure a cathartic effect.

Infusum Taraxaci. U. S. 1870. *Infusion of Dandelion.* "Take of Dandelion, bruised, *two troyounces;* Boiling Water *a pint.* Macerate for two hours in a covered vessel, and strain." *U. S.* 1870. The dose is a wineglassful two or three times a day, or oftener.

† *Infusum Zingiberis.* U. S. 1870. *Infusion of Ginger.* "Take of Ginger, bruised, *half a troyounce;* Boiling Water *a pint.* Macerate for two hours in a covered vessel, and strain." *U. S.* 1870. The dose of this infusion is two fluidounces (60 C.c.).

INJECTIO APOMORPHINÆ HYPODERMICA. *Br.* *Hypodermic Injection of Apomorphine.*

(ĮN-JĔC'TĮ-Ō ĂP-Q-MŎR-PHĪ'NÆ HȲ-PQ-DĔR'MĮ-CĄ—įn-jĕk'shę-ō.)

"Take of Hydrochlorate of Apomorphine *two grains*; Camphor Water *one hundred minims*. Dissolve and filter. The solution should be made as required for use." *Br.* The dose, by subcutaneous injection, is from 2 to 8 minims.

INJECTIO ERGOTINI HYPODERMICA. *Br.* *Hypodermic Injection of Ergotin.*

(ĮN-JĔC'TĮ-Ō ĔR-GQ-TĪ'NĪ HȲ-PQ-DĔR'MĮ-CĄ.)

"Take of Ergotin *one hundred grains*; Camphor Water, *two hundred fluidgrains* (or 3 fluidrachms). Dissolve by stirring them together. The solution should be made as required for use." *Br.* The dose, by subcutaneous injection, is from 3 to 10 minims.

INJECTIO MORPHINÆ HYPODERMICA. *Br.* *Hypodermic Injection of Morphine.*

(ĮN-JĔC'TĮ-Ō MŎR-PHĪ'NÆ HȲ-PQ-DĔR'MĮ-CĄ.)

"A solution of acetate of morphine containing one grain of the acetate in ten minims of the injection." *Br.*

"Take of Hydrochlorate of Morphine *ninety-two grains*; Solution of Ammonia, Acetic Acid, Distilled Water, of each, *a sufficiency*.

"Dissolve the hydrochlorate of morphine in two ounces of distilled water, aiding the solution by gently heating; then add solution of ammonia so as to precipitate the morphine, and render the liquid slightly alkaline; allow it to cool; collect the precipitate on a filter, wash it with distilled water, and allow it to drain; then transfer the morphine to a small porcelain dish with about an ounce of distilled water, apply heat gently, and carefully add acetic acid until the morphine is dissolved, and a very slightly acid solution is formed. Add now sufficient distilled water to make the solution measure exactly two fluidounces. Filter and preserve the product in a stoppered bottle excluded from the light." *Br.*

Properties. "A clear solution free from any solid particles. Very slightly acid to test paper. A fluidrachm of it rendered slightly alkaline by the addition of solution of ammonia yields a precipitate of morphine which, after being washed and dried, should weigh 4·25 grains, corresponding to six grains of acetate of morphine." *Br.* The dose, by subcutaneous injection, is from 1 to 5 minims.

INULA. *U.S.* *Inula.* [*Elecampane.*]

(ĬN'Ū-LĄ.)

"The root of Inula Helenium. Linné. (*Nat. Ord.* Compositæ.)" *U.S.*

Aunée, *Fr.*; Alantwurzel, *G.*; Enula Campana, *It.*, *Sp.*

Gen. Ch. *Receptacle* naked. *Seed-down* simple. *Anthers* ending in two bristles at the base. *Willd.*

Inula Helenium. Willd. *Sp. Plant.* iii. 2089; Woodv. *Med. Bot.* p. 64, t. 26. Elecampane has a perennial root, and an annual stem, which is round, furrowed, villous, leafy, from three to six feet high, and branched near the top. The leaves are large, ovate, serrate, crowded with reticular veins, smooth and deep green upon the upper surface, downy on the under, and furnished with a fleshy midrib. Those which spring directly from the root are petiolate, those of the stem sessile and embracing. The flowers are large, of a golden-yellow color, and stand singly at the ends of the stem and branches. The calyx exhibits several rows of imbricated ovate scales. The florets of the ray are numerous, spreading, linear, and tridentate at the apex. The seeds are striated, quadrangular, and furnished with a simple somewhat chaffy pappus.

This large and handsome plant is a native of Europe, where it is also cultivated for medical use. It has been introduced into our gardens, and has become naturalized in some parts of the country, growing in low meadows, and on the roadsides, from New England to Pennsylvania. It flowers in July and August. The roots, which are the officinal part, should be dug up in autumn, and in their second year. When older they are apt to be stringy and woody.

The fresh root of elecampane is very thick and branched, having whitish cylindrical ramifications, furnished with thread-like fibres. It is externally brown, internally whitish and fleshy; and the transverse sections present radiating lines. The dried root is "in transverse, concave slices or longitudinal sections, with overlapping bark, externally wrinkled and brown, flexible in damp weather; when dry, breaking with a short fracture; internally grayish, fleshy, slightly radiate and dotted with numerous shining, yellowish brown resin-cells; odor peculiar, aromatic; taste bitter and pungent." *U. S.* Its medical virtues are extracted by alcohol and water, the former becoming most strongly impregnated with its bitterness and pungency. A peculiar principle, resembling starch, was discovered in elecampane by Valentine Rose, of Berlin, in 1804, who named it *alantin;* but the title *inulin,* proposed by Dr. Thomson, has been generally adopted. It differs from starch in being deposited unchanged from its solution in boiling water when the liquor cools, and in giving a yellowish instead of a blue color with iodine. It has been found in the roots of several other plants. It may be obtained white and pure by precipitating a concentrated decoction with twice its volume of alcohol, dissolving the precipitate in a little distilled water, treating the solution with purified animal charcoal, and again precipitating with alcohol. (*A. J. P.*, xxxi. 69.) It readily dissolves in about three parts of boiling water; the lævogyre solution is perfectly clear and fluid, not paste-like, but on cooling deposits nearly all the inulin.

Its formula, according to Kiliani (Tollens, *Handbuch der Kohlenhydrate*, 1888, p. 202), is $6C_6H_{10}O_5 + H_2O$. On prolonged heating with water, more rapidly under the influence of dilute acids, it is changed into *levulose* and reduces Fehling's solution. As in the case of starch, intermediate products can be obtained before it is completely changed into reducing sugar. Dragendorff obtained by heating with water for ten hours *metinulin*, and by heating for forty to fifty hours *levulin*, an optically inactive amorphous substance easily changing into *levulose*.

The amount of inulin varies according to the season, but is most abundant in autumn. Dragendorff obtained from the root in October not less than 44 per cent., but in spring only 19 per cent.

A crystallizable substance was long since noticed to collect in the head of the receiver when the elecampane root is submitted to distillation with water. Similar crystals may also be observed after carefully heating a thin slice of the root, and are even found as a natural efflorescence on the surface of a root that has been long kept. They can be extracted from the root by means of alcohol, and precipitated with water.

Kallen (*Deutsch. Chem. Ges.*, 1873, p. 1506, and 1876, p. 154) has found that these crystals consist chiefly of the anhydride, $C_{15}H_{20}O_2$, of *alantic acid*, melting at 66° C., and that what was formerly known as *helenin* was a mixture of these with a liquid, *alantol*, $C_{10}H_{16}O$, boiling at 200° C., the true *helenin** and *alant camphor*. The crystals of *helenin*, C_6H_8O, have a bitterish taste, but no odor, and melt at 110° C. The camphor melts at 64° C., and in taste and smell is suggestive of peppermint.

Medical Properties and Uses. Elecampane is tonic and gently stimulant, and has been supposed to possess diaphoretic, diuretic, expectorant, and emmenagogue properties. By the ancients it was much employed, especially in the complaints

* Dr. Korab (*Lon. Lancet*, vol. i., 1885, p. 672) states that helenin is a powerful antiseptic and bactericide, one part in ten thousand of urine being sufficient to arrest putrefaction, and a few drops of a solution of this strength immediately killing the ordinary bacterial organisms, including the tubercle bacillus. He lauds it as antiseptic in surgery, and has given it with alleged success internally in doses of one-third to one grain in tubercular, infantile, and catarrhal diarrhœas. It is also stated by Dr. J. B. Obiol (*Lancet*, April, 1886) to be an efficient local remedy in the treatment of diphtheria. Every four hours the false membrane is to be dusted over with powdered camphor, and then painted with a two per cent. solution of helenin in oil of sweet almonds. It is affirmed that when the treatment was commenced on the first day of the patches the cure followed in twenty-four hours. The helenin was also given internally. Dose, one and a half grains to children six years of age.

peculiar to females; and it is still occasionally resorted to in amenorrhœa. In this country it is chiefly used in chronic diseases of the lungs, and is sometimes beneficial when the affection of the chest is attended with weakness of the digestive organs, or with general debility. From a belief in its deobstruent and diuretic virtues, it was formerly prescribed in chronic engorgements of the abdominal viscera, and the dropsy to which they so often give rise. It has also been highly recommended both as an internal and external remedy in tetter, psora, and other diseases of the skin. The usual modes of administration are in powder and decoction. The dose of the powder is from a scruple to a drachm (1·3–3·9 Gm.). The decoction may be prepared by boiling half an ounce of the root in a pint of water, and given in the dose of one or two fluidounces (30–60 C.c.).

IODOFORMUM. *U. S., Br.* *Iodoform.*

CHI_3; 392·8. (Ī-Q-DQ-FŌR′MŬM.) C_2HI_3; 392·8.

"Iodoform should be kept in well-stopped bottles, in a cool place." *U. S.* "A product of the action of iodine on a mixture of alcohol and solution of carbonate of potassium." *Br.*

Iodoformium, *P.G.;* Iodoforme, *Fr.;* Iodoform, *G.*

This compound, discovered by Sérullas in 1822, was introduced as a remedy, about the year 1837, by Dr. R. M. Glover, of London, and M. Bouchardat, of Paris, and was first adopted as officinal in the U. S. Pharmacopœia of 1870.

Preparation. Cornélis and Gille published a process in *Journ. de Pharm.*, 1852, p. 196. (See U. S. D., 14th ed., p. 511.) Wittstein's process is an improvement on this. Take two parts of carbonate of potassium, two of iodine, one of 95 per cent. alcohol, and five of water, mix them in a retort, and heat the mixture by means of a water-bath, until perfectly colorless; then, after the cooling of the liquid, pour it into a suitable vessel, and allow it to settle. The yellow scaly mass deposited is collected on a filter, washed thoroughly with water, and dried between folds of bibulous paper. As iodoform is very volatile, it must be prepared in closed vessels. The liquid remaining after the deposition of iodoform contains iodate and iodide of potassium, which may be decomposed with renewed formation of iodoform by adding potassium dichromate 2 to 3 parts, and hydrochloric acid 16 to 24 parts; this liberates iodine. 32 parts of carbonate of sodium, 6 parts of iodine, and 16 parts of alcohol are now added, the liquid is then again poured off from the iodoform produced, and the operation again repeated if necessary. The formation of the iodoform is represented by the following equation: $C_2H_5.OH + 4I_2 + 3K_2CO_3 = CHI_3 + CHKO_2 + 5KI + 2H_2O + 3CO_2$. Other products, such as potassium iodate, are, however, formed. Mr. G. R. Bell (*N. R.*, March, 1882) has practically tried nearly all of the processes for the preparation of iodoform, and recommends Filhol's, which is as follows. Put into a long-necked matrass or flask which is supplied with a perforated cork and long supply-tube, a solution of 200 parts of crystallized carbonate of sodium and 1000 parts of distilled water, and add 100 parts of alcohol, heat in a water-bath from 60° C. to 71·1° C. (140° to 160° F.), then gradually add 100 parts of iodine, about 10 parts at a time. When the liquid has become colorless, remove the flask from the water-bath, and allow it to cool three or four hours, then pour out on a filter; return the filtrate to the flask, add 200 parts of carbonate of sodium, 100 parts of alcohol, heat to 71·1° C. (160° F.), and pass a slow current of chlorine gas through the mixture as long as iodine is separated, continuing until the brown liquid is again decolorized. A small excess of chlorine is of no consequence (Hager states that for every 100 parts of iodine it requires the chlorine which can be evolved from about 200 parts of hydrochloric acid by means of manganese dioxide). Let the flask stand twenty-four hours, then throw the contents on a filter and examine the filtrate with chlorine water to see whether it still contains an appreciable amount of iodine compounds, then if necessary subject the filtrate to a second treatment of chlorine gas, adding previously only 20 parts of carbonate of sodium and 10 parts of alcohol. Collect the iodoform after twenty-four hours. The filtrate may be concentrated and decomposed by excess of nitric acid, according to the method recommended in Bouchardat's process. The collected crystals of iodoform are now well washed with the smallest quantity of cold distilled water, spread out on pieces of bibulous paper, and dried in the open air.

The fact, noticed by Lieben in 1870, that many other compounds besides ethyl alcohol yielded iodoform when treated with iodine and alkali, led Krämer (*Ber. Chem. Ges.*, 1880, p. 1000) to propose the iodoform formation as an exact quantitative test for the presence of acetone in methyl alcohol. This "iodoform test" is now used in testing the purity of methyl alcohol for use in the manufacture of aniline dye colors, as well as the purity of acetone itself. (See article *Acetone*, Part II.) Heinrich Spindler proposes to make iodoform from the chlorides, bromides, or chlorobromides of the paraffin series by reaction with an inorganic iodide; thus if chloroform and *anhydrous* calcium iodide are heated to 120° C. iodoform is produced. (*Amer. Drug.*, 1886, p. 67.)

F. Günther recommends mixing alcohol containing 25 per cent. of aldehyd with ten times its weight of solution of soda, adding the iodine, and passing a current of carbonic acid gas through the mixture. (*Archiv d. Pharm.*, 1887, p. 373.)

Properties. It is in the form of "small, lemon-yellow, lustrous crystals of the hexagonal system, having a saffron-like and almost insuppressible odor, and an unpleasant, slightly sweetish, iodine-like taste. Not perceptibly soluble in water, to which it imparts a slight odor and taste; soluble in 80 parts of alcohol at 15° C. (59° F.), in 12 parts of boiling alcohol, in 5·2 parts of ether, and in chloroform, benzol, benzin, disulphide of carbon, and in fixed or volatile oils. Its solutions have a neutral reaction. Sp. gr. 2.000. It sublimes slightly at ordinary temperatures, and distils slowly with water; at about 115° C. (239° F.) it melts to a brown liquid, and at a higher temperature yields vapors containing iodine and carbonaceous matter. If Iodoform be digested with an alcoholic solution of potassa, the mixture, when acidulated with diluted nitric acid, will give a blue color with gelatinized starch. Distilled water shaken with Iodoform should not change the color of blue litmus paper, and when filtered, should give no precipitate with test-solution of nitrate of silver (abs. of iodide). Upon full combustion, Iodoform should leave no residue." *U. S.* It is a volatile substance, soft to the touch, and totally devoid of corrosive properties. With potassa in solution, it is decomposed, yielding formiate and iodide of potassium. Hence these two principles are incompatible in prescriptions.

Medical Properties and Uses. M. Maitre, who has studied the physiological effects of iodoform on men, states that from a dose of 30 or 40 centigrammes (about 5 or 6 grains) no effects are observed except a slight increase of appetite. Two hours after it has been taken, the presence of iodine can be detected in the urine and the saliva, and nearly three days elapse before the whole is eliminated. (See also Höyges, *Journ. de Pharm.*, Juillet, 1867.) It passes off also with the lacteal secretion. Given to dogs in much larger doses, several grammes for example, it produces narcotic effects; and two stages in its operation have been noticed; the first marked with more or less prostration, with symptoms of intoxication, the animal tottering, inclining to one side with the head falling, with loss of appetite, but without vomiting. The next day, unless a very large dose has been given, complete recovery takes place. A still larger dose induces the second stage, characterized by a remarkably intense excitation, with anxious breathing, strong and short pulse, a true opisthotonus, sometimes very striking, and convulsive movements of the paws, especially the hinder. After death fatty degeneration of the heart, liver, and kidneys may be found. (*A. Höyges.*) The very free use of iodoform in Germany as an antiseptic dressing to wounds, ulcers, etc., has led to many cases of poisoning. In the most characteristic and severe cases the phenomena of iodoform-poisoning resemble somewhat those of meningitis: they are headache, somnolence deepening into stupor, contracted, motionless pupils, abnormal quiet or restlessness ending in active delirium, with, however, a normal temperature and an exceedingly rapid pulse. In cases of this character death almost always follows, although the symptoms may have developed abruptly and the dressing have been removed at once. In other cases the principal symptoms are general malaise and depression, faintness, headache, loss of appetite, and a persistent iodoform taste in the mouth. In some cases there is a slight temporary increase of temperature. Mental depression or excitement is especially noticed. Finally the pulse becomes accelerated, soft, and feeble; in some cases the pulse is very rapid,—150–180,—while the temperature remains normal, or only slightly elevated.

Iodoform, though containing 29 parts in 30 of its weight of iodine, is not locally irritant, but anæsthetic and antiseptic. It is said, when employed as a suppository, to produce unconsciousness of the act of defecation. In the form of vapor, it possesses anæsthetic properties, but inferior to those of chloroform. On account of its large proportion of iodine, it was supposed to be capable of replacing that element and the iodides as a remedy, with the advantages of being non-irritant, and of having an organic nature, qualities which favor its absorption and assimilation. The principal diseases in which it has been tried are goitre, rickets, scrofula, phthisis, amenorrhœa, syphilis, glandular tumors, inflammatory disease of the fauces, with or without venereal taint, etc., and cutaneous eruptions. It may be given in from one to three grains, three or four times a day, in pill form; but it has not met the expectation of its early advocates, and is not much used internally. The chief value of iodoform in practical medicine is as an external application. It has long been used in cases of painful ulcers, especially when of syphilitic origin, but has been found to act almost equally well in indolent leg ulcers and other non-specific abrasions, and will even produce marked relief in open cancers. Within the last few years it has been freely employed as an antiseptic dressing to wounds, and the testimony from surgeons is so strong that it is difficult to avoid believing that it is one of the most certain remedies of the class. The good results which have been achieved have led to a series of studies of its action upon septic organisms, with results which are apparently at variance with practical surgical teachings,* and which seem to prove that the iodoform itself has little power as a bactericide. When, however, it is brought in contact with the living surface of a wound it undergoes a slow chemical change, resulting in the liberation of iodine, which element has a distinct influence upon the development of septic organisms. Moreover, iodoform appears to have a specific influence upon human tissue, by which it prevents the formation of purulent or serous exudation, and greatly diminishes the soil in which the bacteria develop. Iodoform, locally applied, has been found by various clinicians to be especially valuable in tubercular abscesses, and has even been used with asserted good results, dusted upon the surface of the peritoneum, in tubercular peritonitis. In uterine affections vaginal suppositories, made by incorporating 5·5 grains of iodoform with 2·5 drachms of cacao butter, have been largely used, and similar rectal suppositories have been employed with asserted advantage in enlargements of the prostate gland and in fissures of the anus. In surgical dressings with iodoform the powder is usually sprinkled freely upon the wounds and secured in place by a dry dressing. *Iodoform gauze*, or *iodoform cotton wool*, may be made by saturating suitable material with a concentrated ethereal solution and afterwards drying.

The maximum amount of iodoform which may be used with safety as an external application is uncertain. Dr. Langenstein attributes a fatal result to one drachm, whilst one hundred and twenty grains have certainly caused death. In our opinion not more than half a drachm of the iodoform should ever be applied to a wound.

One of the principal obstacles to its employment is the odor, which, to some patients, is unbearable. Many methods of disguising the odor have been recommended, but in our experience the large quantity required of each deodorising agent would preclude its employment. Tannin has been recommended, but, as this operates by decomposing the iodoform, it is not to be thought of in this connection. Probably the best class of substances to use are the volatile oils, such as anise, peppermint, fennel, bergamot, almond, etc., tonka, coffee, and balsam of Peru, although the latter acts by forming a compound, and the aim should be not to destroy the odor,† but so to modify it as to remove its objectionable features.

Off. Prep. Unguentum Iodoformi.

Off. Prep. Br. Suppositoria Iodoformi; Unguentum Iodoformi.

* For a more elaborate discussion of these investigations, the reader is referred to Dr. H. C. Wood's *Treatise on Therapeutics*, 7th edition.

† The pale yellow essential oil of the *Evodia Fraxinifolia* is asserted by Mr. H. Helbing (*P. J. Tr.*, vol. xviii. 249) to have the power of covering the odor of iodoform.

IODUM. *U. S., Br.* *Iodine.*

I; 126·6. (I-Ō'DŬM.) I; 126·6.

"A non-metallic element, obtained from the ashes of sea-weeds and from mineral iodides and iodates." *Br.*

Iodinium, *U. S.* 1870; Iode, *Fr.*; Jod, *G.*; Iodina, *It.*, *Sp.*

The Iodine of the U. S. and Br. Pharmacopœias is considered as pure; and in both, the tests are given by which its purity may be determined. "Iodine should be preserved in glass-stoppered bottles, in a cool place." *U. S.*

Iodine is a non-metallic element, discovered in 1812 by Courtois, a soda manufacturer of Paris. It exists in certain marine vegetables, particularly the fuci or common sea-weeds, which have long been its most abundant natural source. It has been detected in some fresh-water plants, among which are the water-cress, brooklime, and fine-leaved water-hemlock; also in the ashes of tobacco, and of Honduras sarsaparilla. (*Chatin.*) It has been found in the beet-root of the grand-duchy of Baden. (*Lamy.*) Dr. Macadam detected a trace of iodine in 100 gallons of water used for domestic purposes in Edinburgh, in several of the domestic animals, and in man. He detected it also in potatoes, beans, peas, wheat, barley, and oats. (*P. J. Tr.*, Nov. 1854, p. 235.) Iodine is, moreover, found in the animal kingdom, as in the sponge, the oyster, various polypi, cod-liver oil, and eggs; and, in the mineral kingdom, in sea-water in minute quantity, in certain salt springs, as iodide of silver in a rare Mexican mineral, in a zinc ore of Silesia, in native nitrate of sodium, and in some kinds of rock salt. It is now obtained commercially from one of these sources,—viz., from the native sodium nitrate, or Chili saltpetre, with which it occurs as sodium iodate. The production of the province of Tarapaca (Peru) has assumed large dimensions within the last few years, as a result of higher prices established by a combination of Scotch, French, and Peruvian producers. The present production of the Chili saltpetre-works is estimated at 300,000 kilos. annually. The exportations from Iquique in 1881 were 140,000 kilos. and in 1882 205,800 kilos.; from Autofagasta in 1881 4000 kilos., and in 1882 5000 kilos. M. Bussy has obtained iodine, in the proportion of one part in five thousand, from the coal-gas liquor of the gas-works of Paris. It was first discovered in the United States in the water of the Congress Spring, at Saratoga, by Dr. William Usher. It was detected in the Kanawha saline waters by the late Professor Emmet; and it exists in the bittern of the salt-works of Western Pennsylvania, in the amount of about eight grains to the gallon. In sea-weeds the iodine exists in the state probably of iodide of sodium. In different countries, sea-weeds are burned for the sake of their ashes, the product being a dark-colored fused mass called *kelp.* This substance, besides carbonate and iodide of sodium, contains more or less common salt, chloride of potassium, sulphate of sodium, etc. The deep-sea fuci contain the most iodine; and, when these are burned at a low temperature for fuel, as is the case in the island of Guernsey, their ashes furnish more iodine than ordinary kelp. (*Graham.*) According to Dr. Geo. Kemp, the laminarian species, especially *Laminaria digitata*, *L. saccharina*, and *L. bulbosa*, which are deep-water sea-weeds, and contain more potassium than sodium, are particularly rich in iodine.

Preparation. Although most largely produced in South America, iodine is still obtained from kelp, and in Great Britain is manufactured chiefly at Glasgow. The kelp, which on an average contains a 224th part of iodine, is lixiviated with water, in which about half dissolves. The solution is concentrated to a pellicle and allowed to cool; whereby nearly all the salts, except iodide of sodium, are separated, they being less soluble than the iodide. The remaining liquor, which is dense and dark-colored, is made very sour by sulphuric acid, which causes the evolution of carbonic acid, sulphuretted hydrogen, and sulphurous acid, and the deposition of sulphur. The liquor is then introduced into a leaden still, and distilled with manganese dioxide into a series of glass receivers, inserted into one another, in which the iodine is condensed. In this process the iodide of sodium is decomposed, and the iodine evolved according to the reaction $2NaI + 2H_2SO_4 + MnO_2 = MnSO_4 + Na_2SO_4 + 2H_2O + I_2$ which leaves as residue manganous sulphate and sulphate of sodium.*

* The methods formerly practised for obtaining iodine from sea-weeds were accompanied with great loss. A notable improvement over the old kelp processes are the "char" and "wet" pro-

The methods for the separation of the iodine from its combinations in the mother-liquors as practised in South America, may be divided essentially into three classes. (1.) The mother-liquors after the crystallization of the saltpetre without further concentration are treated with a solution of sodium sulphite of strength corresponding to the amount of iodine present; the iodine is liberated according to the reaction: $2NaIO_3 + 4HNaSO_3 + SO_2 = Na_2SO_4 + 4HNaSO_4 + I_2$; the iodine thus separated from the sodium iodate is filtered through linen cloth, washed, pressed, and sublimed. (2.) The mother-liquors are treated with sodium sulphite or bisulphite until the precipitated iodine is converted into HI, and this is precipitated as cuprous iodide by a solution of copper sulphate and sodium sulphite. (3.) The percentage of iodine is increased by fractional evaporation and crystallization of the mother-liquors, and then, after adding the calculated amount of sodium bisulphite, the iodine is distilled off from the acidified liquor. (*Dingler's Polytech. Journ.*, 231, p. 375.)

The British Pharmacopœia of 1864 purified iodine as follows. "Take of Iodine of Commerce *one ounce*. Introduce the Commercial Iodine into a porcelain capsule of a circular shape, cover this as accurately as possible with a glass matrass filled with cold water, and apply to the capsule the heat of boiling water for twenty minutes. Let the matrass be now removed, and should colorless acicular prisms of a pungent odor be found attached to its bottom, let them be separated from it. This being done, the matrass is to be restored to its previous position, and a gentle and steady heat (that of a gas lamp answers well) applied, so as to sublime the whole of the iodine. Upon now allowing the capsule to cool, and lifting off the matrass, the purified product will be found attached to the bottom of the latter. When separated it should be immediately enclosed in a bottle furnished with an accurately ground stopper."

In this process, which is that of the former Dublin Pharmacopœia, a short preliminary sublimation by the heat of a water-bath is ordered, in which the bottom of a glass matrass filled with cold water is the refrigerator. The object of this is to separate any iodide of cyanogen that may happen to be present. This impurity is sometimes present in considerable amount. Klobach obtained from eighty avoirdupois pounds of commercial iodine twelve ounces of this iodide, which is in the proportion of nearly one per cent. (*Chem. Gaz.*, April 15, 1850.) Should the matrass, upon its removal, have attached to its bottom white acicular crystals, these will be the iodide in question, and must be rejected. The matrass having been replaced, heat is again applied until the whole of the iodine has sublimed, and attaches itself to the cool bottom of the matrass.

Water has sometimes been found in iodine to the extent of 15 or 20 per cent. If considerable, it is easily discovered by the iodine adhering to the inside of the bottle. M. Bolley estimates its amount by rubbing together, until the smell of iodine disappears, 30 grains of iodine with about 240 of mercury, in a small weighed porcelain dish, using a small weighed agate pestle. When complete combination has been effected, the whole is placed in a water-bath to dissipate the water. The loss of weight gives the amount of water in the iodine. (*Chem. Gaz.*, March 15, 1853, p. 118.) The presence of water is injurious only as it renders all the preparations of iodine weaker than they should be. In the former Ed. Pharmacopœia, directions were given to dry it, by placing it "in a shallow basin of earthenware, in a small confined space of air, with ten or twelve times its weight of fresh-burnt lime, till it scarcely adheres to the inside of a dry bottle."

Properties. Iodine is described by the U. S. Pharmacopœia as "heavy, bluish black, dry and friable, rhombic plates of a metallic lustre, a distinctive odor, a sharp and acrid taste, and a neutral reaction. Iodine imparts a deep brown, slowly evanescing stain to the skin, and slowly destroys vegetable colors. It is sparingly solu-

cesses of Mr. E. C. C. Stanford (*Jour. Soc. Chem. Ind.*, 1885, p. 518), which show the following results when compared with the old processes. *Kelp process*. Per cent. utilized, 18. Kelp, 18 tons, yield salts 9 tons and iodine 270 lbs. Residuals, kelp waste, 18 tons, valueless. *Char process*. Per cent. utilized, 36. Char, 36 tons, yield salts 15 tons and iodine 600 lbs. Residuals, charcoal, 36 tons, tar and ammonia. *Wet process*. Per cent. utilized, 70. Water extract, 33 tons yield salts 20 tons and iodine 600 lbs. Residuals, algin, 20 tons, cellulose, 15 tons, dextrine, etc.

ble in water, soluble in about 11 parts of alcohol at 15° C. (59° F.); very soluble in ether, disulphide of carbon and chloroform. It is slowly volatilized at ordinary temperatures. When heated to 114° C. (237·2° F.) it melts, and then rises in purple vapor, being gradually dissipated without leaving a residue. With gelatinized starch, in a cold solution, it produces a dark blue color." *U. S.* Its sp. gr. is 4·9. It is a volatile substance, and evaporates even at common temperatures. Its vapor has the sp. gr. 8·7, being the heaviest aëriform substance known. If inhaled mixed with air, it excites cough and irritates the nostrils. When it comes in contact with cool surfaces, it condenses in brilliant steel-gray crystals. Iodine is freely soluble in alcohol and ether, but requires 7000 times its weight of water to dissolve it. If water stands on iodine for some time, especially in a strong light, it apparently dissolves more iodine; but the result depends upon the formation of hydriodic acid, in a solution of which iodine is more soluble than in water. The solution of iodine in water has no taste, a feeble odor, and a light brown color; in alcohol or ether, is nearly black. Its solubility in water is very much increased by the addition of certain salts, as the chloride of sodium, nitrate of ammonium, or iodide of potassium; and the same effect is produced, to some extent, by tannic acid. Its solution in tannic acid is called *iodo-tannin*, of which MM. Socquet and Guillermond make a syrup for internal, and an aqueous solution for external use. For the formulas, see the *B. and F. Medico-Chir. Rev.*, 1854, p. 181. It is also soluble in glycerin, as ascertained by M. Cap in 1854. According to Dr. I. Walz, glacial acetic acid is an excellent solvent of iodine, at least equal to alcohol. When the acid is heated by boiling with excess of iodine, and then allowed to cool slowly, it deposits iodine in beautiful large slender crystals, sometimes half an inch long, much larger and more abundant than those formed from the alkaline solution. (*Chem. News*, May 9, 1873, p. 233; from the *Journal of the Franklin Institute.*) In chemical characters iodine resembles chlorine, but its affinities are weaker. It combines with most of the non-metallic, and nearly all the metallic elements, forming a class of compounds called *iodides*. Some of these are officinal, as the iodides of iron, mercury, lead, potassium, and sulphur. It forms with oxygen one oxide, *iodic oxide*, I_2O_5, and two acids, *iodic** and *periodic*, and with hydrogen a gaseous acid, called *hydriodic acid*.

Tests, etc. Iodine, in most cases, may be recognised by its characteristic purple vapor; but where this cannot be made evident, it is detected unerringly by starch, which produces with it a deep blue color. This test was discovered by Colin and Gaultier de Claubry, and is so delicate that it will indicate the presence of iodine in 450,000 times its weight of water. In order that the test may succeed, the iodine must be free, and the solutions cold. To render it free when in combination, as it always is in the animal fluids, a little nitric acid, free from iodine, must be added to the solution suspected to contain it. Thus, in testing urine for iodine, the secretion is mixed with starch, and acidulated with a drop or two of nitric acid; when, if iodine be present, the color produced will vary from a light purple to a deep indigo-blue, according to the amount of the element present. Sometimes, in mineral waters, the proportion of iodine is so minute that the starch test, in connection with nitric acid, gives a doubtful coloration. In such cases, Liebig recommends the addition to the water of a very small quantity of iodate of potassium, followed by a little starch and hydrochloric acid. Assuming the iodine to be present as hydriodic acid, the liberated iodic acid sets free from the iodine of the mineral water, and becomes itself deoxidized, thus increasing the amount of the free iodine ($HIO_3 + 5HI = 3I_2 + 3H_2O$). This test would be fallacious, if iodic acid, mixed with hydrochloric acid, colored starch; but this is not the case. Still, Liebig's test is inapplicable in the presence of reducing agents, such as sulphurous acid, which would give rise to free iodine from the test itself, independently of the presence of the element in the water tested. (*Dr. W. Knop.*) The U. S. Pharmacopœia furnishes the following tests.

* Dr. R. H. Brett, of Liverpool, has found that when a small portion of the alkaloids, or their salts, is mixed with about an equal portion of iodic acid and a few drops of water, and the mixture gently heated, a succession of distinct explosions, attended by the evolution of gas, takes place. Dr. Brett finds that this phenomenon does not occur with other organic substances, and suggests it as a general test for alkaloids. (*P. J. Tr.*, Nov. 1854.)

"A solution of Iodine in chloroform should be perfectly clear and limpid (abs. of moisture). When shaken with distilled water, it should not communicate to the latter more than a light brownish tinge, and no deep brown color (abs. of chloride of iodine). If the iodine be removed from this dilute aqueous solution by agitation with disulphide of carbon, and, after the separation of the latter, some dilute solution of ferrous sulphate with a trace of ferric chloride be added, finally solution of soda, and the whole supersaturated with hydrochloric acid, no blue precipitate should make its appearance (abs. of cyanide of iodine). If Iodine be dissolved in sulphurous acid, the solution strongly supersaturated with ammonia, and completely precipitated by nitrate of silver, the filtrate, on being supersaturated with nitric acid, should not at once become more than faintly cloudy (abs. of more than traces of chlorine or bromine). If 0·633 Gm. of Iodine, with 1 Gm. of iodide of potassium, be dissolved in 25 C.c. of water, it should require 50 C.c. of the volumetric solution of hyposulphite of sodium to fully decolorize the liquid (corresponding to 100 per cent. of absolute Iodine)." *U. S.* The British Pharmacopœia states that "12·7 grains, dissolved in an ounce [fluidounce] of water containing 15 grains of iodide of potassium, require for complete discoloration 1000 grain-measures of the *volumetric solution of hyposulphite of sodium.*" M. Carey Lea proposes chromic acid as a substitute for the nitric, for the liberation of iodine, as a more delicate test. It may be most conveniently applied by first adding starch to the liquid to be tested, and then a little dilute solution of bichromate of potassium, enough to cause a pale yellow color, followed by a few drops of hydrochloric acid. (*Am. Journ. of Sci. and Arts*, xlii. 109.) Another test for iodine, proposed by M. Rabourdin, is chloroform, by the use of which he supposes that the element may be not only detected in organic substances, but approximately estimated. Thus, if 150 grains of a solution, containing one part in one hundred thousand of iodide of potassium, be treated with 2 drops of nitric and 15 or 20 of sulphuric acid, and afterwards shaken with 15 grains of chloroform, the latter acquires a distinct violet tint. M. Rabourdin applies his test to the detection of iodine in the several varieties of cod-liver oil. For this purpose he incinerates, in an iron spoon, 50 parts of the specimen of oil with 5 of *pure* caustic potassa, dissolved in 15 of water, and exhausts the cinder with the smallest possible quantity of water. The solution is filtered, acidulated with nitric and sulphuric acids, and agitated with 4 parts of chloroform. After a time the chloroform subsides, of a violet color more or less deep according to the proportion of iodine present. M. Lassaigne considers the starch test more delicate than that of chloroform. For detecting iodine in the iodides of the metals of the alkalies, he considers bichloride of palladium as extremely delicate, producing brownish flocks of biniodide of palladium. According to M. Moride, benzin is a good test for free iodine, which it readily dissolves, forming a solution of a bright red color, deeper in proportion to the amount of iodine taken up. As benzin does not dissolve chlorine or bromine, it furnishes the means of separating iodine from these elements. Mr. D. S. Price has pointed out the nitrites as exceedingly sensitive tests of iodine, combined as an iodide. The suspected liquid is mixed with starch paste, acidulated with hydrochloric acid, and treated with solution of nitrite of potassium. The iodine is set free, and a blue color appears, more or less deep, according to the proportion of iodine present. By this test, iodine may be detected in an aqueous solution containing only one in 400,000 parts. A similar test had been previously proposed by M. Grange.

It has been long known that, when a mixture of iodine and starch in water is subjected to heat, the blue color disappears, and, if the heat be not too long continued, so as to volatilize the iodine, or convert it into hydriodic acid, the color will return on the cooling of the liquid. Various explanations have been given of this curious fact by Personne and others, but none quite satisfactory, until that by M. Magnes Lahens, which he supports by experiment, that during the continuance of the heat the particles of starch and iodine separate, to unite again on refrigeration. (*Journ. de Pharm.*, 4e sér., iii. 405.)

Adulterations. Iodine is said to be occasionally adulterated with mineral coal, charcoal, plumbago, and black oxide of manganese. These are easily detected by their fixed nature, while pure iodine is wholly volatilised by heat. Herberger found native sulphide of antimony in one sample, and plumbago in another; and Righini has detected as much as 25 per cent. of chloride of calcium. The presence of iodide of cyanogen and of water has already been referred to, and the modes of detecting and separating them pointed out. (See page 806.) Besides the test given at page 806, the British Pharmacopœia directs that officinal iodine should be soluble in alcohol, ether, and a solution of iodide of potassium, and should sublime without residue, and that the part which first comes over should contain no colorless prisms of a pungent odor.

Medical Properties. Iodine was first employed as a medicine in 1819, by Dr. Coindet, Sr., of Geneva. It operates as a general excitant of the vital actions, especially of the absorbent and glandular systems. Its effects are varied by its degree of concentration, state of combination, dose, etc.; and hence, under different circumstances, it may prove corrosive, irritant, or simply alterative. It is absorbed into the circulation, and may be found in all the secretions, but is chiefly eliminated by the kidneys, not, however, uncombined, but in the state of hydriodic acid or an iodide. Cantu detected it not only in the urine and saliva, but also in the sweat, milk, and blood. According to Dr. John C. Dalton, Jr., of New York, iodine, taken in a single moderate dose, appears in the urine in thirty minutes, and may be detected for nearly twenty-four hours. In two cases in which large doses of iodide of potassium had been taken for six or eight weeks, and the medicine intermitted, all trace of iodine disappeared from the urine in eighty-four hours.

The tonic operation of iodine is evinced by its increasing the appetite, which is a frequent effect of its use. Salivation is occasionally caused by it, and sometimes soreness of the mouth only. In some cases, pustular eruptions and coryza have been produced; especially when the remedy has been given in the form of iodide of potassium. In an overdose it acts as an irritant poison. Doses of two drachms, (7·8 Gm.) administered to dogs, have produced irritation of the stomach, and death in seven days; and the stomach was found studded with numerous little ulcers of a yellow color. From four to six grains (0·26 to 0·4 Gm.) in man, cause a sense of constriction in the throat, sickness and pain at the stomach, and at length vomiting and colic. Even in medicinal doses, it sometimes causes alarming symptoms; such as fever, restlessness, disturbed sleep, palpitations, excessive thirst, acute pain in the stomach, vomiting and purging, violent cramps, frequent pulse, and, finally, progressive emaciation, if the medicine be not laid aside. Such violent symptoms are, however, very rare, but where iodine or iodide of potassium is given freely a mild *iodism* is not unfrequent. It is usually characterised by pain or heaviness in the region of the frontal sinuses, with or without coryza; in some instances soreness of the mucous membrane of the mouth and throat, or a mild ptyalism, is the prominent symptom; or a papular eruption may be the first manifestation of the constitutional action of the remedy.

Testimony is not wanting to the effect, that a long course of the remedy has in some instances occasioned absorption of the mammæ and wasting of the testicles, but such result is extremely rare. Dr. Lebert, who has practised both in Switzerland and France, states that, under his observation, the accidents produced by iodine, with scarcely an exception, were in those cases of goitre in which the remedy acted rapidly in removing the tumor; while in scrofulous, tuberculous, and syphilitic patients, free from goitre, though the medicine was given in considerable doses, no injury to the system ensued. He supposes that the bad effects, in the goitre cases, arose from the too prompt absorption of the abnormal material of the tumor, which, entering the circulation in the course of its elimination, produced the poisonous effect, and not from the iodine itself. (*Ann. de Thérap.*, 1855, p. 228.)

Iodine has been principally employed in diseases of the absorbent and glandular systems. It has been used with success in ascites, especially when connected with diseased liver. It acts most efficiently immediately after tapping. In glandular enlargements and morbid growths, it has proved more efficacious than in any other class of diseases, and instances of its successful use in cases of ovarian tumor have even been reported. Dr. Coindet discovered its extraordinary power in curing goitre;* and it has been used with more or less advantage in enlargements and indurations of the liver, spleen, mammæ, testes, and uterus. In hepatic affections of this kind, where mercury has failed or is inadmissible, iodine is our best resource. Dr. Morell Mackenzie reports very favorably of the effects of iodine injected hypodermically into the thyroid. (*Am. Journ. of Med. Sci.*, Oct. 1873, p. 553.) In chronic diseases of the uterus, with induration and enlargement, and in hard tumors of the cervix and indurated puckerings of the edges of the os tincæ, iodine has occasionally effected cures, administered internally, and rubbed into the cervix, in the form of ointment, for ten or twelve minutes every night. In the form of iodide of potassium, in tertian syphilis, mercurial cachexy, and the poisonous effects of lead, it is one of our best remedies. It is habitually employed in scaly skin affections, and in chronic rheumatism.

But it is in scrofulous diseases that the most striking results have been obtained by the use of iodine. Dr. Coindet first directed attention to its effects in scrofula, and Dr. Manson reported a number of cases of this affection, in a large proportion of which the disease was either cured or ameliorated. We are indebted, however, to Dr. Lugol for the most extended early researches in relation to the use of iodine in scrofula. This physician began his trials in the Hospital Saint Louis, in 1827, and published his results in 1829, 1830, and 1831. The scrofulous affections cured by Dr. Lugol by the iodide treatment were glandular tubercles, ophthalmia, ozæna, lupus, and fistulous and carious ulcers. Since the publication of the three memoirs of Lugol, the use of iodine in scrofulous affections has become universal.

The most eligible form of iodine for internal administration is its solution in water, aided by iodide of potassium. (See *Liquor Iodi Compositus.*) The solutions employed by Dr. Lugol contained one part of iodine, and two of iodide of potassium; and the doses given by him were equivalent to half a grain (0·03 Gm.) of iodine daily for the first fortnight, three-quarters of a grain (0·05 Gm.) daily for the second and third fortnights, one grain (0·065 Gm.) daily during the fourth and fifth, and, in some cases, a grain and a quarter (0·081 Gm.) daily for the remainder of the treatment; always largely diluted. The tincture of iodine is not eligible for internal use; for, when freshly prepared, the iodine is precipitated from it by dilution with water; and, as a consequence, the irritating solid iodine will come in contact with the stomach when the dose is swallowed. The same objection is not applicable to the compound tincture, or to the simple tincture after having been long kept.

A mode of safely bringing and maintaining the system under the influence of iodine, proposed by M. Boinet, and called by him *iodic alimentation*, is to mix the medicine with the food, as with bread and other farinaceous substances, so that the patient may take daily a due quantity, which, with this mode of administration, may be large, if desirable, without inconvenience. (See *Amylum Iodatum.*)†

* M. Chatin, finding, according to his observations, a great variation in the amount of iodine in the air, water, and soil of different localities, has founded on this supposed fact an explanation of the prevalence of goitre and cretinism in some places, and their absence in others. Thus, in certain parts of France, near Paris, which he calls the Paris zone, the amount of iodine thus distributed is comparatively large, and goitre and cretinism are unknown; while, in the Alpine valleys, where only one-tenth the amount of iodine is found, these affections are endemic. These conclusions are contreverted by M. Lohmeyer, of Göttingen, and M. Kletzinsky, of Vienna, who failed to detect iodine in the air of those cities the inhabitants of which are free from goitre.

† *Iodised Oil.* The following is the original process of M. Personne. Five parts of iodine are mixed with a thousand of almond oil, and the mixture is subjected to a jet of steam, until decolorised. The same operation is repeated with five additional parts of iodine. The oil is then washed with a weak alkaline solution, to remove the hydriodic acid, developed in the process. By this mode of proceeding, it may be presumed that the iodine is intimately united with the oil, along with which it would find an easy entrance into the system; and that, while about half of the iodine is lost as hydriodic acid, the remainder takes the place of the hydrogen eliminated from the oil. In 1851, the French Academy appointed MM. Guibourt, Soubeiran, Gibert, and Ricord, to report upon the therapeutic value of a definite combination of iodine and oil. The reporter (Guibourt) approved of M. Personne's process; and MM. Gibert and Ricord reported favorably of the therapeutic effects of the preparation. M. Personne's iodized oil differs little in appearance and taste from almond oil, and is easily taken alone or in emulsion. The dose is two fluidounces (60 C.c.) daily, which may be increased to three fluidounces (90 C.c.) or more. (*Am. Journ. of Med. Sci.*, xxiii. 502.)

M. Berthé and M. Lepage have objected to M. Personne's iodized oil, that it is of variable iodine strength, and that it is liable to become rancid, in consequence of the use of steam in its prepara-

According to M. Hutet, one grain of iodine is deprived entirely of taste and smell by one teaspoonful of a strong infusion of coffee. (*P. J. Tr.*, Dec. 1870.)

The external treatment by iodine may be divided into general and topical. By its use in this way it does not create a mere local effect, but, by its absorption, produces its peculiar constitutional impression. The external treatment, when general, consists in the use of the *iodine bath*. This for adults should contain from two to four drachms of iodine, with double that quantity of iodide of potassium, dissolved in water, in a *wooden* bath-tub; the proportion of the water being about a gallon for every three grains of iodine employed. The quantity of ingredients for the baths of children is one-third as much as for adults, but dissolved in about the same proportional quantity of water. The quantity of iodine and iodide for a bath having been determined upon, it is best to dissolve them in a small quantity of water (half a pint, for example) before they are added to the water of the bath; as this mode of proceeding facilitates their thorough diffusion. The iodine baths, which may be directed three or four times a week, usually produce a slight rubefacient effect, but occasionally a stronger impression, causing the epidermis to peel off, particularly of the arms and legs. The skin at the same time acquires a deep yellow tinge, which usually disappears in the interval between the baths.

The topical application of iodine is made by means of several officinal preparations. (See *Unguentum Iodi* and *Tinctura Iodi.*) Besides these, several others have been employed topically. Lugol's *iodine lotion* consists of from two to four grains of iodine, and double that quantity of iodide of potassium, dissolved in a pint of water. It is used as a wash or injection in scrofulous ophthalmia, ozæna, and fistulous ulcers. His *rubefacient iodine solution* is formed by dissolving half an ounce of iodine and an ounce of iodide of potassium in six fluidounces of water. This is useful for exciting scrofulous ulcers, for touching the eyelids, and as an application to recent scrofulous cicatrices, to render them smooth. The rubefacient solution, added to warm water in the proportion of about a fluidrachm to the gallon, makes a convenient local bath for the arms, legs, feet, or hands; and, mixed with linseed meal or some similar substance, it forms a cataplasm useful in certain eruptions, especially where the object is to promote the falling off of scabs. External applications of iodine have been recommended for the removal even of internal plastic exudations, as to the side, for example, in protracted pleurisy. The rubefacient preparation of iodine at present most commonly employed is the tincture. (See *Tinctura Iodi.*) The preparation called *iodine paint* is a tincture twice as strong as the officinal tincture, and is made by dissolving a drachm of iodine in a fluidounce of alcohol, and allowing the solution to stand in a glass-stoppered bottle for several months before it is used, when it will become thick and syrupy. It is applied with a glass or a camel's-hair brush, in one or more coatings, according to the degree of effect desired. Iodine paint is used as a counter-irritant, with advantage, in pains of the chest; in aphonia, applied to the front of the throat; in chronic pleuritic effusion, or consolidated lung, applied extensively opposite to the diseased part; in periostitis, whether syphilitic, strumous, or the result of injury; in inflammation of the joints; in serous effusion into bursæ; and in the cicatrices of

tion. M. Berthé makes an iodised oil, which he alleges to be free from these objections, by heating, to about 176°, five parts of iodine with a thousand parts of almond oil, in a water-bath, until decoloration shall have taken place. The resulting oil is colorless, perfectly transparent, without odor or rancidity, not acted on by starch, and of a constant composition. To shorten the time in preparing the oil, M. Lepage dissolves the iodine in three times its weight of ether, before adding it to the oil, and briskly shakes the mixture for eight or ten minutes. The preparation is then heated in a water-bath, to decolorize it and drive off the ether. M. Hugounenq objects to this process that, if the oil be completely deprived of the odor of ether, the heating must be continued for several hours. He also objects to any process which requires the continued application of heat, as rendering the oil liable to become quickly rancid. His plan is to rub up the iodine, for five or six minutes, in a porcelain mortar, with a small portion of the oil, and then gradually to add the remainder. A red limpid liquor is obtained, which may be completely decolorized by exposure for fifteen minutes to the sun's rays. Iodised oil, thus prepared, has the odor and taste of almond oil, is not more liable to become rancid than the pure oil, and is free from hydriodic acid. (*Journ. de Pharm.*, Mars, 1856.) From the above statements it is not easy to determine which is the best method of preparing iodised oil; but the preparation may be made with good olive oil, instead of the more expensive almond oil.

burns. When thus used, it must be borne in mind that the iodine acts also by being absorbed. Another valuable application of it is for the removal of cutaneous nævi. Lugol's *caustic iodine solution* is made of iodine and iodide of potassium, each, an ounce, dissolved in two fluidounces of water. This is used to destroy soft and fungous granulations, and has been employed with decided benefit in lupus. The *Liniment of Iodine* of the British Pharmacopœia is intermediate in strength between the two solutions last mentioned. (See *Linimentum Iodi.*) Another caustic solution of iodine, under the name of *iodized glycerin*, is made by dissolving one part of iodide of potassium in two parts of glycerin, and adding the solution to one part of iodine, which it completely dissolves. Dr. Max Richter, of Vienna, to whom the credit belongs of having introduced into practice the solution of iodine in glycerin, found this caustic particularly useful in lupus, non-vascular goitre, and scrofulous and constitutional syphilitic ulcers. The solution is applied by means of a hair-pencil to the diseased surface, which must then be covered with gutta-percha paper, fixed at the edges by strips of adhesive plaster, in order to prevent the evaporation of the iodine. The application produces burning pain, which rarely lasts for more than two hours. The dressing is removed in twenty-four hours, and pledgets dipped in cold water applied. This iodine caustic is too strong for ordinary local use. A weaker solution is recommended by Dr. Szukits, formed of one part of iodine to five of glycerin, for application to the neck, female breast, abdomen, etc. After four or five paintings it causes excoriation, which requires its discontinuance, and the use of cold applications. A mode of applying iodine locally has been suggested by Dr. R. Greenhalgh, of London, which consists in thoroughly impregnating raw cotton with a solution in glycerin of iodide of potassium and of iodine, in the proportion of two ounces of the former and one ounce of the latter to eight ounces of the menstruum, and then drying the "*iodized cotton.*" It is intended for application to the cervix or os uteri, which is effected through a speculum. (*Lancet*, May 26, 1866, p. 582.) Mehn's method of making iodised cotton is as follows. Finely divided iodine (5 to 10 parts) is sprinkled between layers of loose cotton (100 parts) introduced into a tall glass vessel, and the latter placed horizontally on a water or sand-bath. As soon as vapors of iodine are seen to rise, and the air has been expelled from the vessel, the latter is tightly stoppered. On continuing to apply a moderate and uniform heat, the iodine vapors penetrate the cotton, and color it yellow. After about two hours, the cotton will have assumed the color of burnt coffee, and the operation is finished. Cotton iodized in other ways, as by immersion in concentrated solutions of iodine in ether or carbon disulphide, retains merely traces of iodine. (*N. R.*, April, 1867.)

Iodine is used by injection into various cavities. It has been employed in this way for the cure or relief of hydrocephalus, pleuritic effusion, hydropericardium, ascites, ovarian dropsy, hernia, hydrocele, spina bifida, dropsy of the joints, large cystic bronchocele, and chronic abscesses. The discussion of the indications for the use of the injections in these cases, and of the precautions and the methods to be adopted, belongs rather to treatises upon the practice of medicine and surgery than to a work like the present. To such treatises, therefore, the reader is referred.

Enemata containing iodine have been used, by several practitioners, in the chronic dysentery and diarrhœa of both adults and children, with decided benefit, a prominent effect being the relief of tenesmus. They are supposed to act locally on ulcers in the colon and rectum, and generally by absorption. The injection should be made of Lugol's solution, one to ten fluidrachms in one or two quarts of water. It should be preceded by an emollient enema to empty the intestine, and should be repeated once or twice daily, gradually increasing its strength. If the pain be severe, a laudanum injection will bring immediate relief.

Iodine, in the state of vapor, has been employed by inhalation; and the experiments, as yet tried, have been in the treatment chiefly of phthisis and chronic bronchitis. Although very extraordinary results were claimed for the method, yet it has entirely failed to fulfil expectations, and is at present very rarely practised. For details as to methods, the reader is referred to the 14th edition U. S. D.*

* M. Barrère has proposed the use, for inhalations, of *iodized camphor*, which is to be taken like snuff. This is prepared by putting powdered camphor in a snuff-box, with a hundredth part

Iodine or an iodide should not be given in solution with an alkaloid, as it forms insoluble compounds, and in Philadelphia death has been produced by the iodide of strychnine which had crystallized out of a mixture. It has even been suggested by Mr. R. F. Fairthorne (*A. J. P.*, 1856) and Dr. H. W. Fuller (*Lancet*, March 21, 1868, p. 373) as an antidote to alkaloids; but the insoluble compounds of these substances would by no means be inert in the stomach.

In cases of poisoning by iodine, the stomach must be first evacuated, and afterwards drinks administered containing an amylaceous substance, such as flour, starch, or arrow-root.

IPECACUANHA. *U.S., Br.* *Ipecac.*

(ĬP-Ĕ-CĂC-Ū-ĂN′HĂ.)

"The root of Cephaëlis Ipecacuanha. A. Richard. (*Nat. Ord.* Rubiaceæ, Coffeæ.)" *U. S.* "The dried root of Cephaëlis Ipecacuanha." *Br.*

Radix Ipecacuanhæ, *P. G.;* Ipecac; Racine brésilienne, Ipecacuanha, *Fr.;* Ruhrwurzel, Brechwurzel, Ipecacuanha, *G.;* Ipecacuana, *It., Sp.*

The term *ipecacuanha*, derived from the language of the aborigines of Brazil, has been applied to various emetic roots of South American origin.* The U. S. and British Pharmacopœias recognize only that of *Cephaëlis Ipecacuanha;* and no other is known by the name in the shops of this country. Our chief attention will, therefore, be confined to this root, and the plant which yields it; but, as others are employed in South America, are occasionally exported, and may possibly reach our markets mingled with the genuine drug, we shall, in a note, give a succinct account of those which have attracted most attention.

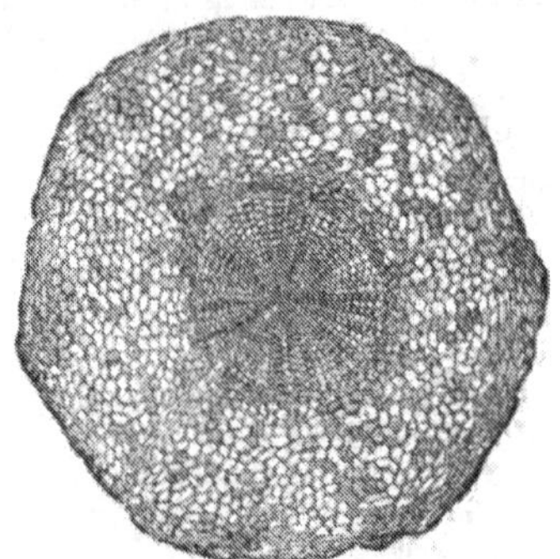

Ipecacuanha, transverse section.

The botanical character of the ipecacuanha plant was long unknown. Pison and Marcgrav, who were the first to treat of this medicine, in their work on the Natural History of Brazil, published at Amsterdam, 1648, described in general terms two plants; one producing a whitish root, distinguished by the name of white ipecacuanha, the other, a brown root, which answers in their description precisely to the officinal drug. But their account was not sufficiently definite to enable botanists to decide upon the character of the plants. The medicine was generally thought to be derived from a species of *Viola*, which Linnæus designated as *V. Ipecacuanha.* Opinion afterwards turned in favor of a plant, sent to Linnæus by Mutis from New Granada, as affording the ipecacuanha of that country and of Peru. This was described in the *Supplementum* of the younger Linnæus, 1781, under the name of *Psychotria emetica*, and was long erroneously considered as the source of the true ipecacuanha. Dr. Gomez, of Lisbon, was the first who accurately described and figured the genuine plant, which he had seen in Brazil, and specimens of which he

in bulk of iodine, contained in a muslin bag. In the course of a few hours, the substances, by occasional shaking, unite, forming a powder resembling iodine in color. The difficulty in practising ordinary iodine inhalation depends chiefly on the irritation caused by the vapor, which excites cough and fatigues the patient. According to M. Barrère, this inconvenience is avoided by the use of the iodized camphor. A pinch of it produces sneezing and some smarting in the nostrils; but when the vapor reaches the lungs, it causes a refreshing sensation, which induces the patient to draw a long and deep breath. (*Ann. de Thérap.*, 1855, p. 232.) M. Hutet recommends the inhalation of hydriodic ether in affections of the lungs.

Dr. Brainard employs the vapor of iodine, with great advantage, in the treatment of indolent ulcers, first dressing the ulcer with simple cerate spread on lint, then applying over this several layers of lint in which from one to four grains of iodine have been folded, and covering the whole with oiled silk and tin foil, secured by a bandage, so as to prevent the escape of the iodine, which is vaporized by the heat of the body. (*Chicago Med. Journ.*, Jan. 1860.)

* M. Weddell states that the word ipecacuanha is nowhere in Brazil used to designate the Cephaëlis, which is generally called *poaya.* (*Journ. de Pharm.*, 3e sér., xvi. 34.)

took with him to Portugal; but Brotero, professor of botany at Coimbra, with whom he had left specimens, having drawn up a description, and inserted it with a figure in the Linnæan Transactions without acknowledgment, enjoyed for a time the credit due to his countryman. In the paper of Brotero the plant is named *Callicocca Ipecacuanha;* but the term *Callicocca*, having been applied by Schreber, without sufficient reason, to the genus already established and named, has been universally abandoned for the *Cephaëlis* of Swartz, though this also, it appears, is a usurpation upon the previous rights of Aublet.

Gen. Ch. Flowers in an involucred head. *Corolla* tubular. *Stigma* two-parted. *Berry* two-seeded. *Receptacle* chaffy. *Willd.*

Cephaëlis Ipecacuanha. Richard, *Hist. Ipecac.* p. 21, t. i.; Martius, *Spec. Mat. Med. Brazil*, t. i. p. 4; *Curtis's Bot. Mag.*, N. S., vol. xvii. pl. 4083, 1844.—*Callicocca Ipecacuanha.* Brotero, *Linn. Trans.* vi. 137. This is a small shrubby plant, with a root from four to six inches long, about as thick as a goose-quill, marked with annular rugæ, simple or somewhat branched, descending obliquely into the ground, and here and there sending forth slender fibrils. The stem is two or three feet long, but, being partly under ground, and often procumbent at the base, usually rises less than a foot in height. It is slender; in the lower portion leafless, smooth, brown or ash-colored, and knotted, with radicles frequently proceeding from the knots; near the summit, pubescent, green, and furnished with leaves seldom exceeding six in number. These are opposite, petiolate, oblong-obovate, acute, entire, from three to four inches long, from one to two broad, obscurely green and somewhat rough on their upper surface, pale, downy, and veined on the under. At the insertion of each pair of leaves are deciduous stipules, embracing the stem, membranous at the base, and separated above into numerous bristle-like divisions. The flowers are very small, white, and collected to the number of eight, twelve, or more, each accompanied with a green bract, into a semi-globular head, supported upon a round, solitary, axillary footstalk, and embraced by a monophyllous involucre, deeply divided into four, sometimes five or six obovate, pointed segments. The fruit is an ovate, obtuse berry, which is at first purple, but becomes almost black when ripe, and contains two small plano-convex seeds.

The plant is a native of Brazil, flourishing over a very wide extent of territory in moist, thick, and shady woods, and abounding most within the limits of the eighth and twentieth degrees of south latitude. According to Humboldt, it grows also in New Granada. It flowers in January and February, and ripens its fruit in May. The root is active in all seasons, but, as it has to be dried rapidly, collection during the rainy season is relaxed. The native collector, or *poayero*, seizes all the stems of a clump, loosens them by a zigzag motion, and then, thrusting a pointed stick under the roots, tears up the whole mass. The roots, freed from dirt by shaking, are then dried. The amount gathered daily varies from 8 to 30 pounds, according to skill and locality. Extirpation does not take place, because, as shown by the Edinburgh gardeners McNab and Lindsay, a very small fragment of the root, or even a petiole of a leaf, will rapidly produce a new plant. Weddell, indeed, many years since, stated that the remains of the root, often purposely left in the ground, serve the purpose of propagation, each fragment giving rise to a new plant. Ipecacuanha of commerce comes chiefly from the interior province of Matto-Grosso, upon the upper waters of the Paraguay, although some is said to be gathered near Philadelphia, north of Rio Janeiro.* The chief places of export are Rio Janeiro, Bahia, and Pernambuco. It is brought to the United States in large bags or bales.

Properties. Genuine ipecacuanha is in pieces two or three lines thick, variously bent and contorted, simple or branched, consisting of an interior slender, light straw-colored, ligneous cord, with a thick, brittle, brownish, finely wrinkled, cortical covering, which presents on its surface a succession of circular, unequal, prominent rings or rugæ, separated by very narrow fissures, frequently extending nearly down to the central fibre. This appearance of the surface has given rise to the term *annelé* or

* Strenuous efforts have been made by the British authorities to establish the cultivation of ipecacuanha in India. Some thousands of plants have been grown, under very varying conditions, but, according to latest reports, the indications of practical success were not very encouraging.

annulated, by which the true ipecacuanha is designated by French pharmaceutists. The cortex is hard, horny, and semi-transparent, breaks with a resinous fracture, and easily separates from the tougher ligneous fibre, which possesses the medicinal virtues of the root in a much inferior degree. On microscopic examination the very thick bark is seen to be formed of uniform parenchymatous cells, without traces of the medullary rays, which are very distinct in the woody central cylinder. Attached to the root is frequently a smoother and more slender portion, which is the base of the stem, and should be separated before pulverization. Pereira has met, in the English market, with distinct bales composed of these fragments of stems, with occasionally portions of the root attached. Much stress has been laid upon the color of the external surface of the ipecacuanha root; and diversity in this respect has even led to the formation of distinct varieties. Thus, the epidermis is sometimes deep brown, or even blackish, sometimes reddish brown or reddish gray, and sometimes light gray or ash-colored. Hence the distinction into *brown*, *red*, and *gray ipecacuanha*. But these are all derived from the same plant, are essentially the same in properties and composition, and probably differ only in consequence of difference in age, place of growth, or mode of desiccation. The colors are often so intermingled that it would be impossible to decide in which variety a particular specimen should be placed. The *brown* is the most abundant in the packages brought to our market. The *red*, besides the color of its epidermis, presents a rosy tint when broken, and is said to be somewhat more bitter than the preceding variety. The *gray* is much lighter-colored externally, usually rather larger, with less prominent rings and wider furrows, and is still more decidedly bitter. Many years ago there was imported from Caraccas into the United States a large gray ipecacuanha with badly-marked rings. This variety disappeared for a time, but is probably the *Colombian* or *Carthagena Ipecacuanha* of modern commerce, which is distinguished from the Brazilian drug by being a little larger, with less conspicuous annuli and more marked medullary rays. According to Lefort, it contains rather less emetine than does the Brazilian ipecacuanha; but this is not at all certain. When the bark in either variety is opaque, with a dull amylaceous aspect, the root is less active. As the woody part is nearly inert, and much more difficult of pulverization than the cortical, it often happens that, when the root is powdered, the portion last remaining in the mortar possesses scarcely any emetic power; and care should be taken to provide against any defect from this cause. The color of the powder is a light grayish fawn.

Ipecacuanha has little smell in the aggregate state, but when powdered has a peculiar nauseous odor, which in some persons excites violent sneezing, in others dyspnœa resembling an attack of asthma. The taste is bitter, acrid, and very nauseous. Water and alcohol extract its virtues, which are injured by decoction. Its emetic property resides in an alkaloid called *emetine*, discovered by Pelletier in the year 1817. The cortical portion of the brown ipecacuanha, analyzed by this chemist under the erroneous name of *Psychotria emetica*, yielded, in 100 parts, 16 of an impure salt of emetine, which was at first considered the pure emetic principle, 2 of an odorous fatty matter, 6 of wax, 10 of gum, 42 of starch, 20 of lignin, with 4 parts loss. The root yields of the alkaloid less than 1 per cent. The formula, according to Lefort and F. Würtz (*Ann. Ch. Phys.*, [5] 12, p. 277), is $C_{28}H_{40}N_2O_5$, while according to Glenard (*Ann. Ch. Phys.*, [5] 8, p. 233) it is $C_{15}H_{22}NO_2$. In addition to these principles, Bucholz found extractive, sugar, and resin; and Erwin Willigk, afterwards, traces of a disagreeably smelling volatile oil, phosphatic salts, and a peculiar acid, *ipecacuanhic acid*, which resembles caffeotannic and quinic acids, and has been shown by Reich (*Arch. Pharm.*, [2] 113, p. 208) to be a glucoside of the formula $C_{14}H_{18}O_7$. (See *A. J. P.*, xxiii. 352.) Good ipecacuanha contains about 80 per cent. of cortical and 20 of ligneous matter.

Attempts have been made to adulterate powdered ipecacuanha with the powder of almonds; but the fraud is readily detected by forming a paste with a little water, and putting it into a hot place for half an hour, when, if the ipecacuanha be pure, only its own odor will be perceived, but, if adulterated, a decided odor of almonds will be noticed. (*Journ. de Pharm.*, Juin, 1874, p. 479.)

Emetine, when perfectly pure, is whitish, inodorous, slightly bitter, pulverulent, unalterable in the air, very fusible, sparingly soluble in cold water, more soluble in hot water, and very soluble in alcohol and chloroform, and in solution of potassa and soda, though less so in water of ammonia. It is readily soluble in ether, acetic ether, amylic alcohol, carbon bisulphide, oil of turpentine. With sulphuric, phosphoric, and acetic acids, it forms very soluble and uncrystallizable salts; but Flückiger prepared a crystallized hydrochlorate; and nitric acid has the remarkable property of forming with it a nitrate, at first bulky, and very slightly soluble in water, but soon agglutinating into a brown, pitch-like matter, very soluble in water, and uncrystallizable. (*Lefort.*) According to Lefort, this insoluble nitrate, which equally forms by double decomposition between the acetate or sulphate of emetine and nitrate of potassium, forms the most distinctive character of emetine. (*Journ. de Pharm.*, 1869, p. 244.) It is precipitated by gallic and tannic acids from its solutions, and contains nitrogen. It is, however, very difficult to procure it in this state of purity, and the proportion afforded by the root is exceedingly small. Dr. F. B. Power has shown that an intense yellow color is produced when emetine is brought in contact with chlorinated lime and acetic acid. *Impure emetine* is in transparent scales of a brownish red color, almost inodorous, of a bitterish acrid taste, deliquescent, very soluble in water and alcohol, insoluble in ether, precipitated from its solutions by gallic acid and the acetates of lead, but not by tartar emetic or the salts of iron.

The taste of its compounds is very bitter. When exposed to light and air, emetine soon turns yellow, but it remains white when protected from the light. On very slowly evaporating its solutions in ether or alcohol, emetine is deposited in thin agglutinating scales, but if the solutions are rapidly evaporated, it is separated in fine uniform granules. It melts at 62° to 65° C. (143·6° to 149° F.), has a strong alkaline reaction, and is neutralized by acids forming salts, which on evaporation *in vacuo* form brilliant, colorless, irregular crystals. Various methods of preparing emetine will be found in U. S. D., 14th edition, but Podwyssotzki's process is probably the best for obtaining it. He recommends to treat the powdered ipecacuanha first with ether and then with petroleum benzin, in order to remove the liquid oil, the white fatty or waxy matter, and those coloring matters which are soluble in the solvents named, then extract the powdered root two or three times successively, at a moderate heat, with 85 per cent. alcohol, without adding any acid; evaporate the mixed tinctures to a syrupy consistence, add after cooling a very concentrated solution of as much ferric chloride as corresponds to from 10 to 13 per cent. of the weight of the powdered ipecac used, mix the mass well, add sodium carbonate in excess, boil the mass in a flask, on a water-bath, with successive small portions of petroleum benzin (in which the emetine dissolves), shaking frequently, and continue to use fresh portions of the menstruum until no more emetine goes into solution; the filtered benzin solutions are mixed, and, if concentrated, the mixture is allowed to stand for twelve hours in a very cool place, when almost all of the emetine will separate pure as a white precipitate. If, however, the mixture is not very concentrated, atmospheric air is blown through it for some time, when pure emetine will separate in white flakes. By concentrating or evaporating the benzin solution, however slowly, pure white emetine is *never* obtained. The emetine should be collected quickly on a filter and dried over sulphuric acid. (*A. J. P.*, April, 1880.)*

* NON-OFFICINAL IPECACUANHAS. When ipecacuanha began to be popular in Europe, the roots of several other plants were imported and confounded with the genuine; and the name came at length to be applied to almost all emetic roots derived from America. Several of these are still occasionally met with, and retain the name originally given to them. The two most worthy of notice are the ipecacuanha of Colombia and Peru, and the white ipecacuanha of Brazil. On each of these we shall offer a few remarks.

1. *Peruvian Ipecacuanha. Striated Ipecacuanha. Black Ipecacuanha.* This is the root of *Psychotria emetica*, a plant belonging to the Rubiaceæ. A description of it, sent by Mutis, was published by Linnæus, the younger, in his Supplement. It has since been described in the *Plant. Æquin.* of Hum. and Bonpl.; and has been figured by A. Richard in his History of the Ipecacuanhas, and by Hayne in the eighth volume of his Medical Botany published at Berlin. It is a small shrub, with a stem twelve or eighteen inches high, simple, erect, round, slightly pubescent, and furnished with opposite, oblong-lanceolate, pointed leaves, narrowed at their base into a short petiole, and accompanied with pointed stipules. The flowers are small, white, and supported in small clusters towards the end of an axillary peduncle. The plant flourishes in Peru and Colombia,

Professor Flückiger (*Pharm. Zeitung*, 1886, p. 30) gives a process for assaying ipecacuanha, which consists in exhausting 10 to 15 grammes of the drug in very fine

and was seen by Humboldt and Bonpland growing in abundance near the river Magdalena. The dried root is said to have been exported from Carthagena. It is cylindrical, somewhat thicker than the root of the Cephaëlis, usually simple, but sometimes branched, not much contorted, wrinkled longitudinally, presenting here and there deep circular intersections, but without the annular rugæ of the true ipecacuanha. The longitudinal direction of the wrinkles has given it the name of *striated ipecacuanha.* It consists of an internal woody cord, and an external cortical portion; but the former is usually larger in proportion to the latter than in the root of the Cephaëlis. The bark is soft and easily cut with a knife, and when broken exhibits a brown, slightly resinous fracture. The epidermis is of a dull reddish gray color, which darkens with age and exposure, and ultimately becomes almost black. Hence the root has sometimes been called *black ipecacuanha.* The ligneous portion is yellowish, and perforated with numerous small holes visible by the microscope. Peruvian ipecacuanha is nearly inodorous, and has a flat taste, neither bitter nor acrid. From 100 parts Pelletier obtained 9 of impure emetine, 12 of fatty matter, with an abundance of starch, besides gum and lignin. The dose, as an emetic, is from two scruples to a drachm.

2. *White Ipecacuanha. Amylaceous Ipecacuanha. Undulated Ipecacuanha.* This variety is produced by different species of *Richardsonia*, the *Richardia* of Linnæus. *R. scabra*, or *R. Brasiliensis* of Gomez, and *R. emetica* are especially indicated by Martius. For the root usually called *white ipecacuanha*, Guibourt has proposed the name of *undulated ipecacuanha*, derived from the peculiar character of the surface, which presents indentations or concavities on one side, corresponding with prominences or convexities on the other, so as to give a wavy appearance to the root. It differs little in size from the genuine; is of a whitish gray color externally; and, when broken, presents a dull white farinaceous fracture, offering by the light of the sun shining points, which are nothing more than small grains of fecula. Like the other varieties, it has a woody centre. It is inodorous and insipid, and contains, according to Pelletier, a very large proportion of starch, with only 6 per cent. of impure emetine, and 2 of fatty matter. Richard found only 3·5 parts of emetine in the hundred. It is said to be sometimes mixed with the genuine ipecacuanha.

According to Martius, different species of *Ionidium* (*Viola*, Linn.) also produce what is called *white ipecacuanha.* The roots of all the species of Ionidium possess emetic or purgative properties. The root of *I. ipecacuanha* is described by Guibourt as being six or seven inches long, as thick as a quill, somewhat tortuous, and exhibiting at the point of flexion semicircular fissures, which give it some resemblance to the root of the Cephaëlis. It is often bifurcated at both extremities, and terminates at the top in a great number of small ligneous stalks. It is wrinkled longitudinally, and of a light yellowish gray color. The bark is thin, and the interior ligneous portion very thick. The root has little taste or smell. According to Pelletier, 100 parts contain 5 of an emetic substance, 35 of gum, 1 of nitrogenous matter, and 37 of lignin. (*Hist. abrégée des Drogues simples*, i. 514.)

The root of a species of Ionidium growing in Quito has attracted some attention as a remedy in elephantiasis, under the South American name of *cuichunchulli.* The plant received from Dr. Bancroft the name of *I. Marcucci;* but Sir W. Hooker found the specimen, received from Dr. Bancroft, to be the *I. parviflorum* of Ventenat. Lindley thinks a specimen he received under the same name from Quito, to be the *I. microphyllum* of Humboldt. If useful in elephantiasis, it is so probably by its emeto-purgative action. (See *A. J. P.*, vii. 186.)

The reader is referred to a paper on Ipecacuanha by the late R. E. Griffith, M.D., in the *Journ. of the Phila. Coll. of Pharm.* (iii. 181), for a more extended account of the roots which have been used under that name.

M. Planchon (*Journ. de Pharm.*, Dec. 1872) finds that there are two distinct striated ipecacuanhas, the *larger* and the *lesser*, of which the first is the product of *Psychotria emetica*, the second being of unknown origin.

1. *Larger striated ipecacuanha.* This presents itself in rather long fragments, sometimes 9 or 10 centimetres (3 or 4 inches), with a thickness of from 5 to 9 millimetres (⅕ to ⅓ of an inch). The pieces are for the most part almost straight, sometimes sinuous, more rarely tortuous. At distant intervals they are marked by contractions, or simply circular furrows. Their whole surface is largely striated longitudinally. At their upper part are often attached one or more remaining portions of the stem, distinguished from the root by their much smoother surface. Their color is a grayish brown, tending sometimes to reddish brown. Like other ipecacuanhas, they have an outer cortical and central ligneous portion. The former is soft, so that it may even be penetrated by the nail. It has a horny aspect, and a variable color, passing from whitish, by shades of rose, violaceous, and blackish violet. Its thickness is at least two-thirds of the root, and becomes still greater when this is immersed in water. The central part is yellowish white. The root has little odor, and a taste scarcely nauseous, sometimes flat, and often sweetish. As to the microscopic characters, the most striking is probably the total absence of the starch granules, and the relatively very small diameter of the vessels in the central part. Chemically this variety is characterized by the presence of a principle capable of reducing the cupro-potassic reagent. It is so abundant in the cortical part, that a simple digestion in water gives a liquid with strong reducing powers, but without deviating action on polarized light. The larger striated ipecacuanha comes from Colombia.

2. *Lesser striated ipecacuanha.* This is in very short fragments, 2 or 3 centimetres at most long, and 2 or 3 millimetres in thickness; some nearly cylindrical, others narrowly fusiform; others again formed of roundish or pyriform segments, somewhat thicker than the preceding, placed end to end. The color is generally of a gray brown, darker than that of the other kind. The longitudinal striæ are fine, and regular on the transverse section. The cortical portion is as it were horny, and its consistence firmer than in the larger kind; the central part is yellowish, and under the microscope exhibits numerous pores. The ligneous centre is at once distinguished by the size of its vessels, which give it a porous appearance. The presence of the starch granules is another of the

powder with boiling chloroform, to which a drop of solution of ammonia has been added; the extraction is continued until the chloroform passing through shows no sign of alkaloid when treated with acidulated water. Upon distilling off the chloroform, the emetine is left in a very pure condition, and may be dried at 100° C. and weighed, or perhaps more conveniently titrated with Mayer's reagent. He found the average quantity of emetine in ipecacuanha root not to exceed 1 per cent. (*P. J. Tr.*, 1886, 643.) H. W. Jones approves of this method, and modifies it by treating the residue from the chloroformic solution with water and dilute sulphuric acid, filtering, and recovering the alkaloid by means of chloroform and ammonia. (*P. J. Tr.*, 1886, p. 277.) For other methods see a paper by Dr. A. B. Lyons, *A. J. P.*, 1885, pp. 531, 542.

Medical Properties and Uses. Ipecacuanha is in large doses emetic, in smaller doses diaphoretic and expectorant, and in still smaller, stimulant to the stomach, exciting appetite and facilitating digestion. In quantities not quite sufficient to vomit, it produces nausea, and frequently acts on the bowels. As an emetic, it is mild but tolerably certain, and, being free from corrosive or narcotic properties and usually thrown from the stomach by one or two efforts, never produces dangerous effects. It was employed as an emetic by the natives of Brazil when that country was first settled by the Portuguese; but, though described in the work of Pison, it was not known in Europe till 1672, and did not come into use till some years afterwards. John Helvetius, grandfather of the famous author of that name, having been associated with a merchant who had imported a large quantity of ipecacuanha into Paris, employed it as a secret remedy, and with so much success in dysentery and other bowel affections, that general attention was drawn to it; and the fortunate physician received from Louis XIV. a large sum of money and public honors on the condition that he should make it public.

As an emetic it is peculiarly adapted, by its mildness and efficiency, to cases in which the object is merely to evacuate the stomach, or where a gentle impression only is desired; and, in most other cases in which emetics are indicated, it may be advantageously combined with the more energetic medicines, which it renders safer by insuring their discharge. It is especially useful where narcotic poisons have been swallowed; as, under these circumstances, it may be given in almost indefinite doses, with little comparative risk of injury. In tropical or typhoid dysentery it is of very great value. As a nauseating remedy it is used in asthma, hooping-cough, and the hemorrhages; as a diaphoretic combined with opium, in numerous diseases. (See *Pulvis Ipecacuanhæ et Opii.*) Its expectorant properties render it useful in catarrhal and other pulmonary affections. It has been given, also, with supposed advantage, in very minute doses, in dyspepsia, and in chronic disease of the gastro-intestinal mucous membrane, and as an antemetic. It has been found especially useful in winter coughs and asthmatic catarrh, inhaled in the form of spray; the wine of ipecacuanha being the preparation used.*

Ipecacuanha is most conveniently administered, as an emetic, in the form of powder suspended in water. The dose is about twenty grains (1·3 Gm.), repeated, if necessary, at intervals of twenty minutes till it operates. In some persons much smaller quantities prove emetic, and we have known an individual who was generally vomited by the fraction of a grain. The operation may be facilitated, and rendered milder, by draughts of warm water, or warm chamomile tea. An infusion in boiling water, in the proportion of two drachms to six fluidounces, may be given in the dose of a fluidounce repeated as in the former case. For the production of nausea, the dose in substance may be two grains (0·13 Gm.), repeated more or less

distinguishing characters of this variety. It contains a larger proportion of emetine than the preceding, yielding, according to the analysis of Pelletier, 9 per cent.

The commercial variety of ipecacuanha examined by Mr. Attfield, of London, which had been sent to London from Bogota, and was no doubt the root of *Psychotria emetica*, was probably identical with the larger variety of M. Planchon, although its highly elastic quality, which induced Mr. Attfield to give it the distinctive name of *elastic striated ipecacuanha*, had not been given as a property of the larger striated by Planchon. In its very small yield of emetine, only 2·75 per cent., it corresponds with the large variety.

* Sidney Ringer, M.D., and Wm. Murrell. The *Lancet*, Sept. 5, 1874, p. 323.

frequently according to circumstances. As a diaphoretic it may be given in the quantity of a grain (0·065 Gm.); as an alterative, in diseases of the stomach and bowels, in that of a quarter or half a grain (0·016–0·03 Gm.) two or three times a day.

Emetine has been used, but its operation on the stomach is more violent and continued than that of ipecacuanha; and, if given in overdoses, it may produce dangerous and even fatal consequences. The dose of impure emetine is about a grain (0·065 Gm.), of the pure not more than an eighth (0·008 Gm.) of a grain, repeated at proper intervals till it vomits. In proportional doses, it may be applied to the other purposes for which ipecacuanha is used. It will excite vomiting when applied to a blistered surface after the removal of the cuticle.

An ointment, made with one part of the powder, one of olive oil, and two of lard, rubbed once or twice a day for a few minutes upon the skin, produces a copious and very permanent eruption, but is at present only very rarely employed as a counter-irritant.

Off. Prep. Extractum Ipecacuanhæ Fluidum; Pulvis Ipecacuanhæ et Opii; Trochisci Morphinæ et Ipecacuanhæ.

Off. Prep. Br. Pilula Conii Composita; Pilula Ipecacuanha cum Scilla; Pulvis Ipecacuanhæ Compositus; Trochisci Ipecacuanhæ; Trochisci Morphinæ et Ipecacuanhæ; Vinum Ipecacuanhæ.

IRIS. *U.S.* *Iris.* [*Blue Flag.*]

(Ī'RĬS.)

The rhizome and rootlets of Iris versicolor. Linné. (*Nat. Ord.* Iridaceæ.)" *U. S.*

Rhizome d'Iris varié, Glaïeul bleu, *Fr.;* Verschiedenfarbige Schwertlilie, *G.*

Gen. Ch. *Corolla* six-parted; the alternate segments reflected. *Stigmas* petal-shaped. *Willd.*

In all the species belonging to this genus, so far as examined, the roots are more or less acrid, and possessed of cathartic and emetic properties. In Europe, *Iris fœtidissima*, *I. Florentina*, *I. Germanica*, *I. pseudo-acorus*, and *I. tuberosa* have at various times been admitted into use, and the unpeeled roots of *I. Germanica* are still sold in the Indian bazaars under the name of *Irisia*. Florentine Iris is of sufficient importance to demand careful consideration.†

* *Iris Florentina.* U. S. Secondary List, 1870. (*Rhizoma Iridis*, P.G.; *Radix Iridis Florentinæ*, *Radix Ireos; Orris Root*, *Iris de Florence*, Fr.; *Florentinische Violenwurzel*, *Veilchenwurzel*, G.; *Ireos*, It.; *Liro Florentina*, Sp.) The root (rhizome) of the Florentine Iris is perennial, horizontal, fleshy, fibrous, and covered with a brown epidermis. The leaves, which spring directly from the root, are sword-shaped, pointed, nerved, and shorter than the stem, which rises from the midst of them more than a foot in height, round, smooth, jointed, and bearing commonly two large white or bluish white terminal flowers. The calyx is a spathe with two valves. The corolla divides into six segments or petals, of which three stand erect, and the remaining three are bent backward, and bearded within at their base with yellow-tipped white hairs. The fruit is a three-celled capsule, containing many seeds. This plant is a native of Italy and other parts of the south of Europe, where it is also cultivated. The root is dug up in spring, and prepared for the market by the removal of its cuticle and fibres. It is cultivated for commerce chiefly in the neighborhood of Florence, and is exported from Leghorn in large casks.

Florentine orris is in pieces of various form and size, often branched, usually about as thick as the thumb, knotty, flattened, white, heavy, of a rough though not fibrous fracture, an agreeable odor resembling that of the violet, and a bitterish, acrid taste. The acrimony is greater in the recent than in the dried root; but the peculiar smell is more decidedly developed in the latter. The pieces are brittle and easily powdered, and the powder is of a dirty white color. Vogel obtained from Florentine orris, gum, a brown extractive, fecula, a bitter and acrid fixed oil or soft resin, a volatile crystallizable oil, and vegetable fibre. According to Landerer, the acrid principle is volatile, separating in the form of a stearopten from water distilled from the root. (*Arch. der Pharm.*, lxv. 302.) The solid oil which is prepared in Europe from orris root by distillation has been examined by Prof. Flückiger. By repeated crystallization from alcohol and treatment with animal charcoal, inodorous crystals were obtained, having the composition ($C_{14}H_{28}O_2$) and the properties of myristic acid, whilst the odorous principle remained in the mother-liquor, so that oil of orris must be regarded as myristic acid, impregnated with some volatile oil. The acid does not pre-exist in orris root, and is probably liberated from a fat by the influence of steam. (*A. J. P.*, 1876, p. 411, also 1885, p. 133.) According to Hager, the commercial oil has the following properties. At the ordinary temperature it is a pea-yellow acid, resembling basilicon ointment (*Phar. Germ.*) in color and consistence. It is lighter than water, fuses at 38° to 40° C. (100·4° to 104° F.) to a transparent liquid, and commences to congeal at about 28° C (82·4° F.). Two drops of the fused oil dissolve in 10 or 12 drops of warm stronger alcohol, and the solution does not separate at a medium temperature. Three drops of the oil and 20 to 25 drops of concen-

der with boiling chloroform, to which a drop of solution of ammonia has
ed; the extraction is continued until the chloroform passing through sh
of alkaloid when treated with acidulated water. Upon distilling off th
rm, the emetine is left in a very pure condition, and may be dried at 10
weighed, or perhaps more conveniently titrated with Mayer's reagent
nd the average quantity of emetine in ipecacuanha root not to exceed 1 per
J. Tr., 1886, 643.) H. W. Jones approves of this method, and modifies
ting the residue from the chloroformic solution with water and dilute sul
, filtering, and recovering the alkaloid by means of chloroform and am
J. Tr., 1886, p. 277.) For other methods see a paper by Dr. A. B. Ly
., 1885, pp. 531, 542.

Medical Properties and Uses. Ipecacuanha is in large doses emetic, i
es diaphoretic and expectorant, and in still smaller, stimulant to the st
ng appetite and facilitating digestion. In quantities not quite suffici
roduces nausea, and frequently acts on the bowels. As an emetic, it
rably certain, and, being free from corrosive or narcotic properties
own from the stomach by one or two efforts, never produces danger
was employed as an emetic by the natives of Brazil when that countr
tled by the Portuguese; but, though described in the work of Pison
own in Europe till 1672, and did not come into use till some years
hn Helvetius, grandfather of the famous author of that name, havin
ted with a merchant who had imported a large quantity of ipecacuanh
ployed it as a secret remedy, and with so much success in dysent
wel affections, that general attention was drawn to it; and the fortu
ceived from Louis XIV. a large sum of money and public hon
tion that he should make it public.

As an emetic it is peculiarly adapted, by its mildness and effi
hich the object is merely to evacuate the stomach, or where a ge
desired; and, in most other cases in which emetics are indicate
geously combined with the more energetic medicines, which
suring their discharge. It is especially useful where narcoti
wallowed; as, under these circumstances, it may be given in alm
ith little comparative risk of injury. In tropical or typho
ery great value. As a nauseating remedy it is used in asthma
he hemorrhages; as a diaphoretic combined with opium, in num
Pulvis Ipecacuanhæ et Opii.) Its expectorant properties ren
hal and other pulmonary affections. It has been given, as
antage, in very minute doses, in dyspepsia, and in chroni
testinal mucous membrane, and as an antemetic. It has
seful in winter coughs and asthmatic catarrh inhaled in
ine of ipecacuanha being the preparation u

Ipecacuanha is most conveniently admi
owder suspended in water. The dose is
necessary, at intervals of twenty minu
naller quantities prove emetic, and we
ly vomited by the fraction of a grain.
ered milder, by draughts of warm w
iling water, in the proportion of
the dose of a fluido
usea, the dose in

tinguishing cha
ing, yielding
The comm
to Lon
with

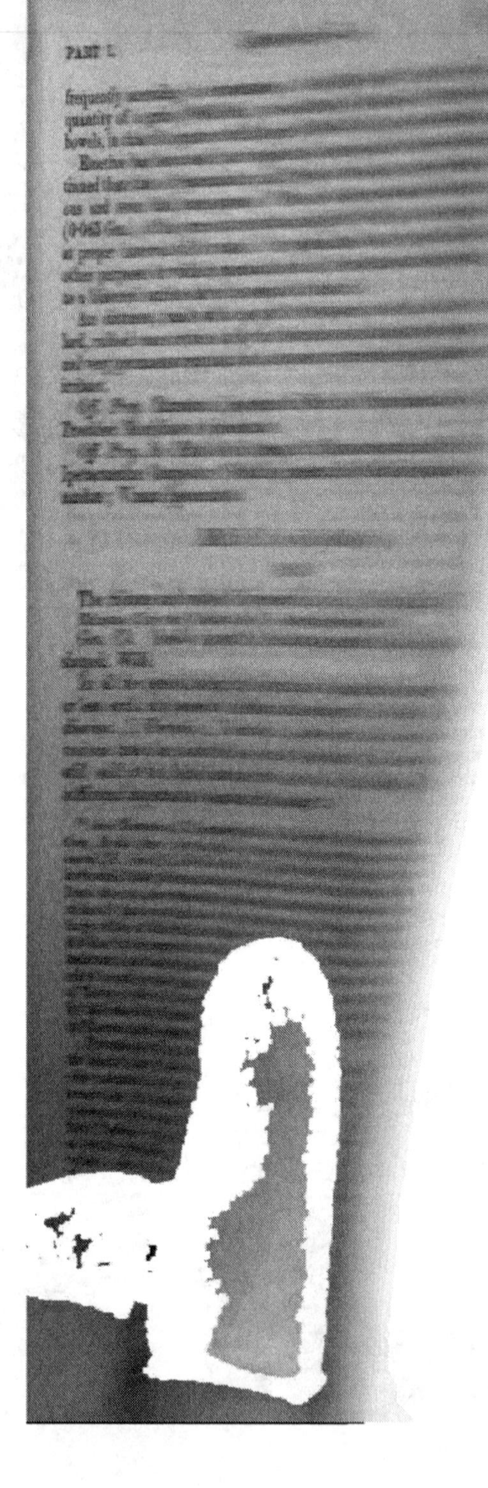

CPSIA information can be obtained
at www.ICGtesting.com
Printed in the USA
LVHW060557260323
742530LV00050B/516